Handbuch der experimentellen Pharmakologie

Handbook of Experimental Pharmacology

Heffter-Heubner New Series

Herausgegeben von / Edited by

O. Eichler A. Farah
Heidelberg Syracuse, N. Y.

Vol. XVIII/1

Springer-Verlag Berlin Heidelberg GmbH 1966

Histamine and Anti-Histaminics

Part 1

Histamine. Its Chemistry, Metabolism and Physiological and Pharmacological Actions

Contributors

S. G. A. Alivisatos · W. H. Bachrach · W. T. Beraldo · H. H. Dale
W. Dias da Silva · N. Emmelin · U. S. von Euler · H. Giertz
F. Hahn · R. D. Higginbotham · A. C. Ivy · R. G. Jones
C. Laborde-Burtin · S. E. Lindell · L. A. J. Lison · F. C. McIntire
E. Mendes · M. Mordelet-Dambrine · I. Mota · H. Moussatché
P. Naranjo · G. Nicot · J. L. Parrot · H. W. Raudonat · J. F. Riley
M. Rocha e Silva · A. M. Rothschild · A. Saindelle · R. W. Schayer
U. Serafini · P. Stern · H. Tabor · J. Thouvenot · B. Vasseur
I. Vugman · G. B. West · H. Westling · T. White

Sub-Editor

Mauricio Rocha e Silva

In Collaboration with Hanna A. Rothschild

With 175 Figures

Springer-Verlag Berlin Heidelberg GmbH 1966

ISBN 978-3-662-12018-7 ISBN 978-3-662-12016-3 (eBook)
DOI 10.1007/978-3-662-12016-3

Originally published by Springer-Verlag · Berlin · Heidelberg · New York in 1966
Softcover reprint of the hardcover 1st edition 1966

Library of Congress Catalog Card Number AGR 25—699

Title No. 5723

Preface

It was an agreable, though strenuous task to edit a book with so many distinguished contributors, on a subject to which I have given half of my life. In 1959, when Prof. O. EICHLER invited me to edit a book on "Histamine and Antihistaminics", as a supplement to HEFFTER's *Handbuch*, I thought the task could be done in three years. Now, five years are gone and only half is fulfilled. Though, so far as the "Histamine" part of the book is concerned, the initial plan has been followed very closely, we had to leave the Anti-histaminics for another volume of unpredictable dimensions. In 1924, eight pages inserted in a Chapter on *Mutterkorn*, by ARTHUR R. CUSHING were considered enough, in vol. II, Part II, pg. 1319—1326, of the *Handbuch*. Now, 922 pages did not suffice to cover all the aspects of the subject. Especially in the last few years the subject has expanded in so many directions, that the antihistaminic part had to be excluded from the present volume. Possibly, another thousand pages will be necessary to cover what remains of the subject.

In planning the book we made great use of the excellent and classical monograph by W. FELDBERG and E. SCHILF on *Histamin*, published by Julius Springer, in 1930. With the invitation to edit the present volume, the recommendation was made that "anything still valid in that book should appear in the volume to be edited". This was the most agreable recommendation I could receive from the Editors of the *Handbuch*, as it gave me a free hand to explore once more the inexhaustible source of historical and fundamental knowledge about histamine contained in FELDBERG and SCHILF's monograph. If making a book of such proportions can be compared to the work of building up a skyscraper, this historical and fundamental knowledge resembles the concrete foundation of the new structure.

The new book was planned in such a way that each Chapter represents a complete survey of a broad sector of the histamine problem.

Chapter I is entirely devoted to the chemistry, isolation and occurrence of histamine. It is subdivided into six sections with a complete survey on the methods of synthesis of histamine and analogs, the relationships between structure and activity and the methods of isolation for biological and chemical estimation in tissues and body fluids; the last two sections give an extensive view of the histochemical aspects of EHRLICH's mast cells, as well as on the association of histamine and heparin in cells and tissues.

Chapter II is entirely devoted to the pharmacology of histamine and is subdivided into eight sections dealing with absorption and toxicity of histamine, actions upon smooth muscles and the cardio-vascular system, on salivary and gastric secretion, and its relationships with the autonomous nervous system.

Chapter III treats in a most exhaustive way the problem of histamine release by venoms and toxins, by physical and chemical agents, by basic compounds, in anaphylaxis, and by macromolecular releasers, such as anaphylatoxin, dextran, egg white, and so forth. The enzymatic mechanism of histamine release in its relationships with respiration, carbohydrate metabolism and phosphorylation is authoritatively discussed in connection with the practical problem of histamine release in anaphylaxis and allergy.

Chapter IV is concerned with the metabolism of histamine and is again subdivided into seven sections dealing with *in vivo* and *in vitro* formation and catabolism of histamine in different species of animals and in man. A special section draws attention to the relationship between histamine and the brain.

Chapter V is subdivided into five sections and is intended to give a survey of the importance of histamine in normal physiology, with an extensive discussion of its possible significance as a normal stimulant of gastric secretion. Small sections are dedicated to the controversial participation of histamine in vascular reflexes, in chronic inflammation. The last two sections deal with the role played by histamine in human and experimental allergy.

In a book to which 38 collaborators contributed to different aspects of the subject, some overlapping was inevitable, but desirable. The diversity of view points on any growing subject of research can be of great advantage to any one working in the field, opening up new pathways to explore the unknown. Only limitations of space should prevent an editor from giving free hand to authors to expand their subjects as desired. Though this authority was exerted during the editing of this book, it was to an astonishingly small extent that any limitation had to be imposed to the contributors. Another factor to diversify the treatments given to the different subjects, was the selection of the authors from different countries: Brazil, Ecuador, France, Germany, Great Britain, Italy, Sweden, the United States and Yugoslavia. This diversity of nationalities adds a new dimension to the discussion of any scientific subject and, combined with the overlapping of individual contributions tends to eliminate cultural fads or local customs that lead to a stereotyped treatment of the subject. I believe that almost every aspect of the histamine problem has been dealt with adequately.

The presentation of some personal views of the problem was even encouraged by the invitation to authors to present short papers on their own work, to a certain extent at the margin of the main lines of the subject. These small contributions were introduced among the main papers as flowers to be gathered *en passant*. This procedure deviates somehow from the style of the great text-books and is more on the line of a Symposium. In so doing, we intended to insufflate fresh air in the dense atmosphere of a massive textbook.

It is a great pleasure to acknowledge the collaboration given by so many distinguished contributors of this volume for their exact and excellent cooperation in bringing the work to its final present form.

The task for editing this volume would be beyond my forces without the collaboration of Dr. Hanna A. Rothschild, in every phase of the preparatory work and especially in checking every single word and name appearing in this volume. To Miss Odete Pizarro and Maria Leticia Fernandes, we are indebted to most of the typing of our own contributions and of the indexes at the end of the volume.

This book is dedicated to all investigators whose work has contributed to the advance of our knowledge of the histamine problem. Two of them, however, deserve a special and honourable mention, namely Sir Henry H. Dale, of London, and Prof. Dankwart Ackermann, of Würzburg. By a fortunate coincidence this is the year of Sir Henry's ninetieth anniversary, and we are happy to have his Foreword to this book.

M. Rocha e Silva

Ribeirão Prêto, São Paulo, February, 1965.

Contributors

S. G. A. Alivisatos, Professor Dr., Division of Enzymology and Experimental Hypersensitivity, Institute of Medical Research, The Chicago Medical School, 2020 West Ogden Avenue, Chicago Ill., 60612/USA.

William Harris Bachrach, Dr., 8733 Beverly Blvd., Los Angeles 48. Calif./USA.

Wilson Teixeira Beraldo, Professor Dr., Departamento de Fisiologia, Faculdade de Medicina, Universidade de Minas Gerais, Belo Horizonte, Minas Gerais/Brasil.

Sir Henry Hallett Dale, The Wellcome Trust, 52, Queen Anne Street, London, W. 1./England.

Wilmar Dias da Silva, Dr., Departamento de Fisiologia, Faculdade de Medicina, Universidade de Minas Gerais, Belo Horizonte, Minas Gerais/Brasil.

Nils Emmelin, Professor Dr., Department of Physiology, University of Lund, Lund/Sweden.

Ulf S. von Euler, Professor Dr., Department of Physiology, Karolinska Institutet, Solnavägen 1, Stockholm 60/Sweden.

H. Giertz, Dozent Dr., Pharmakologisches Institut der Universität, 78 Freiburg i. Br./Deutschland, Katharinenstraße 29.

Fritz Hahn, Professor Dr., Pharmakologisches Institut der Universität, 78 Freiburg i. Br./Deutschland, Katharinenstraße 29.

Robert D. Higginbotham, Professor Dr., Department of Microbiology, The University of Texas-Medical Branch, Galveston, Texas/USA.

Andrew Conway Ivy, Professor Dr., Roosevelt University, 430 So. Michigan Avenue, Chicago 60605, Ill./USA.

Reuben G. Jones, Dr., Organic Chemical Division, The Lilly Research Laboratories, Eli Lilly and Co., Indianapolis 6, Ind./USA.

Claude Laborde-Burtin, Dr. (Madame), Laboratoire de Physiologie pathologique de l'Ecole pratique des Hautes Etudes, Hôpital Boucicaut, 78, Rue de la Convention, Paris XVe/France.

Sven Eric Lindell, Dr., Almänna Sjukhuset, Department of Clinical Physiology, Malmö/Sweden.

Lucien A. J. Lison, Professor Dr., Departamento de Morfologia, Faculdade de Medicina, Universidade de São Paulo, Ribeirão Prêto, São Paulo/Brasil.

Floyd C. McIntire, Dr., Head Biochemical Research, Abbott Laboratories, Scientific Divisions, North Chicago, Ill./USA.

Ernesto Mendes, Dr., Departamento de Microbiologia e Immunologia, Faculdade de Medicina, Avenida Dr. Arnaldo, São Paulo/Brasil.

MADELEINE MORDELET-DAMBRINE, Dr., Laboratoire de Physiologie pathologique de l'Ecole pratique des Hautes Etudes, Hôpital Boucicaut, 78, Rue de la Convention, Paris XVe/France.

IVAN MOTA, Dr., Laboratório de Fisiologia Celular, Departamento de Histologia, Faculdade de Medicina, Avenida Dr. Arnaldo, São Paulo/Brasil.

HAITY MOUSSATCHÉ, Professor Dr., Divisão de Fisiologia e Farmacologia, Instituto Oswaldo Cruz, Rio de Janeiro, Estado da Guanabara/Brasil.

PLUTARCO NARANJO, Professor Dr., Laboratorios „Life", Quito/Ecuador.

GEORGES NICOT, Dr., Ecole de Médecine de Limoges, Limoges (Haute-Vienne)/France.

JEAN-LOUIS PARROT, Professor Dr., Laboratoire de Physiologie pathologique de l'Ecole pratique des Hautes Etudes, Hôpital Boucicaut, 78, Rue de la Convention, Paris XVe/France.

HEINZ-WALTER RAUDONAT, Dr. Wissenschaftlicher Rat, Institut für gerichtliche und soziale Medizin der Universität, 6 Frankfurt a/Main/Deutschland, Kennedy-Allee 104.

JAMES F. RILEY, Professor Dr., Department of Radiotherapy, Royal Infirmary, Dundee/Scotland.

MAURICIO ROCHA E SILVA, Professor Dr., Departamento de Farmacologia, Faculdade de Medicina, Universidade de São Paulo, Ribeirão Prêto, São Paulo/Brasil.

ADOLFO MAX ROTHSCHILD, Dr., Departamento de Farmacologia, Faculdade de Medicina, Universidade de São Paulo, Ribeirão Prêto, São Paulo/Brasil.

ANATOLE SAINDELLE, Dr., Laboratoire de Physiologie pathologique de l'Ecole pratique des Hautes Etudes, Hôpital Boucicaut, 78, Rue de la Convention, Paris XVe/France.

RICHARD W. SCHAYER, Dr., The Merck Institute for Therapeutic Research, Rahway, New Jersey/USA. *Present address:* Laboratory of Chemical Pharmacology, National Heart Institute, Bethesda, Maryland 20014/USA.

UMBERTO SERAFINI, Professor Dr., Istituto di Patologia Speciale Medica e Metodologia Clinica, Università di Sassari, Viale San Pietro 8, Sassari/Italia.

PAUL STERN, Professor Dr., Institute of Pharmacology, Faculty of Medicine, Sarajevo/Yugoslavia.

HERBERT TABOR, Dr., Department of Health Education and Welfare, Public Health Service, National Instional Institutes of Health, Bethesda, Md. 20014/USA.

JOSEPH THOUVENOT, Professor Dr., Faculté de Médecine et de Pharmacie, Chaire de Physiologie, Tours/France.

BERNARD VASSEUR, Dr., Département de Physiologie, Faculté de Médecine, 45, Rue des Saint-Pères, Paris VIe/France.

ITAMAR VUGMAN, Dr., Departamento de Farmacologia, Faculdade de Medicina, Universidade de São Paulo, Ribeirão Prêto, São Paulo/Brasil.

GEOFFREY B. WEST, Professor Dr., Department of Pharmacology, School of Pharmacy, University of London, 29/39 Brunswick Square, London W. C. 1/England.

HÅKAN WESTLING, Dr., Department of Clinical Physiology, Lasarettet, Lund/Sweden.

THOMAS WHITE, Dr., Institute of Physiology, University of Lund, Lund/Sweden.

Contents

Section C: Toxicity of histamine: Lethal doses

By P. Naranjo

Section B: Release of histamine by noxious physical agents, organic compounds and by metals
By I. Vugman

Section C: Histamine release by basic compounds
By Adolfo M. Rothschild

Section D: Release of histamine in anaphylaxis
By M. Rocha e Silva

Chapter 4: Metabolism of histamine

Section A: L'excrétion de l'histamine

Par Jean-Louis Parrot et Madeleine Mordelet-Dambrine

Section B: Catabolism of histamine in vivo

By Richard W. Schayer

Section C: The relation of histamine to inflammation

By P. Stern

Section D: L'histamine dans l'allergie humaine

Par Umberto Serafini

Section E: Histamine and experimental asthma of the guinea pig

By Ernesto Mendes

Foreword

Professor ROCHA E SILVA has honoured me by an invitation to write some kind of introductory note to this volume of more than a thousand pages, which seem now to be required for the review of all the separate aspects of what has so far been discovered and discussed about this one, simple, natural base, histamine – one of the series of "proteinogenous amines," formed by the decarboxylation of the natural amino-acids; and, further, about the synthetic "antihistamines," which antagonize its potent actions. The fact that a book of such proportions should now be appearing as a mere Supplement to the regular volumes of HEFFTER's great Handbuch der experimentellen Pharmakologie, may be regarded, perhaps, as giving some measure of the prodigious growth, during the past half-century, of those areas of scientific knowledge which can properly be regarded now as belonging to the domain of Pharmacology. For it would appear that, until we were well into the first decade of the present century, the recognized range of pharmacology, though never rigidly defined, was still almost restricted in practice to the study of a number of traditional drugs, of which the uses in medicinal treatment had, in a large proportion of cases, no firmer basis than empirical conventions and assumptions; so that no more than a handful of these remedies were being found, in fact, to have actions accessible to experimental analysis, and thus to a scientific interpretation.

Even some years before 1910, however, medicinal therapeutics had begun to receive powerful reinforcements from outside these conventional limits of pharmacology, by its application of discoveries made in such rapidly developing disciplines as immunology, chemotherapy, endocrinology and biochemistry, all of them offering remedies with specific and clearly recognized actions against causes of disease – by the prevention or arrest of known infections on the one hand, and the replacement of known deficiencies, hormonal or nutritional, on the other. Pharmacology, beginning of itself to develop a more direct relation to practical therapeutics, had naturally been bound to admit, to the widening scope of its interests, a general cognizance of these antitoxins, vaccines, chemotherapeutic agents, hormones and vitamins, and of their modes of action; though it was clear that the further development of remedies of these kinds, all of them dealing with primary causes, would largely be the function of the special disciplines in which they had originated.

There would remain, however, as the more particular care of a newly progressive pharmacology, a deeper penetration, with the aid of increasing resources of experimental equipment, into the modes of action of such remedies as could be shown to be genuinely effective in the treatment of symptoms, rather than in the prevention or removal of causes; and such a pharmacology might be expected, in due course, to promote a more consistent effort, in intimate alliance with synthetic chemistry, to discover new remedies of this kind, more specifically potent than those which had been obtained from natural sources, or effective in the relief of symptoms for which no remedy had so far been found. And to make its full contribution to experimental progress on these lines, pharmacology would now have to work in an increasing intimacy of co-operation, with the accelerating growth of relevant knowledge in physiology, biochemistry, pathology and immunology, and, indeed, in any of the more fundamental scientific disciplines. Such a pharmacology would obviously need to be alert for evidence of the occurrence, in normal animal tissues, of substances having activities which would make them likely contributors to the genesis of such symptoms as would call for medicinal treatment. And I think that it could be claimed for histamine that, apart from specifically active hormones, it was the first substance to be chemically identified, among a number now recognized as having such more generally suggestive actions, in relation to potentially remediable symptoms.

It seems to me, indeed, that we may attribute at least some of the great volume and variety of the researches which have since been concerned with histamine, to the fact that its occurrence as a natural, biological product, and the striking and suggestive character of its actions, first began to come to notice in 1910, when, as I have been suggesting, pharmacology and medicinal therapeutics were just beginning to find a new impulse, towards a more adventurous kind of experimental enterprise.

When a particular combination of actions, especially on the small, peripheral branches of the vascular system, was found to be produced by histamine with a remarkable potency, this was also recognized as having at least a general resemblance to one which had been observed with simple extracts from a large proportion of the organs of the animal body. BAYLISS and STARLING, for example, had thus observed that an acid extract from the duodenal mucosa always contained, in addition to the specific hormone secretin, such an unspecific "depressor substance", unless special procedures had been adopted to exclude, or to remove it. POPIELSKI had given the name "vasodilatin" to a hypothetical principle responsible for this widely distributed type of activity. Several observers had also found that the preparation known as "Witte's peptone," which was understood to consist of peptides obtained by the peptic digestion of bovine blood-fibrin, when injected intravenously in relatively large doses, would produce, and especially in the dog, with which most of the experiments on its action had been made, a general vasodilatation, causing a shock-like collapse of the arterial blood pressure. Histamine was found to produce a generally comparable type of effect, though with a dosage which was something like a thousand times smaller than that of the peptone. And then, not long before a more systematic exploration of the actions of histamine had been undertaken, the striking contrast between the actions of this peptone on different animal species, and especially between the general aspects of its effects on the dog and on the guinea-pig, had been described by BIEDL and KRAUS, and had been presented by them as offering presumptive evidence with regard to the meaning of the remarkably similar contrast between the acute anaphylactic reactions in the same two species, which those produced by the peptone resembled, indeed, in highly suggestive detail. All was ready, therefore, for the observation that the actions of histamine, when tested in the appropriately lower order of dosage, reproduced, almost as clearly, these contrasted features of the acute anaphylactic reactions in the dog and the guinea-pig – the vasodilator collapse in the dog, and the rapidly fatal, asphyxiating constriction of the bronchioles in the guinea-pig. The resemblance, however, especially in the dog, was definitely less complete with histamine than with the peptone. A conspicuous feature of both the anaphylactic and the peptone "shock" in the dog was the gross vascular swelling of the liver, with constriction of the outlet through the hepatic veins, and the consequent retrograde congestion of the whole area drained by the portal vein. The general vasodilator effect, on the peripheral branches of all the systemic arterioles and the capillaries, appeared in both these cases to be secondary, indeed, to this primary and direct effect on the liver; whereas, in the shock due to histamine there was little such effect on the liver, and the general, systemic vasodilatation was evidently a primary, direct effect. Neither the anaphylactic nor the peptone shock could, indeed, be produced in a dog unless the liver was in circulation; while the histamine shock, by contrast, was but little affected by its exclusion. For the explanation of these differences it was necessary to wait for much later experiments and discoveries, of which full accounts will be found in the appropriate chapters of this Supplementary Volume. The point to be emphasized here is that the resemblance, between the contrasted actions of histamine and of the anaphylactic antigen, in the dog and the guinea-pig respectively, was still sufficiently impressive to convey a definite suggestion, that the liberation of histamine, in a manner enabling it to produce its intense activities, on the systems or organs most susceptible to them in these two different species, might eventually be found to play a conspicuous, or even a predominant part, in these different manifestations of the anaphylactic reaction. And all the evidence which was to become available in later years, for the presence of histamine itself, in some natural, inactivating association, in most of the organs and tissues of the normal animal body; for its presence in special concentration, and in association with heparin, in the mast cells; and for its liberation from these and other cellular sources so as to produce its characteristic actions, by various physical and chemical injuries, including those inflicted by a specific antigen on cells anaphylactically sensitized to contact with it – all this evidence was to give an impulse to experimental enterprise leading to the discovery of the "antihistamines," which will form one of the important subjects of this Supplementary review, as remedies which have established their value for the relief of the symptoms of many of the manifestations of anaphylactic or allergic conditions, and have therewith greatly strengthened the case for regarding the liberation of histamine as at least a conspicuous factor in the evocation of the corresponding reactions. And I do not think that anybody will doubt that this evidence for the connexion of histamine with allergic phenomena has played an important part, in attracting so large a proportion of more fundamental researches to the study of its occurrence, its metabolism an the mechanism of its actions. When once, however, this resemblance between the effects of histamine and those of the anaphylactic reactions, as seen in certain different species, had been recognized and described, the meaning of the correspondence was the subject of but little further investigation, or even of discussion, for more than another two decades. More convincing chemical evidence for the presence of histamine, as a natural constituent of extracts from normal, sterile animal tissues, was first required, to encourage the production then of further experimental evidence for its release in connexion with anaphylactic reactions. This did not begin to appear till 1932, when Bartosch, Feldberg and Nagel demonstrated the presence of histamine in the saline effluent from the perfused lungs of an anaphylactic guinea-pig, when the specific antigen was added to the arterial inflow, to produce the characteristic constriction of the bronchioles; and it was in the same year that Dragstedt and his collaborators showed that histamine appeared in the lymph, flowing at an increased rate from the thoracic duct of an anaphylactic dog, when an intravenous dose of the specific antigen had produced the characteristic, primary turgescence of the liver.

Meanwhile, however, during the years which had intervened, more attention had been directed to the possibility that the special characters of the vasodilator reactions which had been observed with histamine in certain animal species might have some significance, if only by analogy, for vascular reactions, observed in the human subject, to various kinds of irritation or injury, and without any special reference to the phenomena of anaphylaxis. Soon after the outbreak of the war in 1914, the conditions of shock, resulting from massive battle-injuries of the tissues, had prompted a more detailed study of the effects of histamine, producing evidence of the restriction of its vasodilator action, especially in the cat, to the ultimate arterioles and the capillary network; the full relaxation of the latter, and the abnormal permeability associated therewith, being important factors in the resulting shock-like condition produced by histamine in larger dosage. SOLLMANN in the U.S.A. had observed the oedematous wheal produced by local injection of histamine into the human skin; but the most systematic study of these local effects in man was that which was continued for some years by THOMAS LEWIS, with a series of collaborators, on the reactions of "The blood-vessels of the human skin," the "threefold reaction" of which, to mild local injuries of various kinds, they were led to attribute to the liberation from the injured cells of what, with admirable caution, they referred to as the "H-substance", meaning thereby a chemical agent resembling histamine in its local action on the minute blood-vessels, but not yet identified as histamine itself. Their caution has, of course, been more than justified by the much more recent isolation of peptide "kinins," with vascular actions similar to, though not identical with that of histamine, and rivalling, or even surpassing it in potency. There is now good reason to suppose that such a peptide agent, or agents, in addition to histamine, would be liberated under the conditions of mild injury to the skin studied by THOMAS LEWIS and his team; so that they might, perhaps, even more suitably have described the agent responsible for their threefold reaction as an "H-complex." It may be noted, in passing, that they did include a local, allergic skin-reaction, among the vascular responses to injury which they attributed to the liberation of the H-substance. In general, however, speculations about the functional significance of histamine and its actions, during the two decades following 1910, were mostly concerned with the nature of these local and systemic vascular reactions to injuries of any kind, comparatively little attention being given, at that stage, to the suggestive similarity between its more general activities, and those of the anaphylactic reactions seen in different animal species.

There were already, during that period, two different conceptions available, concerning the nature of the anaphylactic response to the specific antigen. It was generally recognized that the anaphylactic condition was due, in some way, to the appearance in the subject of an antibody of the precipitin type, having, under other conditions, an immunizing function. One of the rival conceptions, encouraged presumably by BIEDL and KRAUS's observation of the close similarity of the different types of anaphylactic shock to those produced by "peptone," supposed that an encounter between antigen and antibody, in the circulating blood, would somehow "trigger off" a proteolysis producing a toxic peptide, or "anaphylatoxin," which would then be directly responsible for the resulting symptoms. The alternative conception – referred to at the time as that of the "sessile receptors" – attributed the anaphylactic condition to the predominant fixation of the antibody to the cells of the particular organ, or tissue, which was specially sensitized in each species – to those of the liver in the dog, and to those of the plain muscle, conspicuously of the bronchioles, in the guinea-pig. A remarkable volume of research was early devoted to the support of the "anaphylatoxin" theory; and the publication of evidence in its favour has, indeed, continued even to quite recent times, as the relevant chapters in this volume will show. It might have been expected, perhaps, that the initiation of a rapid, toxin-producing proteolysis, by the encounter of the antigen with a circulating antibody, would have been easy to demonstrate, *in vitro* or *in vivo*, by producing an appropriate reaction between the specific antigen and serum from an anaphylactic guinea-pig. For some reason, however, such direct evidence for the theory was not available; so that the search for the anaphylatoxin soon began to follow the course – the relevance of which to the theoretical expectation has never yet been clear to me – of finding inert suspensions, or colloidal solutions, the incubation of which with serum from normal guinea-pigs would produce a mixture, in which there was no evidence, indeed, of any proteolytic cleavage, but which, when injected into normal guinea-pigs, would produce a train of symptoms having at least a superficial resemblance to the "Auer-Lewis Phenomenon" – the lethal constriction of the bronchioles forming the most conspicuous feature of the acute anaphylactic shock in the guinea-pig. The fact that even this resemblance was, in fact, only superficial, had seemed to me to have been made clear, by experiments showing that the bronchial obstruction produced by what was then the most potent of these colloidal "anaphylatoxins" – the "agar-anaphylatoxin" of the late Professor JULES BORDET – while sufficient to asphyxiate the guinea-pig, was very much weaker than that produced by the antigen in the true anaphylactic reaction. And it may further be noted that there has yet been no evidence that any of these artificial anaphylatoxins can produce an effect at all resembling the anaphylactic reaction in the dog, or in any species other than the guinea-pig. WITTE's peptone could still, in fact, make a fuller claim, in that respect, to be regarded as an anaphylatoxin, than any of the colloidal complexes so far prepared from the blood sera of guinea-pigs, or of rats. Whatever, therefore, may be the theoretical interest and importance, which may indeed prove to be great, of all the experiments made by distinguished investigators on these anaphylatoxin phenomena, I find it impossible, even yet, to persuade myself that they have any direct relevance to the nature of the anaphylactic reactions.

On the other hand, even before the outbreak of war in 1914, the evidence available in direct support of the rival conception of anaphylaxis, as due to the predominant fixation of an otherwise protective, precipitating antibody, to tissue cells, which this attachment would render specifically sensitive to contact with the antigen, had appeared to me to be not only much stronger, but even practically decisive. It could be shown that, if the antigen was injected into the circulation of a sensitized dog through one branch of the hepatic artery, the immediate, congestive reaction in the liver was practically limited to the part of the organ supplied by that branch. In the guinea-pig, the direct, contractile response of the sensitized plain muscle, to high dilutions of the antigen, had been demonstrated on isolated preparations of a loop of the ileum, or a horn of the virgin uterus; and it had been made clear that the washing of such a preparation, to free it from traces of blood and serum, increased, rather than diminishing, the sensitiveness of its closely specific response to the antigen. Practically every feature, indeed, of the anaphylactic phenomena – sensitization, desensitization, resensitization, the protective effect of excess of antibody in the surrounding medium, etc. – had been demonstrated on such isolated preparations of plain muscle from the guinea-pig. And others had effectively demonstrated the same relation of the distribution of the antibody between the tissues and the circulating blood, to the anaphylactic or immune condition of the living guinea-pig; the experiments of the late RICHARD WEIL being especially complete and convincing in this direction. Dr. WEIL and I had met for the first and, alas, the only time, at an International Medical Congress in London, in 1913, when we had eagerly compared the results of our respective experiments by these different methods, and had shared a great satisfaction from the close agreement of our results and conclusions; but he died all too early, during the war which was so soon to follow. I think that it is probable, indeed, that most of those who have been active in this field of research during more recent years, have likewise become convinced by the available evidence that at least the main, primary cause, of an acute anaphylactic reaction, is in such a meeting of the antigen with a precipitating antibody which has become fixed to, or incorporated by, the protoplasm, or the surface membranes, of the cells which are primarily injured, or stimulated, by the contact; whereas the same antibody, circulating in excess in the blood plasma and encountering the antigen there, forms a harmless precipitate with it, thus performing its teleologically proper, protective, immunizing function.

It may, of course, be assumed that, in many kinds of allergic reaction, the cells thus primarily affected, when this aggregating reaction occurs in their protoplasm or their surface membranes, are not those directly responsible for the overt symptoms of the reaction; their part in it may be only to release such directly vasodilator and plain-muscle stimulating substances as they contain, or can rapidly form – histamine, bradykinin – under the directly injurious effect of the antigen, so that these become, in turn, the direct agents of the pharmacodynamic effects. The demonstrable release of such substances as histamine and heparin from cells of the anaphylactic dog's liver under the primary assault of the specific antigen, and the secondary effects of these on the small blood-vessels of the general system, could be cited as an obvious example of such a stagewise, anaphylactic reaction. An allergic, urticarial skin-reaction may now be similarly regarded as due to the release of histamine and other vaso-active agents – LEWIS's "H-substance" – from sensitized tissue cells, to produce their effects on the tone and permeability of the minute blood-vessels, with a further surrounding area of arteriodilatation due to an axon-reflex; the mast-cells, or other cells primarily involved, being, as in other cases, sensitized to the antigen by "sessile" antibody. We should still have to enquire, however, whether there are not other cases, in which the cells directly involved in an anaphylactic reaction are themselves rendered sensitive to the antigen, by such an incorporation, or attachment, of its specific antibody. The most obvious example is, of course, that of the guinea-pig's plain muscle, the response of which to the intravenous injection of the antigen, together with the valvular action of the folded mucous membrane of the bronchioles, produces the "Auer-Lewis" phenomenon of acute emphysema and asphyxiation, which, in that species, anticipates what might otherwise be an anaphylactic reaction of a more general type. This plain-muscle reaction, to the antigen in high dilution, first came to my own notice in an experiment on an isolated preparation, obtained, through a misunderstanding, from an anaphylactic guinea-pig; and the reaction to the antigen seemed to me then to resemble, in the rapidity of its onset and the steepness of its rise to a maximum, the effect of a powerful stimulant drug such as pilocarpine, or of the then recently discovered histamine, rather than the ingravescent effect which I should then have been inclined to expect – perhaps without adequate reason – from an agent newly produced by proteolysis. It seemed natural to me, in any case, to assume that the presence of the precipitating antibody in the surface membrane of a plain-muscle fibre would act as a specific receptor, conferring upon the contractile fibre a specific sensitiveness to contact with the antigen, and that the consequent aggregating reaction would act by itself as an adequate stimulus; and, accordingly, I discounted the suggestion that something like peptone, or histamine, must first be liberated to account for its effect. In a Croonian Lecture to the Royal Society, in 1919, I presented this interpretation of the evidence as follows*):

"In the case of the anaphylactic cell alone, we are able to obtain a 'receptive substance,' the antibody, apart from the cell, and to study in the test-tube the nature of its reaction with the 'drug,' the specific antigen. We are entitled, I think, to suppose that, when antigen meets antibody in the specifically sensitive cell, the immediate effect is a change in the dispersion of the colloids entering into its

*) Proc. roy. Soc. Lond. **91**, 146 (1919).

structure. It appears to me to be at least a legitimate working hypothesis, to suppose that certain poisonous substances produce similar symptoms, because they also produce a change of this type. We should still have to explain why such a change, occurring in a plain muscle cell, caused it to contract; occurring in an endothelial cell, caused it to become lax and permeable."

It may again be recalled that, at this time, there was still no adequate evidence for the presence of histamine, in some inactivating association, as a constituent of many normal, sterile, animal tissues. Such evidence was not to become available till 1927; and then a further five years elapsed, before the evidence, already mentioned, was obtained by FELDBERG and his colleagues with a perfusate from the guinea-pig's lung, and by DRAGSTEDT and his team with thoracic-duct lymph from the dog, that histamine is actually liberated in connexion with the anaphylactic reaction. In the latter case, the histamine so liberated could clearly be assumed to play its part in the secondary, generalized vascular reaction, seen in the anaphylactic shock of the dog; but, in the guinea-pig, the primary, asphyxiating effect on the bronchioles is so rapidly lethal, that the production of such a more general, secondary reaction is apt to be largely, or even wholly, precluded, and is, in any case, hardly recognized as a necessary component of the anaphylactic shock in that species. And it ought, I think, to be borne in mind, that the observed appearance of histamine in the dog's thoracic duct was the result, not the cause, of the primary effect of the antigen on the cells of the liver. Even in the guinea-pig, the available evidence justifies no conclusion more definite, than that histamine is liberated in the lung at a time not distant from the response of the bronchioles. It might be liberated from cells other than those of the plain muscle, or, on the analogy of the dog's liver, its appearance might be the *result* of a primary effect of the antigen on the plain muscle fibres, rather than the *cause* of their contraction.

These experimental demonstrations, however, of the appearance of histamine in connexion with the anaphylactic shocks of both these contrasted types, undoubtedly caused a swing of opinion, in favour of its participation in all such reactions. I myself, indeed, was induced to relinquish, at least for a time, my own earlier advocacy of an action of the antigen as a direct stimulant of the sensitized plain muscle in the anaphylactic guinea-pig. Much of the more recent evidence on this question has been obtained from experiments on that species; and much of it, indeed, has only been directly relevant to the special nature of its anaphylactic phenomena. And even when difficulties began to appear, in reconciling some of these with the assumed intervention of histamine, I must further confess that I was tempted to explain them away, by a theoretical distinction between "intrinsic" and "extrinsic" histamine – picturing it as liberated, in the former case from the cells actually involved in the overt reaction, such as those of the guinea-pig's plain muscle, and in the latter case from other sensitized but non-contractile cells, such as mast-cells, in the adjacent tissues. On these lines I had proposed to explain the anomaly, that an injection of a potent "agar-anaphylatoxin" was found to liberate much more histamine from a perfused, normal lung, than the specific antigen would liberate from one which was anaphylactic to it; whereas it had been demonstrated that the resulting bronchiolar constriction was much stronger in the latter case. And again, when the antihistamines were discovered, it was found that they readily abolished the constriction of the bronchioles produced by histamine, when this was added as such to the fluid perfusing such a lung; but that they were without any recognizable effect in preventing, or relieving, the constriction produced by the specific antigen. And I was ready, here also, to suggest that, in the latter case, the histamine was inaccessible to the antagonism of an antihistamine, because it was "intrinsically" liberated, by contrast with histamine "extrinsically" applied from the outside, or liberated from other cells. My readiness, however, to accept the assumptions involved in such an explanation began to weaken, when SCHILD and his co-workers discovered that a prolonged exposure of isolated plain muscle from a guinea-pig, to histamine in a higher concentration, would make it completely insensitive to further applications of that substance; but that, if anaphylactic, it would even then still give its normal response to the antigen. And there was further evidence of such a discrepancy between the two kinds of sensitiveness, obtained by subjecting the anaphylactic plain muscle to a temperature some degrees above 40°C. When restored to the physiologically normal temperature, such a preparation was found to be still fully responsive to histamine, but had lost its sensitiveness to the anaphylactic antigen. It could rather obviously have been suggested, that the heating might somehow have just broken the links between the plain-muscle cells and the sensitizing antibody. The results of further experiments appear to show, however, that the effect must be a deeper one than such a mere detachment; for it has been found that, after such treatment, though its response to histamine is intact, the plain muscle has lost the capacity for being resensitized to the antigen, by a renewed exposure to the antibody. Whatever may yet come, however, from following this further clue, it obviously does nothing to reduce the difficulty of attributing the effect of the antigen on sensitized plain muscle to the liberation of histamine.

There was yet, however, at least one other possibility to be considered. As already indicated, there has been much evidence during recent years that, in addition to histamine, one or more peptides of the "bradykinin" type are concerned in reactions to injury of various kinds, including anaphylactic reactions to the antigen. As a direct stimulant of guinea-pig's plain muscle such a peptide may be even more potent than histamine; and its action is unaffected by the antihistamines. Here again, however, we seem to be encountering the same kind of difficulty as with histamine. For it has been known for some time that that *doyen* of the synthetic remedies, aspirin, still unrivalled in the range and variety of the symptoms for the relief of which it is hopefully applied, is an antagonist to the stimulating effects of bradykinin, as effective as the antihistamines are to those of histamine. Here again, however, the most recent evidence indicates that aspirin, like the antihistamines, fails to interfere with the effect of the antigen on the plain muscle of the anaphylactic guinea-pig.

It would not be reasonable to suggest that all the possibilities of a non-specific agent, liberated to produce the plain-muscle reaction in the anaphylactic guinea-pig, have therewith been excluded, or exhausted. It may yet become possible to consider, in that connexion, the claims of some other biogenous amine, such as serotonin (5. HT), of some other kind of peptide, or of such an apparently non-nitrogenous candidate as the 'slowly reacting substance' (SRS · A), found by BROCKLEHURST also to be liberated from the guinea-pig's lung in the anaphylactic reaction. I think, however, that it can fairly be suggested that the only substances which can, so far, be clearly recognized, as having actions which might entitle them to be considered for anything like a complete intermediary function, even in the anaphylactic reaction of the guinea-pig alone, are histamine and bradykinin. At present, therefore, it seems that we have still to deal with the difficulty that the anaphylactic plain muscle can be deprived of its response to either of these, and yet retain, without perceptible diminution, its specific sensitiveness to an antigen. I have, of course, no right to suggest that the distinction between "intrinsic" and "extrinsic" histamine, or bradykinin, should no longer be considered, as providing a possible explanation of this observed indifference of the anaphylactic, plain-muscle reaction, to the antagonists of these substances. I can only hope that it may yet be found possible to put such a theoretical conception to the test of an experiment so crucial, that its result would enable the idea to be more firmly accepted, or finally discarded. I venture now to express a similar hope, however, with regard to the earlier and, for a time, discounted conception, of a direct sensitization of the guinea-pig's plain muscle, by the cell-fixed antibody, to a specific, aggregating effect of the antigen. Perhaps some of the modern resources for the measurement, or observation, of ultramicroscopic changes, might yet be able to bring this idea also, to the test of a direct and decisive experiment.

In any case, and whatever the pattern of interpretation which may for the moment commend itself to the individual judgment, I think that it has to be recognized that, not only in the guinea-pig, but also in the allergic human patient, there is evidence of two components in an allergic reaction, varying in their relative prominence in different individuals, and in the same individual in different manifestations of his allergy; so that the same patient may suffer on one occasion from an urticaria which yields readily to treatment with an antihistamine, and on another occasion from a bronchial asthma, which is hardly, if at all, affected by the same treatment. And it seems to me that, on any theory, it must be recognized as probable that the former would be due to the liberation, from neighbouring tissue cells, of an intermediary agent, with which the treatment could deal by suppressing its vascular effects; whereas the asthmatic attack would be largely due to a more direct effect of the antigen on bronchiolar plain muscle, for which some other kind of remedy would still have to be sought.

So far, I have been using this opportunity to offer certain comments on the evidence suggesting a significance for histamine and its actions, in connexion with the reactions of the body – of its small blood vessels and of other contractile elements – to various kinds of local and systemic injury, including the types of injury caused, in an allergic subject, by contact with the specific antigen. It cannot, indeed, be doubted that it has been with this mainly pathological aspect of its significance, that an overwhelming majority of the experiments dealing with the functions of histamine have hitherto been concerned. There is already, on the other hand, a great accumulation of evidence concerning the origin, distribution and metabolism of histamine, as a natural constituent of many organs and tissues; and such knowledge, whatever may have been the nature of the interest prompting the researches which have produced it, will obviously be available for the consideration of other possible functions of histamine, in connexion with normal, physiological phenomena; most obviously of its possible concern with the fine adjustment of blood-flow to the varying needs of small tissue units. It is obvious that methods permitting measurements in a much finer range, than those which have been used in the classical physiology of the circulation, will be needed to explore such a possibility; but I believe that there will be no lack of the enterprise needed to test it. Meanwhile Professor KAHLSON and his team at LUND, have been finding evidence that the rapid growth of foetal rats *in utero*, of the granulation tissue repairing a wound, and of certain tumors, is accompanied by the presence of an abnormally high amount of histidinase in the cells of the tissues concerned, and the excretion of an abnormal proportion of the metabolites of histamine; while metabolic and pharmacological treatments, which prevent the abnormal excess of histidinase, prevent also the kinds of rapid growth in question. This apparent increase of histamine is not associated with any recognizable symptoms of the kind hitherto associated with its presence, or its liberation. And perhaps it should further be noted that, so far, this phenomenon of the increased, intracellular formation of histamine in tissues undergoing a rapid development, has apparently been observed only in the rat – a species which is conspicuously insensitive to those pharmacodynamic effects which histamine characteristically produces in other species, and which had hitherto attracted so much interest to its occurrence and its functional significance. This, however, may perhaps be regarded as only another of those paradoxes, which the study of histamine and its actions has already appeared to present in an unending series, and which have assuredly not been without their share in producing such an imposing succession of researches, as are here to be brought under detailed review, by the distinguished authors of the special Chapters of this Volume.

HENRY H. DALE

Chapter 1

Chemistry, Isolation and Occurrence of Histamine

Section A

Chemistry of Histamine and Analogs. Relationship between Structure and Pharmacological Activity

By

REUBEN G. JONES

I. Introduction

A. Historical background

The first correlation of the chemical structure of histamine with its powerful physiological effects upon smooth muscle and upon blood pressure was reported by BARGER and DALE (1910a). These workers had isolated histamine from ergot and had shown it to be identical with a specimen of 4 (or 5)-(2-aminoethyl)-imidazole prepared by ACKERMANN (1910) by bacterial decarboxylation of histidine. Indeed, histamine had been chemically synthesized by WINDAUS and VOGT (1907) several years before its physiological actions were recognized. DALE and LAIDLAW (1910, 1912) fully described many of the physiological effects of histamine.

Following the isolation of histamine from ergot by KUTSCHER (1910) and by BARGER and DALE (1910a, b), the occurrence of histamine in intestinal mucosa was demonstrated by BARGER and DALE (1911). MELLANBY and TWORT (1912) confirmed the fact that histamine could be isolated from intestinal mucosa, but they suggested that it was formed by bacterial action on histidine present in the intestinal contents. It remained for ABEL and KUBOTA (1919) to show that histamine was present as a normal constituent of many, if not all, tissues and was not exclusively a product of bacterial decarboxylation of histidine. These authors isolated histamine from pituitary glands, liver, muscle, and other tissues. Later, BEST, et al. (1927) identified histamine in liver and lung tissue, and ACKERMANN and MOHR (1938) described its isolation from liver.

B. Nomenclature

In the realm of natural products, histamine is one of the simplest of chemical compounds. It is 4 (or 5)-(2-aminoethyl)imidazole, $C_5H_9N_3$, and is represented structurally by either formula I or II.

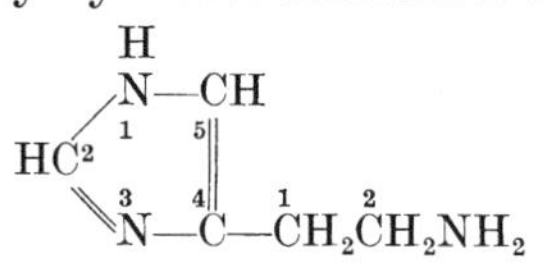

I

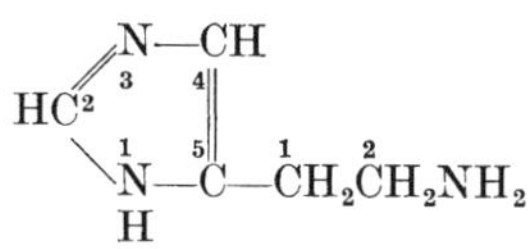

II

The conventional way of numbering the atoms in the imidazole ring is to assign the imino nitrogen (the one carrying hydrogen) position 1, and to follow around the ring in such a way that the other nitrogen atom is given the smallest possible number (3). Thus, structure I is 4-(2-aminoethyl)imidazole and structure II is 5-(2-aminoethyl)imidazole. As is seen in structure I and II, the carbon atoms of the ethyl side chain are numbered 1 and 2 independently of the ring. The imino hydrogen of the imidazole ring is mobile and can shift from one nitrogen atom to the other with a concomitant shift of the double bond. Thus, the two forms, I and II, of histamine coexist. Although tautomeric forms of histamine and certain other compounds may exist, when structural formulas are used hereafter, only one form arbitrarily will be given. The naming of such compounds, however, will indicate the two possible structures. Obviously, when histamine or other similar compounds have substituents on the 1-position of the imidazole ring, tautomerism is no longer possible. Therefore, 1-methyl-4-(2-aminoethyl)imidazole and 1-methyl-5-(2-aminoethyl)imidazole are two separate and distinct compounds.

II. Synthesis of histamine

A. Synthesis from histidine

Bacterial decarboxylation. Ackermann (1910) discovered that histamine is readily obtained by bacterial decarboxylation of histidine, and this method is generally used for the commercial production of histamine. Ackermann's original procedure was as follows: Forty-nine grams of histidine dihydrochloride was dissolved in 4 l. of water to which was added 10 g. of peptone, 20 g. of glucose, several drops of manganese sulfate and sodium phosphate solutions, and an excess of calcium carbonate to maintain the mixture alkaline. The innoculum consisted of the unidentified bacteria growing in small pieces of beef pancreas that had been allowed to stand in an incubator with very dilute sodium carbonate solution for twenty-four hours. Fermentation was allowed to proceed in a closed flask for fifty-two days at 35° C.

The earlier procedure for isolating the histamine from the filtered broth of such a fermentation involved precipitation as the picrate. More recently, Galat and Friedman (1949) have recommended the use of 3,4-dichlorobenzenesulfonic acid, which precipitates histamine as an insoluble salt that is readily purified by recrystallization from water. The filtrate from the fermentation of twenty grams of histidine monohydrochloride is treated with one hundred and twenty grams of 3,4-dichlorobenzenesulfonic acid and allowed to stand overnight. The crystals of histamine bis-3,4-dichlorobenzenesulfonate are collected, washed with water, and recrystallized from four hundred ml. of boiling water. After drying at 100°, the product weighs forty-seven grams which represents a yield of eighty-seven percent.

Histamine dihydrochloride is readily prepared from the 3,4-dichlorobenzenesulfonate by adding the latter to ten times its weight of boiling n-butanol saturated with hydrogen chloride. After cooling the solution to room temperature, the crystalline histamine dihydrochloride is collected on a filter, washed with n-butanol then with benzene and dried. The yield is about ninety percent.

The preparation of histamine diphosphate consists of treating a hot solution of the bis-3,4-dichlorobenzenesulfonate in about five times its weight of water with exactly one equivalent of barium hydroxide in water solution. After the mixture has cooled, the precipitate of barium 3,4-dichlorobenzenesulfonate is removed by filtration, and the filtrate is treated with phosphoric acid in some excess. The solution is then concentrated to small volume, and the histamine diphosphate is precipitated by the gradual addition of methanol. A yield of about ninety percent is realized.

Many different bacteria appear to be able to decarboxylate histidine to form histamine. KOESSLER and HANKE (1919b) studied an *E. coli* strain and observed that the fermentation required a nitrogen source and the presence of oxygen. Of a large number of organisms studied, HANKE and KOESSLER (1922) found six *E. coli* strains that could carry out the decarboxylation. EGGERTH (1939) investigated organisms from the human intestinal tract and found forty-nine strains in fourteen species of seven genera that could decarboxylate histidine. GALE (1940) has studied the optimum conditions for the decarboxylation of histidine by various species of *E. coli* and GALE (1941) has also carried out similar studies with organisms of the Clostridium group. The most active of a number of species and strains of bacteria examined by AISO, et al. (1956) was *Proteus morganii*. PENNIMPEDE, et al. (1957) observed various Klebsiella species that can convert histidine to histamine to the extent of thirteen to sixteen percent in twenty-four hours.

Heat decarboxylation. The preparation of histamine from histidine by heat induced decarboxylation was described by EWINS and PYMAN (1911). Solutions of histidine in concentrated hydrochloric acid, moderately dilute sulfuric acid, or fused potassium acid sulfate were heated in closed vessels to 265—270°. The yields of histamine were about twenty-five percent. Another variation was to heat benzoylhistidine to 240°.

B. From imidazolepropionic acid

The original synthesis of histamine by WINDAUS and VOGT (1907) involved the Curtius degradation of imidazoleproprionic acid hydrazide as indicated in the accompanying reactions:

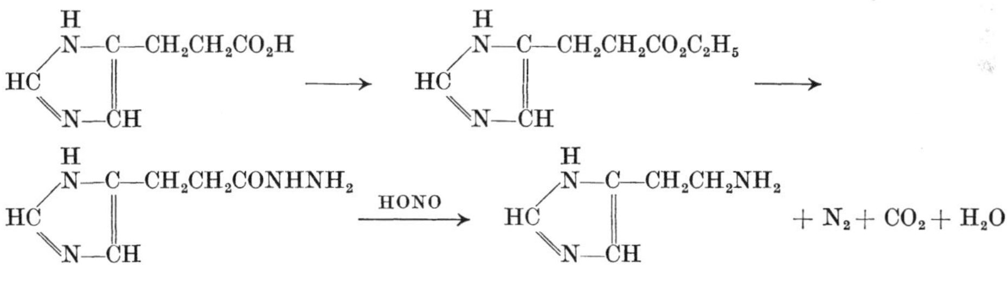

Imidazolepropionic acid can be obtained by deamination of histidine or by a variety of chemical syntheses starting from simpler materials.

C. From α-aminoketones

The greatest problem in the synthesis of histamine has been in the preparation of the imidazole ring with substituents suitable for further chemical transformations. PYMAN (1911a) used diaminoacetone as a starting material. This was allowed to react with thiocyanic acid to form 2-mercapto 4 (or 5)-aminomethylimidazole. The latter, upon treatment with nitric acid, was converted to 4 (or 5)-hydroxymethylimidazole. This key intermediate was converted through the chloride to the nitrile which was reduced with sodium metal and alcohol to histamine. The reactions are outlined in the accompanying chart.

KOESSLER and HANKE (1918) carefully reinvestigated this method and made some improvements in certain of the steps. More recently, PLIML and PROTIVA (1952) have described much better methods of carrying out the last step in the above sequence. Instead of using sodium and alcohol, they have employed lithium aluminum hydride or hydrogen with a nickel catalyst to reduce the nitrile.

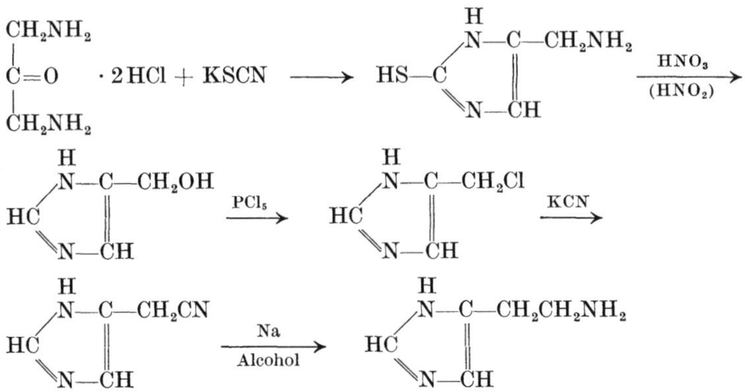

Another histamine synthesis described by PYMAN (1930a) involves 1,4-diamino-2-butanone as the starting material.

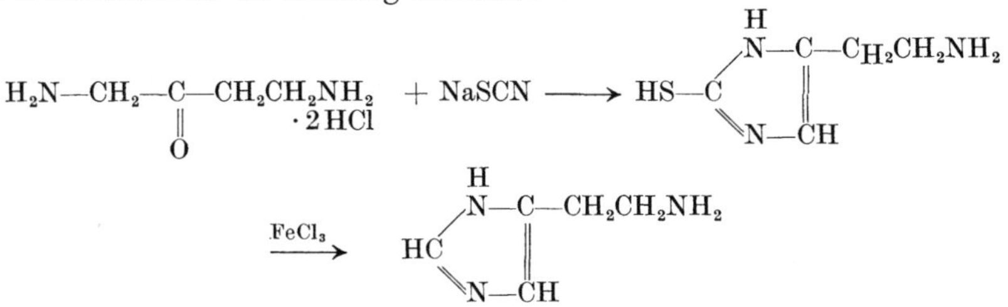

This method has become of more interest recently with the discovery by FRASER and RAPHAEL (1952) of a way to prepare the intermediate 1,4-diamino-2-butanone from the readily available 1,4-dihydroxy-2-butyne.

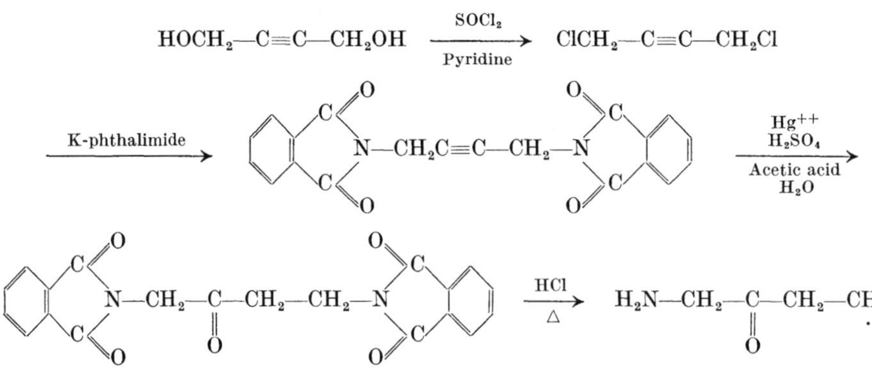

By this series of reactions, FRASER and RAPHAEL (1952) have prepared histamine in an over-all yield of forty percent starting from 1,4-dihydroxy-2-butyne. Should it become necessary to synthesize histamine on a large scale, this chemical method would appear to be the most practical yet devised.

D. From α-aminoaldehydes

α-Aminoaldehydes react with thiocyanic acid just as do α-aminoketones to yield 2-mercaptoimidazoles with substituents in the 4 (or 5) position of the ring. AKABORI (1933) has devised a method for making α-aminoaldehydes from esters of α-amino acids and converting these aldehydes to imidazoles. Starting from an α,γ-diaminobutyric acid ester, AKABORI and NUMANO (1932, 1936) have described a synthesis of histamine by the following series of reactions:

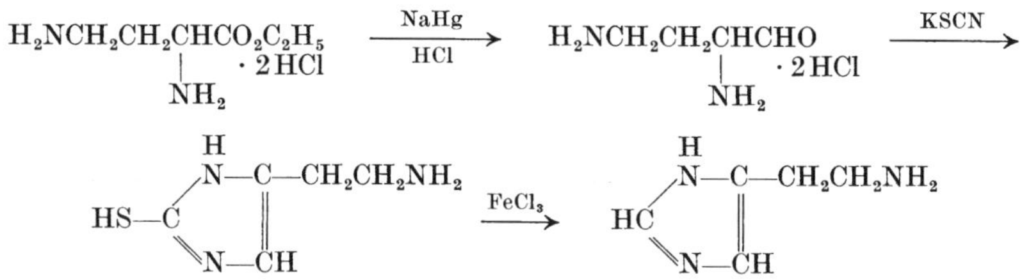

An entirely analogous series of reactions carried out by AKABORI (1933), starting from diethyl glutamate, leads to ethyl 4 (or 5)-imidazolepropionate, the intermediate used in the original histamine synthesis by WINDAUS and VOGT (1907).

E. From α-hydroxyketones

A general method for the synthesis of imidazole compounds consists of a reaction between ammonia, an aldehyde, and an α-hydroxyketone in the presence of cupric acetate which acts as an oxidizing agent. The imidazole is isolated as an insoluble copper salt which is treated with hydrogen sulfide to free the imidazole compound. This reaction was extensively investigated by WEIDENHAGEN and HERRMANN (1935). These workers prepared 4 (or 5)-hydroxymethylimidazole (a key intermediate mentioned above in PYMAN's histamine synthesis) from formaldehyde, ammonia, dihydroxyacetone, and cupric acetate.

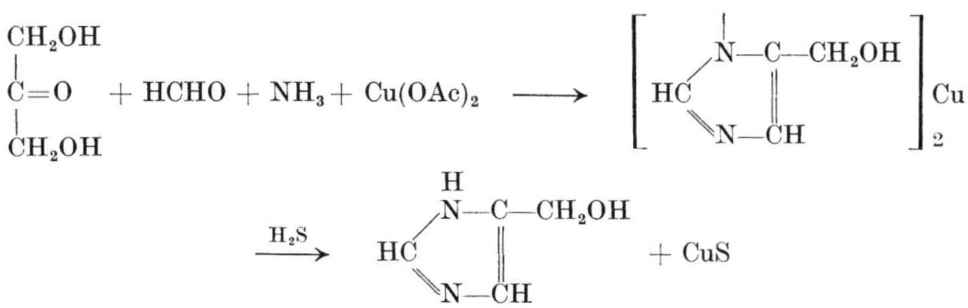

This same hydroxymethylimidazole wapres pared also by WEIDENHAGEN, et al. (1937) using fructose in place of dihydroxyacetone. DARBY, et al. (1942) have developed this reaction of fructose, ammonia, formaldehyde, and cupric acetate into a useful method for preparing 4 (or 5)-hydroxymethylimidazole, and with this intermediate readily available, the method of PYMAN (1911) described above has become more practical for the synthesis of histamine.

A reaction of 1,4-dihydroxy-2-butanone with formaldehyde, ammonia, and cupric acetate has been reported by EBEL, et al. (1951) to give 4 (or 5)-(2-hydroxyethyl)-imidazole. The latter can be converted to the chloroethyl compound which by reaction with ammonia gives histamine. HUEBNER (1951) has investigated this same reaction sequence starting with 1,4-dihydroxy-2-butyne.

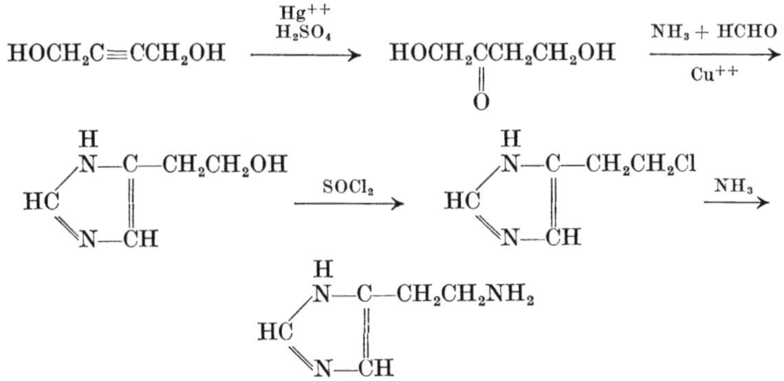

This chemical synthesis, like the others just described, is probably not of practical importance at present. Up until now the commercial needs for histamine have been satisfied by relatively small quantities of material prepared by decarboxylation of histidine using bacterial fermentation.

III. Labeled histidine and histamine

A. Histidine

In recent years there has been considerable interest in the mechanism of formation and the metabolism of histamine in the animal body. Studies along these lines have been greatly facilitated by the use of isotopically labeled compounds. Histidine, as well as histamine, has been employed in this work, and the preparation of both of these compounds labeled in various positions is discussed here.

Histidine containing C^{14} in the carboxyl group was synthesized by BORSOOK, et al. (1952). The starting compound was carboxyl-labeled glycine. This was converted to N-benzoyl glycine which was carried through the standard azlactone synthesis with imidazole aldehyde as shown in the accompanying reactions.

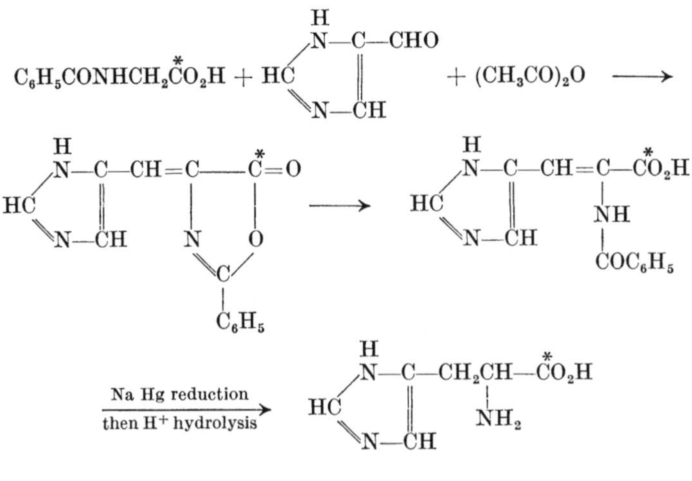

Another synthesis of carboxyl-labeled histidine has been described by BOUTHILLIER and D'IORIO (1950). This preparation starts from C^{14} sodium cyanide and involves another standard amino-acid synthesis.

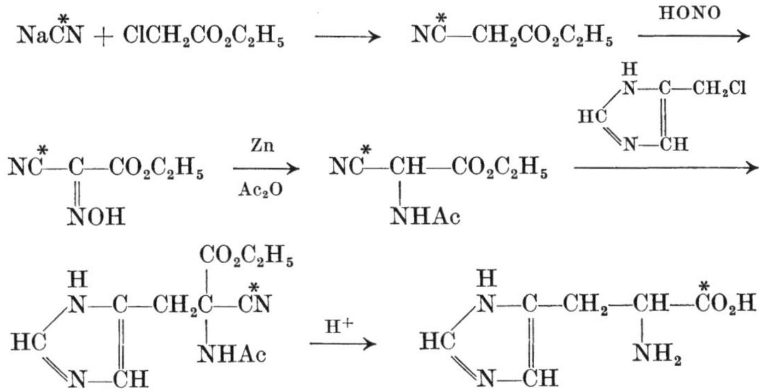

The over-all yield of C^{14} *dl*-histidine was six percent.

The same series of reactions was used by WOLF (1953) to prepare *dl*-histidine labeled with C^{14} in the α-carbon atom. In this case the starting compound was ethyl acetaminocyanoacetate labeled in the α-position.

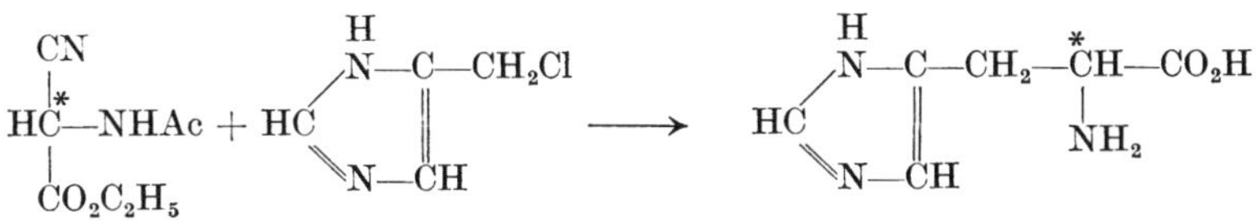

L-histidine labeled with C^{14} in the 2 position of the imidazole ring has been synthesized by BORSOOK, et al. (1950), SPRINSON and RITTENBERG (1952), and by SCHAYER (1952). Each of these groups employed a synthetic method based on the work of ASHLEY and HARRINGTON (1930). The sequence of reactions beginning with cold *L*-histidine is particularly suitable for isotope work because the label is introduced near the end of the process. Furthermore, no racemization of the asymmetric carbon atom takes place so the final product is optically active if optically active histidine is used as starting material.

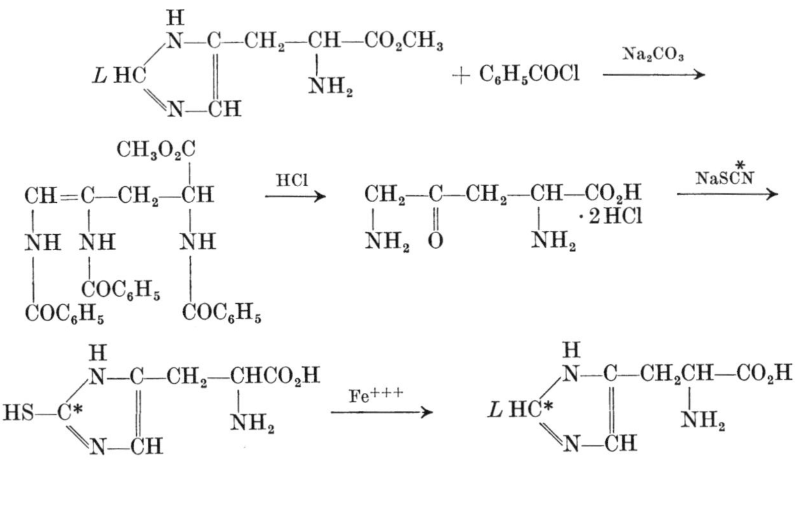

This same procedure of ASHLEY and HARRINGTON (1930) just described has been used by TESAR and RITTENBERG (1947) to prepare histidine in which one of the nitrogen atoms of the imidazole ring was labeled with N^{15}. Potassium thiocyanate containing N^{15} was used.

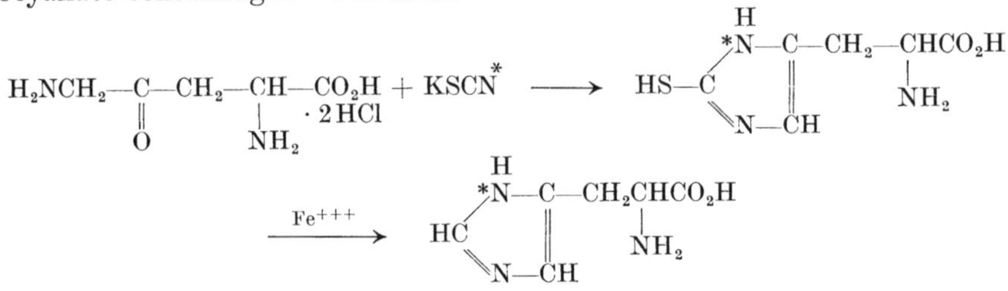

Histidine in which the amino nitrogen of the side chain was labeled with N^{15} has been described by TABOR, et al. (1952). Again, the starting material was naturally occurring histidine. It was treated with nitrous acid in the presence of concentrated hydrochloric acid to give 2-chloro-3-(4 or 5-imidazole)propionic acid. This, in turn, was heated with N^{15}-containing ammonia to yield N^{15}-labeled histidine.

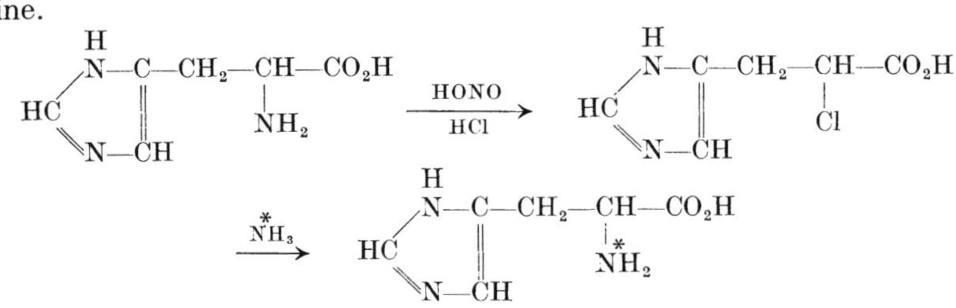

B. Histamine

Histamine labeled with C^{14} in the carbon atom carrying the amino group of the side chain has been prepared by BOUTHILLIER and GOLDNER (1953). The method involved condensation of chloromethylimidazole with C^{14} potassium cyanide followed by reduction of the resulting nitrile with sodium and alcohol.

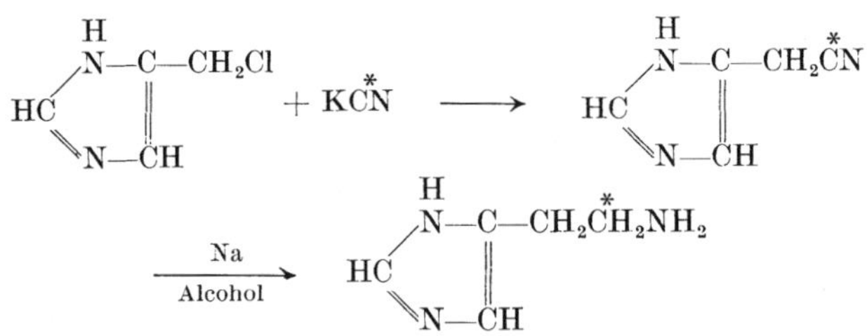

SCHAYER (1952) has prepared histamine labeled with C^{14} at the 2 position of the imidazole ring from the corresponding labeled histidine described above. This was accomplished by use of a decarboxylase enzyme from Lactobacillus. The yield of pure product was sixty-five percent.

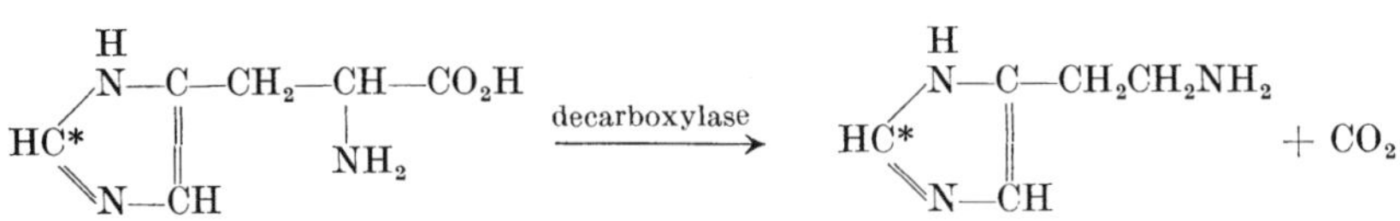

Methylation of the acetyl derivative of histamine labeled at position 2 of the ring was carried out by ROTHSCHILD and SCHAYER (1958) to prepare the histamine analog, 1-methyl-4-(2-aminoethyl)imidazole-2C^{14}. This is one of the mammalian metabolic products of histamine.

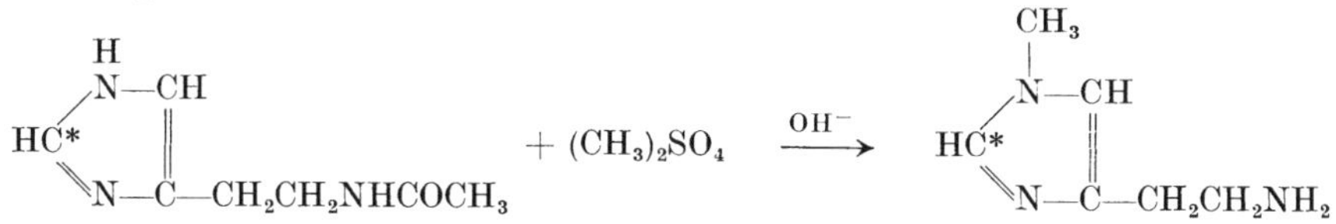

IV. Physical and chemical properties of histamine

A. Physical properties

Histamine base was first isolated by PYMAN (1912), who obtained it by treating an aqueous solution of the dihydrobromide with excess sodium carbonate, evaporation of the mixture to dryness, and extraction of the histamine from the inorganic salts with hot chloroform. The base also has been prepared by TABOR and MOSETTIG (1949) by treatment of a water solution of the dihydrochloride with Amberlite IRA-400 resin.

Free histamine crystallizes as colorless plates and melts at 83—84°. It distills at 209—210° (18 mm.). The base is highly soluble in water and in alcohol, but insoluble in ether or benzene. HATEM (1956) has studied viscosity of histamine solutions in water and has reported that the compound is highly associated by hydrogen bonds. The absorption spectrum in the ultraviolet is of no value as an analytical method for histamine, because, as LEWIS, et al. (1933) observed, the compound does not exhibit an absorption maximum in the 210 to 700 mμ region.

When titrated in water solution, histamine is found to have two basic centers with pK'_a values of 5.94 and 9.80 as reported by HOLMES and JONES (1960). SCHALIEN (1958) reported pK'_a values of 5.79 and 9.76 obtained by titration in aqueous potassium chloride solution at 25°. Two series of salts are formed dependent upon whether one or both of the basic groups are neutralized. In Table 1 are listed the salts of histamine, together with some of their properties.

B. Metal complexes

Histamine forms salts and complexes with a number of heavy metals. The conditions under which these metal compounds can be observed appear to be quite specific, and therefore the literature on this subject is confused. In connection with the original preparation of histamine, WINDAUS and VOGT (1907) observed that the compound gave no precipitate with ammoniacal silver or zinc solutions, but it did give a precipitate with mercuric chloride and potassium hydroxide. This mercury precipitate has not been further investigated.

HATEM (1955) has studied a silver complex of histamine of the composition $[Ag(C_5H_9N_3)_2]NO_3 \cdot XH_2O$. This is obtained as a gel-like precipitate when solutions of histamine and silver nitrate are mixed at pH 7.5.

Contrary to the early observations of WINDAUS and VOGT (1907) and to a more recent statement by EICHLER and MEYER (1948), histamine does form an insoluble zinc complex. ACKERMANN and FUCHS (1939) and KAPELLER-ADLER (1941) have made use of this insoluble compound in the isolation of histamine from urine. The procedure consisted of treating 1 liter of urine with 30 ml. of a saturated solution of zinc hydroxide in ammonium hydroxide. After standing overnight the zinc-histamine precipitate was collected, and the histamine was isolated by appropriate procedures. Weitzel and Fretzdorff (1956) have shown that the composition of the water-insoluble precipitate formed by the reaction of histamine with zinc hydroxide is $C_{10}H_{16}N_6Zn$ which corresponds to (Histamine)$_2$Zn. In acidic solutions zinc and histamine do not form insoluble complexes. A solution containing Histamine · 2HCl and $ZnCl_2$ when evaporated gives crystals of $C_5H_9N_3 \cdot ZnCl_2 \cdot$ · 2HCl which are very water soluble according to Weitzel and Fretzdorff (1956). In connection with other studies, Albert (1952) has measured the formation constant of a zinc-histamine complex in aqueous solution.

Axmacher (1936) found that histamine base with copper sulfate in water solution gave a deep blue color. When the solution was evaporated, a water soluble, amorphous, blue residue was obtained. Histamine dihydrochloride gave no blue color with copper sulfate. Equilibrium constants for the formation of complexes between histamine and copper (II), as well as cobalt (II) and nickel (II), ions in aqueous solution have been measured by Albert (1952), Mickel and Andrews (1955a, b), Hares, et al. (1956), and Holmes and Jones (1960). There is general agreement that the copper-histamine complex involves one cupric ion associated with two histamine molecules while the cobalt and nickel complexes each involve one metal ion associated with three histamine molecules. Albert (1952) and Mickel and Andrews (1955b) have speculated that the copper complex may have a structure like I. An alternative structure II has been suggested by Eichler and Meyer (1948).

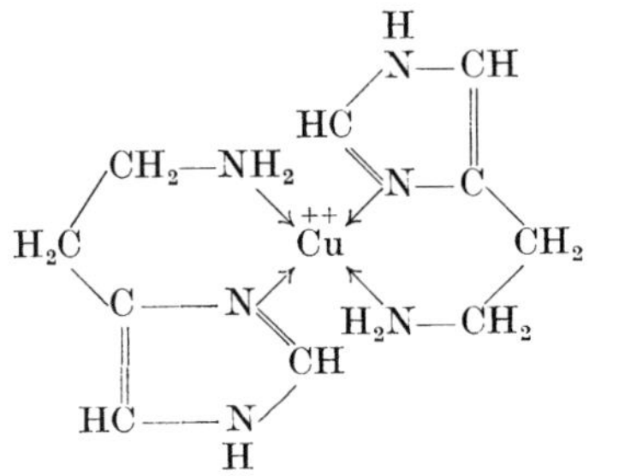

I

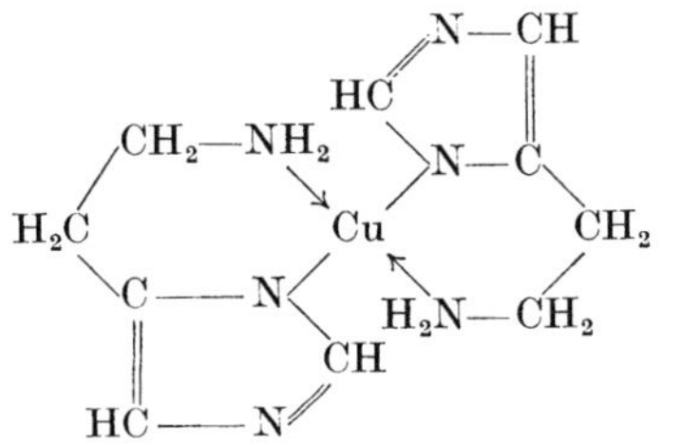

II

The reason for proposing structure II was the observation that copper interferes with the coupling of histamine with diazonium compounds (Pauly color test), and Fargher and Pyman (1919) have stated that for this diazo coupling to take place a free imino hydrogen must be present on the imidazole nucleus.

It is quite possible that a complex of structure I may exist in solution at low and intermediate pH ranges and that it may be converted to structure II as the pH is raised. Andrews and Lyons (1957) have observed the formation of a stable complex *in vitro* between histamine, cupric ion, and bovine serum albumin. The presence of copper is necessary for the binding of histamine to albumin, and this may have some implications relative to the physiological binding and activity of histamine.

Recently Eichler and Höbel (1963) have observed that histamine and copper (II) ions in borate buffer at pH 8.6 to 9.4 formed a blue-violet 1 : 1 complex which was characterized by electrophoresis and by ultra-violet spectrum. In the presence of excess histamine, a brown, less stable 1 : 2 complex also was formed. The 1 : 1 complex did not combine with hog serum albumen. In fact, the albumen decomposed the complex with formation of a copper-albumen compound and liberation of histamine.

A violet precipitate is obtained when a solution of histamine and cobalt nitrate is treated with base, and this reaction has been proposed by ZIMMERMANN (1929) as a specific color test for histamine. REY-BELLET and ERLENMEYER (1954) have reported that a violet crystalline precipitate is obtained when an aqueous solution of histamine dihydrochloride is treated with ammoniacal $Ni(CN)_2$. The composition of the compound is $C_7H_9N_5Ni$ which corresponds to a 1:1 ratio of histamine to $Ni(CN)_2$. This product is quite insoluble even in hot concentrated ammonium hydroxide.

C. Chemical properties

Histamine undergoes the expected chemical reactions characteristic of primary amines and of imidazole compounds. With nitrite in acid solution the primary amino group is replaced by hydroxyl to form 4 (or 5)-(2-hydroxyethyl)imidazole as observed by WINDAUS and OPITZ (1911). GERNGROSS (1919a) carried out an alkylation of the amino group by reaction of histamine with 4-(2-chloroethyl)-phenol to prepare N-2-(4-hydroxyphenyl)ethylhistamine. Another alkylation reaction was reported by VAN DER MERWE (1928). In this case histamine was allowed to react withN-benzoyl-5-chloroamylamine, and the resulting product was hydrolyzed to yield N-5-aminoamylhistamine. VAN DER MERWE (1928) carried out reactions of histamine with potassium cyanate, cyanamide, phenyl isocyanate, and α-naphthyl isocyanate to obtain respectively N-carbamyl-, N-guanyl-, N-phenylcarbamyl-, and N-α-naphthylcarbamylhistamine.

Acylation of the primary amino group of histamine takes place readily. By reaction with acetic anhydride, VAN DER MERWE (1928) and TABOR and MOSETTIG (1949) prepared N-acetyl histamine. N-Benzoylhistamine has been prepared by GERNGROSS (1919b) and by DIEMAIR and FOX (1938) by mild treatment of histamine with benzoyl chloride. Further reaction of this product with benzoyl chloride in benzene solution under carefully controlled conditions leads to 1-benzoyl-4-(2-benzamidoethyl)imidazole as described by GERNGROSS (1919b).

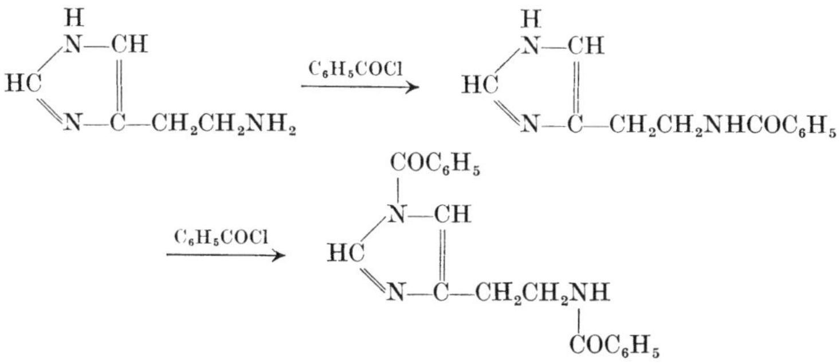

WINDAUS and VOGT (1907) and WINDAUS, et al. (1921, 1922) have found that benzoyl chloride and other acyl chlorides react with histamine in the presence of aqueous sodium hydroxide to bring about opening of the imidazole ring as indicated by the accompanying reaction.

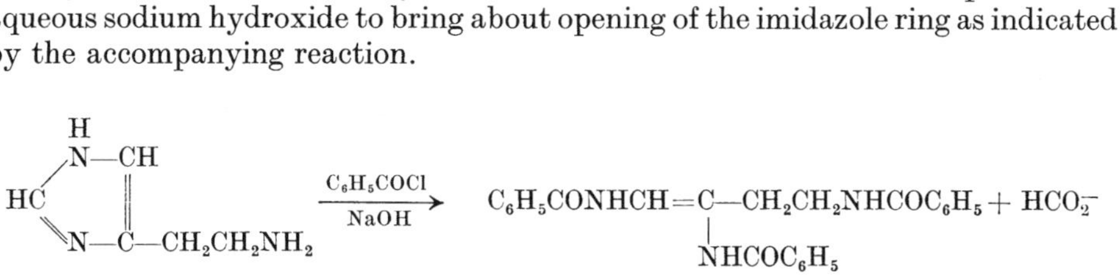

As might be expected, acyl azides, as well as azlactones, acylate the primary amino group of histamine. ROCHA E SILVA (1943) has prepared amino acid derivatives of histamine by reactions of the following types:

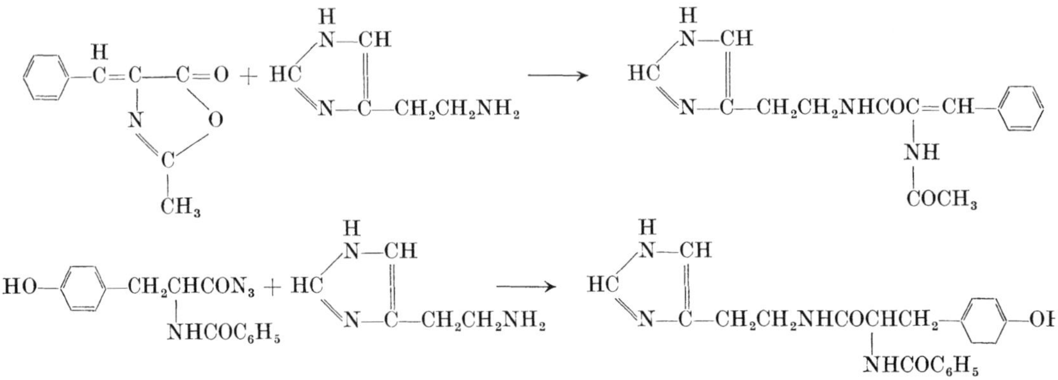

Aromatic aldehydes react with histamine to form Schiff bases which are isolated as yellow or orange crystalline solids. These compounds can be reduced either catalytically or with sodium in alcohol to form N-alkylated histamines. VAN DER MERWE (1928) carried out such reactions with anisaldehyde and 3,4-methylenedioxybenzaldehyde, HEYL, et al. (1948) with pyridoxal, and PLIML and PROTIVA (1953) with benzaldehyde. These latter authors also have described the reaction of histamine with benzophenone to give benzhydrylidinehistamine isolated as a crystalline compound. It did not undergo catalytic reduction.

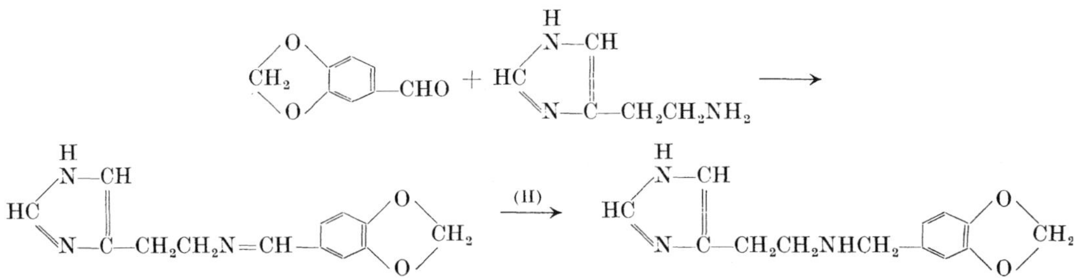

The reaction product obtained by heating an acidic, aqueous solution of histamine and formaldehyde is a bicyclic compound. This was first reported by FRÄNKEL and ZEIMER (1920) to be even more active than histamine on smooth muscle, but later DALE and DUDLEY (1921) found the compound to be practically devoid of histamine-like activity.

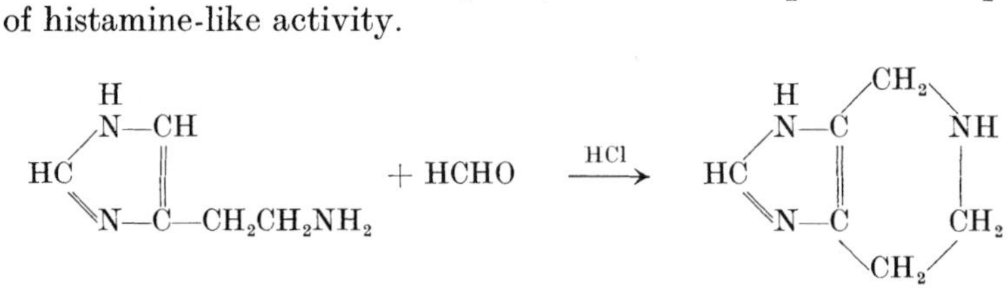

A related bicyclic compound has been described by HEYL, et al. (1948) and HOFFMAN, et al. (1951), obtained from a reaction of histamine with pyridoxal.

A reaction typical of many imidazole compounds, including histamine, is coupling with diazotized aromatic amines in weakly basic solution to form azo dyes. PAULY (1904) first described this as a color test for histidine and related imidazole compounds. KOESSLER and HANKE (1919a) and GEBAUER-FÜLNEGG (1930) developed the diazonium coupling reaction as a color test for histamine. The analytical aspects of the reaction will be discussed in detail in a later section of this monograph. After a careful study of the reactions of diazonium compounds with imidazoles, FARGHER and PYMAN (1919) concluded that in the products the azo group was attached to a carbon atom in the imidazole nucleus. In order for coupling to take place, a free imino group must be present and also a hydrogen atom or some other displaceable group must be in position 2, 4, or 5 of the imidazole ring. KESZTYUS (1948) has described 2-phenylazohistamine, 2-(4-nitrophenyl)azohistamine, and 2-(4-aminophenyl)azohistamine as crystalline products. The latter was diazotized and coupled to horse or cattle serum which, according

Table 1. *Histamine salts and some of their properties*

Salt	M. P. °C.	Solubility in water	Reference
Monohydrochloride . . .	193	very soluble	GERNGROSS (1919b)
Dihydrochloride	240—242	very soluble	WINDAUS and VOGT (1907)
Monohydrobromide . . .	182—183	very soluble	PYMAN (1912)
Dihydrobromide	284	very soluble	EWINS and PYMAN (1911)
Dinitrate	149—150	very soluble	GERNGROSS (1919b)
Di-acid phosphate	132—133	1 part in 4, cold; readily soluble hot	PYMAN (1912)
Dichloraurate	200—206	insoluble cold[1]	ACKERMANN and MOHR (1938)
Chloroplatinate	dec. 200	sparingly cold, readily soluble hot	WINDAUS and VOGT (1907)
Iodoplatinate		insoluble	VAN ITALLIE and STEENHAUER (1925)
Iodobismuthate		insoluble	VAN ITALLIE and STEENHAUER (1925)
Phosphotungstate		insoluble	WINDAUS and VOGT (1907)
Silicotungstate		insoluble	VAN ITALLIE and STEENHAUER (1925)
Monopicrate	233—234	insoluble cold, soluble hot	EWINS and PYMAN (1911)
Dipicrate	238—242	insoluble cold, soluble hot[2]	PYMAN (1911a)
Dipicrolonate	266	insoluble cold, 1 part in 450 hot	WINDAUS and VOGT (1907)
Di-pentachlorophenate . .	177—179	insoluble	IKEDA and IKEDA (1951)
Di-5-nitrobarbiturate . . .		about 7.4 g. per liter, 25°	REDEMANN and NIEMANN (1940)
Monoflavianate[3]	258—260	0.15 g. in 100 ml., 21°	ACKERMANN and MOHR (1938)
Diflavianate[4]	262—263	0.10 g. in 100 ml., 21°	ACKERMANN and MOHR (1938)
Disozoiodolate[5]	241	0.76 g. in 100 ml., 25°	ACKERMANN (1934)
Di-2-nitroindane-1,3-dionate		about 0.8 g. per liter	WANAG and DOMBROWSKI (1942)
Di-3,4-dichlorobenzene-sulfonate	225—227	insoluble cold; very soluble hot	GALAT and FRIEDMAN (1949)
Diaminoquinonesulfonate .		insoluble	GARREAU (1935)

[1] The dichloraurate dissolves to the extent of 0.4 g. in 50 ml. of boiling water, HORN (1932). It undergoes decomposition in water but may be recrystallized without decomposition from strong hydrochloric acid.

[2] According to ACKERMANN and MOHR (1938) the solubility of the dipicrate is 0.10 g. per 100 ml. of water at 16°.

[3] Flavianic acid is 2,4-dinitronaphthol-7-sulfonic acid.

[4] The diflavianate is formed in the presence of excess flavianic acid. According to LANGLEY and ALBRECHT (1935), it easily goes over to the monoflavianate when heated in water.

[5] Sozoiodolic acid is 2,6-diiodophenol-4-sulfonic acid.

to WENT and KESZTYUS (1946), induced the formation of an antihistaminic antibody in rats and guinea pigs.

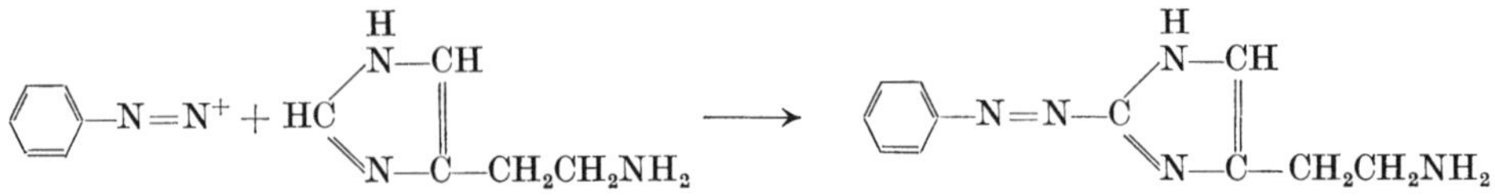

N-Benzoylhistamine also undergoes coupling with benzenediazonium salts, as reported by DIEMAIR and FOX (1938), to give benzeneazobenzoylhistamine. 1,N-Dibenzoylhistamine does not couple with diazotized aniline.

V. Analogs of histamine

Soon after the powerful physiological effects of histamine were observed, chemists began to synthesize analogs and derivatives of it to see how changes in the structure of the molecule might affect its activity. Work along these lines has been carried on, intermittently, over the past fifty years. At first the synthetic analogs were confined to derivatives of imidazole, but in 1941 WALTER, HUNT and FOSBINDER observed that 2-(2-aminoethyl)pyridine exhibited typical histamine activity on smooth muscle. Since then many compounds not containing the imidazole ring have been found to have physiological activities resembling histamine. In Table 2 is presented a comprehensive list of compounds that may be regarded as analogs of histamine. An effort has been made to include all compounds deliberately synthesized and tested for their histamine-like properties. The table also includes compounds that, in the opinion of the author, are chemically analogous to histamine or to other compounds that have been found to possess histamine-like properties. For many of the compounds, no reports on physiological activities are available. Relationships between chemical structure and physiological activity will be discussed in the following section. It is to be noted here, however, that, although many of the histamine analogs possess activities resembling those of histamine, none has yet been discovered that antagonizes any of the activities of histamine. The antihistamine drugs (those compounds that antagonize one or more of the physiological activities of histamine) are not analogs of histamine in a chemical sense.

This book is not the place to discuss the chemistry of the many compounds listed in Table 2. Appropriate references are given so that those who may be interested in methods of synthesis or other chemical aspects of any of the compounds can consult the original literature. The arrangement of Table 2 is based on the chemical structures of the compounds, i.e., imidazole compounds are grouped together and subgrouped according to structural features such as position of substituents, side-chain variations, etc. Physiological activities are given whenever available. The significance of these activities will be discussed in the following section. Three kinds of physiological effects are listed in Table 2 under Relative Activity. In column A are recorded activities of the various compounds in causing contraction of smooth muscle — usually an isolated strip of guinea pig ileum. Column B lists the effects of the compounds on blood pressure — usually of anesthesized cats or dogs. In Column C are listed effects of the compounds on the stimulation of gastric secretion of cats or dogs. Whenever possible quantitative values are given relative to histamine. The references given in the last column of Table 2 relate primarily to the chemistry of the compounds. The literature dealing with pharmacological tests is referred to by superscripts a, b, c, etc., in Columns A, B, and C under Relative Activity.

Table 2. *Analogs of histamine and their physiological activities*

A. Imidazole compounds

1. 4 (or 5)-substituted imidazoles

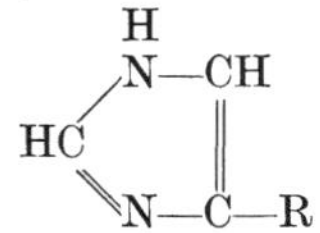

a) Aminomethyl compounds

No.	R	Relative activity histamine = 1			Reference
		A	B	C	
1	$—CH_2NH_2$	0[a]	0[a]	—	TURNER, et al. (1949)
2	CH_2NHCH_3	0.6[a]*	0[a]	—	TURNER, et al. (1949)
3	$CH_2NHC_2H_5$	0.7[a]	active[a]	—	TURNER, et al. (1949)
4	$CH_2N(CH_3)_2$	0.6[a]*	0[a]	0[b, c]	TURNER, et al. (1949)
5	$CH_2N(C_2H_5)_2$	0.25[a]	active[a]	0[b]	TURNER, et al. (1949)
6	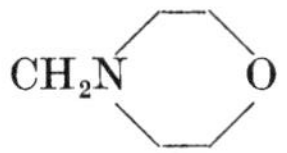	—	—	—	TURNER (1948)
7	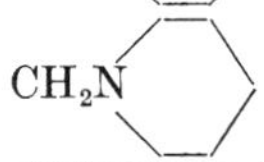	0[a]	active[a]	0[b]	TURNER, et al. (1949)
8	$CH_2NHCH_2C_6H_5$	0.2[a]	0[a]	—	TURNER, et al. (1949)
9	$CH_2N(CH_3)CH_2C_6H_5$	0[a]	0[a]	0[c]	TURNER, et al. (1949)
10	$CH_2N(C_2H_5)CH_2C_6H_5$	0[a]	active[a]	—	TURNER, et al. (1949)
11	$CH_2N(CH_2C_6H_5)CH_2CH_2OH$	—	—	—	CAMPBELL, et al. (1949)
12	$CH_2N(CH_2C_6H_5)CH_2CH_2Cl$	—	—	—	CAMPBELL, et al. (1949)
13	$CH_2N(C_6H_5)CH_2C_6H_5$	0[a]	0[a]	—	TURNER, et al. (1949)
14	$CH_2N(CH_2C_6H_5)_2$	0[a]	active[a]	—	TURNER, et al. (1949)

b) Aminoethyl compounds (histamine derivatives)

No.	R	A	B	C	Reference
15	$CH_2CH_2NH_2$ (Histamine)	1.0	1.0	1.0	
16	$CH_2CH_2NHCH_3$	1.0[d]	0.5[d]	2.5—3.0[c, e]	GARFORTH and PYMAN (1935)
17	$CH_2CH_2NHCONH_2$	0	0	—	VAN DER MERWE (1928)
18	$CH_2CH_2NHC(=NH)NH_2$	0	0	—	VAN DER MERWE (1928)
19	$CH_2CH(CH_3)NH_2$	0.01	0.01	active[b]	ALLES, et al. (1943)

Table 2. (Continued)

No.	R	A	B	C	Reference
20	$CH_2CH(CH_2OH)NH_2$	0.0003	0.001	—	KARRER, et al. (1949)
21	$CH_2CH_2NHC_2H_5$	0.75[a]	active[a]	active[c]	HUEBNER, et al. (1949)
22	$CH_2CH_2N(CH_3)_2$	0.80[a]	0.20[d]	2—3[c, e]	HUEBNER, et al. (1949)
23	$CH_2CH_2NHCOCH_3$	0.002[c]	0[c]	0.001[b, e]	TABOR and MOSETTIG (1949)
24	$CH_2CH_2NHCH_2CH_2CH_3$	0.70[a]	active[a]	0[b]	HUEBNER, et al. (1949)
25	$CH_2CH_2NHCH(CH_3)_2$	0.60[a]	active[a]	—	HUEBNER, et al. (1949)
26	$CH_2CH_2N(CH_3)_3Cl$	0	0[d]	—	GARFORTH and PYMAN (1935)
27	$CH_2CH_2N(C_2H_5)_2$	0.60[a]	0.05[d]	0[b]	HUEBNER, et al. (1949)
28	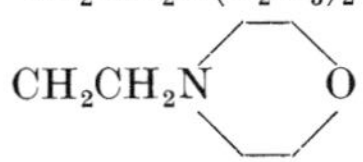	0[a]	0[a]	—	HUEBNER, et al. (1949)
29	$CH_2CH_2NHCOCH(CH_3)_2$	—	—	—	VAN DER MERWE (1928)
30	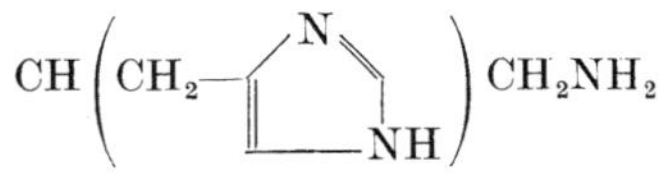	slight		—	PYMAN (1911 b)
31	$CH_2CH_2NH(CH_2)_5NH_2$	0	0	—	VAN DER MERWE (1928)
32	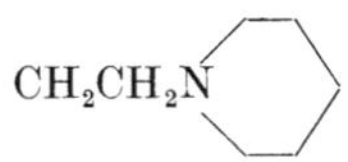	0.20[a]	0[a]	0[b]	HUEBNER, et al. (1949)
33	$CH_2CH_2N(C_3H_7)_2$	0.10[a]	active[a]	—	HUEBNER, et al. (1949)
34	$CH_2CH_2NHCH_2C_6H_5$	0.005[f]	—	active[b]	PLIML and PROTIVA (1953)
35	$CH_2CH_2NHCOC_6H_5$	—	—	—	GERNGROSS (1919 b)
36	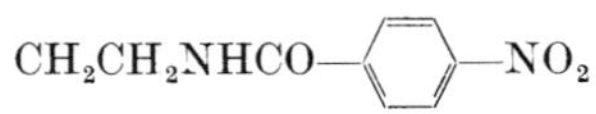	—	—	—	FELL, et al. (1943)
37	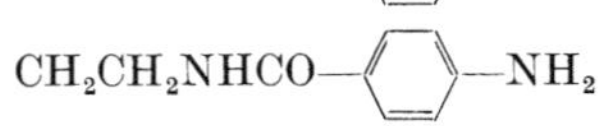	0	—	—	FELL, et al. (1943)

[a] Pharmacological tests on muscle strip and dog blood pressure by CRAVER, et al. (1951).
[b] Tests on gastric secretion by GROSSMAN, et al. (1952).
[c] Pharmacological tests by LIN (1961).
[d] Pharmacological tests by VARTIAINEN (1935).
[e] Tests on gastric secretion by ALPHIN and LIN (1960).
[f] Pharmacological tests by LEE, et al. (1961).

* New samples of these compounds have been prepared recently by Dr. C. AINSWORTH of the Lilly Research Laboratories. They have been tested for their effects on guinea pig ileum strips by Dr. T. M. LIN. Compound 2 was found to be completely inactive while compound 4 had, at most, 1/4000 the activity of histamine.

38	$CH_2CH_2NHCONHC_6H_5$	0	0	—	VAN DER MERWE (1928)
39	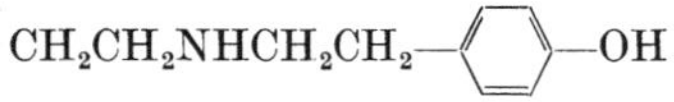	—	—	—	GERNGROSS (1919a)
40	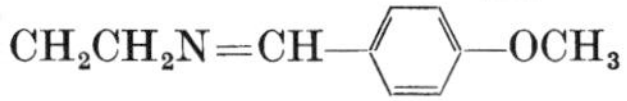	0	0	—	VAN DER MERWE (1928)
41	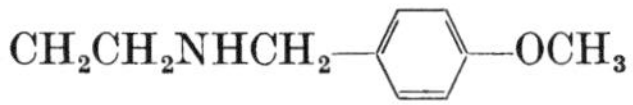	0	0	—	VAN DER MERWE (1928)
42	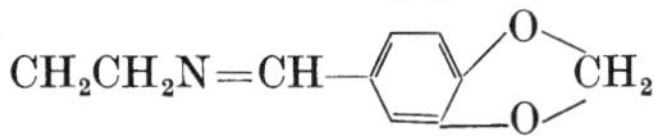	0	0	—	VAN DER MERWE (1928)
43	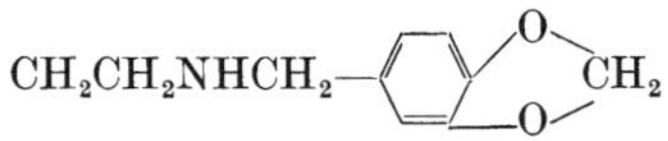	0	0	—	VAN DER MERWE (1928)
44	$CH_2CH_2N(CH_3)CH_2C_6H_5$	0.25[a]	active[a]	—	HUEBNER, et al. (1949)
45	$CH_2CH_2N(C_2H_5)CH_2C_6H_5$	0[a]	0[a]	—	HUEBNER, et al. (1949)
46	$CH_2CH_2NHCOC{=}CHC_6H_5$ │ $NHCOCH_3$	0	0	—	ROCHA E SILVA (1943)
47	$CH_2CH_2NHCOCHCH_2C_6H_5$ │ $NHCOCH_3$	0	0	—	ROCHA E SILVA (1943)
48	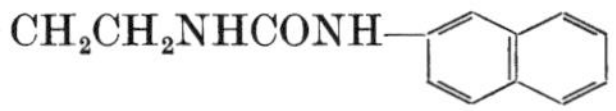	0	0	—	VAN DER MERWE (1928)
49	$CH_2CH_2N{=}C(C_6H_5)_2$	—	—	—	PLIML and PROTIVA (1955)
50	$CH_2CH_2NHCOCHCH_2CH(CH_3)_2$ │ $NHCOOCH_2C_6H_5$	0	0	—	ROCHA E SILVA (1943)
51	$CH_2CH_2N(CH_2C_6H_5)_2$	0.20	0	—	HUEBNER, et al. (1949)
52	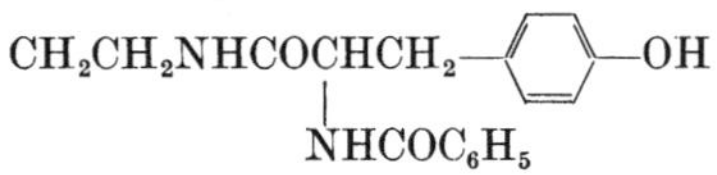	0	0	—	ROCHA E SILVA (1943)

Table 2. (Continued)

No.	R	A	B	C	Reference
53	$CH_2CH_2NHCOCHCH_2$—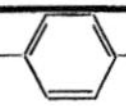—OH, with $NHCOOCH_2C_6H_5$	0	0	—	ROCHA E SILVA (1943)
	c) Miscellaneous 4 (or 5)-substituted imidazoles				
54	CH_2CH_2OH	0.35[a]	0[a]	0[c]	HUEBNER, et al. (1949)
55	CH_2CH_2Cl	0.30[a]	0[a]	—	HUEBNER, et al. (1949)
56	$CH_2CH_2CH_2NH_2$	active ?	—	—	AKABORI and KANEKO (1932)
57	$CH_2CH_2CH(CH_3)NH_2$	0	0	—	PYMAN (1911b)
58	$CH_2CH_2CH_2CH_2NH_2$	0	—	—	AKABORI and KANEKO (1932)
59	$CH_2CH_2CH_2NHC(=NH)NH_2$	—	—	—	AKABORI and KANEKO (1936)
60	C_6H_5	0[g]	—	—	CLEMO, et al. (1938)
61	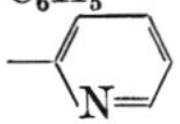	0.001[g]	—	—	CLEMO, et al. (1938)
62	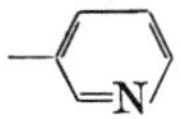	0[g]	—	—	CLEMO, et al. (1938)
63	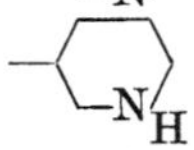	active	—	—	YAMAMOTO (1941)
64	$CH_2CH_2OC_6H_5$	0.40[a]	0[a]	—	HUEBNER, et al. (1949)
65	CH_2CH_2O—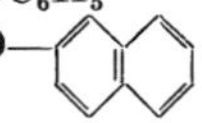	0.50[a]	0[a]	0[b]	HUEBNER, et al. (1949)
	2. 1-substituted imidazoles				
66	$CH_2CH_2NH_2$	0[h]	—	—	LURE, et al. (1939)
67	$CH_2CH_2CH_2NH_2$	—	—	—	LURE, et al. (1939)

2. 1-substituted imidazoles

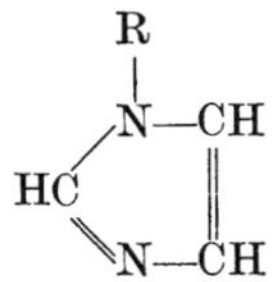

[a] Pharmacological tests on muscle strip and dog blood pressure by CRAVER, et al. (1951).
[b] Tests on gastric secretion by GROSSMAN, et al. (1952).
[c] Pharmacological tests by LIN (1961).
[g] Pharmacological tests by HEATHCOTE (1939).
[h] Pharmacological tests by ACKERMANN and WASMUTH (1939).

3. 2-substituted imidazoles

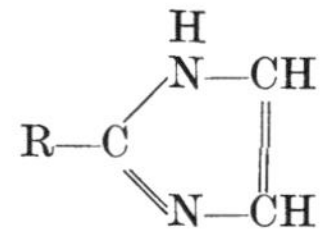

No.	R	A	B	C	Reference
68	$CH_2CH_2NH_2$	0[i]	0[i]	0[b]	JONES (1949a)
69	CH_2CH_2N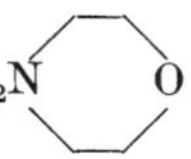	0	0	—	CRAVER, et al. (1951)

4. 1,2-disubstituted imidazoles

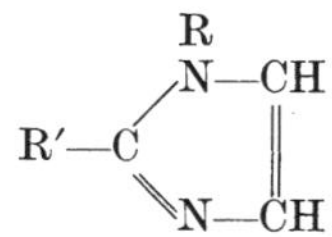

No.	R	R′	A	B	C	Reference
70	$CH_2CH_2NH_2$	CH_3	—	—	—	LURE, et al. (1941)
71	$CH_2C_6H_5$	$CH_2CH_2NH_2$	0[i]	0[i]	0[b]	JONES (1949a)
72	CH_3	$CH_2CH_2NH_2$	0	0	0	JOCELYN (1958)

5. 1,4-disubstituted imidazoles

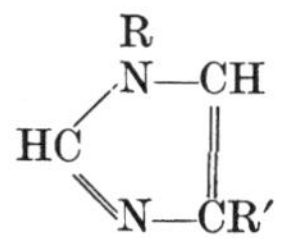

No.	R	R′	A	B	C	Reference
73	CH_3	$CH_2CH_2NH_2$	0.006[i]	0.002[i]	0[b,c]	PYMAN (1911b)
74	COC_6H_5	$CH_2CH_2NHCOC_6H_5$	—	—	—	GERNGROSS (1919b)

Table 2. (Continued)

6. 1,5-disubstituted imidazoles

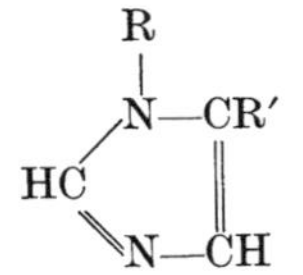

No.	R	R′	A	B	C	Reference
75	CH_3	$CH_2CH_2NH_2$	0[i]	0[i]	0[b,c]	Jones and McLaughlin (1949)
76	$CH_2C_6H_5$	$CH_2CH_2NH_2$	0[f]	0[f]	—	Jones and Mann (1961)

7. 2,4 (or 5)-disubstituted imidazoles

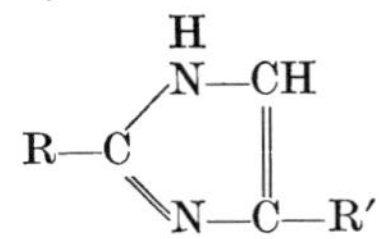

No.	R	R′	A	B	C	Reference
77	—SH	$CH_2CH_2NH_2$	0.0005	0	—	Pyman (1930)
78	CH_2NH_2	CH_3	—	—	—	Ellinger and Goldberg (1949)
79	CH_3	$CH_2CH_2NH_2$	0.30[i]	0.15[i]	active[b]	van der Merwe (1928)
80	$CH_2CH_2NH_2$	CH_3	—	—	—	Ellinger and Goldberg (1949)
81	C_2H_5	$CH_2CH_2NH_2$	—	—	—	van der Merwe (1928)
82	SH	$CH_2CH_2CH_2NHC(=NH)NH_2$	—	—	—	Akabori and Kaneko (1936)
83	SH	$CH_2CH_2CH_2CH_2NH_2$	—	—	—	Akabori and Kaneko (1936)
84	CH_3	CH_2CH_2N 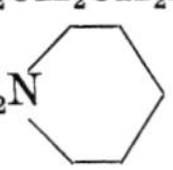	—	—	—	Huebner (1951)
85	C_6H_5	$CH_2CH_2NH_2$	active[j]		—	van der Merwe (1928)
86	$N{=}NC_6H_5$	$CH_2CH_2NH_2$	0	0	—	Kesztyus (1948)
87	N=N— 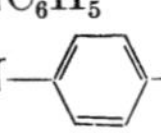 —NO_2	$CH_2CH_2NH_2$	0	0	—	Kesztyus (1948)
88	N=N— 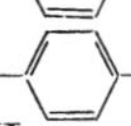 —NH_2	$CH_2CH_2NH_2$	—	—	—	Went and Kesztyus (1946)
89	$CH_2C_6H_5$	$CH_2CH_2NH_2$	—	—	—	van der Merwe (1928)

[b] Tests on gastric secretion by Grossman, et al. (1952).
[c] Pharmacological tests by Lin (1961).
[f] Pharmacological tests by Lee, et al. (1961).
[i] Tests on guinea pig ileum and on cat blood pressure by Lee and Jones (1949).
[j] Tests by Huebner (1951).

90	$CH_2NHCOC_6H_5$	CH_3	—	—	—	Ellinger and Goldberg (1949)
91	C_2H_5	CH_2CH_2N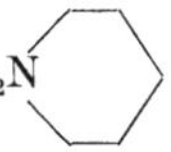	—	—	—	Huebner (1951)
92	C_6H_5	$CH_2CH_2N(CH_3)_2$	active	—	—	Huebner (1951)
93	$CH_2CH_2NHCOC_6H_5$	CH_3	—	—	—	Ellinger and Goldberg (1949)
94	$N{=}N$—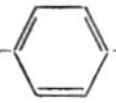—$NHCOCH_3$	$CH_2CH_2NH_2$	—	—	—	Went and Kesztyus (1946)
95	C_6H_5	CH_2CH_2N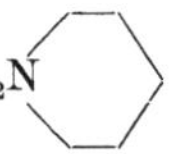	—	—	—	Huebner (1951)
96	$N{=}NC_6H_5$	$CH_2CH_2NHCOC_6H_5$	—	—	—	Diemair and Fox (1938)

8. 4,5-disubstituted imidazoles

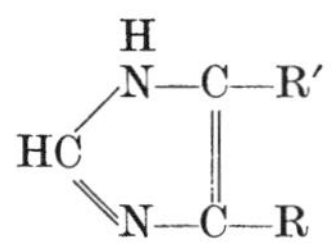

97	CH_2NH_2	CH_3	0	0	—	Ewins (1911)
98	CH_2NHCH_3	CH_3	0	0	—	Ewins (1911)
99	$CH_2CH_2NH_2$	CH_3	0.003	0.01	active[b]	Alles, et al. (1943)
100	$CH_2CH(CH_3)NH_2$	CH_3	0	0.001	active[b]	Alles, et al. (1943)
101	$CH_2CH(CH_3)N(C_2H_5)_2$	CH_3	0	0	—	Sarasin (1923)
102	$CH_2NHC_6H_5$	CH_3	—	—	—	Gerngross (1919a)
103	CH_2NH—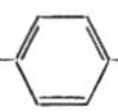—NH_2	CH_3	—	—	—	Gerngross (1919a)
104	$CH_2NHCH_2CH_2C_6H_5$	CH_3	—	—	—	Gerngross (1919a)

Table 2. (Continued)

9. 1,2,4-trisubstituted imidazoles

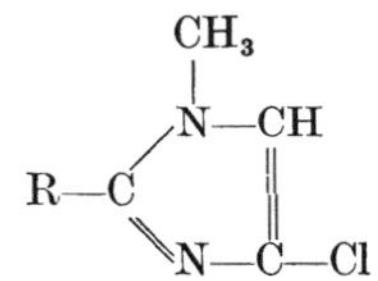

No.	R	A	B	C	Reference
105	CH_2NHCH_3	—	—	—	Sonn, et al. (1924)
106	$CH_2CH_2NH_2$	—	—	—	Sonn, et al. (1924)
107	$CH_2N(CH_3)_2$	—	—	—	Sonn, et al. (1924)
108	$CH_2NHC_6H_5$	—	—	—	Sonn, et al. (1924)
109	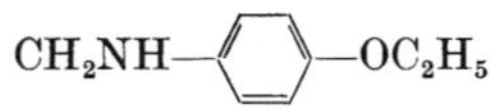	—	—	—	Sonn, et al. (1924)

10. 2,4,5-trisubstituted imidazoles

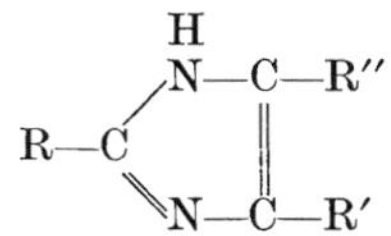

No.	R	R′	R″	A	B	C	Reference
110	CH_3	CH_2NH_2	CH_2NH_2	—	—	—	Tamamushi (1935)
111	C_2H_5	CH_2NH_2	CH_2NH_2	—	—	—	Tamamushi (1937)
112	CH_3	$CH_2CH_2NH_2$	COOH	0.015	—	—	Tamamushi (1933)

11. Miscellaneous imidazoles

No.	Structure	A	B	C	Reference
113	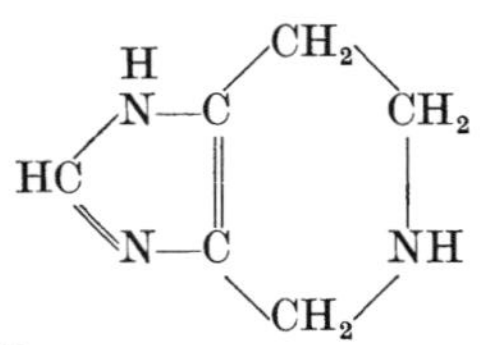	0	0	0[c]	Dale and Dudley (1921)

[b] Tests on gastric secretion by Grossman, et al. (1952).
[c] Pharmacological tests by Lin (1961).

B. Pyrazole compounds

1. 1-substituted pyrazoles

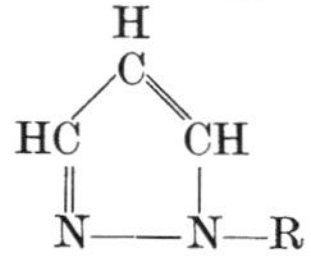

No.	R	A	B	C	Reference
114	$CH_2CH_2NH_2$	0.002	0	0[b]	JONES, et al. (1954)
115	$CH_2CH_2NHCH_3$	0.002	0.01	0[b]	JONES, et al. (1954)
116	$CH_2CH_2N(CH_3)_2$	0.002	0	0[b]	JONES, et al. (1954)

2. 3 (or 5)-substituted pyrazoles

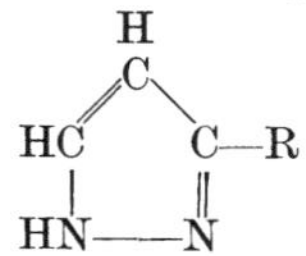

No.	R	A	B	C	Reference
117	$CH_2CH_2NH_2$	0.01[c]	0.0014[k]	0.014[k]	JONES (1949b)
118	$CH_2CH_2CH_2NH_2$	—	—	0[l]	JONES (1961)
119	$CH_2CH_2NHCH_2CH_2$— 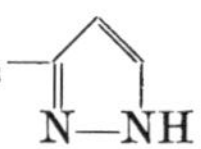	0.002[f]	0[f]	active[b]	JONES and MANN (1953)
120	$CH_2CH_2NHCH_2C_6H_5$	0[f]	—	0[c]	AINSWORTH (1961)
121	$CH_2CH_2NHCH_2$— 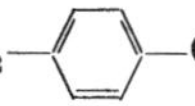 —OCH_3	0[f]	—	—	AINSWORTH (1961)

3. 4-substituted pyrazoles

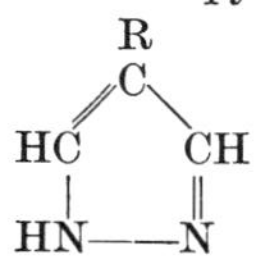

Table 2. (Continued)

No.	R	A	B	C	Reference
122	CH_2CH_2OH	0[f]	0[f]	—	Jones and Mann (1953)
123	$CH_2CH_2NH_2$	0.001[f]	0.001[f]	active[b]	Jones (1949b)
124	$CH_2CH_2CH_2NH_2$	0[f]	0[f]	0[b]	Jones and Mann (1953)

4. 1,3-disubstituted pyrazoles

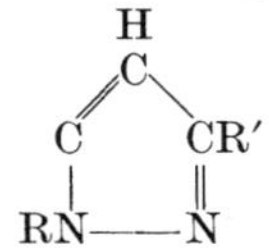

No.	R	R′	A	B	C	Reference
125	$CH_2CH_2NH_2$	C_6H_5	0	0	0	Jones, et al. (1954)
126	$CH_2C_6H_5$	$CH_2CH_2NH_2$	0.002	0	0[b]	Jones, et al. (1954)
127	$CH_2C_6H_5$	$CH_2CH_2NHCH_3$	0.002	0	0[b]	Jones, et al. (1954)
128	$CH_2CH_2N(CH_3)_2$	C_6H_5	0	0	0	Jones, et al. (1954)
129	CH_2CH_2N 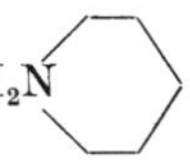	C_6H_5	0	0	0	Jones, et al. (1954)
130	$CH_2CH_2NHCH_2C_6H_5$	C_6H_5	0	0	0	Jones, et al. (1954)

5. 3,5-disubstituted pyrazoles

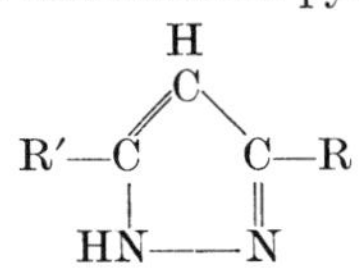

No.	R	R′	A	B	C	Reference
131	$CH_2CH_2NH_2$	CH_3	0	0	0[b,c]	Jones, et al. (1954)
132	$CH_2CH(CH_3)NH_2$	CH_3	0[f]	0[f]	0[f]	Ainsworth and Jones (1954a)
133	$CH_2CH_2N(CH_3)_2$	C_6H_5	0	0	0[b]	Jones, et al. (1954)
134	$CH_2CH(C_6H_5)NH_2$	C_6H_5	—	—	—	Ainsworth and Jones (1954a)

[b] Tests on gastric secretion by Grossman, et al. (1952).
[c] Pharmacological tests by Lin (1961).
[f] Pharmacological tests by Lee, et al. (1961).
[i] Tests on guinea pig ileum and on cat blood pressure by Lee and Jones (1949).
[k] Tests by Rosiere and Grossman (1951).

6. 1,4-disubstituted pyrazoles

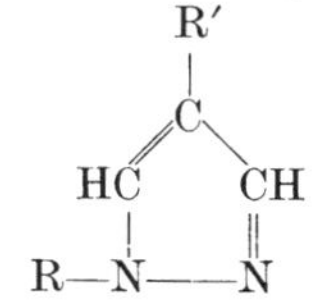

No.	R	R′	A	B	C	Reference
135	$CH_2C_6H_5$	CH_2NH_2	0.002[f)]	0[f)]	0[b, c)]	JONES (1949b)
136	$CH_2C_6H_5$	$CH_2CH_2NH_2$	0[f)]	0[f)]	0[c)]	JONES (1949b)
137	$CH_2C_6H_5$	$CH_2CH_2NHCH_2C_6H_5$	0[f)]	0[f)]	0[f)]	AINSWORTH (1961)

7. 1,5-disubstituted pyrazoles

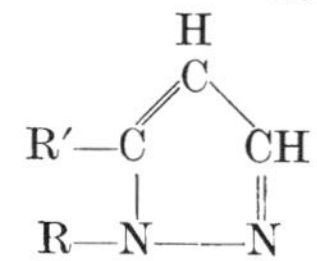

No.	R	R′	A	B	C	Reference
138	C_6H_5	$CH_2CH_2NH_2$	—	—	—	AINSWORTH and JONES (1954a)

C. 1,2,3-triazole compounds

1. 4 (or 5)-substituted 1,2,3-triazoles

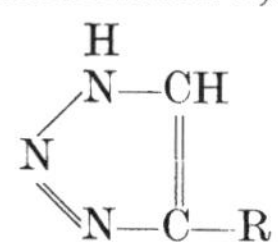

No.	R	A	B	C	Reference
139	CH_2CN	0[f)]	—	—	SHEEHAN and ROBINSON (1949)
140	$CH_2CH_2NH_2$	0.02[f)]	active[f)]	active[c)]	SHEEHAN and ROBINSON (1949)
141	$CH_2CH_2NHCOCH_3$	0[f)]	—	—	SHEEHAN and ROBINSON (1949)
142	$CH_2CH_2NHCH(CH_3)_2$	—	—	—	SHEEHAN and ROBINSON (1949)
143	$CH_2CH_2NHCH_2C_6H_5$	0[f)]	0[f)]	—	AINSWORTH (1961)

Table 2. (Continued)

2. 1,4-disubstituted 1,2,3-triazoles

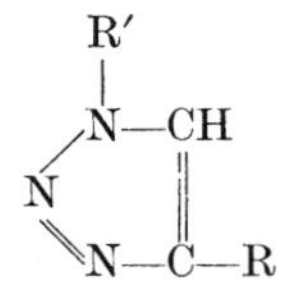

No.	R	R′	A	B	C	Reference
144	$CH_2CH_2NH_2$	CH_3	—	—	—	HUTTEL, et al. (1954)
145	$CH_2CH_2NH_2$	C_6H_5	—	—	—	SHEEHAN and ROBINSON (1951)

3. Miscellaneous 1,2,3-triazoles

No.	Structure	A	B	C	Reference
146	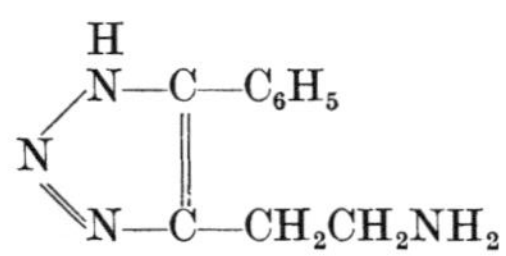	—	—	—	SHEEHAN and ROBINSON (1951)
147	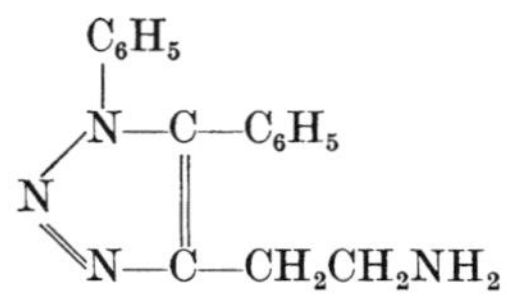	—	—	—	SHEEHAN and ROBINSON (1951)

[b] Tests on gastric secretion by GROSSMAN, et al. (1952).
[c] Pharmacological tests by LIN (1961).
[f] Pharmacological tests by LEE, et al. (1961).

D. 1,2,4-triazoles

1. 3 (or 5)-substituted 1,2,4-triazoles

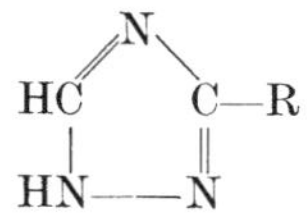

No.	R	A	B	C	Reference
148	CH_2NH_2	0	0	0[c]	AINSWORTH and JONES (1954b)
149	$CH(CH_3)NH_2$	0	0	—	AINSWORTH and JONES (1954b)
150	$CH_2CH_2NH_2$	0.73[l]	0.74[l]	0.60[l]	AINSWORTH and JONES (1953)
151	$CH_2CH_2NHCH_3$	0.07	0.03	—	AINSWORTH and JONES (1954b)
152	$CH_2CH_2NHCONH_2$	0[f]	0[f]	—	AINSWORTH and JONES (1953)
153	$CH(CH_3)CH_2NH_2$	0.0016	0.001	—	AINSWORTH and JONES (1954b)
154	$CH_2CH(CH_3)NH_2$	0.0025	0	0[c]	AINSWORTH and JONES (1954b)
155	$CH_2CH_2CH_2NH_2$	0	0	—	AINSWORTH and JONES (1954b)
156	$CH_2CH_2NHC_2H_5$	0.007	0.008	—	AINSWORTH and JONES (1954b)
157	$CH_2CH_2N(CH_3)_2$	0.04	0.025	—	AINSWORTH and JONES (1954b)
158	$CH_2CH_2NHCOCH_3$	0.025[f]	0.01[f]	active[c]	AINSWORTH and JONES (1953)
159	$CH_2CH_2NHCH(CH_3)_2$	0.005[f]	0.004[f]	active[c]	AINSWORTH and JONES (1953)
160	$CH_2CH_2N(C_2H_5)_2$	0.001	0	—	AINSWORTH and JONES (1954b)
161	$CH_2CH_2NHCH_2C_6H_5$	0.01[f]	0.01[f]	active[c]	AINSWORTH and JONES (1953)
162	$CH_2CH_2NHCOC_6H_5$	0[f]	0[f]	—	AINSWORTH and JONES (1953)
163	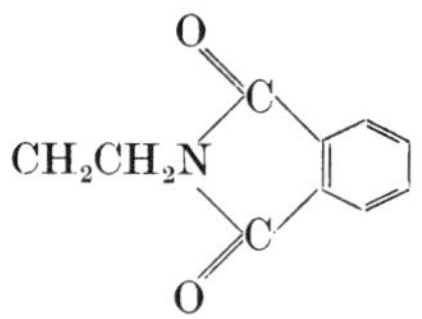	0.002[f]	0[f]	—	AINSWORTH and JONES (1953)

2. 3,5-disubstituted 1,2,4-triazoles

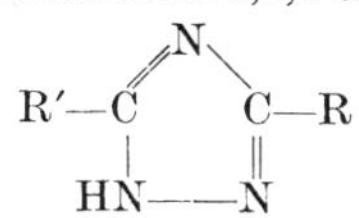

Table 2. (Continued)

No.	R	R′	A	B	C	Reference
164	$CH_2CH_2NH_2$	SH	0[f]	0[f]	0[c]	AINSWORTH and JONES (1953)
165	$CH_2CH_2NH_2$	SCH_3	0[f]	0.006[f]	0[c]	AINSWORTH and JONES (1953)
166	$CH_2CH_2NH_2$	SO_2NH_2	0[f]	0[f]	—	AINSWORTH and JONES (1953)

3. Miscellaneous 1,2,4- and 1,3,4-triazoles

No.	Structure	A	B	C	Reference
167	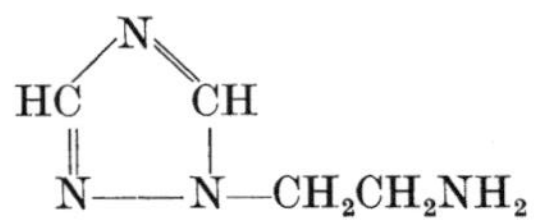	0	0	0[c]	AINSWORTH and JONES (1955)
168	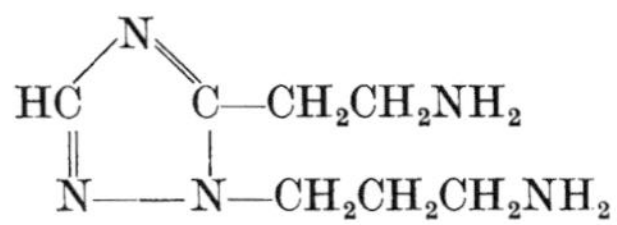	0	0	—	AINSWORTH and JONES (1955)
169	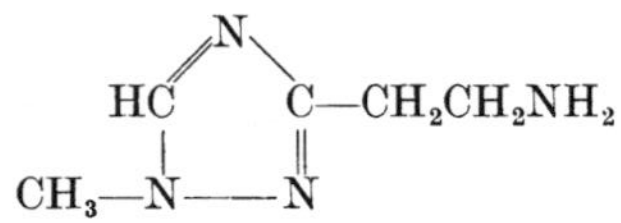	0.0025	0.0014	—	AINSWORTH and JONES (1955)
170	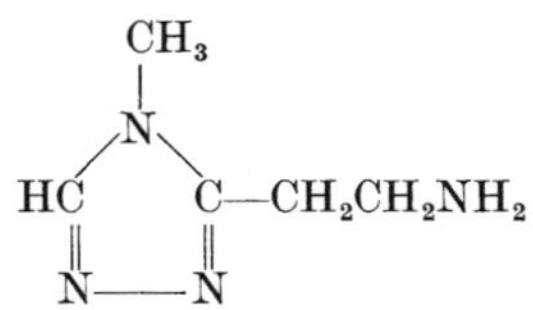	0	0	—	AINSWORTH and JONES (1955)
171	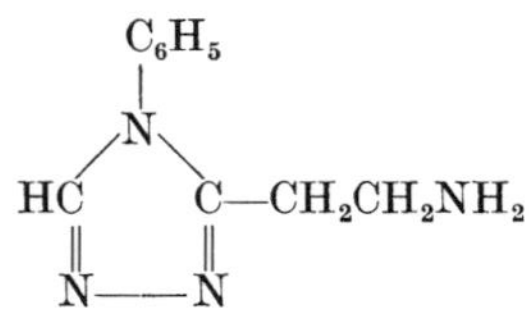	0	0	—	AINSWORTH and JONES (1955)

[c] Pharmacological tests by LIN (1961).
[f] Pharmacological tests by LEE, et al. (1961).
[l] Pharmacological tests by LIN and ALPHIN (1959).

No.	Structure	A	B	C	Reference
172	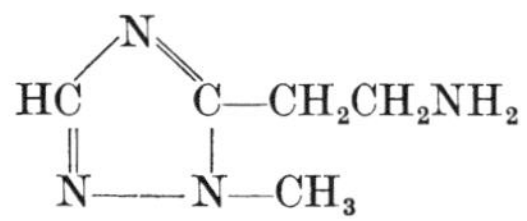	0.0025	0.01	—	AINSWORTH and JONES (1955)

E. Thiazole compounds

1. 2-substituted thiazoles

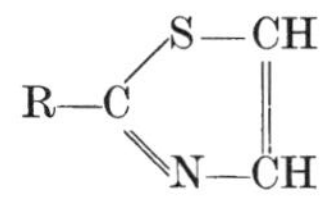

No.	R	A	B	C	Reference
173	CH_2NH_2	—	—	—	JONES, et al. (1950b)
174	$CH_2CH_2NH_2$	0.30[i]	0.08[i]	0[b]	JONES, et al. (1950b)

2. 4-substituted thiazoles

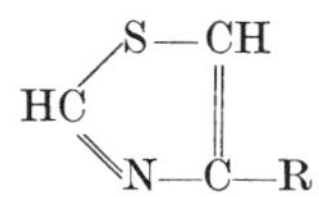

No.	R	A	B	C	Reference
175	CH_2NH_2	—	—	—	JONES, et al. (1950b)
176	$CH_2CH_2NH_2$	0.02[i]	0.006[i]	active[b]	ERLENMEYER and MÜLLER (1945)

3. 2,4-disubstituted thiazoles

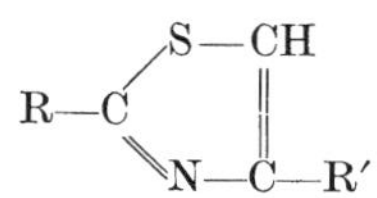

Table 2. (Continued)

No.	R	R′	A	B	C	Reference
177	$CH_2CH_2NH_2$	CH_3	0.15[i]	0.02[i]	0[b]	Goldberg and Kelly (1947)
178	CH_3	$CH_2CH_2NH_2$	0.005[i]	0.003[i]	0[b]	Burger and Ullyot (1947)
179	$CH_2CH_2NH_2$	$CH_2CH_2NH_2$	0[i]	0[i]	0[b]	Jones, et al. (1950b)
180	$CH_2CH_2NH_2$	C_6H_5	0[i]	0[i]	0[b]	Jones, et al. (1950b)
181	$CH_2C_6H_5$	$CH_2CH_2NH_2$	—	—	—	Burger and Ullyot (1947)
182	CH_3	$CH_2CH_2NHCH_2C_6H_5$	—	—	—	Burger and Ullyot (1947)

4. 2,4,5-trisubstituted thiazoles

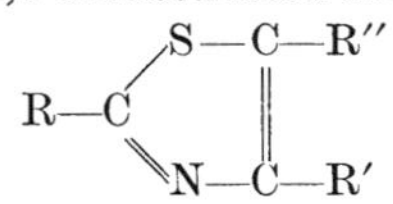

No.	R	R′	R″	A	B	C	Reference
183	CH_3	CH_3	$CH_2CH_2NH_2$	—	—	—	Burger and Ullyot (1947)
184	C_6H_5	CH_3	$CH_2CH_2NH_2$	—	—	—	Burger and Ullyot (1947)

F. Pyridine compounds

1. 2-substituted pyridines

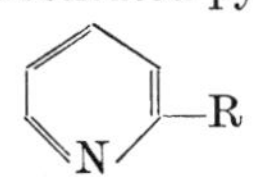

No.	R	A	B	C	Reference
185	$CH_2CH_2NH_2$	0.09[i]	0.02[i]	0[b, c]	Walter, et al. (1941)
186	$CH_2CH_2NHCH_3$	0.20	—	—	Walter, et al. (1941)
187	$CH_2CH(CH_3)NH_2$	0.01[m]	active[m]	0.005[m]	Löffler and Kirschner (1905)
188	$CH_2CH(CH_3)NHCH_3$	0.20	—	—	Walter, et al. (1941)
189	$CH_2CH_2N(CH_3)_2$	—	—	0	Grossman, et al. (1952)

[b] Tests on gastric secretion by Grossman, et al. (1952).
[c] Pharmacological tests by Lin (1961).
[i] Tests on guinea pig ileum and on cat blood pressure by Lee and Jones (1949).
[m] Pharmacological tests by Graham and Tonks (1956).

No.	R	A	B	C	Reference
190	$CH_2CH(CH_3)NHC_2H_5$	—	—	—	Löffler and Kirschner (1905)
191	$CH_2CH_2N(C_2H_5)_2$	0.03	—	—	Walter, et al. (1941)
192	$CH(C_3H_7)CH(CH_3)CH_2NH_2$	—	—	—	Burger and Ullyot (1947)
193	$CH_2CH(CH_3)N(C_2H_5)_2$	—	—	—	Löffler and Kirschner (1905)

2. Miscellaneous pyridine compounds

No.	Structure	A	B	C	Reference
194	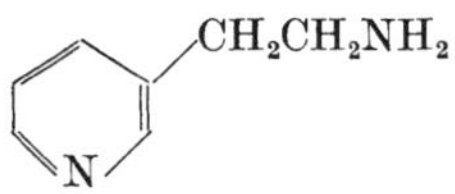	0	pressor	—	Niemann and Hays (1942)
195	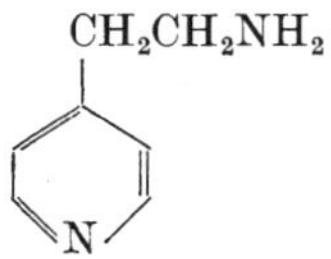	0	pressor	—	Walter, et al. (1941)
196	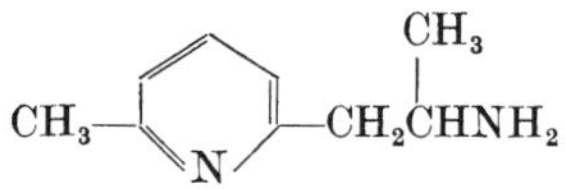	little or no activity	—	—	Burger and Ullyot (1947)

G. Miscellaneous compounds

No.	Structure	A	B	C	Reference
197	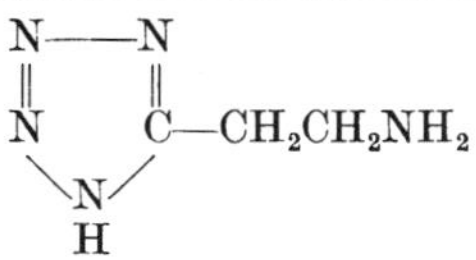	0	0	0[c)]	Ainsworth (1953)
198	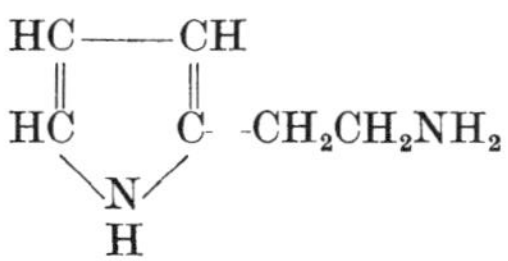	0[i)]	0[i)]	active[b)]	Kutscher and Klamerth (1952)

Table 2. (Continued)

No.	Structure	A	B	C	Reference
199	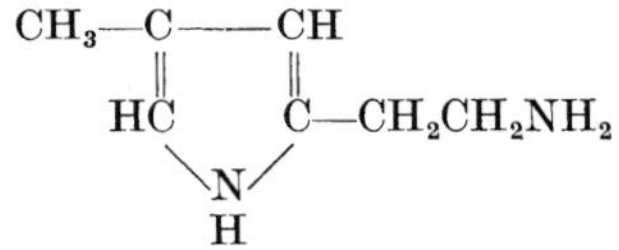	0	0	—	KUTSCHER and KLAMERTH (1951)
200	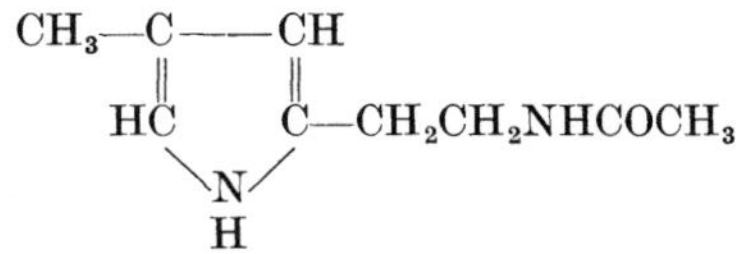	—	—	—	KUTSCHER and KLAMERTH (1951)
201	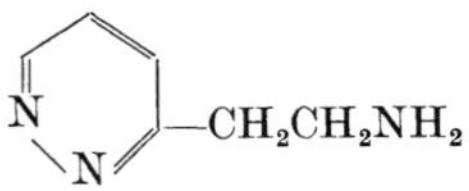	0.002[i]	0.0015[i]	0[b]	JONES, et al. (1950a)
202	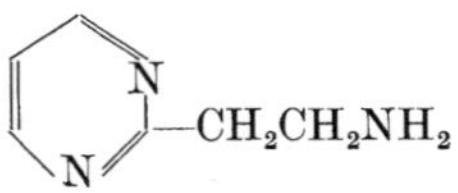	0.05[i]	0.02[i]	active[b]	JONES, et al. (1950a)
203	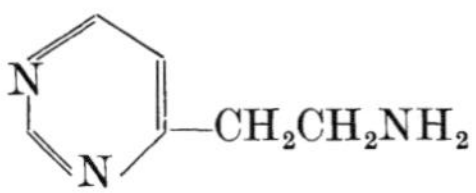	0.0009[i]	0.002[i]	0[b]	JONES, et al. (1950a)
204	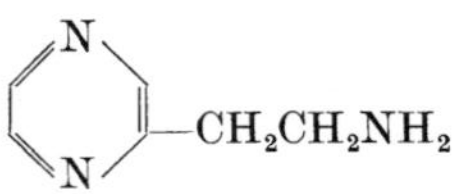	0[i]	0[i]	0[b]	JONES, et al. (1950a)
205	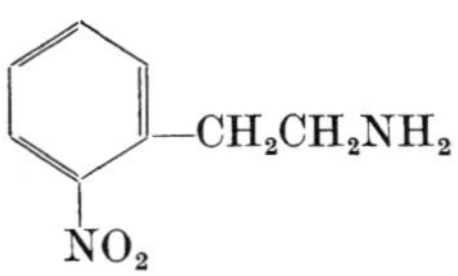	0	0	0[b]	LEE and JONES (1949)

[b] Tests on gastric secretion by GROSSMAN et al. (1952).
[c] Pharmacological tests by LIN (1961).
[i] Tests on guinea pig ileum and cat blood pressure by LEE and JONES (1949).

206	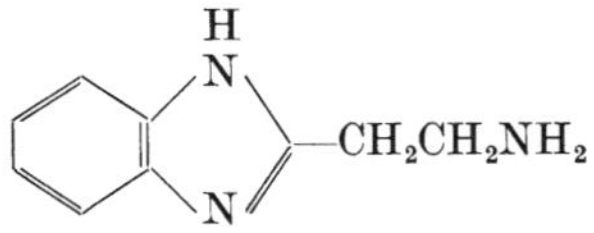	$0^{i)}$	$0^{i)}$	—	CHATTERJEE (1929)
207	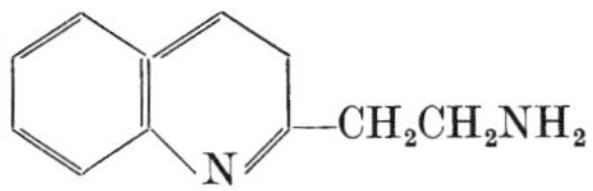	$0^{i)}$	$0^{i)}$	$0^{b)}$	JONES (1952)
208	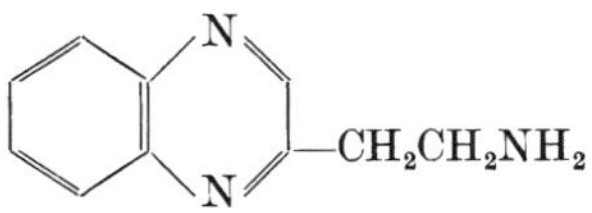	$0^{i)}$	$0^{i)}$	$0^{b)}$	JONES, et al. (1950a)
209	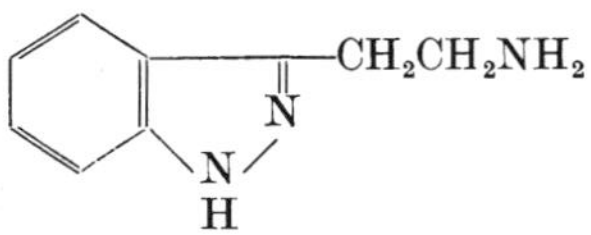	—	—	0	AINSWORTH (1957)
210	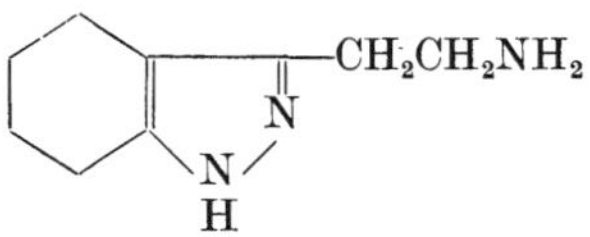	—	—	active[c)]	AINSWORTH (1957)

[b)] Tests on gastric secretion by GROSSMAN et al. (1952).
[c)] Pharmacological tests by LIN (1961).
[i)] Tests on guinea pig ileum and on cat blood pressure by LEE and JONES (1949).

VI. Chemical constitution and pharmacological activity

In this discussion of relationships between chemical structure and physiological activity, three of the well-known effects of histamine are considered. These are (A), the contraction of smooth muscle; (B), the lowering of blood pressure of the anesthesized cat or dog; and (C), the stimulation of gastric secretion in the cat or dog. This data is recorded under columns A, B, and C of Table 2 in the preceding section. The ideal situation would be one in which all of the physiological measurements had been made by the same investigator, using the same methods and the same species of animal for each compound. Unfortunately this ideal condition does not exist. The compounds in Table 2 have been prepared by many different workers over a long period of years, and the physiological measurements are often superficial and unreliable. Indeed, for many of the compounds in Table 2, no pharmacological data are available. The reason for including these compounds is that they are chemically analogous to histamine and may be of interest for future study. In the case of other compounds in Table 2, the reports of pharmacological activities are distressingly vague. Still other compounds have been quite carefully investigated, sometimes by several different workers. The results of these independent investigations occasionally do not agree. For example, GROSSMAN, et al. (1952) reported that compound 54 of Table 2 caused a stimulation of gastric secretion in dogs, whereas SCHNEDORF and IVY (1953) and LIN (1961) found that this compound has no gastric-stimulating activity. LEE and JONES (1949) reported that compound 117 had no activity on the muscle strip or cat blood pressure, but later ROSIERE and GROSSMAN (1951) and LIN (1961) found that the compound definitely did affect blood pressure, and LIN (1961) found that at higher concentrations it also caused contraction of smooth muscle. A major point of disagreement concerns compounds 2 and 4 reported by CRAVER, et al. (1951) to be sixty percent as active as histamine in causing contraction of the guinea pig ileum strip. Recently LIN (1961) has re-examined these two compounds very carefully and has found that they have essentially no activity. Until this discrepancy is cleared up, it may be wise to withhold any judgment about the activities of compounds 2, 3, 4, 5, and 8 reported in column A of Table 2. Several other examples of disagreement concerning the degree of activity of certain compounds can be cited. CRAVER, et al. (1951) reported that compounds 21 and 25 had, respectively, seventy-five and sixty percent the activity of histamine on smooth muscle, but VARTIAINEN (1935) and SHEEHAN and ROBINSON (1949) reported the activities to be only five percent and three percent respectively. These discrepancies may arise from differences in the pharmacological testing methods. Another source of the disagreement may be in the type of tissue or the species of animal used.

Different species of animals may respond quite differently to histamine, and they also may respond differently and unpredictably to histamine analogs. LIN and ALPHIN (1959) have observed that compound 150 has seventy-four percent the activity of histamine in depressing cat blood pressure but only twenty-five percent the activity of histamine on dog blood pressure. LEE, et al. (1961) found that compound 79 caused a sharp and prolonged fall of blood pressure in the cat, but at the same dose in dogs it had no effect at all on blood pressure.

It is not always easy to decide whether a given compound does or does not have histamine-like activity, and the decision may be especially difficult for those compounds that have very low or borderline activity. In the extensive testing done by LEE and JONES (1949) and by LEE, et al. (1961) and LIN (1961), compounds that appeared to have less than one thousandth the activity of histamine arbitrarily were considered to be inactive. Compounds 54, 55, 64, and 65 of Table 2 are reported to be highly effective in causing contraction of the guinea pig ileum strip. This is probably not a typical histamine-like response but is a nonspecific effect. Perhaps these four compounds should not be included in Table 2 as histamine analogs for the reason that their activities on the muscle strip are not inhibited by antihistamine drugs. LEE and JONES (1949) and CRAVER, et al. (1951) have considered that when a compound causes contraction of smooth muscle and lowering of blood pressure this activity is histamine-like only if it is inhibited by one of the typical antihistamine drugs.

In spite of the difficulties of defining and quantitatively measuring histamine-like activity, a surprisingly large number of the chemical analogs of histamine have been found to possess one or more of its physiological properties. About seventy of the two hundred odd compounds included in Table 2 have some histamine-like activity. A number of the compounds mimic histamine in all of its effects while others may possess only one of histamine's activities. Generally all of the analogs are less active than the parent histamine, but there are two exceptions. N-Methylhistamine and N,N-dimethylhistamine (compounds 16 and 22) are more active than histamine as stimulants of gastric secretion in the dog.

Most of the compounds that have histamine-like activities contain in their structures the fragment:

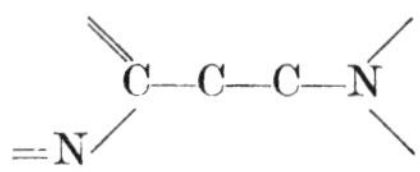 or 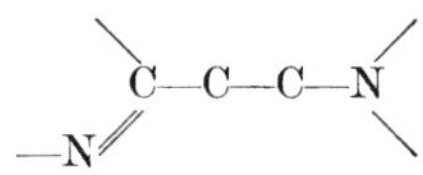

WALTER, et al. (1941) and LEE and JONES (1949) advanced the idea that this arrangement of atoms embodied the minimum requirements for histamine-like activity. This idea had to be abandoned when it was found that not only do many compounds having this structural fragment lack histamine-like activity, as pointed out by LEE and JONES (1949), but a number of compounds having histamine-like activity do not contain this arrangement of atoms in their structures. Examples are compounds 114, 115, 123, and 198. As larger numbers of compounds have been made and tested, it has become increasingly difficult to formulate any general rule relating structure to histamine -like activity. About all that can be said is that compounds possessing appreciable histamine-like activity consist of small nitrogen-heterocyclic aromatic rings to which are attached 2-aminoethyl side chains.

Perhaps the most satisfactory way to discuss the structure-activity relationships is to consider the compounds in groups as they are presented in Table 2.

Imidazoles. Most of the histamine analogs so far synthesized are derivatives of imidazole wherein the structure of histamine has been modified by placing substituents at various points on the ring and on the side chain, shortening or lengthening the side chain, and attaching the side chain to different positions on the ring.

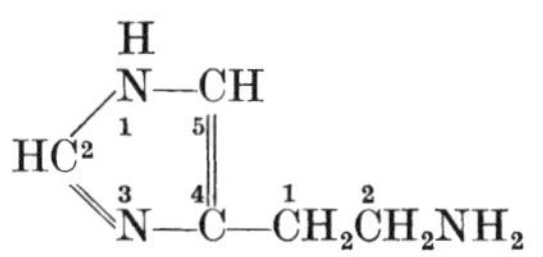

Histamine

Replacement of one or both of the hydrogens on the primary amino group of histamine with small alkyl groups gives compounds that retain activity. Compounds 16 and 22 of Table 2, in which the substituent group is methyl, are the only known compounds that are actually more active than is histamine itself. This enhanced activity of these two compounds is on gastric secretion only. On the muscle strip and on blood pressure they are less active than histamine. Compounds such as 24, 25, 27, 32, 33, and 34, having larger alkyl groups on the amino nitrogen, retain appreciable activity, but, in general, as the size of the substituent group increases the histamine-like activity decreases. The quaternary compound, 26, is inactive. Acyl derivatives of histamine appear to be inactive as exemplified by compounds 17, 29, and 35. An interesting exception is acetyl histamine (compound 23), a naturally occurring metabolic product of histamine. TABOR and MOSETTIG (1949) and LIN (1961) have shown that it has no activity on blood pressure, but LIN (1961) has studied very carefully its effect on isolated muscle and gastric secretion, and in these two tests it appears to have activity at high doses. The possibility that the activity may be due to hydrolysis of the acetyl group with liberation of a little free histamine during the testing procedures has been considered but seems unlikely.

Substituents on the side chain of histamine, as seen in compounds 19 and 20, lower but do not abolish activity. Substituents at positions 2 and 5 of the imidazole ring also lower but do not eliminate activity; examples are compounds 79 and 85. The metabolic product of histamine, 1-methyl-4-(2-aminoethyl)imidazole (compound 73), has slight, but measureable activity on smooth muscle and blood pressure, but the isomeric 1-methyl-5-(2-aminoethyl)imidazole (compound 75) is inactive. The histamine derivatives with multiple substituents on the ring or side chain that have been tested (compounds 100 and 112) are less active than the corresponding compounds 99 and 79 that have fewer substituents.

Lengthening the aminoalkyl side chain of histamine from ethyl to propyl or butyl (compounds 56, 57, and 58) appears to eliminate activity. Likewise, activity is abolished when the side chain is shortened to aminomethyl (compound 1). The very interesting observation was reported by CRAVER, et al. (1951), however, that 4 (or 5)aminomethylimidazoles had activity approaching that of histamine itself on the muscle strip if the amino group was secondary or tertiary. Compounds 2, 3, 4, 5, and 8 are examples. LIN (1961) has been unable to confirm the activity of compounds 2 and 4. He finds them to be essentially inactive on the guinea pig ileum strip. Some of the secondary and tertiary aminomethylimidazoles also affect blood pressure, but none of those tested have any activity at all in stimulating gastric secretion (compounds 4, 5, and 7).

The position at which the aminoethyl side chain is attached to the imidazole ring is of decisive importance for histamine-like activity. When the side chain is moved from the 4 (or 5) position in histamine to the 1 or the 2 position, as in compounds 66, 68, 69, 71, and 72, activity is completely eliminated.

Pyrazoles. The pyrazole analogs of histamine are interesting in several respects. In contrast with the imidazole compounds discussed above, the pyrazole nucleus may have an aminoethyl side chain attached to it in any one of the three possible positions (1,3 or 5, and 4) to give compounds that have histamine-like activities. 1-(2-Aminoethyl)pyrazole (compound 114) has some activity on smooth muscle, and its methyl homolog, 115, has, in addition, appreciable activity on blood pressure. 3 (or 5)-(2-aminoethyl)pyrazole (compound 117) and 4-(2-aminoethyl)-pyrazole (compound 123) are active to some degree on smooth muscle and blood pressure, but they are of special interest as stimulants of gastric secretion. Com-

[1] HISTALOG^{TM}, betazole hydrochloride, Lilly, registered trademark of Eli Lilly and Company, Indianapolis, Indiana, U.S.A., for 3 (or 5)-(2-aminoethyl)pyrazole. As a recent reference to the clinical use of this substance, see CLAYMAN, et al. (1961).

pound 117 has been studied in great detail as a stimulator of gastric secretion. It has clinical usefulness for this purpose and is available on the market as HISTALOG[1]. A dose of fifty milligrams of the hydrochloride salt given either orally or parenterally generally will elicit maximum gastric secretion in the human subject without the usual side effects of flushing and headache that are caused by histamine. Compound 131, which differs from 117 only in that it has a methyl group in position 5 of the pyrazole ring, surprisingly is entirely devoid of activity.

Triazoles. Only a very few 1,2,3-triazoles have been examined for pharmacological activity. The closest analog of histamine, compound 140, has appreciable activity.

The 1,2,4-triazole analogs constitute the most carefully studied and one of the most interesting groups. Compound 150 closely approaches histamine in all of its physiological effects. Unlike histamine, however, 150 is about as active when given orally as parenterally. Structurally, compound 150 is the model in the 1,2,4-triazole series most closely resembling histamine. If the ethyl side chain is shortened (compound 148) or lengthened (compound 155) or if it is moved to position 1 of the nucleus (compound 167), activity is completely lost just as in the imidazole series. Also, activity is lowered or destroyed by placing substituents on the side chain, the primary amino group, or the nucleus.

Thiazoles, pyridines, and miscellaneous compounds. Of the several thiazoles for which pharmacological data are available, compound 174 is the most potent in causing smooth muscle contraction and in lowering blood pressure. It has no activity, however, as a stimulant of gastric secretion. The isomeric compound 176, in which the side chain is attached to position 4 instead of position 2 of the thiazole nucleus, also has histamine-like properties. As in the other series, substitution of additional groups onto the nucleus lowers or eliminates activity.

In the pyridine series, histamine-like activity is found only in those compounds with an aminoethyl group in the position adjacent to the nitrogen atom of the ring (position 2). The pyridazine and pyrimidine compounds 201, 202, and 203, having the aminoethyl side chain attached adjacent to a ring nitrogen, also possess histamine-like activity. By analogy with these and other compounds one would confidently expect the pyrazine compound 204 and the tetrazole compound 197 to be active. It is surprising to find them both totally inert. Compounds with larger molecular structures like 206, 207, 208, and 209, even though they have the aminoethyl group attached adjacent to a nitrogen of the aromatic ring, have no activity.

Optical activity and pharmacological properties. Histamine has no asymmetric centers in its structure, and therefore the question of optical activity vs. pharmacological activity seems not to be very relevant. Nevertheless, CHAPMAN and WILLIAMS (1953) have resolved the histamine analog, 2-(2-aminopropyl) pyridine (compound 187), which does have an asymmetric center. GRAHAM and TONKS (1956) have carefully studied the isomers pharmacologically. Both have histamine-like properties, but on smooth muscle, blood pressure, and gastric secretion, as well as in several other test, the *d*-isomer is consistently three times as active as the *l*-isomer.

Histaminase and the histamine analogs. In recent years many of the histamine analogs have been examined for their ability to act as substrates for histaminase or diamine oxidase. The results of an *in vitro* study by LINDELL and WESTLING (1957) on seven compounds are presented in Table 3. LIN (1961) has confirmed the results presented in Table 3 with the exception that he finds compound 73 to be a much less effective substrate than is indicated in the table. About forty additional histamine analogs have been examined by LIN (1961). Of these, only compounds 75, 131, 140, and 167 are oxidized to any appreciable extent by histaminase *in vitro*.

ARUNLAKSHANA, et al. (1954), LINDELL and WESTLING (1956), LIN, et al. (1959), and others have shown that the *in vivo* effects of histamine are potentiated by inhibitors of histaminase such as aminoguanidine. The effects of certain histamine analogs also may be potentiated by aminoguanidine. 4 (or 5)-(2-Aminoethyl)-1,2,3-triazole (compound 140) is particularly interesting in this connection. LIN (1961) has observed that it has only moderate activity as a stimulator of gastric secretion in the dog, but when the animal is given aminoguanidine along with compound 140 the activity is very greatly enhanced. This is the only clearcut example so far discovered where the *in vivo* activity of a histamine analog, like that of histamine itself, is markedly enhanced by the presence of a diamine oxidase inhibitor. Many of the most active analogs, such as compounds 16, 21, 22, 150, and 185, are not affected by histaminase. The fact that they are not destroyed by this enzyme may, in part, account for their high and prolonged activity. Compounds 68, 75, 131, and 167 that have no measureable activity on smooth muscle, blood pressure, or gastric secretion do act as diamine oxidase substrates.

Table 3. *Oxidation of histamine analogs by histaminase*

No.	Name	Degree of oxidation
15	Histamine	100
68	2-(2-Aminoethyl)imidazole	10
117	3 (or 5)-(2-Aminoethyl)pyrazole . .	9
73	1-Methyl-4-(2-aminoethyl)imidazole	150
176	4-(2-Aminoethyl)thiazole	0
150	3-(2-Aminoethyl)-1,2,4-triazole . .	0
185	2-(2-Aminoethyl)pyridine.	0
202	2-(2-Aminoethyl)pyrimidine . . .	0

Separation of histamine activities. Perhaps the most significant finding that has come from the studies on histamine analogs is that certain compounds can mimic histamine in only one of its several physiological effects. That is, some compounds may stimulate gastric secretion quite effectively but have relatively less activity on smooth muscle or blood pressure. Others may be highly active on muscle or blood pressure but have no activity at all on gastric secretion. Still other compounds may resemble histamine in all of its pharmacological activities. Some of the more outstanding examples have been taken from Table 2 and are presented in Table 4.

Table 4. *Relative physiological activities of some histamine analogs*[1]

Compound number	Smooth muscle A	Blood pressure B	Gastric secretion C
15 (Histamine)	1.0	1.0	1.0
150	0.73	0.74	0.60
174	0.30	0.08	0
185	0.09	0.02	0
115	0.002	0.01	0
16	1.0 (.79)	0.50 (.70)	2.5—3
22	0.80 (.18)	0.20 (.33)	2—3
117	0.01	0.0014 (0.001)	0.014 (.02—.025)

[1] The values given in parentheses were determined by LIN (1961).

Compound 150 closely resembles histamine in most of its various activities; compounds 174 and 185 are active on smooth muscle and blood pressure but not on gastric secretion; and compound 115 has its greatest relative activity on blood pressure. Compounds 16, 22, and 117 are, relative to histamine, about five to twenty times as effective in stimulating gastric secretion as in decreasing blood pressure.

Literature

ABEL, J., J., and S. KUBOTA: Presence of histamine (4-imidazoleethylamine) in the hypophysis cerebri and other tissues of the body and its occurrence among the hydrolytic decomposition products of proteins. J. Pharmacol. exp. Ther. **13**, 243 (1919).
ACKERMANN, D.: Über den bacteriellen Abbau des Histidins. Hoppe-Seylers Z. physiol. Chem. **65**, 504 (1910).
— Die Sozojodosäure als Basenfällungsmittel. Hoppe Seylers Z. physiol. Chem. **225**, 46 (1934).
— u. H. G. FUCHS: Zur Frage des Vorkommens von Histamin im normalen Harn. Hoppe-Seylers Z. physiol. Chem. **259**, 32 (1939).
—, u. M. MOHR: Präparative Sicherstellung des Vorkommens von Histamin im normalen Säugetierkörper. Hoppe-Seylers Z. physiol. Chem. **255**, 75 (1938).
—, u. W. WASMUTH: Zur Wirkungsweise des Histamins. Hoppe-Seylers Z. physiol. Chem. **259**, 28 (1939).
AINSWORTH, C.: 5-β-Aminoethyltetrazole. J. Amer. chem. Soc. **75**, 5728 (1953).
— Indazole analog of tryptamine: A new synthesis of indazoles. J. Amer. chem. Soc. **79**, 5242 (1957).
— Work done at Lilly Research Laboratories, unpublished (1961).
—, and R. G. JONES: 1,2,4-Triazole analogs of histamine. J. Amer. chem. Soc. **75**, 4915 (1953).
— — Reactions of hydrazines with gamma-pyrones. J. Amer. chem. Soc. **76**, 3172 (1954).
— — 3-Aminoalkyl-1,2,4-triazoles. J. Amer. chem. Soc. **76**, 5651 (1954).
— — Isomeric and nuclear-substituted beta-aminoethyl-1,2,4-triazoles. J. Amer. chem. Soc. **77**, 621 (1955).
AISO, K., H. TOYOURA and K. NAKANO: The specificity of histidine decarboxylation in Proteus morganii. II. Nippon Saikingaku Zarshi **11**, 517 (1956); Chem. Abstr. **51**, 14002 (1957).
AKABORI, S.: Synthese von Imidazol-derivaten aus α-Aminosäuren, I. Mitteil.: Eine neue Synthese von Desamino-histidin und ein Beitrag zur Kenntnis der Konstitution des Ergothioneins. Ber. **66**, 151 (1933).
—, and T. KANEKO: Amino acids and their derivatives. V. 3. Synthesis of two higher homologs of histamine. J. chem. Soc. Japan **53**, 207 (1932); Chem. Abstr. **27**, 293 (1933).
— — Synthesis of imidazole derivatives from α-amino acids. III. Synthesis of two higher homologs of histamine. Bull. chem. Soc. Japan **11**, 208 (1936); Chem. Abstr. **30**, 5985 (1936).
—, and S. NUMANO: Amino acids and their derivatives. VI. 4. A new synthesis of histamine. J. chem. Soc. Japan **53**, 213 (1932); Chem. Abstr. **27**, 293 (1933).
— — Synthesis of imidazole derivatives from α-amino acids. IV. New synthesis of histamine. Bull. chem. Soc. Japan **11**, 214 (1936); Chem. Abstr. **30**, 5986 (1936).
ALBERT, A.: Quantitative studies of the avidity of naturally occurring substances for trace metals. Biochem. J. **50**, 690 (1952).
ALLES, G. A., B. B. WISEGARVER and M. A. SHULL: Comparative physiological actions of some β-(imidazolyl-4)alkylamines. J. Pharmacol. exp. Ther. **77**, 54 (1943).
ALPHIN, R. S., and T. M. LIN: Effect of histamine metabolites and histaminase inhibitor on gastric secretion in dogs. Fed. Proc. **19**, 192 (1960).
ANDREWS, A. C., and T. D. LYONS: Binding of histamine and antihistamine to bovine serum albumin by mediation with Cu (II). Science **126**, 561 (1957).
ARUNLAKSHANA, O., J. L. MONGAR and H. O. SCHILD: Potentiation of pharmacological effects of histamine by histaminase inhibitors. J. Physiol. (Lond.) **123**, 32 (1954).
ASHLEY, J. N., and C. R. HARRINGTON: Synthesis of 1-2-thiolhistidine. J. Chem. Soc. **1930**, 2586.
AXMACHER, F.: Über eine Farbreaktion des Histamins und Schwermetallkomplexsalze des Methylimidazols. Biochem. Z. **284**, 339 (1936).
BARGER, G., and H. H. DALE: The presence in ergot and physiological activity of β-imidazolylethylamine. J. Physiol. (Lond.) **40**, XXXVIII (1910).
— — CCLXV.-4-β-Aminoethylglyoxaline (β-iminazolylethylamine) and the other active principles of ergot. J. chem. Soc. **97**, 2592 (1910).
— — β-Iminazolylethylamine, a depressor constituent of intestinal mucosa. J. Physiol. (Lond.) **41**, 499 (1911).
BEST, C. H., H. H. DALE, H. W. DUDLEY and W. V. THORPE: The nature of the vaso-dilator constituents of certain tissue extracts. J. Physiol. (Lond.) **62**, 397 (1927).
BORSOOK, H., C. L. DEASY, A. J. HAGEN-SMIT, G. KEIGHLEY and P. H. LOWY: Metabolism of C^{14}-labeled glycine, L-histidine, L-leucine, and L-lysine. J. biol. Chem. **187**, 839 (1950).
— — — — — Incorporation *in vitro* of labeled amino acids into proteins of rabbit reticulocytes. J. biol. Chem. **196**, 669 (1952).
BOUTHILLIER, L. P., and A. D'IORIO: Synthesis of radioactive DL-histidine ($C^{14}OOH$). Rev. can. biol. **9**, 382 (1950); Chem. Abstr. **45**, 6192 (1951).
—, and M. GOLDNER: The metabolism of histamine-β-C^{14}. Arch. Biochem. **44**, 251 (1953).

BURGER, A., and G. E. ULLYOT: Analgesic studies. β-Ethyl and β-isopropylamine derivatives of pyridine and thiazole. J. Org. Chem. **12**, 342 (1947).

CAMPBELL, K. N., J. F. ACKERMAN and B. K. CAMPBELL: The preparation of β-chloroethylamines containing heterocyclic nuclei. J. Amer. chem. Soc. **71**, 2905 (1949).

CHAPMAN, N. B., and J. F. A. WILLIAMS: Optically active forms of 1-methyl-2,2′-pyridylethylamine. J. chem. Soc. **1953**, 2797.

CHATTERJEE, B.: CCCC-Attempts to find new antimalarials. Part IV. β-Benziminazolylethylamine and β-5(or 6)-ethoxybenziminazolylethylamine. J. chem. Soc. **1929**, 2965.

CLAYMAN, C. B., J. B. KIRSNER, and H. FORD: A simple oral gastric secretory stimulant (Betazole hydrochloride). J. Amer. med. Ass., **175**, 908 (1961).

CLEMO, G. R., T. HOLMES and G. C. LEITCH: The synthesis of phenyl- and pyridyl-glyoxalines. J. chem. Soc. **1938**, 753.

CRAVER, B. N., W. BARRETT, A. CAMERON and E. HERROLD: Histamine-like drugs. Pharmacological actions of thirty-five derivatives of 4-methyl, 5-ethyl, or 2-substituted imidazoles. Arch. int. Pharmacodyn. **87**, 33 (1951).

DALE, H. H., and H. W. DUDLEY: The physiological action of N-methylhistamine and of tetrahydropyrido-3,4-iminazole (imidazolisopiperidin of FRÄNKEL). J. Pharmacol. exp. Ther. **18**, 103 (1921).

—, and P. P. LAIDLAW: The physiological action of β-iminazolylethylamine. J. Physiol. (Lond.) **41**, 318 (1910).

— — Further observation on the action of β-iminazolylethylamine. J. Physiol. (Lond.) **43**, 182 (1912).

DARBY, W. J., H. B. LEWIS and J. R. TOTTER: The preparation of 4 (or 5)-hydroxymethylimidazole. J. Amer. chem. Soc. **64**, 463 (1942).

DIEMAIR, W., and H. FOX: Über einige neue Azoverbindungen und Jod-derivate des Histidins und Histamins. Ber. **71**, 2493 (1938).

EBEL, F., H. PASEDACH and O. V. SCHICKH: Ger. Pat. 805,523 (May 21, 1951); Chem. Abstr. **46**, 1051 (1952).

EGGERTH, A. H.: The production of histamine by bacterial cultures. J. Bact. **37**, 205 (1939).

EICHLER, O., u. M. HÖBEL: Über die Reaktion von Kupfer (II) mit Histamin und die Wechselwirkung von Schweinserumalbumin mit Kupfer (II)-Histamin. Unpublished (1963).

—, u. G. MEYER: Über Komplexe von Histamin mit Schwermetallsalzen. Naturwissenschaften **1948**, 93.

ELLINGER, L. P., and A. A. GOLDBERG: A new route to iminazoles: Synthesis of 2-ω-aminoalkyl derivatives of 4-methyliminazole. J. chem. Soc. **1949**, 263.

ERLENMEYER, H., u. M. MÜLLER: Zur Kenntnis des β-(4-thiazolyl)-äthylamine. Helv. chim. Acta **28**, 922 (1945).

EWINS, A. J.: CCXXXII. — Some derivatives of 4(or 5)-methylglyoxaline. J. chem. Soc. **99**, 2052 (1911).

—, and F. L. PYMAN: XLIII. — Experiments on the formation of 4(or 5)-β-aminoethylglyoxaline from histidine. J. chem. Soc. **99**, 339 (1911).

FARGHER, R. G., and F. L. PYMAN: XXVI. — Nitro-arylazo- and aminoglyoxalines. J. chem. Soc. **115**, 217 (1919).

FELL, N., G. RODNEY and D. E. MARSHALL: Histamine-protein complexes: Synthesis and imunologic investigation. J. Imunol. **47**, 237 (1943).

FRÄNKEL, S., u. K. ZEIMER: Über das Imidazolisopiperidin und seine Derivate. Biochem. Z. **110**, 234 (1920).

FRASER, M. M., and R. A. RAPHAEL: A synthesis of histamine from but-2-yne-1,4-diol. J. chem. Soc. **1952**, 226.

GALAT, A., and H. L. FRIEDMAN: A new method for the isolation of histamine. J. Amer. chem. Soc. **71**, 3976 (1949).

GALE, E. F.: The production of amines by bacteria. I. The decarboxylation of amino acids by strains of bacterium coli. Biochem. J. **34**, 392 (1940).

— 4. The decarboxylation of amino acids by organisms of the groups clostridium and proteus. Biochem. J. **35**, 66 (1941).

GARFORTH, B., and F. L. PYMAN: 4(5)-β-Alkylaminoethylglyoxalines. J. chem. Soc. **1935**, 489.

GARREAU, Y.: Quelques sels organiques d'un acide diaminoquinone-disulfonique. Compt. rend. **201**, 1515 (1935).

GEBAUER-FÜLNEGG, E.: Zur Kenntnis der Paulyschen Diazoreaktion. Hoppe-Seylers Z. physiol. Chem. **191**, 222 (1930).

GERNGROSS, O.: Über einige an der Aminogruppe arylierte Derivate des 4(5)-methyl-5(4)-aminomethyl-imidazoles und die Synthese des [β-p-oxyphenyl-äthyl]-[β-4-(5)-imidazolyläthyl]-amines. Ber. **52**, 2304 (1919).

— Über Benzoylderivate des Histidins und Histamins. Hoppe-Seylers Z. physiol. Chem. **108**, 50 (1919).

GOLDBERG, A. A., and W. KELLY: Synthesis of the 2-ω-aminoalkyl and 2-ω-sulfanilamido-alkyl derivatives of thiazole and pyrimidine. J. chem. Soc. **1947**, 1372.
GRAHAM, J. D. P., and R. S. TONKS: Stereoisomerism and activity in a congener of histamine. Arch. int. Pharmacodyn. **106**, 457 (1956).
GROSSMAN, M. I., C. ROBERTSON and C. E. ROSIERE: The effect of some compounds related to histamine on gastric acid secretion. J. Pharmacol. exp. Ther. **104**, 277 (1952).
HANKE, M. T., and K. K. KOESSLER: Studies on proteinogenous amines. XII. The production of histamine and other imidazoles from histidine by the action of microorganisms. J. biol. Chem. **50**, 131 (1922).
HARES, G. B., W. C. FERNELIUS and B. E. DOUGLAS: Equilibrium constants for the formation of complexes between metal ions and polyamines. J. Amer. chem. Soc. **78**, 1816 (1956).
HATEM, S.: Complexe histamine-argent. Compt. rend. **241**, 1392 (1955).
— L'état hautement associé de l'histamine. Compt. rend. **243**, 801 (1956).
HEATHCOTE, R. S. A.: A note on the pharmacological actions of some new derivatives of glyoxaline. Quart. J. Pharm. **12**, 260 (1939).
HEYL, D., E. LUTZ, S. A. HARRIS and K. FOLKERS: Chemistry of vitamin B_6. VII. Pyridoxylidene- and pyridoxylamines. J. Amer. chem. Soc. **70**, 3669 (1948).
HOFFMAN, D. H., S. A. HARRIS and K. FOLKERS: Pyridoxal-histamine and homologs. U.S. Pat. 2,540,946 (Feb. 6, 1951); Chem. Abstr. **45**, 6663 (1951).
HOLMES, F., and F. JONES: Metal complexes of histamine and some structural analogs. Part. I. J. chem. Soc. **1960**, 2398.
HORN, F.: Über Chloraurate des Histamins und Imidazols. Hoppe-Seylers Z. physiol. Chem. **207**, 111 (1932).
HUEBNER, C. F.: Studies of imidazole compounds. V. A new and improved synthesis of 4-(2-substituted aminoethyl)imidazoles. J. Amer. chem. Soc. **73**, 4667 (1951).
— R. A. TURNER and C. R. SCHOLZ: Studies of imidazole compounds. IV. Derivatives of 4-ethylimidazole. J. Amer. chem. Soc. **71**, 3942 (1949).
HÜTTEL, R., T. SCHNEIDERHAN, H. HERTWIG, A. LEUCHS, V. REINCKE, u. J. MILLER: Synthese einiger Äthylamine und Alanine der Pyrazol- und 1,2,3-Triazol-Reihe. Ann. **585**, 115 (1954).
IKEDA, H., and H. IKEDA: Amine polyhalophenoxides. J. Sci. Res. Inst. (Tokyo) **45**, 207 (1951); Chem. Abstr. **47**, 6891 (1953).
ITALLIE, L. VAN, and A. J. STEENHAUER: Microchemical reactions to distinguish between tyramine and histamine. Pharm. Weekblad **62**, 429 (1925); Chem. Abstr. **19**, 1873 (1925).
JOCELYN, P. C.: The pharmacological significance of 1-methyl-2-(β-aminoethyl)imidazole. Arch. int. Pharmacodyn. **113**, 251 (1958).
JONES, R. G.: Studies on imidazole compounds. I. A synthesis of imidazoles with functional groups in the 2-position. J. Amer. chem. Soc. **71**, 383 (1949).
— The synthesis of some amines and amino acids containing the pyrazole nucleus. J. Amer. chem. Soc. **71**, 3994 (1949).
— 2-β-Aminoethylquinoline. J. Amer. chem. Soc. **74**, 4207 (1952).
— Work done at Lilly Research Laboratories, unpublished (1961).
— E. C. KORNFELD and K. C. MCLAUGHLIN: The synthesis of some β-aminoethyldiazines as histamine analogs. J. Amer. chem. Soc. **72**, 3539 (1950).
— — — The synthesis of some analogs of histamine and histidine containing the thiazole nucleus. J. Amer. chem. Soc. **72**, 4526 (1950).
—, and M. J. MANN: New methods of synthesis of β-aminoethylpyrazoles. J. Amer. chem. Soc. **75**, 4048 (1953).
— — and K. C. MCLAUGHLIN: Substituted β-aminoethylpyrazoles. J. Org. Chem. **19**, 1428 (1954).
— — Work done at Lilly Research Laboratories, unpublished (1961).
—, and K. C. MCLAUGHLIN: Studies on imidazoles. III. 1-Substituted analogs of histamine and histidine. J. Amer. chem. Soc. **71**, 2444 (1949).
KAPELLER-ADLER, R.: Histidine metabolism in toxaemia of pregnancy. Isolation of histamine from the urine of patients with toxaemia of pregnancy. Biochem. J. **35**, 213 (1941).
KARRER, P., M. SUTER and P. WASER: L. Histidinol. Helv. chim. Acta **32**, 1936 (1949).
KESZTYUS, L.: Azo compounds of histamine. Naunyn-Schmiedeberg's Arch. exp. Path. Pharmak. **205**, 287 (1948); Chem. Abstr. **43**, 5058 (1949).
KOESSLER, K. K., and M. T. HANKE: Studies on proteinogenous amines. I. The synthesis of β-imidazolylethylamine (histamine). J. Amer. chem. Soc. **40**, 1716 (1918).
— — Studies on proteinogenous amines. II. A microchemical method for estimating imidazole derivatives. J. biol. Chem. **39**, 497 (1919).
— — Studies on proteinogenous amines. IV. The production of histamine from histidine by bacillus coli communis. J. biol. Chem. **39**, 539 (1919).
KUTSCHER, F.: The physiological action of a secal base and of imidazolylethylamine. Zbl. Physiol. **24**, 163 (1910); Chem. Abstr. **4**, 2504 (1910).

KUTSCHER, W., u. O. KLAMERTH: Darstellung von histaminähnlichen Substanzen aus der Pyrrolreihe. Hoppe-Seylers Z. physiol. Chem. **286**, 190 (1951).
— — Darstellung von histaminähnlichen Substanzen aus der Pyrrolreihe. II. Mitteilung: Die Synthese von 2-[β-amino-äthyl]-pyrrol. Hoppe-Seylers Z. physiol. Chem. **289**, 229 (1952).
LANGLEY, W. D., and A. J. ALBRECHT: The identification of the flavianates of various organic bases. J. biol. Chem. **108**, 729 (1935).
LEE, H. M., W. G. DINWIDDIE and F. G. HENDERSON: Work done at Lilly Research Laboratories, unpublished (1961).
—, and R. G. JONES: The histamine activity of some β-aminoethyl heterocyclic nitrogen compounds. J. Pharmacol. exp. Ther. **95**, 71 (1949).
LEWIS, B., E. VON GEBAUER-FUELNEGG and C. J. FARMER: A spectroscopic study and assay of histamine. J. Amer. chem. Soc. **55**, 2025 (1933).
LIN, T. M.: Work done at Lilly Research Laboratories, unpublished (1961).
—, and R. S. ALPHIN: Comparative study of histamine and 3-β-aminoethyl-1,2,4-triazole on gastric secretion. Fed. Proc. **18**, 416 (1959).
— — F. G. HENDERSON and K. K. CHEN: Effect of histamine derivatives and histiminase inhibitors on gastric secretion in dogs. Abstracts of Communications, XXI Int. Congress Physiol. Sci., **1959**, page 164.
LINDELL, S. E., and H. WESTLING: Potentiation by histaminase inhibitors of the blood pressure responses to histamine in cats. Acta physiol. scand. **37**, 307 (1956).
— — Enzymatic oxidation of some substances related to histamine. Acta physiol. scand. **39**, 370 (1957).
LÖFFLER, K., u. M. KIRSCHNER: Derivate des α-Picolyl- und α-Picolylmethyl-alkins [III. Theil]. Ber. **38**, 3329 (1905).
LURE, S. I., M. G. KULESHOVA and N. K. KOCHETKOV: Nitrogen derivatives of imidazole (glyoxaline). J. gen. Chem. (U.S.S.R.) **9**, 1933 (1939); Chem. Abstr. **34**, 4387 (1940).
—, O. I. STAROBOGATOV, and E. S. NIKITSKAYA: The problem of hydrolysis of acetylsulfanilic acid derivatives. III. J. gen. Chem. (U.S.S.R.) **11**, 545 (1941); Chem. Abstr. **35**, 6938 (1941).
MELLANBY, E., and F. W. TWORT: On the presence of β-imidazole-ethylamine in the intestinal wall; with a method of isolating a bacillus from the alimentary canal which converts histidine into this substance. J. Physiol. (Lond.) **45**, 53 (1912).
MERWE, P. VAN DER: Über einige neue Derivate des Histamins. Hoppe-Seylers Z. physiol. Chem. **177**, 301 (1928).
MICKEL, B. L., and A. C. ANDREWS: Complexes of histamine with CO^{II}, Ni^{II}, and Cu^{II}. J. Amer. chem. Soc. **77**, 323 (1955).
— — Stability of histamine chelates. J. Amer. chem. Soc. **77**, 5291 (1955).
NIEMANN, C., and J. T. HAYS: The relation between structure and histamine-like activity. J. Amer. chem. Soc. **64**, 2288 (1942).
PAULY, H.: Über die Konstitution des Histidines. Hoppe-Seylers Z. physiol. Chem. **42**, 508 (1904).
PENNIMPEDE, F. C., I. S. M. DE ISSALY and A. S. DE ISSALY: Klebsiella studies. VI. Metabolism of histidine. Rev. Asoc. bioquim. argent. **22**, 72 (1957); Chem Abstr. **52**, 16468 (1958).
PLIML, J., and M. PROTIVA: Synthetic experiments in the histamine series. III. New methods of the reduction of 4(5)-(cyanomethyl)-imidazole to histamine. Chem. Listy **46**, 772 (1952); Chem. Abstr. **47**, 11182 (1953).
— — Synthetic experiments in the histamine series. IV. 4(5)-(2-Benzylaminoethyl)imidazole. Chem. Listy **47**, 1874 (1953); Chem. Abstr. **49**, 1016 (1955).
PYMAN, F. L.: LXXIV. — A new synthesis of 4(or 5)-β-aminoethyl-glyoxaline, one of the active principles of ergot. J. chem. Soc. **99**, 668 (1911).
— CCXLV. — Aminoalkylglyoxalines. J. chem. Soc. **99**, 2172 (1911).
— LXI. — The synthesis of glyoxaline derivatives allied to pilocarpine. J. chem. Soc. **101**, 530 (1912).
— 2-Thiol-4-(5)-β-aminoethylglyoxaline (2-thiolhistamine). J. chem. Soc. **1930**, 98.
— Synthetic drugs. Brit. Pat. 325,151 (March 22, 1929); Chem. Abstr. **24**, 3861 (1930).
REDEMANN, C. E., and C. NIEMANN: The diliturates (5-nitrobarbiturates) of some physiologically important bases. J. Amer. chem. Soc. **62**, 590 (1940).
REY-BELLET, H., u. H. ERLENMEYER: Beiträge zum Problem der Ähnlichkeit bei Komplexverbindungen. II. Helv. chim. Acta **38**, 533 (1954).
ROCHA E SILVA, M.: Pharmacological properties of simple compounds of histamine with amino acids. J. Pharmacol. exp. Ther. **77**, 198 (1943).
ROSIERE, C. E., and M. I. GROSSMAN: An analog of histamine that stimulates gastric acid secretion without other actions of histamine. Science **113**, 651 (1951).

ROTHSCHILD, Z., and R. W. SCHAYER: Synthesis and metabolism of a histamine metabolite, 1-methyl-4-(β-aminoethyl)imidazole. Biochem. biophys. Acta (Amst.) **30**, 23 (1958).
SARASIN, J.: Nouvelles synthèses dans le groupe de l'imidazol. Helv. chim. Acta **6**, 377 (1923).
SCHALIEN, S. N. R. v.: Potentiometric studies on histamine and its metal chelates. I. Ionization constants of histamine in aqueous potassium chloride solutions. Suomen Kemistilchti, **31 B**, 372 (1958): Chem. Abstr. **53**, 12798 (1959).
SCHAYER, R. W.: Synthesis of histamine-2-C^{14}-imidazole. J. Amer. chem. Soc. **74**, 2440 (1952).
SCHNEDORF, J. G., and A. C. IVY: Effects of methyl histamine and hydroxyethylglyoxaline on gastric secretion and blood pressure in the dog. Proc. Soc. exp. Biol. (N.Y.) **32**, 777 (1935).
SHEEHAN, J. C., and C. A. ROBINSON: The synthesis of triazole analogs of histamine and related compounds. J. Amer. chem. Soc. **71**, 1436 (1949).
— — The synthesis of phenyl-substituted triazole analogs of histamine. J. Amer. chem. Soc. **73**, 1207 (1951).
SONN, A., E. HOTES u. H. SIEG: Synthetische Versuche in der Imidazolgruppe. Ber. **57**, 953 (1924).
SPRINSON, D. B., and D. RITTENBERG: The metabolic reactions of carbon atom 2 of L-histidine. J. biol. Chem. **198**, 655 (1952).
TABOR, H., A. H. MEHLER, O. HAYAISHI and J. WHITE: Urocanic acid as an intermediate in the enzymatic conversion of histidine to glutamine and formic acids. J. biol. Chem. **196**, 121 (1952).
—, and E. MOSETTIG: Isolation of acetylhistamine from urine following oral administration of histamine. J. biol. Chem. **180**, 703 (1949).
TAMAMUSHI, Y.: Synthesis of homologs of histamine and their pharmacological actions. J. Pharm. Soc. Japan **53**, 1080 (1933); Chem. Abstr. **29**, 7328 (1935).
— Synthesis of 2-methylimidazole derivatives. II. The synthesis of 2-methyl-4,5-bis(aminomethyl)imidazole. J. Pharm. Soc. Japan **55**, 1053 (1935); Chem. Abstr. **31**, 6654 (1937).
— Synthesis of 2-ethylimidazole derivatives. Synthesis of 2-ethyl-4,5-diaminomethylimidazole. J. Pharm. Soc. Japan **57**, 1023 (1937); Chem. Abstr. **32**, 3394 (1938).
TESAR, C., and D. RITTENBERG: The metabolism of L-histidine. J. biol. Chem. **170**, 35 (1947).
TURNER, R. A., C. F. HUEBNER and C. R. SCHOLZ: Studies on imidazole compounds. I. 4-Methylimidazole and related compounds. J. Amer. chem. Soc. **71**, 2801 (1949).
TURNER, R. J.: Some new derivatives of 4-methylimidazole. J. Amer. chem. Soc. **70**, 3523 (1948).
VARTIAINEN, A.: The action of certain new histamine derivatives. J. Pharmacol. exp. Ther. **54**, 265 (1935).
WALTER, L. A., W. H. HUNT and R. J. FOSBINDER: β-(2- and 4-Pyridylalkyl)amines. J. Amer. chem. Soc. **63**, 2771 (1941).
WANAG, G., u. A. DOMBROWSKI: Verwendung von 2-Nitro-indandion-(1,3) für die Isolierung und Identifizierung organischer Basen, II. Mitteilung. Ber. **75**, 82 (1942).
WEIDENHAGEN, R., u. R. HERRMANN: Eine neue Synthese von Imidazolderivaten. Ber. **68**, 1953 (1935).
— — u. H. WEGNER: Über neue Abkömmlinge des Imidazols (IV. Mitteil. Über Imidazole). Ber. **70**, 570 (1937).
WEITZEL, G., u. A. M. FRETZDORFF: Zink-Imidazol-Verbindungen. Hoppe-Seylers Z. physiol. Chem. **305**, 1 (1956).
WENT, I., and L. KESZTYUS: Synthetic preparation of histamine antigen (histamine azobenzeneazoprotein). Orvosok Lapja Nepegeszsegugy **2**, 257 (1946); Chem. Abstr. **42**, 3062 (1948).
WINDAUS, A., W. DÖRRIES u. H. JENSEN: Über das Verhalten einiger aus Imidazolen bereiteter bis[Acyl-amino]-äthylen-derivate. Ber. **54**, 2745 (1921).
—, u. W. LANGEBECK: Über das Verhalten einiger aus Imidazolen bereiteter bis[Benzoylamino]-äthylene-derivate gegenüber Säure-anhydriden. Ber. **55**, 3706 (1922).
—, u. H. OPITZ: Synthese einiger Imidazol-derivate. Ber. **44**, 1721 (1911).
—, u. W. VOGT: Synthese des Imidazolyl-äthylamins. Ber. **40**, 3691 (1907).
WOLF, G.: The metabolism of α-C^{14}-histidine in the intact rat. I. Radioactivity in amino acids from protein. J. biol. Chem. **200**, 637 (1953).
YAMAMOTO, T.: The pharmacological actions of some imidazole derivatives. Folia Pharmacol. Japan **31**, 145 (1941); Chem. Abstr. **35**, 5992 (1941).
ZIMMERMANN, W.: Über eine spezifische Farbreaktion für Histamin. Hoppe-Seylers Z. physiol. Chem. **186**, 260 (1929).

Section B

Die Isolierung von Histamin aus biologischem Material

Von

Heinz Walter Raudonat

Mit 3 Abbildungen

A. Einleitung

Histamin ist eine kleinmolekulare, in Wasser, Alkohol und heißem Chloroform gut lösliche Base, hingegen ist seine Löslichkeit in wasserfreiem Äther nur gering. Ein ähnliches Lösungsverhalten zeigt auch sein Chlorhydrat, jedoch löst sich dieses kaum noch in heißem Chloroform. Gegen Erhitzen bei saurer Reaktion ist Histamin stabil und wird selbst durch kurzes Kochen mit 3 n-Salzsäure nicht zerstört. Wie alle Amine bildet es mit zahlreichen Alkaloidfällungsmitteln schwerlösliche Komplexsalze. Diese wichtigen Eigenschaften des Histamins sind die Grundlage aller Isolierungs-Methoden. Der erste Schritt jeder Reinigung ist die Abtrennung von Begleitstoffen. Schwierigkeiten treten dabei auf, wenn die Base aus fett- und eiweißreichen Organhomogenaten, aus Blut, Urin oder aus pflanzlichem Gewebebrei zu isolieren ist. Selten wird es dann gelingen, in ein oder zwei Reinigungsstufen das für biologische und biochemische Untersuchungen oder für eine sich anschließende Kristallisation geeignete Rohprodukt zu erhalten, vielmehr wird man durch eine sinnvolle Kombination von verschiedenen Fällungsmethoden mit Extraktionen oder Dialysen von Fall zu Fall einen geeigneten Weg für jedes spezielle Rohmaterial zu suchen haben. In diesem Abschnitt wird anhand von erprobten Beispielen dem Untersuchenden gesagt werden, welche Möglichkeiten einer Isolierung von Histamin aus biologischem Material sich bieten, jedoch läßt sich der Wunsch nach einer allgemein gültigen Arbeitsvorschrift naturgemäß nicht erfüllen.

B. Allgemeine Aufarbeitungsverfahren

1. Extraktion

a) Eine der ältesten, für die Histamin-Isolierung bedeutsamen Methoden ist die Anreicherung des Histamins nach dem Silber-Baryt-Verfahren, das auf Arbeiten von Kossel und Kutscher (1900) fußt. Der vorgeschlagene Aufbereitungsgang ist relativ umständlich und auch verlustreich, sei hier jedoch wiedergegeben, da — wie später gezeigt wird — er die Grundlage für zahlreiche Isolierungsversuche geworden ist.

Der zu untersuchende Gewebebrei wird mit 5%iger Schwefelsäure versetzt und unter Rühren mit einer Lösung von 500 g Phosphorwolframsäure (PWS) in 1 l 5%iger Schwefelsäure langsam vermischt (Überschuß vermeiden!). Nach längerem Stehen (12—14 Std) bei +4°C setzt sich ein gut filtrierbarer Niederschlag ab, der mit 5%iger Schwefelsäure gewaschen werden muß. Nach kräftigem Abnutschen wird dieser Niederschlag in einer Reibschale mit festem Bariumhydroxid verrieben, bis sich an der Oberfläche eine weiße Haut bildet ($BaCO_3$). Man saugt ab und wiederholt den Vorgang mit dem Rückstand unter Umständen ein zweites Mal. Beide Filtrate werden vereinigt und durch Einleiten von Kohlendioxyd vom überschüssigen Barium befreit. Die kongosaure Reaktion wird dann mit Silbernitrat, besser noch mit Silbersulfat (fest) oder Silbercarbonat (fest) gefällt. Den erhaltenen Niederschlag bezeichnet man als Purin-Fraktion, er soll kein Histamin enthalten.

Dem Filtrat, das noch genügend Ag-Ionen enthalten soll, fügt man dann erneut festes Bariumhydroxid hinzu, bis eine entnommene, klare Probe mit ammoniakalischer Silbernitratlösung keine Fällung mehr gibt. Dieser Niederschlag, die sog. Histidin-Fraktion, enthält das meiste Histamin, ein weiterer Anteil, Arginin-Fraktion, fällt nach Zugabe eines Überschusses an Barium zum Filtrat der Purin-Fraktion aus. Durch CO_2 kann ein möglicher Silber*überschuß* entfernt werden. Die Freisetzung der Amine aus der Silberbindung erfolgt leicht durch Einleiten von Schwefelwasserstoff in die angesäuerte Lösung. Abschließend sei bemerkt, daß die Umsetzung der Phosphorwolframfällung ebenso schnell und vollständig in einer gut filtrierbaren Aceton-Wasser-Mischung (3:4) erfolgen kann. Man erhält in jedem Fall einen von großmolekularen und stickstofffreien Ballaststoffen gereinigten Extrakt, der sich leicht — wie nun gezeigt werden wird — bis zum reinen Histamin weiterverarbeiten läßt.

b) Ein verbessertes Verfahren brachten später KOESSLER und HANKE (1919) heraus. In eigenen Untersuchungen trafen sie die Feststellung, daß Histamin aus alkalischer Lösung mittels Amylalkohol quantitativ extrahierbar ist. Sie benutzten hierzu eine einfache apparative Versuchsanordnung, die in Abb. 1 wiedergegeben ist. Eine wesentliche Steigerung der möglichen Histaminausbeute erzielten sie außerdem durch Totalhydrolyse des Untersuchungsmaterials.

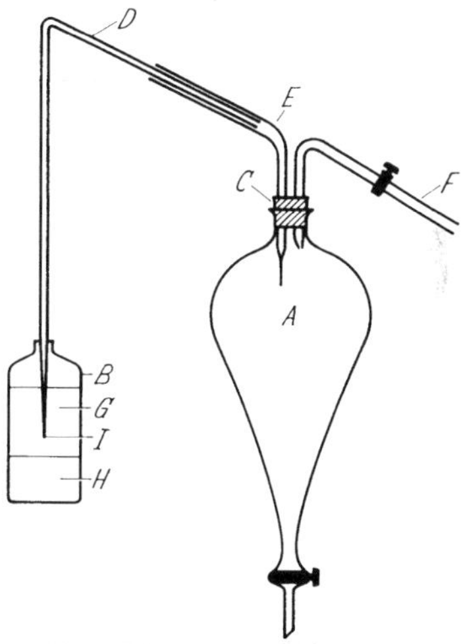

Abb. 1. Heber zum Abtrennen von Amylalkohol nach K. K. KOESSLER and M. T. HANKE (1919). *A* Scheidetrichter; *B* Vorlage mit zwei Phasenlösungsmitteln (*H* wäßrig, *G* Amylalkohol); *C* Gummistopfen; *E* weiteres —, *D* engeres Glasrohr; *F* Anschluß für Wasserstrahlpumpe; *I* Capillare. Durch Anlegen eines leichten Vakuums an *F* ist es möglich, den Amylalkohol *G* durch die Capillare *I* (kein Aufwirbeln!) nach *A* zu saugen

Methode: Das auf Histamin zu untersuchende Material wird mit 10—20 Teilen seines Gewichtes mit 37%iger Salzsäure gemischt und 30 Std auf dem Sandbad gekocht (Rückfluß). Hierbei bilden sich Huminstoffe, die zu Histaminverlusten führen können, wenn man vom Unlöslichen abfiltriert. Es ist ratsam, hierauf zu verzichten, da die Histaminausbeute hiervon wesentlich beeinflußt wird. Die Salzsäure wird nach beendeter Hydrolyse durch Vakuum-Destillation (60° C) entfernt. Der Rückstand wird mit dem 10—20fachen Volumen Wasser aufgenommen und mit Calciumhydroxid versetzt. Dann wird ein doppeltes Volumen reinen Alkohols mit der Kalkaufschwemmung des Extraktes gemischt und erneut im Vakuum destilliert, um allen Ammoniak zu entfernen. Der Rückstand wird in Wasser gelöst und filtriert. Auf dem Filter verbleiben u. a. die im Laufe der Hydrolyse entstandenen Huminstoffe. Das Filtrat selbst ist gleichfalls stark gefärbt, doch stört die Farbe nicht, sie ist später durch Quecksilbersulfid-Fällung leicht zu entfernen.

Das alkalische Filtrat wird mit Salzsäure angesäuert. Hierbei schlägt die Färbung meist von Rotbraun nach Gelbbraun um. Die Lösung wird auf dem Wasserbad eingeengt und mit Phosphorwolframsäure behandelt. Die Fällung wird abfiltriert, gewaschen und in kleinen Anteilen in einem großen Mörser mit überschüssiger, heißer, konzentrierter Bariumhydroxidlösung behandelt. Dadurch kommt es zu einer sehr vollständigen Reaktion des Phosphorwolframates mit dem Bariumhydroxid, wobei alles gebundene Histamin freigesetzt wird. Es wird anschließend filtriert und im Filtrat das Barium mit Schwefelsäure gefällt. Nach erneuter Filtration wird auf dem Wasserbad eingeengt, alkalisch gemacht und mittels Amylalkohol extrahiert, der das Histamin quantitativ aufnimmt.

Die vereinigten Amylalkoholextrakte werden 5mal mit 1 n-Salzsäure geschüttelt, wobei das Histamin quantitativ in die wäßrige Phase übertritt. Mittels Bariumhydroxid wird die Schwefelsäure entfernt und der jetzt neutrale Histaminextrakt auf dem Wasserbad eingeengt und erneut mit Bariumhydroxid versetzt.

Wie oben beschrieben, wird diese Amylalkoholextraktion 3 mal wiederholt, um das Histamin quantitativ vom Histidin zu trennen, da durch die Aminosäure eventuelle colorimetrische Histaminbestimmungen gefälscht würden. Die mehrfache Amylalkoholextraktion setzt die Histaminausbeute nicht herab, wenn man die Versuchsbedingungen genau einhält!

Oft enthalten Gewebsextrakte Störsubstanzen, die sich durch Wolframatfällung allein nicht entfernen lassen. In solchen Fällen muß vor die Amylalkoholextraktion ein zusätzlicher Reinigungsschritt eingeschoben werden: Die schon vorgereinigte Lösung (letzte Phosphorwolframat-Fraktion) wird mit einem Überschuß an Silbernitrat und anschließend mit Bariumhydroxid versetzt, der Niederschlag filtriert und mit kaltgesättigter Barytlauge gewaschen. Anschließend suspendiert man ihn in verdünnter Salzsäure und erhitzt die Mischung eine Stunde auf dem siedenden Wasserbad unter Hinzugabe von 20%iger Natriumsulfatlösung, um das Barium auszufällen. Silberchlorid und Bariumsulfat werden anschließend abfiltriert, das Filtrat mit NaOH neutralisiert und eingeengt. Schließlich erfolgt, wie oben beschrieben, die Amylalkoholextraktion. So sind fast alle starkfärbenden Störsubstanzen entfernt worden; sollte jedoch noch eine Restfärbung verblieben sein, so kann man durch Zugabe von 1 g Quecksilberchlorid und anschließender H_2S-Fällung auch diese ohne Histaminverlust noch entfernen.

2. Elektrodialyse

a) An Substrat-Modellen haben GEBAUER-FUELNEGG und KENDALL (1931) den Versuch unternommen, die Elektrodialyse zur Trennung und Isolierung organischer Basen anzuwenden. Diese Arbeiten hatten Erfolg. Sie konnten nicht nur aus Gemischen von Histamin mit Histidin oder Histamin mit Cholin und Eiklar das Amin bei p_H 7,5 im Kathodenraum ansammeln, sondern sie zerlegten auch mit Hilfe handelsüblicher 3-Zellen-Elektrodialysatoren Chloroplatinate und Pikrate des Histamins. Damit war es nicht mehr unbedingt erforderlich, solche Doppelsalze durch Ausschütteln mit Äther oder Benzol umzusetzen.

b) Wesentlich vervollkommnet haben MACGREGOR und THORPE (1933) die E.-Dialysetechnik. Sie erprobten ein sehr brauchbares und einfaches Verfahren zur Isolierung des Histamins aus Gewebsextrakten. Alkohol-Extrakte nach der Methode von BEST et al. (1927) waren gelb gefärbt und nicht frei von Biuret-Substanzen. Letztere extrahierten das Gewebe zuerst 24 Std mit 96%igem Alkohol und wiederholten die Extraktion des Rückstandes mit 60%igem Alkohol. Die vereinigten Auszüge wurden eingeengt und durch Schütteln mit Äther entfettet. Demgegenüber waren alle Elektrodialysate von MACGREGOR und THORPE wasserklar und farblos. Die Trennung ist nach 2 Std beendet. Während des Versuches steigt die Temperatur nicht über 40° C.

In Vergleichsuntersuchungen haben diese Autoren außerdem Extrakte nach der Methode von BEST und MCHENRY (1930) gefertigt. Hierzu wurde Gewebe mit 10%iger HCl eine Stunde auf 95° C erhitzt und anschließend im Vakuum eingeengt. Die biologische Aktivität solcher Extrakte war größer als jener nach Elektrodialyse; dies ist leicht erklärlich wenn man bedenkt, daß bei Hydrolysen auch „gebundenes“ Histamin freigesetzt wird.

Methode: MACGREGOR und THORPE verwendeten 3-Zellen-Apparate, die sie selbst aus paraffingetränktem Holz gebaut hatten oder sich aus Glas anfertigen ließen. Das Gesamtvolumen schwankte von 100 ml bis zu 500 ml Inhalt je Zelle. Es dürfte jeder handelsübliche Apparat brauchbar sein, da die Form selbst von untergeordneter Bedeutung ist. Zur Dialyse von Lunge und Blutproben waren

Membranen aus Pergament oder Cellophan ausreichend, jedoch nicht für Herzmuskel oder Leber-Homogenate. Bei letzteren wanderten biuretpositive Substanzen in den Kathodenraum. Dafür erwiesen sich Collodium-Membranen als brauchbarer. Als Kathode wurde ein Nickelblech verwendet, als Anode eine Kohleplatte. Während des ganzen Versuches mußte die Gewebssuspension in der Mittelzelle kräftig *gerührt* werden, da sich sonst leicht fest haftende Belege an der Kathoden-Membran bildeten – besonders bei Herzmuskel –, die den elektrischen Widerstand des Systems beträchtlich heraufsetzen. Ein zu dicker Belag ließ sich mit Hilfe eines Glasstabes entfernen. Als *Stromquelle* diente 230 V Gleichstrom. Die Zelle

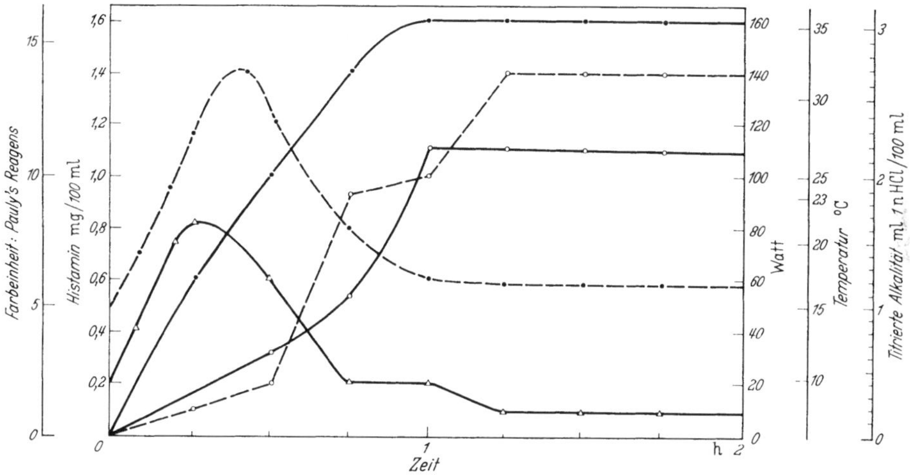

Abb. 2. Elektrodialyse von 20 g Lunge in 100 ml verdünntem Homogenat nach R. G. MacGregor and W. V. Thorpe (1933).

- Histaminwert in der Kathodenflüssigkeit
- Farbintensität nach Paulys Reagens
- Titrierbare Alkalität (kathodenrein)
- Temperatur (Mittelraum)
- Stromaufnahme in Watt

Ergebnis: 1. Die Intensität der Paulyschen Farbreaktion erreicht *nie* vor Eintritt maximaler Histaminkonzentration im Kathodenraum ihr Maximum. 2. Die titrierbare Alkalität der Zelle erreicht immer ihr Maximum vor maximaler Histaminkonzentration im Kathodenraum. 3. Die Stromaufnahme der Zelle fällt bei Erreichung des Histaminmaximums stark ab

wurde parallel mit 4 Kohlenfadenlampen geschaltet, die jede einen Strom bis 1 Ampere liefert. Je nach Größe der jeweiligen Dialyse-Zelle wurden 1–3 Lampen abgeschaltet. Die Leistungs-Aufnahme einer 100 ml-Zelle betrug etwa 50 Watt/Std, die einer 250 ml Zelle 120 Watt/Std. Um die Temperatur nicht über 40° C ansteigen zu lassen, wird die Zelle mittels Kühlschlange und kaltem Wasser gekühlt. Nur in der ersten halben Stunde (Stromspitze!) entsteht viel Wärme, später fällt die Temperatur auf 20° C.

Die p_H-Änderung während des Versuches war gering, in extremen Fällen fiel der Wert von p_H 7,4 auf p_H 4,6, doch nur bei Muskel-Homogenaten. Bei Versuchen mit Blut bleibt der p_H-Wert oberhalb von 6.

Der Versuch ist beendet, wenn der Widerstand der Zelle sich nicht mehr ändert und wenn die Alkaliabscheidung an der Kathode konstant wird (Titration). Trotzdem ist es ratsam, den Verlauf der Histamin-Wanderung durch laufende Farbteste der Kathoden-Flüssigkeit (Pauly-Reaktion) zu kontrollieren. Dialysiert man zu lange, so muß man Histamin-Verluste mit in Kauf nehmen (s. Abb. 2).

Versuchsbeispiel: Ein Dialyseapparat von 750 ml Gesamtvolumen wird im Kathodenraum und im Anodenraum mit je 250 ml destilliertem Wasser gefüllt. Der Mittelraum erhält 200 ml Wasser mit 50 g Gewebe. Ein Elektrolyt zur Erhöhung der Leitfähigkeit ist nicht erforderlich! Nach Einschalten der Kühlung und des Rührwerkes wird der Strom eingeschaltet. Nur in der Mittelzelle steigt die Temperatur schnell an und erreicht spätestens nach 1 Std ihren Höhepunkt. Nach Erreichung des Endpunktes (s. o.) wird abgeschaltet. Das Histamin befindet sich *quantitativ* in Kathodenraum. Durch Zugabe einer bekannten Menge Histamin zum Homogenat konnte dies bestätigt werden.

Versuchsergebnisse von Reihenversuchen

Gewebe	Tierart	Zahl der Exper.	Extrem. Hist. Wert in mg/kg
Herz	Rind	8	8—25
Leber	Hund	2	13—40
	Rind	2	10—20
	Schwein	2	13
	Schaf	3	2,5— 6
Lunge	Hund	3	10—13
	Rind	11	30—60

3. Papierelektrophorese

Im Gegensatz zur präparativen Elektrodialyse ist die Elektrophorese eine analytische Methode. Alle bisher hier aufgeführten Trennverfahren haben den Nachteil, daß nach mehr oder minder umständlicher Vorreinigung ein kleines Volumen Flüssigkeit verbleibt, aus dem das Histamin mit unspezifischen Fällungsmitteln gefällt wird. Da meist gleichzeitig andere Amine zugegen sind, erhält man auch nach mehrmaliger Umkristallisation nie ein reines Histamin. Durch Anwendung der Elektrophorese läßt sich die Reinigung von Extrakten wesentlich verbessern und beschleunigen. Als Puffer für die Elektrophorese histaminhaltiger Rohextrakte schlagen CLOTTEN und CLOTTEN (1962) eine Mischung aus 40 ml Pyridin, 20 ml Eisessig, 20 g Citronensäure und 940 ml Wasser vor. Es ist ratsam, mit Hochspannung zu arbeiten.

Im folgenden sei ein Arbeitsvorgang von CODE (1937) wiedergegeben, der in wenigen Arbeitsgängen einen für die Elektrophorese brauchbaren Rohextrakt liefert.

Versuchsbeispiel: 5 g Gewebe (Lunge, Leber, Muskel) werden mit (evtl. unter Zugabe von Quarzsand) 10—15 ml 10%iger Trichloressigsäure homogenisiert. Das Homogenat wird zentrifugiert und der Niederschlag mit 10 ml 5%iger Trichloressigsäure gewaschen. Um in Lösung gegangene Lipoide zu entfernen, werden die vereinigten Auszüge 3mal mit dem gleichen Volumen Äther ausgeschüttelt, wobei auch ein Teil des Trichloressigsäureüberschusses mit entfernt wird. Hiernach fügt man 5 ml konz. HCl hinzu (in dieser Form ist der Auszug wochenlang ohne Histamineinbuße haltbar). Zur Hydrolyse wird die Lösung auf einem Sandbad oder auf offener Flamme (kein Wasserbad!) 90 min in stetem Sieden gehalten, möglichst unter Anwendung eines Rückflußkühlers. Hierbei darf am Rande keine Verkohlung eintreten, da sich sonst aus anwesendem Histidin Histamin bilden könnte.

Nach beendeter Hydrolyse wird die Flüssigkeit im Vakuum bei 70°C zur Trockene eingeengt. Histaminverluste treten hierbei nicht auf. Der Rückstand wird mit 10 ml Äthanol versetzt und zur Vertreibung von Salzsäureresten und Wasser erneut eingeengt, wobei darauf zu achten ist, daß alle festen Bestandteile in der alkoholischen Lösung fein suspendiert werden. Nicht unbedingt erforderlich, aber ratsam ist eine nochmalige Alkoholdestillation, wobei vorher durch Zentrifugation unlösliche, histaminfreie Ballaststoffe entfernt werden können. Der nach der letzten Alkoholdestillation verbleibende Rückstand ist unbegrenzt haltbar.

4. Papierchromatographie

Ebenso wie die Papierelektrophorese ist auch die Papierchromatographie zur Auftrennung von vorgereinigten Gewebsextrakten brauchbar. Nach Untersuchungen von WEST und RILEY (1954), die Histamin aus Trichloressigsäure-Extrakten verschiedener Gewebe papierchromatographisch in n-Butanol-Essigsäure-Wasser (4:1:5) abtrennen konnten, ist der Einfluß des Extraktionsmittels von erheblicher Bedeutung. Reste überschüssiger Trichloressigsäure führen dazu, daß das Histamin in 2 Flecken (mit biol. Aktivität) von $R_f = 0,11$ und $R_f = 0,65$ wandert. Erst bei einer Rechromatographie beider Eluate zerfällt die Substanz mit dem $R_f = 0{,}65$ und läuft nur noch mit niederem R_f-Wert. Man kann diesen Mißstand weitgehend beseitigen, wenn man die zur Extraktion verwendete Trichloressigsäure sehr sorgfältig mit Äther ausschüttelt, doch scheinen für die papierchromatographische Wanderungsgeschwindigkeit auch noch andere Substanzen, wie z. B. basische Aminosäuren, von Bedeutung zu sein.

5. Neuere Fällungsmittel für Histamin

Bei den meisten hier beschriebenen Isolierungsmethoden schließt sich an die Vorreinigung durch Silberbaryt-Fällung, Bleiacetat, Tannin etc. eine Fällung der Stickstoffbasen mit Pikrinsäure, Pikrolonsäure oder Flaviansäure an. Diese letztere Fällung ist nur sinnvoll, wenn die Amine mit anorganischen Begleitsalzen gemischt sind. Die eben genannten klassischen Fällungsmittel lassen sich anschließend leicht wieder zerlegen und geben dadurch das Amin frei. Daneben haben in neuerer Zeit u. a. zwei Komplexbildner eine gewisse Bedeutung erlangt, die mit Histamin sehr schwer lösliche Verbindungen eingehen. REDEMANN und NIEMANN (1939) stellten das Histaminsalz der 5-Nitrobarbitursäure (Dilitursäure) dar. Seine Löslichkeit in Wasser liegt bei nur 17 mMol/l. ZEIDLER (1952) fällte Histamin mit Hilfe des Tetraphenylborkomplexes, dessen Löslichkeit in Wasser bei 0,01% liegt. Die Fällung ist nur in neutralem oder schwach saurem Medium möglich. Suspendiert man den Histamin-Komplex in Salzsäure, so läßt sich durch Ausäthern das Fällungsmittel leicht vollständig entfernen. Das Amin verbleibt als Chlorhydrat in der wäßrigen Phase.

C. Spezielle Aufarbeitungsverfahren

1. Isolierung von Histamin aus Pflanzen und Bakterien

a) Histamin aus Bakterien

Eine der ältesten Arbeiten von ACKERMANN (1910) befaßt sich mit der Isolierung von Histamin aus Bakterien in faulendem Pepton. Er beimpfte einen Versuchsansatz, bestehend aus 49 g Histidinchlorhydrat in 4 l Wasser, versetzt mit 10 g Pepton (WITTE), 20 g Traubenzucker, einigen Tropfen einer Magnesiumsulfatlösung und Natriumphosphat, sowie einem Überschuß von Calciumcarbonat, um eine bleibende alkal. Reaktion zu garantieren. Beimpft wurde mit einer Spur zerkleinertem Rinderpankreas, die vorher in Sodalösung bebrütet wurde.

Nach einer Fäulniszeit von 52 Tagen bei 35° C im Brutschrank wurde der Ansatz filtriert und schwach phosphorsauer nach KUTSCHER (1910) aufgearbeitet. Restliches Pepton wurde mittels Tannin entfernt. Nach der Phosphorwolframsäurefällung (s. o.) wurde der Niederschlag mit Baryt zerlegt, die salpetersaure Lösung der Amine mit Silbernitrat versetzt und so lange Bariumhydroxid hinzugefügt, bis die Flüssigkeit gegen ammoniakalische Silbernitratlösung nur noch eine ganz schwache Trübung zeigte. Der Niederschlag wurde abfiltriert und mit Salzsäure zerlegt. Im Filtrat des Silberchlorid-Niederschlages wurden die Amine erneut mit Phosphorwolframsäure gefällt und die Fällung mit 5%iger H_2SO_4 völlig nitratfrei gewaschen. Der Niederschlag wurde mit Baryt zerlegt und nach Einengen mit Pikrinsäurelösung gefällt. Ausbeute: 53,8 g Pikrat.

b) Histamin aus gefaulten Sojabohnen (Glycine hispida)

YOSHIMURA (1910) gelang die weitgehende Anreicherung (Pikrat) des Histamins aus faulenden Sojabohnen. Als Versuchsansatz dienten ihm 1 kg gekochter und stark zerkleinerter Sojabohnen in 4 l Wasser. Dieser milchige Brei wurde bei Zimmertemperatur für die Dauer von 4 Monaten sich selbst überlassen, dann durch ein Tuch koliert, die Flüssigkeit mit Bleiessig versetzt und filtriert. Dem Filtrat wurde das überschüssige Blei durch H_2S-Fällung entzogen.

Die klare Flüssigkeit wurde mit Phosphorwolframat gefällt, der Niederschlag mit Baryt zerlegt und das stark saure Filtrat mit Silbernitrat behandelt. Ein geringer Niederschlag (Purinfraktion) wurde verworfen. Das Filtrat wurde mit Silbernitrat im Überschuß sowie mit Bariumhydroxid behandelt. Dieser Niederschlag wurde mit H_2S zerlegt und das restliche Barium als Carbonat gefällt. Im Vakuum wurde das Filtrat des Silbersulfides eingeengt, mit Salzsäure neutralisiert und im Vakuum-Exsiccator zur Sirupdicke eingetrocknet. Nach Zugabe eines Überschusses an absolutem Äthylalkohol kristallisiert Histaminchlorhydrat in farblosen, dünnen Prismen. Ausbeute: 0,3 g Histamin. Die gefundenen und die berechneten Analysendaten des gleichzeitig hergestellten Pikrates sowie des Chloroplatinates stimmten praktisch überein.

c) Isolierung von Histamin aus Faeces-Bakterien

Hanke und Koessler (1924 b, c, d) beimpften ein synthetisches Substrat mit Faeces-Bakterien, um die Decarboxylierung des Histidins zu Histamin verfolgen zu können. Das Substrat bestand aus einer sterilen Nährlösung, die in 200 ml folgende Substanzen enthielt:

0,20 g Histidin	0,02 g Natriumsulfat (wasserfrei)
0,20 g Ammoniumchlorid	0,40 g Natriumbicarbonat
0,10 g Kaliumnitrat	0,01 g Calciumchlorid (wasserfrei)
0,40 g Kaliumdihydrogenphosphat	4,0 g Glycerin
0,80 g Natriumchlorid	

Das mit Faeces beimpfte Substrat blieb für 14 Tage bei 37° C im Brutschrank und wurde dann wie folgt aufgearbeitet:

Die Suspension wurde durch ein Berkefeldfilter gesaugt, der Rückstand gewaschen und die vereinigten Filtrate mit 1 ml konz. Schwefelsäure versetzt. Auf dem Wasserbad wurde die Lösung schließlich zur Sirupdicke eingeengt und in 25 ml Wasser gelöst. Von dieser Lösung wurden je 10 ml mit 3 g festem Natriumhydroxid versetzt und 6mal mit dem doppelten Volumen Amylalkohol ausgeschüttelt. Auf diese Weise gelingt die Trennung von Histidin, das in der wäßrigen Phase verbleibt.

Mittels 1 n-Schwefelsäure konnte das Roh-Histamin aus den Amylalkoholauszügen zurückgewonnen werden. Der die colorimetrische Bestimmung des Histamins störende Amylalkohol läßt sich durch Ausschütteln der Lösung mit etwas Chloroform leicht entfernen.

d) Verfahren zur Isolierung von Histamin aus Pflanzen

Um die Verbreitung des Histamins in der Pflanzenwelt zu untersuchen, prüften Werle und Raub (1944) zahlreiche Pflanzenfamilien auf ihren Gehalt an Histamin. Sie verwendeten zur Anreicherung des Histamins das Verfahren von Barsoum und Gaddum (1935) mit geringen Abänderungen:

Die zur Untersuchung auf ihren Histamingehalt bestimmten Pflanzen wurden sorgfältig gewaschen, mit Filtrierpapier getrocknet und als solche, oder getrennt in ihre einzelnen Organe, unter Zerreiben mit Seesand im Mörser extrahiert. Zu 1 g Pflanze wurden 2 ml Wasser gegeben. Diese Auszüge waren selbst für biologische, orientierende Blutdruckversuche unbrauchbar. Deshalb erfolgte die

Extraktion später nur noch mit 10%iger Trichloressigsäurelösung (2 ml TCE/1 g Pflanze). Nach dieser ersten Extraktion wurde das Material noch einmal mit 5%iger und ein zweites Mal mit 1%iger Trichloressigsäure ausgezogen. Aus den vereinigten Extrakten wurde die Trichloressigsäure ausgeäthert. Nach Zugabe von 1 ml 25%iger Salzsäure wurde der Extrakt $1^1/_2$ Std gekocht und im Vakuum zur Trockene eingeengt. Zur Entfernung von HCl-Resten wurde noch viermal mit NaCl-gesättigtem Alkohol abgedampft und dann das Histamin sechsmal mit 5 ml NaCl-gesättigtem Alkohol extrahiert. Der filtrierte Auszug wurde im Vakuum eingedampft und in Ringerlösung aufgenommen, wobei der p_H-Wert mit NaOH auf 7,0 eingestellt wurde. Diese Extrakte eigneten sich vorzüglich für die pharmakologische Prüfung.

e) Darstellung von Histamin aus der Lederkoralle (Alcyonium digitatum)

In jüngster Zeit gelang Ackermann und Menssen (1959) die Isolierung einer kleinen Histaminmenge aus der Lederkoralle auf papierchromatographischem Wege. Sie arbeiteten den Gewebsbrei nach dem klassischen Silberbaryt-Verfahren auf, indem sie die zerlegte Silber-Barium-Fraktion mit Flaviansäure ausfällten. Die aus den Flavianaten zurückgewonnenen Amine wurden dann papierchromatographisch in n-Butanol-Eisessig-Wasser (6:1:2) aufgetrennt.

2. Isolierung aus Körperflüssigkeiten und aus tierischen Geweben

a) Verfahren zur Abtrennung des Histamins aus Blut

Zum pharmakologischen, quantitativen Nachweis des Histamins im Blut haben Barsoum und Gaddum (1935) eine einfache Methode geschaffen, die, ohne Pikratfällung o. ä., auf direktem Wege eine weitgehend gereinigte Histaminfraktion liefert. Die Herstellung des Extraktes geschieht wie folgt:

10 ml Blut werden langsam in 15 ml einer 10%igen Trichloressigsäurelösung gegossen und nach frühestens einer Stunde durch Papier filtriert. Der abgetrennte Niederschlag wird nun 4mal mit je 5 ml Trichloressigsäurelösung gewaschen und die vereinigten Filtrate 4–5mal mit kleinen Portionen Äther im Scheidetrichter ausgeschüttelt, bis die wäßrige Lösung gegen Kongo-Papier neutral reagiert. Danach werden der Lösung 10 ml 1 n-Salzsäure zugefügt und der Extrakt 90 min auf offener Flamme gekocht, wobei verdampfendes Wasser laufend ersetzt werden soll. Nach Beendigung der Hydrolyse wird auf dem Wasserbad im Vakuum eingeengt (bis zur Trockene) und der Rest durch zweimalige Destillation mit je 10 ml Alkohol (96%) von Salzsäureresten befreit. Der verbleibende Rückstand wird schließlich 3mal (2 + 2 + 2 ml) mit einem an Natriumchlorid gesättigtem Alkohol (enthält etwa 1,4% Wasser) extrahiert. Die filtrierten Extrakte werden eingedampft, in etwa 2 ml Wasser aufgenommen und mit x ml 1 n-NaOH gegen Lackmus neutralisiert. Nach Zugabe von $(0{,}28 - x)$ ml 1 n-NaCl wird auf 2,5 ml aufgefüllt.

Dieser vorgereinigte eingeengte Extrakt eignet sich auch zur Fraktionierung auf der Hochspannungselektrophorese nach Clotten und Clotten (1962).

b) Verfahren zur Abtrennung des Histamins aus menschlichem Urin nach Dunér *und* Pernow *(1956)*

1924 hatten Hanke und Koessler (1924a) sich bemüht, Histamin und histaminähnliche Substanzen aus Urin zu isolieren. Sie erhielten nach Blei-Acetatfällung eine Imidazol-Fraktion, die stark positiv Paulysche Reaktion zeigte, jedoch in Alkohol unlösliche Ba-Salze bildete und sich aus natronalkalischer Lösung nicht mit Amylacetat extrahieren ließ. Vielleicht hatte man unberücksichtigt gelassen, daß Histamin meist konjugiert ausgeschieden wird und sich auf diese Weise dem Nachweis entzog. Zur Extraktion des gesamten Histamins – freies und Acetyl – aus Urin haben deshalb DUNÉR und PERNOW (1956) eine einfache Methode erprobt, die wie folgt ausgeführt wird:

100 ml Urin werden bei p_H 6,5 mit dem doppelten Volumen Aceton geschüttelt und filtriert. Die resultierende, klare Lösung wird im Vakuum eingeengt und in 10 ml 10 n-Salzsäure aufgenommen. Anschließend erfolgt eine 90 min dauernde Hydrolyse auf dem Wasserbad. Nach mehrmaligem Abdampfen der Flüssigkeit zur Entfernung des Salzsäureüberschusses wird der Rückstand in wenig Wasser aufgenommen. Die Abtrennung des Histamins aus diesem Rohextrakt erfolgt dann entweder papierchromatographisch (empfohlen) oder durch weitere Extraktionen mit Amylalkohol.

c) Extraktion von freiem und konjugiertem Histamin aus Urin nach ROBERTS *und* ADAM *(1950)*

Das Prinzip ist einfach; das freie Histamin des Urins wird bei p_H 8,0 an *Decalso*[1], einem Ionenaustauscher, absorbiert und durch wechselndes Waschen mit Ammoniak und Chloroform extrahiert. Das vom Austauscher nicht gebundene, acetylierte Histamin wird an Kohle absorbiert und von dieser mit saurem Alkohol heruntergewaschen.

Methode: Extraktion des freien Histamins: In einer Säule von 6 cm Höhe befinden sich 3 g Austauscher, die vor dem Versuch mit Wasser gewaschen werden. Nach Durchlauf des Harnes (p_H 8,0) wird mit 25 ml 0,9%iger NaCl-Lösung nachgewaschen und das Wasser mit 15 ml absolutem Alkohol verdrängt. Zur Elution wird die Säule kurz mit 3 ml konz. Ammoniak gespült und anschließend mit Chloroform (NH_3-gesättigt, wasserfrei!) das Histamin heruntergewaschen. Das ammoniakalische Chloroform-Eluat wird eingeengt, der Rückstand in Alkohol (3% Salzsäure) aufgenommen, erneut eingeengt und in Alkohol gelöst.

Extraktion des konjugierten Histamins: Eine 6 cm lange und 1 cm dicke Säule wird mit Kohle gefüllt. Die Kohle muß vorher mit konz. Salzsäure aktiviert (10 ml Säure/1 g Kohle, 15 min 100° C), mit destilliertem Wasser säurefrei gewaschen und getrocknet werden (ROBERTS und ADAM 1950). Dieser Kohle wird außerdem 1% Quarzsand zugesetzt. Der aus der *Decalso*-Säule kommende Harn wird über die Kohlesäule gegeben und nach Waschen mit destilliertem Wasser mit 30 ml salzsaurem Alkohol (3%) eluiert. Diese Lösung wurde mit 10 ml 20%iger Salzsäure gemischt und 1 Std unter Rückfluß auf offener Flamme hydrolysiert. Das Hydrolysat wird eingeengt, mit Alkohol mehrmals abgedampft und in Wasser aufgenommen. Zur Abtrennung des Histamins müssen beide Extrakte, der des freien und der des konjugierten Amines, noch papierchromatographisch oder papierelektrophoretisch weiter aufgearbeitet werden.

d) Verfahren zur Gewinnung von Histamin aus Hypophysen nach ABEL *und* KUBOTA *sowie nach* DUDLEY

ABEL und KUBOTA (1919) suspendierten etwa 500 gepulverte Hypophysen in 8 ml einer 2%igen Lösung von Quecksilberchlorid in 0,8%iger Salzsäure. Von der Fällung wurde abfiltriert und der Überschuß an Quecksilber durch H_2S entfernt. Das Filtrat wurde mit Phosphorwolframsäure, wie oben beschrieben, behandelt und der Niederschlag mit Bariumhydroxid zerlegt. Nach mehrfacher wiederholter Alkoholextraktion wurde der Extrakt mit gepulvertem Soda (wasserfrei) versetzt und

[1] *Decalso*-Hersteller: Permutit Comp. 330 W., 42nd Street New York 18. NY. Techn. Name = Folin *Decalso*.

mittels heißem Chloroform extrahiert. Aus diesem Chloroformauszug kristallisierte das Histamin beim Stehen als sehr aktives Material aus. Der nach Eindampfen der Mutterlauge verbleibende Rückstand wurde mit schwefelsaurem Alkohol aufgenommen und in eine Mischung Alkohol-Äther (1:2) getropft. Dabei fiel reines Histaminsulfat aus, das als Pikrat identifiziert wurde.

Etwa zu gleicher Zeit hatte auch DUDLEY (1919) Hypophysen auf Amine untersucht und die Ergebnisse von ABEL und KUBOTA teilweise bestätigen können. Er verwandte nicht, wie diese, heißes Chloroform als Extraktionsmittel für Rohextrakte, sondern benutzte einen einfachen Apparat zur kontinuierlichen Extraktion mit Butylalkohol (s. Abb. 3). Er fand, daß die Löslichkeit für Histamin in heißem Chloroform gering ist, dafür aber keine oxytocischen Substanzen mit in Lösung gehen. Bei der Verwendung von n-Butanol in „saurer" Lösung fand er jedoch (damals noch unbekannte) fremde, uterustimulierende Substanzen. DUDLEY gebrauchte zum Enteiweißen seiner Rohextrakte Ferrihydroxid (kolloidal), das er tropfenweise seiner Lösung zusetzte.

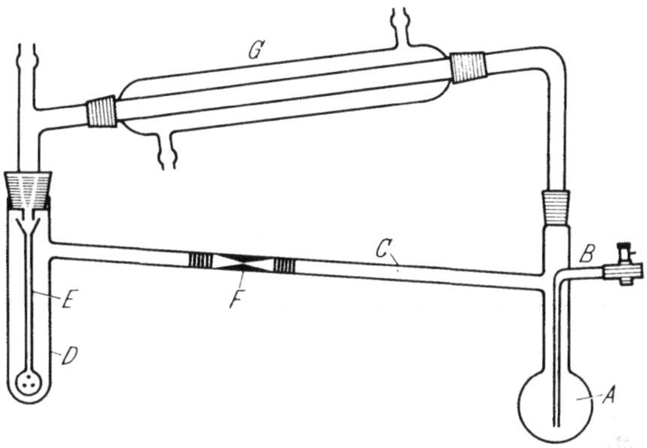

Abb. 3. Apparat zur kontinuierlichen Amin-Extraktion mittels *n*-Butanol nach H. W. DUDLEY (1919). *A* Kochflasche; *B* Gaseinleitungsrohr; *C* Seitenrohr; *D* Extraktionsglas; *E* Perforationsrohr; *F* Verbindungsstück von *A* und *D*; *G* Kühler. Durch Anlegen eines Wasserstrahlpumpenvakuums an *B* ist es möglich, einen in *D* befindlichen Histamin-Rohextrakt kontinuierlich mit *n*-Butanol bei niederer Temperatur (70° C) zu extrahieren. Das Lösungsmittel verdampft bei *A*, kondensiert bei *G*, und tropft in den Perforator *E*. Über *F* und *C* läuft das mit Amin gesättigte Butanol nach *A* zurück und verdampft dort erneut unter Zurücklassen des Histamins

e) Verfahren zur Abtrennung des Histamins aus Dünndarmschleimhaut nach BARGER *und* DALE *(1911)*

Dünndarm des Rindes – frisch vom Schlachthaus – wird in fließendem Wasser gewaschen und bei 2°C aufbewahrt. Am nächsten Tag wird die Schleimhaut abgeschabt und mit Sand verrieben. Mit Salzsäure wird die dickflüssige Masse auf 0,1% HCl gebracht, kurz gekocht und mittels Wasserstrahlpumpe filtriert. So erhält man von jedem Kilo „Geschabtem" 750 ml Extrakt (Filtrat). Nach dem Kurzerhitzen des Extraktes wurden durch langsames Hinzufügen von 20% Tanninlösung die Proteine ausgeflockt und abfiltriert. Das Filtrat wird anschließend nach der Methode von KUTSCHER (1910) behandelt und das gewonnene Silber-Präcipitat, erhalten nach Zugabe eines Überschusses an „Baryt" in Gegenwart von $AgNO_3$, gesammelt. Die vorgereinigten Basen wurden schließlich mit heißem Äthylalkohol (absolutem) extrahiert. Nach Abdestillieren des Alkohols verbleibt ein sirupartiger Rückstand. Dieser wurde mit einer wäßrigen, gesättigten Pikrinsäurelösung versetzt, wobei ein gut kristallisierendes Pikrat ausfiel (etwa 19 mg), das bei 228°C schmolz. Nach einmaligem Umkristallisieren schmolzen die gelben Nadeln oder rhombischen Tafeln erst bei 232°C. Sie verhielten sich hierin dem Histamindipikrat sehr ähnlich.

Um das Histamin zurückzugewinnen, wurden 10 mg des Dipikrates in verdünnter Salzsäure gelöst und die Pikrinsäure durch Ausäthern entfernt. Die Ausbeute an Histamin beträgt nach dieser Prozedur nur noch 0,5 mg.

f) Verfahren zur Isolierung von Histamin aus Rinderleber nach Best, Dale, Dudley *und* Thorpe *(1927)*

66 kg frischer Rinderleber werden kleingeschnitten und unter Rühren in 95%igen Alkohol (2,25 l/kg Gewebe) gegeben. Nach 24stündigem Stehen wird der Extrakt filtriert und der Rückstand erneut 24 Std mit 60%igem Alkohol (2 l/kg Gewebe) ausgezogen. Danach wird abermals filtriert, beide Filtrate vereinigt und mit 0,18 ml Schwefelsäure pro Liter versetzt, um inaktives Material auszuflocken. Gleichzeitig wird durch diese Präcipitation ein Schäumen beim nachfolgenden Einengen im Vakuum (bei höchstens 50°C) verhindert. Dem verbleibenden sirupartigen Rückstand wird dann Alkohol, bis zu einer Endkonzentration der Lösung von 80% Äthanol hinzugefügt und erneut filtriert. Dem klaren Filtrat setzt man 3 Volumen Aceton unter Rühren hinzu und sammelt das entstehende Präcipitat, welches 70% der im Extrakt vorhandenen pressorischen Substanz enthält. Den Verlust von 30% nimmt man gern in Kauf, da man durch diese Prozedur der Fällung sehr schnell zu einem weitgehend vorgereinigten Material kommt.

Nun wird die Aceton-Fällung in Wasser gelöst, mit Natriumhydroxid neutralisiert und mit basischem Bleiacetat behandelt, bis kein Niederschlag mehr ausfällt. Danach wird das überschüssige Blei mit Schwefelwasserstoff entfernt, die Lösung vom Bleisulfid abfiltriert und im Vakuum auf 1050 ml eingeengt. Nunmehr werden 5% Schwefelsäure zugesetzt und mit Phosphorwolframsäure (25% in 5%iger Schwefelsäure) vollständig gefällt. Man benötigt etwa 5 l Reagens. Der Niederschlag wird abfiltriert und mit 5%iger H_2SO_4 gewaschen. Das Filtrat ist frei von pressorischen Substanzen. Das Phosphorwolframat wird durch Verreiben mit einem Überschuß von Bariumhydroxid bei 60°C im Wasserbad zerlegt und im Filtrat das überschüssige Barium mit Schwefelsäure entfernt. Schließlich wird die Lösung im Vakuum auf 400 ml eingeengt.

190 g Silbernitrat in 400 ml Wasser werden dann unter Rühren der schwach sauren Lösung beigegeben und vom Niederschlag abfiltriert. Der Niederschlag ist histaminfrei. Das Filtrat wird mit Baryt gesättigt und, nach Stehen in Eiswasser, von der entstehenden Fällung abgetrennt, diese nun 2mal mit gesättigter Barytlauge gewaschen.

Anschließend wird der Niederschlag in verdünnter Schwefelsäure gelöst (schwach Kongo-sauer!) und das Silber als Sulfid gefällt. Vom Silbersulfid und Bariumsulfat wird abfiltriert, mit Baryt neutralisiert und im Vakuum auf 25 ml eingeengt. 25 g kristallines Bariumhydroxid werden zur Lösung gegeben und nach gutem Durchmischen wird der so erhaltene Brei im Exsiccator unter Vakuum über Schwefelsäure getrocknet. Das trockene Pulver wird anschließend im Soxhlet-Apparat mit absolutem Alkohol 3 Std extrahiert. Der Extrakt wird mit Wasser verdünnt und mit Schwefelsäure neutralisiert, wobei gleichzeitig etwa in Lösung gegangenes Barium als Sulfat entfernt wird. Der Alkohol wird im Vakuum abdestilliert, der Rückstand mit wasserfreiem Calciumsulfat verrieben und erneut extrahiert. Dieser Extrakt wird im Vakuum auf 25 ml eingeengt und mit Natriumpikrat gefällt.

Ausbeute: 608 mg Pikrat, nach zweimaliger Umkristallisation 431 mg.

α) Verfahren zur Isolierung von Histamin aus Lunge nach Best, Dale, Dudley und Thorpe (1927). 10 kg frischer Lunge werden zerkleinert und mit Alkohol extrahiert (s. Leber). Die Acetonfällung unterbleibt jedoch. Der Auszug wird im Vakuum weitgehend eingeengt und durch mehrmaliges Schütteln mit Äther entfettet. Schließlich wird auf ein Volumen von 2 l eingeengt und wie unter Leber angegeben aufgearbeitet.

Ausbeute: 146 mg Histamindipikrat.

β) Die Isolierung von Histamin aus der Lunge nach Ackermann und Fuchs (1939). 15 Rinderlungen (38 kg) wurden in kochendem Wasser zerkleinert und das Filtrat mit Tannin und Phosphorwolframsäure behandelt. Nach Zerlegen des Wolframates mit Bariumhydroxid wurde entstandenes K_2SO_4 mittels Methanol ausgefällt und nach Filtration der Methylalkohol abgedampft. Überschüssige Schwefelsäure wurde als $BaSO_4$ entfernt und die Lösung mit $Zn(OH)_2$ in konz. Ammoniak versetzt. Am anderen Tag wurde der Niederschlag abgesaugt und mit H_2S zerlegt. H_2SO_4, H_2S und Ammoniak wurden wie üblich entfernt und das Histamin als Flavianat gefällt.

Ausbeute: 2,7 g Histamindiflavianat.

g) Isolierung von Histamin aus Muskel nach Thorpe *(1927)*

35 kg Rindermuskelgewebe wurden mit 79 l 95%igem Alkohol 24 Std extrahiert. Diese Extraktion wurde mit 72 l 60%igem Alkohol wiederholt. Die Filtrate wurden angesäuert, erneut filtriert, und im Vakuum auf 4 l eingeengt. Durch Abkühlung auf 0° C schied sich das Fett quantitativ an der Oberfläche ab und wurde entfernt. Nach Neutralisation mit NaOH wurden Ballaststoffe durch Zusatz von basischem Bleiacetat gefällt und der Rückstand auf 700 ml im Vakuum eingeengt. Nach Ansäuern mit Schwefelsäure wurde für die weitere Verarbeitung das Verfahren von Kossel und Kutscher (1900) angewendet.

Diese Aufstellung von Verfahren zur Isolierung von Histamin aus biologischem Material erhebt nicht den Anspruch auf Vollständigkeit. Viele Methoden sind einander sehr ähnlich und unterscheiden sich vielleicht nur durch die Wahl verschiedener Fällungsmittel (z. B. Bleiacetat oder Zinkhydroxid). Das Histamin besitzt kein charakteristisches Molekül. Ein spezifisches Analysenverfahren zu schaffen ist deshalb nicht möglich. So muß man im Laufe der Aufarbeitung dem Histamin verwandte Begleitstoffe mit durch den Analysengang schleppen. Deshalb wird sich jeder Analytiker selbst, mit Fingerspitzengefühl, seinen für ihn geeigneten Weg suchen müssen. Die hier angeführten Methoden mögen ihm als Stütze dienen.

Literatur

Abel, J. J., and S. Kubota: On the presence of histamine (β-imidazolylethylamine) in the hypophysis cerebri and other tissues of the body and its occurence among the hydrolytic decomposition products of proteins. J. Pharmacol. exp. Ther. **13**, 243 (1919).

Ackermann, D.: Über den bakteriellen Abbau des Histidins. Hoppe Seylers Z. physiol. Chem. **65**, 505 (1910).

—, u. H. G. Fuchs: Über das Vorkommen von Histamin und anderen Basen in der Rinderlunge. Hoppe Seylers Z. physiol. Chem. **257**, 153 (1939).

—, u. H. G. Menssen: Niedrigmolekulare Inhaltsstoffe der Lederkoralle. Hoppe Seylers Z. physiol. Chem. **317**, 144 (1959).

Barger, G., and H. H. Dale: β-Imidazolylethylamine, a depressor constituent of intestinal mucosa. J. Physiol. (Lond.) **41**, 499 (1911).

Barsoum, G. S., and J. H. Gaddum: The pharmacologic estimation of adenosine and histamine in blood. J. Physiol. (Lond.) **85**, 1 (1935).

Best, C. H., H. H. Dale, H. W. Dudley, and W. V. Thorpe: The nature of the vasodilator constituents of certain tissue extracts. J. Physiol. (Lond.) **62**, 397 (1927).

—, and E. W. McHenry: The inactivation of histamine. J. Physiol. (Lond.) **70**, 349 (1930).

Clotten, R., u. A. Clotten: Hochspannungselektrophorese. Stuttgart: Georg Thieme Verlag 1962.

Code, C. F.: The quantitative estimation of histamine in the blood. J. Physiol. (Lond.) **89**, 257 (1937).

Dudley, H. W.: Some observations on the active principles of the pituitary gland. J. Pharmacol. exp. Ther. **14**, 295 (1919).

Dunér, H. C., u. B. Pernow: Quantitative Bestimmung von Aminen mit Ninhydrin. Scand. J. clin. Lab. Invest. **5**, 296 (1956).

GEBAUER-FUELNEGG, E., u. A. I. KENDALL: Die Trennung und Isolierung organischer Basen durch Elektrodialyse. Ber. dtsch. chem. Gesellsch. **64**, 1067 (1931).
HANKE, M. T., and K. K. KOESSLER: Studies on proteinogenous amines. XVI. The excretion of imidazoles in the urine under normal conditions with special consideration of nephritis. J. biol. Chem. **95**, 803 (1924a).
— — Studies on proteinogenous amines. XVII. On the faculty of normal intestinal bacteria to form toxic amines. J. biol. Chem. **59**, 835 (1924b).
— — Studies on proteinogenous amines. XIX. On the factors involved in the production of phenol by the colon group. J. biol. Chem. **59**, 867 (1924c).
— — Studies on proteinogenous amines. XX. On the presence of histamine in the mammalian organism. J. biol. Chem. **59**, 879 (1924d).
KOESSLER, K. K., and M. T. HANKE: Studies on proteinogenous amines. III. A quantitative method for separating histamine from histidine. J. biol. Chem. **39**, 521 (1919).
KOSSEL, A., u. F. KUTSCHER: Beiträge zur Kenntnis der Eiweißkörper. Hoppe-Seylers Z. physiol. Chem. **31**, 165 (1900).
KUTSCHER, F.: Zit. nach ACKERMANN (1910).
MACGREGOR, R. G., and W. W. THORPE: The quantitative extraction of histamine from tissues by electrodialysis. J. biol. Chem. **27**, 1394 (1933).
REDEMANN, C. E., and C. NIEMANN: The diliturates (5-nitrobarbiturates) of some physiologically important bases. J. Amer. chem. Soc. **62**, 590 (1939).
ROBERTS, M., and H. M. ADAM: New methods for the quantitative estimation of free and conjugated histamine. Brit. J. Pharmacol. **5**, 526 (1950).
THORPE, W. V.: XV. Vasodilator constituents of tissue extracts. Isolation of histamine from muscle. J. biol. Chem. **22**, 94 (1927).
WERLE, E., u. A. RAUB: Über Vorkommen, Bildung und Abbau biogener Amine bei Pflanzen unter besonderer Berücksichtigung des Histamins. Biochem. Z. **318**, 538 (1944).
WEST, G. B., and J. F. RILEY: Chromatography of tissue histamine. Nature (Lond.) **174**, 882 (1954).
YOSHIMURA, K.: Über Fäulnis-Basen (Ptomaine) aus gefaulten Sojabohnen (Glycine hispida). Biochem. Z. **28**, 16 (1910).
ZEIDLER, L.: Tetraphenylbor-Verbindungen zum Nachweis von Histamin und anderen Basen. Hoppe Seylers Z. physiol. Chem. **291**, 177 (1952).

Section C

Determination of Histamine by Chemical Means

By

F. C. McIntire

With 3 Figures

I. Introduction

The lack of useful light absorption or emission properties of histamine (Lewis, Gebauer-Fuelnegg and Farmer, 1933) has required that non-biological methods of measuring it be based upon the properties of derivatives prepared by various chemical reactions. Pure histamine in solution may be quantified by each of several different chemical methods, but the assay of biological materials usually requires the purification of histamine before any chemical determination can be satisfactorily applied. Moreover, purification of the histamine derivative before measurement is necessary in some methods. In this discussion the preliminary purification procedures will be considered separately from the principles of reactions and reagents employed in the various chemical determinations. Finally representative procedures for each of the more useful methods will be presented in detail.

While currently the recent fluorometric method (Shore, Burkhalter and Cohn, 1959) appears by far the most promising of all, the other methods are included because each method might be the one of choice for some special problem, and a complete account might help set the stage for future advances. The author has attempted to mention all of the important modifications of the useful methods, but not all of the minor variations and applications.

II. Principles of chemical methods

A. Diazo methods

In preparing benzenazoimidazole, Rung and Behrend (1892) first demonstrated the coupling between imidazole and a diazotized aromatic amine. Burian (1904) prepared many arylazoimidazoles from diazotised p-sulfanilic acid and observed that 1-substituted imidazoles would not couple. Pauly (1904) studied the coupling of diazotized sulfanilic acid to histidine and suggested that the azo imidazoles were C-azo compounds. The quantitative determination of histidine (Weiss and Ssobolew, 1914) was the first reported use of the diazo reaction in quantitative colorimetry, but Koessler and Hanke (1919) were first to use this reaction for the quantitative determination of histamine and imidazoles in general. Later (Hanke and Koessler, 1920) these authors published the first procedure where histamine purification preceded the diazo reaction in an attempt to achieve specificity.

The position of coupling between histamine and the different diazotized amines is not clear. Fargher and Pyman (1919) found that imidazole and azobenzene, in equal molar portions, will couple to give almost exclusively 2-benzeneazoimidazole. They further showed that under the same circumstances 4-methyl imidazole will yield equal amounts of 2-, 5-, and 2,5-bis(benzeneazo)-4-methyl imidazole. Diemair and Fox (1938a and b) found that histamine forms only a single monoazo derivative with each diazotized aromatic amine but they did not determine the position of coupling. Kesztyüs (1948) cited the work of Fargher and Pyman (1919) and *assumed* that the azo coupling was in the 2 position of histamine.

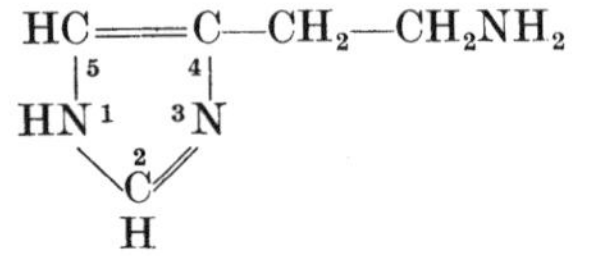

For the determination of histamine in biological materials, methods based upon the diazo coupling have two major obstacles to overcome: (1) the instability of the colored products and (2) the nonspecificity of the reaction. The diazotized aromatic amines couple with imidazoles, phenols and several other classes of compounds (Rosenthal and Tabor, 1948) including aliphatic amines (Peesez and Poirier, 1953). The achievement of adequate specificity in the diazo methods demands much of procedures to purify histamine before coupling and also the colored histamine derivative. Fortunately extraction of the histamine azo derivatives into alcohols, ketones and esters serves to partially stabilize the colored compounds and to increase the specificity of the methods. Rosenthal and Tabor (1948) achieved further specificity by a pH 7.7 barbital buffer washing of the methyl isobutyl ketone solution of p-nitrophenylazo histamine. The colored derivative remains in the ketone. In this solution the light absorption decreases by 7 per cent in one hour and 25 per cent in 24 hours.

The number of different "methods" listed in Table 1 indicates the general recognition of difficulties in achieving specificity for histamine and stability of the azo derivatives. Hanke and Koessler (1920) went far toward achieving specificity, but their method involved numerous steps. Some of the authors listed were concerned with conditions of the coupling reaction and stabilization of the color, not with the application to biological materials (Gebauer-Fuelnegg, 1930; Halpern, Viennet and Pattee, 1946; Havinga, Seekles and Strengers, 1947; Andrews and Lyons, 1957; Stefanović, Cirković and Bresjaneć, 1959). The methods which employ paper chromatography probably are most nearly specific for histamine, but these procedures are only roughly quantitative, because of difficulties in measurement on the paper or in removing the azo derivatives from the paper for quantification.

Among non-chromatographic methods that of Rosenthal and Tabor (1948) was the first to come close to satisfactory specificity with reasonable convenience. Most of the subsequently published diazo methods for histamine have used the Rosenthal and Tabor procedure for the diazo coupling and the purification and quantification of the histamine derivative (Lubschez, 1950; Kantor, Levine and Fischbach, 1951; Sager and Horowitz, 1957; Thouvenot, Flavian and Weber, 1957). Lubschez (1950) scaled down the procedure to increase the sensitivity five fold — a lower limit of 0.1 microgram of histamine free base. The important features of the Rosenthal and Tabor procedure are (1) the use of p-nitroaniline, (2) extraction of the coupling products from the alkaline solution with a small volume of methyl isobutyl ketone, and (3) washing the ketone solution with pH 7.7 barbital buffer to remove interference by ammonia and other compounds.

Table 1. *Diazo methods for histamine determination*

Authors	Amine diazotized	Histamine purification	Azo derivative purification
URBACH and GISCAFRE (1948)	p-bromoaniline	BuOH ext., p.c. BuOH—NH_4OH	
BARAUD, GENEVOIS, MANDILLON and RINGENBACH (1946)	p-bromoaniline	TCA ext., AmOH ext.	iso-BuOH ext.
HANKE and KOESSLER (1920)	p-sulfanilic acid	PTA pptn. AmOH ext.	
SCHWARTZ and RIEGERT (1936a, b)	p-sulfanilic acid	Permutit	
SCHWARTZ (1952)	p-sulfanilic acid	Permutit	
MACAIG and SCHOENTAL (1938)	p-sulfanilic acid	Permutit	
HALPERN, VIENNET and PATTEE (1946)	p-sulfanilic acid		EtOH to stabilize color stabilizers
HAVINGA, SEEKLES and STRENGERS (1947)	p-sulfanilic acid		
ANDREWS and LYONS (1957)	p-sulfanilic acid		
SCHMIDT and VORHEISOR (1955)	p-sulfanilic acid	p.c. BuOH—AcOH—H_2O, BuOH—NH_4OH	
DUTTA (1956)	p-sulfanilic acid	ion exchange, p.c. BuOH-i-PrOH—NH_4OH	
SHIFRINE, OUSTERHOUT, GRAU and VAUGHN (1959)		p.c. i-PrOH—NH_4OH	
STEFANOVIC, CIRKOVIC and BRESJANEC (1959)	p-aminobenzoic acid		
GEBAUER-FUELNEGG (1930)	p-nitroaniline		BuOH ext.
ROSENTHAL and TABOR (1948)	p-nitroaniline	BuOH ext. CS or TCA ext.	MIK ext.
LUBSCHEZ (1950)	p-nitroaniline	MPA ext., BuOH ext. Amberlite IRC-50	MIK ext.
KANTOR, LEVINE, and FISCHBACH (1951)	p-nitroaniline	Benzaldehyde, benzene — BuOH, CS	MIK ext.
SAGER, and HOROWITZ (1957)	p-nitroaniline	MeOH ext benzaldehyde, benzene — BuOH, CS	MIK ext.
THOUVENOT, FLAVIAN and WEBER (1957)	p-nitroaniline		MIK ext.
FUYUO (1958)	p-nitroaniline	TCA	EtOAc
STEPANYAN (1954)	p-nitroaniline	BuOH ext., H_2SO_4 ext., BuOH ext. p.c. BuOH—NH_4OH	
SCHMIDT and GRUHN (1955)	p-nitroaniline		EtOH stabilization

Abbreviations:

p.c.	= paper chromatography	ext.	= extraction
BuOH	= n-butanol	pptn.	= precipitation
AmOH	= n-amyl alcohol	CS	= cotton acid succinate
MIK	= methylisobutyl ketone	MPA	= meta phosphoric acid
TCA	= trichloroacetic	EtOAc	= ethyl acetate
PTA	= phosphotungstic acid	AcOH	= acetic acid
i-PrOH	= isopropanol	MeOH	= methanol

The authors of this procedure made a careful study of all known potentially interfering compounds and they applied the procedure to tissue extracts before and after histaminase treatment. This method, preceded by suitable purification steps which will be discussed later, seemed adequately specific for histamine in the biological materials examined.

B. 2,4-Dinitrofluorobenzene (DNFB) methods

Soon after SANGER (1945) reported the quantitative labeling of free amino groups with DNFB, two different laboratories independently used this reagent for the quantitative determination of histamine (McINTIRE, WHITE and SPROULL, 1950; LOWRY, GRAHAM, HARRIS, PRIEBAT, MARKS and BREGMAN, 1954). The two methods are identical in principle and very similar in specificity but they are quite different in manipulations. The method of LOWRY and colleagues, employing micro technique, measures the light absorption of .05 ml. of solution and is correspondingly the more sensitive with a lower limit of 0.01 microgram of histamine. The original method of McINTIRE, WHITE and SPROULL was designed for the handling of many samples simultaneously; it required materials not commercially available, which might be difficult to prepare in some laboratories. WEISSBACH, WAALKES and UDENFRIEND (1958) combined features from both of the earlier methods. ISHIHARA (1957) published a method which appears almost identical to the one of McINTIRE, WHITE and SPROULL (1950). The method of LOWRY and colleagues has been used successfully without modification in several laboratories and has been simplified somewhat by DODGE (1952) for measuring the histaminolytic power of serum. DNFB affords a simple and very reliable method for determining histamine in pure solutions (McINTIRE, 1952).

Histamine reacts with DNFB to yield two different derivatives (McINTIRE, WHITE and SPROULL, 1950): Nα-(2,4-dinitrophenyl) histamine (I), and Nα, N′-bis(2,4-dinitrophenyl) histamine (II), where Nα refers to the β-ethylamino nitrogen and N′ is the substituted ring nitrogen.

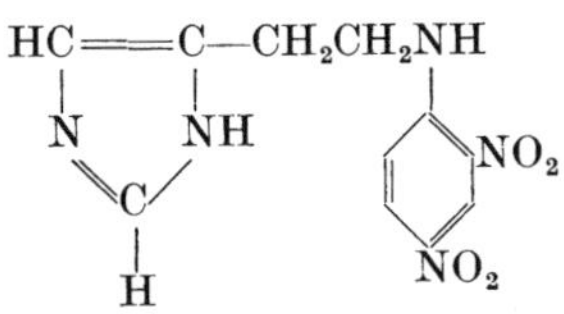

I

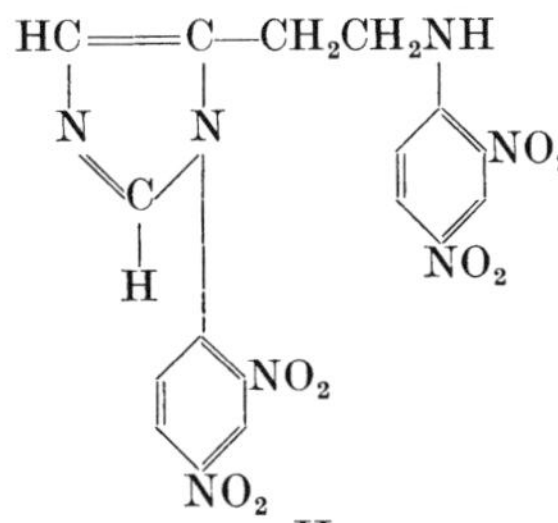

II

The success of the methods depends on the control of conditions — primarily pH and DNFB concentration — so that Nα-(2,4-dinitrophenyl) histamine (I) is obtained almost exclusively. This is a very stable yellow compound with an intense light-absorption maximum at 355—360 mμ. Retaining the basic character of the imidazole ring, I is preferentially soluble in water under acid conditions and is extracted from water by organic solvents under alkaline conditions. Thus it may be separated from excess reagent, dinitrophenol, and the dinitrophenyl derivatives of the monoamino acids and simple amines by partition between certain organic solvents and water under acid conditions; it may be separated from dinitrophenol and the monodinitrophenyl derivatives of the basic amino acids by partition under alkaline conditions. Diamines, such as cadaverine and putrescine, and polyamines, such as spermine and spermidine, give negligible interference; all of the amino groups on these molecules react with DNFB under the specified conditions, and the products are not soluble in aqueous acid solutions. Imidazoles which have no free primary or secondary amino group on a side chain, for example, imidazole and N α-acetylhistamine, do not interfere. All of the potentially interfering compounds known to occur in natural products have been tested, and only histidinol and agmatine gave considerable "false histamine" values (Lowry, Graham, Harris, Priebat, Marks and Bregman, 1954; McIntire, White, and Sproull, 1950). Fortunately these two compounds do not appear in significant amounts in the animal fluids and tissues to which this method has been applied. The DNFB method has been used successfully for the determination of histamine in guinea-pig lung; rabbit lung, spleen, whole blood, plasma, and blood cell fractions; dog liver; and human whole blood, serum and blood cells.

The types of compounds which might give false histamine values in DNFB methods are: (1) ethylenediamine or its derivatives in which both amino groups are either primary or secondary aliphatic amines; under the conditions of the histamine assay, such compounds react with DNFB to yield largely monodinitrophenyl derivatives which follow along with the histamine derivative in the purification procedure; (2) diamines in which one basic group either does not react or reacts relatively slowly with DNFB, for example, histidinole, N,N-dimethylethylenediamine, and agmatine; (3) primary or secondary amines which do not react with DNFB, but which form water-soluble hydrochlorides and which absorb light strongly in the near ultraviolet; (4) tertiary amines which absorb light strongly in the near ultraviolet and which form water soluble hydrochlorides.

Interference by ethylenediamine itself can be eliminated by the use of either phenylisocyanate or nitrous acid immediately following the histamine-DNFB reaction, and interference by most compounds of types (1) and (3) might be eliminated similarly. Elimination of the interference by types (2) and (4), if such interference is ever encountered, must await further refinements of the purification procedures either before or after the DNFB-histamine reaction. Very likely compounds of type (4) and the DNFB derivatives of compounds of type (2) could be separated from dinitrophenylhistamine by paper chromatography. Many compounds of type (4) can be separated from histamine by solvent partition prior to histamine purification.

The reaction between histamine and DNFB can be controlled so that the yield of the desired derivative, I, is highly reproducible at 80—85% of theoretical. Under certain conditions, the reaction is complete in 10—15 minutes at room temperature (McIntire, White, and Sproull, 1950). Under other conditions (Lowry, Graham, Harris, Priebat, Marks and Bregman, 1954), a longer time and higher temperature are required to give a maximal yield of I. In both cases the relative yields of I and II depend primarily on the pH and the excess of DNFB, so that these two factors must be controlled carefully. The yield of I is directly proportional to the amount of histamine originally present, and day-to-day variation in the per cent yield is slight.

Recent results (McIntire unpublished) indicate that 1-methyl-4(β-aminoethyl) imidazole may be determined in the presence of histamine by a modification of the DNFB method.

C. The fluorometric method

Currently the most promising quantitative chemical method for histamine is unquestionably the fluorometric method of Shore, Burkhalter and Cohn (1959).

Comparing favorably with the best bioassays, this method has at least a 10-fold advantage in sensitivity and it is more specific than even the DNFB method. While the fluorometric method requires essentially the same degree of histamine purification prior to preparation of the derivative, the fluorophore formation and quantification are simpler than in either the diazo or the DNFB method. The fluorescent histamine derivative lacks the stability of the monodinitrophenyl histamine (DNFB method) but with a recent minor modification the stability is adequate for most purposes (KREMZNER and WILSON, 1961; THOMPSON, 1961; BRAENDLE, 1961). In several laboratories the Shore method has replaced the previous method of choice, the DNFB method. There have been a few modifications of the histamine purification procedure, but the original procedure for the development of the fluorophore has not seen serious change. GRAHAM and collaborators scaled down the method and used the histamine purification procedure of LOWRY et al. (1954) to measure the histamine in 1 ml. of human serum (NOAH and BRAND, 1961).

SHORE, BURKHALTER and COHN observed that o-phthalaldehyde would condense with histamine under strongly alkaline conditions to give a product which, at a very low pH, had an activation spectrum with a sharp peak at 350 mμ and a fluorescence spectrum with a sharp peak at about 450 mμ. They suggested the following structure for the fluorescent compound but gave no supporting evidence.

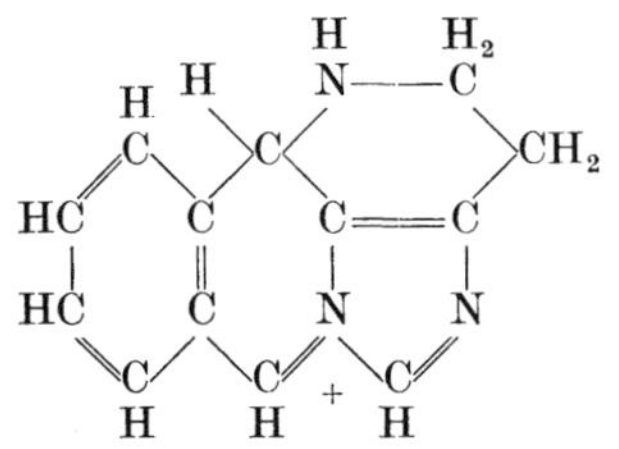

They found the fluorescence intensity proportional to the histamine concentration between 0.005 and 0.5 micrograms per ml. The reaction is of sufficient specificity that purification of the histamine derivative is not necesarry — an advantage of simplicity as compared to other methods.

Ammonia, histidine, and peptides where histidine is N-terminal might interfere, but there are special procedures for their separation from histamine prior to the condensation with o-phthalaldehyde (OATES, 1961; WEISSBACH, LOVENBERG and UDENFRIEND, 1961; KREMZNER and WILSON, 1961). SHORE et al. investigated many amines and imidazoles and they found the reaction remarkably specific for N-unsubstituted 4-(β-aminoethyl) imidazoles — histamine, histidine and probably histidinol (although the latter was not tested). Methylation of histamine either on the ring or on the side chain prevents formation of the fluorophore — the main specificity advantage over the DNFB method. Specificity of the method for histamine in several different animal tissues was demonstrated by the following criteria where the tissue histamine and authentic histamine appeared identical in direct comparison: (1) Activation and fluorescence spectra, (2) bioassay, (3) partition between butanol and water at several different pH values, (4) rate of destruction by diamine oxidase. Although the fluorometric method seems to have relatively few faults it is a new method and one can anticipate some improvements. One desired improvement would be the stabilization of the fluorescent derivative to allow additional manipulations, e.g. column chromatography, paper chromatography or countercurrent distribution.

D. The radioisotope method

KESTON, UDENFRIEND and CANNON (1946) introduced radioactive (I^{131}) p-iodosulfonyl chloride (pipsyl chloride) for the quantitative labeling of amino groups in the analysis of amino acid mixtures. SCHAYER, KOBAYASHI and SMILEY (1955) utilized the same reagent in developing a method for the quantitative determination of histamine. The sample is treated with radioactive pipsyl chloride under conditions which give a 93 to 96 per cent yield of dipipsyl histamine. The radioactive derivative is extracted from the reaction medium, mixed with a large known amount of cold dipipsyl histamine, and the mixture purified and crystallized to constant specific radioactivity. The total histamine in the samples may be calculated from the following known quantities: specific activity of the pipsyl chloride, constant specific activity of the dipipsyl histamine, the amount of cold dipipsyl histamine added, and the final amount of the crystallized compound.

While this method can be made extremely sensitive and, with adequate purification and recrystallization of the dipipsyl histamine, very specific, it is so laborious and time consuming that its use is not justified for most purposes.

E. Miscellaneous methods

The following methods have found very limited use:

SCHMALL, WOLLISH and GALENDER (1952) published a procedure for determining histamine gravimetrically by precipitation with nitranilic acid.

MADER, STERNE, ROSIN and FREDIANI (1950) reported that histamine in pure solution may be assayed by the red color it forms with 1,2 naphthoquinone-4-sodium sulfonate. This would not be suitable for determining histamine in biological materials because of interference from ammonia and organic bases in general.

Extending the KNOOP test for histidine to a study of the reactions of halogens with histamine and histidine, NEWMAN and TURNBULL (1960) proposed a quantitative method for these compounds based upon their reaction with iodine (KI_3) in the presence of pyridine at a pH of 11.0 to 12.0. A purple color with a maximum at 560 mμ develops to full value in a few minutes. The lower sensitivity limit is 1 microgram of histamine. The chemistry of this reaction has not been clarified.

The precipitation of amines with tetraphenyl borate and separation of them by high voltage paper electrophoresis was reported by GAYER (1956). He compared ninhydrin, diazotized sulfanilic acid and a triketo-piperidein derivative for detecting the amine spots on the paper. The latter reagent gave some color differentiation among the amines separated — histamine, arginine, tyramine, tryptamine, adrenaline and serotonin.

High voltage paper electrophoresis was also used by FISCHER and BONN (1957) for the separation and estimation of histamine, spermine, spermidine, cadaverine, putrescine, trimethylenediamine and colamine. For quantification the paper was treated with ninhydrin and copper nitrate. The ninhydrin copper complexes of the amines were eluted from the paper with methanol and their light absorption was measured at 506 mμ. As little as 0.5 microgram of amine could be detected.

III. Inhibitors of histamine reactions

Certain heavy metal ions have a strong affinity for histamine and thereby inhibit some of the reactions used for the quantitative assay for histamine (Table 2).

The histamine-DNFB reaction is inhibited completely by 1 μg-ion of Cu^{++} or Cu^{+} per μmole of histamine. Because the degree of inhibition follows closely the ratio of metal ions to histamine molecules and is independent of the DNFB concentration, the inhibition probably is a result of coordination between histamine and the metal ions. The inhibition by copper can be nullified by the use of chelating agents — 2 μmoles of 8-hydroxyquinoline or 4 μmoles of sodium diethyldithiocarbamate per microgram-ion of Cu^{++}, 7 μmoles of sodium diethyldithiocarbamate per microgram-ion of Cu^{+}. All versions of the DNFB method use this chelating agent.

Table 2. *Inhibition of the histamine-DNFB reaction by ions of the heavy metals*

Ion[1]	Inhibition, %	Ion[1]	Inhibition, %
Ag^{+}	12	Fe^{+++}	0
Au^{+}	45	Mn^{++}	2
Co^{++}	28	Ni^{++}	70
Cu^{++}	98	Sn^{++}	0
Cu^{+}	100	Zn^{++}	4

[1] One μg.-ion per μmole of histamine.

ANDREWS and LYONS (1957) reported heavy metal inhibition of the histamine diazo coupling, and they recommended diethylenetriaminepentaacetic acid (Chel 330) for preventing this inhibition. KREMZNER and WILSON (1961) recommended the use of ethylenediaminetetraacetic acid during the coupling of histamine with o-phthalaldehyde in the fluorometric method.

Aldehydes also inhibit the histamine-DNFB reaction and they may cause a low recovery through the butanol extraction and ion exchange purification of histamine. On the other hand KANTOR, LEVINE and FISCHBACH (1951) made good use of its reaction with benzaldehyde for the purification of histamine.

ROSENTHAL and TABOR (1948) found that uric acid inhibits the coupling of histamine to p-nitrodiazobenzene. They were able to eliminate this inhibition by a mild nitrous acid treatment.

IV. Purification of histamine for chemical assay

A. Acid hydrolysis

Much of the histamine in the body is not held by a covalent bond and it may be extracted from tissues by various procedures which coagulate or precipitate proteins and other macro-molecules (McINTIRE, 1956). Dog, hog, beef and sheep liver, guinea pig skin and some other mammalian tissues contain considerable amounts of histamine which is not released by trichloroacetic acid extraction but is set free by acid hydrolysis — 1.2 N HCl in boiling water 3 hrs (JOHNSON, 1955; GRAHAM, HANNEGAN, and NOURSE, 1956). AKERBLOM (1941) and SCHMITERLÖW (1949) reported that acid hydrolysis of tissues and blood may decarboxylate histidine and thus lead to erroneous histamine values. EMMELIN, KAHLSON and WICKSELL (1941) could not confirm these findings. HUGHES, SALVIN and WOOD (1951) concluded that the error from acid decarboxylation of histidine is not serious unless the histidine level is 0.5 mg. per ml. or more. They suggested that trichloroacetic acid in extracts during hydrolysis is responsible for histidine decarboxylation.

B. Protein precipitants

Precipitation of protein and other macromolecules is useful as a first step, but in most cases it does not provide adequate purification of histamine for chemical assay. HANKE and KOESSLER (1920) were perhaps the first to use heavy metals and acids, such as phosphotungstic, in an attempt to purify histamine. Currently the favored reagents for extracting histamine from tissues are trichloroacetic acid (ROSENTHAL and TABOR, 1948; LOWRY, GRAHAM, HARRIS, PRIEBAT, MARKS and BREGMAN, 1954; SCHAYER, KOBAYASHI and SMILEY, 1955), perchloric acid (SHORE, BURKHALTER and COHN, 1959), metaphosphoric acid (LUBSCHEZ, 1950), zinc hydroxide (WEISSBACH, WAALKES and UDENFRIEND, 1958) and high salt concentration (MCINTIRE, ROTH and SHAW, 1947).

C. Alcohol extraction

While histamine may be extracted from tissues with methanol (SAGER and HOROWITZ, 1957) and ethanol (MCINTIRE, 1956) the butyl and amyl alcohols have found the most use in assay procedures. KOESSLER and HANKE (1919) were first to purify histamine by extraction with amyl alcohol from water at a high pH where histamine exists as the free base and the amino acids are largely undissociated sodium salts. This extraction separates histamine from all but small amounts of the amino acids. KOESSLER and HANKE removed histamine from the amyl alcohol by a simple extraction with dilute aqueous sulphuric acid. Although the KOESSLER and HANKE procedure requires several extractions with amyl alcohol to remove all of the histamine from the aqueous phase, several different laboratories employed this method until MCINTIRE, ROTH and SHAW showed that one extraction with butanol is adequate if the aqueous solution has a high pH and a high salt concentration. With a weak base such as histamine, salt formation favors solubility in water and the free base is more soluble in organic solvents. Therefore the distribution between water and an immiscible alcohol is a function of pH, salt concentration and the volume of each solvent. Data for equal volumes of water and

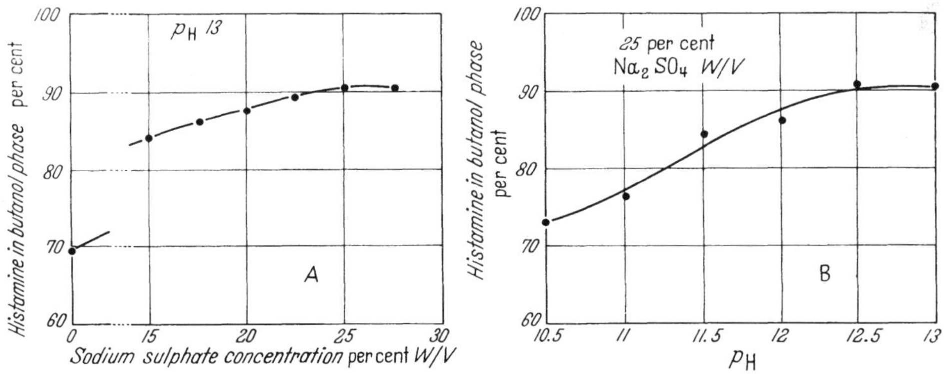

Fig. 1. The effect of salt concentration and pH on the distribution of histamine between water and butanol

n-butanol with varying pH and sodium sulphate concentration are shown in Fig. 1 (MCINTIRE, ROTH and SHAW, 1947). The conditions required for a maximum of histamine in the butanol phase are pH 12.5 and 25 per cent (w/v) sodium sulphate.

D. Ion exchangers

Cation exchangers (free acid form) are very useful for the quantitative removal of histamine (free base) from solution in butyl or amyl alcohol. The cation exchanger is conveniently employed as a small column through which the alcohol solution is filtered. The weak (carboxy) acid type is much preferred over the strong sulfonic cation exchanges for two main reasons: (1) histamine is difficult to remove from the latter, and (2) the weak acid type is the more selective for histamine.

The exchanger most commonly used is cotton acid succinate, CS, (McINTIRE, WHITE and SPROULL, 1950; ROSENTHAL and TABOR, 1948; KANTOR, LEVINE and FISCHBACH, 1951; WEISSBACH, WAALKES and UDENFRIEND, 1958) which was originated specifically for the removal of histamine from butanol solution at a time when no other satisfactory cation exchanger was available (McINTIRE, ROTH and SHAW, 1947). Carboxy acid resins and carboxy methyl cellulose which are now available may be satisfactory. CS has the disadvantage of not being available commercially. Finding it difficult to prepare, LUBSCHEZ (1950) turned to Amberlite IRC-50 which required a batch style of operation (shaking with the butanol extract) and was thereby less convenient than CS. Attractive features of CS are its high ion-binding capacity and its fine texture. With proper care, avoidance of strong alkali, it can be used almost indefinitely without replacement.

Histamine may be eluted from CS with salt solutions or dilute acids; only small amounts of strong mineral acids or their salts are required. ROSENTHAL and TABOR (1948) separated histamine from acetyl histamine by treating the CS column with 1 ml. of 0.014 M Na_3PO_4, which removed the acetyl histamine and left the histamine on the CS. These authors also found that certain salts (chlorides, trichloroacetates and probably others) are sufficiently soluble in butanol to prevent CS from taking histamine out of the butanol solution.

Under the conditions of the butanol extraction, aldehydes react with histamine to yield a product which has less affinity than histamine for CS, probably a Schiff base involving the primary amino group. In the butanol, quantities of salt which will not prevent histamine uptake by CS will prevent the Schiff base uptake. Faced with this difficulty in determining histamine in streptomycin, KANTOR, LEVINE and FISCHBACH (1951) found that the reaction product of benzaldehyde and histamine can be extracted from water by a mixture of benzene and butanol, that the very low salt content of the benzene butanol permits "benzylidine histamine" to be removed quantitatively by CS, and that benzylidine histamine can be removed from CS quantitatively and measured by the ROSENTHAL and TABOR method. The histamine purification thus proposed by KANTOR et al. has been applied to other tissues and has been adequately confirmed (McINTIRE, unpublished; SAGER and HOROWITZ, 1957; YUSEM, 1961). For many purposes this procedure is superior to the butanol extraction CS method.

OATES (1961) applied urine directly to amberlite IRC-50 to separate histamine from ammonia and other interfering substances, preparatory to assay by the fluorometric method.

Strong base anion exchangers have been employed to remove amino acids and other anions prior to the fluorometric assay. WEISSBACH, LOVENBERG and UDENFRIEND (1961) used Dowex-1 carbonate and KREMZNER and WILSON (1961) used Dowex-1X8, Bio Rad-1X8, or IRA-410. In both methods amino acids and other anions are retained by the anion exchanger while histamine is not retained at all. KREMZNER and WILSON applied trichloroacetic acid extracts of tissue directly to the exchanger column and treated the filtrate with o-phthalaldehyde in the fluorometric histamine assay.

E. Permutit (Decalso)

Permutit was introduced by WHITEHORN (1923) as a reagent for purifying amines. It has been the key to the purification of histamine in assay methods developed or modified by SCHWARTZ and RIEGERT (1936a and b), MACAIG and SCHOENTAL (1938), ROBERTS and ADAM (1950), WEDENISSOW (1949), SCHWARTZ (1952), and LOWRY, GRAHAM, HARRIS, PRIEBAT, MARKS and BREGMAN (1954). By careful control of such conditions as Decalso pretreatment and particle size, flow rate, pH and salt concentration during adsorption, adsorption "load", and elution temperature, LOWRY and colleagues developed a very reproducible procedure with an 80 to 85 per cent recovery of histamine. The excellence of their method is attested by its adoption with success in several other laboratories.

According to LOWRY et al. Decalso adsorbs histamine and other amines most efficiently in the pH range of 3 to 5 where the adsorption is 95 to 97 per cent complete. Elution is never complete; it is achieved best with saturated salt solutions and at a temperature of 75—80° C. Sodium hydroxide, strong ammonium hydroxide and chloroform saturated with ammonia have also been used. Decalso will adsorb histamine directly from pH-adjusted trichloroacetic acid tissue extracts, a distinct advantage over the carboxy cation exchangers. Decalso has the disadvantage that it must be renewed for each assay.

The Decalso procedure of LOWRY et al. is unquestionably the method of choice in purifying histamine from human blood plasma for the fluorometric assay. In a careful study GRAHAM (1961) has shown that human plasma contains a substance which gives very high false histamine values in the fluorometric assay. This interference is eliminated by the Decalso purification but not by either the butanol extraction (SHORE et al.) or the benzylidine histamine purification (KANTOR et al.).

F. Paper chromatography

URBACH and GISCAFRE (1948) were the first to publish a method for paper chromatography of histamine. The various methods (Table 1) differ mainly with regard to the solvent system for developing the chromatogram and the diazo reagent employed for locating the histamine spot. In some procedures, quantification of the histamine depends upon comparison of color intensity of spots on paper — the unknown quantity of histamine compared visually with a series of known amounts. SCHMIDT and VORHEISOR (1955) and DUTTA (1956) eluted the histamine from the paper before coupling with the diazo reagent. This, of course, requires a diazo sprayed control chromatogram for precisely locating the histamine before the paper section is cut and eluted.

Not listed in Table 1, but worth mentioning are studies by WEST and RILEY (1954) and RAUTENBURG (1957) who used butanol-acetic acid-water systems for developing the paper chromatogram. WEST and RILEY, chromatographing trichloroacetic acid extracts of tissues, found two bands with histamine activity by bioassay. The faster moving histamine band was dependent upon the presence of trichloroacetic acid and a basic amino-acid. RAUTENBURG, chromatographing urine, found that the sulfate concentration affected the rate of histamine migration. Such difficulties were not encountered by URBACH and GISCAFRE (1948) who purified the histamine through two successive butanol extractions and spotted the second butanol extract on the paper. BODÁNSZKY, HÁLLOS and NÉMETH (1957) used a solvent system of ethanol-butanol-water (1:4:5). Using ninhydrin to develop their chromatograms, BREMNER and KENTEN (1951) did an extensive study of paper chromatography of amines in which they compared 29 different amines in 7 different solvent systems.

If one requires specificity at a cost of time and a sacrifice of quantification and sensitivity, perhaps he should choose paper chromatography even over SHORE's fluorometric method. Improvements in quantification with paper chromatography might be forthcoming. Its use for the identification of monodinitrophenyl histamine (Weissbach, Waalkes and Udenfriend, 1958), suggests one possible avenue for future developments. Chromatography of a stable colored derivative, applicable to all or most of the biogenic amines would be most useful.

G. Electroseparations

High voltage paper electrophoresis has been mentioned under II E. This technique has limitations and virtues analogous to paper chromatography; it was used by Bohmer and Giersberg (1956) for separating histamine from histidine and tyramine. High voltage paper electrophoresis should have a timewise advantage and may achieve some separations more easily than paper chromatography.

Electrodialysis has been used for the purification of histamine from tissue extracts (MacGregor and Thorpe, 1933) and from blood serum (Minard, 1941). This technique has not been widely used because other extraction and purification procedures offer more selective purification with less effort.

V. Procedures

The procedures which follow are quoted directly from the original authors wherever practical.

A. The fluorometric determination of histamine

(Shore, Burkhalter and Cohn, 1959)

"*Solvents and reagents.* n-Butanol, reagent grade. n-Heptane, pure grade such as Phillips 99 mol-%. o-Phthalaldehyde (OPT) reagent, 1% in reagent grade absolute methanol. Commercially obtained o-phthalaldehyde, if not pure, may be recrystallized from ligroin. The methanolic solution is stable for at least two weeks when kept in a dark bottle under refrigeration. (o-Phthalaldehyde may be obtained from K & K Laboratories, Inc., 177-10 93rd Ave., Jamaica 33, N.Y.; California Corp. for Biochemical Research, 3625 Medford St., Los Angeles 63, Calif.; or Mann Research Laboratories, Inc., 136 Liberty St., New York 6, N.Y.) Salt-saturated 0.1 N NaOH. Sufficient solid NaCl is added to 0.1 N NaOH so that an excess of solid NaCl remains.

Extraction of histamine from tissues. Tissues are homogenized in 9 volumes of 0.4 N perchloric acid using a motor-driven glass homogenizer. The homogenate is allowed to stand for 10 minutes and is then centrifuged. A 4-ml aliquot of the supernatant fluid is transferred to a 25-ml glass-stoppered shaking tube containing 0.5 ml of 5 N NaOH, 1.5 g of solid NaCl and 10 ml of n-butanol. The tube is shaken for 5 minutes to extract the histamine into the butanol, and after centrifugation, the aqueous phase is removed by aspiration. The organic phase is then shaken for about 1 minute with 5 ml of salt-saturated 0.1 N NaOH. This wash removes any residual amounts of histidine which may be present.

The tube is then centrifuged and an 8 ml aliquot of the butanol is transferred to a 40-ml glass-stoppered shaking tube containing 2.5 to 4.5 ml of 0.1 N HCl and 15 ml of n-heptane. After shaking for about 1 minute the tube is centrifuged and the histamine in the aqueous phase is assayed fluorometrically as described below.

For the analysis of blood of species such as the dog which contain only small amounts of histamine in blood, 5 ml of oxalated blood are hemolyzed by the addition of 4.5 ml water, and 0.5 ml of concentrated (10—12 N) perchloric acid is added. The tube is then shaken for 10 minutes. The subsequent steps are similar to those described above.

The solubility characteristics of histamine are such that in the initial extraction about 92% of the histamine is extracted into the butanol. After the additional wash of the butanol with salt-saturated 0.1 N NaOH, a total of about 85% of the histamine remains in the butanol phase. There are also small volume changes in the various phases due to the relative solubility of water in butanol. To correct for these factors, standards are prepared by carrying known amounts of histamine added to 0.4 N perchloric acid through the procedure. Recoveries of histamine added to tissue homogenates range from 90 to 100%.

Fluorometric assay. After extraction from tissues the histamine is condensed with OPT in strongly alkaline solution. The resulting rather labile fluorescent product is stabilized upon acidification.

To estimate histamine in the acid extract a 2-ml aliquot containing 0.005 to 0.5 μg histamine per ml is transferred to a test tube and 0.4 ml of 1 N NaOH is added followed by 0.1 ml of OPT reagent. After 4 minutes, 0.2 ml of 3 N HCl is added. The contents of the tubes are thoroughly mixed after each addition. The solution is then transferred to a cuvette and the fluorescence at 450 mμ resulting from activation at 360 mμ is measured in a spectrofluorometer (wavelengths uncalibrated, American Instrument Co., Silver Spring, Md., or Farrand Optical Co., New York 70, N.Y.). The fluorescence of the acidified solution is stable for at least one-half hour. The fluorescence intensity is proportional to histamine concentration over the range 0.005 to 0.5 μg/ml.

The small fluorescence blanks in tissues or reagents may be corrected for by omission of the condensation step. This is accomplished by adding all the reagents to a separate aliquot of tissue extract, but reversing the order of addition of OPT and 3 N HCl. The resulting solution contains tissue and reagent blanks, but not the fluorophore resulting from condensation of OPT and histamine, since the reaction does not proceed in acid".

Shore (1961) indicated that the interfering fluorophore from OPT and ammonia may be removed from the acidified reaction mixture by extraction with an equal volume of isoamyl alcohol. The histamine fluorophore remains in the aqueous phase with only slight loss.

B. Modifications of the Shore method

Oates (1961) developed the following procedure for removing interfering substances from human urine preparatory to assaying for histamine by the method of Shore, Burkhalter and Cohn:

"*Ion exchange resin.* The resin used is IRC-50, 100—200 mesh, obtained in the hydrogen form (Fisher Scientific Co., CG-50, Type I). After addition of one volume of distilled water to the resin and agitating, the mixture is adjusted to pH 9 with 10 N NaOH. The resin is then washed with water and cycled back to the hydrogen form by adjusting the pH to less than 3 with 12 N HCl. After additional washing with water, it is brought to pH 7.5 by addition of 10 N NaOH, and washed twice with 0.5 M sodium phosphate buffer, pH 7.5. Volumes approximately equivalent to that of the wet resin are used for all washes. The resin may be stored in the pH 7.5 buffer at 2° C.

Preparation of the urine for assay. Urine samples are collected in bottles containing 15 ml 6 N HCl or 30 ml toluene. Because of the relatively large amounts of histamine which may be formed rapidly by decarboxylation of histidine in urine, such bacteriostatic precautions are imperative. If more than a few days are to elapse before assay, the urine should be frozen. Twenty-five to 30 ml samples of urine are adjusted to pH 7.5 (using a pH meter) by dropwise addition of 10 N NaOH, and filtered through Whatman No. 1 paper. A twenty-ml aliquot of the filtered urine is mixed thoroughly with 10 ml of 0.25 M sodium phosphate buffer, pH 7.5, and buffer-urine mixture is applied to the column.

Preparation of the ion exchange column. The outflow of the chromatographic column (Scientific Glass Co., No. JT-7390, 200 mm length, 6 mm bore) is plugged with a small amount of glass wool. The resin is pipetted into the column to a height of 55 mm with care taken to avoid trapping of air within the resin bed. It is then washed with 10 ml 0.5 M sodium phosphate buffer, pH 7.5, followed by 15 ml distilled water.

Ion exchange separation. The 30 ml of urine-buffer mixture should be applied to the column before the meniscus of the distilled water disappears into the resin. After application of the urine, a 10 ml and a 5 ml portion of 0.5 M sodium acetate buffer, pH 6.5, are passed through the column in succession, with care taken to wash the glass above the resin bed. This differential elution with buffer removes the impurities, and histamine may now be eluted from the column with 5 ml 1 N HCl. The acid eluate is collected in a 35 ml glass-stoppered centrifuge tube with tapered bottom (Kontes No. K8-9475).

Extraction procedure. The eluate is made alkaline by addition of 0.75 ml of 10 N NaOH, and is saturated with NaCl. Twelve ml n-butanol are added and the histamine is extracted into the butanol phase during a 2 minute period of shaking. After centrifugation the aqueous phase is removed by aspiration and discarded. The butanol phase is then washed once by shaking with 5 ml of salt and butanol-saturated 0.1 N NaOH. After centrifugation, 10 ml of the butanol layer are transferred to a 50 ml tapered, glass-stoppered centrifuge tube containing 20 ml n-heptane and 3 ml 0.1 N HCl. After shaking for 2 minutes the tube is centrifuged and the butanol-heptane phase removed by aspiration. A 2 ml aliquot of the acid extract is then transferred to a test tube for fluorometric assay." (By the procedure of Shore, Burkhalter and Cohn).

Weissbach, Lovenberg and Udenfriend (1961) and Kremzner and Wilson (1961), studying histidine decarboxylases, devised ion exchange column procedures for separating histamine from a great excess of histidine.

Weissbach et al.: "At various time intervals 0.5 ml of the incubation mixture was transferred to a test tube containing 0.2 ml 5% trichloroacetic acid and heated at 100° C for 1 min. After cooling 1.5 ml of water were added and the precipitated protein was removed by centrifugation. The clear supernatant fraction was passed over a 0.5×3 cm Dowex-1 carbonate column to remove the histidine and the column was then washed with 1 ml of water. The effluent and washings were combined and assayed for histamine by the method of Shore et al."

Kremzner and Wilson purified histamine over a column of anion exchanger under their own conditions and they omitted the butanol extraction step of Shore et al. Applying their procedure to different animal tissues they obtained results within the range reported by other workers. They reported excellent recovery of different amounts of histamine added to the protein fraction of animal tissue homogenates.

"*Preparation of resin:* The anion-exchange resin (Dowex-1-X8, Bio Rad-1-X8, and IRA-410 were used and found satisfactory), 50—100 mesh, is converted to the acetate-hydroxide form in a large column with several volumes of 0.75 M sodium acetate –0.05 M NaOH. The resin is then washed with distilled water and stored under refrigeration. If the resin is stored at room temperature it is satisfactory if it is washed with several volumes of distilled water.

Column preparation: The columns used were 10-ml graduated pipettes in which the upper constriction was removed so as to facilitate the introduction of resin slurry. The column is fitted with a glass-wool plug. The resin slurry is then added, allowed to settle and the resin volume adjusted to approx. 6 ml. Before the sample is added, the water above is lowered to the resin surface.

Preparation of tissue extract and assay: 1 g of tissue is homogenized with 4 ml 5% trichloroacetic acid and the mixture centrifuged. (The solution volume is considered to be 4.8 ml.) One ml of the supernatant is added to a 10 ml volumetric flask containing 0.50 ml 0.50 N NaOH and several ml 0.01 M pH 7.0 phosphate buffer and brought to the mark with water.

Five ml of this solution is applied to the column by pipette. When the sample reaches the top surface, phosphate buffer (0.05—0.01 M) is added as a wash. The flow rate is controlled at approximately 1 ml/min with a screw clamp. The first 1—2 ml are discarded and the effluent is collected to approximately the mark in a 10-ml volumetric flask containing 0.1 ml of 10^{-2} M ethylenediaminetetra-acetic acid (EDTA) and made to volume. To 2 ml of this solution are added 0.40 ml 0.5 N NaOH and 0.1 ml 1% o-phthalaldehyde. After 3.5 ($\pm$0.5) min. 0.20 ml 2.5 M H_3PO_4 are added. The fluorescence is measured at 445 mμ with excitation at 345 mμ (in these studies the Aminco Bowman spectrophotofluorometer was used with the 1 P 21 tube and slit arrangement No. 3).

In solutions where histamine is not bound as in the assay of histidine decarboxylase, it is advantageous to use the following procedure: 2 ml of solution (salt 0.05 M) containing histamine (0.001—0.5 μg/ml) is applied to a 3 ml column, the first ml is discarded and a little less than 4.5 ml of effluent is collected in a 5.0-ml volumetric flask containing 0.5 ml 30% trichloroacetic acid and 0.05 ml of 10^{-2} M EDTA, and the solution brought to the mark. The solution is centrifuged and a 2-ml aliquot is taken; 0.40 ml 1.5 N NaOH is added and 0.10 ml o-phthalaldehyde (1%) is added. After (3.5 $\pm$ 0.5) min, 0.20 ml 2.5 M H_3PO_4 is added. The fluorescence is measured at 445 mμ with excitation at 345 mμ.

Standard curves are prepared by using suitable dilutions of histamine in 0.03% trichloroacetic acid (TCA) when measuring bound histamine, and histamine in 3% TCA in the procedure for the assay of free histamine. All dilutions should be 10^{-4} M with EDTA. The fluorescence intensity is proportional to the concentration of histamine in the range 0.003—0.5 μg/ml.

As there is no loss of histamine in the procedures outlined, the use of internal standards is not required. The small non-histamine fluorescence in tissue or reagents is corrected by omission of the condensation step, i.e. all the reagents are added to a separate aliquot of the unknown, but the order of addition of o-phthalaldehyde and acid is reversed.

In this procedure the fluorescence is measured at pH 2.0 rather than at pH 0.85 as described by Shore et al. because, the intensity is greater at this pH."

Using Graham's (1961) scaled-down version of Shore's fluorometric assay, Noah and Brand (1961) determined histamine in 1 ml of human plasma. Applied to TCA extracts of plasma, the procedure gave high false histamine values, which could be corrected only by purifying the TCA extracts through the Decalso procedure of Lowry and associates (see under DNFB methods).

Noah and Brand: "To 500 microliters of Decalso eluate was added 0.2 gm NaCl, 60 microliters of 5 N NaOH, and 1.25 ml of n-butyl alcohol. The addition of each material was followed by thorough buzzing. After standing to permit separation of the aqueous and alcoholic layers, the aqueous layer was removed and discarded. The butanol portion was then washed twice with 1.0 ml. amounts of 0.1 N NaOH saturated with NaCl. After the second NaOH-NaCl wash, 1.0 ml. of the butanol layer was added to 1.5 ml of n-heptane and 380 microliters of 0.1 N HCl. After buzzing and standing long enough to permit separation of layers, 300 microliters of the acid layer were withdrawn, and to this were added 60 microliters of 1 N NaOH, and after mixing, 14 microliters of 0.1% o-phthalaldehyde (OPT). After standing at room temperature for 4 minutes, 25 microliters of 3 N HCl were added. Within 30 minutes, this mixture was placed in a small cuvette and the intensity of fluorescence determined in a fluorometer. A Turner Fluorometer, Model 110, was used for these determinations. To read samples of 250 microliter volume, a special adapter, generously supplied by Dr. Robert E. Phillips, of G. K. Turner Associates, Palo Alto, California, was installed in place of the regular cuvette holder. This permits the use of 6 mm. × 50 mm. standard Pyrex tubes as cuvettes. The primary filter used (color specification No. 7—60) and the secondary filter (color specification No. 2-A) are those routinely supplied with this instrument.

Because of the ubiquity of interfering fluorophores, all reagents used must be of the highest obtainable purity. Distilled water must be triple-distilled, in glass. Exposure of any of the materials involved to rubber, plastics, or silicones may produce erratic results. All glassware, after conventional cleaning with detergent and water, is boiled in 50% nitric acid and further cleansed with distilled water. After 4 to 7 days, blank readings usually increase and new reagent solutions must be prepared."

The pH to which the reaction is acidified after the alkaline OPT condensation is important. Kremzner and Wilson acidified the alkaline reaction mixture to pH 2.0 instead of pH 0.85, with phosphoric instead of hydrochloric acid, and thereby they increased both the stability and the intensity of the fluorescence. These same findings were reported by Thompson (1961), who used only half of the amount of hydrochloric acid called for in Shore's directions. Braendle (personal communication) used half of the amount of phosphoric acid prescribed by Kremzner and Wilson and found that the fluorescence was stable at 25° C for at least four hours; in 24 hours there was a 20 to 25 per cent loss at 25° C but no loss at 4° C.

Because the condensation of o-phthalaldehyde with histamine is quite sensitive to temperature, Braendle prefers to run the reaction in a water bath at 25 ± 0.5° C for 4 minutes.

C. DNFB procedures

Lowry and associates (1954) presented the following method for the assay of histamine in blood plasma and cells. The procedure is applicable generally to 5 per cent TCA extracts of tissues:

"*Reagents.* 1. Water, redistilled from glass, is used throughout. 2. Trichloroacetic acid (TCA), redistilled. 3. Sodium acetate, 4 M. 4. Potassium bromide, 40 gm. per 100 ml. 5. Carbonate buffer (pH 10) containing per liter 21 gm. (0.2 mole) anhydrous Na_2CO_3, and 8.4 gm. (0.1 mole) $NaHCO_3$. 6. Sodium diethyldithiocarbamate (Distillation Products Industries, Rochester, N.Y.) 12.5 mgm. per cent solution prepared from stock 1.25 per cent solution. Both solutions keep well at 5° C. 7. 2,4-Dinitrofluorobenzene (DNFB) (e.g., Jasonols Chemical Corporation, 1085 Myrtle Avenue, Brooklyn 6, N. Y.) 2 per cent (by volume) in absolute ethanol. Contact of DNFB with the skin may produce a severe rash. However, at 2 per cent concentration little trouble has been encountered even with sensitized individuals. 8. Methyl-n-hexyl ketone (2-octanone), practical grade. If turbidity is encountered in the last step of the analysis, it may be minimized by redistillation and/or acid washing of the ketone. 9. Hydrochloric acid, 2 N. 10. Histamine standards, 1 to 100 microgm. histamine base (1.66 to 166 microgm. histamine dihydrochloride) per ml. in 0.01 N HCl. Such standards are stable over long periods when frozen at −20° C. 11. Decalso (The Permutit Company, New York, N.Y.). This is boiled with 3 per cent acetic acid, washed in H_2O and dried. The 40 to 60 mesh portion is used.

Apparatus. 1. Hot box (Fig. 2) with lamp heaters and thermal control switch maintaining temperature at 75° to 80° C. The box is designed to keep the eluting fluid hot.

2. Adsorption column (Fig. 2) (A.S. Aloe Company, St. Louis). This is composed of an upper reservoir, a long tube to provide a sufficient head of pressure, a third narrower segment to hold the adsorbent (this portion is made very slender to reduce to a minimum the amount of adsorbent and thereby the required eluting volume), a constriction to hold back sand and adsorbent and a tapered tip. For satisfactory elution the third (adsorbent) segment must fall entirely within the hot box. Columns that are too long may be raised to the proper position with a rubber collar (not shown). With the aid of flowing redistilled water, a layer of acid washed sand (40 to 60 mesh) a few mm. thick is introduced into a tube, followed by sufficient Decalso to make a column 3 cm. ± 0.3 cm. high after it is packed down lightly by tapping the tube. The height rather than the weight of Decalso is critical. The flow through a column so prepared should be 0.1 to 0.5 ml. per minute. Bubbles of air above the absorbing material which slow or stop the flow may be removed with aid of stainless steel wire. If particles of sand block the constriction they can be loosened with a very fine wire inserted through the tip.

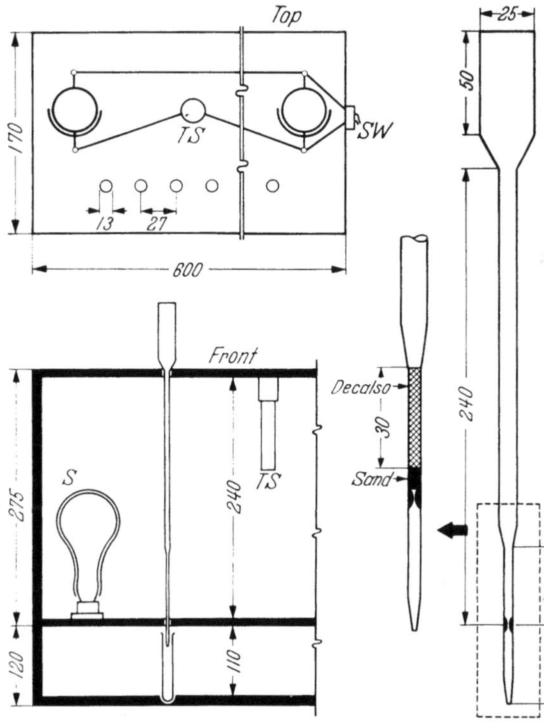

Fig. 2. Adsorption column and hot box. Numbers give dimensions in millimeters. Inner diameter middle segment of column, 8 mm.; Decalso segment, 1.8 mm.; constriction, 0.3 mm. *TS* = Fenwal thermal switch, *SW* = on-off switch, *S* = 100-watt lamp, partially surrounded by aluminumfoil shield to prevent local overheating

3. Buzzer for rapid mixing (and extraction) of solutions (Bessey, Lowry and Brock, 1946b). This is a slightly bent 1/4 inch rod clamped in the chuck of a rather high speed — 2,000 or more r.p.m. — motor or stirrer. The rod is oriented horizontally. When a tube is held at an angle against the rotating rod, the contents whirl vigorously.

4. Micro cuvettes, 1 to 1.4 mm. inner width with 10 mm. light path (Pyrocell Mfg. Co., 507 East 84th Street, New York, N.Y.) are used in the Beckman spectrophotometer adapted to give readings with a minimum sample of 25 to 30 microliters (Lowry and Bessey, 1946).

5. Acid-cleaned tubes for collecting eluate and for all later steps. These are boiled for half an hour in concentrated nitric acid diluted 1:1, rinsed and boiled with distilled water, then rinsed finally with glass-distilled water.

6. Lang-Levy constriction pipettes [Microchemical Specialities Company, Berkeley, California; The Carlsberg Laboratory, Copenhagen, Denmark; or Arthur H. Thomas Co., Philadelphia. See BESSEY, LOWRY, BROCK and LOPEZ (1946a), in reference to construction of such pipettes.] These are used for measuring all volumes less than 1 ml. Special constriction pipettes, 0.5 ml. capacity, long enough (25 cm.) to reach almost to the Decalso are used for adding the KBr eluting fluid.

Preparation of extracts. One-tenth volume of isotonic potassium oxalate (1.7 per cent $K_2C_2O_4$) is used as anticoagulant (BESSEY, LOWRY and BROCK, 1947). Plasma must be separated quickly at low temperature to avoid a positive error from release of leukocyte histamine. To 10 ml. of plasma (equivalent to 8.3 ml. of original plasma) is added 2 ml. of 30 per cent TCA with prompt vigorous mixing. After 30 minutes this is centrifuged at the highest speed to obtain a maximum yield of supernatant fluid (about 10 ml. which would be equivalent to 7.25 ml. of original plasma, since about 6 per cent of the original plasma volume consisted of solids). Whole blood, 2 ml., is treated with 2 ml. of 10 per cent TCA and centrifuged. Because of the blood solids present (about 14 per cent of the blood volume), 2 ml. of the extract is equivalent to 1.07 ml. of blood. Extracts of buffy coat suspensions are similarly prepared (5 per cent final TCA concentration) except that due to the higher histamine concentrations it is feasible to use greater dilution.

Adsorption and elution. To a measured volume of the supernatant fluid (about 10 ml. of plasma extract or 2 ml. of blood extract), 1/10 volume of 4 M sodium acetate is added to bring the pH to about 4. With a little water, this mixture is rinsed into a Decalso column. After this flows through at not over 0.5 ml. per minute, the column is washed with 5 ml. water. The last drops of wash-water are blown out, the column is placed in the hot box, and 0.5 ml. of 40 per cent KBr is introduced just above the Decalso. The eluate is collected in a tube (6 ml., 11 × 100 mm., No. 9450 Arthur H. Thomas Co., Philadelphia) containing about 40 microliters of sodium diethyldithiocarbamate (0.0008 M). The last drops of eluate (blown out) are included.

Color development and extraction. To each eluate are added 0.25 ml. carbonate buffer and immediately before mixing with the buzzer, 20 microliters of 2 per cent DNFB. (In the analysis of whole blood there may be advantage in using three times the recommended amount of DNFB reagent. Although this decreases the readings with histamine by 15 per cent, it reduces to about half the color from non-histamine interfering substances in red cells.) The tubes are heated in a constant temperature bath at 60° C. for 30 minutes. After the introduction of 0.4 ml. of methyl-n-hexyl ketone, each tube is buzzed vigorously and centrifuged. An aliquot (0.30 or 0.35 ml.) of the ketone is transferred into a 1 ml. tube (7 × 70 mm. Kimble No. 45060-S181, A.S. Aloe Co., St. Louis) containing 50 microliters of 2 N HCl. This mixture is buzzed for 10 seconds or long enough to produce maximum fading, and centrifuged for 5 minutes at 3,000 r.p.m.

Reading and standardization. The ketone layer is sucked off carefully and discarded, and the acid layer is read at λ 360 mμ in a micro cuvette.

The procedure may be interrupted overnight or longer either (1) at the stage when the histamine is adsorbed in the Decalso column, or (2) after the histamine is in the final acid solution. In the latter case, in order to prevent evaporation, the overlying ketone is not removed and the samples are refrigerated.

Standards containing 0.05 to 0.2 microgram histamine, and blanks, each with a volume of 5 per cent TCA equal to the volume of sample extract used, are carried through the whole process with the samples to be analyzed. The reading of the blank is usually as low as that of 0.02 microgram histamine. With amounts of histamine too high to read, appropriate dilution with 2 N HCl will yield satisfactory readings at least up to 10 micrograms of histamine."

Weissbach, Waalkes and Udenfriend (1958) combined the histamine purification of McIntire, White and Sproull (1950) with the Lowry conditions for the DNFB reaction. They used this method on blood plasma or tissue extracts prepared by HCl extraction and $Zn(OH)_2$ precipitation of proteins.

Tissue extraction (Weissbach, Waalkes and Udenfriend, 1958): "Tissues were homogenized in at least 2 times their volume of 0.1 N HCl. An aliquot of the homogenate (corresponding to no more than 2 gm.) was made up to 8 ml. with 0.9 per cent saline. The proteins were then precipitated by the addition of 1 ml. of 10 per cent $ZnSO_4$ followed by 0.5 ml. of 1 N NaOH. After thorough shaking, the tubes were centrifuged at 2500 r.p.m. for 20 minutes."

Histamine purification(McIntire, White and Sproull, 1950):

"*Reagents:* Salt mixture of reagent grade anhydrous Na_2SO_4, and $Na_3PO_4H_2O$. The $Na_3PO_4H_2O$ may be prepared by drying reagent grade $Na_3PO_4 12H_2O$ at 100° C for 48 hours, then at 300° C for 2—3 hours. The salts should be finely powdered and mixed in a ratio of 6.25 g. of Na_2SO_4 to 1 g. of $Na_3PO_4H_2O$.

n-Butanol reagent grade is refluxed overnight with Raney nickel catalyst (roughly 3 g. catalyst/l. butanol), redistilled, and kept under nitrogen. Raney nickel catalyst supplied by the Harshaw Chemical Company is suitable.

Sodium diethyldithiocarbamate (NaDi) (Eastman, or Distillation Products Industries) 0.04 M (6.84 mg./ml.) in low-copper distilled water.

Cotton acid succinate (CS) prepared as follows: Dissolve 5 g. of fused sodium acetate and 40 g. of succinic anhydride in 300 ml. of glacial acetic acid. Immerse 10 g. of cotton in this solution, attach a drying tube to the flask and maintain the temperature at 100° C for 48 hours. (Absorbent cotton is not satisfactory. A grade of cotton to be recommended is coil cotton, pharmaceutical grade A, Kendall Mills, Walpole, Massachusetts.) Filter off the partially esterified cotton, and wash well with water, dilute hydrochloric acid, water, and finally with alcohol. Dry the product preferably in a vacuum oven.

Apparatus: Glass-stoppered test tubes, 16—16.5 mm. O.D., 120 mm. long without stopper, 13/14 standard taper joint with solid flathead stoppers. When many extractions are to be carried out, these tubes will fit into multiple carriers for use in a No 240 International centrifuge head.

Shaking rack for shaking a large number of glass-stoppered tubes simultaneously, illustrated in Fig. 3.

Mechanical shaker for adequate shaking of a rack full of tubes during the butanol extraction. A precision heavy-duty equipoise shaker proved satisfactory.

Pipetting bulb with bead valve, illustrated in Fig. 3. Bulbs of 10—20 ml. capacity are a convenient size.

Metal cup for measuring salt mixture. A small cup, preferably stainless steel, approximate inside dimensions: 7 mm. deep, 13 mm. diameter. Such a device will save time and is sufficiently accurate for measuring the 1.33 g. portions of salt mixture.

A cotton succinate tube is shown in Fig. 3. Each tube contains 100 mg. of CS packed firmly but not tightly. If the CS pads are washed well with alcohol after each experiment, and protected from dust, they should require replacment only once every 2—3 months, with moderate use.

Histamine purification: Into a glass-stoppered test tube, place 5 ml. of aqueous tissue extract to be assayed; add 1.33 g. of the salt mixture, 0.05 ml. of 0.04 M

NaDi solution and a small lead sphere (air-rifle shot). Stopper the tube and shake thoroughly.

To each tube add 5 ml. of butanol; shake vigorously for a few seconds; let stand a few minutes, and then shake briefly to break the protein gel. Shake vigorously in a mechanical shaker for 1/2 hour, and then centrifuge at about 2000 r.p.m. for 15—20 minutes.

Using the pipetting bulb attached to a 5-ml. serologic pipet, transfer 4.6 ml. of butanol solution from each test tube to a CS tube. Be sure that no droplets of the aqueous phase are transferred to the CS pad. After the butanol extract has

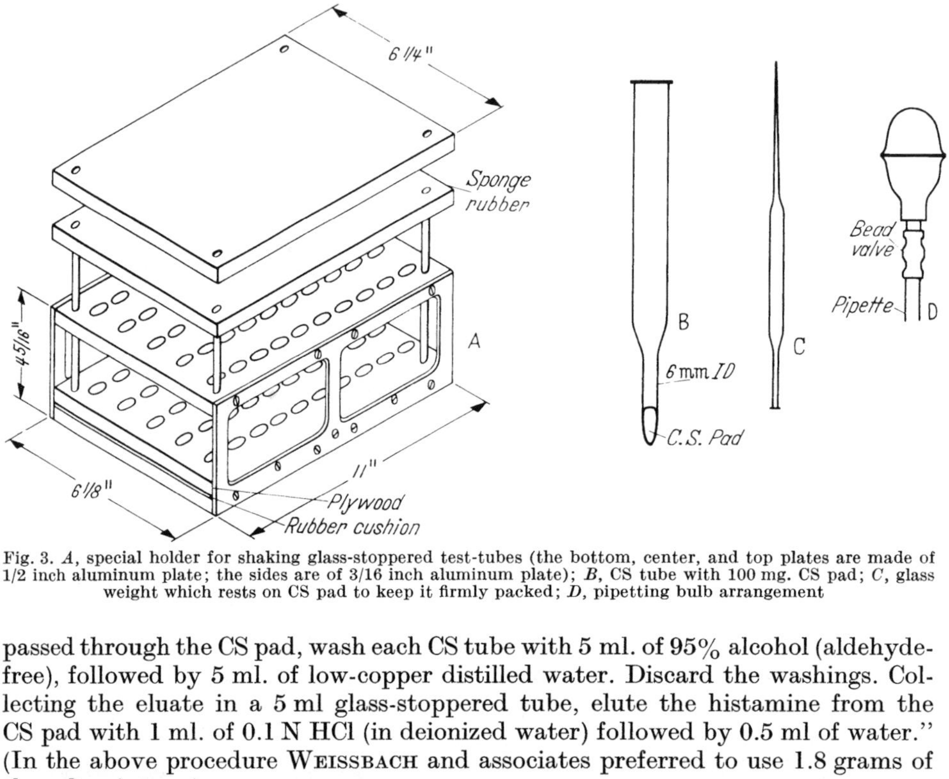

Fig. 3. *A*, special holder for shaking glass-stoppered test-tubes (the bottom, center, and top plates are made of 1/2 inch aluminum plate; the sides are of 3/16 inch aluminum plate); *B*, CS tube with 100 mg. CS pad; *C*, glass weight which rests on CS pad to keep it firmly packed; *D*, pipetting bulb arrangement

passed through the CS pad, wash each CS tube with 5 ml. of 95% alcohol (aldehyde-free), followed by 5 ml. of low-copper distilled water. Discard the washings. Collecting the eluate in a 5 ml glass-stoppered tube, elute the histamine from the CS pad with 1 ml. of 0.1 N HCl (in deionized water) followed by 0.5 ml of water." (In the above procedure Weissbach and associates preferred to use 1.8 grams of the salt mixture.)

Histamine assay (Weissbach, Waalkes and Udenfriend, 1958): "The following reagents were prepared as described previously by Lowry, Graham, Harris, Priebat, Marks and Bregman (1954): Sodium diethyldithiocarbamate (12.5 mg. per cent in deionized water). 2,4-Dinitrofluorobenzene (DNFB), 2 per cent (by volume) in absolute ethyl alcohol. 2-Octanone (practical grade). Carbonate buffer, pH 10, containing 21 gm. anhydrous sodium carbonate and 8.4 gm. of sodium bicarbonate per liter of solution.

To the 5 ml. glass-stoppered centrifuge tubes containing the acid eluate from the CS columns were added 0.04 ml. of sodium diethyldithiocarbamate, 0.6 ml. of carbonate buffer, and the 2 per cent DNFB solution (0.05 ml. for plasma and 0.1 ml. for blood and tissues). After mixing, the tubes were heated at 60° for 30 minutes and cooled. 1 ml. of 2-Octanone was added to each tube; the tubes were shaken for 1 minute and centrifuged. 0.9 ml. of the ketone layer was removed and added to 0.3 ml. of 2 N HCl in a small test tube. After mixing by swirling, the tubes were centrifuged, the ketone layer was carefully removed by aspiration, and the acid layer read at 360 mμ on the Beckman spectrophotometer.

Standards and internal recoveries as well as reagent blanks, were carried through the entire procedure with each experiment. Histamine, when added to tissue extracts, was recovered to the extent of about 80 to 95 per cent."

KANTOR, LEVINE *and* FISCHBACH *histamine purification:* Although it was published for use with the ROSENTHAL and TABOR (1948) diazo assay, this procedure is very satisfactory for the DNFB assay (MCINTIRE, unpublished; YUSEM, 1961).

"*Reagents in copper-free water:* Sodium hydroxide, 5 N. Sulfuric acid 0.4 N. benzaldehyde, chlorine-free. Solvent mixture, benzene-n-butanol (3:2). Cotton acid succinate (CS), prepared according to MCINTIRE, WHITE and SPROULL (1950). Standard histamine solutions. Prepare aqueous solutions of histamine dihydrochloride equivalent to 1.0, 2.0, 3.0, 4.0 and 5.0 micrograms of free base per ml. When kept in the refrigerator, they are stable for at least one month.

Procedure: Transfer 200 mg. of the streptomycin or dihydrostreptomycin salt to a glass-stoppered test tube. Dissolve in 4 ml. of water and cool in an ice bath. (In the case of the streptomycin calcium chloride double salt, dissolve in 3 ml. of water and add 1 ml. of the sodium citrate solution to prevent the precipitation of calcium hydroxide.) Add 1 drop of benzaldehyde and 0.2 ml. of 5 N sodium hydroxide, and shake vigorously for 10—15 seconds. Keep in the ice bath for two minutes, during which time 5 ml. of the benzene-butanol mixture is added. Shake vigorously for 15 seconds. Centrifuge at 2000—2500 r.p.m. for one to two minutes. Pipette the organic phase into the prepared CS (150 mg) column, carefully avoiding the aqueous phase. Re-extract with 5 ml. of the solvent mixture. After the solvent has passed through the CS pad, wash with 3 ml. of ethyl alcohol, followed by two washings of 2—3 ml. of water each. Elute the histamine with 2 ml. of 0.4 N sulfuric acid, followed by 1 ml. of water; collect the acid and water eluates in a glass-stoppered test tube. To prepare the CS pad for re-use, wash it immediately free of acid with water and then with alcohol." The CS eluate is ready for the diazo coupling by the ROSENTHAL and TABOR procedure quoted later.

Applied to perchloric acid extracts of blood and tissues, the KANTOR procedure is superior to the butanol extraction in purifying histamine for the chemical assays. For such applications the following modifications are recommended: (1) In addition to the specified 0.2 ml. 5 N NaOH use enough to neutralize all acid present; (2) as much as 5 drops of benzaldehyde may be used if the solution to be extracted contains a considerable quantity of amino compounds; (3) one extraction with 20 ml. of benzene-butanol may be used in place of the two 5 ml. extractions.

D. The Rosenthal and Tabor diazo method

Reagents, in copper-free water: 1—0.1 per cent p-nitroaniline in 0.1 N HCl in dark glass bottle, 2-diazo reagent, freshly prepared, 1 ml. 4 per cent sodium nitrite added to 10 ml. of ice-cold p-nitroaniline solution, 3—20 per cent sodium carbonate, 4—5 N sodium hydroxide, 6—M/20 barbital buffer, pH 7.7—10 g. sodium barbital dissolved in 975 ml. water, adjusted to pH 7.7 with 6 per cent acetic acid, 7-methyl isobutyl ketone.

Procedure: Chill the CS eluate and wash (3 ml. from KANTOR procedure) in the ice bath; add 0.5ml. of diazo reagent and mix well. Add 0.3 ml. sodium carbonate, mix; add 0.2 ml. sodium carbonate, mix. Keep reaction on ice one minute and add 0.12 ml. 5 N sodium hydroxide and mix. Add 5 ml. of methyl isobutyl ketone; stopper, and shake 25 times. Place in ice bath while ketone layer separates. Centrifuge briefly if necessary.

With a capillary pipette and rubber bulb transfer most of the ketone layer to a glass stoppered test tube containing 5 ml. of barbital buffer; shake vigorously. After 20 to 30 minutes measure the optical density of the ketone solution at 516 mμ.

E. Paper chromatography

Procedure of URBACH *and* GISCAFRE (1948): "2—20 ml of plasma are diluted with an equal amount of water and the pH and salt concentration are adjusted according to the procedure used by McINTIRE, ROTH and SHAW (1947) for the extraction of histamine with butanol. The histamine is then extracted from the butanol with a small amount of 0.5 N sulfuric acid which is, in turn, brought to the proper salt concentration and pH and re-extracted with approximately 3 ml of butanol. The final butanol extract is then applied to the filter paper strip by means of capillary pipettes with a very slow flow rate. Control strips with known amounts of histamine are prepared in a similar manner. A set of strips is then suspended in a closed chamber from a trough containing butanol saturated with 10% ammonium hydroxide as the solvent mixture. After 12—15 hours the strips are removed, dried and treated with an alkaline diazotized solution of p-bromaniline employed as a color reagent for histamine by BARAUD, GENEVOIS, MANDILLON and RINGENBACH (1946). Histamine, in excess of 1 μg can be detected as a red band on the strips. Its presence and identity are established by the color of the band and more critically by the position of the colored band on the strips. Approximate estimation of the amount of histamine is possible by comparison with a standard series of strips".

Literature

AKERBLOM, E.: Zur Histaminbestimmung in Gewebsextrakten. Acta physiol. scand. **2**, 378 (1941).

ANDREWS, A. C., and T. D. LYONS: Quantitative determination of histamine in presence of certain interfering metallic ions. Anal. Chem. **29**, 1325 (1957).

BARAUD, J., L. GENEVOIS, G. MANDILLON and G. RINGENBACH: Determination of histamine in blood during poisoning. C. R. Acad. Sci. (Paris) **222**, 760 (1946); Chem. Abstr. **40**, 4099 (1946).

BESSEY, O. A., O. H. LOWRY, M. J. BROCK and J. L. LOPEZ: The determination of vitamin A and carotene in small quantities of blood serum. J. biol. Chem. **166**, 177 (1946).

— — — A method for the rapid determination of alkaline phosphatase with five cubic millimeters of serum. J. biol. Chem. **164**, 321 (1946).

— — — The quantitative determination of ascorbic acid in small amounts of white blood cells and platelets. J. biol. Chem. **168**, 197 (1947).

BODÁNSZKY, M., J. HALLÓS and O. NÉMETH: Determination of small amounts of histamine in histidine preparations. Magyar Kem. Folyoirat. **62**, 317 (1957); Chem. Abstr. **52**, 15630ᵉ (1958).

BOHMER, U., u. H. GIERSBERG: Untersuchungen über Histamin und eine pharmakologisch histaminähnlich wirkende Substanz und ihr Verhalten nach Bestrahlung mit UV. Naturwissenschaften **43**, 303 (1956).

BRAENDLE, C.: Unpublished 1961.

BREMNER, J. M., and R. H. KENTEN: Paper chromatography of amines. Biochem. J. **49**, 651 (1951).

BURIAN, R.: Diazoaminoverbindungen der Imidazole und der Purinsubstanzen. Ber. **37**, 696 (1904).

DIEMAIR, W., u. H. FOX: Über einige neue Azoverbindungen und Jod-Derivate des Histidins und Histamins. Ber. **71**, 2493 (1938a).

— — Zur Zubereitung der Nahrung und deren ernährungsphysiologischen Bedeutung. IV. Mitteilung: Untersuchungen über die Vorgänge bei der Kuppelung des Histidins und Histamins mit Diazoniumsalzen. Biochem. Z. **298**, 38 (1938b).

DODGE, A. C.: A test for pregnancy based on the histaminolytic activity of serum. Amer. J. Obstet. Gynec. **63**, 1212 (1952).

DUTTA, S. K.: Microestimation of histamine in protein hydrolysate. Sci. and Culture (India) **21**, 610 (1956).

EMMELIN, N., G. KAHLSON and F. WICKSELL: Histamine in plasma and methods for its estimation. Acta physiol. scand. **2**, 123 (1941).

FARGHER, R. G., and F. L. PYMAN: Nitro-, Arylazo-, and Amino-glyoxalines. J. chem. Soc. **115**, 217 (1919).
FISCHER, F. G., u. H. BONN: Über die Bestimmung von Spermin, Spermidin und anderen biogenen Aminen nach papierelektrophoretischer Abtrennung und ihre Mengenverhältnisse in tierischen Organen. Hoppe-Seylers Z. physiol. Chem. **308**, 108 (1957).
FUYUO, O.: Formation of amine in fish muscle. IV. Rapid method for the determination of histamine in fish muscle. Bull. Jap. Soc. Sci. Fisheries **24**, 37 (1958); Chem. Abstr. **53**, 7454e (1959).
GAYER, J.: Zum Nachweis biogener Amine (Eine methodische Mitteilung). Biochem. Z. **328**, 39 (1956).
GEBAUER-FUELNEGG, E.: Zur Kenntnis der Paulyschen Diazoreaktion. Hoppe-Seylers Z. physiol. Chem. **191**, 222 (1930); Chem. Abstr. **24**, 5735 (1930).
GRAHAM, H. T.: Personal communication. (1961).
— T. W. HANNERGAN and C. M. NOURSE: Dependence of tissue histamine content on local histidine decarboxylase activity. Biochem. biophys. Acta (Amst.) **20**, 243 (1956).
HALPERN, B. N., S. VIENNET and S. PATTEE: Kinetic photometric study of the diazotization reactions of histamine and histidine. Utilization of this technique for differentiation of the two substances. C. R. Soc. Biol. (Paris) **140**, 212 (1946); Chem. Abstr. **41**, 3153[a] (1947).
HANKE, M. T., and K. K. KOESSLER: Studies on proteinogenous amines. VIII. A method for the quantitative colorimetric estimation of histamine in protein and protein-containing matter. J. biol. Chem. **43**, 543 (1920).
HAVINGA, E., L. SEEKLES and TH. STRENGERS: The extinctiometric determination of small quantities of histamine. Rec. Trav. **66**, 605 (1947).
HUGHES, D. E., E. SALVIN and D. R. WOOD: Decarboxylation of histidine as a source of error in extracting histamine from tissues. J. Physiol. (Lond.) **113**, 218 (1951).
ISHIHARA, J.: Role of histamine in inflammation. I. Estimation of histamine with 2,4-dinitrofluorobenzene (DNFB). Nippon Saikingaku Zasshi **12**, 183 (1957); Chem. Abstr. **52**, 20362[h]. (1958).
JOHNSON, H. H.: Microchemical method for the determination of histamine. Arch. Derm. **72**, 307 (1955).
KANTOR, N., J. LEVINE and H. FISCHBACH: Chemical determination of histamine in streptomycin and dihydrostreptomycin. Antibiot. and Chemother. **1**, 579 (1951).
KESTON, A. S., S. UDENFRIEND and R. K. CANNON: Micro-analysis of mixtures (amino acids) in the form of isotopic derivatives. J. Amer. chem. Soc. **68**, 1390 (1946).
KESZTYÜS, L.: Über die Azoverbindungen des Histamins. Naunyn-Schmiedeberg's Arch. exp. Path. Pharmak. **205**, 287 (1948).
KOESSLER, K. K., and M. T. HANKE: Studies on proteinogenous amines. III. A quantitative method for separating histamine from histidine. J. biol. Chem. **39**, 521 (1919).
— — Studies on proteinogenous amines. II. A microchemical colorimetric method for estimating imidazole derivatives. J. biol. Chem. **39**, 497 (1919).
KREMZNER, L. T., and I. B. WILSON: A procedure for the determination of histamine. Biochem. biophys. Acta (Amst.) **50**, 364 (1961).
LEWIS, B., E. VON GEBAUER-FUELNEGG and C. J. FARMER: A spectroscopic study and assay of histamine. J. Amer. chem. Soc. **55**, 2025 (1933).
LOWRY, O. H., and A. O. BESSEY: The adaptation of the Beckman Spectrophotometer to measurements on minute quantities of biological materials. J. biol. Chem. **163**, 633 (1946).
— H. T. GRAHAM, F. B. HARRIS, M. K. PRIEBAT, A. R. MARKS and R. U. BREGMAN: The chemical measurement of histamine in blood plasma and cells. J. Pharmacol. exp. Ther. **112**, 116 (1954).
LUBSCHEZ, R.: Chemical determination of histamine in human blood. J. biol. Chem. **183**, 731 (1950).
MACGREGOR, R. G., and W. V. THORPE: The quantitative extraction of histamine from tissues by electrodialysis. Biochem. J. **27**, 1394 (1933).
MCINTIRE, F. C.: The mode of histamine binding in animal tissues. In: Ciba Symposium on Histamine. p. 170. Little, Brown (1956).
— The determination of histamine in pharmaceutical products by means of 2,4-dinitrofluorobenzene. J. Amer. pharm. Ass. sci. Ed. **41**, 277 (1952).
— L. W. ROTH and J. L. SHAW: Purification of histamine for bioassay. J. biol. Chem. **170**, 537 (1947).
— F. B. WHITE and M. SPROULL: The determination of histamine with 2,4-dinitrofluorobenzene. Arch. Biochem. **29**, 376 (1950).
MACAIG, A., and R. SCHOENTAL: Modifikation der Reaktion von PAULY, im Zusammenhang mit der mikro-kolorimetrischen (photometrischen) Bestimmung der Imidazolkörper (Histamin). Mikrochemie **24**, 243 (1938).
MADER, W. J., H. S. STERNE, JR., J. ROSIN and H. A. FREDIANI: Colorimetric determination of histamine in histamine phosphate injection, U.S.P. J. Amer. pharm. Ass. sci. Ed. **39**, 175 (1950).

MINARD, D.: The presence and distribution of histamine in the blood. Amer. J. Physiol. **132**, 327 (1941).
NEWMAN, P. M., and J. H. TURNBULL: New colorimetric method for the estimation of histidine and histamine. Biochem. J. **74**, 379 (1960).
NOAH, J. W., and A. BRAND: A fluorometric method to determine levels of histamine in human plasma. J. Allergy **31**, 236 (1961).
OATES, J. A.: Personal communication (1961).
PAULY, H.: Über die Konstitution des Histidins. I. Mitteilung. Hoppe-Seylers Z. physiol. Chem. **42**, 508 (1904).
PEESEZ, M., et P. POIRIER: Sur la recherche et le dosage des amines aliphatiques primaires par réaction colorée. Bull. Soc. chim. Fr. **20**, 754 (1953).
RAUTENBURG, H. W.: Zur Papierchromatographie der basischen Aminosäuren und des Histamins in Gegenwart von Sulfat und Selenat. Biochem. Z. **329**, 255 (1957).
ROBERTS, M., and H. M. ADAM: New methods for the quantitative estimation of free and conjugated histamine in body fluids. Brit. J. Pharmacol. **5**, 526 (1950).
ROSENTHAL, S. M., and H. TABOR: An improved colorimetric method for the estimation of histamine. J. Pharmacol. exp. Ther. **92**, 425 (1948).
RUNG, F., u. M. BEHREND: Notizen über Glyoxalin. Annalen **271**, 28 (1892).
SAGER, O. S., and W. HOROWITZ: A chemical method for the determination of histamine in canned tuna fish. J. Ass. Offic. Agr. Chem. **40**, 892 (1957).
SANGER, F.: The free amino groups of insulin. Biochem. J. **39**, 507 (1945).
SCHAYER, R. W., Y. KOBAYASHI and R. L. SMILEY: Determination of histamine as an isotopic derivative. J. biol. Chem. **212**, 593 (1955).
SCHMALL, M., E. G. WOLLISH and J. GALENDER: Gravimetric determination of histamine. J. Amer. pharm. Ass. sci. Ed. **41**, 138 (1952).
SCHMIDT, F., u. I. GRUHN: Eine Methode zur Erfassung kleinster Histaminmengen. Naturwissenschaften **42**, 391 (1955).
—, u. D. VORHEISOR: Über die Isolierung und Bestimmung des Histamins mit Hilfe der Papierchromatographie. Naturwissenschaften **42**, 392 (1955).
SCHMITERLÖW, C. G.: Some remarks on determination of histamine with special reference to horse blood. Acta physiol. scand. **19**, 260 (1949).
SCHWARTZ, A., et A. RIEGERT: Le dosage de traces d'histamine dans le sang par le procédé de la permutite. Simplification de la technique primitive. C. R. Soc. Biol. (Paris) **123**, 801 (1936b).
— — Un procédé simple d'isolement quantitatif de l'histamine et de la tyramine dans le sérum (et le plasma) sanguin. C. R. Soc. Biol. (Paris) **123**, 219 (1936a).
— Technique du dosage de l'histamine dans le plasma et le sérum sanguins par la méthode de la permutite. Bull. Soc. chim. Biol. **34**, 835 (1952).
SHIFRINE, M., L. E. OUSTERHOUT, C. R. GRAU and R. H. VAUGHN: Toxicity to chicks of histamine formed during microbial spoilage of tuna. Appl. Microbiol. **7**, 45 (1959).
SHORE, P. A., A. BURKHALTER and V. H. COHN, JR.: A method for the fluorometric assay of histamine in tissues. J. Pharmacol. exp. Ther. **127**, 182 (1959).
— Personal communication (1961).
STEFANOVIC, V., D. CIRKOVIC and M. BRESJANEC: New color reaction for the identification and determination of histamine. Acta pharm. jugosl. **9**, 153 (1959); Chem. Abstr. **54**, 12480 (1960).
STEPANYAN, E. P.: Paper chromatographic method of estimating the amount of free histamine in the blood of normal and hypertensive persons. Klin. Med. (U.S.S.R.) **32**, 42 (1954); Chem. Abstr. **49**, 5562 (1955).
THOMPSON, W. L.: Measurement of plasma histamine concentration. Fed. Proc. **20**, 257 (1961).
THOUVENOT, J., N. FLAVIAN et R. WEBER: Sur une methode colorimetrique du dosage de l'histamine, mise au point. Bull. Soc. Chim. biol. (Paris) **39**, 1511 (1957).
URBACH, K. F., and L. GISCAFRÉ: Identification of histamine in blood by paper chromatography. Proc. Soc. exp. Biol. (N.Y.) **68**, 430 (1948).
WEDENISSOW, U.: New chemical method of testing blood histamine. Bull. Soc. Ital. Biol. Sper. **25**, 78 (1949); Chem. Abstr. **44**, 8405 (1950).
WEISS, M., u. N. SSOBOLEW: Über ein colorimetrisches Verfahren zur quantitativen Bestimmung des Histidins. Biochem. Z. **58**, 119 (1914); Chem. Abstr. 8, 1597 (1914).
WEISSBACH, H., W. LOVENBERG and S. UDENFRIEND: Characteristics of mammalian histidine decarboxylating enzyme (SC 1779) Biochem. biophys. Acta (Amst.) **50**, 177 (1961).
— T. P. WAALKES and S. UDENFRIEND: A simplified method for measuring serotonin in tissues; simultaneous assay of both serotonin and histamine. J. biol. Chem. **230**, 865 (1958).
WEST, G. B., and J. F. RILEY: Chromatography of tissue histamine. Nature (Lond.)**174**, 882 (1954).
WHITEHORN, J. C.: "Permutit" as a reagent for amines. J. biol. Chem. **56**, 751 (1923).
YUSEM, M.: Chemical estimation of histamine in "gastrin". Fed. Proc. **20** (1) 250, (1961).

Section D

Biological Determination of Histamine in Living Tissues and Body Fluids

By

I. Vugman and M. Rocha e Silva

With 5 Figures

The amounts of histamine that can be extracted from tissues and mammalian blood can be so small and the earliest methods of extraction and purification so laborious that they could not allow a satisfactory recovery for a quantitative chemical titration. Therefore, up to very recent times, the only accepted method for histamine estimation was the biological assay. By choosing appropriate conditions, the preparation could be rendered highly discriminative to estimate histamine in presence of other pharmacologically active principles which might contaminate the extracts.

In order to obtain a high level of discrimination, three main possibilities should be considered:

I. refinements in the methods of extraction;

II. choice of conditions to increase the specificity of the biological structure to be utilized in the assay;

III. application of statistically sound designs to operate the assay.

I. Methods of extraction suitable for the bio-assay

The methods of extraction to be presented in this Section differ from those described by McIntire in Chapter I, Section C, because they never attain such a high degree of purification as to allow a chemical titration of histamine. Nevertheless, since the biological structures to be used respond to other pharmacologically active materials which are likely to occur in the extracts, special care should be taken to avoid interference of such principles, either by destroying them, or blocking their action with suitable inhibitors previously added to the reacting biological structures. The commonest endogenous pharmacologically active agents to be found in tissue extracts and body fluids are acetylcholine, serotonin (5-HT), polypeptides (oxytocin, vasopressin, angiotensin, bradykinin, substance-P), catecholamines, and adenyl compounds. In many circumstances the amounts of histamine present in the extracts far exceed those of other agents in such a way that rather crude methods of extraction are suitable for a fairly good estimation of histamine, even without taking any special care to exclude other principles. Furthermore, prolonged boiling with concentrated HCl, after deproteinization of the extracts with trichloroacetic acid (TCA), will certainly eliminate all the active materials indicated above, with the exception of histamine itself.

Another aspect of the subject that greatly impressed earlier workers in the field was the idea that histamine being bound to tissues, drastic methods of extraction should be used in order to release it entirely from the inert material (mainly proteins) present in the extracts. This idea justified the complicated methods of deproteinization or total hydrolysis of the proteins to make sure the release of the whole activity for the assay. For instance, KUTSCHER (see ACKERMANN, 1910) made large use of a 50% tannin solution in an acid medium to coagulate the proteins and set free the amine. Also, lead acetate and other protein precipitants have been used in the past to deproteinize tissue extracts until it was verified that histamine appears quantitatively in the supernatant after precipitation of the proteins with a 10 to 15% TCA solution (BARSOUM and GADDUM, 1935; CODE, 1937a). Wide use was made in the past of the drastic and dangerous procedure of destroying the whole protein content of the extracts by total hydrolysis; for this purpose, the tissue was suspended in a 10 to 20% solution of HCl and refluxed for 30 hours in an electric heater. Though fastidious, this procedure and the subsequent steps to separate the active material from the voluminous bulk of inert material, were considered safe to avoid losses of the amine and the method was utilized in many physiological laboratories as a routine procedure for histamine extraction. With small improvements, this method was still the one preconized by BEST and MCHENRY (1930). However, any method involving prolonged boiling of large amounts of protein digests in concentrated HCl is likely to produce histamine by decarboxylation of the free histidine generated in the process of hydrolysis (ÅKERBLOM, 1941; SCHMITERLÖW, 1949). This inconvenience was to a large extent overcome by BARSOUM and GADDUM's method of boiling the extracts after removal of the bulk of proteins by TCA.

A further aspect of the problem which hindered progress in earlier days was the suspicion that all histamine extracted from tissues and body fluids resulted from a putrefaction process by which histidine would be decarboxylated by enzymes deriving from germs or from the tissues themselves. In 1919, ABEL and KUBOTA claimed to have demonstrated that histamine was a common constituent of extracts from several organs and tissues, and might account for their lowering effect on blood pressure and oxytocic activity upon the guinea pig uterus. This claim as applied to pituitary extracts was the object of a live controversy with DALE (see DALE, 1953) who concluded that the presence of histamine in the extracts obtained by ABEL and KUBOTA (1919) was mainly due to a partial putrefaction process occurring in the glands. Especially the assumption that histamine could be identified with the essential oxytocic principle of the pituitary gland was strongly opposed by DALE and shown to be grossly incorrect in the following years. But even the claim by ABEL and KUBOTA (1919) that histamine could be obtained in the form of a pure salt (picrate) by extraction from the pituitary gland or the earliest finding of BARGER and DALE (1911) of the presence of small amounts of histamine extracted from the gastro-intestinal mucosa, could not be accepted as convincing evidence that it was a normal constituent of the tissues and not an occasional product of some putrefactive alteration (BEST et al., 1927; DALE, 1953). These criticisms explain the caution of LEWIS (1924–1927) calling histamine-like (H-substance) any material obtained from the skin and displaying the pharmacological actions of histamine. It was only in 1927 that BEST et al. demonstrated beyond doubt that histamine as such is a natural constituent of tissues (spleen and liver). With similar methods of extraction, THORPE (1928) gave a first survey of the histamine content in several organs, showing that especially the lung, the skin, the liver and the spleen were rich sources of histamine. At the same time, HARRIS (1927) had no difficulty in showing that histamine itself and no hypothetical

H-substance was present in extracts of the skin of man and other mammals, in amounts that might explain LEWIS's triple response in the case of its release by noxious agents (see Chapter III, Section B).

A. Earlier methods of extraction

As indicated above early methods developed for the extraction and assay of histamine from tissues as those described by ABEL and KUBOTA (1919), HANKE and KOESSLER (1920) and BEST et al. (1927) were all rather laborious and time consuming. Actually they were neither sensitive nor quantitative. These methods were thus of little avail for detecting histamine in biological materials. The next important step was the method devised by BEST and MCHENRY (1930) which consisted in boiling the tissue in 10% HCl, removing the acid *in vacuo*, extracting the residue with alcohol, removing it by distillation and suspending the residue in water and, after neutralizing the remaining acid, assaying for histamine upon the cat's blood pressure.

B. Methods for extraction of histamine from blood

Barsoum and Gaddum's method: A decisive improvement was the method described by BARSOUM and GADDUM (1935) which was sufficiently sensitive to detect quantitatively minute amounts of the amine and was especially fitted for the assay of the histamine present in blood:

1. 10 ml of blood are added to 15 ml of 10% TCA and after standing from half to one hour are filtered by suction. The precipitate and filter paper are carefully washed twice with 5% TCA and the acid removed from the filtrate by repeated extraction with ethyl ether.

2. After evaporation of the ether, 10 ml of concentrated HCl are added to the filtrate which is boiled for 90 minutes with the aid of a reflux air condenser, water being added to prevent desiccation. Towards the end of the boiling period the volume is reduced to less than 5 ml, and following several additions of absolute alcohol, the residue is dried *in vacuo* on a hot water bath.

3. The residue is extracted three times with alcohol previously saturated with NaCl. The alcoholic extract is filtered, and then evaporated to dryness. The residue is taken up in about 2 ml of water, neutralized to litmus with N NaOH and the total volume is made up to 2.5 ml.

In step 1 proteins are precipitated by TCA and the histamine held inside the cells is liberated. When the blood is added to the precipitating acid, agitation should be sufficiently vigorous so as to prevent the formation of crusts of precipitate over the blood cells the interior of which might not be reached by the acid. When amounts of blood different from those stated are used for histamine extraction TCA should be added until precipitation is complete. Excess acid ensures a low pH in which histamine is stable and may be stored at room temperature for long periods.

In step 2, boiling of the filtrate with concentrated HCl is intended to destroy other pharmacologically active substances which may interfere with the accurate biological assay of histamine (BARSOUM and GADDUM, 1935).

Step 3 is primarily designed for the extraction of histamine from the dry residue. The purpose of the extraction with alcohol saturated with NaCl is to remove excess of inorganic salts, especially potassium salts. This is an important step since potassium ions in concentration higher than that in the perfusion fluid interfere with the assay of histamine (BARSOUM and GADDUM, 1935; CODE, 1937a).

Code's Method: Alterations in Barsoum and Gaddum's method have been introduced by CODE (1937a) especially in step 1 by suppressing the laborious extraction of TCA with ether. As TCA is destroyed by the prolonged boiling in concentrated HCl, the second step of the method provides already for the complete removal of TCA which is transformed into CO_2 and HCl. The other phases of Code's method are the same as in the original Barsoum and Gaddum method. However, since some histamine may be lost during the alcohol extraction in step 3, CODE proposed a direct extraction of the dry residue with water whenever the amount of potassium present in the residue is not high enough as to interfere with the biological assay. It may be enough to increase the potassium chloride concentration in the Tyrode utilized for the perfusion, when the guinea pig ileum is used for the assay, since high concentrations of potassium render the gut less sensitive to further additions of the ion. When the alcohol extraction is to be included in the procedure, histamine losses can be avoided and a good recovery obtained by repeating several times the extraction with absolute alcohol (ANREP et al., 1939; ZON et al., 1939; KWIATKOWSKI, 1941; CODE et al., 1947). According to Code's modification, in step 3 the dry residue is extracted 3 times with 2 ml of distilled water and the combined extracts are neutralized using bromothymol blue as indicator. For estimation upon the isolated guinea pig gut the final volume should be the same as that of blood taken for the extraction.

Criticisms have been raised against Barsoum and Gaddum's and Code's methods of extraction of histamine from blood, especially regarding the rather drastic procedure in step 2 of boiling with strong acid that might give anomalous high values, as some or even all histamine eventually found in extracts might come from the histidine originally present in the tissue and transformed into histamine by the chemical treatment. CODE and ING (1937) tried to meet this criticism by comparing the histamine content of boiled (with HCl) and unboiled TCA filtrates from blood and found the same histamine values after either treatment. Likewise EMMELIN et al. (1941), adding from 0.1 μg to 10 mg histidine to different 5 ml samples of Tyrode's solution, and then submitting them to combined TCA precipitation and boiling with concentrated HCl, could find no histamine-like activity in the final extracts. These findings were once more confirmed by EMMELIN (1945) by comparing the histamine content of plasmas of several animal species after ultrafiltration and after extraction according to Code's method and finding complete agreement between the values obtained by either procedure.

At variance with these findings, ÅKERBLOM (1941) found that by treating a 1 mg/ml histidine solution by Code's method, histamine appeared in the final solution in a concentration of 1 μg/ml. Such a transformation of histidine into histamine was confirmed by SCHMITERLÖW (1949) by submitting 1 mg/ml solutions of histidine to Code's method: the extracts induced a strong contraction of the guinea pig ileum and caused a marked fall in the cat's blood pressure, both effects being abolished by the antihistamine drug Lergitin. It should be stressed, however, that the yield of histamine from the extracted histidine solutions was fairly inconstant; sometimes two samples of histidine treated in exactly the same way gave widely different results. In 1949 SCHMITERLÖW developed a method for histamine extraction which avoided the boiling acid extraction and consisted of extracting the histamine solution with 2 volumes of alcohol at pH about 4, filtering, washing the precipitate with alcohol and final reduction of the combined alcohol extracts to a small volume by evaporation *in vacuo*. After dilution with water and adjusting the pH to neutrality the extract was tested biologically. Extraction of histamine from blood by this method yielded 0.065 μg/ml contrasting with 0.13 μg/ml obtained by Code's method. SCHMITERLÖW accounts for the differences in histamine yield between the two treatments by a transformation of histidine into histamine, which would not occur in his method.

The recovery of histamine in Barsoum and Gaddum's method and in its modification by CODE has been tested. CODE (1937a) added histamine to water and to blood and compared the values obtained by his extraction procedure. From water, the histamine was quantitatively recovered. For estimation of the recovered histamine CODE used blood that had previously been perfused through dog's kidney, a method which BEST and MCHENRY (1930) and STEGGERDA et al. (1935) had shown to remove practically all histamine. After the perfusion, histamine was added in varying amounts to the blood before submitting it to the extraction procedure. Ninety percent or more of the added histamine was recovered by Code's method. ANREP et al. (1939) also added histamine to Tyrode's solution and extracted it following the method proposed by BARSOUM and GADDUM and according to Code's modification. In both procedures the recovery was between 92 and 108%, although some differences were found. While 92 to 108% of the added histamine were recovered by Code's water extraction, only 92% were recovered by Barsoum and Gaddum's alcohol extraction. ANREP et al. (1939) have shown that such differences might be reduced by repeating the alcohol extraction twice, the histamine recovery being then of the same level as that by Code's method. On the other hand KWIATKOWSKI (1941) found that only 75–80% of the histamine added to blood could be recovered by Barsoum and Gaddum's method, inspite of four successive alcoholic extractions. The accuracy of Code's modified procedure was also tested by EMMELIN et al. (1941) who added histamine to blood plasma before precipitation with TCA. After the extraction procedure the histamine was assayed and the "observed values" compared to "calculated figures". Such comparison showed that an error of less than 11% occurs in Code's procedure. CODE et al. (1947) also found a satisfactory recovery (79–81%) of the histamine added to gastric juice and extracted by the same method, although the alcohol extraction was employed because of the high amount of potassium present in gastric juice.

C. Methods of histamine extraction from tissues

As rather great amounts of histamine are frequently present in tissues, and other pharmacologically active substances usually occur in minute quantities or are wholly absent, simpler methods of extraction can be used instead of the complex methods needed for the extraction from blood. A simplified method was introduced in 1937 (a) by FELDBERG and KELLAWAY. The tissue is cut into small pieces and thoroughly ground up in a mortar with quartz powder and a little Tyrode. Several times during the grinding the supernatant fluid is pipetted off and replaced by fresh Tyrode. The combined supernatant fluids are then brought to boiling, cooled and tested on the guinea pig ileum. TRETHEWIE (1938) used this method to extract histamine from dog's liver and has shown that boiling after grinding is a very important step in order to release the whole activity from the tissue. This method, as modified by DOUGLAS et al. (1951) and by FELDBERG and TALESNIK (1953), is at present widely used for the extraction of histamine from tissues: The tissue is cut into pieces in N HCl (about 2 ml/g) and ground up with a little sand in a mortar. During the grinding about 10 ml/g of distilled water are added. The extract is put into a flask, the mortar washed several times with a little saline solution and the washings added to the flask, the content of which is boiled for a minute or two and filtered through cotton wool. The filtrate can be either kept in the refrigerator or tested at once for histamine on the guinea pig ileum preparation after neutralization with N NaOH, using bromothymol blue as indicator, and then making up to a given volume. The acidification of the extract avoids histamine losses which would otherwise occur during the boiling at an alkaline pH. No substances which may interfere with the assay of histamine on the guinea pig ileum are usually present in tissues extracted according to this method.

II. Biological assay of histamine

Advantage had been taken of some of the pharmacological actions of histamine for the development of methods for its biological assay. Thus, methods based on the effects of histamine on the blood pressure and on smooth muscle rendered possible the identification and estimation of the histamine present in extracts from blood and tissues. Since the chemical assay of histamine is comparatively laborious and frequently not very sensitive, the simpler biological methods for the assay of histamine are still widely used. Furthermore, the more recent introduction of anti-histamine drugs acting rather specifically against histamine made the biological identification of histamine quite easy. On the other hand, the use of atropine and anti-serotonin drugs makes possible the inhibition of the action of acetylcholine and serotonin which eventually can be concomitantly released during experimental procedures.

A. Blood pressure assay

It has long been recognized that extracts from some organs are able to depress the blood pressure of several animal species when injected intravenously. When DALE and LAIDLAW (1910–1911) described the pharmacological actions of histamine it soon became apparent that the hypotensive action of organ extracts could be due to a contamination with histamine. Indeed, in the first attempts to demonstrate the presence of histamine bound to tissues as in the work of ABEL and KUBOTA (1919), ABEL and NAGAYAMA (1920), or when this demonstration was actually made (BEST et al., 1927; DALE and DUDLEY, 1929; THORPE, 1928) besides the chemical extraction and identification of pure histamine salts the main biological assay used was the action on blood pressure.

For the assay the animal, preferably the cat because of its smaller size, is anesthetized with ether, chloralose (80–100 mg/kg) or pentobarbital sodium (30 mg/kg). Careful attention should be paid to the level of the anesthesia, which should be kept at a constant and not very deep level, since changes in the depth of the anesthesia will change the sensitivity of the preparation to histamine. The blood pressure changes are recorded continuously from the carotid or femoral artery. The injections are given through a systemic vein to which a polythene tubing is tied. The tubing is connected to a burette from which 2 or 3 ml of physiological saline solution are delivered into the vein following each test injection.

B. Guinea pig ileum

In 1904 MAGNUS developed a technique for the study of the pharmacological actions of drugs upon isolated smooth muscle. Employing plain muscle from different organs, this technique has been widely used in the study of the pharmacological actions of histamine and in methods for its identification and estimation in tissue and blood extracts. SCHULTZ (1911) introduced the use of the guinea pig ileum, a great improvement in MAGNUS's technique, because of the great sensitivity of this preparation to histamine and because the fast muscle contraction and relaxation enable frequent additions of the test solution. The great sensitivity to histamine of the guinea pig ileum which is able to react to concentrations between 2.5×10^{-9} to 10^{-9} as shown by WATANABE (see FELDBERG and SCHILF, 1930), led GUGGENHEIM and LOEFFLER (1916) to analyze the quantitative relationship between concentration of histamine and intensity of contraction of the gut. Thus the basis for a method of quantitative assay of histamine by comparing the contractions of the guinea pig gut induced by the extracts and those induced by a standard solution of histamine was established.

Setting the preparation. For the assay, the classical apparatus of DALE (1912 to 1913), a perfusion bath designed for the use of isolated smooth muscle, is employed. A medium sized guinea pig (180–250 g) is killed with a blow on the head and bled from the jugular vein. The abdomen is opened through a midline incision, the abdominal contents exposed and the ileocecal junction identified. The terminal portion of the ileum is taken out (about 10–15 cm) and its lumen carefully washed with warm Tyrode solution (37° C). After washing, a small piece of the gut (2–3 cm) is cut and one of its ends is tied in position to the bottom of the perfusion chamber, while the other end is tied to a simple lateral writing lever or, preferably, a frontal writing lever (SCHILD, 1944). The remainder of the piece of gut is set aside and kept in Tyrode solution at room temperature or in a refrigerator at 4° C; if necessary another piece may be taken later and used for the assay. Before attaching the gut to the chamber, the openings at the ends of the gut should be enlarged through lateral cutting with scissors so that the perfusion fluids may flow freely in and out the gut when the liquid is changed. During the manipulation procedure, undue stretching or handling of the gut should be avoided. The length of the piece of gut should be the longest possible, but the wholly relaxed gut should always be fully immersed in the perfusion fluid, otherwise irregular contractions will ensue. The perfusion chamber should be of small capacity, about 3 ml, so that the test solution added will not be unduly diluted. It is also important that a constant level be kept inside the chamber so that all additions will be equally diluted. When large volumes are added the fluid level inside the chamber should have previously been lowered so as to avoid overspilling. Whenever the concentration of histamine in the extract differs to any great extent from that of the standard solution a previous dilution of the strongest sample will render possible the use of comparable volumes of both solutions.

Air or oxygen, delivered through a small opening at the bottom of the chamber should be continuously bubbled throughout the experiment. This aids to keep the gut in good living conditions and also ensures a fast mixing of the solution added to the perfusion fluids. Under these conditions contractions of the smooth muscle induced by histamine are fast and reproducible throughout the experiment. Air can be supplied by a small pump or by a simple system comprised of two Mariotte bottles standing at different levels. The intensity of the bubbling is regulated by a clamp placed on the rubber tubings.

Ionic influences. The fluid used in the perfusion bath is Tyrode solution as suggested by BARSOUM and GADDUM (1935). Modifications have been introduced in the original composition of Tyrode solution since it was shown that alterations in the concentration of calcium, potassium and magnesium ions improved the sensitivity of the gut to histamine.

Calcium is essential since when it is omitted from the solution no response to histamine is observed, while increasing two or three times its normal concentration diminishes the tonus and enhances the muscle sensitivity to histamine (KWIATKOWSKI, 1941). High concentrations of potassium induce spontaneous contractions and indeed if such concentrations are reached by adding the extracts, misleadingly high histamine values may be obtained (CODE, 1937a; ANREP et al., 1939; KWIATKOWSKI, 1941; CODE et al., 1947). High concentrations of magnesium decrease the sensitivity of the ileum to histamine (KOCHMANN, 1923) although its presence in the perfusion fluid is important for abolishing the spontaneous contractions of the gut. It can be wholly omitted if atropine is present in the Tyrode solution (FELDBERG and TALESNIK, 1953).

The total ion concentration of the perfusion fluid is also an important factor to the ileum response as shown by DALE (1913): an increase in the ion concentration diminishes the sensitivity of the gut to histamine, while a decrease of it increased the sensitivity. BUCHER (1951) compared the effect of different osmotic concentrations of Tyrode solution on the estimation of histamine using an inverted gut preparation. Alterations of $\pm$ 20% of the normal Tyrode osmotic pressure did not affect appreciably the assay, but hypertonic solutions seemed to affect more the histamine estimation than hypotonic solutions.

In Table 1 a modified Tyrode solution, as routinely used in this laboratory, is given. This solution may be prepared from stock solutions, the composition of which is also given in Table 1. From the amounts given, 20 liters of Tyrode solution may be prepared. These stock solutions may be kept at room temperature for several weeks.

Table 1. *Composition of modified Tyrode solution*

NaCl	8.00 g
KCl	0.20 g
$CaCl_2$	0.20 g
$MgCl_2$	0.10 g
$NaHCO_3$	1.00 g
NaH_2PO_4	0.05 g
Glucose	1.00 g
Distilled water	1,000 ml
Stock solution A	
NaCl	160.0 g
KCl	4.0 g
$CaCl_2$	4.0 g
$MgCl_2$	2.0 g
Distil. water to	1,000 ml
Stock solution B	
$NaHCO_3$	20.0 g
NaH_2PO_4	1.0 g
Distil. water to	1,000 ml

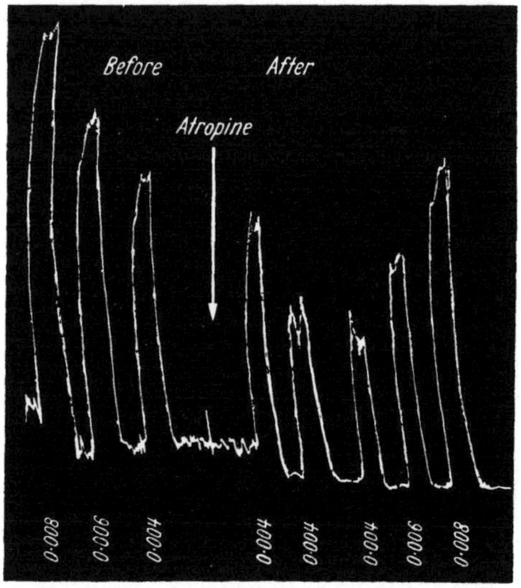

Fig. 1. Consecutive contractions of segment of guinea-pig ileum in response to 0.004—0.008 μg histamine before and after atropine is added to Tyrode's perfusion fluid to make concentration of 0.2 μg atropine sulfate per milliliter Tyrode's solution. Histamine is added each minute except during 2—3 minutes required for addition of atropine. After addition of atropine, note decline in sensitivity of gut to histamine, lowered base line, indicating increased relaxation, and more regular base line, indicating less spontaneous activity of gut. (According to CODE and MCINTIRE, 1956)

To prepare 1 liter of Tyrode solution 50 ml of stock solution *A* are mixed to about 800 ml of glass distilled water; 50 ml of stock solution *B* and 1 g of glucose are then added and the volume made up to 1 liter. The concentrated stock solutions should not be mixed together without previous dilution, otherwise some precipitation occurs.

Atropine sulfate is usually added to the Tyrode solution at a concentration of 0.1 to 0.2 μg/ml. The presence of atropine in the perfusion fluid helps the assay of histamine by abolishing spontaneous contractions, shortening the relaxation time of the gut, and blocking acetylcholine when present in the extracts. These advantages are counteracted by a reduction in the sensitivity of the ileum to histamine. Fig. 1 from CODE and MCINTIRE (1956) ilustrates the action of atropine on the gut. In the blood pressure assay, atropinization of the animal (1–2 mg of atropine sulfate injected intravenously) should also be used especially when acetylcholine is suspected to be present as a contaminant in the extract.

Influence of temperature. The temperature of the perfusion bath is usually maintained at 35° C. ZADINA (1939) has shown that from 20° C on, the height of contraction of the ileum by histamine increases when the temperature is raised, reaching its maximum at 31–32° C. The speed of contraction of the gut also increases by raising the temperature but reaches its maximum at 35° C only. CRABS (1962) has recently suggested the use of 30° C as the temperature of the bath; this would render the ileum free of spontaneous contractions and keep its sensitivity constant for long hours. However, the experience in this laboratory is that the sensitivity of the ileum can be kept constant at 35° C for more than 5 hours (ROCHA E SILVA, 1960).

Influence of pH. The interpretation of the results on the influence of pH on the reactivity of the ileum to histamine is frequently difficult because in such studies the effect of the hydrogen ion concentration is usually intermingled with the effect of the CO_2 concentration. Thus, GARAN (1938) has shown that by increasing the partial pressure of CO_2 in Tyrode the response of the ileum to histamine would be decreased even to the point of being abolished. GARAN (1938) demonstrated that at pH 7.5–8.0 the response of the ileum to histamine was maximal, this response decreasing at lower pH, and attributed this loss of reactivity to the formation of a carbamate compound, though SÖRENSENS's phosphate buffer instead of carbonate was used in the perfusion fluid. KIESE (1940) confirmed the inhibitory action of CO_2 on the guinea pig gut and showed that this inhibition could neither be due to formation of a histamine carbamate nor to electric changes in the histamine molecule itself but to changes in the tissue receptors. More recently, HALPERN (1956a, b) confirmed the reversible CO_2 inhibitory action and showed that this inhibition is not due to the anoxia indirectly created. This action of CO_2 would be rather specific upon the tissue receptors for histamine without influencing very much the receptors for acetylcholine and KCl. According to HALPERN et al. (1959) the lowered sensitivity of the ileum to histamine would be due to the increased concentration of carbonic acid in the Tyrode solution and not to the decrease in pH because when the bicarbonate buffer was replaced by a maleate buffer the sensitivity to histamine remained the same in spite of pH changes. ROCHA E SILVA (1960), using maleate buffered Tyrode as well as Tyrode with different concentrations of CO_2 was led to the conclusion that the loss in sensitivity of the ileum at lower pH is actually due to changes in pH and not to different CO_2 concentrations. However, since the curve of optimum activity of histaminase is very similar to that followed by the loss of reactivity of the ileum as caused by pH changes, and since histaminase inhibitors potentiate the effect of histamine upon the gut (ARUNLAKSHANA et al. 1954), the loss of sensitivity of the ileum could well be due to an increasing effect of the enzyme present in the gut. This possibility was tested by ROCHA E SILVA (1960) by adding to the Tyrode the powerful histaminase inhibitor aminoguanidine (SCHÜLLER, 1952) at a concentration of 2×10^{-6} M. Under these conditions, variations in gut sensitivity to histamine between pH 8.3 to 7.0 disappeared, but the fact that in some experiences the pH effect has been irreversible and that when the pH was lowered to 6.8 a sharp loss in sensitivity of the ileum was observed, ruled out the possibility of the sensitivity changes of the ileum to histamine being entirely caused by the activation of histaminase (see Chapter II, Section D II).

Dose-response curves. Within a certain range of doses the extent of contraction of the gut is linearly related to the logarithm of the dose of histamine added to the bath. For the assay the doses of histamine producing minimal responses as well as those producing maximal or near maximal responses should not be used, for the greatest differences in gut response to small dose variations are obtained when such extremes are avoided. According to EMMELIN et al. (1941) the most reliable results are obtained if the gut is allowed to contract between 10 and 60% of its maximal response. Below and above these limits the curves tend to bend upwards or downwards in a typical sigmoid curve.

Another way to rectify the dose-response curve is to make use of the reciprocals of the effects plotted against the reciprocals of the doses or concentrations. The theoretical basis for this procedure can be found in the inversion of CLARK's equation, which is obeyed over a large range of doses (ROCHA E SILVA, 1959). In Fig. 2a the responses in triplicate or quadruplicate to 4 doses of histamine are indicated and in Fig. 2b and c, the 3 kinds of plots (arithm., log-dose and reciprocals) are given for comparison.

The double reciprocal plot can give a better insight into the intimate mechanism of the phenomenon of drug-receptor interaction and especially a theoretical value

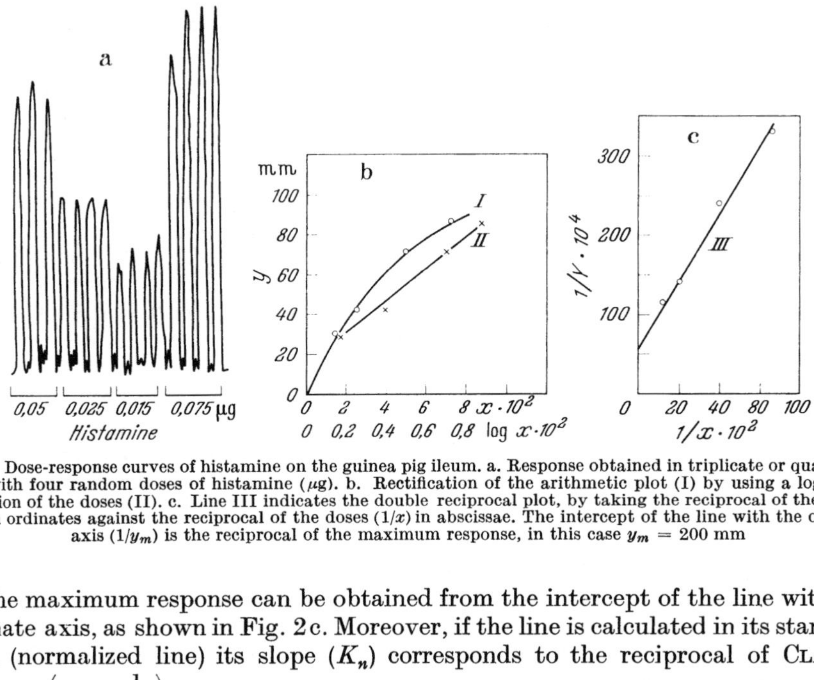

Fig. 2. Dose-response curves of histamine on the guinea pig ileum. a. Response obtained in triplicate or quadruplicate, with four random doses of histamine (μg). b. Rectification of the arithmetic plot (I) by using a log-transformation of the doses (II). c. Line III indicates the double reciprocal plot, by taking the reciprocal of the effects ($1/y$) in ordinates against the reciprocal of the doses ($1/x$) in abscissae. The intercept of the line with the ordinate axis ($1/y_m$) is the reciprocal of the maximum response, in this case $y_m = 200$ mm

for the maximum response can be obtained from the intercept of the line with the ordinate axis, as shown in Fig. 2c. Moreover, if the line is calculated in its standard form (normalized line) its slope (K_n) corresponds to the reciprocal of CLARK's constant $\left(K_n = \frac{1}{K_c}\right)$. For details see ROCHA E SILVA (1959, 1961) and Chapter II, Section D II.

Performance of the assay. A rather rigid time schedule of additions of doses to the bath should be followed for this helps to avoid changes in sensitivity of the gut to histamine. The contraction of the gut to histamine is usually complete in 30 seconds or less. Upon completion of the contraction the gut should be washed two or three times by changing the Tyrode solution which fills the bath. There follows the relaxation of the gut and a rest period, about one minute being allowed for both. Additions can then be made each $1^1/_2$ minutes. By keeping rigidly to this time schedule alternate doses of the standard histamine solution and unknown solution are added to the bath until equal contractions are obtained. Usually the doses of the standard are kept fixed and by varying the amounts of the unknown it is possible to bracket with two doses of the standard a certain equivalent dose of the unknown. Illustrations of this method can be found in many papers on the subject and especially in CODE (1937a), and CODE and MCINTIRE (1956).

Under the conditions described, when employing a 2–3 ml chamber, the gut is usually sensitive to less than 0.04 ml of a 1:5,000,000 histamine (base) standard solution. Addition of such volumes containing 0.008 μg of histamine base produces minimal contractions suitable for the assay. Extracts should be concentrated during the preparation whenever they contain less than 0.08 μg of histamine per ml, since volumes of extracts greater than 0.4 ml when added to the bath are liable to cause changes in ionic concentration, in pH, and in osmotic pressure which may affect the gut (CODE, 1937b). Large doses of histamine should be avoided for they produce a long lasting spasm of the gut that subsides slowly and makes the muscle refractory to further additions of small doses of histamine (BARSOUM and GADDUM, 1935). A depressed response of the gut to standard doses of histamine is also observed after maximal contractions produced by smooth muscle stimulating substances like acetylcholine and pilocarpine, this refractoriness being suppressed by KCl (CANTONI and EASTMAN, 1946). The intensity of this refractoriness is also dependent on the concentration of the stimulating substances previously applied (BERALDO and ROCHA E SILVA, 1949).

Since the common salts of histamine – the dihydrochloride ($C_5H_9N_3 \cdot 2\,HCl$) and the diphosphate ($C_5H_9N_3 \cdot 2\,H_3PO_4$) with molecular weights of 184 and 307 – contain 60.4 and 36.2% of the base respectively, it is necessary to express the results of the assay in terms of histamine base or mention the histamine salt used. Otherwise the quantitative comparison between the results of different authors becomes impossible. As the dihydrochloride salt of histamine is hygroscopic the diphosphate is usually preferred.

C. Superfusion techniques

When assaying extracts containing very low amounts of histamine the problem of reaching suitable concentrations of the amine in contact with the gut has led to the development of special techniques, since neither great volumes of the extract can be added nor the bath can conveniently be made much smaller than 2 ml. In order to solve this problem advantage had been taken of the method described by FINKLEMAN (1930) in which a piece of intestine is suspended in air and kept in good condition by a stream of nutrient fluid running over its surface. Such a preparation has been used for the assay of histamine by KWIATKOWSKI (1941) by injecting the drug into the stream of fluid as used by GADDUM et al. (1939). GADDUM (1953a) described an improved apparatus and showed that greater sensitivity can be obtained by applying the active solution undiluted to the surface of the muscle. GADDUM has called this technique superfusion, since the fluid runs over the tissue, by analogy with perfusion in which the fluid runs through the tissue. The apparatus, as described by GADDUM (1953) and shown in Fig. 3 can be described as follows.

The guinea pig ileum is suspended in air in the middle of a glass tube which is immersed in a water bath kept at a constant temperature. The water bath is attached to a vertical rod with the writing lever. The whole apparatus is subjected to slight vibration to diminish friction of the point on the drum. The Tyrode solution is kept in a reservoir 20–40 cm above the bath, and is warmed up before flowing to the gut. The rate of flow is controlled by a fine point of a capillary tube inside a wider glass tube both held by a rubber cap. The fluid drips at a rate of 1–5 ml per minute from a glass tube along the thread which attaches the gut to the writing lever. The end of this tube has been filed off at an acute angle in order to facilitate the administration of drugs. The height of the glass tube should be sufficient ($>$ 10 cm) for allowing each drop of the fluid to be broken up on reaching the tissue and thus wet it evenly and avoid drying one of its sides.

For the assay the flow of fluid is stopped for a standard time. The solutions to be tested are warmed before use and added by means of a teat pipette to the filed off end of the glass tube where the fluid form drops on falling off. A standard number of drops is added, generally 5 drops or about 0.2 ml in a short time (3–4 seconds). The size of the drops running down the thread does not depend on the pipette and their exact volume is not critical. The test solution is left in contact with the surface of the gut for a standard time (10 seconds) and then the normal flow is restarted. Since the fluids are applied directly to the tissue their pH and salt concentration should be the same of the superfusion fluid. Small differences in their composition may affect the result. For example, superfusion fluid diluted with only 5% of water has been found to cause a contraction of the guinea pig ileum.

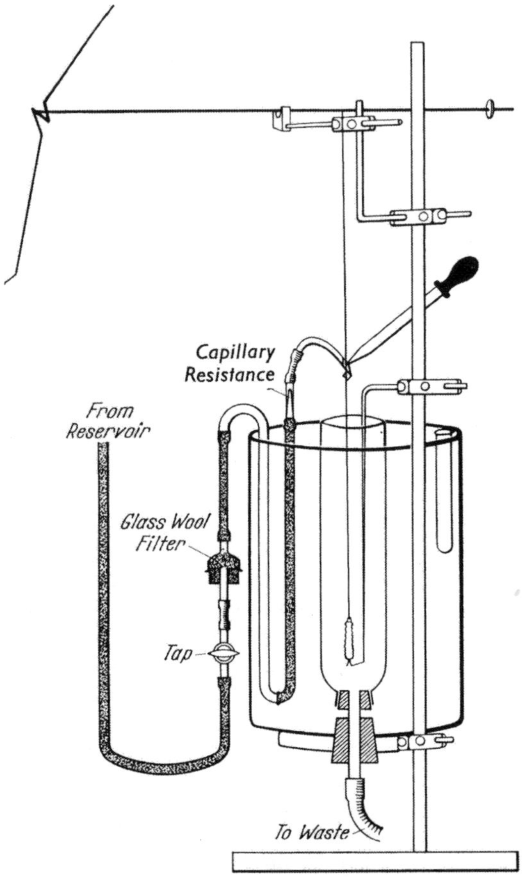

Fig. 3. Apparatus for superfusion technique (according to GADDUM, 1953)

When histamine is applied to the gut the contraction begins in less than 15 seconds but does not reach its maximum until about 20–30 seconds after the addition of the drug. By that time, the muscle has already been superfused with the drug-free fluid for a while. Addition of histamine can be made at intervals of 2 minutes. The contraction of the gut does not depend so much on the amount of fluid added but on the concentration of active drug in the solution applied to the muscle. The sensitivity of this method is similar to that which might be achieved with an usual 2 ml bath.

Another technique for assaying solutions containing low amounts of histamine has been described by BUCHER (1951) based on the demonstration made by FEIGEN and CAMPBELL (1946) that isolated intestinal strips respond to smooth muscle stimulating drugs only when the muscle comes into contact with them through the peritoneal surface. BUCHER uses small pieces of inverted gut, whose lumen constitutes a small chamber with 0.2 ml capacity. The gut with the mucosal surface turned outside is placed in a bath with Tyrode solution, while 3 to 5 ml of oxygenated Tyrode per minute run continuously through its lumen. For the assay, the flux of Tyrode is stopped and the histamine containing Tyrode is allowed to fill the inside of the gut. Upon reaching maximum contraction the solution is washed away by restarting the Tyrode flux. The sensitivity of the gut thus prepared is similar to that obtained with an usual bath.

D. Bronchiolar constriction

Histamine induced bronchiolar tone alterations can be measured by recording lung air volume changes. KONZETT and RÖSSLER (1940) developed a method in which the alterations of bronchiolar resistance are measured by recording the pressure in a semi-closed system connected with the lungs. EMMELIN et al. (1941) studied the sensitivity of the bronchiolar plain muscle using Konzett and Rössler's method. The histamine can be injected intravenously when the experiment is performed on the anesthetized animal or into the perfusion fluid when using the isolated lung. DELAUNOIS et al. (1956) developed a method for administering micromicelar aerosols to the isolated lungs of the guinea pig. Improvements in this method have also been described by JENDEN and TUREMAN (1956) and by JIMÉNEZ VARGAS (1951) increasing its sensitivity and making possible quantitative measurements of changes in bronchiolar tone.

III. A Four-point assay for histamine estimation

The standard method as described above of bracketing any addition of the unknown with two doses of the standard solutions, if suitable for practical purposes, does not allow any accurate calculation of the error of the method. In order to evaluate the confidence limits from the standard error of the mean rather complicated statistical designs can be applied. For the sake of simplicity, only a description of a four-point assay first employed by SCHILD (1942) for histamine estimations on the basis of the previous work by BLISS and MARKS (1939a, b) is going to be given. For the performance of the assay 2 doses of the standard (S_1 and S_2) and 2 doses of the unknown (U_1 and U_2) are selected to produce effects falling in the 20–80% range of the dose-response line and presenting the same ratio (D):

$$\frac{S_1}{S_2} = \frac{U_1}{U_2} = D \quad \text{Log } S_1 - \log S_2 = \log U_1 - U_2 = \log D \,.$$

Each random sequence of additions of the four doses will form a group, and at least four groups will constitute the whole assay. Instead of a complete randomized sequence, a Latin square (L^2) design which might be useful to identify any systematic variation due to the "order of additions" is selected. Examples of a L^2 Latin square design and a fully randomized one (5 groups of 4 doses) are presented in Table 2.

Table 2. *Examples of sequence of additions of 4 doses in $k = 4$ groups (L^2) and $k = 5$ groups (fully random)*

Groups	Sequence of additions: $L^2(k = 4)$ (Latin square)		Fully randomized ($k = 5$)
I	A B C D	I	B D C A
II	B C D A	II	C A D B
III	C D A B	III	A C B D
IV	D A B C	IV	C A D B
		V	D B A C

Note: The symbols A = U_1, B = S_1, C = U_2, D = S_2, represent the higher and lower doses of the unknown and the higher and lower doses of the standard.

From all values, the means of the responses ($\overline{Y}_{S_1}$, $\overline{Y}_{S_2}$, $\overline{Y}_{U_1}$ and $\overline{Y}_{U_2}$) corresponding to the higher and lower doses of the standard and the higher and lower doses of the unknown are plotted against the common logarithm interval of the doses (log D), as shown in Fig. 4. The individual responses (Y) and the total average ($\overline{Y}_t$) are utilized to calculate the total sum of squares [$(Y - \overline{Y}_t)^2$.]

If the totals for each dose are represented by the corresponding letters S_1, S_2, U_1 and U_2 and using orthogonal coefficients the three important contrasts

$$\theta = -S_1 - S_2 + U_1 + U_2$$
$$\varphi = +S_1 - S_2 + U_1 - U_2$$
$$\psi = +S_1 - S_2 - U_1 + U_2$$

will permit the calculation of the three parts into which the sum of squares corresponding to the variation due to "Doses" can be split:

"Between samples" $= \theta^2/4\,k = A^2$,

"Slope" $= \varphi^2/4\,k = B^2$ and

"Deviation from parallelism" $= \psi^2/4\,k = C^2$,

where k indicates the number of groups. The validity of the assay corresponds to an expectation $\psi = 0$, or to a variance ratio C^2/s^2 smaller than 5.12 (F) at a probability level of 5% and 9 degrees of freedom or in general $3(k-1)$ degrees of freedom. Contrariwise, the variance B^2 must be as large as possible when compared with the error variance (s^2) of the assay. The value of A^2 will of course depend upon the dilutions of standard and unknown. A preliminary assay should be done to make the potencies of both samples as near as possible by dilution in order to reduce the value of A^2 appearing in the expression of S_M. In fact the assay must be understood as providing for a "correction term" to be applied to that preliminary estimation of the ratio of potency.

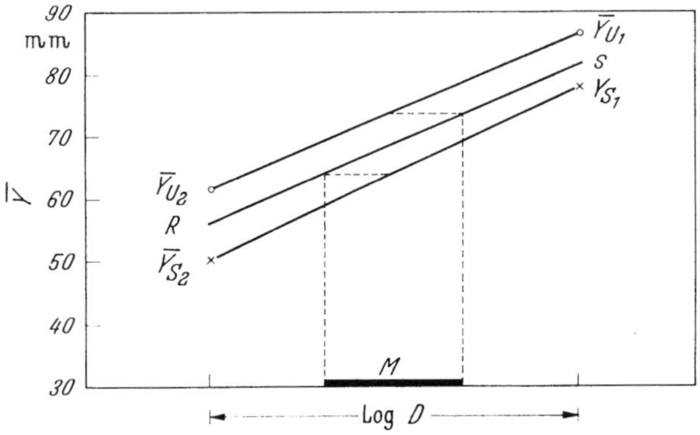

Fig. 4. The horizontal distance (M) of the lines to the mean regression line (RS) is the graphical representation of the log ratio of potency $M = \log U - \log S$

The first two contrasts presented above permit the calculation of the logarithmic ratio of potency

$$M = \frac{\theta \log D}{\varphi} = \frac{A \log D}{B} \qquad \log D = 0.301$$

and antilog $M = \frac{U}{S}$ will give the desired ratio of potency and therefore the estimation of histamine in μg/ml of the unknown. The expression log D equals 0.301, when the ratio of the doses $\left(\frac{U_1}{U_2} = \frac{S_1}{S_2}\right)$, equals 2.00. The slope of the mean regression line will be given by the formula

$$b = \frac{2\,\varphi}{4\,k \log D}$$

and the variance of the slope $s_b^2 = \frac{2\,s^2}{4\,k (\log D)^2}$ the standard deviation in terms of log dose indicated by $\lambda = s/b$ can measure the efficiency of the assay (GADDUM, 1953b); alternatively, the reciprocal of its square $1/\lambda^2$ is taken as the "inherent precision" of the assay.

The value of M (log ratio of potency) can be measured graphically on the horizontal distance of the two regression lines as indicated in Fig. 4.

For the calculation of the error of M, the simplified formula

$$S_M = \frac{s \log D \sqrt{A^2 + B^2}}{B^2}$$

can be used and the fiducial limits of the ratio of potency calculated in the conventional way by taking the antilogs ($M \pm S_M t$) where t is taken from a STUDENT'S table for a probability level of 5% and (n) degrees of freedom (those corresponding to the error of the assay in the analysis of variance). When the ratio b/s_b is lower than 7.8 the exact formula for S_M should be employed (BLISS, 1952) and the fiducial limits calculated by the formula:

$$CM \pm t\, S_M \sqrt{C}$$

where $C = B^2/(B^2 - s^2\, t^2)$ and the values of A and B are those appearing in the analysis of variance (Table 3).

Table 3. *Analysis of variance of data obtained in a 4-point assay*

Sources of variation	Degrees of freedom	Sum of squares	Variances	F
Total	$(N - 1)$	$\Sigma(Y - \bar{Y})^2 = H^2$	—	—
Between groups	$(k - 1)$	$\frac{\Sigma T_g^2}{4} - \frac{T^2}{N} = G^2$	$G^2/(k - 1)$	G^2/s^2
Between doses	3	$A^2 + B^2 + C^2 = E^2$	$E^2/3$	E^2/s^2
a) Between samples . . .	1	A^2	A^2	A^2/s^2
b) Slope (regression) . . .	1	B^2	B^2	B^2/s^2
c) Deviation from parallelism	1	C^2	C^2	C^2/s^2
Error (by difference) . . .	$3(k - 1)$	$H^2 - (G^2 + E^2)$	s^2	—

st. dev. $= \sqrt{s^2} = s$

An example of a four point assay is given below. The concentrations of the solutions were $U = 1 \times 10^{-6} = 1$ µg/ml and $S = 0.75 \times 10^{-6} = 0.75$ µg/ml. In Table 4 the contractions in mm of the guinea pig upon the different additions are given.

Table 4. *Responses (in mm height) of a piece of guinea pig ileum in a 4-point assay of histamine estimation*

Doses \ Groups	I	II	III	IV	V	Totals (Td)	Averages
0.20 ml U_1	93	90	88	75	92	438 (U_1)	87.6
0.10 ml U_2 . . .	67	65	57	56	66	311 (U_2)	62.2
0.20 ml S_1	81	78	80	70	84	393 (S_1)	78.6
0.10 ml S_2	50	50	49	46	57	252 (S_2)	50.4
Totals (Tg)	291	283	274	247	299	T = 1394	69.7

Table 5 gives the analysis of variance of data presented in Table 4, with details of calculation of the main statistics pertinent to the experiment. The final histamine estimation is given in µg/ml.

Table 5. *Analysis of variance of data of Table 4*

Sources of variation	Degrees of freedom	Sum of squares	Mean squares	F	P
Total	19	4,642.2	—	—	—
Between groups . .	4	402.2	100.5	12.28	<0.001
Between doses . .	3	4,141.8	—	—	—
a) between samples	1	—	540.8	66.11	<0.001
b) slope	1	—	3,591.8	439.09	<0.001
c) parallelism. . .	1	—	9.8	1.19	>0.20
Error (by difference)	12	98.2	$s^2 = 8.18$	—	—

Contrasts:

$$\theta = -393 - 252 + 438 + 311 = 104$$
$$\varphi = +393 - 252 + 438 - 311 = 268$$
$$\psi = +393 - 252 - 438 + 311 = 14$$

Log ratio of potency:

$$M = \frac{\theta \log D}{\varphi} = \frac{104 \times 0.301}{268} = 0.1168$$

$$\text{Antilog } M = \frac{U}{S} = 1.31 \text{ (found)}$$

$$\frac{U}{S} = 1.33 \text{ (real)}$$

Slope of the mean regression line: $b = \frac{2\varphi}{20 \log D} = 89.03$

Variance of the slope: $s_b^2 = \frac{2 s^2}{20 (\log D)^2} = 9.03$

Standard deviation of the assay: $s = \sqrt{8.18} = 2.86$

Standard deviation in term of log-dose: $\lambda = \frac{s}{b} = \frac{2.86}{89.03} = 0.032$

Standard error of the log ratio of potency (M):

$$S_M = \frac{S \log D \sqrt{A^2 + B^2}}{B^2} = 0.014$$

Confidence limits ($P = 0.05$):

$$FL = M \pm tS_M = \begin{cases} 0.1168 + 2.18 \times 0.014 = 0.1494 \\ 0.1168 - 2.18 \times 0.014 = 0.0840 \end{cases}$$

Antilog FL $= \begin{cases} 1.410 \\ 1.213 \end{cases}$ 1.31 (found) 5 % probability

Limits of error in % $\begin{cases} 107\,\% \\ 94\,\% \end{cases}$

Histamine content in ml of the unknown = 0.99 μg to compare with the theoretical 1.00 μg/ml.

Automatic assay of histamine. An apparatus designed for assay work on isolated organs and especially fitted to be used in a four-point assay has been described by Boura et al. (1954). This apparatus adds and removes the drug solutions, washes the tissue and controls rotation of the drum automatically. The different test solutions can be added to the tissue chamber in any pre-selected sequence. Fig. 5 shows the drug reservoirs, warming tube and isolated-organ chamber of this apparatus. The test solutions are kept in the drug reservoirs in their final dilution.

When air is allowed into the drug reservoir, the test solution runs through the warming jacket filling the organ chamber. The filling and emptying of this chamber with the different test solutions are controlled by electromagnetic valves, while the timing of the operations is controlled by a switching unit.

For a four-point assay the sensitivity of the gut is established and the concentrations of the test solutions to be used in the assay determined by a preliminary assay. If necessary the solutions are diluted so that their concentration will fall

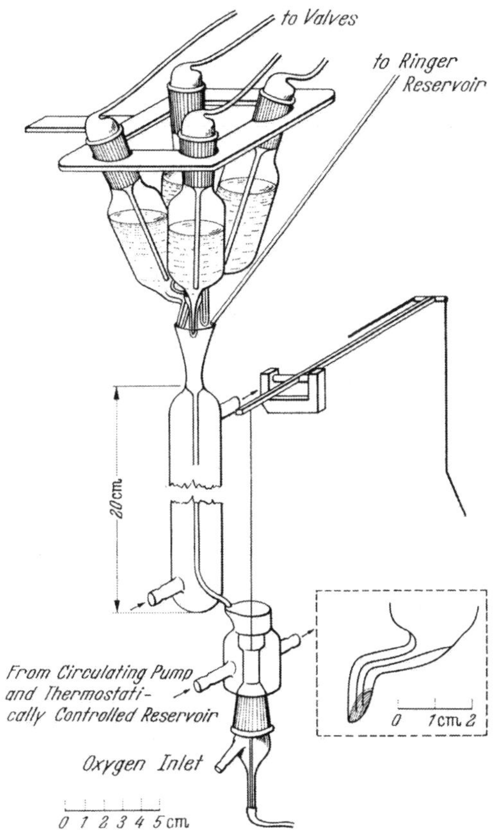

Fig. 5. Drug reservoirs, warming tube and isolated-organ bath. Inset illustrates the bevelled end of the drug delivery tube. For explanation, see text. (According to BOURA et al. 1954)

within the range of sensitivity of the gut and have approximately the same activity as that of the standard solution. Half diluted standard and test solutions are prepared and the higher and lower concentrated solutions are then filled into the four drug reservoirs. The assay is then conducted automatically in the manner previously described.

IV. Histamine content of organs and body fluids

Table 6 gives the histamine content of organs and body fluids determined using the methods of extraction and biological assay previously described.

Table 6. *Histamine content of organs and body fluids* (μg of histamine base per g or ml)

Material	Range of histamine content	Authors
Appendix		
rat	10.0	Rose and Browne (1938)
Aqueous humour		
guinea pig	0.095—0.300	Emmelin (1945)
rat	0.100—0.350	Emmelin (1945)
cat	0.025—0.150	Emmelin (1945)
Bile		
dog	0.75	Ungar and Pocoulé (1937)
Blood		
whole		
rabbit	9.60—12.00	Barsoum and Gaddum (1935)
rabbit	0.59—2.66	Code (1937a)
rabbit	0.22	Riesser (1937)
rabbit	7.30	Tarras-Wahlberg (1937)
rabbit	0.96—3.75	Zon et al. (1939)
rabbit	0.54—2.34	Dragstedt and Rocha e Silva (1941)
rabbit	1.80—5.00	Minard (1941)
rabbit	0.90—8.60	Wilson (1941)
rabbit	2.40—3.80	Rocha e Silva and Essex (1942)
rabbit	0.07—2.80	Rocha e Silva, Graña and Porto (1945)
rabbit	0.40—3.15	Graña and Rocha e Silva (1945)
rabbit	2.20—3.51	Code et al. (1953)
man	0.03—0.04	Barsoum and Gaddum (1935)
man	0.027—0.050	Barsoum and Gaddum (1936)
man	0.050—0.11	Barsoum and Smirk (1936a)
man	0.01—0.08	Haworth and Macdonald (1937)
man	0.15—0.20	Riesser (1937)
man	0.016—0.042	Ungar et al. (1937)
man	0.025—0.08	Rose and Browne (1940)
man	0.057—0.090	Valentine and Lawrence (1948)
man	0.082	Lowry et al. (1954)*
man	0.045—0.084	Nilzén (1947)
infant (at birth)	0.025—0.130	Mitchell and Cass (1959)
child ($1^1/_2$—12 years)	0.020—0.080	Mitchell and Cass (1959)
cat	<0.013	Barsoum and Gaddum (1935)
cat	0.015	Tarras-Wahlberg (1937)
cat	0.042—0.052	Code and Jensen (1941)
dog	0.040—0.075	Barsoum and Gaddum (1935)
dog	0.000—0.016	Code (1937b)
dog	0.000—0.040	Code (1939)
dog	0.025—0.035	Minard (1941)
guinea pig	1.00—1.50	Barsoum and Gaddum (1935)
guinea pig	0.08—0.19	Riesser (1937)
guinea pig	0.066—0.184	Code (1939)
guinea pig	0.05—0.30	Rocha e Silva and Essex (1942)
guinea pig	0.13—0.90	Giertz and Hahn (1955)
rat	0.05	Rose and Browne (1938)
rat	0.03	Rose and Browne (1941)
horse	0.028—0.033	Code and Hester (1939)
horse	0.027—0.033	Code and Jensen (1941)
calf	0.000—0.027	Code and Hester (1939)
cow	0.015	Code and Jensen (1941)
bullock	0.05	Code (1937b)
goat	0.127—0.162	Code (1937b)
swine	1.0	Baxter et al. (1954)
platelets		
rabbit	1.20—3.80	Minard (1941)
man	0.038	Parrot and Gabe (1945)
dog	0.70—0.50	Minard (1941)
horse	0.50	Code (1937c)

Table 6 (Continuation)

Material	Range of histamine content	Authors
plasma		
man	0.004—0.008	Barsoum and Smirk (1936a)
man	0.002—0.010	Barsoum and Smirk (1936b)
man	0.001—0.005	Anrep et al. (1944b)
man	0.017	Parrot and Gabe (1945)
man	0.0014	Lowry et al. (1954)*
man (foetal)	<0.01—0.067	Wicksell (1949)
infant (at birth) . . .	<0.005—0.020	Mitchell and Cass (1959)
child ($1^1/_2$—12 years) .	<0.003—0.014	Mitchell and Cass (1959)
rabbit	0.019—0.056	Code (1937b)
horse	0.000—0.069	Code (1937b)
cat	<0.10	MacIntosh and Paton (1949)
cat	0.01	Smith (1953a)
cat	0.005—0.05	Smith (1953b)
dog	0.000—0.05	Code (1939)
rat	0.03	Mota (1958)
guinea pig.	0—0.22	Mota and Vugman (1956)
guinea pig.	0.03—0.25	Giertz and Hahn (1955)
serum		
guinea pig.	0.10—0.45	Giertz and Hahn (1955)
buffy coat		
man	0.076—0.080	Lowry et al. (1954)*
rabbit	1.34—2.04	Code (1937b)
dog	0.00—0.07	Code (1939)
horse	0.024—0.052	Code (1937b)
erythrocytes		
man	0.11—0.18	Barsoum and Smirk (1936a)
man	0.05—0.20	Barsoum and Smirk (1936b)
man	0.000—0.004	Lowry et al. (1954)*
rabbit	0.012—0.049	Code (1937b)
horse	0.000—0.014	Code (1937b)
dog	0.000	Code (1939)
eosinophile		
man	0.007	Parrot and Gabe (1945)
mononucleocyte		
man	0.002	Parrot and Gabe (1945)
lymphatic leukemia		
man	0.021—0.10	Code and Macdonald (1937)
myeloid leukemia		
man	1.70—17.5	Code and Macdonald (1937)
eosinophilia		
man	0.40—1.00	Code and Macdonald (1937)
Blood vessels		
aorta		
man	4.2	Stone et al. (1955)*
ox	10.0	Riley and West (1953)
pig	0.7	Riley and West (1953)
inferior vena cava		
ox	20.0	Riley and West (1953)
Bone marrow		
man	3.3	Stone et al. (1955)*
guinea pig.	10.4—22.1	Code and Jensen (1941)
rabbit	6.66—11.05	Code and Jensen (1941)
cat	3.05—13.12	Code and Jensen (1941)
dog (reddish)	0.384—0.958	Code and Jensen (1941)
dog (yellowish) . . .	0.070—0.781	Code and Jensen (1941)
horse (reddish). . . .	2.00—2.06	Code and Jensen (1941)
horse (yellow)	0.00—0.017	Code and Jensen (1941)
cow (yellow)	0.027	Code and Jensen (1941)

Table 6 (Continuation)

Material	Range of histamine content	Authors
Caecum		
rat	13.0—15.0	MARSHALL (1943)
Cartilage		
ear		
hog	2.0	RILEY and WEST (1956)
ox	5.5	RILEY and WEST (1956)
Colon		
cat	8.0—16.0	SMITH (1953b)
Duodenum		
man	14.0	STONE et al. (1955)*
cat	29.0—50.0	SMITH (1953b)
mucosa		
dog	35.0—112.0	FELDBERG and HARRIS (1953)
Embryo		
chick (4 days)	traces	MISRAHY (1946)
chick (9 days)	0.020	MISRAHY (1946)
chick (11—13 days)	0.052—0.104	MISRAHY (1946)
chick (14—16 days)	0.204—0.304	MISRAHY (1946)
chick (17—18 days)	0.520—0.712	MISRAHY (1946)
chick (19—20 days)	0.912—1.040	MISRAHY (1946)
chick (just hatched)	1.144	MISRAHY (1946)
chick (24 hours after hatching)	1.360	MISRAHY (1946)
chick (48 hours after hatching)	1.640	MISRAHY (1946)
rat (9 days)	0.68	MISRAHY (1946)
rat (11 days)	1.60	MISRAHY (1946)
rat (14 days)	2.80	MISRAHY (1946)
rat (15 days)	3.20	MISRAHY (1946)
rat (16 days)	3.40	MISRAHY (1946)
rat (18 days)	3.76	MISRAHY (1946)
rat (19 days)	4.24	MISRAHY (1946)
rat (20 days)	5.48	MISRAHY (1946)
rat (at birth)	6.32	MISRAHY (1946)
Gastric juice		
dog	0.20—0.50	UNGAR and POCOULÉ (1937)
cat	0.006—0.055	EMMELIN and KAHLSON (1944)
Heart		
rat	1.70—2.50	FELDBERG and TALESNIK (1953)
rat	4.28—5.50	MARSHALL (1943)
man	1.60	STONE et al. (1955)*
Hypophysis		
man	3.50—4.65	WERLE and WEICKEN (1949)
ox	6.30—7.70	WERLE and WEICKEN (1949)
Ileum		
rat	5.5	MOTA et al. (1956)
dog	28.0	FELDBERG and HARRIS (1953)
cat	14.0—32.0	SMITH (1953b)
guinea pig	8.5—20.0	SCHILD (1939)
Jejunum		
rat	5.0—6.00	ROSE and BROWNE (1938)
rat	1.09—4.80	ROSE and BROWNE (1941)
rat	6.30—8.78	MARSHALL (1943)
rat	19.0	EISEN, ELLIS and WILSON (1956)
rat (adult)	35.0	BEAUMARIAGE and LECOMTE (1958)
cat	11.0—55.0	HAEGER and KAHLSON (1952)
cat (gl. layer)	3.5—41.2	HAEGER and KAHLSON (1952)
cat (musc. layer)	3.1—15.3	HAEGER and KAHLSON (1952)
cat	19.0—38.0	SMITH (1953b)
cat (before birth)	0.1—1.0	WATON (1963)

Table 6 (Continuation)

Material	Range of histamine content	Authors
cat (at birth)	1.0—5.0	WATON (1963)
cat ($2^1/_4$ days old) . .	1.0—5.0	WATON (1963)
rabbit	0.4—2.7	ROSE (1941)
rabbit	8.4	BEAUMARIAGE and LECOMTE (1958)
chicken	71.9	BEAUMARIAGE and LECOMTE (1958)
Kidney		
rat	0.00—0.40	ROSE and BROWNE (1938)
rat	1.04—1.86	MARSHALL (1943)
cat	0.02—0.77	HAEGER and KAHLSON (1952)
cat	0.80—2.00	SMITH (1953b)
cat (before birth) . .	0	WATON (1963)
cat (at birth)	0	WATON (1963)
cat ($2^1/_4$ days old) . .	0	WATON (1963)
dog	1.0	CASS et al. (1954)
man	2.5	STONE et al. (1955)*
Liver		
rat	2.0—4.0	ROSE and BROWNE (1938)
rat	<0.2—2.8	GOTZL and DRAGSTEDT (1940)
rat	1.0—4.3	ROSE and BROWNE (1941)
rat	2.43—7.72	MARSHALL (1943)
rat	0.30	RILEY and WEST (1953)
rat	0.50	MOTA et al. (1956)
rabbit	1.0—4.0	TRETHEWIE (1939)
rabbit	0.8—3.0	ROSE (1941)
man	2.5	STONE et al. (1955)*
dog	20.0—110.0	FELDBERG and KELLAWAY (1937b)
dog	31.0—62.0	TRETHEWIE and DAY (1949)
dog	25.0	CASS et al. (1954)
dog	13.0—108.0	MOTA, FERRI and JUNQUEIRA (1956)
dog (foetal)	5.0	DRAGSTEDT et al. (1940)
guinea pig.	1.0—3.3	GIERTZ and HAHN (1955)
cock	3.0—10.0	BEAUMARIAGE and LECOMTE (1956)
cat (before) birth) . .	0—1.0	WATON (1963)
cat (at birth)	0.1—1.0	WATON (1963)
cat ($2^1/_4$ days old) . .	0.1—1.0	WATON (1963)
capsule		
dog	24.0	RILEY and WEST (1953)
ox	40.0	RILEY and WEST (1953)
cow	22.0	RILEY and WEST (1953)
cow (young)	5.0	RILEY and WEST (1953)
sheep.	35.0	RILEY and WEST (1953)
pig	10.0	RILEY and WEST (1953)
cat	1.0	RILEY and WEST (1953)
parenchyma		
dog	22.0	RILEY and WEST (1953)
ox	5.0	RILEY and WEST (1953)
cow	5.0	RILEY and WEST (1953)
cow (young)	1.0	RILEY and WEST (1953)
sheep.	6.0	RILEY and WEST (1953)
pig	8.0	RILEY and WEST (1953)
cat	1.0	RILEY and WEST (1953)
Lung		
rat	4.0—10.0	ROSE and BROWNE (1938)
rat	3.6—10.9	GOTZL and DRAGSTEDT (1940)
rat	5.5—9.1	ROSE and BROWNE (1941)
rat	4.38—5.4	MARSHALL (1943)
rat (adult)	10.5	BEAUMARIAGE and LECOMTE (1958)
dog	20.0—220.0	FELDBERG and KELLAWAY (1937b)
dog	25.0	CASS et al. (1954)
monkey	80.0—100.0	FELDBERG and KELLAWAY (1938)

Table 6 (Continuation)

Material	Range of histamine content	Authors
guinea pig	5.0—95.0	FELDBERG and KELLAWAY (1937a)
guinea pig	3.3—50.0	MACKAY (1937)
guinea pig	5.0—22.8	GIERTZ and HAHN (1955)
guinea pig	19.0	MONGAR and SCHILD (1953)
guinea pig (at birth)	39.0—83.0	TRETHEWIE (1947)
guinea pig (1—4 days)	133.0—300.0	TRETHEWIE (1947)
guinea pig (8 weeks)	43.0—90.0	TRETHEWIE (1947)
guinea pig (20 weeks)	14.0—105.0	TRETHEWIE (1947)
guinea pig (40 weeks)	48.0—138.0	TRETHEWIE (1947)
guinea pig (foetal)	<0.02	TRETHEWIE (1947)
guinea pig	17.5—54.2	MOTA and VUGMAN (1956)
cock	8.0—51.0	BEAUMARIAGE and LECOMTE (1956)
chicken	15.4	BEAUMARIAGE and LECOMTE (1958)
rabbit	7.0—26.6	ROSE (1941)
rabbit	13.9	BEAUMARIAGE and LECOMTE (1957)
rabbit	13.3	BEAUMARIAGE and LECOMTE (1958)
cat	8.0—175.0	FELDBERG and KELLAWAY (1937a)
cat	15.0—48.0	SMITH (1953b)
cat (kitten)	<10.0	FELDBERG and KELLAWAY (1937b)
cat (1.5—3 kg)	10.0—60.0	FELDBERG and KELLAWAY (1937b)
cat (3—6 kg)	10.0—175.0	FELDBERG and KELLAWAY (1937b)
cat (young)	4.0	RILEY and WEST (1953)
cat (adult)	36.0	RILEY and WEST (1953)
cat (before birth)	0—1.0	WATON (1963)
cat (at birth)	1.0—5.0	WATON (1963)
cat ($2^1/_4$ days old)	1.0—5.0	WATON (1963)
cow (young)	8.0	RILEY and WEST (1953)
cow (adult)	25.0	RILEY and WEST (1953)
man (young)	6.0	RILEY and WEST (1953)
man (adult)	25.0	RILEY and WEST (1953)
man	33.0	STONE et al. (1955)*
pleura		
ox	200.0	RILEY and WEST (1953)
sheep	80.0	RILEY and WEST (1953)
pig	40.0	RILEY and WEST (1953)
cat	38.0	RILEY and WEST (1953)
cow	25.0	RILEY and WEST (1953)
dog	35.0	RILEY and WEST (1953)
parenchyma		
ox	80.0	RILEY and WEST (1953)
sheep	60.0	RILEY and WEST (1953)
pig	20.0	RILEY and WEST (1953)
cat	32.0	RILEY and WEST (1953)
cow	25.0	RILEY and WEST (1953)
dog	20.0	RILEY and WEST (1953)
Lymph node		
rabbit	1.60—3.30	CODE (1937c)
dog	4.0	CASS et al. (1954)
Mast cell tumour		
dog	277.0—1.290	CASS et al. (1954)
man	950	RILEY and WEST (1953)
man	555	RILEY and WEST (1953)
Mesentery		
rat	12.0	RILEY and WEST (1953)
guinea pig	7.70—20.0	MOTA and VUGMAN (1956)
Muscle		
guinea pig	3.0—5.0	ROCHA E SILVA and DRAGSTEDT (1941)
rat	8.7	MARSHALL (1943)
man	0.97	STONE et al. (1955)*
dog (foetal)	0.10	DRAGSTEDT et al. (1940)

Table 6 (Continuation)

Material	Range of histamine content	Authors
diaphragm		
rat	11.0—24.2	ROCHA E SILVA and SCHILD (1949)
rat	6.4—11.0	FELDBERG and TALESNIK (1953)
rat	7.0—41.0	VUGMAN (1961)
cat	1.9—4.0	SMITH (1953b)
gastrocnemius		
dog	2.7—6.1	ANREP et al. (1939)
rat	2.2—3.0	FELDBERG and TALESNIK (1953)
cat	1.4—2.8	SMITH (1953b)
Nervous tissue		
brachial plexus		
cat	0.56—2.5	KWIATKOWSKI (1943)
dog	2.10—2.3	KWIATKOWSKI (1943)
dog	7.7	WERLE and PALM (1950)
man	1.30—1.7	KWIATKOWSKI (1943)
man	1.4	WERLE and WEICKEN (1949)
guinea pig.	1.40—5.0	KWIATKOWSKI (1943)
guinea pig.	6.3	WERLE and WEICKEN (1949)
monkey	1.4	KWIATKOWSKI (1943)
rat	3.0—6.5	KWIATKOWSKI (1943)
rabbit	0.3—0.6	KWIATKOWSKI (1943)
sciatic nerve		
cat	0.9—3.0	KWIATKOWSKI (1943)
dog	2.4—2.5	KWIATKOWSKI (1943)
dog	4.9—7.7	WERLE and PALM (1950)
man	2.2—3.0	KWIATKOWSKI (1943)
ox	7.3—12.6	WERLE and WEICKEN (1949)
ox	11.9	EULER (1956)
guinea pig.	1.6—5.0	KWIATKOWSKI (1943)
guinea pig.	16.1—28.0	WERLE amd WEICKEN (1949)
monkey	2.2	KWIATKOWSKI (1943)
rat	3.4—13.0	KWIATKOWSKI (1943)
rabbit	0.3—0.95	KWIATKOWSKI (1943)
tibial nerve		
man	3.5—7.0	WERLE and WEICKEN (1950)
median nerve		
man	9.1	WERLE and WEICKEN (1950)
motor nerves		
man	<0.1—2.8	KWIATKOWSKI (1943)
man	1.5—4.3	KWIATKOWSKI (1943)
cat	0.34—1.8	KWIATKOWSKI (1943)
cat	2.0—2.7	KWIATKOWSKI (1943)
sensory nerves		
man	<0.1	KWIATKOWSKI (1943)
cat	<0.1	KWIATKOWSKI (1943)
dog	<0.1	KWIATKOWSKI (1943)
rabbit	<0.1	KWIATKOWSKI (1943)
sensory nerves (from skin)		
man	1.0—11.0	KWIATKOWSKI (1943)
cat	1.6—11.0	KWIATKOWSKI (1943)
rabbit	1.4—6.5	KWIATKOWSKI (1943)
skin nerves		
ox	8.4	WERLE and WEICKEN (1949)
phrenic nerve		
dog	2.9—4.9	WERLE and PALM (1950)
ox	19.6	EULER (1956)
intercostal nerve		
dog	4.2—4.9	WERLE and PALM (1950)
man	1.4—2.8	WERLE (1956)
ox	13.5—20.0	WERLE (1956)

Table 6 (Continuation)

Material	Range of histamine content	Authors
vagus nerve		
cat	2.1—4.5	Kwiatkowski (1943)
dog	4.5	Kwiatkowski (1943)
dog	9.1—12.6	Werle and Palm (1950)
man	2.25—2.1	Kwiatkowski (1943)
man	1.4—2.1	Werle (1956)
guinea pig.	6.7	Kwiatkowski (1943)
rabbit	0.7	Kwiatkowski (1943)
ox	10.5—14.0	Werle and Weicken (1949)
ox	16.8	Euler (1956)
monkey	0 <0.3	Kwiatkowski (1943)
splancnic nerve		
dog	5.6—11.9	Werle and Palm (1950)
ox	32.9—35.0	Werle (1956)
ox	65.0	Euler (1956)
man	3.5—7.0	Werle (1956)
splenic nerve		
dog	8.4—13.3	Werle (1956)
brain		
ox	0.07—0.7	Euler (1956)
rat	traces	Marshall (1943)
rat	0.053	Carlini and Green (1963)
rat	0.246	Carlini and Green (1963)*
cortex		
cat	0 <0.2	Kwiatkowski (1943)
dog	0.1—0.16	Kwiatkowski (1943)
guinea pig.	0.05	Kwiatkowski (1943)
rabbit	0.05	Kwiatkowski (1943)
ox	0.7—1.05	Werle and Weicken (1949)
cerebellum		
cat	1.5—2.0	Kwiatkowski (1943)
dog	1.5	Kwiatkowski (1943)
gray matter		
ox	1.4	Werle and Weicken (1949)
white matter		
ox	1.4—2.1	Werle and Weicken (1949)
spinal cord		
dog	0.1—0.56	Werle and Palm (1950)
man	0.0—0.14	Werle (1956)
ox	0.98	Euler (1956)
lumbar region		
cat	0 <0.1	Kwiatkowski (1943)
dog	0 <0.2	Kwiatkowski (1943)
guinea pig.	0 <0.2	Kwiatkowski (1943)
monkey.	0 <0.2	Kwiatkowski (1943)
man	0 <0.1	Kwiatkowski (1943)
rabbit	0 <0.05	Kwiatkowski (1943)
anterior root		
man	4.0—0.7	Werle (1956)
ox	1.05—1.5	Werle (1956)
ox	4.2—6.3	Euler (1956)
posterior root		
man	0—0.7	Werle (1956)
ox	1.05—1.5	Werle (1956)
ox	2.8—7.7	Euler (1956)
thoracic region		
grey matter		
ox	0.10—0.7	Werle (1956)
posterior white collumn		
ox	0.14—0.42	Werle (1956)

Table 6 (Continuation)

Material	Range of histamine content	Authors
anterior collumn		
ox	0.10—0.14	WERLE (1956)
sympathetic trunk		
dog	4.2—7.7	WERLE (1956)
man	3.15—5.6	WERLE (1956)
ox	65.1	EULER (1956)
ox	17.5—28.0	WERLE (1956)
sympathetic (lumbar)		
cat	1.0—1.4	KWIATKOWSKI (1943)
dog	1.25	KWIATKOWSKI (1943)
rabbit	<0.2	KWIATKOWSKI (1943)
sympathetic (neck)		
preganglionar		
ox	23.1	EULER (1956)
postganglionar		
ox	42.0	EULER (1956)
ganglia		
sympathetic		
man	4.2—5.6	WERLE (1956)
ox	21.0—70.0	WERLE (1956)
stellate		
dog	4.2—9.1	WERLE and PALM (1950)
ox	47.6—77.0	WERLE (1956)
man	4.9—6.3	WERLE (1956)
superior cervical		
man	6.3—8.4	WERLE (1956)
ox	24.5—47.6	WERLE (1956)
middle cervical		
man	5.6—7.0	WERLE (1956)
superior mesenteric		
dog	8.4—13.5	WERLE and PALM (1950)
inferior (vagus)		
dog	5.6—9.1	WERLE and PALM (1950)
peripheral (vagus)		
ox	31.9	WERLE (1956)
gasserian		
man	1.4—2.8	WERLE (1956)
inferior (glossopharingeal)		
dog	4.9—7.0	WERLE (1956)
spinal		
man	2.8—6.3	WERLE (1956)
ox	22.4—36.4	WERLE (1956)
meninges		
ox	42.0—44.1	WERLE and WEICKEN (1949)
dura mater		
man	1.4—2.8	WERLE and WEICKEN (1949)
pia mater		
man	traces	WERLE and WEICKEN (1949)
Nose		
mucosa		
man (2—12 years) . .	5.4—54.0	BAXTER and ROSE (1953)
man (18—42 years) . .	4.2—29.8	BAXTER and ROSE (1953)
woman (3—12 years) .	6.0—48.4	BAXTER and ROSE (1953)
woman (15—39 years)	6.25—38.5	BAXTER and ROSE (1953)
Oesophagus		
dog	10.0—24.0	DOUGLAS et al. (1951)
Omentum		
rat	18.0	RILEY and WEST (1955)

Table 6 (Continuation)

Material	Range of histamine content	Authors
Pancreas		
man	4.8	Stone et al. (1955)*
cat	1.2—5.8	Smith (1953b)
pineal gland		
ox	10.0	Giarman and Day (1958)
Placenta		
cat (before birth) . .	0	Waton (1963)
man	0.16—1.5	Wicksell (1949)
Rectum		
rat	2.5	Mota et al. (1956)
Skin		
rat	10.9—16.5	Gotzl and Dragstedt (1940)
rat	40.5—53.2	Marshall (1943)
rat	40.0	Perry (1956)
rat (abdomen)	26.5—47.0	Feldberg and Talesnik (1953)
rat (abdomen)	32.6	Eisen, Ellis and Wilson (1956)
rat (abdomen)	24.0—37.0	Eisen and Wilson (1957)
rat (dorsum).	27.9	Mota et al. (1956)
rat (ear)	45.0	Riley and West (1955)
rat (flank)	7.0—57.9	Geiringer and Hardwick (1953)
rat (flank, at birth) . .	18.5—39.0	Hardwick (1954)
rat (flank, 2—14 days)	17.5—22.4	Hardwick (1954)
rat (flank, 20—24 days)	36.9—61.5	Hardwick (1954)
rat (flank, 31 days) . .	28.5—35.3	Hardwick (1954)
rat (foetal)	4.0—8.1	Hardwick (1954)
rat (young)	48.3	Beaumariage and Lecomte (1958)
rat (adult)	35.7	Beaumariage and Lecomte (1958)
rat (foot)	65.0	Feldberg and Talesnik (1953)
rat (foot)	61.0	Mota et al. (1956)
rat (inn. surf.)	35.0	Riley and West (1956)
rat (out. surf.)	8.0	Riley and West (1956)
rat (tigh)	29.0	Feldberg and Talesnik (1953)
rabbit	3.5—5.6	Riesser (1957)
rabbit	14.7	Tarras-Wahlberg (1937)
rabbit	0.43—2.9	Rose (1941)
rabbit	4.0	Perry (1956)
rabbit	2.0	Riley and West (1956)
rabbit (young) . . .	3.0—17.1	Rocha e Silva (1940)
rabbit (adult)	1.5—6.0	Rocha e Silva (1940)
rabbit (abdomen) . .	7.2	Beaumariage and Lecomte (1957)
rabbit (ear)	15.3	Beaumariage and Lecomte (1957)
dog	9.0	Cass et al. (1954)
dog (abdomen). . . .	8.6—15.0	Feldberg and Miles (1953)
dog (back)	15.0	Feldberg and Miles (1953)
dog (bristle area) . .	20.0—62.0	Feldberg and Miles (1953)
dog (ear)	22.2—32.0	Feldberg and Miles (1953)
dog (lids)	15.6—33.0	Feldberg and Miles (1953)
dog (lips)	20.0	Feldberg and Miles (1953)
dog (lips-hairless) . .	4.2	Feldberg and Miles (1953)
dog (nipples)	20.0	Feldberg and Miles (1953)
dog (areola around nipples)	18.0	Feldberg and Miles (1953)
dog (front paw, dorsum)	16.0	Feldberg and Miles (1953)
dog (above foot) . . .	5.2—9.4	Feldberg and Talesnik (1953)
dog (middle of leg) . .	4.4—10.6	Feldberg and Talesnik (1953)
dog (knee).	4.4—16.4	Feldberg and Talesnik (1953)
dog (submental) . . .	6.3—17.0	Feldberg and Miles (1953)
dog	8.0	Perry (1956)
cat	30.8	Tarras-Wahlberg (1937)
cat (young)	1.0	Riley and West (1953)

Table 6 (Continuation)

Material	Range of histamine content	Authors
cat (adult)	20.0	RILEY and WEST (1953)
cat (inn. surf.)	6.0	RILEY and WEST (1953)
cat (out. surf.)	20.0	RILEY and WEST (1953)
cat (ear)	71.0—136.0	SMITH (1953b)
cat (ear)	95.0—120.0	FELDBERG and MILES (1953)
cat (abdomen)	18.0—27.0	SMITH (1953b)
cat (abdomen)	18.2—28.0	FELDBERG and MILES (1953)
cat (back)	10.0—19.0	FELDBERG and MILES (1953)
cat (lid)	36.0—50.0	FELDBERG and MILES (1953)
cat (lid)	32.0—40.0	SMITH (1953b)
cat (lid, upper) . . .	42.0	FELDBERG and MILES (1953)
cat (submental) . . .	42.0—44.0	FELDBERG and MILES (1953)
cat (bristle area) . . .	32.0—40.0	FELDBERG and MILES (1953)
cat (nasal area) . . .	36.0—52.0	SMITH (1953b)
cat (throat)	31.0—34.0	FELDBERG and MILES (1953)
cat (vertex)	28.0—30.0	FELDBERG and MILES (1953)
cat (nipple, areola) . .	40.0	FELDBERG and MILES (1953)
cat (nipple)	28.0	FELDBERG and MILES (1953)
cat (anal margin) . .	25.0—27.0	FELDBERG and MILES (1953)
cat (tail, proximal) . .	25.0	FELDBERG and MILES (1953)
cat (tail, distal) . . .	35.0	FELDBERG and MILES (1953)
cat (thigh)	33.0	FELDBERG and MILES (1953)
cat (foreleg)	25.0	FELDBERG and MILES (1953)
cat (paws and toes) .	25.0—30.0	FELDBERG and MILES (1953)
cat	20.0	PERRY (1956)
cat (before birth) . .	0	WATON (1963)
cat (at birth)	0.1—1.0	WATON (1963)
cat ($2^1/_4$ days old) . .	0.1—1.0	WATON (1963)
man (abdomen) . . .	1.8—26.7	FELDBERG and LOESER (1954)
man (breast)	5.2—13.6	FELDBERG and LOESER (1954)
man (neck)	11.5—17.6	FELDBERG and LOESER (1954)
man	5.0—24.0	NILZÉN (1947)
man	6.6	STONE et al. (1955)*
man	4.0—8.0	PERRY (1956)
man (inn. surf.) . . .	3.0	RILEY and WEST (1956)
man (out. surf.) . . .	10.0	RILEY and WEST (1956)
man (dermis)	5.0—8.0	MONGAR (1956)
man (epidermis) . . .	0.6—5.0	MONGAR (1956)
hog (ear)	7.1—13.6	SMITH (1953b)
hog (ear, upper surface)	25.0—31.0	RILEY and WEST (1956)
hog (ear, lower surface)	10.0—18.0	RILEY and WEST (1956)
ox (ear, upper surface)	15.0—28.0	RILEY and WEST (1956)
ox (ear, lower surface)	15.0—22.0	RILEY and WEST (1956)
ox (ear, tip)	32.0	RILEY and WEST (1956)
guinea pig	2.0	RILEY and WEST (1956)
guinea pig (abdomen) .	2.1—4.0	FELDBERG and MILES (1953)
guinea pig (abdomen) .	3.0	PERRY (1956)
guinea pig (abdomen, young)	3.1—8.8	JOHNSON (1956)
guinea pig (abdomen, adult)	2.2—5.0	JOHNSON (1956)
guinea pig (back) . .	1.5—4.2	FELDBERG and MILES (1953)
guinea pig (back, young)	3.1—7.6	JOHNSON (1956)
guinea pig (back, adult)	1.5—3.7	JOHNSON (1956)
guinea pig (ear, margin)	14.0—18.5	FELDBERG and MILES (1953)
guinea pig (ear, base) .	10.3—12.5	FELDBERG and MILES (1953)
guinea pig (lid)	8.9—11.0	FELDBERG and MILES (1953)
guinea pig (lid, young)	8.6—14.5	JOHNSON (1956)
guinea pig (lid, adult)	2.9—10.8	JOHNSON (1956)

Table 6 (Continuation)

Material	Range of histamine content	Authors
guinea pig (submental)	10.5—17.2	FELDBERG and MILES (1953)
guinea pig (submental, young)	11.7—27.5	JOHNSON (1956)
guinea pig (submental, adult)	4.1—11.6	JOHNSON (1956)
guinea pig (bristle area)	7.3—13.0	FELDBERG and MILES (1953)
guinea pig (vertex) . .	5.8—10.0	FELDBERG and MILES (1953)
guinea pig (vertex, young)	4.5—14.4	JOHNSON (1956)
guinea pig (vertex, adult)	2.5—7.6	JOHNSON (1956)
guinea pig (head) . .	8.6—10.3	MOTA and VUGMAN (1956)
guinea pig (lips, nose) .	6.0—11.5	FELDBERG and MILES (1953)
guinea pig (cheek) . .	5.0—8.5	FELDBERG and MILES (1953)
guinea p. (nipples, areola)	14.2—15.5	FELDBERG and MILES (1953)
guinea pig (anal margin)	6.0—11.7	FELDBERG and MILES (1953)
guinea pig (foreleg) .	5.0—6.7	FELDBERG and MILES (1953)
guinea pig (foreleg) .	4.3—10.3	MOTA and VUGMAN (1956)
guinea pig (foreleg, upper, young) . . .	3.1—11.8	JOHNSON (1956)
guinea pig (foreleg, upper, adult) . . .	2.5—5.9	JOHNSON (1956)
guinea pig (foreleg, paws)	5.8—11.4	FELDBERG and MILES (1953)
guinea pig (thigh) . . .	1.2—2.9	FELDBERG and MILES (1953)
guinea pig (thigh, young)	2.0—5.5	JOHNSON (1956)
guinea pig (thigh, adult)	1.7—3.4	JOHNSON (1956)
guinea pig (calf) . . .	2.0—4.0	FELDBERG and MILES (1953)
guinea pig (hindleg, paws)	4.3—8.0	FELDBERG and MILES (1953)
guinea pig (scrotum) .	5.0—6.5	FELDBERG and MILES (1953)
mouse	15.3—18.1	DEKANSKY (1945)
mouse	40.0	PERRY (1956)
mouse (out. surface) .	45.0	RILEY and WEST (1956)
mouse (inn. surf.) . .	28.0	RILEY and WEST (1956)
mouse (young) . . .	19.25—23.1	BEAUMARIAGE (1960b)
mouse (male, 4 m. old, dorso lumbar) . . .	37.18	BEAUMARIAGE (1960a)
mouse (male, 4 m. old, lumbo sacral) . . .	42.66	BEAUMARIAGE (1960a)
mouse (male, 6 m. old, dorso lumbar) . . .	45.96	BEAUMARIAGE (1960a)
mouse (male, 6 m. old, lumbo sacral) . . .	62.00	BEAUMARIAGE (1960a)
mouse (female, 4 m. old, dorso lumbar) . . .	53.13	BEAUMARIAGE (1960a)
mouse (female, 4 m. old, lumbo sacral) . . .	69.33	BEAUMARIAGE (1960a)
mouse (female, 6 m. old, dorso lumbar) . . .	74.63	BEAUMARIAGE (1960a)
mouse (female, 6 m. old, lumbo sacral) . . .	83.11	BEAUMARIAGE (1960a)
chicken	5.7	BEAUMARIAGE and LECOMTE (1958)
cock (head)	3.0—15.0	BEAUMARIAGE and LECOMTE (1956)
cock (abdomen) . . .	1.8—4.7	BEAUMARIAGE and LECOMTE (1956)
cock (dorsal)	1.16	GONÇALVES and LAURE (pers. comm.)
cock (comb)	0.16—1.0	GONÇALVES and LAURE (pers. comm.)
cock (wattle)	0.26—1.5	GONÇALVES and LAURE (pers. comm.)
ferret	3.0	PERRY (1956)
monkey	4.0	PERRY (1956)

Table 6 (Continuation)

Material	Range of histamine content	Authors
Spleen		
rat	2.0—5.0	Rose and Browne (1938)
rat	2.65—3.09	Marshall (1943)
cat	4.8—14.0	Smith (1953b)
dog	5.0	Cass et al. (1954)
man	3.4	Stone et al. (1955)*
rabbit	30.0—65.0	Rose (1941)
cock	0.8—6.0	Beaumariage and Lecomte (1956)
capsule		
dog	6	Riley and West (1953)
ox	7	Riley and West (1953)
sheep	6	Riley and West (1953)
cow	5	Riley and West (1953)
pig	3	Riley and West (1953)
cat	2	Riley and West (1953)
parenchyma		
dog	7	Riley and West (1953)
ox	7	Riley and West (1953)
sheep	6	Riley and West (1953)
cow	5	Riley and West (1953)
pig	3	Riley and West (1953)
cat	2	Riley and West (1953)
Stomach		
man (gl. layer) . . .	0.09—37.50	Neves et al. (1956)
man (musc. layer) . .	0—11.36	Neves et al. (1956)
man (mucosa, fundus)	3.5—24.1	Trach et al. (1944)
man (mucosa, antral) .	3.0—12.5	Trach et al. (1944)
man	14.0	Stone et al. (1955)*
rat	9.0	Rose and Browne (1938)
rat	8.0—20.0	Rose and Browne (1941)
rat	35.2—43.7	Marshall (1943)
rat (cardia)	3.0	Mota et al. (1956)
rat (fundus)	15.1	Mota et al. (1956)
rat (pylorus)	23.4	Eisen, Ellis and Wilson (1956)
dog (gl. layer, body) .	48—133	Feldberg and Harris (1953)
dog (gl. layer, pylorus)	32—57	Feldberg and Harris (1953)
dog (fundus)	48.0—180.0	Emmelin and Kahlson (1944)
dog (pylorus)	24.0—80.0	Emmelin and Kahlson (1944)
dog (pylorus)	24—32	Douglas et al. (1951)
dog (fundus)	69	Douglas et al. (1951)
dog (body)	57—70	Douglas et al. (1951)
dog (fundus, mucosa) .	120—133	Douglas et al. (1951)
dog (fundus, submucosa)	56—60	Douglas et al. (1951)
dog (fundus, musc. externa)	23—41	Douglas et al. (1951)
dog (body, mucosa) .	65—100	Douglas et al. (1951)
dog (body, submucosa)	86—109	Douglas et al. (1951)
dog (body, musc. externa)	25—42	Douglas et al. (1951)
dog (pylorus, mucosa)	40—63	Douglas et al. (1951)
dog (pylorus, submuc.)	46—50	Douglas et al. (1951)
dog (pylorus, musc. externa)	12.5—15	Douglas et al. (1951)
cat (before birth) . .	0	Waton (1963)
cat (at birth)	1.0—5.0	Waton (1963)
cat ($2^1/_4$ days old) . .	1.0—5.0	Waton (1963)
cat	12.4—57.0	Haeger and Kahlson (1952)
cat (gl. layer)	7.6—40.1	Haeger and Kahlson (1952)
cat (musc. layer) . . .	3.1—16.4	Haeger and Kahlson (1952)
cat (fundus)	5.3—34.0	Emmelin and Kahlson (1944)

Table 6 (Continuation)

Material	Range of histamine content	Authors
cat (pylorus)	4.3—16.0	EMMELIN and KAHLSON (1944)
cat (body, mucosa) . .	11.0—40.0	SMITH (1953b)
cat (body, submucosa + m. mucosae) . .	8.0—26.0	SMITH (1953b)
cat (body, musc. externa)	5.0—19.0	SMITH (1953b)
cat (pylorus, mucosa) .	7.0—32.0	SMITH (1953b)
cat (pylorus, submucosa + m. mucosae) . .	6.0—27.0	SMITH (1953b)
cat (pylorus, musc. externa)	4.0—15.0	SMITH (1953b)
rabbit	2.9—4.0	ROSE (1941)
Subcutaneous tissue		
rat	16.0	RILEY and WEST (1953)
rat	32.0	RILEY and WEST (1955)
Testis		
man	4.6	STONE et al. (1955)*
Thyroid		
man	1.0	STONE et al. (1955)*
Tongue		
cat (ventral surf.) . .	18.0	FELDBERG and MILES (1953)
cat (distal surf.) . . .	9.5	FELDBERG and MILES (1953)
dog	3.6—10.6	MOTA, FERRI and JUNQUEIRA (1956)
rat	14.5	MOTA et al. (1956)
rat	35.0—40.0	WEST (1956)
Urine		
man	0.032—1.8	ANREP et al. (1944a)
man (free)	0.008—0.01	ADAM (1950)
man (conjugated) . .	0.01—0.027	ADAM (1950)
man (child, free) . . .	6.7—17.3	MITCHELL et al. (1954)**
man (child, free) . . .	0.3—2.8	ADAM and MITCHELL (1953)**
man (child, conj.) . .	<2—<6	ADAM and MITCHELL (1953)**
man (child, free) . . .	7.7—29.2	MITCHELL and CODE (1954)**
man (child, conj.) . .	11—149	MITCHELL and CODE (1954)**
man	0.02—0.06	DUNÉR et al. (1961)
dog	0.054—25.2	ANREP et al. (1944a)
rat	0.036—3.68	ANREP et al. (1944a)
cat	0.10—5.4	ANREP et al. (1944a)
mouse	0.08—0.24	DEKANSKY (1945)
Uterus		
guinea pig	9.0—20.0	SCHILD (1939)

*Chemical method of extraction and assay.
**μg/24 hours.

References

ABEL, J. J., and S. KUBOTA: On the presence of histamine in the hypophysis, cerebri and other tissues of the body and its occurrence among the hydrolytic decomposition products of proteins. J. Pharmacol. exp. Ther. **13**, 243 (1919).

—, and T. NAGAYAMA: On the presence of histamine in extracts of the posterior lobe of the pituitary gland and on the preliminary experiments with the pressor constituent. J. Pharmacol. exp. Ther. **15**, 347 (1920).

ACKERMANN, D.: Über den bakteriellen Abbau des Histidins. Z. physiol. Chem. **65**, 504 (1910).

ADAM, H. M.: Excretion of histamine in human urine. Quart. J. exp. Physiol. **35**, 281 (1950).

—, and R. G. MITCHELL: The urinary excretion of histamine in children. Arch. Dis. Child. **28**, 61 (1953).

ÅKERBLOM, E.: Zur Histaminbestimmung in Gewebeextrakten. Acta physiol. scand. **2**, 378 (1941).

ANREP, G. V., M. S. AYADI, G. S. BARSOUM, G. R. SMITH and M. M. TALAAT: The excretion of histamine in urine. J. Physiol. (Lond.) **103**, 155 (1944a).
— G. S. BARSOUM, S. SALAMA and Z. SOUDIAN: Liberation of histamine during reactive hyperaemia and muscle contraction. J. Physiol. (Lond.) **103**, 297 (1944b).
— — M. TALAAT and E. WIENINGER: Determination of histamine in blood. J. Physiol. (Lond.) **95**, 476 (1939).
ARUNLAKSHANA, O., J. L. MONGAR and H. O. SCHILD: Potentiation of pharmacological effects of histamine by histaminase inhibitors. J. Physiol. (Lond.) **123**, 32 (1954).
BARGER, G., and H. H. DALE: β-iminazolylethylamine a depressor constituent of intestinal mucosa. J. Physiol. (Lond.) **41**, 499 (1911).
BARSOUM, G. S., and J. H. GADDUM: The pharmacological estimation of adenosine and histamine in blood. J. Physiol. (Lond.) **85**, 1 (1935).
— — The effect of cutaneous burns on the blood histamine. Clin. Sci. **2**, 357 (1936).
—, and F. H. SMIRK: Observations on histamine yielding substance in plasma and red cells of normal human subjects and of patients with congestive heart failure. Clin. Sci. **2**, 337 (1936a).
— — Observations on increase in concentration of histamine-like substance in human venous blood during period of reactive hyperaemia. Clin. Sci. **2**, 353 (1936b).
BAXTER, H., J. A. DRUMMOND, B. ROSE, L. G. STEPHENS-NEWSHAM and R. G. RANDALL: Blood histamine levels in swine following total body x-radiation and a flash burn. Ann. Surg. **139**, 179 (1954).
BAXTER, J. D., and B. ROSE: The histamine content of allergic and non-allergic human nasal mucous membrane with simultaneous observations on the eosinophilia. J. Allergy **24**, 18 (1953).
BEAUMARIAGE, M. L.: Teneur en histamine de la peau chez la souris adulte exposée au rayonnement X. C. R. Soc. Biol. (Paris) **154**, 1533 (1960a).
— Teneur en histamine de la peau du Souriceau et irradiation par rayons X. C. R. Soc. Biol. (Paris) **154**, 2135 (1960b).
—, et J. LECOMTE: Teneur en histamine de quelques organes du coq. C. R. Soc. Biol. (Paris) **150**, 227 (1956).
— — Teneur en histamine des tissus du lapin irradié par rayons X. C. R. Soc. Biol. (Paris) **151**, 1976 (1957).
— — Irradiation par rayons X et libération de l'histamine tissulaire. Arch. int. Pharmacodyn. **116**, 257 (1958).
BERALDO, W. T., and M. ROCHA E SILVA: Biological assay of antihistaminics, atropine and antispasmodics upon the guinea pig gut. J. Pharmacol. exp. Ther. **97**, 388 (1949).
BEST, C. H., H. H. DALE, H. W. DUDLEY and W. V. THORPE: The nature of vasodilator constituents of certain tissue extracts. J. Physiol. (Lond.) **62**, 397 (1927).
—, and E. W. McHENRY: The inactivation of histamine. J. Physiol. (Lond.) **70**, 349 (1930).
BLISS, C. I.: Statistics of Bioassay. New York: Academic Press Inc. 1952.
—, and H. P. MARKS: Biological assay of insulin. I. Increasing the precision of the curve relating dosage and graded response. Quart. J. Pharm. **12**, 82 (1939a).
— — Biological assay of insulin. II. Estimation of drug potency from a graded response. Quart. J. Pharm. **12**, 182 (1939b).
BOURA, A., J. L. MONGAR and H. O. SCHILD: Improved automatic apparatus for pharmacological assays on isolated preparations. Brit. J. Pharmacol. **9**, 24 (1954).
BUCHER, K.: Eine einfache und empfindliche Methode zur biologischen Histaminbestimmung in kleinen Flüssigkeitsmengen. Experientia (Basel) **7**, 111 (1951).
CANTONI, G. L., and G. EASTMAN: Smooth muscle stimulants. J. Pharmacol. exp. Ther. **87**, 392 (1946).
CARLINI, E. A., and J. P. GREEN: The subcellular distribution of histamine, slow reacting substance and 5-hydroxytryptamine in the brain of the rat. Brit. J. Pharmacol. **20**, 264 (1963).
CASS, R., J. F. RILEY, G. B. WEST, K. W. HEAD and S. W. STROUD: Heparin and histamine in mast cell tumours from dog. Nature (Lond.) **174**, 318 (1954).
CODE, C. F.: The quantitative estimation of histamine in the blood. J. Physiol. (Lond.) **89**, 257 (1937a).
— The source in blood of the histamine-like constituent. J. Physiol. (Lond.) **90**, 349 (1937b).
— The histamine-like activity of white blood cells. J. Physiol. (Lond.) **90**, 485 (1937c).
— The histamine content of the blood of guinea pigs and dogs during anaphylactic shock. Amer. J. Physiol. **127**, 78 (1939).
— P. B. DEWS and G. M. HIGGINS: The relationship of the adrenal gland to concentration of histamine and the number of leucocytes in the blood of rabbits. J. Physiol. (Lond.) **121**, 487 (1953).
— G. A. HALLENBECK and R. A. GREGORY: Histamine content of canine gastric juice. Amer. J. Physiol. **151**, 593 (1947).
—, and H. R. HESTER: The blood histamine during anaphylactic shock in the horse and calf. Amer. J. Physiol. **127**, 71 (1939).

CODE, C. F., and H. R. ING: The isolation of histamine from the white cell layer of centrifuged rabbit blood. J. Physiol. (Lond.) **90**, 501 (1937).
—, and J. L. JENSEN: A comparison of the histamine content of blood and bone marrow. Amer. J. Physiol. **131**, 768 (1941).
—, and A. D. MACDONALD: The histamine-like activity of blood. Lancet **1937 II**, 730.
—, and F. C. MCINTIRE: Quantitative determination of histamine. Methods of Biochemical Analysis. vol. 111. Inc. New York: Interscience Publishers 1956.
CRABS, L.: Contribution à la pathogénie de l'anaphylaxie cutanée chez le rat. Int. Arch. Allergy **20**, suppl. 2 (1962).
DALE, H. H.: The anaphylactic reaction of plain muscle in the guinea pig. J. Pharmacol. exp. Ther. **4**, 167 (1912—1913).
— The effect of varying tonicity on the anaphylactic and other reactions of plain muscle. J. Pharmacol. exp. Ther. **4**, 517 (1913).
— Adventures in Physiology. Oxford: Pergamon Press 1953.
—, and H. W. DUDLEY: The presence of histamine and acetylcholine in the spleen of the ox and the horse. J. Physiol. (Lond.) **68**, 97 (1929).
—, and P. P. LAIDLAW: The physiological action of beta-iminazolylethylamine. J. Physiol. (Lond.) **41**, 318 (1910—1911).
DEKANSKY, J.: The effect of cutaneous burns on histamine in mice. J. Physiol. (Lond.) **104**, 151 (1945).
DELAUNOIS, A. L., L. DAUTREBANDE and C. HEYMANS: Method for administering micromicellar aerosols to guinea pig isolated lungs. Arch. int. Pharmacodyn. **108**, 238 (1956).
DOUGLAS, W. W., W. FELDBERG, W. D. M. PATON and M. SCHACHTER: Distribution of histamine and substance P in the wall of the dog's digestive tract. J. Physiol. (Lond.) **115**, 163 (1951).
DRAGSTEDT, C. A., M. R. ARELLANO and A. H. LAWTON: Peptone shock in fetal dogs and its significance in the metabolism of histamine. Proc. Soc. exp. Biol. (N. Y.) **43**, 28 (1940).
—, and M. ROCHA E SILVA: Effect of trypsin upon blood histamine of rabbits. Proc. Soc. exp. Biol. (N. Y.) **47**, 420 (1941).
DUNÉR, H., S. O. LILJEDAHL and B. PERNOW: Does the urinary excretion of imidazole acetic acid reflect the endogenous histamine metabolism in man? Acta physiol. scand. **51**, 41 (1961).
EISEN, V. D., R. E. ELLIS and C. W. M. WILSON: The effect of X-irradiation on tissue histamine in the rat. J. Physiol. (Lond.) **133**, 506 (1956).
—, and C. W. M. WILSON: Effect of β-irradiation on skin histamine and vascular responses in the rat. J. Physiol. (Lond.) **136**, 122 (1957).
EMMELIN, N.: On the presence of histamine in a physiologically active form. Acta physiol. scand. **11**, suppl. 34 (1945).
—, and G. S. KAHLSON: Histamine as a physiological excitant of acid gastric secretion. Acta physiol. scand. **8**, 289 (1944).
— — and F. WICKSELL: Histamine in plasma and methods for its estimation. Acta physiol. scand. **2**, 123 (1941).
EULER, U. S. VON: Histamine and Nerves. Ciba Foundation Symposium on Histamine, page 235. London: Churchill 1956.
FEIGEN, G. A., and D. H. CAMPBELL: The relative sensitivity of the mucosal and peritoneal surfaces of guinea pig ileum to histamine, acetylcholine and specific antigens. Amer. J. Physiol. **145**, 676 (1946).
FELDBERG, W., and G. W. HARRIS: Distribution of histamine in the mucosa of the gastrointestinal tract of the dog. J. Physiol. (Lond.) **120**, 352 (1953).
—, and C. H. KELLAWAY: Liberation of histamine from perfused lung by snake venoms. J. Physiol. (Lond.) **90**, 257 (1937a).
— — The circulatory and pulmonary effects of the venom of Australian copperhead (Denisonia superba). Aust. J. exp. Biol. med. Sci. **15**, 81 (1937b).
— — Liberation of histamine and formation of lysocithin-like substances by cobra venom. J. Physiol. (Lond.) **94**, 187 (1938).
—, and A. A. LOESER: Histamine content of human skin in different clinical disorders. J. Physiol. (Lond.) **126**, 286 (1954).
—, and A. A. MILES: Regional variations of increased permeability of skin capillaries induced by a histamine liberator and their relation to the histamine content of the skin. J. Physiol. (Lond.) **120**, 205 (1953).
—, und E. SCHILF: Histamin. Berlin: Julius Springer 1930.
—, and J. TALESNIK: Reduction of tissue histamine by compound 48/80. J. Physiol. (Lond.) **120**, 550 (1953).
FINKLEMAN, B.: Inhibition of the intestine. J. Physiol. (Lond.) **70**, 145 (1930).
GADDUM, J. H.: The technique of superfusion. Brit. J. Pharmacol. **8**, 321 (1953a).
— Simplified mathematics for bioassay. J. Pharm. Pharmacol. **5**, 345 (1953b).

GADDUM, J. H., C. S. JANG and H. KWIATKOWSKI: The effect on the intestine of the substance liberated by adrenergic nerves in a rabbit's ear. J. Physiol. (Lond.) **96**, 104 (1939).
GARAN, R. S.: Inaktivierung von Histamin durch Kohlensäure. Naunyn-Schmiedeberg's Arch. exp. Path. Pharmak. **188**, 247 (1938).
GEIRINGER, E., and D. C. HARDWICK: Changes in skin histamine after remote injury. J. Physiol. (Lond.) **119**, 410 (1953).
GIARMAN, N. J., and M. DAY: Presence of biogenic amines in the pineal body. Biochem. Pharmacol. **1**, 235 (1958).
GIERTZ, H., u. F. HAHN: Die inverse Anaphylaxie vom Standpunkt der Histamintheorie der Anaphylaxie. Int. Arch. Allergy **6**, 23 (1955).
GONÇALVES, J. M., and C. J. LAURE: Personal communication.
GOTZL, F. R., and C. A. DRAGSTEDT: Effect of thyroidectomy and experimental hyperthyroidism upon histamine content of rat tissues. Proc. Soc. exp. Biol. (N. Y.) **45**, 688 (1940).
GRAÑA, A., and M. ROCHA E SILVA: Effect of hydatic fluid on histamine content of rabbit blood. Amer. J. Physiol. **143**, 314 (1945).
GUGGENHEIM, M., u. W. LÖFFLER: Biologischer Nachweis proteinogener Amine in Organextrakten und Körperflüssigkeiten. Biochem. Z. **72**, 303 (1916).
HAEGER, K., and G. KAHLSON: Distribution of histamine and histaminase in the gastrointestinal mucosa of fed and starved cats. Acta physiol. scand. **25**, 230 (1952).
HALPERN, B. N.: Inhibition réversible de la contraction histaminique et anaphylactique des muscles lisses de cobaye par la substitution dans le milieu de survie de l'anhydride carbonique à l'oxygène moléculaire. C. R. Soc. Biol. (Paris) **150**, 505 (1956a).
— Modalité et spécificité de l'action inhibitrice de l'anhydride carbonique sur la contraction histaminique des organs à muscles lisses. C. R. Soc. Biol. (Paris) **150**, 897 (1956b).
— R. BINAGHI, M. MAYER and C. BUGNARD: The mechanism of the inhibition of carbonic acid of the smooth muscle contraction produced by histamine and oxytocin. Brit. J. Pharmacol. **14**, 19 (1959).
HANKE, N. T., and K. K. KOESSLER: Studies on proteinogenous amines. VIII. A method for the quantitative colorimetric estimation of histamine in protein and protein-containing matter. J. biol. Chem. **43**, 543 (1920).
HARDWICK, D. C.: Age changes in the histamine content of rat skin. J. Physiol. (Lond.) **124**, 157 (1954).
HARRIS, K. E.: Observations upon a histamine-like substance in skin extracts. Heart **14**, 161 (1927).
HAWORTH, E., and A. D. MACDONALD: On histamine in cotton dust, and in the blood of cotton workers. J. Hyg. (Lond.) **37**, 234 (1937).
JENDEN, D. J., and J. R. TUREMAN: New technique for study of drug actions on bronchial resistance in isolated lung. Proc. Soc. exp. Biol. (N. Y.) **91**, 275 (1956).
JIMÉNEZ-VARGAS, J.: Nuevo método de registro del espasmo bronquial experimental. Rev. esp. Fisiol. **7**, 197 (1951).
JOHNSON, H. H., JR.: Variations in histamine levels in guinea pig skin related to skin region, age (or weight), and time after death of animal. J. invest. Derm. **27**, 159 (1956).
KIESE, M.: Wirkungen des Kohlendioxyds. Biochem. Z. **305**, 22 (1940).
KOCHMANN, M.: Zur Wertbestimmung der Hypophysenpräparate. Hoppe-Seylers Z. physiol. Chem. **129**, 95 (1923).
KONZETT, H., u. R. RÖSSLER: Versuchsanordnung zu Untersuchungen an der Bronchialmuskulatur. Naunyn-Schmiedeberg's Arch. exp. Path. Pharmak. **195**, 71 (1940).
KUTSCHER, F.: See ACKERMANN (1910).
KWIATKOWSKI, H.: Observations on the relation of histamine to reactive hyperaemia. J. Physiol. (Lond.) **100**, 147 (1941).
— Histamine in nervous tissues. J. Physiol. (Lond.) **120**, 32 (1943).
LEWIS, T.: Vascular reactions of the skin to injury. I. Reaction to stroking. Heart **11**, 119 (1924).
— Vascular reactions of the skin to injury. IV. An irresponsive condition of the vessels. Heart **13**, 153 (1926).
— Blood vessels of the human skin and their responses. London: Shaw and Sons Ltd. 1927.
LOWRY, O. H., H. T. GRAHAM, F. B. HARRIS, M. K. PRIEBAT, A. R. MARKS and R. U. BREGMAN: The chemical measurement of histamine in blood plasma and cells. J. Pharmacol. exp. Ther. **112**, 116 (1954).
MACINTOSH, F. C., and W. D. M. PATON: The liberation of histamine by certain organic bases. J. Physiol. (Lond.) **109**, 190 (1949).
MACKAY, M.: The effects of histidine on the histamine content of the lungs and on histamine reactions. Aust. J. exp. Biol. med. Sci. **16**, 137 (1937).
MAGNUS, R.: Cit. in Feldberg and Schilf. (1930)
MARSHALL, P. B.: The influence of adrenal cortical deficiency on the histamine content of rat tissues. J. Physiol. (Lond.) **102**, 180 (1943).

MINARD, D.: The presence and distribution of histamine in blood. Amer. J. Physiol. **132**, 327 (1941).
MISRAHY, G. A.: The metabolism of histamine and adenylic compounds in the embryo. Amer. J. Physiol. **147**, 462 (1946).
MITCHELL, R. G., and R. CASS: Histamine and 5-hydroxytryptamine in the blood of infants and children. J. clin. Invest. **38**, 595 (1959).
—, and C. F. CODE: Urinary excretion of histamine after administration of cortisone. J. clin. Endocr. **14**, 707 (1954).
— G. B. LOGAN, G. PETERS and L. L. HENDERSON: Urinary excretion of histamine in patients having asthma and hay fever: observations on changes produced by administration of cortisone. J. Allergy **25**, 504 (1954).
MONGAR, J. L.: Ciba Foundation Symposium on Histamine, page 406. London: Churchill 1956.
—, and H. O. SCHILD: Quantitative measurement of the histamine-releasing activity of a series of mono-alkylamines using minced guinea pig lung. Brit. J. Pharmacol. **8**, 103 (1953).
MOTA, I.: Mast cell and histamine in rat anaphylaxis: the effect of Haemophilus pertussis. Nature (Lond.) **182**, 1021 (1958).
— W. T. BERALDO, A. G. FERRI and L. C. U. JUNQUEIRA: Action of 48/80 on the mast cell population and histamine content of the wall of the gastro-intestinal tract of the rat. Ciba Foundation Symposium on Histamine, page 47. London: Churchill 1956.
— A. G. FERRI and L. C. U. JUNQUEIRA: Action of peptone on the mast cells and histamine content of dog tissues. Acta haemat. (Basel) **15**, 409 (1956).
—, and I. VUGMAN: Action of compound 48/80 on the mast cells and histamine content of guinea pig tissues. Brit. J. Pharmacol. **11**, 304 (1956).
NEVES, D. P., L. R. TRABULSI, S. R. MONSÃO e J. F. PONTES: Distribuição da histamina na mucosa gástrica humana e seu possível papel no mecanismo da secreção clorídrica. Rev. Hosp. Clín. **11**, 25 (1956).
NILZÉN, Å.: Studies in histamine (H substance) with special reference to the conditions obtaining in urticaria and related skin changes. Acta dermato-venereol. (Stockh.) **27**, suppl. 17 (1947).
PARROT, J. L., et M. GABE: Sur la répartition de l'histamine dans les éléments constitutifs du sang humain. C. R. Soc. Biol. (Paris) **139**, 965 (1945).
PERRY, W. L. M.: Skin Histamine. Ciba Foundation Symposium on Histamine, page 242. London: Churchill 1956.
RIESSER, O.: Histaminstudien. Naunyn-Schmiedeberg's Arch. exp. Path. Pharmakol. **187**, 1 (1937).
RILEY, J. F., and G. B. WEST: The presence of histamine in tissue mast cells. J. Physiol. (Lond.) **120**, 528 (1953).
— — Studies with a histamine liberator of low toxicity (compound 48/80). J. Path. Bact. **69**, 269 (1955).
— — Skin histamine, its location in the tissue mast cells. Arch. Derm. **74**, 471 (1956).
ROCHA E SILVA, M.: Histamine in the rabbit skin. Proc. Soc. exp. Biol. (N. Y.) **45**, 586 (1940).
— Concerning the theory of receptors in pharmacology. A rational method of estimation of pAx. Arch. int. Pharmacodyn. **118**, 74 (1959).
— Influence of pH on the interaction of histamine with its receptors in the guinea pig ileum. Arch. int. Pharmacodyn. **128**, 355 (1960).
— On the nature of the receptors for histamine. Chemotherapia **5**, 544 (1961).
— and C. A. DRAGSTEDT: Nature of the capillary permeability factor present in extracts of normal tissues. Proc. Soc. exp. Biol. (N. y.) **46**, 303 (1941).
—, and H. E. ESSEX: The effect of animal poisons (rattlesnake venom and trypsin) on the blood histamine of guinea pigs and rabbits. Amer. J. Physiol. **135**, 372 (1942).
— A. GRAÑA and A. PORTO: Inhibitory effect of glycogen upon anaphylactic shock in the rabbit. Proc. Soc. exp. Biol. (N. Y.) **59**, 57 (1945).
—, and H. O. SCHILD: The release of histamine by D-tubocurarine from the isolated diaphragm of the rat. J. Physiol. (Lond.) **109**, 448 (1949).
ROSE, B.: Studies on the histamine content of the blood and tissues of the rabbit during anaphylactic shock. J. Immunol. **42**, 161 (1941).
—, and J. S. L. BROWNE: Distribution and rate of disappearance of intravenously injected histamine in rat. Amer. J. Physiol. **124**, 412 (1938).
— — Changes in the blood histamine in shock. Proc. Soc. exp. Biol. (N. Y.) **44**, 182 (1940).
— — The effect of adrenalectomy on histamine content of the tissues of the rat. Amer. J. Physiol. **131**, 589 (1941).
SCHILD, H. O.: Histamine release in anaphylactic shock from various tissues of the guinea pig. J. Physiol. (Lond.) **95**, 393 (1939).
— A method of conducting a biological assay on a preparation giving repeated responses illustrated by the estimation of histamine. J. Physiol. (Lond.) **101**, 119 (1942).
— An approximately linear and isotonic frontal writing lever. J. Physiol. (Lond.) **103**, 11 P (1944).

SCHMITERLÖW, C. G.: Some remarks on the determination of histamine with special reference to horse blood. Acta physiol. scand. **19**, 260 (1949).
SCHÜLLER, W.: Zur Hemmung der Diaminoxydase (Histaminase). Experientia (Basel) **8**, 230 (1952).
SCHULTZ, W. H.: Reaction of smooth muscle from guinea pigs rendered tolerant to large doses of serum. J. Pharmacol. exp. Ther. **2**, 221 (1911).
SMITH, A. N.: The effect of compound 48/80 on acid gastric secretion in the cat. J. Physiol. (Lond.) **119**, 233 (1953a).
— Release of histamine by the histamine liberator compound 48/80 in cats. J. Physiol. (Lond.) **121**, 517 (1953b).
STEGGERDA, F. R., H. E. ESSEX and F. C. MANN: The inactivation of histamine in perfused organs. Amer. J. Physiol. **112**, 70 (1935).
STONE, J. L., J. M. MERRILL and G. R. MENEELY: Distribution of histamine in human tissues. Fed. Proc. **14**, 147 (1955).
TARRAS-WAHLBERG, B.: Über den Histamingehalt der Haut nach Ultraviolettbestrahlung. Klin. Wschr. **16**, 958 (1937).
THORPE, W. V.: Vasodilator constituents of tissue extracts; isolation of histamine from muscle. Biochem. J. **22**, 94 (1928).
TRACH, B., C. F. CODE and O. H. WANGENSTEEN: Histamine in human gastric mucosa. Amer. J. Physiol. **141**, 78 (1944).
TRETHEWIE, E. R.: Experiments on the problem of "free" and "bound" histamine and acetylcholine. Aust. J. exp. Biol. med. Sci. **16**, 225 (1938).
— Comparison of haemolysis and liberation of histamine by two Australian snake venoms. Aust. J. exp. Biol. med. Sci. **17**, 145 (1939).
— Age and lung histamine. J. Immunol. **56**, 211 (1947).
—, and A. J. DAY: Tissue injury by Australian black snake venom and "bound" histamine. Aust. J. exp. Biol. med. Sci. **27**, 385 (1949).
UNGAR, G., J.-L. PARROT et A. POCOULÉ: Sur la présence de l'histamine dans le sang humain normal. C. R. Soc. Biol. (Paris) **124**, 1202 (1937).
—, et A. POCOULÉ: Sur les vies d'élimination de l'histamine et son absence dans les urines normales. C. R. Soc. Biol. (Paris) **124**, 1204 (1937).
VALENTINE, W. N., and J. S. LAWRENCE: Studies on blood histamine. Partition of blood histamine before and after clotting in health and disease states. Amer. J. med. Sci. **216**, 619 (1948).
VUGMAN, I.: Fatores que influem na libertação da histamina do diafragma isolado de rato pelo composto 48/80. Thesis, Ribeirão Preto 1961.
WATON, N. G.: Histamine metabolism in foetal and very young cats. J. Physiol. (Lond.) **169**, 919 (1963).
WERLE, E.: Histamine in Nerves. Ciba Foundation Symposium on Histamine, page 264. London: Churchill 1956.
—, u. D. PALM: Histamin in Nerven. II. Biochem. Z. **320**, 322 (1950).
—, u. G. WEICKEN: Über das Vorkommen von Histamin in Nerven. Biochem. Z. **319**, 457 (1949).
WEST, G. B.: Ciba Foundation Symposium on Histamine, page 404. London: Churchill 1956.
WICKSELL, F.: Observations on histamine and histaminolysis in pregnancy. Acta physiol. scand. **17**, 395 (1949).
WILSON, A.: Effect of adrenalectomy on blood histamine of rabbits. J. Physiol. (Lond.) **99**, 241 (1941).
ZADINA, R.: Influence de la température sur la contraction histaminique de l'intestin du cobaye. C. R. Soc. Biol. (Paris) **132**, 28 (1939).
ZON, L. E., E. T. CEDER and C. W. CRIGLER: The presence of histamine in the platelets of the rabbit. U. S. Pub. Hlth. Rep. **54**, 1978 (1939).

Section E

The Occurrence of Histamine in Mast Cells

By

J. F. Riley and G. B. West

With 4 Figures

I. Introduction

Through the discovery of the high histamine content of the mast cells of Ehrlich, the decade 1950—1960 has seen a fresh orientation of knowledge concerning the location of histamine in blood and tissues. Looking back on events, it is now apparent that several independent lines of research were converging on this common point. In Scotland, Riley (1952; 1953a; 1953b) had traced a fluorescent histamine liberator (stilbamidine) to its target in the mast cells of the peritoneum of the rat, and with West (1952; 1953) had provided the first pharmacological correlation between mast cell content and histamine value for a number of tissues including human skin rich in mast cells. In Brazil, Mota et al. (1953) using a more specific histamine liberator (compound 48/80) had noted its characteristic disruptive effects on rat mast cells. Meanwhile, in the United States, Graham and her colleagues (1952) had traced the histamine in human blood to the few basophils or blood mast cells which are normally present; later (1955) they confirmed the correlation between histamine values and mast cell content in tissues.

There was yet another line of approach. Grossberg and Garcia in Montreal (1954) and Hagen in Oxford (1954) had become interested in the location of histamine in the subcellular particles of dog liver homogenates, first described by Trethewie in 1938. Thought to be mitochondria, these particles were ultimately found to be granules of disrupted mast cells (Mota et al., 1954).

There is now no longer room for doubt that most, though not all, of the histamine in the body is located in the granules of mast cells. The details of this knowledge and the mode of its discovery form the main topic of the present section. Brief mention will also be made of the occurrence of heparin in mast cells generally, and of 5-hydroxytryptamine in the mast cells of mouse and rat. These various items are perhaps best described in historical sequence.

II. Discovery of mast cells

There are two types of mast cell, both of which were discovered by Paul Ehrlich (1877; 1898). The first and more common is the tissue mast cell, so called because of its abundance in well-nourished connective tissue ("Mästung" = feeding); the second is the blood mast cell or basophil which stems from precursors in the bone marrow and thereafter circulates in the peripheral blood. Both types of mast cell are characterized by cytoplasmic granules which stain metachromatically with certain basic dyes. EHRLICH believed that mast cells are concerned functionally with the connective tissues, an hypothesis which still finds a measure of support (RILEY, 1959).

III. Heparin in mast cells

Sixty years after EHRLICH's discovery, Scandinavian histologists (HOLMGREN and WILANDER, 1937) used the metachromatic reaction of LISON (1935) to show that the mast cell content of a tissue corresponds closely to its yield of extractable heparin. The reader is referred to the monograph by JORPES (1946) for a full account of the work of this period.

A. Normal tissues

In their original paper, HOLMGREN and WILANDER (1937) described ox liver capsule as a "pure culture" of mast cells. This curious predilection of mast cells for the fibrous capsule enabled comparisons to be made between capsule and parenchyma of various organs, of which a striking example is beef lung, the usual source of commercial heparin. Histologically, the mast cells are situated predominantly in, and immediately under, the pleura (RILEY and WEST, 1953, and see Figs. 1 and 2) and it is here that high yields of heparin are obtained.

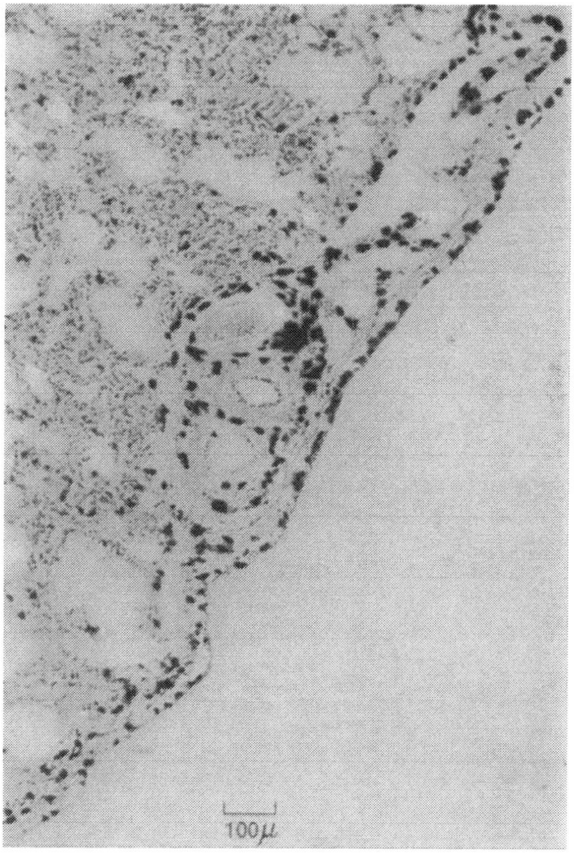

Fig. 1. Section of ox lung. Mast cells are large and numerous in the pleura, small and few in the parenchyma. Section stained with toluidine blue

Although mast cells can be stained supravitally by running 0.5 per cent aqueous toluidine blue on to a fresh tissue spread, it is generally desirable to make permanent preparations by fixing, dehydrating and defatting the tissue before it is stained, as described by RILEY (1953a). When sufficiently large sheets of tissue are available, the spread is draped over the edges of the microscope slide to prevent further shrinkage and is fixed at once in 80 per cent alcohol for 24 hours. If gross amounts of fat are present, they are trimmed away with a sharp scalpel before as much as possible of the remaining fat is removed by immersing the slide for at least one hour in xylol. The preparation is then taken back to alcohol prior to staining it with 0.5 per cent aqueous toluidine blue (or 1 per cent in alcohol 2.5 per cent) for 1—3 minutes. Excess stain is thereafter removed with 80 per cent alcohol and the tissue is thoroughly dehydrated with a final rinse in absolute alcohol before being cleared in xylol and mounted in B.P.S. (dibutyl polystyrene). Sometimes it is necessary to weight the coverslips to prevent the entry of air bubbles into the mountant while it is drying. The solid organs are examined by routine paraffin sections. Material for sectioning is fixed in 10 per cent neutral formalin or in formol-corrosive and is stained with toluidine blue. ZENKER's solution is an unsatisfactory fixative for mast cells. It is well to remember that mast cells stain poorly, or not at all, with the routine haematoxylin-eosin method, even when the material is well fixed.

In certain lower species, the mast cell granules are so water-soluble that the tissues must be fixed in absolute alcohol and stained with strongly alcoholic stains (MICHELS, 1938). Further reference to the handling of mast cells in lower organisms will be found in various papers by ARVY (1955a; 1955b).

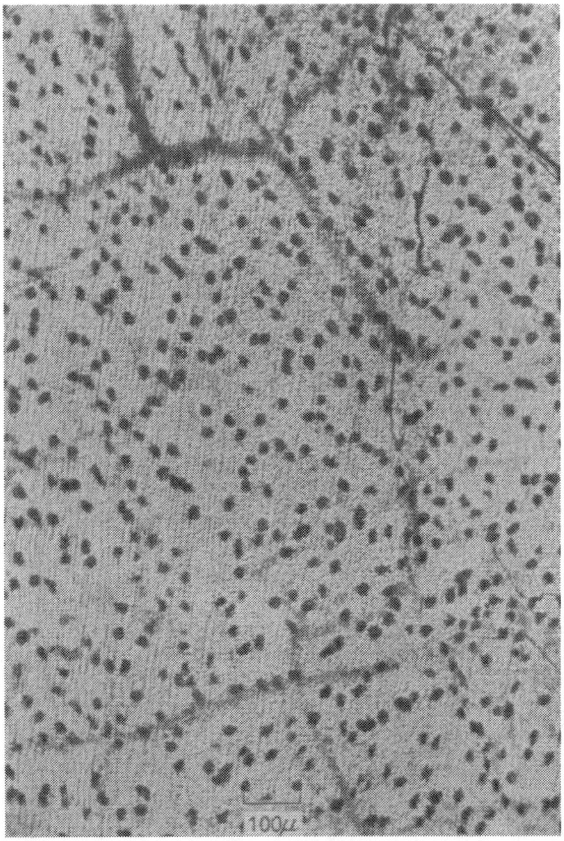

Fig. 2. Fresh spread of ox pleura. Note the enormous number of mast cells filled with metachromatic granules scattered throughout the collagenous pleura. This tissue contained proportionately more histamine than any other normal tissue. Spread stained with methylene blue. (After RILEY and WEST, 1953)

B. Pathological tissues

Any doubts as to the cytological location of heparin in mast cells were removed when OLIVER et al. (1947) found that a small mast cell tumour in a dog may contain more heparin than the entire liver, the organ from which heparin received its name. It is fortunate that the majority of mast cell tumours in domestic animals are composed of slowly-growing, well-differentiated cells which closely resemble normal mast cells in their morphology (HEAD, 1958; ORKIN and SCHWARTZMAN, 1959).

Later studies amply confirmed the high heparin content of mast cell tumours from dogs (Cass et al., 1954; Ringertz, 1960), though it is of interest that the heparins of other species, assayed as anticoagulant, fall well below the potency of dog heparin. Bell and Jaques (1956) record a progressive decline in anticoagulant potency in the series — dog, beef, sheep, pig. Recent work suggests that cat heparin is a yet weaker anticoagulant (Riley, 1959).

The only common human lesions rich in mast cells are seen in the skin disease, *urticaria pigmentosa* (Unna, 1896), which occasionally also involves the internal organs (Sagher, 1956). Up to the present, little information is available on the heparin content of these lesions. Working with tissue rich in mast cells obtained from a case of *elephantiasis scroti*, Ehrich et al. (1949) were able to extract and characterize human heparin.

C. Location of heparin

The metachromatic staining reaction suggests that heparin is formed or stored in the granules of mast cells. Indeed, it has been known since the time of Ehrlich that granules scattered by trauma before fixation or by the microtome knife after fixation continue to stain metachromatically. Hedbom and Snellman (1955), following on the work of Julen et al. (1949) extracted heparin from ox liver capsule and suggested that the heparin is associated with the microsome fraction in the intergranular cytoplasm. On the other hand, Köksal (1953) found that the metachromatic anticoagulant material from mast cells in mouse skin chiefly accompanies the granules on isolation. The discrepancy may lie in the different methods of extraction. According to Benditt (1958), once the heparin has been removed, the remainder of the granule exhibits strongly thromboplastic properties.

D. Synthesis of heparin

Three recent advances in technique have stimulated fresh interest in the ability of mast cells to synthesize heparin and other substances. First is the availability of transplantable mast cell tumours in mice; second is the improvement in methods of maintaining mast cells in tissue culture; and third is the introduction and availability of isotopically-labelled substrates.

Using a transplantable mastocytoma which originated in a mouse subjected to ionizing radiation, Furth et al. (1957) localized the heparin to the large-granule fraction (Barrnett et al., 1958) which is distinct from the mitochondria (Hagen et al., 1959). This particular tumour can be propagated in solid form, in ascites form, or as a mast-cell leukaemia (Ono et al., 1959).

Synthesis of heparin in slices of the Furth mastocytoma has been studied by Korn (1959a and b). Recently it has been found (Day and Green, 1960) that labelled sulphur and glucosamine-1-C^{14} are incorporated in the heparin of the mastocytoma at the same rate, and that cells grown in tissue culture are more active than the parent tissue (Green and Day, 1960).

A second transplantable mast-cell tumour arose in the skin of a mouse painted with a carcinogenic hydrocarbon (Dunn and Potter, 1957). Although this tumour is somewhat less well differentiated than the Furth tumour, nevertheless it rapidly incorporates and stores sulphur, as do normal mast cells (Jorpes et al., 1953; Lagunoff et al., 1960). Spolter and Marx (1959) find that the tumour mast cells avidly accept "active" sulphate from phosphoadenosine phosphosulphate (Lipmann, 1958). The uptake of sulphur by heparin exceeds that of any other tissue mucopolysaccharide (Ringertz, 1960).

For much detailed information on the synthesis of heparin in mast cells, the reader is referred especially to the summarizing reports of BLOOM (1960) and RINGERTZ (1960). These authors have studied the cytological and biochemical properties of mast cells in a wide variety of normal and pathological material including both mouse tumours referred to above.

It is thus concluded that the tissue mast cells are not only the main source of extractable heparin but that the heparin is synthesized in the cells and stored in the cytoplasmic granules to which it imparts their characteristic staining properties. Much of the above work is of significance, and will be referred to again, when histamine in mast cells is under consideration.

IV. Histamine in mast cells

Experimental evidence for the occurrence of histamine in mast cells has been derived from two main sources, both of which rest ultimately upon a comparison between the histamine content of a given tissue, as measured by pharmacological assay, and its mast-cell population. The first is essentially an adaptation and an extension of the work which led to the demonstration of heparin in the mast cells — simple comparisons using both normal and pathological tissues with clearly defined mast-cell populations. The second, which has so far proved to be of little value in tracing heparin to the mast cells, involves alteration in the mast-cell population or alteration in the histamine content, such as occurs in the course of anaphylaxis or in tissues subjected to the influence of chemical histamine-liberators.

A. Normal tissues

The same comparative tests used by JORPES (1946) for heparin and mast cells were adopted by RILEY and WEST (1952) in their original investigation of histamine in relation to mast-cell population.

Inspection of Table 1 indicates that as good a parallelism exists between histamine and mast cells as between heparin and mast cells in these tissues. This finding has been the basis of much subsequent work. RILEY and WEST (1953) then estimated histamine not only in organs of widely differing mast-cell populations but also in parts of the same organ where microscopic examination revealed strongly marked regional variations in the distribution of the mast cells.

Table 1. *Histamine content* (μg/g) *of tissues compared with heparin content* (mg standard heparin/kg) *and the relative mast-cell content*

Tissue	Histamine	Heparin[1]	Mast cells
Rat liver	0·3	0	0
Pig aorta	0·7	0	0
Ox-liver parenchyma .	4·5	56—75	+
Ox aorta	10·0	5—65	+
Rat subcutaneous tissue	16·0	63	++
Ox inferior vena cava .	20·0	100—120	++
Ox-liver capsule . . .	40·0	540—830	+++

[1] Data of JORPES (1946).

For the pharmacological assay, weighed amounts of fresh tissue are placed at once in 5 volumes of 10% v/v trichloroacetic acid and then ground in a mortar with a little sand. After a minimum period of two hours, the extract is centrifuged and the clear supernatant shaken four times with 4 vol. of ether to remove excess acid. The histamine content of the neutralized supernatant is determined using either the isolated guinea-pig ileum suspended in Tyrode solution containing atropine (10^{-7}) or the blood pressure of the atropinized cat (1 mg./kg.) under chloralose anaesthesia. Specificity of the reaction is checked by using mepyramine (10^{-8} for the guinea-pig ileum, or 2 mg./kg. for the cat). The result is expressed in terms of histamine base.

The strong positive correlation for mast cells and histamine is clearly seen when the *liver* of various mammalian species is examined. It will be noted from Table 2 that only the liver of the dog has many mast cells and much histamine in its parenchyma. In the remaining species, the mast cells and histamine are located mainly in the capsule of the liver.

The striking association of mast cells and histamine can likewise be demonstrated when the *lung* is divided in two parts and examined in a similar way. Here, however, the capsule — the visceral pleura — must be removed by sharp dissection before selected areas can be mounted as tissue spreads (Fig. 1 and 2 and Table 3).

Table 2. *Histamine content* (μg/g tissue) *and the relative mast-cell content of the liver of different species*

Species	Capsule		Parenchyma	
	Histamine	Mast cells	Histamine	Mast cells
Ox	40	+++	5	+
Sheep	35	++	6	+
Dog	24	++	22	++
Cow	22	++	5	+
Pig	10	+	8	+
Cat	1	0	1	0

Table 3. *Histamine content* (μg/g tissue) *and the relative mast-cell content of the lung of different species*

Species	Pleura		Parenchyma	
	Histamine	Mast cells	Histamine	Mast cells
Ox	200	++++	80	+++
Sheep	80	+++	60	+++
Pig	40	+++	20	++
Cat	38	++	32	++
Dog	35	+++	20	++
Cow	25	++	25	++

Finally a comparison was made between the same organs of animals at *different ages*, taking advantage of the fact, well known to Ehrlich, that mast cells are generally sparse in the embryo or very young animal, irrespective of the mast-cell population of the organ or tissue in adult life (Table 4). Inspection of Table 4 shows that there is less histamine in a very young or *embryonic tissue* poor in mast cells and that the final histamine content is proportional to the mast-cell population in the adult state.

About the time that Riley and West were carrying out their histological investigations on the distribution of mast cells, Feldberg and Harris (1953) were endeavouring to locate histamine in the *gut* wall of the dog by their technique

Table 4. *Histamine content* (μg/g tissue) *and the relative mast-cell content of organs of young and adult animals*

Organ	Species	Young		Adult	
		Histamine	Mast cells	Histamine	Mast cells
Lung	Cow	8	+	25	++
	Man	6	+	25	++
	Cat	4	+	36	++
Liver capsule	Cow	5	+	22	++
Liver parenchyma . . .	Cow	1	0	5	+
Skin	Cat	1	0	20	++

of the "histamine profile". This is a regional map of the local distribution of histamine, obtained by subdividing frozen sections cut at different levels in the gastro-intestinal tract and comparing them with the corresponding histological picture at that level. Their material was stained only with the routine haematoxylin-eosin method which fails to stain the mast cell granules. When the appropriate comparisons are made, however, a good correlation exists between the histamine content and mast-cell population (ARVY and QUIVY, 1955). Data for the distribution of mast cells and histamine in the gastro-intestinal tract of other laboratory animals are presented by MOTA et al. (1956). LINDHOLM (1960) has also described the distribution of mast cells in the gastro-intestinal tract of hamster and rat.

Early work by HARRIS (1927), separating epidermis from dermis by heat, had suggested that most of the histamine in *skin* is located in the epidermis. FELDBERG and MILES (1953) constructed a regional map of the histamine in whole skin of the guinea-pig and found their highest values in the skin of the ears, snout, lids and in the well-vascularized areas around the nipples and in the perineum. Recognition of the mast cell as the main source of tissue histamine at once clarified the problem of histamine in the skin, for when well-fixed sections of skin of guinea-pig are examined under the microscope it is clear that the mast cells occur entirely in the dermis and especially in the well-vascularized regions mentioned above: horizontal subdivision of such skin indicates that both the histamine and the mast cells occur together in the same tissue plane. MILES and MILES (1952), arguing from a presumed release of histamine around the blood vessels in the skin of the guinea-pig as shown by the outward diffusion of the dye, pontamine sky blue, had suggested that much of the histamine in skin resides in the perivascular areas. This is perhaps the commonest site for the accumulation of tissue mast cells.

In their analysis of the relationship of mast cells to histamine in skin, RILEY and WEST (1956) carried out detailed investigations on whole skin and on sections of skin in many species, including man. Whereas histamine and mast cells occur mainly in the more superficial dermis of the cat, they are both situated more deeply in the dermis of the rat. The mouse, on the other hand, has two layers of mast cells in the skin and a high concentration of histamine in each. Using the "histamine-profile" method of FELDBERG and HARRIS (1953), RILEY and WEST found an excellent correspondence between mast cells and histamine in serial slices of cat skin cut on the freezing microtome parallel to the skin surface. Meanwhile, GRAHAM and her associates (1955a) had carried out a meticulous investigation on the distribution of mast cells and histamine in the skin of the dog in which, like the cat, the majority of the mast cells are situated near the epidermis. They find that the mast cells "which constitute less than 0.2 per cent of the tissue mass, account for most, if not all of the histamine". JOHNSON (1955) on the other hand believes that acid hydrolysis reveals more histamine in skin than the free histamine which is contained in the mast cells; nevertheless, the regional distribution still agrees closely with the topographical data of FELDBERG and MILES (1953). An excellent illustration of the close correlation between mast cell count and histamine content in whole skin of foetal and neo-natal rats is presented by DIXON (1959). A somewhat similar distribution of histamine in mouse skin is described by BEAUMARIAGE and RADIVOJEVIC (1960).

Whether any histamine occurs normally in the *epidermis* of any species is not yet entirely settled. Mast cells are often found close to the epidermis and procedures such as those used originally by HARRIS (1927) and later by MONGAR (1956) lead to the diffusion of some of the histamine from its normal site. It would be interesting to know whether histamine, or a capacity to form histamine, can be detected in pure samples of epidermis grown in tissue culture. However, the general conclusion remains clear; the bulk of the histamine in the normal tissue listed above is located in the tissue mast cells.

Although individual mast cells readily lose or gain histamine and vary in size in different regions, it is of interest to have some idea of the average load of histamine carried by the mast cell in various species and localities. GRAHAM et al. (1955a) carried out a careful comparison of mast cell population and histamine content in dog skin, lung, liver, heart and skeletal muscle, and in beef liver capsule and parenchyma. They used alternate tissue sections for counting mast cells and for assaying histamine. According to these workers histamine values range from 7 $\mu\mu$g per cell for dog skin to 32 $\mu\mu$g per cell for beef liver capsule. The remaining dog tissues had intermediate values for histamine. A value of 25 $\mu\mu$g histamine in mast cells of beef liver capsule was found by RILEY (1959) who used the simpler method of counting mast cells in tissue spreads. BORÉUS and CHAKRAVARTY (1960) state that guinea-pig mast cells contain 21—34 $\mu\mu$g histamine, and these authors mention that other workers have found rat peritoneal mast cells to contain 15—30 $\mu\mu$g histamine per cell. It will be noted that the values so far available are of the same order.

B. Pathological tissues

The sole pathological condition in man outstandingly rich in mast cells is seen in the skin disease, *urticaria pigmentosa*, first described clinically by NETTLESHIP (1869) as 'chronic urticaria leaving brown stains', and histologically by UNNA (1896) who pointed out that the individual skin lesions are almost entirely composed of tissue mast cells. Characteristically it is a disease of infancy and clears up spontaneously in later life: more rarely it manifests itself as a single solitary nodule which can be readily excised. The salient feature of *urticaria pigmentosa* is that even slight trauma to a skin lesion elicits a grossly exaggerated 'triple response' (LEWIS, 1927), visible evidence of a local release of histamine in the skin (DALE, 1929). On occasion the release of histamine is so great as to produce systemic effects (BLOOM et al., 1958; BRINKMANN, 1959; ASBOE-HANSEN, 1960).

It was thus the more curious that no attempt was made to estimate histamine in a skin lesion of urticaria pigmentosa until RILEY and WEST (1952) reported that a biopsy specimen from a case of generalized *urticaria pigmentosa* contained two and a half times more histamine than did skin immediately adjacent to the lesion. Further investigations which included examples of the solitary type (RILEY, 1959) reveal that the greater the number of mast cells in the tissue block the higher is the histamine content, reaching in a solitary nodule packed with mast cells almost 1 mg. histamine per 1 g. wet weight of tissue (Table 5).

Table 5. *Mast cells and histamine in normal human skin and in skin lesions of urticaria pigmentosa of varying extent*

Case No.	Type of lesion	Histamine content (μg/g)	Mast-cell content of specimen
1	Solitary	950	Whole thickness occupied by mast cells
2	Solitary	555	Approximately half thickness occupied by mast cells
3	Generalized (active)	50·0	Thin layer of mast cells under epidermis
4	Generalized (quiescent)	35·0	Thin layer of mast cells under epidermis
5	Generalized ("bullous")	56·4	Thin layer of mast cells under epidermis
6	Generalized (adult type)	39·0	Thin layer of mast cells under epidermis
7	Skin adjacent to active lesion (same patient as No. 3)	20·0	Many scattered mast cells
8—17	Specimens of normal skin	5—10	Few scattered mast cells in each

Tumours composed of mast cells (mastocytomas) occasionally arise spontaneously in domestic animals and, as described earlier, have been induced in mice by x-irradiation and by painting the skin with a carcinogenic hydrocarbon. However, it remains to be explained why spontaneous mastocytomas arise more often in dogs, which are not especially well endowed with tissue mast cells, than in rats whose connective tissue is extraordinary rich in mast cells.

The histamine-mast cell hypothesis was clinched, as was the heparin-mast cell hypothesis, by a pharmacological investigation of mast cell tumours in the *dog*. Providing the tissue is reasonably fresh and has not been in contact with a

Table 6. *Histamine content* (μg/g) *of tissues compared with heparin content* (I.U./g) *and relative mast cell content: 10 y.o. Golden Cocker Spaniel with a mast cell tumour and metastases*

Tissue	Histamine	Heparin	Mast cells
Tumour (biopsy 10.1.54)	1,290	110	++++
Tumour (recurrence 13.3.54)	650	357	++++
Lymph node	600 (4)	293 (9)	++++
Spleen	90 (5)	88 (7)	+++
Liver	60 (25)	50 (20)	++
Lung	30 (25)	29 (13)	++
Skin	10 (9)	8 (11)	+
Kidney	1 (1)	5 (6)	0

Figures in brackets represent control values obtained from normal dogs.

preservative such as formaldehyde, it can readily be shown that mastocytomas in dogs are as rich in histamine as they are in heparin (Cass et al., 1954). A striking example is cited by West (1956) of a dog in which the primary tumour recurred twice after excision and which, at autopsy, was found to have metastases in lymph nodes, spleen and liver (Table 6).

Very high values were found both for histamine and for heparin in the primary tumour and lower values elsewhere in proportion to the local population of tissue mast cells. One sample from the primary site yielded no less than 1,290 μg./g. histamine. The general range of values in this type of tumour has been confirmed by Larsson (1957). Further data on mast cell tumours in dogs may be found in papers by Head (1958) and Lindell et al. (1959). Only one mast cell tumour low in histamine has so far been reported: this is the dog mastocytoma of Williams et al. (1959) which has also been propagated successfully in tissue culture.

Other species in which mast cell tumours have been studied include horse, cow, cat and mouse. Histamine values are available for repeated biopsies from a cow with multiple mast cell lesions of the skin and for three examples of mastocytoma in cats (West, 1958; Riley, 1959). Histamine data for two transplantable mast cell tumours in mice will be found in papers by Furth et al. (1957), Sjoerdsma et. al. (1957), Barrnett et al. (1958), Ono et al. (1959), Schindler et al. (1959), Day and Green (1960) and Green and Day (1960).

To sum up. Apart from a single example of a dog mastocytoma poor in histamine cited by Williams et al. (1959), the findings strongly support the view that the tumour mast cell, like the normal mast cell, is extraordinarily rich in histamine.

C. Location of histamine

Once it was clearly established that the mast cell is the chief repository of the tissue histamine, it became of interest to determine more precisely the location of histamine within the cell. Two methods suggest themselves, chemical and histochemical, both of which are limited by the tendency of the histamine to diffuse rapidly from its primary site.

Despite these difficulties, WEST (1955) found that mast cell granules, isolated by KÖKSAL's method from the subcutaneous tissue of mice, have a higher content of histamine than any other fraction. MOTA et al. (1954) report similar findings for histamine in the mast-cell granules of the rat.

SCHAUER and WERLE (1959) demonstrated histamine histochemically in the granules of mast cells in rat mesentery by treatment of the tissue with Reinecke salt and subsequent diazotization, as described in detail in Section 1F. The discovery by UVNÄS and THON (1959) that diffusion of histamine is minimized if the cells are isolated in the polysaccharide 'Ficoll' may be useful in further work of this nature.

D. Synthesis of histamine

As with the corresponding studies on heparin, the concentration of mast cells which occurs naturally in mastocytomas and the ability of such cells to grow in tissue culture, have proved of value in investigating the synthesis and storage of histamine by the mast cell. Normal mast cells isolated from the peritoneal fluid of rats (PADAWER and GORDON, 1955) may be used for comparison.

Mast granules isolated from the Furth mouse mastocytoma (FURTH et al., 1957) are rich in histamine and in histidine decarboxylase (BARRNETT et al., 1958; HAGEN et al., 1959) and similar findings are reported for the Dunn and Potter tumour by SJOERDSMA et al. (1957). Using the ascites form of the Furth mastocytoma, SCHINDLER et al. (1959) propagated tumour mast cells in tissue culture and found them capable of synthesizing histamine in vitro. GREEN and DAY (1960) separated three distinct clones of cells from the Dunn and Potter mouse mastocytoma, each with its own biochemical characteristics, and confirmed the ability of these cells to convert C^{14}-labelled histidine into histamine. Tumour mast cells from the dog behave similarly (LINDELL et al., 1959).

Comparable studies on mast cells from the peritoneal cavity of normal rats and in the skin of rats both normal and depleted of their histamine following injection of compound 48/80 are described by SCHAYER (1956) and by SCHAYER et al. (1959). SCHAYER (1960) makes the interesting observation that the histidine-decarboxylase is an adaptive enzyme, reaching high levels of activity in regenerating mast cells and vessel walls and in the mast cells of tissues subjected to stress. The requisite co-enzyme, pyridoxal-5'-phosphate, is thought to be located in the intergranular cytoplasm (BENDITT, 1958).

E. Effects of histamine liberators

Comparative studies indicate that a tissue rich in mast cells is also rich in histamine. Evidence will now be presented which shows that the mast cell can be induced to shed its histamine in response to a specific stimulus and that, should the cell survive, it can again accumulate a high concentration of histamine. Experiments of this kind followed the discovery of the chemical histamine-liberators (MACINTOSH and PATON, 1949) whose mode of action is discussed in detail elsewhere and whose effects in some species closely resemble the syndrome of anaphylaxis.

The simplest histamine-liberator is water which induces an osmotic disruption of the mast cell — an entirely non-specific effect. Nevertheless, once it had been envisaged that tissue histamine is normally concentrated within the mast cells, the osmotic effect of water, well known to EHRLICH, was used effectively by

Fawcett (1954, 1955) to show first, that an intraperitoneal injection of water can temporarily remove the mast cells from the peritoneum of the rat and, secondly, that as this occurs, assayable histamine now appears in the peritoneal fluid.

In his original study of the effects of chemical histamine-liberators Riley (1953b) traced the fluorescent liberator stilbamidine, to the mast cells in the peritoneum of the rat. Following an acute injection in which the animal dies within a matter of seconds, the mast cells appear normal, apart from a golden fluorescence of the granules. However, if a similar injection be given more slowly

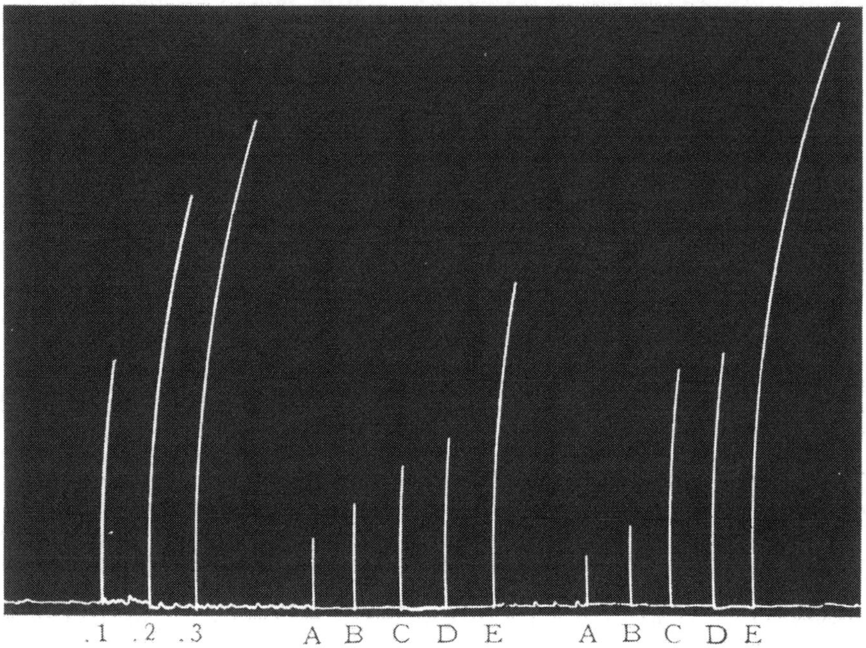

Fig. 3. Kymographic record of an experiment demonstrating a graded pharmacological response to a graded dose of compound 48/80. The first three contractions represent the responses of the guinea-pig ileum to 0,1, 0,2 and 0,3 ml of histamine solution, 1/100000. Five rats, A to E, received intraperitoneal injections of 20 ml of Tyrode solution containing respectively 0, 20, 100, 500 and 1000 μg. of 48/80. The set of contractions labelled A to E represents the responses of the ileum to 0,3 ml of fluid recovered from each of the 5 rats 30 min after injection. An increasing concentration of histamine with increasing dosage of 48/80 is clearly shown. The final set of contractions represents responses to 0·6 ml of fluid from each animal 60 min. after 48/80.

to another rat, permitting the animal to survive for some minutes, it is now seen that the mast cells are swollen, vacuolated and disrupted. Their fluorescence has largely disappeared. This is especially so in those large pericapillary mast cells which are normally packed with strongly metachromatic granules and are regarded as fully developed mast cells (Riley, 1953a).

With the introduction of compound 48/80, a more specific histamine-liberator for the rat (Paton, 1951), these observations were confirmed and extended. Mota et al. (1953) describe and illustrate the acute effects of compound 48/80 and stilbamidine as seen under the phase-contrast microscope. Smith (1958) suggests that the initial loss of brilliance of the granules signifies the actual freeing of histamine from its binding sites in the mast-cell. This recalls the earlier observation of Zollinger (1950) on the effect of water on the granules.

Fawcett (1954), following up his histological observations (1955) and combining them with pharmacological assay for histamine, produced convincing evidence not only for a release of histamine from the mast cells in the rat, but also for the graded action of compound 48/80 with increasing dosage (Figs. 3 and 4). Whereas TYRODE's fluid causes no morphological change in the mast cell and no release of histamine, water, on the other hand, disrupts the cells and gives rise to a rapid, though transient, release of histamine. Compound 48/80 in TYRODE's fluid releases histamine more slowly, but in greater quantity. However, compound 48/80 proved to be quite ineffective in rats previously injected with water, its target, the mast cells, having been destroyed. These findings were thoroughly

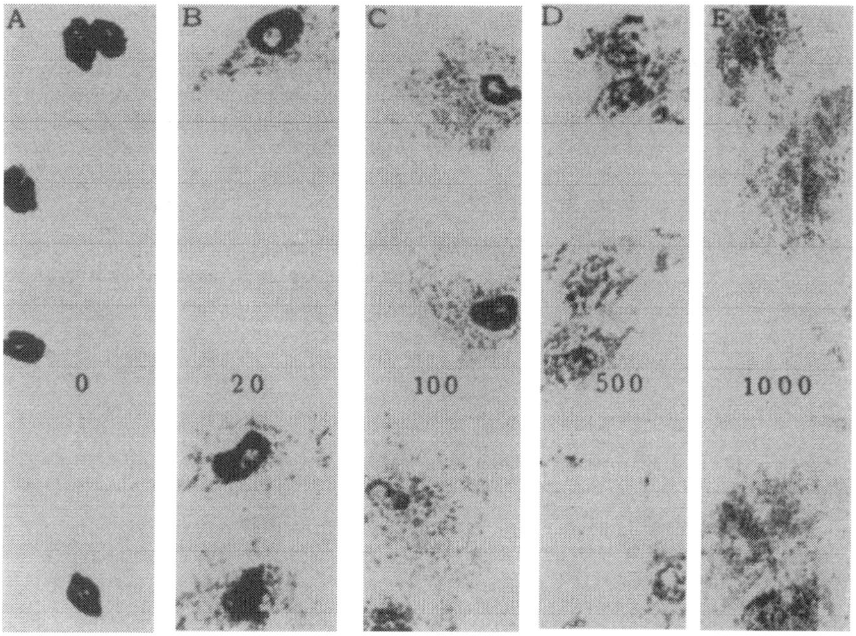

Fig. 4. Photomicrographs showing the condition of the mesenteric mast cells in the 5 animals whose histamine release is recorded in Fig. 3. There is a graded morphological response in the mast cells ranging from release of occasional granules in the rat receiving Tyrode solution alone to the discharge of nearly all the granules in the one which received 1000 μg of 48/80. (After FAWCETT, 1954).

confirmed by KELLER and BURKARD (1956) in an almost identical series of experiments.

A more extensive study of the effects of compound 48/80 on mast cells at various sites in the rat (RILEY and WEST, 1955a) indicates clearly the close positive correlation between mast cell damage and the level of tissue histamine. Compound 48/80 was injected intraperitoneally in increasing dosage until, by the end of a week daily doses as high as 1 mg. were readily tolerated. The tissues taking the brunt of the liberator were affected first and here the mast cells mainly suffered irreversible damage, new mast cells arising later from undifferentiated mesenchymal precursors. In the second (seen in tissues at some distance from the site of injection) the mast cells were not destroyed but showed a sequence of swelling and degranulation, followed in the recovery phase by contraction and re-granulation of the cells. Repeated assays for histamine in subcutis, ears, mesentery and omentum faithfully reflected the changing histological picture as judged by the disappearance and reappearance of the mast cells. BENDITT et al. (1955) described a similar sequence of changes in rats treated with ovomucoid.

According to WATSON and KENNEDY (1960), recovery of the mast cell follows immediately upon removal of the chemical agent.

LARSSON (1957) injected compound 48/80 into normal dogs and into dogs bearing mastocytomas. The tumour-bearing animals suffered the more severe shock (comparable to peptone or anaphylactic shock) and, on occasion also showed signs of a release of heparin into the blood (PATON, 1951; QUIVY, 1956). However, the loss of histamine from the tumours was never complete. LARSSON (1957) believes that the precipitous fall in blood pressure may prevent much of the liberated histamine from being flushed from the site of its release.

Compound 48/80 is also an effective histamine-liberator in the *cat*. Here again it is possible to recognize its effects first, by studying the ability of compound 48/80 to liberate histamine either from locally perfused regions of skin and muscle (FELDBERG and PATON, 1951), or from chopped skin in vitro (WESTERHOLM, 1960).

In contrast to the rat, cat, and dog, both the mouse and, especially, the guinea-pig are resistant to the action of compound 48/80 (RILEY and WEST, 1955b; FEINBERG and STERNBERGER, 1955). The guinea-pig on the other hand is well suited for studies on anaphylaxis.

F. Effects of anaphylaxis

The clinical syndrome of anaphylaxis differs considerably from one species to another. Nevertheless, there is clear evidence that in some species the pharmacologically-active substances responsible for the syndrome are released enzymatically from mast cells. To this extent at least it is profitable to compare histamine levels and mast-cell changes during anaphylaxis, as with the chemical histamine-liberators, and so obtain further information on the occurrence of histamine in mast cells. Three examples will be cited — the dog, the guinea-pig and the rat.

Interest in the dramatic syndrome of peptone shock in the dog (SCHMIDT-MÜLHEIM, 1880), in which the blood pressure falls and the blood becomes temporarily incoagulable, was stirred when it was shown that an identical syndrome occurs during anaphylaxis (PORTIER and RICHET, 1902). With the discovery of heparin and its location in the mast cells, WILANDER (1938) showed that anaphylaxis in the dog is accompanied by damage to the mast cells in the liver, the shock organ of this species and the source of its heparin. However, experiments on the perfused isolated organ indicate that not only does the heparin come from the liver but also the histamine (JAQUES and WATERS, 1941; ROCHA E SILVA et al., 1947; SCROGGIE and JAQUES, 1949; JAQUES et al., 1954). Indeed, this was one of the considerations which led to a search for both heparin and histamine within the same cell, the mast cell. It is thus pertinent to enquire to what extent the findings of anaphylaxis in the dog are applicable to other species and to the problem of the cellular location of histamine in general (SMITH, 1959).

As early as 1952 STUART had published a note on the occurrence of mast-cell disruption during anaphylaxis in several additional species — guinea-pig, rabbit, mouse. Similar changes have been observed in the hamster (WEGELIUS et al., 1955). However, STUART's attention was focussed on the common factor of heparin, which was thought to play a defensive role in the reaction. We now recognize the mast cell rather as the source of the pharmacologically-active substances which cause the shock in certain species. It is perhaps worth reiterating here that whereas the chemical liberators can release histamine from isolated granules, the anaphylactic reaction requires intact, living cells (MONGAR and SCHILD, 1955; MACINTOSH, 1956).

As is well known, the guinea-pig is the experimental animal of choice for studies on anaphylaxis, thanks to the exquisite sensitivity of its plain muscle to the mediators of the anaphylactic syndrome, especially histamine. MOTA and VUGMAN (1956) compared the effects of anaphylaxis and compound 48/80 on the mast cells in the lungs of guinea-pigs. As stated earlier, the chemical histamine-liberator, compound 48/80, is almost ineffective in the guinea-pig and has little effect upon its mast cells: on the other hand, the changes during anaphylaxis include swelling and disruption of the mast cells and a release of histamine, as seen in the dog. The mechanism of the anaphylactic reaction and the changes in the mast cells have been studied in detail by MOTA (1959) and HUMPHREY and MOTA (1959). BORÉUS (1960) used samples of nasal mucosa as test material in place of the more usual intact or chopped lung (MONGAR and SCHILD, 1955; AUSTEN and BROCKLEHURST, 1960).

In contrast to the guinea-pig, the rat can be rendered anaphylactic only with difficulty. In his original study RILEY (1953b) endeavoured to imitate the conditions of anaphylaxis in the rat by injecting agar-activated serum, the so-called 'anaphylatoxin' of BORDET (1913) as described by ROCHA E SILVA (1952 and see section 3D). Swelling and degranulation of the mast cells were seen, as with the chemical liberators. However, MOTA (1957) was unable to reproduce these results. More recently true anaphylaxis has been elicited in the tissues of the rat, both in vivo (KELLER, 1957; SANYAL and WEST, 1958) and in vitro (MOTA and DA SILVA, 1960), especially where additional sensitization has been obtained by adjuvant treatment with *H. pertussis* vaccine. HÖGBERG and UVNÄS (1960) have compared the effects of compound 48/80 and the antigen-antibody reaction on the mast cells of rat mesentery and find them very similar. MOTA and ISHII (1960) describe and depict typical changes in sensitized rat peritoneal mast cells treated with the specific antigen in vitro. In studying the release of histamine from such a preparation, GARCIA (unpublished) finds that a critical concentration of antibody is necessary to ensure that a maximal release of histamine is obtained. This may account for some of the previous failures in this type of experiment.

In summary, therefore, we can say that injections of chemical histamine-liberators or anaphylaxis cause changes in the histamine content and in the appearances of the mast cells which are consistent with the view that much of the releasable histamine resides in the mast cells (PERRY, 1956).

G. Blood mast cells

In contrast to our knowledge of the location of histamine in the tissues, comparatively few data are available for the location of histamine in blood. The findings of normal and pathological blood will therefore be considered together.

Up to 1952 it was generally agreed that most of the histamine in blood is associated with the leucocytes, the eosinophil in particular being suspect as the main carrier of blood histamine though subject to variations in its 'load' (CODE, 1952). In the following year, Hungarian workers (BIKICH et al., 1953) once more attempted to define the main repository of histamine in the blood of patients with chronic myeloid leukaemia without being able to conclude more than that in this condition the total cellular histamine may be so high as to constitute a diagnostic criterion for the disease: it was known that the histamine value is not raised in a leukocytosis of non-leukaemic origin (VALENTINE and LAWRENCE, 1948). Meanwhile GRAHAM and her associates (1952) had discovered the essential clue that "the unique feature of the blood picture in chronic myeloid leukaemia, marked basophilia, has apparently been overlooked as a possible explanation of the equally unique histaminemia." This new approach at once showed that the basophil "in spite of its scarcity, accounts for half of the histamine in normal blood" (GRAHAM et al., 1955b). GRAHAM and co-workers segregated the various leukocytes in specific gravity gradient columns consisting of concentrated albumen mixed with leukocyte-containing plasma. Centrifugation then distributed the white cells according to their specific gravities. Histamine was measured by a modification of the dinitrofluorobenzene method of MCINTIRE (1950). From their analysis of blood from normal subjects and from patients with polycythaemia vera and chronic myeloid leukaemia, GRAHAM et al. (1955b) conclude that in normal blood "the basophils contain histamine at a concentration 20,000 times that of platelets and a million times that of plasma" . . . "in chronic myelocytic leukaemia the basophils are poorer and the eosinophils and neutrophils richer than normal in histamine."

Following the initial publication of these findings (GRAHAM et al., 1952) and the evidence that tissue histamine resides in the mast cells (RILEY and WEST, 1952; RILEY, 1953c), EHRICH (1953) analyzed previous data of VALENTINE and LAWRENCE (1948) to demonstrate the correlation which exists between the basophils of the blood and its histamine content. In due course VALENTINE and co-workers themselves supplied convincing evidence that in man "the basophil is the predominant and perhaps exclusive carrier of histamine in the formed elements of the peripheral blood" (VALENTINE et al., 1955).

However, the situation with respect to histamine in the blood of other species is somewhat less clear. In rabbits the platelet contains most, if not all, of the histamine (MINARD, 1937) and, as CODE and MITCHELL (1957) have stressed, the eosinophil may yet play a part, long suspected, in carrying histamine in the blood of many species: in the dog and to some extent in the guinea-pig, the eosinophil appears to play the dominant role in this respect. In dealing with cells so few in number, CODE and MITCHELL rightly insist on the importance of expressing all values in terms of the absolute basophil count (MOORE and JAMES, 1953), that is, the number of cells per c.mm. blood.

The general conclusion from the above work is that the basophil — the counterpart of the mast cell in the tissues (BOSEILA, 1959) — provides the main cytological depot for histamine in the blood of man. In other species this role is taken over by the platelet or the eosinophil. The only reliable attempt to estimate the histamine content of the blood basophil is that of GRAHAM et al. (1955b) who report a value of 1 $\mu\mu$g histamine, about one-twentieth the amount in a tissue mast cell.

V. 5-hydroxytryptamine in mast cells

The presence of a second amine, 5-hydroxytryptamine (serotonin, 5-HT) in peritoneal mast cells of the rat was discovered by BENDITT et al. (1955) and confirmed by KELLER (1958). Unlike histamine, however, 5-HT is not a universal constituent of mast cells being restricted to the mast cells of the mouse and rat (PARRATT and WEST, 1957). The formation of 5-HT in rat skin, a tissue rich in mast cells, has been shown by LAGUNOFF et al. (1957). In parallel with the development of a mastocytosis induced by dietetic methods, 5-HT was found to accumulate in the bones of rats (CASS et al., 1958).

Mast cell tumours from mice (they are unknown in the rat) have also proved as useful a tool for investigating the problem of 5-HT as they have for similar studies on heparin and histamine in mast cells. BENDITT (1958) believes that 5-HT and the coenzyme of the 5-hydroxytryptophan decarboxylase (pyridoxal phosphate) may both reside in the cytoplasm of the mast cell in the rat. However,

Barrnett et al. (1958) and Ono et al. (1959) working with cells from the mouse mastocytoma isolated by Furth et al. (1957) find 5-HT in the granules, together with 5-hydroxytryptophan decarboxylase (Hagen and Lee, 1958; Hagen et al., 1960). Using similar cells in tissue culture, Schindler et al. (1959) have shown that the initial precursor may be tryptophan itself. Sjoerdsma et al. (1957) have likewise demonstrated 5-HT in the granules of the Dunn and Potter (1957) mouse mastocytoma. On the other hand, pathological specimens of mast cell lesions of the dog, cat, cow and man have failed to reveal a 5-HT reaction, even when the mast cell count and tissue histamine content have been exceptionally high (West, 1959).

A curious feature of chemical carcinogenesis in the skin of the mouse is the mast cell reaction which develops under an epidermis rendered hyperplastic by surface applications of a carcinogenic hydrocarbon. Many of these mast cells display under the microscope a golden-brown fluorescence in ultra-violet light, providing that the skin has been previously fixed in formaldehyde. Riley (1958) and Coupland and Riley (1960) have recently shown that the fluorescence is due to 5-HT which is present in high concentration.

VI. Conclusions

The work reviewed above indicates decisively that most of the tissue histamine assayed in the past has been mast-cell histamine. This is not to deny that there are other, and possibly more important, depots of tissue histamine from the standpoint of normal physiology (Kahlson, 1960). Nevertheless, recognition of the mast cell as a concentrated source of histamine in blood and tissues has led to a deeper understanding of the location of histamine and the mechanism of its liberation both by chemical substances and in the course of anaphylaxis in some species.

Histamine is formed in the mast cell and it is held in the mast cell granule. These facts are beyond dispute. The biological significance of the histamine in mast cells is at present unknown.

References

Asboe-Hansen, G.: Urticaria pigmentosa with generalized tissue mastocytosis and blood basophilia. Arch. Derm. **81**, 198 (1960).
Arvy, L.: Particularités histologiques des labrocytes chez quelques Batraciens. C.R. Ass. Anat. XLII Réunion **217** (1955a).
— Les labrocytes (Mastzellen). Rev. Hémat. **10**, 55 (1955b).
—, and D. Quivy: Relation entre la richesse en labrocytes et la teneur en histamine des divers segments du tube digestif chez le Chien. C.R. Soc. Biol. (Paris) **149**, 658 (1955).
Austen, K. F., and W. E. Brocklehurst: Inhibition of the anaphylactic release of histamine from chopped guinea-pig lung by chymotrypsin substrates and inhibitors. Nature (Lond.) **186**, 866 (1960).
Barrnett, R. J., P. Hagen and F. L. Lee: Mast-cell granules containing 5-hydroxytryptamine, histamine and heparin, morphologically and biochemically distinct from mitochondria. Biochem. J. **69**, 36P (1958).
Beaumariage, M. L., et D. V. Radivojevic: Teneur en histamine de la peau chez la Souris. C.R. Soc. Biol. (Paris) **154**, 1493 (1960).
Bell, H. J., and L. B. Jaques: Species differences in heparin. Bull. Soc. chim. Belg. **65**, 36 (1956).
Benditt, E. P.: Morphology, chemistry and function of mast cells. Ann. N. Y. Acad. Sci. **73**, 204 (1958).
—, S. Bader and K. B. Lam: Studies of the mechanism of acute vascular reactions to injury. I. The relationship of mast cells and histamine to the production of oedema by ovo-mucoid in rats. Arch. Path. **60**, 104 (1955).
—, R. L. Wong, M. Arase and E. Roeper: 5-hydroxytryptamine in mast cells. Proc. Soc. exp. Biol. (N. Y.) **90**, 303 (1955).

Bikich, G., J. Borbola, B. Tanos and E. Kelemen: The histamine content of granulocytes as a possible characteristic of myelocytic leukaemia. Acta med. Acad. Sci. hung. **4**, 17 (1953).

Bloom, G.: Studies on the cytology, cytochemistry and pathology of the Mast Cell. Stockholm: Roos Boktryckeri 1960.

—, H. Dunér, B. Pernow, J. Winberg and R. Zetterstom: Spontaneous histamine shocks in urticaria pigmentosa. Acta paediat. (Uppsala) **47**, 153 (1958).

Bordet, J.: Le méchanisme de l'anaphylaxie. C.R. Soc. Biol. (Paris) **74**, 225 (1913).

Boréus, L. O.: Quantitative studies on the antigen-antibody mast-cell reaction 'in vivo' in the guinea-pig lung. Acta physiol. scand. **48**, 431 (1960).

—, and N. Chakravarty: The histamine content of guinea-pig mast cells. Experientia (Basel) **16**, 192 (1960).

Boseila, A. W. A.: The basophil leucocyte and its relationship to the tissue mast cell. Copenhagen: Munksgaard 1959.

Brinkmann, E.: Mastzellenreticulose (Gewebsbasophilom) mit histaminbedingtem Flush und Übergang in Gewebsbasophilen-Leukämie. Schweiz. med. Wschr. **89**, 1046 (1959).

Cass, R., P. B. Marshall and J. F. Riley: 5-hydroxytryptamine and histamine in mast cells of the mouse and rat. J. Physiol. (Lond.) **141**, 510 (1958).

—, J. F. Riley, G. B. West, K. W. Head and S. W. Stroud: Heparin and histamine in mast-cell tumours from dogs. Nature (Lond.) **174**, 318 (1954).

Code, C. F.: Histamine in blood. Physiol. Rev. **32**, 47 (1952).

—, and R. G. Mitchell: Histamine, eosinophils and basophils in the blood. J. Physiol. (Lond.) **136**, 449 (1957).

Coupland, R. E., and J. F. Riley: Mast cells and 5-hydroxytryptamine in precancerous mouse skin. Nature (Lond.) **187**, 1128 (1960).

Dale, H. H.: Some chemical factors in the control of the circulation. Lecture II. Local vasodilator reactions — histamine. Lancet **1929 I**, 1233.

Day, M., and J. P. Green: Heparin, histamine and 5-hydroxytryptamine in neoplastic mast cells in culture. Fed. Proc. **19**, 133 (1960).

Dixon, J. B.: Histamine, 5-hydroxytryptamine and serum globulins in the foetal and neonatal rat. J. Physiol. (Lond.) **147**, 144 (1959).

Dunn, T. B., and M. Potter: A transplantable mast-cell neoplasm in the mouse. J. nat. Cancer Inst. **18**, 587 (1957).

Ehrich, W. E.: Histamine in mast cells. Science **118**, 603 (1953).

— J. Seifter, H. E. Alburn and A. J. Begany: Heparinocytes in elephantiasis scroti. Proc. Soc. exp. Biol. (N. Y.) **70**, 183 (1949).

Ehrlich, P.: Beiträge zur Kenntnis der Anilinfärbungen und ihrer Verwendung in der mikroskopischen Technik. Arch. mikr. Anat. **13**, 263 (1877).

—, and A. Lazarus: Normale und pathologische Histologie des Blutes. Die Anämie, vol. 1. Wien: Holder (Revised and Republished, 1909) 1898.

Fawcett, D. W.: Cytological and pharmacological observations on the release of histamine by mast cells. J. exp. Med. **100**, 217 (1954).

— An experimental study of mast-cell degranulation and regeneration. Anat. Rec. **121**, 29 (1955).

Feinberg, S. M., and L. A. Sternberger: Action of histamine-liberator compound 48/80 in the guinea pig. J. Allergy **26**, 170 (1955).

Feldberg, W., and G. W. Harris: Distribution of histamine in the mucosa of the gastrointestinal tract of the dog. J. Physiol. (Lond.) **120**, 352 (1953).

—, A. A. Miles: Regional variations of increased permeability of skin capillaries induced by a histamine-liberator and their relation to the histamine content of the skin. J. Physiol. (Lond.) **120**, 205 (1953).

—, and W. D. M. Paton: Release of histamine from skin and muscle in the cat by opium alkaloids and other histamine liberators. J. Physiol. (Lond.) **114**, 490 (1951).

Furth, J., P. Hagen and E. I. Hirsch: Transplantable mastocytoma in the mouse containing histamine, heparin, 5-hydroxytryptamine. Proc. Soc. exp. Biol. (N. Y.) **95**, 824 (1957).

Graham, H. T., O. H. Lowry, N. Wahl and M. K. Priebat: Mast cells as sources of tissue histamine. J. exp. Med. **102**, 307 (1955a).

— —, F. Wheelwright, M. A. Lenz and H. H. Parish jr.: Distribution of histamine among leucocytes and platelets. Blood **10**, 467 (1955b).

—, F. Wheelwright, H. H. Parish jr., A. R. Marks and O. H. Lowry: Distribution of histamine among blood elements. Fed. Proc. **11**, 350 (1952).

Green, J. P., and M. Day: Heparin, 5-hydroxytryptamine and histamine in neoplastic mast cells. Biochem. Pharmacol. **3**, 190 (1960).

Grossberg, A. L., and H. Garcia-Arocha: Histamine liberation 'in vitro' and mode of binding of histamine in tissues. Science **120**, 762 (1954).

HAGEN, P.: The intracellular distribution of histamine in dog's liver. Brit. J. Pharmacol. **9**, 100 (1954).

—, R. J. BARRNETT and F. L. LEE: Biochemical and electron microscope study of particles isolated from mastocytoma cells. J. Pharmacol. exp. Ther. **126**, 91 (1959).

—, and F. L. LEE: Amino acid decarboxylases of mouse mast cells. J. Physiol. (Lond.) **143**, 7P (1958).

—, N. WEINER, S. ONO and F. L. LEE: Amino acid decarboxylases of mouse mastocytoma tissue. J. Pharmacol. exp. Ther. **130**, 9 (1960).

HARRIS, K. E.: Observations on a histamine-like substance in skin extracts. Heart **14**, 161 (1927).

HEAD, K. W.: Cutaneous mast-cell tumours in the Dog, Cat and Ox. Brit. J. Derm. **70**, 389 (1958).

HEDBOM, A., and O. SNELLMAN: Isolation and analysis of the large cytoplasmic granules of tissue mast cells. Exp. cell Res. **9**, 148 (1955).

HÖGBERG, B., and B. UVNÄS: Further observations on the disruption of rat mesentery mast cells caused by compound 48/80, antigen-antibody reaction, lecithinase A and decylamine. Acta physiol. scand. **48**, 133 (1960).

HOLMGREN, H., and O. WILANDER: Beitrag zur Kenntnis der Chemie und Funktion der Ehrlichschen Mastzellen. Z. mikr.-anat. Forsch. **42**, 242 (1937).

HUMPHREY, J. H., and I. MOTA: The mechanism of anaphylaxis: specificity of antigen-induced mast cell damage in anaphylaxis in the guinea pig. Immunology **2**, 31 (1959).

JAQUES, L. B., H. J. BELL and M. H. CHO: The physiology of heparin. Proc. 1st Int. Conf. Thrombosis and Embolism, Basel, 281 (1954).

—, E. T. WATERS: The identity and origin of the anticoagulant of anaphylactic shock in the dog. J. Physiol. (Lond.) **99**, 454 (1941).

JOHNSON, H. H. JR.: A microchemical method for the determination of histamine. Arch. Derm. **72**, 307 (1955).

JORPES, J. E.: Heparin in the treatment of thrombosis, 2nd ed. London: Oxford University Press 1946.

—, E. ODEBLAD and H. BOSTRÖM: An autoradiographic study on the uptake of S^{35} labelled sodium sulphate in the mast cells. Acta haemat. (Lpz.) **9**, 273 (1953).

JULEN, C., O. SNELLMAN and B. SYLVÉN: Cytological and fractionation studies on the cytoplasmic constituents of tissue mast cells. Acta physiol. scand. **196**, 289 (1949).

KAHLSON, G.: A place for histamine in normal physiology. Lancet **278**, 67 (1960).

KELLER, R.: Tissue mast cells in anaphylactic shock and anaphylactoid reactions. Int. Arch. Allergy **11**, 328 (1957).

— Zur Bindung von Histamin und Serotonin in den Mastzellen. Arzneimittel-Forsch. **8**, 390 (1958).

—, und W. BURKARD: Die Bedeutung der Gewebemastzellen für die Histaminfreisetzung. Helv. physiol. pharmacol. Acta **14**, 289 (1956).

KÖKSAL, M.: Extraction of heparin-like substance from mast-cell granules in connective tissues. Nature (Lond.) **172**, 733 (1953).

KORN, E. D.: The synthesis of heparin by slices of mouse mast cell tumour. J. biol. Chem. **234**, 1321 (1959a).

— The isolation of heparin from mouse mast cell tumour. J. biol. Chem. **234**, 1325 (1959b).

LAGUNOFF, D., and E. P. BENDITT: Mast cell degranulation and histamine release observed in a new 'in vitro' system. J. exp. Med. **112**, 571 (1960).

—, R. CALHAM and E. P. BENDITT: Direct measurement of radio-active sulphate by rat mast cells. Proc. Soc. exp. Biol. (N. Y.) **104**, 575 (1960).

—, K. B. LAM, E. ROEPER and E. P. BENDITT: 5-hydroxytryptamine formation from 5-hydroxytryptophan by mast cells. Fed. Proc. **16**, 363 (1957).

LARSSON, B.: Effects of compound 48/80 on blood pressure and plasma histamine level of normal dogs and dogs with mastocytoma. Acta physiol. scand. **39**, 12 (1957).

LEWIS, T.: The blood vessels of the human skin and their responses. London: Shaw 1927.

LINDELL, S. E., H. RORSMAN and H. WESTLING: Formation of histamine in a canine mastocytoma. Experientia (Basel) **15**, 31 (1959).

LINDHOLM, S.: The occurrence of connective tissue mast cells in the alimentary canal wall of hamster and rat. Acta path. microbiol. scand. **48**, 328 (1960).

LIPMANN, F.: Biological sulphate activation and transfer. Science **128**, 575 (1958).

LISON, L.: Etudes sur la métachromasie. Colorants métachromatiques et substances chromotropes. Arch. Biol. (Paris) **46**, 599 (1935).

MCINTIRE, F. C., F. B. WHITE and M. SPROULL: Determination of histamine with 2,4-dinitrofluorobenzene. Arch. Biochem. **29**, 376 (1950).

MACINTOSH, F. C.: Histamine and intracellular particles. Ciba Symposium. pp. 20—35. London: Churchill 1956.

—, and W. D. M. PATON: The liberation of histamine by certain organic bases. J. Physiol. (Lond.) **109**, 190 (1949).

MICHELS, N. A.: The mast cells. In H. DOWNEY, Handbook of haematology, vol. 1, pp. 232—254. New York: Hoeber; London: Hamilton 1938.
MILES, A. A., and E. MILES: Vascular reactions to histamine, histamine-liberator and leukotaxine in the skin of guinea pigs. J. Physiol. (Lond.) **118**, 228 (1952).
MINARD, D.: The presence and distribution of histamine-like substances in blood. Amer. J. Physiol. **119**, 375 (1937).
MONGAR, J. L.: Discussion to RILEY. Ciba Symposium. pp. 404—406. London: Churchill 1956.
—, and H. O. SCHILD: Inhibition of histamine release in anaphylaxis. Nature (Lond.) **176**, 163 (1955).
MOORE, J. E., and G. W. JAMES: A simple direct method for absolute basophil leucocyte count. Proc. Soc. exp. Biol. (N. Y.) **82**, 601 (1953).
MOTA, I.: Action of anaphylactic shock and anaphylatoxin on mast cells and histamine in rats. Brit. J. Pharmacol. **12**, 453 (1957).
— Effect of antigen and octylamine on mast cells and histamine content of sensitized guinea-pig tissues. J. Physiol. (Lond.) **147**, 425 (1959).
—, W. T. BERALDO, A. G. FERRI and L. C. U. JUNQUEIRA: Intracellular distribution of histamine. Nature (Lond.) **174**, 698 (1954).
— — and L. C. U. JUNQUEIRA: Protamine-like property of compound 48/80 and stilbamidine and their action on mast cells. Proc. Soc. exp. Biol. (N. Y.) **83**, 455 (1953).
—, and W. D. DA SILVA: Antigen-induced damage to isolated sensitized mast cells. Nature (Lond.) **186**, 245 (1960).
—, A. G. FERRI and L. C. U. JUNQUEIRA: Action of peptone on the mast cells and histamine contents of dog tissues. Acta haemat. (Lpz.) **15**, 409 (1956).
— — and S. YONEDA: The distribution of mast cells in the digestive tract of laboratory animals: its bearing on the problem of the localization of histamine in tissues. Quart. J. micr. Sci. **97**, 251 (1956).
—, and T. ISHII: Inhibition of mast cell disruption and histamine release in rat anaphylaxis 'in vitro'. Comparison with compound 48/80. Brit. J. Pharmacol. **15**, 82 (1960).
—, L. C. U. JUNQUEIRA, W. T. BERALDO and A. G. FERRI: Action of peptone on mast cells of the dog. Nature (Lond.) **173**, 547 (1954).
—, and I. VUGMAN: Effects of anaphylactic shock and compound 48/80 on the mast cells of the guinea-pig lung. Nature (Lond.) **177**, 427 (1956).
NETTLESHIP, E.: Rare forms of urticaria. I. Chronic urticaria, leaving brown stains: nearly two years duration. Brit. med. J. 1869 II, 323.
OLIVER, J., F. BLOOM and C. MANGIERI: On the origin of heparin. An examination of the heparin content and the specific cytoplasmic particles of neoplastic mast cells. J. exp. Med. **86**, 107 (1947).
ONO, S., and P. HAGEN: Pyridoxal phosphate: a coenzyme of histidine decarboxylase. Nature (Lond.) **184**, 1143 (1959).
—, L. ZOMPETTI, P. HAGEN and J. FURTH: Relation of mastocytoma to mast cell leukaemia and of heparin, histamine and serotonin to mast cells. Blood **14**, 770 (1959).
ORKIN, M., and R. M. SCHWARTZMAN: A comparative study of canine and human dermatology. *ii.* Cutaneous tumours — the mast cell and canine mastocytoma. J. invest. Derm. **32**, 451 (1959).
PADAWER, J., and A. S. GORDON: Isolation of mast cells from other cellular elements of rat peritoneal fluid. Proc. Soc. exp. Biol. (N. Y.) 88, 29 (1955).
PARRATT, J. R., and G. B. WEST: 5-hydroxytryptamine and tissue mast cells. J. Physiol. (Lond.) **137**, 169 (1957).
PATON, W. D. M.: Compound 48/80: a potent histamine-liberator. Brit. J. Pharmacol. **6**, 499 (1951).
PERRY, W. L. M.: Skin histamine. Ciba Symposium. pp. 242—247. London: Churchill 1956.
PORTIER, P., et C. RICHET: De l'action anaphylactique de certains venins. C.R. Soc. Biol. (Paris) **54**, 170 (1902).
QUIVY, D.: La coagulation sanguine chez le chien au cours de divers chocs libérateurs d'héparine ou d'histamine. Arch. int. Pharmacodyn. **105**, 429 (1956).
RILEY, J. F.: Morphology and functions of mast cells in the rat. Proc. Scot. Soc. exp. Med., Dundee Meeting, 9th February (1952).
— The relationship of the tissue mast cells to the blood vessels in the rat. J. Path. Bact. **65**, 461 (1953a).
— The effects of histamine-liberators on the mast cells of the rat. J. Path. Bact. **65**, 471 (1953b).
— Histamine in tissue mast cells. Science **118**, 332 (1953c).
— Fluorescent mast cells in precancerous mouse skin. Experientia (Basel) **13**, 141 (1958).
— The mast cells. Edinburgh: Livingstone 1959.
—, and G. B. WEST: Histamine in tissue mast cells. J. Physiol. (Lond.) **117**, 72P (1952).

RILEY, J. F., and G. B. WEST: The presence of histamine in tissue mast cells. J. Physiol. (Lond.) **120**, 528 (1953).
— — Tissue mast cells. Studies with a histamine-liberator of low toxicity (compound 48/80). J. Path. Bact. **69**, 269 (1955a).
— — Histamine-liberation in the rat and mouse. Arch. int. Pharmacodyn. **102**, 304 (1955b).
— — Skin histamine: its location in the tissue mast cells. Arch. Derm. **74**, 471 (1956).
RINGERTZ, N. R.: Acid polysaccharides of mast cell tumours. Uppsala: Almquist and Wiksell's Boktryckeri 1960.
ROCHA E SILVA, M.: Concerning the mechanism of anaphylaxis and allergy. Brit. med. J. **1952 I**, 779.
—, A. E. SCROGGIE, E. FIDLAR and L. B. JAQUES: Liberation of histamine and heparin by peptone from the isolated dog's liver. Proc. Soc. exp. Biol. (N. Y.) **64**, 141 (1947).
SAGHER, F.: Milestones in dermatology. XX. Mast-cell disorders: the changing aspects of urticaria pigmentosa from a pure cutaneous to a systemic disease. Excerpta med. (Amst.) Sect. XIII **10**, 311 (1956).
SANYAL, R. K., and G. B. WEST: The relationship of histamine and 5-hydroxytryptamine to anaphylactic shock in different species. J. Physiol. (Lond.) **144**, 525 (1958).
SCHAUER, A. E., and E. WERLE: Zur histochemischen Darstellung des Histamins der Mastzellen. Z. ges. exp. Med. **131**, 100 (1959).
SCHAYER, R. W.: Formation and binding of histamine by free mast cells of rat peritoneal fluid. Amer. J. Physiol. **186**, 199 (1956).
— Relationship of stress-induced histidine decarboxylase to circulatory homeostasis and shock. Science **131**, 226 (1960).
—, Z. ROTHSCHILD and P. BIZONY: Increase in histidine decarboxylase activity of rat skin following treatment with compound 48/80. Amer. J. Physiol. **196**, 295 (1959).
SCHINDLER, R., M. DAY and G. A. FISCHER: Culture of neoplastic mast cells and their synthesis of 5-hydroxytryptamine and histamine 'in vitro'. Cancer Res. **19**, 47 (1959).
SCHMIDT-MÜLHEIM, A.: Beiträge zur Kenntnis des Peptons und seiner physiologischen Bedeutung. Arch. Anat. Physiol. (Lpz.) 33 (1880).
SCROGGIE, A. E., and L. B. JAQUES: A release of histamine and heparin by antigen from the isolated perfused liver of the sensitized dog. J. Immunol. **62**, 103 (1949).
SJOERDSMA, A., T. P. WAALKES and H. WEISSBACH: Serotonin and histamine in mast cells. Science **125**, 1202 (1957).
SMITH, D. E.: Nature of the secretory activity of the mast cell. Amer. J. Physiol. **193**, 573 (1958).
SMITH, W. E.: Mast cell population of lung of the guinea-pig and other tissues. Nature (Lond.) **184**, 1154 (1959).
SPOLTER, L., and W. MARX: Transfer of radioactive sulphate from phosphoadenosine phosphosulphate to heparin. Biochim. biophys. Acta (Amst.) **32**, 291 (1959).
STUART, E. G.: Mast-cell responses to anaphylaxis. Anat. Rec. **112**, 394 (1952).
TRETHEWIE, E. R.: "Free" and "bound" histamine and acetylcholine. J. Physiol. (Lond.) **94**, 11P (1938).
UNNA, P. G.: The histopathology of the diseases of the skin. Edinburgh: Clay; New York: Macmillan 1896.
UVNÄS, B., and I.-L. THON: Isolation of 'biologically intact' mast cells. Exper. Cell Res. **18**, 512 (1959).
VALENTINE, W. N., and J. S. LAWRENCE: Studies in blood histamine. Partition of blood histamine before and after clotting in health and disease states. Amer. J. med. Sci. **216**, 619 (1948).
— —, M. L. PEARCE and W. S. BECK: The relationship of the basophil to blood histamine in man. Blood **10**, 154 (1955).
WATSON, W. C., and J. S. KENNEDY: Regeneration of the tissue mast cell: an autoradiographic study. Brit. J. exp. Path. **41**, 385 (1960).
WEGELIUS, O., G. HJELMMAN and C. WASASTJERNA: Morphological changes caused by antihamster serum in the mast cells of the hamster. Acta path. microbiol. scand. **36**, 309 (1955).
WEST, G. B.: Histamine in mast-cell granules. J. Pharm. Pharmacol. **7**, 80 (1955).
— Histamine in mast cells. Ciba Symposium. pp. 14—19. London: Churchill 1956.
— Pharmacology of the tissue mast cell. Brit. J. Derm. **70**, 409 (1958).
— Tissue mast cells and tissue amines. J. Pharm. Pharmacol. **11**, 513 (1959).
WESTERHOLM, B.: 'In vitro' release of histamine from cat skin by compound 48/80. Acta physiol. scand. **50**, 41 (1960).
WILANDER, O.: Studien über Heparin. Skand. Arch. Physiol. **81**, Suppl. 15 (1938).
WILLIAMS, W. J., E. LARSON and T. L. PHILLIPS: A neoplastic connective tissue mast cell capable of continuous growth in tissue culture. J. biophys. biochem. Cytol. **6**, 361 (1959).
ZOLLINGER, H. U.: Gewebsmastzellen und Heparin. (Phasenmikroskopische Untersuchung.) Experientia (Basel) **6**, 384 (1950).

Section F

Histochimie des mastocytes

Par

LUCIEN A. J. LISON

I. Introduction

Il y a d'excellentes preuves (voir section 1 E du présent Handbuch) que les mastocytes[1] sont la source principale de l'histamine des tissus. Une meilleure connaissance de l'organisation chimique de ces cellules peut aider à résoudre les problèmes que posent la synthèse, la libération et la signification biologique de l'histamine dans les mastocytes.

Dans le présent exposé, on passera en revue quelques aspects de l'Histochimie des mastocytes. Tous ne seront pas traités avec la même profondeur. Les preuves indirectes de l'existence de l'histamine et d'autres substances pharmacologiquement importantes dans les mastocytes, preuves obtenues principalement en comparant contenus en substances actives et nombre de mastocytes dans les tissus, sont exposées dans une autre section (section 1 E) de cet ouvrage et ne seront rappelées ici qu'en cas de nécessité. D'un autre côté, certains aspects de l'organisation chimique des mastocytes ont paru n'avoir que des relations très indirectes avec les problèmes traités dans cet ouvrage, et on s'est limité à des citations bibliographiques, que permettront au chercheur, le cas échéant, d'approfondir sa documentation.

L'énorme masse des données sur les mastocytes est extrêmement confuse, et il n'est pas aisé de se faire une image claire de l'histochimie de ces cellules. Une partie des contradictions apparentes est due à des erreurs d'observation ou à des fautes techniques, mais à notre avis, la plus grande part est due aux causes suivantes:

1) Les mastocytes, qui jusqu'à présent ont été trouvés chez tous les Vertébrés où ils ont été recherchés avec des techniques adéquates, ne sont nullement un type cellulaire de constitution et de propriétés constantes. Il n'y a qu'un petit nombre de réactions histochimiques fondamentalement semblables dans toutes les espèces examinées. A notre connaissance, deux réactions seulement, la basophilie et la métachromasie, se présentent avec pratiquement toutes les mêmes caractéristiques quelle que soit l'espèce animale. Par conséquent, il ne faut pas parler de l'histochimie *du* mastocyte, mais bien de celle *des* mastocytes.

[1] De la dénomination originale de Ehrlich „Mastzellen", que les anglais traduisent, correctement, «Mast cells», on a dérivé en français l'hybride germano-grec «Mastocytes». Le terme est malheureux, personne n'en doute, parce que sa dérivation philologique est incorrecte et parce que la flexion, «Masto», imitée de l'allemand «mästen» = engraisser, suggère irrésistiblement le terme grec «mastos» = mamelle. Des autres termes proposés pour le remplacer — labrocytes, sitistocytes, basocytes, héparinocytes — seul le premier est encore quelquefois employé. Quelques auteurs utilisent «mastgranules» pour désigner les granulations des mastocytes; on peut faire des réserves sur la dérivation du terme, mais il est commode; nous l'utiliserons.

2) La plus grande part de nos connaissances sur les mastocytes a été obtenue à partir d'études effectuées chez le rat. Le rat est le plus commun des animaux de laboratoire et ses mastocytes sont très favorables à l'observation histologique et histochimique, à cause de la facilité de leur conservation et de leur fixation par les fixateurs histologiques courants. Cependant, ces caractéristiques favorables sont tout-à-fait exceptionelles, et les mastocytes du rat ne peuvent en aucun cas être considérés comme représentant typique des mastocytes en général.

II. Identification, préservation et fixation des mastocytes

Deux conditions préalables doivent être remplies pour que puisse être effectuée l'étude histochimique des mastocytes: 1⁰) l'identification des cellules étudiées comme étant réellement des mastocyctes; 2⁰) leur préservation adéquate durant les prétraitements exigés par l'investigation histochimiques. Comme la réalisation de ces deux conditions a fréquemment été cause de déboires et d'erreurs dans les études sur les mastocytes, il convient que nous lui consacrions quelques lignes préliminaires.

A. L'identification des mastocytes

Quand les mastocytes ont été correctement préservés (voir paragraphe suivant), leur identification ne présente généralement pas de difficultés majeures. Les méthodes les plus courantes font appel à des colorants basiques, les plus employés étant actuellement le bleu de toluidine et la thionine. Ils peuvent être utilisés en solution alcoolique, (c'était le procédé original de *Ehrlich*, 1879), en solution aqueuse, généralement à pH bas (pH 2.5-3, obtenu par addition de 1 % d'acide acétique), suivi ou non de différenciation par des solutions acides, ou encore dans d'autres solvants, comme le tétraméthylèneglycol-éther à 50 % (PADAWER, 1959). Avec ces méthodes, la substance fondamentale du cartilage et certains mucus se colorent comme les granulations des mastocytes, mais l'aspect morphologique en est tellement différent qu'aucune confusion n'est possible. Dans les tissus très riches en substance fondamentale métachromatique, le contraste entre mastocytes et substance fondamentale est insuffisant; un prétraitement par l'hyaluronidase fait apparaître les mastocytes (PRAKKEN et WOERDEMANN, 1952).

Un certain nombre de méthodes ont été proposées spécifiquement pour la coloration élective des mastocytes; ce sont en réalité des modalités de coloration par colorants basiques, mais elles peuvent rendre des services dans des cas particuliers. Telles sont les méthodes à l'érythrosinate de pinacyanol (BENSLEY, 1952), à la chrysoïdine (HARADA, 1957), à l'hématoxyline-rouge neutre et au Feulgen-vert de méthyle (ALLEN, 1960). Une méthode basée sur un principe tout différent a été proposée par BUJARD (1930) et serait tout-à-fait spécifique pour les granules des mastocytes; elle repose sur un traitement successif par la fuchsine acide et par l'eau de brome; son mécanisme est inconnu.

La seule véritable difficulté d'identification des mastocytes réside dans une confusion possible avec les leucocytes basophiles. Les granulations de ces derniers offrent en effet des caractères très voisins de ceux des mastocytes et les deux types cellulaires peuvent coexister: d'une part, les leucocytes basophiles peuvent migrer dans les tissus comme les autres types de leucocytes sanguins; d'autre part, dans la moelle osseuse, les mastocytes, normalement absents ou très rares, peuvent apparaître au cours de diverses myélopathies (UNDRITZ, 1946; LEITNER, 1949; BREMY, 1950; FADEM, 1951; MESSERSCHMITT, 1954; JOHNSTONE, 1956), et pourraient être confondus avec des myélocytes. La morphologie permet d'effectuer la distinction (le leucocyte basophile est plus petit, son noyau polymorphe, ses granulations plus grosses et plus irrégulières), mais non les caractères histochimiques, que les recherches de TURCHINI et KHAU van KIEN (1954) et de TURCHINI (1959) ont montré être très voisins dans les deux types cellulaires. L'histochimie comparée des mastocytes et des leucocytes basophiles demande des nouvelles recherches.

B. Préservation et fixation

Dès 1891, WESTPHAL et son maitre EHRLICH avaient attiré l'attention sur la grande labilité des granulations des mastocytes chez certaines espèces. Beaucoup sont hydrosolubles; pour les préserver, il faut, d'après ces auteurs, fixer dans l'alcool à 50 % et colorer par des solutions alcooliques de colorants. Il est certain, comme l'indique MICHELS (1938), que beaucoup de temps et de travail ont été perdus pour ne pas avoir pris garde aux difficultés de préservation correcte des granulations des mastocytes. Malgré les progrès de la technique, la difficulté persiste encore aujourd'hui.

A ce point de vue, il y a entre espèces animales des différences considérables, pour des raisons inconnues. Les granulations les plus stables sont celles du rat, que n'importe quel fixateur histologique préserve sans difficultés. Plus difficiles à fixer sont celles de l'homme, du chien, du chat, plus difficiles encore celles du lapin et des Ongulés. Celles des Amphibiens et plus encore celles des Poissons sont les plus difficiles de toutes. Il pourrait y avoir en outre des différences chez la même espèce. Chez le chat, les mastocytes sous-cutanés auraient des granules résistant à l'eau, tandis que ceux de l'épiploon seraient hydrosolubles (VARICAK, 1938).

Au sujet des fixateurs histologiques courants, les plus grandes contradictions existent entre les auteurs. Certains (ARVY, 1955 c) estiment que les fixateurs à base de formol, de picro-formol ou de bichromate (BOUIN, HELLY, MAXIMOW) conservent bien les mastocytes, tandis que d'autres sont d'opinion contraire (HOLMGREN, 1938; FERRI, 1955).

Le premier des procédés proposés spécifiquement pour les mastocytes, à savoir la fixation par l'*alcool à* 50 %, paraît effectivement conserver les mastgranules dans la plupart des cas, mais, comme l'indiquaient déjà Ehrlich et Westphal, tous les traitements ultérieurs, y compris la coloration, doivent se faire en milieu anhydre, car les granules se redissolvent au contact de milieux aqueux. Aujourd'hui, la préservation par l'alcool n'est plus que rarement employée. *L'acétate de plomb* à 4 % a été proposé par HOLMGREN (1938), partant du fait que l'acétate de plomb précipite l'héparine. Il a été largement utilisé par l'école suédoise et paraît efficace, bien qu'il ne fixe que médiocrement les tissus. Meilleur du double point de vue de la préservation des mastgranules et de la fixation générale des tissus est le *fixateur de Ferri et Motta* (1954): c'est une solution à 1 % de sous-acétate de plomb dans l'alcool à 50 % contenant 0,5 % d'acide acétique. D'après notre expérience, ce procédé donne des résultats très satisfaisants et devrait substituer les techniques antérieures comme procédé de routine pour l'étude des mastocytes.

III. Héparine et autres mucopolysaccharides

L'héparine ou des mucopolysaccharides voisins de l'héparine sont les constituants histochimiques les plus constants des mastocytes. La découverte de leur localisation a été effectuée par voie histochimique (HOLMGREN et WILANDER, 1937). Ceci, et le fait qu'on a supposé que l'héparine serait liée à l'histamine dans la cellule (sous la forme d'«héparinate d'histamine»), justifie que nous les étudions en premier lieu. Nous décrirons successivement les diverses réactions histochimiques dues à ces composés, ou attribuables à eux.

A. Basophilie

Tous les colorants basiques essayés jusqu'ici colorent intensément les granulations des mastocytes. Quand le colorant est susceptible de donner lieu à des colorations métachromatiques, la coloration est métachromatique. Basophilie et métachromasie sont les deux caractères fondamentaux des granulations des mastocytes, positifs chez toutes les espèces étudiées, du moment que les prétraitements ont conservé les granulations. La métachromasie, dans les mastocytes, est étroitement associée à la basophilie.

Les colorants basiques utilisés pour la coloration des mastocytes sont des thiazines (p. ex. bleu de toluidine, thionine, azur A et B de méthylène, bleu de méthylène), oxazines (bleu de crésyl brillant) et dérivés du triphénylméthane (dahlia, violet de méthyle), mais en fait tous les colorants basiques donnent les mêmes résultats. Il est inutile d'en dresser une liste complète. Cependant, quelques-uns doivent être mentionnés en particulier, à cause de leurs applications spéciales.

Le *Vert Janus*, colorant supravital des mitochondries, colorerait les granulations des mastocytes supravitalement chez le Rat (JORDAN, 1926; ARVY, 1955 c), mais non chez le Hamster, où il ne révélerait d'ailleurs pas de mitochondries (COMPTON, 1952). Sur préparations fixées, il colore les mastgranules, comme n'importe quel autre colorant basique.

Le *Rouge Neutre* colore les granulations aussi bien en coloration supravitale que sur pièces fixées.

Le *Vert de méthyle*, que divers auteurs ont consideré, -erronément-, comme un réactif histochimique spécifique des acides nucléiques (POLLISTER et LEUCHTENBERGER, 1949) colore les granulations des mastocytes (TAFT, 1951; LISON, 1953, 1960).

La *Pyronine*, utilisée généralement en conjunction avec le vert de méthyle (mélange de Unna) pour la coloration sélective des ribonucléines (BRACHET, 1940), colore les granulations des mastocytes, aussi bien seule que dans le mélange de Unna. Cette coloration n'est pas modifiée par un prétraitement par la ribonucléase (ARVY, 1955 c; LISON, 1960), ce qui prouve qu'elle n'est pas due à une ribonucléine.

La coloration des granulations des mastocytes par les colorants basiques se produit dans une gamme de pH très étendue, et se produit même à des pH très bas, inférieurs à 2,0. Bien que la basophilie ne constitue pas une réaction spécifique d'un groupement particulier, il est généralement reconnu qu'elle a un signification histochimique définie: elle démontre la présence de composés dont l'élément macromoléculaire est porteur d'une fonction acidique (voir LISON, 1960). Entre les quatre types de groupements électronégatifs susceptibles de se présenter dans les préparations histochimiques, -carboxyle, phosphorique, céto-acide et sulfurique, - en général, seuls les deux derniers sont basophiles à des pH inférieurs à 3. Comme on le verra plus loin, les caractères de la métachromasie pointent vers le radical sulfurique.

B. Métachromasie

La métachromasie des mastocytes a été découverte par EHRLICH en 1877 (bien que les cellules aient été dénommées «Plasmazellen» dans ce travail, et bien que l'adjectif «metachromatisch» aie été proposé seulement deux ans plus tard). Suivant la définition originale d'EHRLICH (1879) une coloration est métachromatique lorsque la couleur produite est différente de celle du colorant utilisé.

Dans l'expérience de 1877, Ehrlich avait coloré avec une solution alcoolique de dahlia acidifié par 8 % d'acide acétique et observé une coloration rouge-violacée des mastocytes.

Chez toutes les espèces de Vertébrés étudiées, les mastgranules présentent une forte métachromasie lorsqu'ils ont été colorés par des colorants appropriés. En plus du dahlia, originairement utilisé par Ehrlich, plus de deux douzaines de colorants basiques ont été actuellement reconnus capables de colorer métachromatiquement les mastocytes. La plupart sont des oxazines, thiazines, azines et triarylméthanes; le plus utilisé aujoud'hui est le bleu de toluidine, qui colore les mastgranules en rouge-violet foncé.

La métachromasie des mastocytes a été intensément étudiée. Dans les mastocytes, le matérial colorable métachromatiquement est localisé dans les granules, tandis que le cytoplasme intergranulaire ne réagit pas. Ce fait, déjà décrit par Ehrlich, a été confirmé au moyen des techniques les plus variées: observations *in vitro* (Hill, 1957; Arvy, 1955 c), dans des coupes de tissus fixés (Zollinger, 1950; Friberg et coll. 1951; Wislocki et Fawcett, 1951; Ungar et Damgaard, 1955), sur des granules isolés par centrifugation (Köksal, 1953); la conclusion contraire de Julén, Snellman et Sylvén (1949), Sylvén (1957), pour qui la substance métachromatique hydrosoluble serait localisée dans le cytoplasme intergranulaire, se base sur des expériences de centrifugation fractionnée, et s'explique par le déplacement de la substance au cours des violents prétraitements adoptés.

Il y a des différences considérables entre individus et entre espèces quant à l'intensité de la coloration métachromatique. Elles ont été attribuées à des différences fonctionnelles (Wislocki et Fawcett, 1951). C'est probablement le cas pour les mastocytes de l'hypophyse antérieure du rat, qui se colorent toujours beaucoup plus faiblement que les autres (Castiglioni, 1947). De nombreux facteurs techniques influencent la coloration métachromatique, et c'est pourquoi les résultats de divers auteurs sur un même matériel peuvent différer. Après séjour prolongé dans les solutions de bleu de toluidine, les mastgranules se colorent orthochromatiquement, tandis que le cytoplasme intergranulaire se colore métachromatiquement; ce phénomène serait dû à une migration du matériel des granules dans le cytoplasme (Zollinger, 1950). La fixation au formol provoque, surtout lorsqu'on la prolonge, une perte progressive du matériel métachromatique; les granules montrent alors une tendance à se colorer orthochromatiquement (Michels, 1938; Saal et Riek, 1958; Kelly et Bloom, 1959). Le pH de la solution colorante et sa concentration influencent le résultat; la coloration est plus intense (Castiglioni, 1947) et plus rapide (Radden, 1961) à pH bas (3 - 4) qu'à pH plus élevés, au contraire de ce qui se produit avec d'autres éléments histologiques.

On ne peut guère douter aujourd'hui que la coloration métachromatique des mastgranules ne soit due à la présence d'héparine. Il a été démontré il y a longtemps (Lison, 1935) que la métachromasie indique la présence de composés macromoléculaires contenant des radicaux ester sulfurique. Cette conclusion ne serait plus valide aujourd'hui dans sa forme primitive absolue, car d'autres groupements fortement électronégatifs peuvent aussi provoquer la métachromasie (voir les revues de Vitry, 1958; Bergeron et Singer, 1958; Lison, 1960), mais elle vaut encore pour les conditions particulières de la coloration métachromatique des mastocytes (coloration par des solutions très diluées, à pH bas ou en solution alcoolique). En accord avec cette conclusion, il avait été prévu dès 1935, à une époque où la présence d'héparine dans les mastocytes n'était pas encore connue, que le mastgranule devait contenir «un ester sulfurique de poids moléculaire élevé, probablement d'un polysaccharide» (LISON, 1935). Après que JORPES (1936) eut identifié l'héparine comme un polysaccharide fortement estérifié par des radicaux sulfate et observé qu'il est précipité et se colore métachromatiquement par le bleu de toluidine, HOLMGREN et WILANDER (1937), JORPES et coll. (1937), démontrèrent que la teneur en héparine des tissus varie en proportion de leur richesse en mastocytes et admirent l'hypothèse que la métachromasie des mastocytes est due à la présence d'héparine. Nous ne citerons pas ici les nombreuses recherches du type indirect qui ont confirmé ce point de vue. Des arguments plus directs sont les suivants: 1°) De préparations pures de mastocytes du rat, BENDITT (1958) a isolé un matériel qui a les propriétés pharmacologiques de l'héparine, qui a la même mobilité en chromatographie et qui présente la métachromasie avec les caractères observés dans les granules des mastocytes. 2°) Les granules isolés par HEDBOOM et SNELLMAN (1955) à partir des mastocytes du Boeuf ne contenaient pas d'héparine (probablement par suite de dissolution durant l'isolement) et ne se coloraient pas métachromatiquement. Les granules «fantômes» isolés par BENDITT (1958) des mastocytes du rat se comportent de même. 3°) ISIDOR (1954) a démontré que les mastgranules ne se colorent plus métachromatiquement aprés un prétraitement par l'héparinase de JAQUES (1940); le granule persiste, mais se colore orthochromatiquement.

Il a été prétendu par ASBOE-HANSEN (1950, 1951) que la métachromasie des mastgranules est supprimée par un prétraitement par l'hyaluronidase, ce qui entraîne la conclusion qu'elle serait due à l'acide hyaluronique. Le fait n'a été confirmé par aucun des auteurs qui ont fait ou refait cette expérience (DAVIES, 1952; WISLOCKI et DEMPSEY, 1946; WISLOCKI et coll. 1947; COMPTON, 1952; PRAKKEN et WOERDEMANN, 1952; DEGOS et COTTENOT, 1953; ARVY, 1955 c), et il n'existe aucun fait positif prouvant ou suggérant la présence d'acide hyaluronique dans les mastgranules. Les théories qui prétendent que le mastocyte produit la substance métachromatique de la substance fondamentale du conjonctif (SYLVÉN, 1941, 1957; ASBOE -HANSEN, 1951, 1954) ne sont pas appuyées par les constatations histochimiques.

C. Autres réactions de mucopolysaccharides acides

L'aldéhyde-fuchsine, qui parait être un réactif de corps porteurs de groupes électronégatifs (LISON, 1960), colore les mastgranules (ARVY, 1955 c). La coloration est parallèle à la basophilie métachromatique et ne se produit plus après désulfatation au moyen de méthanol-HCl (VALERI, VOZZA et LISON, 1960).

Le bleu Alcian 8 *GS et le bleu Astra*, colorants du groupe des phtalocyanines, sont utilisés pour la recherche des mucopolysaccharides acides. D'après BLOOM et KELLY (1959), le bleu Astra colore intensément les mastgranules, même à un pH aussi bas que 0,2; le bloquage de cette réaction par le chlorure de cétylpyridinium serait une preuve qu'elle est due à l'héparine. SPICER (1960, 1963) déclare que les mastocytes n'ont pas d'affinité pour le bleu Alcian, mais en présentent après méthylation qui retirerait le groupe sulfurique. Nous avons constaté (observations inédites) qu'une proportion relativement petite des mastocytes, dans la langue du Rat, se colore par le bleu Alcian; les mastocytes qui se colorent ainsi sont différents de ceux qui se colorent par le PAS (voir paragraphe suivant).

D. Réactions des α glycols (réaction à l'acide periodique-Schiff et réactions apparentées)

Les mastgranules ont été généralement décrits comme PAS («Periodic Acid-Schiff») négatifs ou faiblement positifs, chez la plupart des animaux (JORPES et coll. 1948; WISLOCKI et coll. 1949; PEARSE, 1960; FRIBERG et coll. 1951; MONTAGNA et coll. 1954). Chez les Batraciens, les mastgranules se colorent intensément (ARVY, 1955 a). Il a été dit que les mastgranules chez le Rat et la Souris (JORPES et coll. 1948; LEBLOND, 1950; KIRKMAN, 1950) se colorent intensément. En réalité, chez ces animaux, les granules d'une minorité de mastocytes se colorent, tandis que les autres ne donnent pas la réaction (LILLIE, 1950; WISLOCKI et FAWCETT, 1951); il en est de même chez le Hamster (COMPTON, 1952). BUÑO (1953) a pensé que les colorations positives par le PAS sont dues à la diffusion de la fuchsine recolorée; bien que le phénomène puisse se produire, nous ne croyons pas qu'elle s'applique aux cas de PAS-positivité reconnus. JORPES, WERNER et ABERG (1948) ont admis que les mastocytes PAS positifs contiennent, non pas l'héparine ordinaire, - qui est l'héparine trisulfurique-, mais l'héparine monosulfurique ou un autre précurseur analogue de l'héparine; l'héparine trisulfurique n'est pas oxydée par l'acide periodique, car 3 des 4 hydroxyles sont bloqués par des radicaux sulfates et elle ne contient donc pas le 2 hydroxyles adjacents sur lequels agit l'acide periodique. L'explication des auteurs est séduisante mais il n'en existe pas de preuve.

E. Conclusion

La basophilie, la métachromasie et la coloration par l'aldéhydefuchsine sont des caractères constants de tous les mastocytes et sont presque certainement dues à la présence d'héparine. D'autres réactions de mucopolysaccharides, comme le PAS et la coloration par le bleu Alcian, sont positives seulement au niveau de certains mastocytes. Elles semblent indiquer la présence d'autres mucopolysaccharides que l'héparine. Il serait tentant de les considérer comme des précurseurs de celle-ci, mais il n'existe pas de fait positif à l'appui de cette hypothèse.

IV. Histamine

Les preuves indirectes, -très nombreuses-, de la présence d'histamine dans les mastocytes, ne seront pas indiquées ici et nous examinerons seulement les méthodes de visualisation directe de cette substance. Tout indique que l'histamine, dans les mastocytes, est très faiblement liée au substrat cellulaire; en conséquence, on éprouve les plus grandes difficultés à la conserver *in situ*, étant données sa grande solubilité dans les solvants aqueux et organiques et son extrême diffusibilité. Avec les procédés usuels de fixation, l'histamine se solubilise.

SCHAUER et WERLE (1959) ont préconisé de précipiter l'histamine par le sel de Reinecke; le reineckate peut être identifié soit grâce à sa biréfringence en lumière polarisée, soit par copulation avec le diazotate de l'acide sulfanilique. Nous avons essayé cette réaction sur des mastocytes de diverses espèces animales et nous n'avons jamais réussi à obtenir les réactions indiqués par les auteurs. LAGUNOFF, PHILLIPS et BENDITT (1961) préparent les tissus par congélation-dessication, de manière à empêcher l'évasion de l'histamine, puis traitent les coupes par les vapeurs de formaldéhyde. L'histamine réagit lentement avec la formaldéhyde pour former le 1. 2. 5. 6 tétrahydro-pyrido-3.4-imidazol, peu soluble, qui probablement se polymérise et s'attache à des protéines par des ponts méthylène. Le produit ainsi formé peut être identifié par la formation d'un composé orange par traitement au moyen du diazotate de p-bromoaniline, par la réduction du ferricyanure ferrique et du nitrate d'argent-méthenamine, et par la fluorescence en lumière ultraviolette. Ces réactions ne sont pas entièrement spécifiques, mais les conditions dans les quelles elles sont appliquées suggèrent qu'elles sont bien dues à l'histamine. Les auteurs ont trouvé les réactions qui précèdent positives pour les mastocytes du rat, de la souris et de l'homme, mais il a été impossible de les produire chez ceux du chien, dont la richesse en histamine est cependant prouvée. Il est difficile d'expliquer cette réaction négative des mastocytes du chien.

V. Protéases: Chymase et tryptase

De même que l'héparine, la découverte de protéases dans les mastocytes a été effectuée par voie histochimique. L'histoire de cette découverte est assez curieuse. En 1953, GOMORI, cherchant de nouveaux substrats pour la recherche des estérases, avait observé que les mastocytes, aprés fixation formolée, contiennent un enzyme hydrolysant intensément l'anilide de l'acide 3-chloroacetoxy-2-naphtoïque (= chloroacétate du naphtol AS), à un pH aussi élevé que 7.4. Chose inattendue, les images histochimiques de la distribution de l'enzyme hydrolysant ce substrat étaient totalement différentes de celles obtenues avec les substrats communs pour les estérases (acetates de naphtol AS et autres). FRENCH et BENDITT (1953) observèrent que l'anilide de l'acide 3-acétoxy-2-naphtoïque, proche voisin du substrat de Gomori, est hydrolysé par la chymotrypsine in vitro et par les mastgranules dans les préparations histochimiques. Peu après, BENDITT et ARASE (1959), travaillant sur des suspensions hautement purifiées de mastocytes prouvèrent que l'enzyme des mastocytes actif sur le substrat de Gomori est homospécifique de l'α-chymotrypsine, et est inhibé de la même manière par le di-isopropylfluorophosphate. LAGUNOFF et BENDITT (1961) prouvèrent en outre que divers dérivés 3-phényl-alkylcarboxyliques de l'anilide de l'acide 2-naphtoïque présentent des activités exactement parallèles sur l'enzyme des mastocytes et sur l'α-chymotrypsine. D'après LAGUNOFF et BENDITT (1963), l'enzyme des mastocytes hydrolyse la caséine, l'albumine et l'insuline, avec un optimum d'activité en milieu alcalin (pH 8,0 - 8,7). A la différence du pancréas, dans lequel on sait que la chymotrypsine est présente sous forme inactive (chymotrypsinogène), le mastgranule contient l'enzyme sous forme active. LAGUNOFF et BENDITT (1963) ont proposé d'appeler «chymase» l'enzyme des mastocytes homospécifique de l'α -chymotrypsine.

Outre la chymase, les mastocytes de l'homme et du chien contiennent un autre enzyme, homospécifique de la trypsine, pour lequel le nom de «tryptase» a été suggéré (LAGUNOFF et BENDITT, 1963). GLENNER et COHEN (1960) l'ont découverte en utilisant comme substrat, dans des préparations histochimiques, la N-benzoyl arginine β-naphtylamide. Plus récemment, GLENNER, HOPSU et COHEN (1962) et LAGUNOFF, BENDITT et WATTS (1962) ont utilisé l'ester ε-amino caproïque du naphtol AS comme substrat pour la recherche histochimique de cet enzyme.

Il n'est pas exclu que la chymase et la tryptase ne soient qu'une seule et même «biprotéase», mais certains faits tendent à montrer que ce sont deux enzymes séparés: le mastocyte du rat contient de la chymase et ne présente pas d'activité tryptasique, tandis que le leucocyte basophile du même animal contient de la tryptase et pas de chymase (LAGUNOFF, BENDITT et WATTS, 1962).

Un troisième enzyme protéolytique, la leucine aminopeptidase, a soit-disant été démontrée dans les mastocytes par une technique utilisant la leucyl-β-naphtylamide comme substrat (BRAUN-FALCO et SALFELD, 1959; EDER et SCHAUER, 1961). Cependant, il est douteux que l'enzyme ainsi révélée soit vraiment la leucine aminopeptidase (PATTERSON, KEPPEL et HSIAO, 1961).

La fonction des protéases dans le mastocyte est inconnue. D'après des calculs de BENDITT et ARASE (1959), la chymase représente une fraction considérable de la masse totale du mastgranule et doit être considérée comme aussi importante fonctionnellement que l'histamine, l'héparine et les autres substances puissamment actives identifiées dans ces cellules.

VI. Autres composés

Nous ne mentionnerons que pour mémoire un certain nombre de substances identifiées dans les mastocytes, mais dont l'importance apparait bien moindre que celle des produits cités plus haut. Ce sont principalement: 1⁰ Des *lipides*. Les donnée de la littérature au sujet de la présence ou de la non-présence de lipides colorables par le Sudan sont très contradictoires (voir discussion plus complète dans COMPTON, 1952). Le test de Baker à l'hématéine acide, considéré comme spécifique pour les phospholipides, est positif dans les mastgranules (MONTAGNA et NOBACK, 1948; MONTAGNA et PARKS, 1948; KIRKMAN, 1950), ce qui est en accord avec le fait que l'analyse chimique des mastgranules isolés a permis d'y trouver des quantités importantes de phospholipides (HEDBOM et SNELLMAN, 1955); 2⁰ des *enzymes divers:* Oxydases (M nadi-indophénoloxydase); données assez contradictoires (discussion approfondie, voir MICHELS, 1938; COMPTON, 1952); Reductases (ARVY, 1955 b); Phosphatase acide (WISLOCKI et FAWCETT, 1951).

Conclusions

De l'ensemble des recherches histochimiques sur les mastocytes, il résulte clairement que les substances pharmacologiquement actives et les constituants spécifiques de ces cellules sont localisés au niveau des granules. La compréhension des mécanismes gouvernant l'accumulation et la libération de ces substances nécessite évidemment une connaissance approfondie de l'organisation des granules. Trois grands groupes de substances puissamment actives y ont été identifiés: 1⁰) l'héparine, et éventuellement des corps apparentés; 2⁰) l'histamine et d'autres amines pharmacologiquement actives; 3⁰) la chymase et la tryptase, enzymes protéolytiques. Ce sont des méthodes histochimiques qui ont révélé pour la première fois les substances du premier et du troisième groupe. Cependant, de que l'on sait de l'organisation des mastgranules ne permet pas encore de comprendre les relations réciproques entre ces substances, ni leur mode de liaison avec les constituants protéiques et lipidiques des granules. Ce sujet demande de nouvelles recherches.

Bibliographie

ALLEN, A. M.: Two methods for coloring mast cells of mammalian tissues. Amer. J. clin. Path. **33**, 461 (1960).

ARVY, L.: Particularités histologiques des labrocytes chez quelques batraciens. C. R. Ass. Anat. Congr. Paris, 218 (1959a).

— Caractères histologiques et réactions des labrocytes linguaux chez Rana esculenta. Modifications de ces éléments sous l'influence d'un libérateur d'histamine. C. R. Soc. Biol. (Paris) **149**, 528 (1955b).

— Les labrocytes (Mastzellen). Rev. Hémat. **10**, 55 (1955c).

ASBOE-HANSEN, G.: A survey of the normal and pathological occurrence of mucinous substances and mast cells in the dermal connective tissue in man. Acta derm.-venereol. (Stockh.) **30**, 338 (1950).

— Om Bindevaevets Mucinøse Substanser. Copenhagen: Rosenkilde & Bagger 1951.

— The mast cell. Int. Rev. Cytol. **3**, 399 (1954).

BENDITT, E. P.: Morphology, chemistry and function of mast cells. Ann. N. Y. Acad. Sci. **73**, 204 (1958).

—, and M. ARASE: An enzyme in mast cells with properties like chymotrypsin. J. exp. Med. **110**, 451 (1959).

BENSLEY, S. H.: Pinacyanol erythrosinate as a stain for mast cells. Stain Technol. **27**, 269 (1952).

BERGERON, J., and M. SINGER: Metachromasy: an experimental and theoretical reevaluation. J. biophys. biochem. Cytol. **4**, 433 (1958).

BLOOM, G., and J. W. KELLY: Absorption characteristics of a new phtalocyanine dye in concentrated solution and in stained mast cells. J. Histochem. Cytochem. **7**, 286 (1959).

BRACHET, J.: La détection histochimique des acides pentosenucléiques. Arch. Biol. (Liège) **51**, 167 (1940).
BRAUN-FALCO, O., and K. SALFELD: Leucine aminopeptidase activity in mast cells. Nature (Lond.) **183**, 51 (1959).
BREMY, P.: Die Gewebsmastzellen im menschlichen Knochenmark. Stuttgart: Georg Thieme 1950.
BUJARD, E.: Une coloration strictement élective des granulations basophiles des mastocytes. Bull. Histol. Techn. micr. **7**, 264 (1930).
BUÑO, W.: Algunas reacciones histoquimicas y funcionales de los mastocitos. Acta physiol. lat.-amer. **3**, 60 (1953).
CASTIGLIONI, G.: Osservazioni sulla cromotropia delle Mastzellen. Ann. Biol. norm. pat. **3**, 3 (1947).
COMPTON, A. S.: A cytochemical and cytological study of the connective tissue mast cells. Amer. J. Anat. **91**, 301 (1952).
DAVIES, D. V.: Specificity of staining methods for mucopolysaccharides of the hyaluronic acid. Stain Technol. **27**, 65 (1952).
DEGOS, R., et F. COTTENOT: Physiologie du mastocyte tissulaire. C. R. Soc. Derm. Syph. **60**, 228 (1953).
EDER, M., u. A. SCHAUER: Fermenthistochemische und experimentelle Untersuchungen an Gewebsmastzellen. Beitr. path. Anat. **124**, 251 (1961).
EHRLICH, P.: Beiträge zur Kenntnis der Anilinfärbungen und ihrer Verwendung in der mikroskopischen Technik. Arch. mikr. Anat. **13**, 263 (1877).
— Beiträge zur Kenntnis der granulierten Bindegewebszellen und der eosinophilen Leucocyten. Arch. Anat. Physiol. (Lpz.) **3**, 166 (1879).
FADEM, R. S.: Tissue mast cells in bone marrow. Blood **6**, 614 (1951).
FERRI, A. G.: Contribuição para o estudo da citofisiologia do mastócito. Tese, S. Paulo (1955).
—, et I. MOTA: Loc. cit. MOTA et coll. (1956).
FRENCH, J. E., and E. P. BENDITT: Histochemistry of connective tissue. J. Histochem. Cytochem, **1**, 321 (1953).
FRIBERG, U., W. GRAF, and B. ÅBERG: On the histochemistry of the mast cells. Acta path. microbiol. scand. **29**, 197 (1951).
GLENNER, G. G., and L. A. COHEN: Histochemical demonstration of a species specific trypsin-like enzyme in mast cells. Nature (Lond.) **185**, 846 (1960).
— V. K., HOPSU, and L. A. COHEN: Histochemical demonstration of a trypsin-like esterase activity in mast cells. J. Histochem. Cytochem. **10**, 109 (1962).
GOMORI, G.: Chloroacyl esters as histochemical substrates. J. Histochem. Cytochem. **1**, 469 (1953).
HARADA, K.: Selective staining of mast cell granules with chrysoidin. Stain Technol. **32**, 183 (1957).
HEDBOM, A., and O. SNELLMAN: Isolation and analysis of the large cytoplasmic granules of tissue mast cells. Exp. Cell. Res. **9**, 148 (1955).
HILL, M.: Secretion of heparin in mast cells. Nature (Lond.) **180**, 654 (1957).
HOLMGREN, H.: Eine neue Methode zur Fixierung der Ehrlichschen Mastzellen mit besonderer Berücksichtigung der Chemie der Zellgranula. Z. wiss. Mikr. **55**, 419 (1938).
—, u. O. WILANDER Beitrag zur Kenntnis der Chemie und Funktion der Ehrlichschen Mastzellen. Z. mikr.-anat. Forsch. **42**, 242 (1937).
ISIDOR, P.: Etude sur la caractérisation histologique et histochimique de l'héparine. Bull. micr. appl. 2ᵉ série **4**, 41 (1954).
JAQUES, L. B.: Heparinase. J. biol. Chem. **133**, 447 (1940).
JOHNSTONE, J. M.: The tissue mast cell in human bone marrow. Amer. J. clin. Path. **26**, 60 (1956).
JORDAN, H.: On the nature of the basophilic granulocytes of the blood and tissues. Anat. Rec. **33**, 89 (1926).
JORPES, J. E.: On heparin: its chemical nature and properties. Acta med. scand. 88, 427 (1936).
— HOLMGREN H. u. O. WILANDER: Über das Vorkommen von Heparin in den Gefäßwänden und in den Augen. Z. mikr.-anat. Forsch. **42**, 279 (1937).
— B. WERNER, and B. ABERG: The fuchsinsulphurous acid test after periodate oxidation of heparin and allied polysaccharides. J. biol. Chem. **176**, 277 (1948).
JULÉN, C., O. SNELLMAN, and B. SYLVÉN: Cytological and fractionation studies on the cytoplasmic constituents of tissue mast cells. Acta physiol. scand. **196**, 289 (1949).
KELLY, J. W., and G. BLOOM: A quantitative spectrophotometric study of the mast cell. Exp. Cell. Res. **16**, 538 (1959).
KIRKMAN, H.: A comparative morphological and cytochemical study of globule leucocytes of the urinary tract and of possibly related cells. Amer. J. Anat. **86**, 91 (1950).

Köksal, M.: Extraction of a heparin like substance from mast cell granules in mouse connective tissue. Nature (Lond.) **172**, 733 (1953).
Lagunoff, D., and E. P. Benditt: Histochemical examinations of chymotrypsin-like esterases. Nature (Lond.) **192**, 1198 (1961).
— — Proteolytic enzymes of mast cells. Ann. N. Y. Acad. Sci. **103**, 185 (1963).
— —, and R. Watts: Histochemical study of esterases homospecific with trypsin. J. Histochem. Cytochem. **10**, 672 (1962).
— M. Phillips, and E. P. Benditt: The histochemical demonstration of histamine in mast cells. J. Histochem. Cytochem. **9**, 534 (1961).
Leblond, C. P.: Distribution of periodic-acid reactive carbohydrates in the adult rat. Amer. J. Anat. **86**, 1 (1950).
Leitner, S. J.: Bone Marrow Biopsy. New York: Grune and Stratton 1949.
Lillie, R. D.: Further exploration of HIO_4-Schiff reaction with remarks on its significance. Ant. Rec. **108**, 239 (1950).
Lison, L.: Etudes sur la métachromasie. Colorants métachromatiques et substances chromotropes. Arch. Biol. **46**, 599 (1935).
— Histochimie et Cytochimie animales. 2ᵉ éd. Paris: Gauthier-Villars 1953.
— Histochimie et Cytochimie animales. 3ᵉ éd. Paris: Gauthier-Villars 1960.
Messerschmitt, J.: Fréquence des mastzellen dans les frottis de moelle osseuse chez l'homme. Rev. Hémat. **9**, 189 (1954).
Michels, N. A.: The mast cells. In Handbbook of Hematol. **1**, 231. Edited by I. Downey. New York: Paul B. Hoeber Inc. 1938.
Montagna, W., A. Z. Eisen, and A. S. Goldman,: The tinctorial behaviour of human mast cells. Quart. J. micr. Sci. **95**, 1 (1954).
—, and C. R. Noback: Localization of lipids and other chemical substances in the mast cells of man and laboratory animals. Anat. Rec. **100**, 535 (1948).
—, and H. F. Parks: A histochemical study of the anal sac of the dog. Anat. Rec. **100**, 297 (1948).
Mota, I., A. G. Ferri, and S. Yoneda: The distribution of mast cells in the digestive tract of laboratory animals: its bearings on the problem of the location of histamine in tissues. Quart. J. micr. Sci. **97**, 251 (1956).
Padawer, J.: A stain for mast cells and its application in various vertebrates and in a mastocytoma. J. Histoch. Cytochem. **7**, 352 (1959).
— Dynamic aspects of mast cell morphology in aging. Anat. Rec. **134**, 622 (1959).
Patterson, E. K., A. Keppel, and S. Hsiao: Evidence from purification procedures that the enzyme which hydrolyzes L-leucyl-β-naphtylamide is not the classical leucine aminopeptidase. J. Histochem. Cytochem. **9**, 609 (1961).
Pearse, A. G. E.: Histochemistry. 2nd. Ed. London: J. A. Churchill Ltd. 1960.
Pollister, A. W., and C. Leuchtenberger: Nucleotide content of the nucleus. Nature (Lond.) **163**, 260 (1949).
Prakken, J. R., and M. J. Woerdeman: Mast cells in diseases of the skin; their relation to tissue eosiniphilia. Dermatologica (Basel) **105**, 116 (1952).
Radden, B. G.: An investigation of the factors influencing the metachromatic staining of mast cell granules. J. Histochem. Cytochem. **9**, 165 (1961).
Saal, J. R., and R. F. Riek: Studies on bovine mast cells: The effect of formalin fixation. Stain Technol. **33**, 123 (1958).
Schauer, A. E., u. E. Werle: Zur histochemischen Darstellung des Histamins der Mastzellen. Z. ges. exp. Med. **131**, 100 (1959).
Spicer, S. S.: A correlative study of the histochemical properties of Rodent acid mucopolysaccharides. J. Histochem. Cytochem. **8**, 18 (1960).
— Histochemical properties of mucopolysaccharides and basic proteins in mast cells. Ann. N. Y. Acad. Sci. **103**, 322 (1963).
Sylvén, B.: Über das Vorkommen von hochmolekularen Esterschwefelsäuren im Granulationsgewebe und bei der Epithelregeneration. Acta chir. scand. **87**, suppl. 66 (1941).
— On the topographical cytochemistry of tissue mast cells. In: Tunbridge R. E.: Connective Tissue; a symposium organized by the Council for international organizations of medical sciences. London: Blackwell 1957.
Taft, E. B.: The specificity of the methyl green-pyronin stain for nucleic acids. Exp. Cell. Res. **2**, 312 (1951).
Turchini, J.: Les mastocytes à la lumière de recherches récentes. C. R. Ass. Anat. 46° Réunion **3**, 30 (1959).
—, et L. Khau van Kien: Etude des basophiles du sang dans quelques conditions où leur nombre se trouve augmenté. V° Congr. Internat. Hematol. (1954).
Undritz, E.: Die nicht zur Blutkörperchenbildung gehörenden Zellen intravitaler Knochenmarkpunktate nebst Auszählungschema für Myelogramme. Schweiz. med. Wschr. **76**, 333 (1946).

UNGAR, G., and E. DAMGAARD: Tissue reactions to anaphylactic and anaphylactoid stimuli, proteolysis and release of histamine and heparin. J. exp. Med. **101**, 1 (1955).

VALERI, V., J. A. VOZZA, et L. LISON: Observations inédites. (Voir LISON 1960).

VARICAK, T. D.: Zur Frage der Darstellung und Wasserresistenz der Mastzellengranula bei der Katze. Z. wiss. Mikr. **55**, 274 (1938).

VITRY, G.: La réaction métachromatique et son utilisation pour l'étude des polysaccharides. Ann. Histochim. **3**, 279 (1958).

WESTPHAL, E.: Über Mastzellen. In: EHRLICH P., Farbanalytische Untersuchungen. Berlin: Hirschweld 1891.

WISLOCKI, G. B., H. BUTING, and E. W. DEMPSEY: Metachromasy in mammalian tissue and its relationship to mucopolysaccharides. Amer. J. Anat. **81**, 1 (1947).

—, and E. W. DEMPSEY: Observations on the chemical cytology of normal blood and hemopoietic tissues. Anat. Rec. **96**, 249 (1946).

—, and D. W. FAWCETT: Some histochemical properties of mast cells and tissue eosinophils in stained spreads of normal rat mesentery. J. Anat. Cancer Inst. **12**, 258 (1951).

— J. J. RHEINGOLD, and E. W. DEMPSEY: Occurrence of periodic acid-Schiff reaction in various normal cells of blood and connective tissue. Blood **4**, 562 (1949).

ZOLLINGER, H. U.: Gewebsmastzellen und Heparin (Phasenmikroskopische Untersuchung). Experientia (Basel) **6**, 384 (1950).

Chapter 2

Pharmacology of Histamine

Section A

Absorption de l'histamine par l'appareil digestif

Par

JEAN-LOUIS PARROT et GEORGES NICOT

Avec 7 figures

La clinique nous apprend que certaines intoxications sont dues à l'histamine du tube digestif. Bien que cette conception soit en contradiction avec les données de la pharmacologie classique, les arguments qualitatifs et quantitatifs des cliniciens sont assez solides pour faire réviser la notion selon laquelle l'histamine contenue dans le milieu intestinal est dépourvue de toxicité pour l'organisme. On sait, en effet, que dans le tube digestif se trouvent normalement des bactéries qui peuvent produire de l'histamine par décomposition de certaines protéines riches en histidine.

BERTHELOT et BERTRAND (1912), MELLANBY et TWORT (1912), KOESSLER et HANKE (1919) isolant du milieu intestinal certains microorganismes *(B. aminophilus, B. coli)* réussirent à provoquer la formation d'histamine, *in vitro*, par décarboxylation de l'histidine. LÉVY-BRUHL, UNGAR et LEVILLAIN (1937) trouvent une substance pharmacologiquement identique à l'histamine, formée sous l'influence du Pneumobacille et du *B. coli*, dans un milieu de culture où l'urée constitue la seule source d'azote. KENDALL et SCHMITT (1926) isolent à partir des selles de 41 individus, 72 échantillons de *B. welchii* et trouvent que 66 d'entre eux sont capables de former une substance pharmacologiquement identique à l'histamine. Bien d'autres auteurs étudient le rôle de la flore intestinale dans la formation de l'histamine, presque tous trouvent dans l'intestin des bactéries susceptibles de décarboxyler certains acides aminés, qui sont alors transformés en amines toxiques; ces dernières s'opposeraient à l'acidité du milieu (ROSKE, 1928), ce qui fait dire à GALE et EPPS (1942) que ces enzymes décarboxylantes, dont le pH optimal se situe entre 2,5 et 5,5, sont peut-être en rapport avec un système d'adaptation destiné à éviter une acidité trop importante du milieu.

L'intestin contient donc normalement des substances toxiques, en particulier l'histamine, qui peuvent être à l'origine de syndromes pathologiques.

I. Les données classiques de la clinique et de la médecine expérimentale

Dès 1922, GERARD considérait l'histamine et les autres produits de putréfaction engendrés par les microbes intestinaux comme responsables du syndrome toxique de l'occlusion intestinale aiguë. Dans le cadre de la spécificité chimique en séméiologie LOEPER et PERRAULT (1937) rendent l'histamine responsable de certaines intoxications alimentaires. Selon NEVOT (1942) les bactéries rencontrées dans les denrées toxiques agissent plus par les produits qu'elles forment dans l'aliment que par elles-mêmes ou par leurs prétendues toxines. LEGROUX, LEVADITI, BOUDIN et BOVET (1946) démontrèrent le rôle pathogène de l'histamine dans l'intoxication consécutive à l'ingestion de thon frais: la chair de thon, responsable des phénomènes toxiques, est à peu près dépourvue de germes, mais elle contient une substance que ces auteurs ont dosée et qui présente les propriétés pharmacologiques de l'histamine; c'est ainsi que les manifestations toxiques peuvent être atténuées ou supprimées par un antagoniste de l'histamine, le N-p-méthoxybenzyl-N-diméthylaminoéthyl aminopyridine (2786 R P ou Néo-antergan). BOYER, DEPIERRE, TISSIER et JACOB (1956) rapportent d'autres intoxications histaminiques collectives provoquées par l'ingestion de thon; les différents échantillons examinés par ces auteurs contenaient tous, sauf un, des quantités d'histamine qui paraissaient suffisantes pour expliquer les manifestations toxiques observées; d'autre part ces échantillons contenaient des germes en plus ou moins grande quantité qui auraient pu former cette substance par décarboxylation de l'histidine. BOYER et JACOB (1961) insistent encore une fois sur la toxicité des aliments vecteurs d'histamine, en évoquant non seulement le rôle de l'histamine exogène et de l'histamine endogène, mais aussi celui des diamines qui facilitent le passage de cette amine à travers la barrière intestinale. Nous aurons du reste l'occasion de revenir sur cette dernière notion et de fournir des arguments expérimentaux. Dans tous les cas évoqués par ces auteurs les antihistaminiques améliorent le tableau clinique de ces intoxications. GOUNELLE et POINTEAU-POULIQUEN (1961) retiennent, eux aussi, le rôle de l'histamine dans l'étiologie des intoxications alimentaires après consommation de poisson. NEVOT (1949) arrive aux mêmes conclusions dans l'étude des troubles provoqués après alimentation carnée.

La clinique vétérinaire fournit aussi un certain nombre d'observations très sérieuses où l'histamine intestinale est considérée comme toxique. ÅKERBLOM (1934) dans ses travaux sur la fourbure du cheval provoquée par le fourrage donne une preuve expérimentale de la toxicité de l'histamine digestive. Ce syndrome toxique se manifeste par des lésions inflammatoires de l'extrémité inférieure des membres de l'animal: il s'agit d'hyperhémie et d'épanchement séreux dans la couche lamellaire avec petites hémorragies; il y a un véritable oedème inflammatoire, avec infiltration cellulaire; d'abord aseptique, il peut ensuite se compliquer d'ostéites et d'arthrites purulentes.

Bien que le plus souvent les signes généraux soient assez discrets, ils peuvent être très intenses; la température dépasse alors 40° C avec tachycardie, polypnée et tremblements musculaires. Ce tableau clinique est pour une part en rapport avec une augmentation du taux d'histamine dans l'intestin. En effet, l'auteur réussit à reproduire expérimentalement le syndrome toxique en faisant ingérer à l'animal de l'histidine ou des aliments riches en histidine, et des bactéries capables de décarboxyler l'histidine (*B. coli* dans ces recherches). C'est la présence ou l'absence d'une telle flore qui explique, d'après ÅKERBLOM, pourquoi après ingestion d'un même fourrage certains chevaux sont atteints de fourbure et d'autres non; les animaux qui reçoivent les microbes histaminogènes avec affouragement consécutif ont des signes de fourbure. Il s'agit bien d'une intoxication histaminique car cette amine donne chez le cheval une affection des articulations et des gaines tendineuses avec lésions hépatique et intestinale.

Les travaux de KOCHAN (1948) devaient confirmer la pathogénie toxique de ce syndrome et montrer l'efficacité d'un antagoniste de l'histamine dans la thérapeutique de la maladie. Récemment d'autre part (Bourle, 1959) l'histamine fut considérée comme jouant un rôle très important dans l'étiologie des indigestions chez les ruminants.

Ces quelques observations nous font envisager le rôle toxique des produits de désintégration protéiques, lié à la présence de certains germes de l'alimentation ou de l'intestin normal. Le problème est de savoir si l'histamine, cantonnée dans le tube digestif, peut passer dans la circulation générale et intoxiquer l'organisme.

II. Les données classiques de la pharmacologie

Les expériences des pharmacologistes paraissaient contredire les données des cliniciens. En effet, l'histamine, administrée par voie digestive, est très bien tolérée chez l'animal et chez l'homme. Les travaux pharmacologiques ou toxicologiques suggèrent qu'un obstacle s'oppose au passage de l'histamine du tube digestif dans le milieu intérieur; seules des doses très élevées de la substance peuvent le déborder. Les recherches de Kendall et Varney (1927) de Feigen et Campbell (1946) sur des préparations d'estomac et d'intestin, *in situ* ou isolées, confirment l'existence de cette barrière que le tube digestif oppose au passage de cette substance. Au contact de la muqueuse intestinale de l'iléon isolé de cobaye l'histamine provoque une contraction lente, après une période de latence de 30 à 60 secondes, alors que la même dose, appliquée directement sur la séreuse, donne une réponse immédiate et rapide (Kendall et Varney, 1927).

L'homme tolère des doses importantes d'histamine *per os*, de 200 à 500 mg au moins, sans modifications du pouls ni de la pression artérielle; alors que la dose minimale injectée dans les veines pouvant produire des modifications circulatoires est de 0,02 mg de phosphate d'histamine correspondant à 0,007 mg d'histamine base (Ivy et Javois, 1925, Weiss et coll., 1932). L'animal peut ingérer, sans subir aucun effet durable, 200 à 500 fois, selon l'espèce, la dose qui est minimale léthale par voie intra-veineuse. Oehme (1913) donne 500 mg d'histamine aux lapins par voie digestive sans observer de troubles; alors que par voie intraveineuse la dose demi-léthale est de 0,6 à 0,7 mg par kg (Giscafré et Espanés, 1948). Le cobaye est tué par des doses aussi faibles que 0,3 à 0,4 mg/kg par voie intra-veineuse (Karády, 1941; Wilcox et Seegal, 1942), mais il supporte très facilement 100 mg/kg de dichlorhydrate d'histamine par voie digestive sans manifestations toxiques durables (Koessler et Hanke, 1924).

Wangensteen et Loucks (1928) placent 50 à 100 mg dans le duodenum du chien et n'observent rien d'anormal, alors que 3 à 10 mg injectés dans les veines mésentériques provoquent toujours une chute de la pression artérielle. Pourtant cette amine disparaît en partie de la lumière intestinale. Mellanby (1916) trouve que la vitesse de disparition de l'histamine de l'intestin du chat augmente en allant de l'origine du grêle au coecum. Meakins et Harrington (1923), qui avaient noté la présence d'histamine dans le coecum et le côlon transverse de l'homme, étudièrent eux aussi sur le chat l'absorption intestinale de cette amine; ils remarquent alors que l'absorption du phosphate acide d'histamine utilisé est très importante dans l'iléon, beaucoup moins dans le coecum, le duodénum et l'estomac. Koessler et Hanke (1924), dans une série d'expériences sur le cobaye et sur le chien, remarquent, par exemple, que si le cobaye reçoit 100 mg de dichlorhydrate d'histamine par voie digestive, 61,8 p. 100 de la substance disparaît de l'intestin en deux heures; on retrouve 33,5 mg dans l'intestin, 4,7 mg dans la paroi intestinale et 4,5 mg dans le foie. La quantité de dichlorhydrate absorbée, 57,3 mg, ne peut pas être passée sans modifications dans la circulation car cette dose équivaudrait à une injection intra-veineuse de 0,5 mg par minute. Les chiens reçoivent 500 mg de dichlorhydrate d'histamine; 53 p. 100 disparaissent en deux heures sans provoquer de troubles; au bout de ce laps de temps 147 mg sont dans l'estomac et 88,6 mg dans l'intestin; la vitesse d'absorption est alors de 2,2 mg par minute; dans ce dernier cas, on ne peut envisager un passage de la substance inchangée dans la circulation, car il suffit d'injecter 0,0054 mg par minute et par kg au chien dans la veine saphène pour obtenir une chute de la pression artérielle.

Le rôle du foie ne semble pas être très important pour la majorité des auteurs. Ivy et Javois (1925) introduisent 500 à 750 mg d'histamine dans l'estomac du chien, porteur d'une fistule d'Eck sans observer de troubles.

L'étude des urines apporte une nouvelle preuve du passage de l'histamine. Anrep, Ayadi, Barsoum, Smith et Talaat (1944) montrent qu'il existe un rapport entre l'alimentation carnée et la quantité d'histamine éliminée par le rein. Plus le régime est riche en viande et plus l'élimination d'histamine est abondante, plus grande aussi est la proportion d'histamine éliminée sous forme conjuguée, dépourvue d'action pharmacologique. La quantité d'histamine conjuguée (exprimée en phosphate acide) que le chien excrète en 24 heures varie, suivant le régime, de moins de 0,1 mg à plus de 30 mg. Chez l'homme l'histamine urinaire totale est de 0,1 à 6,2 mg/l; 3 à 5 p. 100 de l'histamine ingérée se retrouve dans l'urine sous forme conjuguée. D'une façon générale les herbivores excrètent l'histamine sous forme libre et en petites quantités, les carnivores excrètent de fortes proportions sous forme conjuguée. Cette histamine conjuguée, qui est de l'acétylhistamine (Urbach, 1949, Tabor et Mosettig, 1949), se forme sous l'influence de la flore bactérienne de l'intestin, est absorbée à travers la paroi intestinale et passe ensuite dans l'urine (Urbach, 1949). Le contenu du milieu intestinal peut, *in vitro*, transformer l'histamine en composé acétylé, ce qui n'exclut pourtant pas le rôle d'autres organes, en particulier du foie. Cette dernière hypothèse, qui n'est pas rejetée par Urbach, a été vérifiée et prouvée en particulier par Millican, Rosenthal et Tabor (1949), qui ont démontré que des préparations de foie de diverses espèces acétylent l'histamine en présence de coenzyme A et d'A.T.P. Millican (1953) a étudié l'acétylation *in vivo* de l'amine et a pu montrer que chez des rats entérectomisés le pourcentage d'histamine acétylée peut être important. Par contre la preuve de cette détoxication extra-digestive n'a pas été faite chez l'homme. Adam (1950) remarque que chez l'homme après ingestion d'histamine (133 mg) on retrouve dans l'urine de l'histamine conjuguée dont le taux varie de 0,17 à 1 p. 100 de la dose ingérée en 24 heures; par contre si l'injection a lieu par voie intra-veineuse (3,3 à 5 mg, en plusieurs heures) il apparaît dans l'urine des quantités accrues d'histamine libre, l'élimination représente 0,6 à 2,6 p. 100 de la dose.

L'histamine du tube digestif peut donc être absorbée, le plus souvent sous forme inactive, mais aux doses utilisées par les auteurs son action toxique est quasiment nulle.

III. Recherches nouvelles

Il existe pourtant une limite à la tolérance de l'intestin; des manifestations pathologiques peuvent se produire dans certaines conditions expérimentales. Il est possible de tuer un cobaye en lui faisant ingérer des doses élevées d'histamine (Parrot, Gabe et Herrault, 1947a). L'étude toxicologique permet de préciser un certain nombre de points importants.

A. Toxicologie

Les doses inférieures à 100 mg de dichlorhydrate d'histamine par kg, introduites par voie digestive, sont habituellement bien supportées par l'animal; au-dessus de

400 mg/kg la mortalité est égale à 100 p. 100, la dose semi-léthale étant de 250 mg par kg (PARROT, GABE et HERRAULT, 1947b). Cette dernière dose fut retrouvée plus tard par MILLICAN, ROSENTHAL et TABOR (1949).

La courbe de toxicité est représentée par la fig. 1.

On voit donc que par voie digestive la toxicité de l'histamine ne se manifeste que pour des quantités très élevées, supérieures à celles qui sont utilisées dans les travaux pharmacologiques habituels.

Cette intoxication aiguë ainsi réalisée avec de l'histamine seule, sur des animaux à jeun depuis 8 à 18 heures, se manifeste 30 à 45 minutes après l'administra-

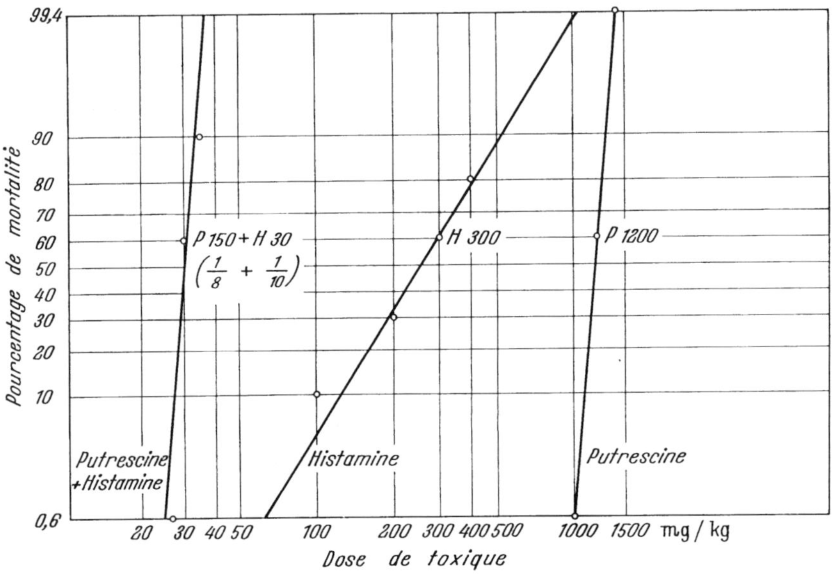

Fig. 1. Courbes de toxicité pour le Cobaye. En ordonnées: pourcentage de mortalité sur une échelle «probabilité». En abscisses: les doses (en mg/kg) sur une échelle logarithmique. De droite à gauche: — dichlorhydrate de putrescine seul. — dichlorhydrate d'histamine seul. — dichlorhydrate d'histamine précédé d'une dose 5 fois plus forte de dichlorhydrate de putrescine. Les substances ont été administrées par voie gastrique. Les points correspondant à une mortalité de 60 p. 100 se sont trouvés fournis par l'expérience pour les 3 essais: les doses respectives sont inscrites en regard de chacun de ces points. Pour l'ensemble des données numériques voir PARROT, GABE et HERRAULT (1947).

tion de la solution par sonde œsophagienne. Elle est caractérisée par des troubles respiratoires, digestifs et nerveux; la mort survient deux à quatre heures après le début de l'expérience, souvent par ulcération aiguë et perforation de l'estomac, sinon, vraisemblablement, par fuite extravasculaire de liquide plasmatique.

B. Passage de l'histamine dans le sang et dans les organes

Pour analyser le mécanisme de ce syndrome toxique, la répartition de l'histamine dans le sang et dans les organes de cobayes qui avaient ingéré cette substance a été étudiée (PARROT, 1948, 1949). Les dosages ont été effectués après extration selon la méthode de BARSOUM et GADDUM, modifiée par CODE, sur l'iléon isolé de Cobaye.

Si l'on fait ingérer 200 mg de dichlorhydrate d'histamine par kg à des cobayes, la barrière intestinale est forcée: on observe une hyperhistaminémie qui est maximale environ 50 minutes après l'ingestion. Pour des quantités inférieures à la dose minimale mortelle (60 mg/kg) les dosages révèlent une hypohistaminémie paradoxale qui apparaît au bout de deux heures. Cette baisse du taux de l'histamine est peut-être en rapport avec l'accumulation dans la muqueuse digestive de certains éléments figurés riches en histamine qui se trouvent ainsi soustraits du sang circulant. En effet, GABE remarque que les leucocytes sont très abondants dans les vaisseaux, les espaces interstitiels et la sous-muqueuse de l'estomac.

La fig. 2 résume les résultats fournis par les dosages d'histamine dans le sang total.

Les organes fixent une quantité importante d'histamine, si l'on administre des doses énormes capables de forcer la barrière intestinale; les cobayes reçoivent 400 mg de dichlorhydrate d'histamine par kg; la survie est alors de 40 minutes à 3 heures. La comparaison avec la valeur moyenne trouvée chez les témoins permet d'évaluer approximativement la quantité d'histamine fixée en μg de dichlorhydrate par gramme d'organe:

Intestin	premier quart	500
	deuxième moitié	120
Foie et poumons		60
Reins		25
Surrénales		10

soit environ 10 mg de dichlorhydrate d'histamine fixés dans l'ensemble de ces organes. Ce premier résultat montre qu'au moins dans ces conditions la destruction enzymatique de l'histamine n'est pas importante dans le délai de ces expériences et qu'un autre processus intervient avant cette oxydation.

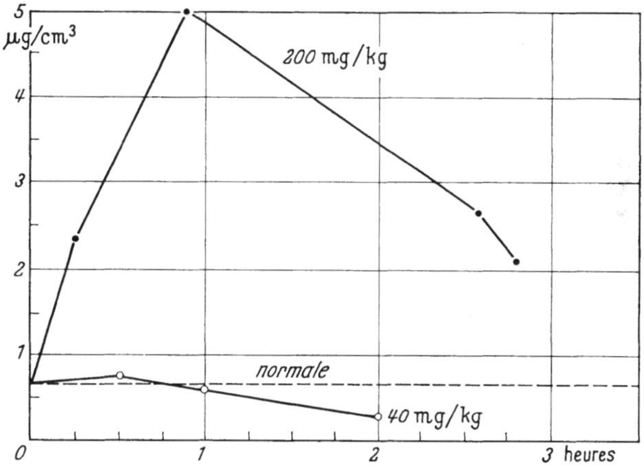

Fig. 2. Histaminémie chez le Cobaye. Au temps 0 les animaux ont reçu par voie gastrique respectivement: dichlorhydrate d'histamine (40 mg/kg); dichlorhydrate d'histamine (200 mg/kg). En ordonnées: histamine exprimée en μg de dichlorhydrate par ml de sang total (valeurs moyennes sur 5 dosages pour 200 mg/kg et 6 dosages pour 40 mg/kg). En abscisse: temps en heures. La moyenne normale est indiquée. (Selon PARROT, 1949).

L'étude histophysiologique (GABE, 1952) permet de retrouver d'une part des lésions analogues à celles que l'on observe après injection d'histamine et d'autre part des lésions assez particulières à l'ingestion de cette amine. La congestion très intense des organes splanchniques et la stimulation des glandes digestives, en particulier de l'estomac et du pancréas exocrine, correspondent à ce que l'on observe dans le choc histaminique classique. Au contraire la lésion du parenchyme pulmonaire est différente, l'aspect «soufflé» si caractéristique après injection parentérale est en partie masquée par la congestion intense. A l'examen de l'estomac, du duodénum et des premières anses grêles on note un afflux leucocytaire extravasculaire très important. Cet afflux leucocytaire est semblable à celui que l'on observe dans les premières phases de la digestion; il résiste aux anti-histaminiques, comme l'action même de l'histamine sur les glandes gastriques; enfin, il est surtout marqué dans la zone des ulcères. Cette étude a permis à GABE de suivre le processus ulcéreux qui évolue de la façon suivante: rupture des anses capillaires sous-épithéliales, exfoliation de l'épithélium de surface; la couche glandulaire sous-jacente n'est plus alors protégée contre l'action du suc gastrique hyperacide, d'où attaque de la surface vers la profondeur avec perforation dans tous les cas où la survie des animaux est suffisante.

C. La traversée de la paroi intestinale par l'histamine *in vitro*

Cette étude toxicologique devait amener à étudier, *in vitro*, le passage de l'histamine à travers la paroi de l'intestin (PARROT, 1948, 1949). Des doses considérables furent utilisées d'emblée. Une anse grêle de cobaye ayant été isolée et

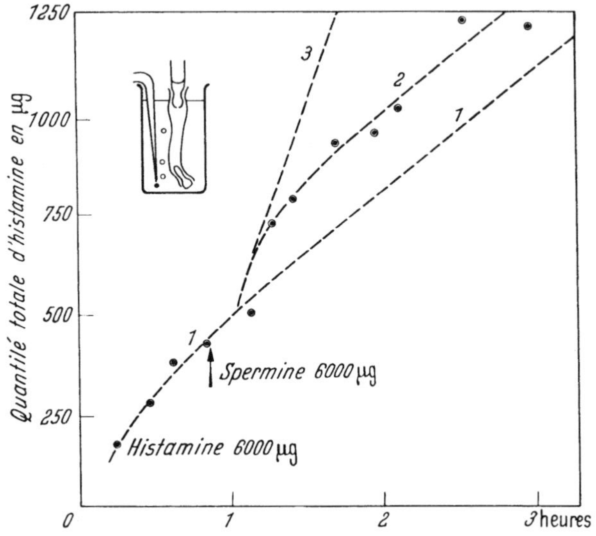

Fig. 3. Traversée de l'histamine étudiée «in vitro». Le cartouche indique le dispositif expérimental. Le fragment initial de l'intestin grêle de cobaye est de 6 cm environ, température 35°. A l'intérieur de l'intestin, on introduit 1,5 ml d'une solution de dichlorhydrate d'histamine à 4 p. 1000 au temps initial. L'histamine est dosée à l'extérieur de l'anse. En ordonnées: quantité totale d'histamine dans le bain extérieur. En abscisses: temps de prélèvement après le début de l'expérience (PARROT, 1948).

conservée en survie, on place à l'intérieur une solution d'histamine à forte concentration et on dose à intervalles réguliers la quantité de substance dans le bain extérieur. La fig. 3 (courbe 1) résume le résultat des recherches.

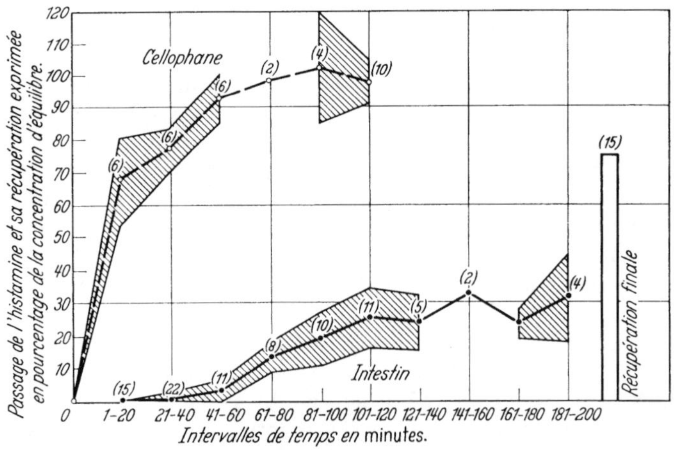

Fig. 4. Comparaison du passage de l'histamine à travers la paroi de l'iléon isolé de Cobaye et à travers la cellophane. Les valeurs moyennes sont représentées par des points. Le nombre d'échantillons est indiqué entre parenthèses à chaque point. Les zones pointillées délimitent une déviation standard au-dessus et au-dessous de la moyenne. La colonne à droite indique la récupération procentuelle moyenne de l'histamine qui est placée à l'intérieur des fragments d'intestin; déviation standard de cette dernière valeur: 9,4. (DWORETZKY et CODE, 1951).

On remarque que, même avec des doses très importantes (6 mg), il y a toujours un temps de latence de 10 à 15 minutes, comme si un substrat devait être saturé avant de permettre le passage de l'histamine. Confirmation de ce fait devait être donnée quelques années plus tard par DWORETZKY et CODE (1951). Pratiquant des expériences semblables sur des segments d'iléon de cobaye isolés, avec des doses plus faibles de substance, au plus 0,01 mg, ces auteurs devaient observer un temps de latence de 30 à 60 minutes. Au bout de 200 minutes environ 30 p. 100 de la quantité d'histamine, contenue dans le segment intestinal au temps 0, se trouve dans le bain extérieur. En utilisant un sac de cellophane de même calibre que le segment intestinal, ces auteurs notent que 67 p. 100 de l'histamine passe dans le bain extérieur en 20 minutes et 100 p. 100 en 41 à 60 minutes (fig. 4).

L'intestin oppose donc une barrière au passage de l'histamine; le temps de latence observé dans les expériences *in vitro* extériorise le phénomène et l'étude de l'action des diamines sur l'absorption intestinale de cette amine va nous aider à l'élucider.

D. Action des diamines sur l'absorption intestinale de l'histamine

La première hypothèse qui venait à l'esprit était qu'il pouvait s'agir d'une action enzymatique de l'histaminase au cours de la traversée intestinale; on sait, en effet, que la paroi intestinale est particulièrement riche en histaminase. C'est pour bloquer cette enzyme que des diamines, telles que la putrescine, la cadavérine ou la spermine ont été utilisées dans les expériences qui vont être décrites.

a) Toxicologie

Dans une première série d'expériences la toxicité de la putrescine, administrée isolément par voie gastrique, a été évaluée (PARROT, GABE et HERRAULT, 1947b). La dose demi-mortelle de putrescine est 5 à 6 fois plus grande que celle de l'histamine. La mortalité de 60 p. 100 est obtenue avec 1200 mg/kg de dichlorhydrate de putrescine ou avec 300 mg/kg de dichlorhydrate d'histamine (fig. 1).

Tableau 1. *Données toxicologiques — Mortalité obtenue par l'association de dichlorhydrate de putrescine (P) et de dichlorhydrate d'histamine (H) administrés par voie œsophagienne*

Dose en mg/kg		Nombre d'animaux	Nombre de morts	Pourcentage de morts
H	P			
15	15	8	0	0
20	100	6	0	0
25	150	10	0	0
30	150	10	6	60
35	175	10	9	90

Les produits sont administrés par sonde œsophagienne aux cobayes, afin d'éviter leur absorption par la muqueuse buccale. Si l'on donne, par cette même voie, de la putrescine, 40 minutes avant l'histamine, on remarque que des doses d'histamine et de putrescine très inférieures aux doses mortelles, lorsque ces substances sont administrées seules, entraînent la mort des animaux par leur association (voir tableau 1).

Tous les cobayes survivent à 30 mg de dichlorhydrate d'histamine ou à 150 mg de dichlorhydrate de putrescine; ces deux doses représentent chacune environ le huitième de la dose demi-mortelle; or leur association entraîne la mort de 6 cobayes sur 10.

Avec les données précédentes, la représentation des isoboles pour la mortalité 60 p. 100 met en valeur l'accroissement considérable de la toxicité de l'histamine sous l'influence de la putrescine (fig. 5).

On voit que s'il y avait simple addition de toxicité, pour la mortalité 60 p. 100, à 150 mg/kg de putrescine, il devrait être associé une dose d'histamine égale à 250 mg/kg; or elle est seulement de 30 mg/kg, c'est-à-dire huit fois moindre.

Comparée à la toxicité de l'histamine par voie intrapéritonéale, dont la dose 60 p. 100 mortelle est de 10 mg/kg, on remarque que l'histamine par voie digestive,

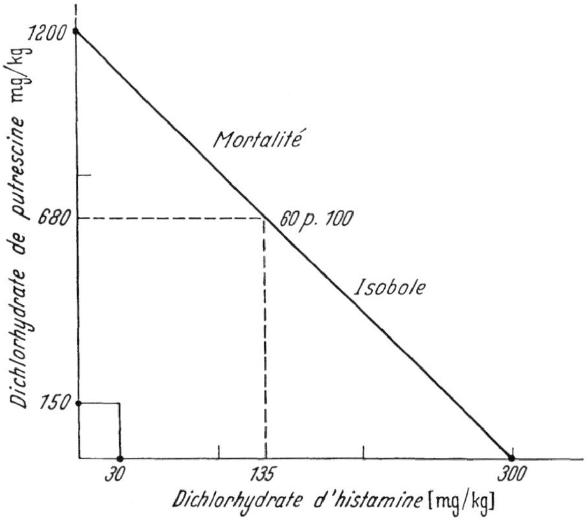

Fig. 5. Toxicités du dichlorhydrate d'histamine (H) et du dichlorhydrate de putrescine (P) administrés au Cobaye par voie œsophagienne; doses en mg/kg. Représentation des isoboles pour la mortalité de 60p. 100 d'après les données de PARROT, GABE et HERRAULT (1947). La mortalité 60p. 100 est obtenue soit avec 300 de H seule, soit avec 1200 de P seule, soit avec 30 de H associée à 150 de P. S'il y avait simple addition de toxicité, la même mortalité de 60p. 100 pourrait être obtenue n'importe par quelle combinaison de doses indiquées par la droite oblique, soit par exemple, pour prendre les mêmes proportions, 135 de H et 680 de P. La toxicité a donc été considérablement accrue: il a suffi environ de 4 fois moins de H et de 4 fois moins de P.

précédée de putrescine, est seulement trois fois moins toxique. Le rapport de toxicité de l'histamine $\left(\frac{\text{voie digestive}}{\text{voie parentérale}}\right)$ devient normal, il est de l'ordre de celui que l'on trouve pour les substances absorbées sans obstacle par voie digestive.

Les animaux intoxiqués de cette façon présentent des manifestations cliniques analogues à celles que l'on obtient avec l'histamine seule à doses beaucoup plus élevées; l'évolution est toutefois plus longue, toujours supérieure à 2 heures; la mort est annoncée par des convulsions.

b) Le dosage d'histamine dans le sang et dans les organes

Les animaux reçoivent 200 mg de dichlorhydrate de putrescine par kg et, 20 minutes après, 40 mg de dichlorhydrate d'histamine par kg. Ces valeurs correspondent à peu près à la plus petite dose qui provoque la mort dans 100 p. 100 des cas. Il y a une élévation du taux d'histamine dans le sang, pour une dose de cette substance qui, seule, ne provoque aucune hyperhistaminémie. Les dosages révèlent une histaminémie maximale au bout de 30 minutes, elle est alors de 2,8 μg/ml environ (fig. 6).

Le taux d'histamine fixé par les organes au bout d'une heure est plus important, après ingestion d'histamine précédée de putrescine, dans les poumons et dans le premier quart de l'intestin; il est égal dans la deuxième moitié de l'intestin.

En revanche le foie, au bout du même laps de temps, fixe deux ou trois fois moins d'histamine. Au bout de deux heures, intestin et poumons contiennent la même quantité d'histamine fixée, qu'on administre l'histamine seule ou précédée de putrescine; le foie en capte alors environ quatre fois plus qu'après ingestion d'histamine à la même dose (fig. 7).

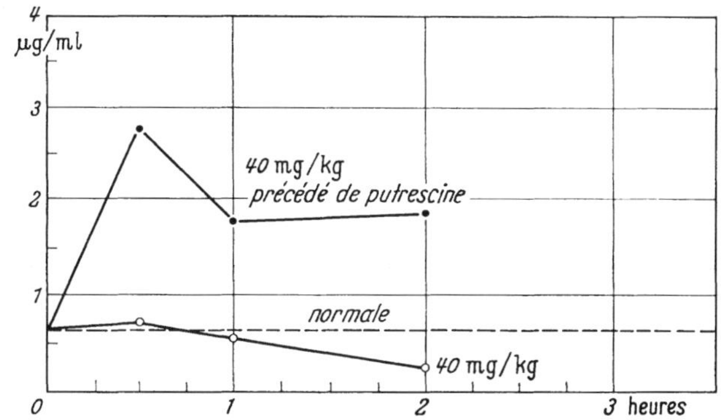

Fig. 6. Histaminémie chez le Cobaye. Au temps 0 les animaux ont reçu par voie gastrique: dichlorhydrate d'histamine (40 mg/kg) précédé ou non de dichlorhydrate de putrescine (200 mg/kg). En ordonnées: histamine exprimée en μg de dichlorhydrate par ml de sang total (moyennes sur 8 cobayes). En abscisses: temps en heures. La moyenne normale est indiquée. (Selon PARROT, 1949).

Les données histologiques (GABE et PARROT, 1951, 1952; GABE, 1952), montrent qu'il s'agit bien de lésions caractéristiques de l'histamine; elles correspondent à celles que l'on avait notées avec des doses 8 à 10 fois plus élevées d'histamine

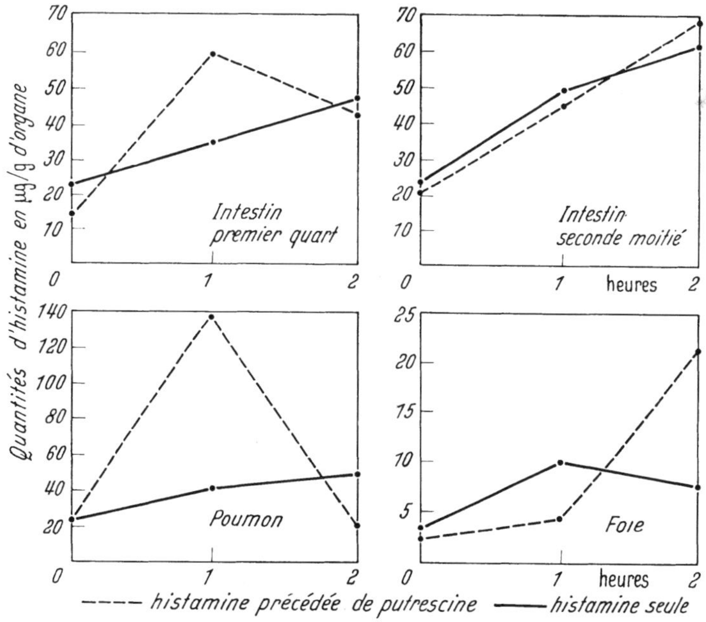

Fig. 7. L'histamine des organes chez le Cobaye après ingestion d'histamine. Valeurs moyennes. Méthode de Barsoum et Gaddum. Test: iléon isolé Cobaye. Au temps 0, les animaux ont tous reçu, par sonde œsophagienne, 40 milligrammes de dichlorhydrate d'histamine par kilogramme. Ceux du premier groupe n'ont rien reçu d'autre: traits pleins. Ceux du second groupe avaient reçu par la même voie, 20 minutes avant, 200 milligrammes de dichlorhydrate de putrescine par kilogramme: trait interrompu. Les valeurs initiales ont été fournies par des animaux qui n'avaient reçu aucune ingestion (1er groupe) et par des animaux qui avaient reçu 20 minutes auparavant la putrescine seule à la même dose (2e groupe). Le foie fixe 2 ou 3 fois moins d'histamine, sous l'influence de la putrescine, au bout d'une heure. (PARROT, 1950, données numériques inédites).

seule. Le foie présente une stéatose qui est sans doute en rapport avec une action de la putrescine sur cet organe, car cette lésion hépatique se retrouve chez les cobayes témoins qui ont reçu uniquement de la putrescine à dose élevée.

IV. Mécanisme d'action de la diamine associée à la putrescine

La putrescine lève donc l'obstacle qui s'oppose normalement au passage de l'histamine à travers l'intestin. En sa présence, de faibles doses d'histamine déterminent une importante hyperhistaminémie; il en résulte une intoxication histaminique caractéristique. Ce premier résultat est intéressant pour expliquer les observations cliniques, mais il reste à examiner le mécanisme de cette potentiation.

Cette action peut être analysée, *in vitro*, par l'étude de la traversée intestinale de l'histamine sur l'iléon isolé de cobaye, en présence d'une diamine (Parrot, 1948).

L'introduction d'une diamine, la spermine (4 mg de phosphate), dans un fragment (6 cm) d'intestin grêle de Cobaye qui contient déjà une solution de dichlorhydrate d'histamine à 4 p. 1000, ne modifie pas la pente générale de la courbe de passage de l'histamine à travers la paroi, mais lui fait subir un décalage vers le haut. Autrement dit la spermine a mis en liberté une certaine quantité d'histamine.

Un exemple des résultats obtenus est représenté par la fig. 3. La courbe 1 correspond à la quantité d'histamine qui passe dans le bain extérieur, si l'intestin contient seulement de l'histamine. La courbe 2, parallèle à la précédente nous montre qu'en introduisant de la spermine dans le segment intestinal, on augmente la quantité d'histamine qui passe dans le bain extérieur, mais la vitesse de passage n'est pas changée; en effet la pente de la courbe est la même que celle de la courbe témoin. Si, normalement, une fraction importante de l'histamine subissait une destruction enzymatique au cours de la traversée intestinale, la spermine, en bloquant l'enzyme, devrait accélérer son passage, selon, par exemple, la courbe 3; en effet, il y aurait alors une augmentation de débit et celle-ci se manifesterait par un changement de pente. Or il n'en est rien, la spermine a simplement mis en liberté une certaine quantité d'histamine.

La quantité d'histamine ainsi libérée par la spermine est de l'ordre de 100 à 300 μg. Une telle quantité ne peut venir de l'intestin lui-même; l'intestin contient environ 15 à 30 μg de dichlorhydrate d'histamine par gramme. Autrement dit la quantité d'histamine libérée ne peut venir que d'un stock qui s'est constitué au début de l'expérience. Dès lors s'explique l'existence du temps de latence que nous avons déjà mis en valeur: au début de l'expérience il y a une captation de l'histamine par un substrat; ensuite lorsque celui-ci est saturé l'histamine traverse l'intestin. Un temps de latence initial a été aussi noté par Dworetzky et Code (1951).

Quel est le substrat de cette captation ? Sans doute l'intestin du cobaye peut se charger d'histamine et cette charge peut aller *in vivo* jusqu'à 0,5 mg par gramme d'organe frais; mais ni la spermine, ni la putrescine ne peuvent libérer ce stock d'histamine, ni s'opposer à sa constitution. Il doit donc exister un autre lieu de stockage et nous avons étudié de nouveau (Parrot, 1949b) le passage de l'histamine à travers la paroi de l'intestin de Cobaye (les 6 premiers centimètres environ) mais selon une technique différente. Un dispositif permettait de laver d'une manière continue l'intestin isolé, à l'aide d'une solution contenant de l'histamine; le suc intestinal se trouve ainsi éliminé à mesure qu'il est sécrété. On s'aperçoit alors que l'addition de spermine au bain intérieur ne met plus en liberté aucune quantité d'histamine supplémentaire. On peut donc conclure que dans les premières expériences la quantité libérée avait été retenue par le suc intestinal.

La méthode pharmacologique et les équilibres de dialyse ont permis de montrer que l'histamine est captée par les sucs gastriques et intestinaux (PARROT, 1949 b).

Parmi les constituants des sucs digestifs capables de capter l'histamine, nous avons retenu la mucine. Trois sacs de collodion sont baignés, intérieur et extérieur, par une solution de dichlorhydrate d'histamine dans un mélange tampon à pH 8,1. Le premier de ces dispositifs de dialyse sert de témoin, le second contient de la mucine dans le bain extérieur, le troisième également et à la même concentration, mais du dichlorhydrate de putrescine y est ajouté. Les trois lots sont placés à 5° C et les dosages sont effectués dans le bain intérieur au bout de 24 à 48 heures. On remarque alors a) que la quantité d'histamine augmente du côté de la mucine, le rapport des deux concentrations pouvant atteindre 2 ou même dépasser cette valeur; b) la putrescine limite ce déplacement et le rapport tombe par exemple de 1,3 à 1,1 ou de 2,7 à 1,5. Ces expériences d'équilibre de dialyse ont été reprises pour étudier les variations de la captation en fonction du pH (PARROT, NICOT et LABORDE, 1961): dans tous les cas la mucine gastrique fixe l'histamine, avec un maximum à pH 3. Les essais pharmacologiques mettent en évidence la captation de l'histamine et l'action de la putrescine qui limite cette captation.

Les travaux de COHEN (1953, 1954) réalisés sur l'intestin grêle de Rat, en utilisant une technique de perfusion vasculaire des anses intestinales, ont montré que l'intestin de l'animal s'oppose au passage de l'histamine dans la circulation sanguine. Dans les premières expériences réalisées par l'auteur, le liquide de perfusion utilisé était une solution de 3,5 p. 100 de polyvinylpyrrolidone dans du liquide de TYRODE glucosé et bicarbonaté; or cette solution provoque une lyse de l'épithélium intestinal, détruit les cellules mucigènes chez l'animal à jeun; et la mucine ainsi libérée était probablement, comme le remarque COHEN, le facteur responsable de la captation.

Le rôle protecteur de la mucine du tube digestif contre l'histamine contenue dans la lumière intestinale semble évident à la suite de ces diverses expériences et montre que le rôle joué par la diamino-oxydase est, sans doute, secondaire dans cette protection. Si l'on admet que l'action de cette enzyme se manifeste *in vivo* avec la même lenteur qu'*in vitro*, on comprend qu'elle se trouve débordée par un brusque apport d'histamine. La captation, au contraire, agit d'une manière quasi instantanée et précède l'attaque enzymatique. Les diamines interviendraient donc beaucoup plus par leur fixation sur la mucine que sur la diamino-oxydase; autrement dit elles agiraient à l'égard de l'histamine d'abord comme compétiteurs de fixation ayant saturé le substrat de captation; elles permettent à l'histamine de rester libre et, par conséquent, d'être absorbée en abondance.

Résumé et conclusion

Normalement le milieu intestinal contient de l'histamine. Une part, très faible, est absorbée sous forme libre et active. La plus grande part se trouve soit inactivée, soit retenue dans l'intestin. L'inactivation se fait par acétylation: l'acétylhistamine, inactive, passe dans le milieu intérieur; elle est excrétée par le rein: c'est l'histamine conjuguée des urines. D'autre part il existe un mécanisme qui retient l'histamine dans l'intestin: c'est sa captation par la mucine.

Dans certaines conditions, l'histamine libre passe dans le milieu intérieur en quantité suffisante pour provoquer des troubles. Sans doute un excès d'histamine dans l'intestin favorise ce passage car les mécanismes protecteurs, acétylation et pexie sont alors débordés. Mais on peut concevoir aussi qu'ils cessent de fonctionner et que la quantité d'histamine normalement présente dans l'intestin soit alors suffisante pour être pathogène. Excès d'histamine et absence de protection peuvent fort bien d'ailleurs intervenir simultanément.

A notre connaissance on n'a pas établi dans quelles circonstances l'acétylation pourrait être contrecarrée. En revanche, le pouvoir histaminopexique de la mucine est inhibé par l'action de certaines diamines, comme la putrescine, la cadavérine, la spermine. De telles substances même à des doses où elles ne sont pas toxiques par elles-mêmes libèrent l'histamine qui, absorbée, exerce alors ses actions caractéristiques. Ainsi agiraient les bases aminées que les anciens auteurs, avec ARMAND GAUTIER, avaient étudiées sous le nom de ptomaïnes et de leucomaïnes.

D'autres mécanismes ont pu être invoqués; par exemple les «modifications dégénératives» de la muqueuse intestinale observées au cours de la réaction d'alarme favoriseraient, selon SELYE, l'absorption de l'histamine. Quant à l'histaminase de la paroi intestinale nous ne pensons pas qu'elle soit capable de protéger efficacement l'organisme contre l'histamine contenue dans l'intestin; nous croyons en effet que son action n'est pas assez rapide; son inhibition par conséquent ne jouerait pas de rôle important dans l'intoxication histaminique d'origine intestinale.

Bibliographie

ÅKERBLOM, E.: Über die Ätiologie und Pathogenese der Futterrehe beim Pferde. Skand. Arch. Physiol., Suppl. 68, 164 (1934).
ADAM, H. M.: Excretion of histamine in human urine. Quart. J. exp. Physiol. **35**, 281 (1950).
ANREP, G. V., M. S. AYADI, G. S. BARSOUM, J. R. SMITH and M. M. TALAAT: The excretion of histamine in urine. J. Physiol. (Lond.) **103**, 155 (1944).
BERTHELOT, A., et D. BERTRAND: Contribution à l'étude de la β-imidazol-éthylamine. C. R. Acad. Sci. (Paris) **155**, 360 (1912).
BOURLE, M.: Rôle de l'histamine dans l'étiologie des indigestions chez les Ruminants. Traitement par les antihistaminiques. Thèse Vét., Alfort (1959).
BOYER, J., F. DEPIERRE, M. TISSIER et J. JACOB: Intoxications histaminiques collectives par le thon. Presse méd. **64**, 1003 (1956).
—, et J. JACOB: Les aliments vecteurs d'histamine. Presse méd. **89**, 35 (1961).
COHEN, Y.: Étude du processus d'inactivation de l'histamine dans l'intestin grêle du Rat. J. Physiol. (Paris) **45**, 86 (1953).
— Sort de l'histamine dans l'intestin grêle du Rat. J. Physiol. (Paris) **46**, 305 (1954).
DWORETZKY, M., and C. CODE: Passage of histamine across the wall of the small bowel of guinea pig. Amer. J. Physiol. **166**, 462 (1951).
FEIGEN, G. A., and O. H. CAMPBELL: The relative sensitivity of the mucosal and peritoneal surfaces of the guinea pig ileum to histamine, acetylcholine and specific antigens. Amer. J. Physiol. **145**, 676 (1946).
GABE, M.: Données histophysiologiques sur l'intoxication histaminique aiguë par voie gastrique. Arch. Mal. Appar. dig. **41**, 10 (1952).
—, et PARROT, J.-L.: Afflux leucocytaire extravasculaire dans la paroi de l'estomac après administration intragastrique d'histamine chez le Cobaye. J. Physiol. (Paris) **43**, 734 (1951).
— — Augmentation de l'absorption intestinale de l'histamine par l'action de certaines diamines. Presse méd. **60**, 1779 (1952).
GALE, E. F., and H. M. R. EPPS: The effect of the pH of the medium during growth on the enzymic activities of bacteria (*Escherichia coli* and *Micrococcus lysodeiticus*) and the biological significance of the changes produced. Biochem. J. **36**, 600 (1942).
GERARD, R. W.: Chemical studies on intestinal intoxication. I. The presence and significance of histamine in an obstructed bowel. J. biol. Chem. **52**, 111 (1922).
GISCAFRÉ, L. Y., and E. M. DE ESPANÉS: Toxicity of histamine in rabbits. Arch. int. Pharmacodyn. **76**, 25 (1948).
GOUNELLE, R., et M. A. POINTEAU-POULIQUEN: Les intoxications alimentaires après consommation de poisson. Rev. Hygiène médecine sociale (nov. 1961).
IVY, A. C., and A. J. JAVOIS: The stimulation of gastric secretion by amines and other substances. Amer. J. Physiol. **71**, 604 (1925).

Karády, E. S.: Histamine tolerance and anaphylactic death in sensitized guinea pigs. J. Immunol. **41**, 1 (1941).
Kendall, A. I., and O. F. Schmitt: Physiologic action of certain cultures of the gaz bacillus. J. infect. Dis. **39**, 250 (1926).
—, and P. L. Varney: The physiologic action of histamine applied directly to the mucosa of the isolated surviving intestine of the guinea pig. J. infect. Dis. **41**, 143 (1927).
Kochan, W. F.: Laminitis and its treatment by a new anti-histaminic: "Anthisan". Vet. Rec. **60**, 257 (1948).
Koessler, K. K., and M. T. Hanke: Studies on proteinogenous amines. IV. The production of histamine from histidine by *Bacillus coli communis*. J. biol. Chem. **39**, 539 (1919).
— — Studies on proteinogenous amines. XXI. The intestinal absorption and detoxication of histamine in the mammalian organism. J. biol. Chem. **59**, 889 (1924).
Legroux, R., J. C. Levaditi, G. Boudin et D. Bovet: Intoxications histaminiques collectives consécutives à l'ingestion de thon frais. Presse. méd. **54**, 545 (1946).
Lévy-Bruhl, M., G. Ungar et A. Levillain: Production par voie bactérienne, à partir de l'urée, d'une substance physiologiquement identifiable à l'histamine. C. R. Acad. Sci. (Paris) **204**, 1222 (1937).
Loeper, M., et M. Perrault: Traitement des intoxications alimentaires. Paris: J. B. Baillière, 1937.
Meakins, J., and G. R. Harrington: The absorption of histamine from the intestine. J. Pharmacol. exp. Ther. **20**, 45 (1923).
Mellanby, E.: An experimental investigation on diarrhoea and vomiting of children. Quart. J. Med. **9**, 165 (1916).
—, and F. Twort: On the presence of β-imidazol-ethylamine in the intestinal wall; with a method of isolating a bacillus from the alimentary canal which converts histidine into this substance. J. Physiol. (Lond.) **45**, 53 (1912).
Millican, R. C.: The acetylation of histamine in normal and enterectomized rats. Arch. Biochem. **42**, 399 (1953).
—, M. S. Rosenthal and H. Tabor: On the metabolism of histamine. A. Urinary excretion following oral administration. β-conjugation *in vitro*. J. Pharmacol. exp. Ther. **97**, 4 (1949).
Nevot, A.: Les test de salubrité des denrées alimentaires. Recueil de l'Ecole d'Alfort, (no. 11) (1942).
— Intoxications alimentaires d'origine carnée observées dans la région parisienne en 1948. Bull. Acad. nat. Méd. (Paris) **133**, 219 (1949).
Oehme, C.: (1913). Cité d'après Ivy and Javois (1925).
Parrot, J.-L.: La fixation de l'histamine par les tissus du Cobaye. Sa libération par une diamine. C. R. Soc. Biol. (Paris) **142**, 631 (1948).
— L'histaminémie du Cobaye après ingestion d'histamine. J. Physiol. (Paris) **41**, 251 A (1949a).
— Nouvelles recherches sur la pénétration de l'histamine par voie intestinale. Rôle protecteur du suc intestinal et de la mucine gastrique. C. R. Soc. Biol. (Paris) **143**, 1553 (1949b).
— Histaminolyse et histaminopexie. Actualités pharmacol. **11**, 233 (1958).
— M. Gabe et A. Herrault: Intoxication histaminique du Cobaye par voie gastrique. C. R. Soc. Biol. (Paris) **141**, 484 (1947a).
— — — Intoxication aiguë du Cobaye par l'administration simultanée d'histamine et de putrescine. C. R. Soc. Biol. (Paris) **141**, 486 (1947b).
— G. Nicot et C. Laborde: Le pouvoir histaminopexique de la mucine gastrique. C. R. Soc. Biol. (Paris) **155**, 1212 (1961).
Rosenthal, S. M., and H. Tabor: An improved colorimetric method for the estimation of histamine. J. Pharmacol. exp. Ther. **92**, 425 (1948).
Roske, G.: Über Bedingungen der Aminbildung durch *Bact. coli*. Jb. Kinderheilk. **120**, 186 (1928).
Tabor, H., and E. Mosettig: Isolation of acetylhistamine from urine following oral administration of histamine. J. biol. Chem. **180**, 703 (1949).
Urbach, K. F.: Nature and probable origin of conjugated histamine excreted after ingestion of histamine. Proc. Soc. exp. Biol. (N. Y.) **70**, 146 (1949).
Wangensteen, O. H., and M. Loucks: Studies in intestinal obstruction; the absorption of histamine from obstructed bowel. Arch. Surg. **16**, 1089 (1928).
Weiss, S., G. P. Robb and L. B. Ellis: The systemic effects of histamine in man. Arch. intern. Med. **49**, 360 (1932).
Wilcox, H. B. jr., and B. C. Seegal: Influence of an ethylenediamine derivative on histamine intoxication or anaphylactic shock in the intact guinea pig and the isolated guinea pig heart. J. Immunol. **44**, 219 (1942).

Section B

Captation de l'histamine par les protéines sériques

Par

Jean-Louis Parrot, Madame Claude Laborde-Burtin et Anatole Saindelle

Avec 3 Figures

L'étude du terrain allergique a conduit à mettre en évidence la captation de diverses amines biologiques par le sérum normal de l'Homme et de diverses espèces animales, et l'absence d'une telle captation par le sérum de sujets allergiques. Ces recherches étaient la suite logique de travaux antérieurs; ceux-ci avaient montré que l'histamine est captée par la mucine du suc intestinal (Parrot, 1949), puis que l'histamine est captée par l'héparine (Parrot et Laborde, 1951).

Ce phénomène de captation de l'histamine en général a reçu le nom d'histaminopexie; le présent exposé sera limité au pouvoir histaminopexique du sérum sanguin[1].

L'histaminopexie sérique — son absence chez l'Homme allergique

Le sérum de l'Homme normal contient une γ-globuline particulière qui est absente ou inactive dans le sérum de l'Homme allergique. Elle a été étudiée grâce à sa propriété de capter diverses amines biologiques et elle a été appelée plasmapexine I.

In vitro la captation de l'histamine est maximale dès la première seconde de contact. A concentration constante de plasmapexine I, la proportion d'histamine captée s'élève quand la quantité totale d'histamine diminue (voir notamment Wallenfels et coll., 1958).

A. Techniques

La mesure peut se faire sur le sérum ou sur le plasma. Dans ce dernier cas on utilisera l'héparine, en employant le minimum de cette substance capable d'éviter la coagulation.

Voici les diverses techniques qui permettent aujourd'hui d'évaluer l'histaminopexie sérique (v. tableau 1 qui indique les références).

I. Techniques physiques

Diverses épreuves physiques ont établi l'existence de l'histaminopexie du sérum humain normal et ont permis de la mesurer. Les mêmes expériences ont

[1] Toute une équipe de collaborateurs a pris part à ces recherches. L'histaminopexie a été étudiée par Mme Mordelet-Dambrine grâce à l'ultrafiltration, et par Thouvenot et Mme Flavian grâce à un équilibre de dialyse suivi du dosage colorimétrique.

Tableau 1. *Les techniques qui permettent d'évaluer l'histaminopexie sérique chez l'Homme*

Techniques		Résultats non allergiques	Résultats allergiques	Références
Physiques *Equilibres de dialyse* suivis de dosages d'histamine par:	Colorimétrie	+	0	PARROT, FLAVIAN et THOUVENOT, 1957. PARROT et LABORDE, 1961 b
	Spectrophotométrie	+		KLAMERTH, 1955
	Mesure de radioactivité	+	0	PARROT, FLAVIAN, BONET-MAURY et PROVOST, 1962
	Dosage biologique	+	0	PARROT, URQUIA et LABORDE, 1951
Ultrafiltration		+	0	PARROT et MORDELET-DAMBRINE, 1961 a
Ultracentrifugation		+	0	WALLENFELS et coll., 1958. SUND et KERP, 1958. KERP et SUND, 1958
Pharmacologique: Appareil	manuel	+	0	LABORDE, PARROT et URQUIA, 1953
	automatique	+	0	FLAVIAN, VASSEUR et PARROT, 1961
Sérologique		+	0	MIKOL, RENOUX et MERKLEN, 1961. PARROT, LABORDE et LEBEL, 1963

+ indique l'activité de la plasmapexine I; 0 indique l'absence d'activité de cette substance.

montré l'absence d'histaminopexie sérique chez l'Homme allergique. Ces expériences se ramènent à trois principes: équilibre de dialyse, ultrafiltration, ultracentrifugation.

1. Equilibre de dialyse

L'histamine, introduite à égale concentration de part et d'autre d'une membrane dialysante[1], se déplace vers le compartiment où se trouve le sérum quand celui-ci provient d'un sujet normal; à l'équilibre, au bout de 4 heures, avec un sac de collodion, le déplacement D de l'histamine peut atteindre 50 p. 100 ($D = 100 \frac{I-E}{E}$, I, concentration de l'histamine à l'intérieur du sac, où se trouve le sérum, c'est-à-dire la somme de l'histamine libre et de l'histamine fixée; E, concentration de l'histamine à l'extérieur du sac, c'est-à-dire l'histamine libre).

Au contraire, si le sérum provient d'un sujet allergique, aucun déplacement appréciable de l'histamine n'est noté.

Les concentrations finales de l'histamine peuvent être évaluées par différentes techniques.

a) *Dosage biologique:*

L'histamine est dosée par la méthode pharmacologique sur l'iléon isolé de Cobaye (PARROT, URQUIA et LABORDE, 1951). Voici un exemple numérique: à l'extérieur d'un sac en collodion se trouvent 10 ml de liquide de TYRODE contenant 50 μg de dichlorhydrate d'histamine par millilitre. A l'intérieur du sac, dans un même volume de 10 ml, se trouvent 2 ml de sérum et l'histamine à la même concentration. A l'équilibre, au bout de 4 heures, un prélèvement de 1 ml est effectué à l'intérieur et à l'extérieur du sac. Afin de pouvoir évaluer la concentration de l'histamine dans les deux lots, il est nécessaire de diluer 200 fois, d'une part pour se placer dans la meilleure zone de sensibilité différentielle de l'iléon, d'autre part pour

[1] Utiliser une membrane suffisamment perméable, par exemple Dialyser Tubing, Arthur H. Thomas Co., Philadelphia 5 Pa. USA. Diamètre 5/8 inch, Epaisseur: 0,0008 inch.

diluer le sérum de façon à annuler son histaminopexie. Ainsi, avec un sérum normal, on peut trouver 40 μg/ml à l'extérieur et 60 μg/ml à l'intérieur; $D = 100 \frac{I - E}{E} = 100 \frac{60 - 40}{40} = 50$. Dans ce cas, le déplacement de l'histamine atteint 50 p. 100.

b) Dosage spectrophotométrique:

KLAMERTH (1955) dose l'histamine au spectrophotomètre (2 115 Å) dans un équilibre de dialyse et conclut notamment à une liaison de cette substance avec les gamma-globulines comme nous l'avions précédemment établi.

c) Dosage colorimétrique:

L'histamine est dosée par la méthode de ROSENTHAL et TABOR (1948). On évalue au colorimètre la coloration rose obtenue en milieu alcalin par copulation de l'histamine avec le chlorure de diazonium de la *para*nitraniline (PARROT, FLAVIAN et THOUVENOT, 1957).

La présence de sérum dans le lot intérieur nécessite de nombreuses purifications avant de pouvoir faire la mesure colorimétrique. Afin de supprimer ces temps opératoires, il est possible de faire l'équilibre de dialyse avec une fraction purifiée du sérum, la plasmapexine I (voir plus loin sa préparation). On peut alors faire la diazotation, même en présence de protéines (PARROT et LABORDE, 1961 b; PARROT, LABORDE, NICOT et FLAVIAN 1961). Mais comme la préparation de la plasmapexine I, telle qu'elle est codifiée, ne s'applique pour le moment qu'au sérum humain, la technique colorimétrique ne peut être utilisée pour le plasma humain ou le sérum des animaux.

d) Mesure de la radio-activité β:

Si dans l'équilibre de dialyse on utilise de l'histamine marquée au carbone 14, au terme de l'équilibre, il suffira de mesurer la radio-activité β de l'histamine (BONET-MAURY, FLAVIAN et coll., 1960; PARROT, FLAVIAN et coll., 1962) — (voir tableau 2).

Quand le sérum utilisé provient d'un sujet normal, on voit que la proportion d'histamine fixée est plus grande si la concentration d'histamine au début de l'équilibre est plus faible.

Tableau 2. *Fixation de l'histamine marquée par le sérum humain normal et le sérum de malade allergique* (PARROT, FLAVIAN et coll., 1962)

	Concentration initiale (μg/ml)	Concentration finale (μg/ml)		Déplacement
		I	E	D
Sérums humains normaux	3	4,0	2,5	60
	6	7,8	4,8	62
	20	20,1	17,0	18
	30	35,8	29,4	22
	40	41,0	36,0	14
Sérums de malades allergiques	3	3	3	0
	3	3,1	3,0	2
	6	5,3	5,8	—9
	12	12,3	12,0	2

Le déplacement D de l'histamine est donné par la formule:

$$D = 100 \frac{I - E}{E}$$

2. Ultrafiltration

Si on ajoute de l'histamine à un sérum humain normal, et qu'on soumette ce mélange à l'ultrafiltration (2 kg/cm^2 pendant 10 à 15 heures), on constate qu'une partie de l'histamine ne traverse pas l'ultrafiltre. La concentration de l'histamine est plus élevée dans le résidu d'ultrafiltration que dans l'ultrafiltrat. Au contraire si le sérum provient d'un malade allergique, il n'y a pas de différence de concentration entre les deux compartiments. Dans cette technique, l'histamine a pu être dosée par méthodes biologique et colorimétrique (PARROT et MORDELET-DAMBRINE, 1961 a).

3. Ultracentrifugation

Si l'on ajoute de l'histamine au sérum humain normal et qu'on le soumette ensuite à l'ultracentrifugation (40 000 tours par minute pendant 8 h à 0° C), l'histamine liée se trouve entraînée avec les protéides; telle est la constatation qui a été faite par WALLENFELS et coll. (1958). Ces auteurs dosent dans le surnageant l'histamine qui est restée libre et calculent la quantité qui est liée. Par extrapolation ces auteurs établissent que la capacité histaminopexique des sérums humains normaux peut atteindre 10 à 24 μg/ml. Si au contraire le sérum provient de sujets allergiques aucune quantité d'histamine n'est entraînée par les protéides.

II. Technique pharmacologique

Le test utilisé est l'iléon isolé de Cobaye qui baigne dans 12 à 15 ml de liquide de TYRODE maintenu à 37° C, sous barbotage d'air. L'iléon est attelé à un myographe isotonique à inscription frontale, sous une tension de 2 grammes. Le coefficient d'amplification du levier est de 20. Le liquide de TYRODE a la composition suivante pour 1000 ml: ClNa 8 g, Cl_2Mg 0,1 g, ClK 0,2 g, Cl_2Ca 0,2 g, CO_3HNa 1 g. Habituellement, ce liquide de TYRODE n'est pas glucosé; on évite ainsi les contractions spontanées. Cependant, quand la sensibilité de l'iléon est faible, on peut travailler en présence de glucose à 0,25 p. 1000 et de sulfate d'atropine à $0,5 \times 10^{-7}$ (poids/vol.)

On compare les contractions déclenchées par une solution donnée d'histamine aux contractions produites par un mélange contenant de l'histamine à la même concentration et du sérum humain dilué au 1/20. Quand le sérum utilisé provient d'un sujet normal, on constate qu'une partie de l'histamine est devenue incapable d'agir sur le test biologique (voir figure 1).

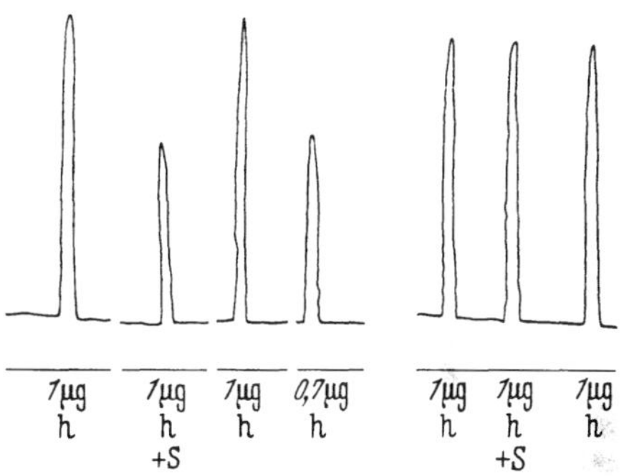

Figure 1. Le pouvoir histaminopexique du sérum humain normal et du sérum d'un malade allergique. Le pouvoir histaminopexique représente le pourcentage de l'histamine fixée. Dans l'exemple ci-dessus, pour le sérum normal il est de $100 \frac{1-0,7}{1} = 30$. Au contraire, pour le sérum d'un sujet allergique, les contractions sont toutes de la même hauteur; il n'y a pas d'histamine fixée et le pouvoir histaminopexique est nul (LABORDE, PARROT et URQUIA, 1953)

Naturellement, on aura choisi, pour de tels essais, une concentration d'histamine qui se place dans la zone de plus grande sensibilité différentielle (de 10^{-6} à 10^{-7} poids/vol. selon les tests dans le tube ou le mélange est préparé): si on utilisait une concentration supramaximale, le phénomène ne pourrait se manifester.

Cette technique se prête au mieux à la recherche et peut s'adapter à la routine; les divers auteurs qui, après nos publications, ont étudié le pouvoir histaminopexique du sérum, ont utilisé presque exclusivement cette technique; le nombre des déterminations ainsi effectuées dans le domaine de la routine et de la recherche se chiffre par dizaines de mille (DANELATOS, 1955; BODIN, 1956; CARRON et coll., 1957; PELLERAT et coll., 1957; SIDI et coll., 1958; TAPPEINER et coll., 1958; LEVRAT et coll., 1959; JEUNE et coll., 1959; HURIEZ et coll., 1960; CARRÉ, 1962). La reproductibilité des résultats a été statistiquement établie par WODNIANSKY

(1961, 1962). Cette technique peut êtreem ployée sur un appareil automatique (FLAVIAN, VASSEUR et PARROT, 1961) tel que celui de BOURA, MONGAR et SCHILD (1954).

Naturellement la technique pharmacologique exige par exemple que le sérum soit débarrassé des substances qui pourraient exercer une action sur le test biologique; une dialyse préalable de 24 heures (1 ml de sérum sur 150 ml de ClNa à 9 p. 1000 changés trois fois dans les 24 h) permet d'obtenir ce résultat. Mais si cette dialyse est insuffisante la captation de l'histamine peut être masquée: le sérum ajoute son action propre à celle de l'histamine libre; ainsi s'expliquerait peut-être l'insuccès de CRAPS et INDERBITZIN (1957).

D'autres difficultés peuvent provenir de certaines impuretés de l'eau qui est utilisée pour composer le liquide de TYRODE.

Dès le début on s'est assuré que la diminution d'activité de l'histamine observée en présence de sérum ne résulte ni d'une destruction partielle de la substance, ni d'une diminution de sensibilité du test sous l'influence du sérum: par exemple on peut rendre son activité à une partie de l'histamine pharmacologiquement masquée en ajoutant un compétiteur de fixation tel que la putrescine; on peut aussi précipiter les protéides par acidification: on retrouve alors la totalité de l'histamine qui avait été ajoutée au sérum; plus simplement encore, si on dilue le sérum additionné d'histamine, on libère la totalité de celle-ci. D'autre part PARROT et LABORDE ont contrôlé la technique pharmacologique par les techniques physiques (équilibre de dialyse ou ultrafiltration) et ont toujours trouvé des résultats parallèles.

Les quelques résultats non reproductibles publiés par PAUTRIZEL et coll. (1960) auraient sans doute été expliqués si ces auteurs avaient réalisé la même étude critique.

III. Séro-agglutination du complexe histamine-polystyrène

MIKOL, RENOUX et MERKLEN (1961), MIKOL et RENOUX (1962) ont ajouté de l'histamine à une suspension de polystyrène-latex; le sérum humain normal agglutine ce mélange, même quand il est ajouté à des dilutions très élevées. Au contraire, quand le sérum utilisé provient d'un malade allergique, il n'y a pas d'agglutination ou bien elle n'existe qu'à des dilutions très faibles. Nous avons mesuré le pouvoir histaminopexique de 120 sérums par la méthode pharmacologique et recherché la dilution limite donnant encore une agglutination avec le mélange polystyrène-latex-histamine. Au moins pour les sérums étudiés, il semble exister une corrélation entre ces deux séries de mesures (PARROT, LABORDE et LEBEL, 1963), et la séro-agglutination du complexe histamine-polystyrène devient une nouvelle technique simple de mesure du pouvoir histaminopexique.

Cette technique permet de mettre en évidence la présence de plasmapexine I, car les gamma-globulines ou l'extrait purifié de sérum agglutinent le complexe à la même dilution que le sérum initial. Le pouvoir histaminopexique du sérum des animaux peut être étudié par cette nouvelle technique. En revanche, elle ne convient pas pour étudier le pouvoir histaminopexique acquis chez les malades allergiques à la suite d'un traitement par les gamma-globulines ou par le mélange gamma-globulines-histamine. En effet, chez les malades ainsi traités, le pouvoir histaminopexique acquis est thermolabile; or la technique au latex comporte un chauffage à 56° C pendant deux heures.

Bien entendu, pour un même sérum étudié par une technique physique ou sérologique et par la technique pharmacologique, les chiffres obtenus ne sont pas les mêmes, car les conditions expérimentales sont très différentes: concentration du sérum, concentration de l'histamine, temps de contact, etc. . . . Mais si plusieurs sérums sont étudiés par des méthodes différentes on observe une corrélation satisfaisante entre les deux séries de résultats.

B. Resultats

1. Sujets normaux

Le sérum des sujets normaux capte l'histamine (PARROT, URQUIA et LABORDE, 1951), la 5-hydroxytryptamine (PARROT et FLAVIAN, 1959) et l'acétylcholine (FLAVIAN, 1963). En raison de sa comodité c'est l'histaminopexie, évaluée par la technique pharmacologique qui a servi de test dans les statistiques suivantes.

a) *Données statistiques*

La figure 2 représente une population de sujets normaux comparée à une population de sujets allergiques (PARROT et LABORDE, inédit).

Chez l'adulte normal la technique pharmacologique, telle qu'elle a été codifiée, a fourni les résultats suivants: chez 79 sujets examinés et interrogés sur les manifestations allergiques qu'eux-mêmes ou leurs ascendants pouvaient avoir présentées, la moyenne est de 33,0 (écart-type 1,08, variance 4,9) et aucun de ces sujets n'a un pouvoir histaminopexique nul. Plus tard ont été étudiés les sérums de 225 sujets qui n'étaient pas aussi soigneusement sélectionnés: dans cette seconde statistique sont alors apparues quelques valeurs nulles ou très basses qui atteignaient 7,1 p. 100 des mesures (PARROT et LABORDE, 1961 *a*).

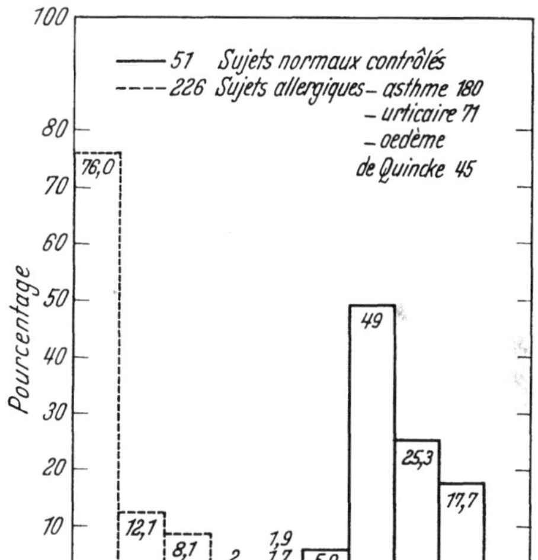

Fig. 2. Répartition des valeurs du pouvoir histaminopexique dans une population de sujets normaux et dans une population de sujets allergiques (PARROT et LABORDE, inédit)

Chez la Femme, au cours de l'accouchement, il existe normalement une chute importante mais brève de l'histaminopexie sérique (VIGNES, 1962).

Pendant la première année de la vie, selon VIALATTE et coll. (1962), l'histaminopexie sérique serait très basse. Cependant JEUNE et coll. (1959) ont enregistré des valeurs normales chez les nourrissons non allergiques; et cette constatation est confirmée par HURIEZ et coll. (voir VIALATTE et coll. 1962).

Chez l'enfant sain sans antécédent allergique personnel ni familial, CARRON et coll. (1957), JEUNE et coll. (1959) trouvent une distribution analogue à celle que l'on relève chez l'adulte normal (109 sujets).

b) *Données chimiques*

L'histaminopexie du sérum normal est due à la présence d'une gammaglobuline, la plasmapexine I qui représente 0,4 à 0,7 p. 1000 des protéides totaux, soit environ 1 p. 1000 des globulines totales (LABORDE, PARROT et SANDOR, 1959). Cette fraction qui est précipitée totalement entre pH 6,5 et pH 5,2 est beaucoup trop faible pour apparaître à l'électrophorèse. Mais elle suffit cependant à justifier toute l'activité histaminopexique du sérum. La plasmapexine I capte aussi la 5-hydroxytryptamine (PARROT et FLAVIAN, 1959), la putrescine, l'histidine, l'acétylcholine, mais non la bradykinine.

En l'absence d'ions minéraux, la plasmapexine I ne fixe pas l'histamine. Le rôle de ceux-ci sera étudié plus loin (voir p. 171).

2. Sujets allergiques

a) Données statistiques

Le sérum de l'Homme allergique ne capte ni l'histamine, ni l'acétylcholine, ni la 5-hydroxytryptamine. C'est presque toujours l'histaminopexie qui a été recherchée dans les données qui vont suivre.

Deux grandes catégories doivent être distinguées selon que l'histaminopexie sérique est absente d'une manière permanente ou seulement par épisodes.

α) L'histaminopexie est absente en permanence. C'est dans cette catégorie que se trouve l'allergie au sens le plus classique et le plus restreint du mot (asthme, rhinite spasmodique, urticaire, œdème de Quincke). Les cas où les anticorps circulants sont abondants se rencontrent ici. Les effets de l'allergie portent sur les muscles lisses ou sur la perméabilité des membranes; ce sont des manifestations immédiates; l'histamine joue un rôle dans certaines d'entre elles: spasme et œdème des bronches, vasodilatation et œdème de la peau. Il ne semble pas qu'il y ait destruction cellulaire.

D'autre part nous classerons dans cette catégorie certaines migraines et l'eczéma constitutionnel parce que dans ces cas aussi l'histaminopexie sérique est nulle en permanence. Un ensemble de résultats trouvés dans la littérature est récapitulé dans le tableau 3.

Tabelau 3. *Tableau recapitulatif. Ensemble de résultats relevés dans la littérature (les auteurs sont cités dans le texte, les références se trouvent à la bibliographie).*

	Nombre de cas	Pourcentage de pouvoirs histaminopexiques faibles ou nuls
Adultes normaux ou malades non allergiques	1237	10
Enfants normaux ou malades non allergiques	201	4
Urticaire et oedème de Quincke	517	91
Asthme	1070	89
Migraine	270	81
Eczéma constitutionnel	185	81

Au cours de recherches systématiques, des histaminopexies nulles ont parfois été notées alors que le sujet n'avait jamais présenté de manifestations cliniques d'allergie. Mais quelques mois ou quelques années plus tard, sont apparues des crises d'asthme typiques ou des accès de migraine caractérisés. Il paraît donc probable que, dans cette catégorie de sujets, l'absence d'histaminopexie sérique préexiste généralement aux manifestations cliniques. Si l'on joint à ce fait la notion d'hérédité, on peut admettre qu'il s'agit là d'un génotype.

β) L'histaminopexie disparaît seulement lorsque la lésion évolue. Ici, il ne s'agit pas seulement de muscles lisses qui se contractent ou de membranes qui deviennent plus perméables. Des cellules sont lésées ou même détruites. L'anticorps, quand il existe, ne passe qu'en faible quantité dans le milieu intérieur. L'histamine ne joue qu'un rôle accessoire, si même elle en joue un. Quant à la disparition de l'histaminopexie sérique, elle semble être ici un caractère acquis et pourrait bien être consécutive à la lésion. Dans cette catégorie le mot «allergie» prend son sens le plus étendu. Nous y trouvons en effet non seulement l'eczéma de contact et l'allergie tuberculeuse, mais aussi l'ulcère gastrique et duodénal (PARROT, LABORDE, DEBRAY et ROURE, 1956; PELLERAT et coll., 1957), la rectocolite hémorragique (PARROT, LABORDE, DEBRAY et GASTARD, 1960), le rhumatisme articulaire aigu (PARROT, MOZZICONACCI et coll., 1957), la polyarthrite chronique évolutive et la goutte (PARROT, GALMICHE et SAINDELLE, 1961). Lorsque nous avons eu l'occasion de mesurer l'histaminopexie de ces malades hors des poussées, nous avons vu, en général, les valeurs s'élever et même atteindre la normale.

Ce fait a été confirmé par BODIN (1956) pour l'ulcère gastrique ou duodénal, et par DANELATOS (1955) pour le rhumatisme articulaire aigu.

b) *Données chimiques*

Les données chimiques ont été étudiées par LABORDE, PARROT et SANDOR (1959).

Le sérum des malades allergiques à pouvoir histaminopexique nul ne possède pas de plasmapexine I. En revanche il contient des protéides qui n'existent pas chez le sujet normal:

1°/ l'antipexine: c'est une globuline qui inhibe la captation de l'histamine par la plasmapexine I;

2°/ la plasmapexine II: c'est une gamma-globuline qui peut capter l'histamine mais qui n'exerce pas cette action dans le plasma sanguin.

Lorsque l'histaminopexie reparaît entre les crises, le fractionnement du sérum fournit des résultats comparables à ceux du sérum normal[1].

3. Sujets malades mais non allergiques

L'histaminopexie sérique existe et sa valeur est le plus souvent normale (voir cependant plus loin le cas où les gamma-globulines plasmatiques se trouvent perturbées, par exemple, au cours de l'insuffisance hépatique).

L'histaminopexie sérique a été mesurée chez 100 malades atteints d'affections aussi diverses que: emphysème, dilatation des bronches, diabète, hypothyroïdie, dermatoses diverses mais non allergiques, glaucomes, cancers du sein, du poumon, de l'estomac . . . Il s'agit ici d'une sélection (PARROT et LABORDE); les auteurs ont eux-mêmes interrogé les sujets: aucun de ces 100 malades ne présentait une affection allergique ou un antécédent allergique. Aucun n'a un pouvoir histaminopexique nul, et la moyenne du pouvoir histaminopexique est de 26,6 (écart-type 1,58, variance 7,9).

Un autre groupe de malades adultes, que les auteurs n'ont pu interroger eux-mêmes, mais dont l'affection en cours n'était pas de nature allergique, réunit 133 malades. Là, des histaminopexies nulles ou faibles apparaîssent, et cela chez 11 p. 100 des malades.

Chez l'enfant malade, une étude a été faite chez 160 sujets non allergiques; treize seulement ont un pouvoir histaminopexique nul; la moyenne calculée sur l'ensemble est de 21,8 (RAHMAN et MOZZICONACCI, 1963).

On voit toute l'importance d'étudier avec soin et de caractériser correctement chaque cas clinique; s'il n'en était pas ainsi une telle statistique perdrait de sa valeur, de nombreuses erreurs risqueraient d'être commises et notamment des états allergiques demeureraient ignorés: ce n'est pas parce qu'un diagnostic «non

---

[1] Les cas du rhumatisme chronique et de la goutte sont peut-être différents et seront l'objet de recherches particulières.

allergique» est inscrit sur la fiche d'un malade que celui-ci n'est pas, en outre, un homme allergique. Une enquête clinique plus approfondie aurait sans doute rendu plus discriminative la statistique de CRUCHAUD et coll. (1961).

4. Cas où les gamma-globulines sériques sont modifiées

a) *Insuffisance hépatique*

L'histaminopexie sérique peut s'annuler au cours de l'insuffisance hépatique (PARROT, MORDELET-DAMBRINE et LABORDE, 1959). Ces auteurs ont tout d'abord étudié 32 malades chez lesquels on avait reconnu ou discuté l'existence d'une insuffisance hépatique; ils ont comparé chez chacun d'eux le pouvoir histaminopexique et le test au thymol de MACLAGAN. Pour cette population, il existe entre ces deux tests une corrélation hautement significative.

Dans une nouvelle série de recherches, ils ont étudié 3 groupes de 15 sujets chacun:

a) sujets normaux
b) sujets allergiques sans insuffisance hépatique
c) sujets atteints d'insuffisance hépatique.

Les trois groupes de sujets peuvent être complètement séparés à l'aide des deux réactions sériques utilisées (thymol en unités Vernes et histaminopexie en p. 100):

a) sujets normaux: histaminopexie $\geqq 15$
thymol < 6
b) sujets atteints d'insuffisance hépatique:
histaminopexie $\leqq 10$
thymol > 6
c) sujets allergiques:
histaminopexie $\leqq 10$
thymol < 6

C'est donc là une première méthode qui permet de distinguer l'Homme allergique du malade atteint d'insuffisance hépatique.

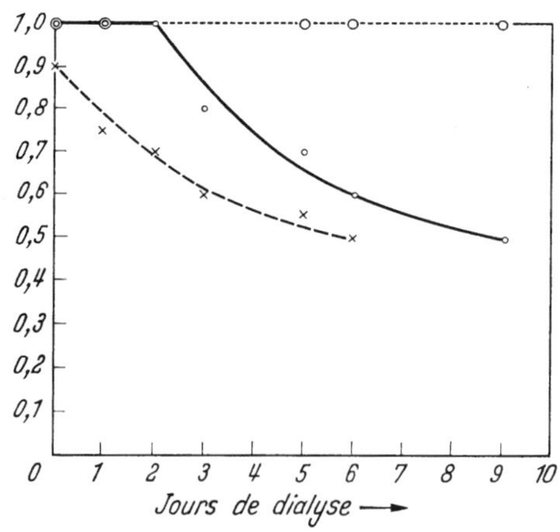

Fig. 3. Activité biologique de l'histamine mise en présence de sérum humain et ses modifications sous l'influence de la dialyse. Cinq ml de sérum sont mis à dialyser aux environs de 0° C dans un sac de collodion qui baigne dans 25 ml d'eau distillée additionnée de 9 p. 1000 de ClNa. Le bain est renouvelé 3 fois par jour. En abscisses: jours de dialyse; au temps 0, sérum non dialysé. En ordonnées: activité biologique de l'histamine titrée sur l'iléon isolé de Cobaye. La valeur 1 représente l'activité totale de la solution de dichlorhydrate d'histamine à 10^{-6} (pds/vol). Les lots d'expérience contiennent le sérum à la concentration de $^{1}/_{20}$ et le dichlorhydrate d'histamine à la concentration de 10^{-6} (pds/vol). Sérum d'allergique: trait plein et cercles. Sérum normal: trait pointillé et croix. Sérum de malade atteint d'insuffisance hépatique: trait pointillé et cercles (PARROT, URQUIA et LABORDE, 1952; PARROT, MORDELET-DAMBRINE et LABORDE 1959)

L'autre procédé repose sur la dialyse prolongée du sérum sur une solution de chlorure de sodium à 9 p. 1000: s'il s'agit d'un sujet allergique (voir fig. 3) le sérum au bout de quelques jours devient capable de capter l'histamine. Au contraire s'il s'agit d'insuffisance hépatique, aucune histaminopexie n'apparaît, ou, du moins, aucune histaminopexie importante.

On remarquera que si allergie et insuffisance hépatique se rencontrent chez le même individu, l'un et l'autre de ces procédés le classera dans la catégorie de l'insuffisance hépatique.

En somme, l'étude de l'histaminopexie sérique permet de caractériser le sujet normal par la présence de plasmapexine I, le sujet allergique par la présence de plasmapexine II, et le malade atteint d'insuffisance hépatique par l'absence de l'une et de l'autre de ces deux gamma-globulines à la fois, ou par leur diminution.

b) *Abondante formation de gamma-globulines anticorps*

α) Sensibilisation. On sensibilise des cobayes par une injection intrapéritonéale de 4 mg d'ovalbumine pure cristallisée. Ces animaux sont sacrifiés trois semaines aprés cette injection et on vérifie pour chacun d'eux que la réaction de SCHULTZ-DALE avec l'ovalbumine est positive pour l'iléon. Chez tous les animaux, le pouvoir histaminopexique du sérum est nul, et la dialyse prolongée ne le restitue pas. Cette absence de restitution par longue dialyse pourrait être expliquée par une modification profonde des gammaglobulines du sérum des animaux sensibilisés (PARROT et LABORDE, 1956).

β) Immunisation. Des lapins immunisés contre la variole ont un sérum dépourvu de pouvoir histaminopexique. Il en est de même pour les gammaglobulines extraites de ces sérums (PARROT et LABORDE, inédit).

Tableau 4. *Histaminopexie sérique du Cheval* (moyennes)

	Immunisation lente	rapide
Avant	24,5	26,6
Demi-immunisation	5	11
Fin d'immunisation		11

Des chevaux ont été soumis à deux sortes d'immunisation: une immunisation rapide, antitétanique, à raison de trois injections d'anatoxine par semaine pendant cinq semaines, suivies d'une injection de toxine tétanique; une immunisation lente, au venin de serpent, *Echis naja* ou *bitis* suivant le cas.

L'installation de l'immunité, quelle que soit sa nature ou la fréquence des injections, a pour corrolaire un abaissement du pouvoir histaminopexique moyen des animaux en expérience (travail inédit en collaboration avec GRANDADAM) (voir tableau 4). La dialyse prolongée du sérum n'élève généralement pas son histaminopexie.

c) *Formation diminuée des gamma-globulines*

L'histaminopexie sérique peut être normale dans les cas dits d'agammaglobulinémie, qui sont en réalité des cas d'hypogammaglobulinémie (LABORDE, inédit).

Un tel fait s'explique car la plasmapexine I représente une proportion si faible des gamma-globulines qu'elle ne donne aucune bande visible à l'électrophorèse même si le sérum est concentré 100 fois.

5. Intervention des ions minéraux

Cette étude a comporté trois étapes. Tout d'abord, *in vitro* la présence d'ions minéraux, et notamment de calcium ou de magnésium est indispensable pour que l'histaminopexie se manifeste. Un excès de potassium au contraire inhibe l'histaminopexie du sérum normal (PARROT, LABORDE et DAMBRINE, 1955; PARROT et MORDELET-DAMBRINE, 1959, 1960).

Puis, d'autres essais in *vitro* mirent en évidence des transformations du système histaminopexique sans doute par la fixation des cations minéraux sur les protides responsables. Par l'action du potassium *in vitro*, un sérum humain normal perd sa propriété de capter l'histamine et les fractionnements caractéristiques d'un sérum allergique ont pu alors être mis en evidence. Inversement, en faisant agir *in vitro* le calcium sur le sérum d'un sujet allergique, on fait apparaître le pouvoir de capter l'histamine et on peut retrouver alors les fractions caractéristiques d'un sérum normal (PARROT et MORDELET-DAMBRINE, 1961b). Ces deux transformations inverses sont observées alors même que le sérum a été ramené par dialyse à une composition saline normale: ainsi dans l'un et l'autre cas, les modifications des protéides sériques survivent à l'excès transitoire d'un ion diffusible.

Enfin des essais ont été entrepris sur le vivant (PARROT, MORDELET-DAMBRINE et TRINQUET, 1962). Après l'injection d'un sel de potassium au Cobaye ou au Rat, l'histaminopexie sérique disparaît. Chez le Rat, où le phénomène a été suivi, l'histaminopexie sérique reste nulle ou faible plusieurs semaines après une seule injection d'un sel de potassium. Pendant cette période, l'injection de chlorure de calcium rétablit l'histaminopexie sérique. Il en est de même chez le Rat dont l'histaminopexie sérique a été préalablement annulée à la suite de la surrénalectomie. Une seule injection de chlorure de calcium rétablit l'histaminopexie sérique pour plusieurs semaines.

Enfin, chez plusieurs malades asthmatiques, dont, comme c'est la règle, l'histaminopexie sérique était nulle ou faible, celle-ci a été rétablie par une injection intraveineuse lente de gluconate de calcium. Parallèlement, s'installait une importante amélioration clinique.

Ces constatations posent de nouveaux problèmes: il est difficile présentement d'expliquer pourquoi ces actions durent aussi longtemps. D'autre part, lorsque chez un malade l'absence de plasmapexine I est épisodique et qu'elle semble liée à l'évolution même de l'affection, on peut se demander si des lésions ayant initialement un caractère banal et portant sur la peau, sur une muqueuse, sur un endothélium ou sur une séreuse, ne peuvent pas, dans certains cas, entraîner soit une décharge de potassium dans les humeurs, soit toute autre modification du milieu intérieur capable de transformer les protéides du système histaminopexique; dès lors l'évolution des lésions s'en trouverait modifiée: de «normergique» elles deviendraient «hyperergiques», aboutissant, selon les cas à l'eczéma, à l'ulcère gastrique ou duodénal, à la rectocolite hémorragique, à l'endocardite ou à l'atteinte articulaire du rhumatisme articulaire aigu, ou de la polyarthrite chronique évolutive.

Enfin, semblable hypothèse est peut-être valable pour d'autres cas où nous avons noté l'absence d'histaminopexie sérique: néphrites aiguës, purpuras thrombopéniques ou non, psoriasis . . .

Ainsi, nous nous sommes éloignés de plus en plus de la notion classique de l'allergie. Dans tous ces cas, il est vraisemblable que le terrain est modifié, mais cette fois il s'agit d'un caractère acquis par l'individu. Au point de vue terminologie, on sera peut-être en droit de parler de terrain allergique acquis lorsqu'à l'absence d'histaminopexie sérique s'ajoute le caractère hyperergique de la lésion.

6. Facteurs humoraux

a) Hypophyse

Des rats mâles et femelles (de 150 à 180 g) ont été hypophysectomisés par voie parapharyngienne, puis maintenus à 22°C, et ont reçu un régime riche en protéides. Neuf rats (3 mâles et 6 femelles) ont été sacrifiés 19 jours après l'intervention. Le sérum de tous les animaux était dénué de pouvoir histaminopexique[1]. Une dialyse longue fait réapparaitre le pouvoir histaminopexique.

Il est possible de restituer partiellement le pouvoir histaminopexique chez le Rat hypophysectomisé par des injections sous-cutanées de corticostimuline (65 u/animal/jour pendant 5 jours et sacrifice le 6ème jour), ou de cortisone (5 mg/animal/jour pendant 5 jours, sacrifice le 6ème jour). Chez ces animaux, on constate que le poids des surrénales a augmenté par rapport aux témoins hypophysectomisés non traités, et que la bande soudanophobe de la zone fasciculée des surrénales est amincie. Il y a donc une compensation partielle de l'hypofonctionnement des surrénales.

En revanche, l'injection d'acétate de désoxycorticostérone (5 mg/ jour pendant 2 jours, puis 2,5 mg/jour pendant 3 jours, sacrifice le 6ème jour) ou celle d'hormone somatotrope (0,5 mg, 48 heures avant le sacrifice) n'entraîne pas d'augmentation du pouvoir histaminopexique. Parallèlement, il n'y a pas de modifications histologiques des surrénales par rapport aux témoins, (Tuchmann-Duplessis, Parrot et Laborde, 1954).

b) *Cortex surrénal*

Surrénalectomie. Des rats mâles, d'un poids moyen de 160 grammes ont été surrénalectomisés et leur survie a été assurée par l'addition de 9 p. 1000 de ClNa à leur eau de boisson[2]. Les animaux sont sacrifiés à des délais différents après l'intervention. Le pouvoir histaminopexique de leur sérum est encore normal 24 heures après, mais s'annule au bout de 3 jours et reste nul pendant au moins trois mois. Des animaux ayant subi une intervention fictive et sacrifiés 3 jours plus tard avaient toujours un pouvoir histaminopexique normal. Ainsi donc, chez le Rat, l'ablation des surrénales annule le pouvoir histaminopexique du sérum (Parrot et Laborde, 1952a).

Si l'on soumet le sérum de Rat surrénalectomisé à une dialyse prolongée sur une solution de ClNa à 9 p. 1000, on voit apparaître au bout de trois jours un certain pouvoir histaminopexique; celui-ci atteint au bout de 9 jours une valeur maximale de 50 p. 100. On obtient le même résultat, rappelons-le, en opérant avec un sérum de malade allergique.

Si, à des rats surrénalectomisés depuis 3 ou 8 jours, on injecte par voie intrapéritonéale de l'acétate de cortisone ou de l'acétate de désoxycorticostérone à la dose de 0,5 mg/100 g, 4 heures avant le sacrifice, le pouvoir histaminopexique revient à des valeurs presque normales (Parrot et Laborde, 1952b, 1953). Avec une seule injection de cortisone, le pouvoir histaminopexique se maintient à sa valeur maximale de 25 p. 100 pendant un délai d'au moins 15 jours, puis diminue et s'annule entre trois semaines et un mois (Parrot et Laborde, inédit).

Excès de cortisone. Des rats normaux reçurent de l'acétate de cortisone à la même dose (0,5 mg/100 g) par voie intrapéritonéale. Quatre heures après, le pouvoir histaminopexique est diminué de moitié. Une étude systématique a été entreprise avec des doses croissantes (0,5 mg, 5 mg et 10 mg par 100 g). Le pouvoir histaminopexique diminue en quatre heures, s'annule vers 12 à 18 heures et s'inverse même, pour les doses les plus fortes, au bout de 1, 2 et 3 jours (Parrot et Laborde, 1954). Le mécanisme d'une telle transformation est inconnu; peut-être cette annulation du pouvoir histaminopexique est-elle en relation avec une diminution des gammaglobulines. Avec une injection d'une forte dose de cortisone (10 mg/ 100 g) à des rats normaux, on a pu reproduire expérimentalement l' «histaminosthénie». Nous proposons de donner ce nom au renforcement de l'activité biologique

[1] Le sérum de Rat normal a un pouvoir histaminopexique de 20 à 30 p. 100 environ.

[2] L'absence de ClNa dans cette eau modifie l'histaminopexie.

de l'histamine. Déjà, le fait avait été observé avec le sérum de certains malades allergiques ou avec celui de malades atteints d'insuffisance hépatique (PARROT et LABORDE, 1954; PARROT, MORDELET-DAMBRINE et LABORDE, 1959).

c) *Hormones sexuelles*

Ces recherches ont été faites chez le Rat par PARROT, TUCHMANN-DUPLESSIS et LABORDE (1957).

α) Mâles. Le pouvoir histaminopexique est nul ou faible 3 et 6 jours aprés castration. Mais 2 semaines après l'intervention le pouvoir histaminopexique est remonté à des valeurs normales.

β) Femelles. Chez les rattes, la castration annule le pouvoir histaminopexique. Cette annulation survient 3 jours après l'intervention et se maintient encore 3 semaines après. Si dix jours après la castration, on injecte aux animaux du benzoate de folliculine tous les jours pendant 5 jours et qu'on les sacrifie le 6ème jour, l'histaminopexie du sérum reste nulle si la dose est de 5 μg/animal/jour; elle reparaît si la dose atteint la valeur considérable de 250 μg/animal/jour. Des essais témoins avec de l'acétate de désoxycorticostérone ou de l'acétate de testostérone n'ont pas permis de modifier le pouvoir histaminopexique qui reste nul chez ces rattes castrées.

Une étude du cycle oestral a été entreprise par des frottis vaginaux quotidiens. Le sérum de 7 rattes en oestrus a un pouvoir histaminopexique moyen de 23, alors que le sérum de 8 rattes en dioestrus a un pouvoir histaminopexique moyen de 4.

Chez trois rattes sacrifiées à la veille de la mise bas (le 20ème jour de la gestation), le pouvoir histaminopexique du sérum a été trouvé nul.

d) *Rate*

Des rats mâles, d'un poids compris entre 90 et 120 g ont été splénectomisés et l'histaminopexie plasmatique a été mesurée 2 jours à deux mois après l'intervention. Le pouvoir histaminopexique est nul ou fortement abaissé.

e) *Rôle de l'acide L-ascorbique*

Le sérum de Cobaye a un pouvoir histaminopexique de 30 p. 100 environ. On soumet des cobayes mâles à un régime scorbutigène composé de son et avoine préalablement autoclavé et de complément vitaminique (thiamine, riboflavine, amide nicotinique, huile de foie de morue). Au bout de 12 jours de ce régime, un prélèvement sanguin est effectué au coeur; le pouvoir histaminopexique du sérum est nul. On donne alors aux mêmes animaux, soumis au même régime de base, 50 mg d'acide L-ascorbique per os, par animal et par jour, pendant 5 jours. Une nouvelle prise de sang est alors effectuée 6 heures après la dernière ingestion d'acide ascorbique. Le pouvoir histaminopexique est restitué à la moitié de sa valeur normale.

Comme les sérums de rats surrénalectomisés ou hypophysectomisés le sérum de Cobaye scorbutique retrouve un pouvoir histaminopexique après une dialyse prolongée.

L'annulation du pouvoir histaminopexique chez le Cobaye scorbutique peut avoir comme origine une certaine insuffisance corticosurrénale; en effet, malgré l'hyperplasie cortico-surrénale du scorbut, la sécrétion et l'efficacité des corticostéroïdes sont diminuées (PARROT et LABORDE, 1953).

7. Etude pharmacologique

On utilise des rats dont l'histaminopexie plasmatique a été annulée par surrénalectomie ou par hypophysectomie et on cherche à restituer le pouvoir histaminopexique; telle a été la méthode employée d'abord par PARROT et LABORDE (1960).

Les rats utilisés sont des mâles de 80 à 120 g, soit surrénalectomisés, soit surrénalectomisés et castrés, soit hypophysectomisés. Ces animaux reçoivent une solution de ClNa à 9 p. 1000 comme eau de boisson. Les substances étudiées sont injectées par voiei ntra-péritonéale.

α) Salicylate de sodium. Le salicylate de sodium injecté à la dose de 5 mg/100 g à de tels animaux 4 heures avant le sacrifice restitue le pouvoir histaminopexique. La restitution est maximale si la dose de salicylate est de 20 mg/100 g.

β) Antipyrine. La dose de 20 mg/100 g permet de restituer environ la moitié du pouvoir histaminopexique deux, quatre, huit et seize heures après l'injection. L'efficacité disparaît à peu près complètement au bout de 24 heures.

γ) Une phénothiazine, non antihistaminique, mais anti-inflammatoire et anti-choc, le 4909 RP[1], aux doses de deux, cinq et dix mg/100 g a permis de restituer, 4 heures après l'injection, une certaine histaminopexie sérique.

δ) La mépyramine (ou néoantergan), antihistaminique spécifique, une heure après l'injection, s'est montrée 50 fois moins active que le corps précédent.

ε) Tripropyl-thiophène-sulfonate de magnésium. Un dérivé magnésien du thiophène, le tripropyl-thiophène-sulfonate de magnésium, à la dose de 100 mg/100g, une heure avant le sacrifice, a été le corps le plus efficace qui ait été étudié au cours de tous ces essais.

ζ) La colchicine, à la dose de 40 μg/100 g, restitue une certaine histaminopexie; l'action est lente et durable, avec un maximum de 48 heures après l'injection et une durée supérieure à 8 jours. Nous supposons que cette lenteur d'action est due à l'activité d'un métabolite de la colchicine (PARROT et SAINDELLE, 1961).

η) La phénylbutazone à la dose de 5 mg/100 g restitue l'histaminopexie; cette action passe par un maximum 6 heures après l'injection pour disparaître 8 heures après (SAINDELLE et PARROT, 1961).

Ainsi, le salicylate de sodium, l'antipyrine, la phénylbutazone, la colchicine, un dérivé magnésien du thiophène, une phénothiazine restituent l'histaminnopexie sérique du Rat surrénalectomisé.

Ces corps agissent comme la cortisone. C'est une action périphérique qui n'a pas besoin de la présence des hormones cortico-surrénales pour s'exercer. Enfin, c'est une action distincte de l'activité anti-histaminique.

Conclusion

Ainsi, à la notion clinique de terrain allergique, répond maintenant une notion chimique, l'absence de plasmapexine I, et un test biologique, l'absence d'histaminopexie sérique. Dans le cas du terrain allergique héréditaire, le sérum est dépourvu de pouvoir histaminopexique, que l'organisme se trouve ou non exposé aux agressions qui déclenchent les crises. Il paraît très vraisemblable que l'histaminopexie sérique était déjà nulle avant toute manifestation clinique. On retrouve souvent, parmi les ascendants du sujet, d'autres personnes dont le sérum présente les mêmes caractéristiques; l'existence de transmetteurs sains a même été décelée dans quelques cas (PARROT, SCLAFER et LABORDE, inédit).

---

[1] Le 4909 RP est le chlorhydrate de chloro-3 (diéthylamino-3′ propyl)-10 phénothiazine.

Cependant le terrain n'est que l'un des deux facteurs étiologiques généraux; l'autre est l'agression déclenchante, et celle-ci peut être de natures fort diverses. Ce qui détermine les manifestations cliniques c'est à la fois l'agressivité des causes extérieures et la prédisposition héréditaire.

Au point de vue chimique, la plasmapexine I est une gammaglobuline qui capte non seulement l'histamine mais aussi d'autres amines biologiques. Ce protéide est absent chez les sujets allergiques. En revanche, leur sérum contient deux protéides qui n'existent pas chez le sujet normal: la plasmapexine II et l'antipexine.

La présence de calcium ou de magnésium permet à la plasmapexine I de manifester son pouvoir histaminopexique. Au contraire, le potassium inhibe la captation.

L'étude des facteurs hormonaux est dominée par deux faits:

1°) L'hypophysectomie, chez le Rat, fait disparaître l'histaminopexie sérique, et l'administration de corticostimuline peut alors la restituer.

2°) L'histaminopexie sérique s'annule chez le Rat surrénalectomisé recevant comme boisson de l'eau salée. Elle peut alors être restituée par certains corticoïdes, et aussi par divers agents anti-inflammatoires tels que le salicylate de sodium, l'antipyrine, la colchicine et la phénylbutazone.

L'importance pharmacologique de l'histaminopexie apparaît peut-être dans le fait suivant. Dans un certain nombre de circonstances, on observe parallèlement la diminution ou la disparition de l'histaminopexie sérique et l'augmentation de la sensibilité à l'histamine: tels sont les cas de l'Homme allergique, du Cobaye scorbutique, et du Rat surrénalectomisé.

Bibliographie

Bodin, H.: Le pouvoir histaminopexique des ulcéreux au cours de la poussée douloureuse et après traitement par le sérum de convalescent. Arch. Mal. Appar.dig. **45**, 621—625 (1956).

Bonet-Maury, P., N. Flavian, J.-L. Parrot et M. Provost: Démonstration de l'histaminopexie sérique à l'aide de l'histamine marquée au C^{14}. J. Physiol. (Paris) **52**, 29—30 (1960).

Boura, A., J. L. Mongar and H. O. Schild: Improved automatic apparatus for pharmacological assays on isolated preparations. Brit. J. Pharmacol. **9**, 24—30 (1954).

Carré, J.: Etude du pouvoir histaminopexique du sérum sanguin dans l'allergie (à propos de quatre cents mesures). Thèse Méd. Paris, n° 968, 41 (1962).

Carron, R., J. Pellerat, M. Jeune et M. Murat: Le pouvoir histaminopexique du sérum. Son intérêt diagnostique et thérapeutique en pédiatrie. Lyon méd. **198**, 85—94 (1957).

Craps, L., et T. Inderbitzin: A propos d'un test sérologique nouveau des états allergiques: l'absence de pouvoir histaminopexique du sérum sanguin. Int. Arch. Allergy **11**, 285—291 (1957).

Cruchaud, A., J.-P. Girard, E. Domine et M. Micheli: Etude critique du pouvoir de fixation de l'histamine et de la sérotonine par le sérum sanguin. Int. Arch. Allergy **19**, 65—85 (1961).

Danelatos, C.: Le pouvoir histaminopexique du sérum au cours de la maladie de Bouillaud. Mémoire pour le titre d'assistant étranger, Fac. Méd. Paris (1955).

Flavian, N.: Fixation des diverses amines biologiques par le sérum humain. Thée Sci. Paris (1963).

—, B. Vasseur et J.-L. Parrot: Histaminopexie plasmatique. Démonstration par la technique biologique à l'aide d'un appareil automatique. J. Physiol. (Paris) **53**, 499—500 (1961).

Huriez, C., F. Desmons et J. C. Cartier: Le pouvoir histaminopexique en dermatologie. Bull. Soc. Fr. Dermatol. Syphilig., **67**, 510—525 (1960).

Jeune, M., R. Carron, J. Pellerat et M. Murat: Le pouvoir histaminopexique du sérum. Son intérêt en pédiatrie. Sem. Hôp. Paris **35**, 2867—2871 (1959).

Klamerth, O.: Zur Frage der Histaminbindung an Plasmaproteine. Biochem. Z. **327**, 62—71 (1955).

Kerp, L., and H. Sund: The binding of histamine in the serum of normal and allergic persons. Excerpta med., p. C 81. (3ème Cong. int. Allergol., Paris) (1958).

Laborde, C., J.-L. Parrot et G. Sandor: Le pouvoir histaminopexique du sérum sanguin chez l'Homme. Etude de ses facteurs protéidiques. C. R. Acad. Sci. (Paris) **248**, 3060—3071 (1959).

— — et D. A. Urquia: Le pouvoir histaminopexique du sérum sanguin chez l'Homme. Technique de mesure. Presse méd. **61**, 1151—1152 (1953).

LEVRAT, M., R. BRETTE, J. PELLERAT, H. RIVES et M. MURAT: Le pouvoir histaminopexique du sérum et du liquide gastrique dans les affections gastro-intestinales. Sem. Hôp. Paris **35**, 31—35 (1959).
MIKOL, C., et M. RENOUX: Réaction personnelle de séro-agglutination à l'histamine sur latex. Rev. franc. Allerg. **2**, 133—139 (1962).
— et F. P. MERKLEN: Séro-agglutination à l'histamine sur latex et allergie. Bull. Soc. méd. Hôp. (Paris) **77**, 441—446 (1961).
PARROT, J.-L.: Nouvelles recherches sur la pénétration de l'histamine par voie intestinale. Rôle protecteur du suc intestinal et de la mucine gastrique. C. R. Soc. Biol. (Paris) **143**, 1553 (1949).
—, et N. FLAVIAN: Captation de la 5-hydroxytryptamine par le sérum humain normal. Absence de cette captation chez les sujets allergiques. C. R. Acad. Sci. (Paris) **240**, 463—465 (1959).
— — P. BONET-MAURY and M. PROVOST: Binding of C^{14} labeled histamine by normal human serum. Proc. Soc. exp. Biol. (N. Y.) **109**, 459—460 (1962).
— — et J. THOUVENOT: Pouvoir histaminopexique du sérum. Etude colorimétrique. C. R. Acad. Sci. (Paris) **49**, 329—332 (1957).
— P. GALMICHE et A. SAINDELLE: Le pouvoir histaminopexique du sérum et des épanchements articulaires chez les rhumatisants (premiers résultats). Rev. Rhum. **28**, 637—642 (1961).
—, et C. LABORDE: Captation de l'histamine par l'héparine. C. R. Soc. Biol. (Paris) **145**, 1047 (1951).
— — Le pouvoir histaminopexique du sérum chez le Rat normal et surrénalectomisé. C. R. Soc. Biol. (Paris) **146**, 1049—1051 (1952a).
— — Action du cortex surrénal sur le pouvoir histaminopexique du sérum. C. R. Soc. Biol. (Paris) **146**, 1662—1665 (1952b).
— — Le pouvoir histaminopexique du sérum. Recherches sur sa régulation. J. Physiol. (Paris) **45**, 211—214 (1953).
— — Augmentation de l'action biologique de l'histamine *in vitro* sous l'influence de certains sérums sanguins. J. Physiol. (Paris) **46**, 492—495 (1954).
— — Le pouvoir histaminopexique du sérum sanguin. Sa disparition chez le Cobaye sensibilisé à l'ovalbumine. J. Physiol. (Paris) **48**, 677—679 (1956).
— — Restitution de l'histaminopexie sérique par divers agents anti-inflammatoires chez le Rat surrénalectomisé. J. Physiol. (Paris) **52**, 183 (1960).
— — L'histaminopexie plasmatique en allergie. Méd. et Hyg. (Genève) **19**, 27—29 (1961a).
— — A routine test of the allergic background. Colorimetric estimation of histamine-binding action of serum. Excerpta med. (Amst.) **42**, p. 7 (1961b).
— — et M. DAMBRINE: Recherches sur le pouvoir histaminopexique du sérum sanguin. Etude de l'inhibiteur sérique. C. R. Soc. Biol. (Paris) **149**, 2094 (1955).
— — C. DEBRAY et J. GASTARD: L'histaminopexie plasmatique au cours de la rectocolite hémorragique et ulcéreuse. Presse méd. **68**, 1820—1822 (1960).
— — — et H. ROURE: Le pouvoir histaminopexique du sérum sanguin et du suc gastrique dans les ulcères gastro-duodénaux. Arch. Mal. Appar. dig. **45**, 612—620 (1956).
— — et B. LEBEL: Le séro-agglutination du complexe histamine-polystyrène, nouvelle méthode pour évaluer l'histaminopexie sérique. Rev. franç. Allerg. **3**, 1—6 (1963).
— — G. NICOT et N. FLAVIAN: Mesure de l'histaminopexie sérique. Equilibre de dialyse et dosage colorimétrique de l'histamine. Pharm. biol. **3**, 177—180 (1961).
—, et M. MORDELET-DAMBRINE: Recherches sur le pouvoir histaminopexique du plasma sanguin. Influence de l'ion K. C. R. Soc. Biol. (Paris) **153**, 750 (1959).
— — Rôle du Ca dans le mécanisme de l'histaminopexie sérique. J. Physiol. (Paris) **52**, 184—185 (1960).
— — Etude de l'histaminopexie par l'ultrafiltration. Arch. int. Pharmacodyn. **130**, 425—435 (1961a).
— — Action *in vitro* des ions potassium et calcium sur l'histaminopexie sérique. J. Physiol. (Paris) **53**, 439 (1961b).
— — et C. LABORDE: Disparition de l'histaminopexie plasmatique au cours de l'insuffisance hépatique. Presse méd. **67**, 451—452 (1959).
— — et G. TRINQUET: Le terrain allergique et l'absence d'histaminopexie sérique. Action du potassium et du calcium. Bull. Acad. Méd. (Paris) **146**, 335—340 (1962).
— P. MOZZICONACCI, C. DANELATOS et C. LABORDE: Le pouvoir histaminopexique du sérum au cours du rhumatisme articulaire aigu. Sem. Hôp. Paris **33**, 2157—2159 (1957).
—, et A. SAINDELLE: Restitution du pouvoir histaminopexique par la colchicine chez le Rat surrénalectomisé. C. R. Soc. Biol. (Paris) **155**, 2075—2077 (1961).
— H. TUCHMANN-DUPLESSIS et C. LABORDE: Modifications du pouvoir histaminopexique du sérum sanguin chez le Rat sous l'influence des hormones sexuelles. J. Physiol. (Paris) **49**, 333—335 (1957).

PARROT, J.-L., D. A. URQUIA et C. LABORDE: Captation de l'histamine par le sérum humain normal. Défaut de captation par le sérum d'asthmatique. C. R. Soc. Biol. (Paris) **145**, 1045 (1951).

— — — Action histaminopexique du sérum humain et son pouvoir protecteur à l'égard de l'histamine. Modifications par la dialyse ou par l'addition d'histamine. C. R. Soc. Biol. (Paris) **146**, 1052 (1952).

PAUTRIZEL, R., A. RIVASSEAU, J. BEZIAN et F. SZERSNOVICZ: Que faut-il attendre de la mesure du pouvoir histaminopexique du sérum? Ann. Biol. clin. **18**, 661—668 (1960).

PELLERAT, J., M. MURAT et H. RIVES: Pouvoir histaminopexique du sérum et dermatoses allergiques. Bull. Soc. Fr. Dermat. Syph. **64**, 450—451 (1957).

RAHMAN, S., et P. MOZZICONACCI: Le pouvoir histaminopexique du sérum chez les enfants atteints de rhumatisme articulaire aign. Ann. Pédiat. **39**, 467—474 (1963).

ROSENTHAL, S. M., and H. TABOR: An improved colorimetric method for the estimation of histamine. J. Pharmacol. exp. Ther. **92**, 425—431 (1948).

SAINDELLE, A., et J.-L. PARROT: Restitution du pouvoir histaminopexique par la phénylbutazone chez le Rat surrénalectomisé. C. R. Soc. Biol. (Paris) **155**, 2118—2119 (1961).

SIDI, E., A. REINBERG, M. HINCKY et J. BOURGEOIS-SPINASSE: Les variations du pouvoir histaminopexique du sérum sanguin au cours de l'évolution des eczémas de l'adulte. Presse méd. **66**, 343—345 (1958).

SUND, H., and L. KERP: The chemistry of histamine binding in the serum. 3ème Cong. int. Allergol., Paris. Excerpta med. (Amst.) p C 81 (1958).

TAPPEINER, J., H. TIRSCHEK u. P. WODNIANSKY: Bestimmung der Histaminopexie zur Feststellung des allergischen Terrains. Arch. klin. exp. Derm. **207**, 261—267 (1958).

TUCHMANN-DUPLESSIS, H., J.-L. PARROT et C. LABORDE: Action de l'hypophyse sur le pouvoir histaminopexique du sérum sanguin chez le Rat. J. Physiol. (Paris) **46**, 841—844 (1954).

VIALATTE, J., J. REY, D. BRUNET et A. LEBEL: Le pouvoir histaminopexique du sérum chez le nourrisson. Rev. franç. Allerg. **2**, 50—51 (1962).

VIGNES, P.: Le pouvoir histaminopexique au cours de la gravido-puerpéralité. Gynéc. et Obstét. **61**, 543—555 (1962).

WALLENFELS, K., L. KERP u. H. SUND: Über die Histaminbindung in Serum von Normalen und Allergikern. Klin. Wschr. **36**, 772—773 (1958).

WODNIANSKY, P.: Statistically significant results on the different histaminopexic power in serum of normals and allergics. Excerpta med. (Amst.) **42**, p. 8 (1961).

— Zur Fehlerbreite und Interpretation der Histaminopexiebestimmung. Auswertung einer Untersuchungsreihe von 650 Personen. Klin. Wschr. **40**, 975—979 (1962).

Section C

Toxicity of Histamine: Lethal Doses

By

PLUTARCO NARANJO

With 10 Figures

I. Toxic and lethal effects

For a substance, such as histamine, whose normal physiological role has not been completely established (FELDBERG, 1954; GADDUM, 1948; JANCSO, 1947; KAHLSON, 1960; PARROT and REUSE, 1954; ROCHA E SILVA, 1955; SCHAYER, 1961), it is difficult to delimit when the effects should be considered toxic. On the other hand, there is no problem in qualifying as toxic the effects when represented by histological alterations or irreversible biochemical reactions, which ultimately produce death.

The effects to be described herein will refer to severe intoxication unless otherwise stated.

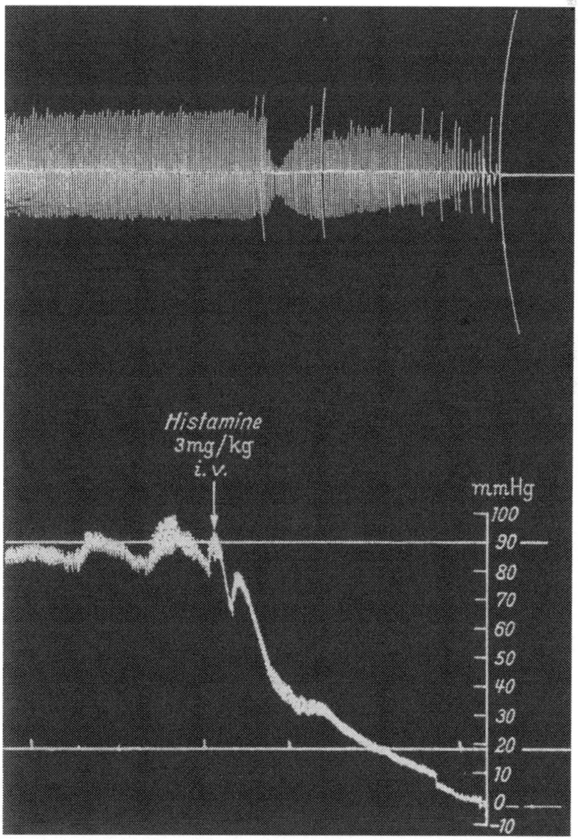

Fig. 1. *Histamine shock in the cat.* Cat, 2.8 kg, anesthetized with a mixture of urethan (700 mg/kg) and sodium pentobarbital (20 mg/kg) intraperitoneally, and prepared for recording of respiration (upper tracing) and measurement of carotid blood pressure (lower tracing). Time in one minute intervals (bottom line). At the arrow, histamine dihydrochloride, 3 mg/kg, was rapidly injected by a jugular vein. Observe the inmediate and precipitous fall of blood pressure until the animal died (original tracing)

A. Cat and dog

The toxic symptoms in these two species are very similar. In unanesthetized animals, after receiving histamine intravenously, the following symptoms can be observed: intense salivation, vomit, diarrhea, dyspnea of a variable degree and finally the animal's collapse.

Since the early works of BARGER and DALE (1910a), DALE and LAIDLAW (1911, 1919), it is well known that in the cat and the dog the circulatory changes are dominant during the histamine shock. The arterial blood pressure falls precipitously and proportionally to the dose. With sublethal and lethal doses blood pressure falls inmediately to a level equivalent to 1/3 or less of the original value. Afterwards, in the first case, it recovers slowly, in minutes or hours, depending of the dose, and in the second case, the blood pressure continues to fall gradually until the animal's death (fig. 1).

The details and sequency of the changes that characterize the experimental histamine shock have been discussed by Dale and Laidlaw (1919), and reviewed by Best and MacHenry (1931). The fall of the systemic blood pressure is due to the great dilatation of the capillaries caused by the direct action of histamine on the contractile mechanism of these vessels (Feldberg and Miles, 1953; Stead and Warren, 1944). The increased capillary permeability allows plasma to escape from the circulation and results in a marked increase in hematocrit and in a diminished circulating blood volume.

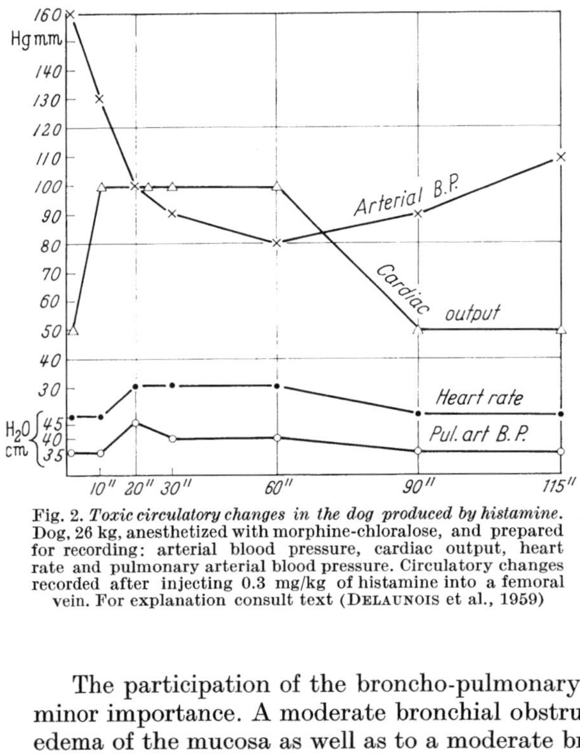

Fig. 2. *Toxic circulatory changes in the dog produced by histamine.* Dog, 26 kg, anesthetized with morphine-chloralose, and prepared for recording: arterial blood pressure, cardiac output, heart rate and pulmonary arterial blood pressure. Circulatory changes recorded after injecting 0.3 mg/kg of histamine into a femoral vein. For explanation consult text (Delaunois et al., 1959)

In dogs, with sublethal doses, as has been demonstrated by Delaunois et al. (1959), the fall of the blood pressure is accompanied by a moderate increase in the pulmonar arterial pressure, the cardiac frequency and the cardiac output (fig. 2), which indicates that the rapid fall of the blood pressure is not primarily due to cardiac failure but rather to the peripheral vasodilatation.

The participation of the broncho-pulmonary tree in the histamine shock is of minor importance. A moderate bronchial obstruction is observed which is due to edema of the mucosa as well as to a moderate broncho-constriction. But the alterations responsible for death are of circulatory nature.

During the histamine intoxication there is also: contraction of the smooth muscles of the hollow viscera, an increase in the intestinal peristalsis and even spasmodic contractions; intense contractions of the uterus and also contraction of the iris.

In these as well as in the other animal species, histamine produces gastric hypersecretion (Wells et al, 1941). Gastric and duodenal ulcers (Hay et al, 1942; Walpole et al, 1940) may appear.

B. Guinea pig

The guinea pig has been the preferred animal for experiments with antihistamine drugs, mainly due to the extreme sensitivity of this animal to histamine.

When a guinea pig is injected, intravenously, with a lethal dose of histamine, before the first minute is completed, the animal becomes dyspneic, jumps a few times and then falls down. When the drug is administered as an aerosol the first symptoms observed appear between 30 and 40 seconds after the animal started to inhale the aerosol. At the beginning the animal becomes restless, then it shows signs of dyspnea at the same time that it begins to masticate. After this the

a

b

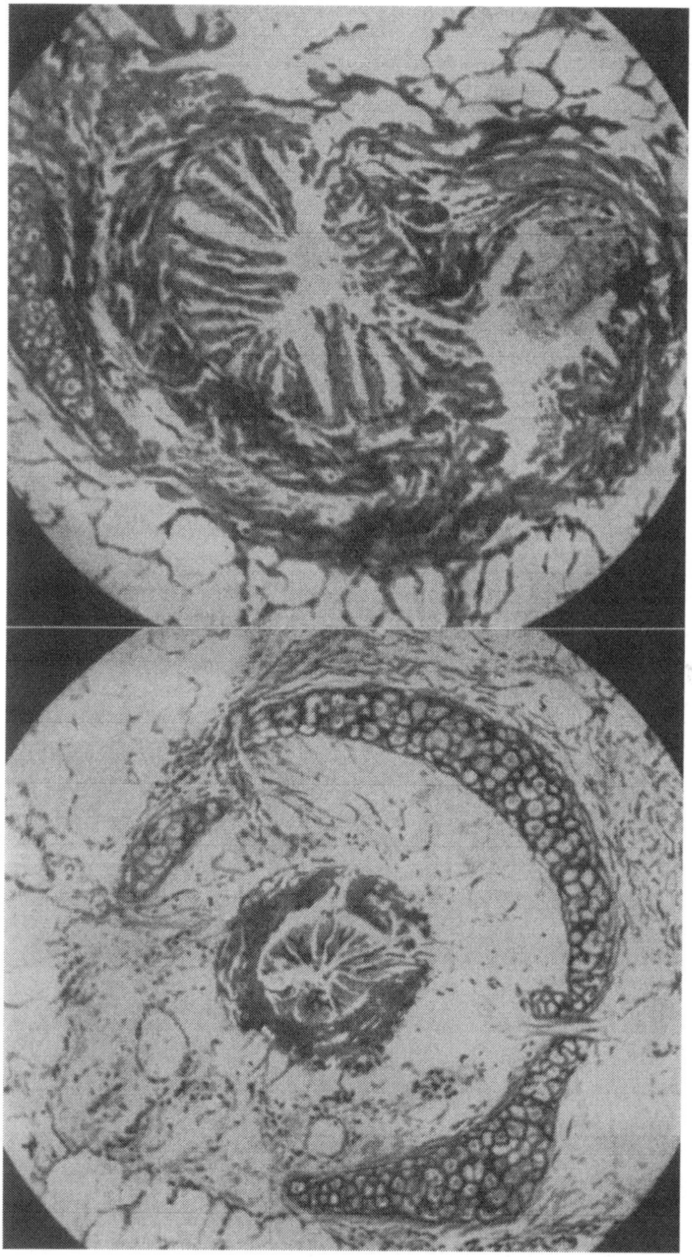

Fig. 3 a and b. ***Bronchial changes produced by histamine and anaphylactic shock in guinea pigs.*** a, a bronchus of a guinea pig that died during histamine shock. Bronchospasm, absence of edema. b, a bronchus of a guinea pig that died during anaphylactic shock. Bronchospasm, but specially marked edema of the connective layer, accompanied by eosinophilic infiltration. (HALPERN, 1949)

animal sits on its hinds and with the forlegs scratches its nose. These symptoms are accompanied by sneezing. As the dyspnea becomes more intense the animal gives small jumps, gets excited and finally falls into a clonic convulsive phase.

From this moment on the pathological changes are similar to those observed when the histamine is given intravenously. Cyanosis becomes very severe. The animal makes deep respiratory movements, even opens its mouth. If the circulation of air through the trachea is still being graphically recorded it is observed that these respiratory movements are totally inefficient since the air cannot be mobilized through the trachea because of the bronchospasm. The abdominal wall becomes very tense, and there is spasm of the diaphragm (NARANJO, 1951), and regurgitation may even take place. The last convulsive movements are of tonic character, the animal urinates, its sphincters and muscles are relaxed and then the guinea pig dies of asphyxia.

The most outstanding feature is the intense broncho-constriction that is produced (fig. 3). In fact the bronchioles start to contract along the time when the animal is making the last 10 to 20 respiratory movements which are predominantely of inhalatory nature. This means that the animal is able to introduce some air into its lungs in spite of the bronchiolar constriction. Since expiration is almost a passive phenomenon with less participation of the respiratory muscles, most of the inhaled air is retained in the lungs, until the fine bronchial ducts are closed and the animal dies of asphyxia. The lungs remain in a high degree of emphysema. In the histopathologic preparations it is observed that the bronchioles are reduced in calibre and completely obstructed by the folds formed by the mucous membrane.

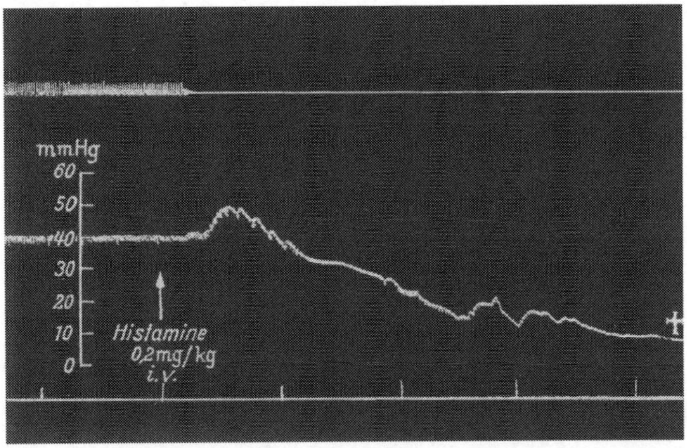

Fig. 4. ***Histamine shock in the guinea pig.*** Guinea pig, 320 gm, anesthetized with ether, and prepared for recording respiration (upper tracing) and measurement of carotid blood pressure (lower tracing). Time in one-minute intervals (bottom line). At the arrow, histamine diphosphate, 0.2 mg/animal, was rapidly injected by a jugular vein. Observe the immediate annulment of the respiratory tracing despite the animal's efforts to continue making deep respiratory movements which are an indication that the bronchi were strongly constricted. Blood pressure reaches a value of zero 4 min later. (Original tracing)

In the larger bronchi a slight edema may be seen between the muscular and cartilaginous layers, but in general, in the histaminic asthma the bronchospasm predominates and is the fundamental cause of death, whereas in the anaphylactic shock, in the same species of animal, even though bronchospasm is also produced, edema and eosinophilic infiltration, which are very intense, contribute greatly to the obstruction of the bronchi (fig. 3), (HALPERN, 1942 and 1949).

Emphysema of the lungs is of the maximal possible intensity, there is no other pathological or toxic condition that produces such strong emphysema. The normal lung sinks in water if a weight equal to its own is added, but when there is emphysema the weight that must be added to sink the lung is greater and in the case of histamine shock, it may require twice its weight (NARANJO and NARANJO, 1961).

Contrary to what happens in the dog and in the cat, in the guinea pig, circulatory changes are less important than the respiratory ones and they are partially dependent on the latter. A few seconds after intravenous injection of histamine the systemic blood pressure rises 50 to 80 per cent above the normal level; asphyxia and an increase in CO_2 concentration in the blood being only in part responsible for this phenomenon. Following this rise, the blood pressure falls progressive- and irreversibly (fig. 4). The heart continues to beat with the sinusal rythm even one or two minutes after the pressure has fallen to zero. Peripheral vasodilatation and congestion of the abdominal viscera are observed, and the intestines contract violently. In pregnant females, sublethal doses will produce abortion.

An increase in the gastric secretion which is rich in hydrochloric acid is observed after the injection of histamine. When histamine is administered intravenously or as an aerosol the shock and its lethal effects are so fast that there is no time for the ulceration of the stomach or duodenum. But when lethal or sublethal doses are administered subcutaneously, gastric ulcers are frequently produced which at last may perforate the wall (CRANE et al., 1947; HAY et al., 1942).

Gastric ulceration is more evident when doses 10, 50 or more times the LD_{50} are administered to guinea pigs that have previously been protected with an antihistamine drug, since this class of drugs protect guinea pigs against the bronchospasm and other effects of histamine, but does not prevent the histaminic gastric hypersecretion (GRAHAM, 1947; HALPERN and HAMBURGER, 1948; LEHMANN and YOUNG, 1945).

It has been stated that histamine administered by oral route is not toxic, but according to GABE (1952) when histamine is given by means of a stomach tube, the toxic effets produced are very similar to those described when the drug is administered parenterally. Of course, the symptoms appear somewhat later, between 45 and 60 minutes after the administration. By this route a dose hundreds of times greater is required to produce similar systemic effects as by intravenous injection, the reason for this is the high histaminase content of the gastric and intestinal mucosae (BEST and MACHENRY, 1930) (See Chapter 2, Section A).

Both in animals that die (some 3 hours after the administration) as well as particularly in those that survive and are later sacrificed for histopathological examination, the following alterations are found (GABE, 1952): a marked congestion of the stomach, duodenum and the proximal part of the ileum; an intense leucocitary infiltration, hypersecretion of the gastric and pancreatic exocrine glands likewise alterations of the gastric mucosa, which permit a study of the ulceration process, from the early exfoliation of the epithelium to the perforation of the gastric wall.

C. Rabbit

When a lethal dose of histamine is administered intravenously, the animal loses its equilibrium within a minute, falls on its side and begins to make movements with the extremities as if it were running. Soon after this a state of opisthotonos, apnea and intense contraction of the abdominal wall (specially with doses 2 times or more the LD_{50}) is produced. This phase lasts from 30 to 60 seconds, when the animal begins to make deep respiratory movements, finally dying within $2^1/_2$ and 3 minutes after the injection. At the beginning there is a contraction of the pupil which dilates toward the end. There is also fasciculation of some muscles and during the last moments the animal may defecate and urinate.

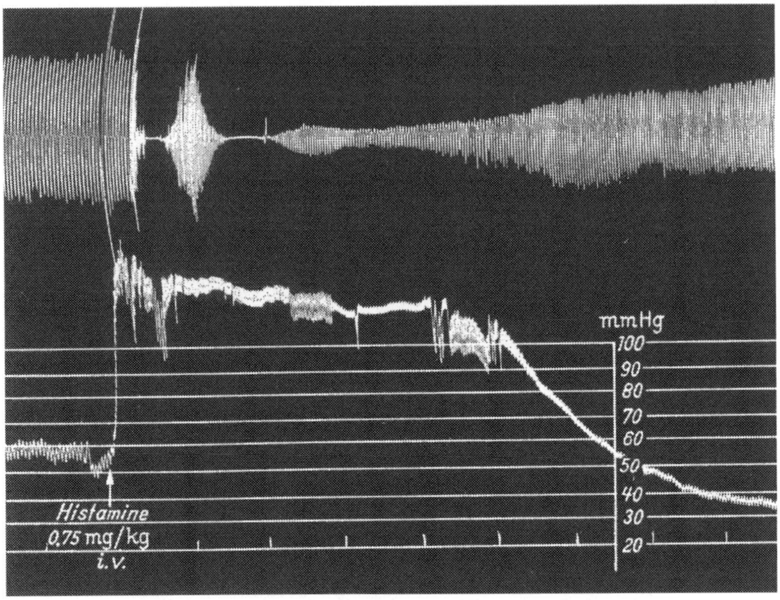

a

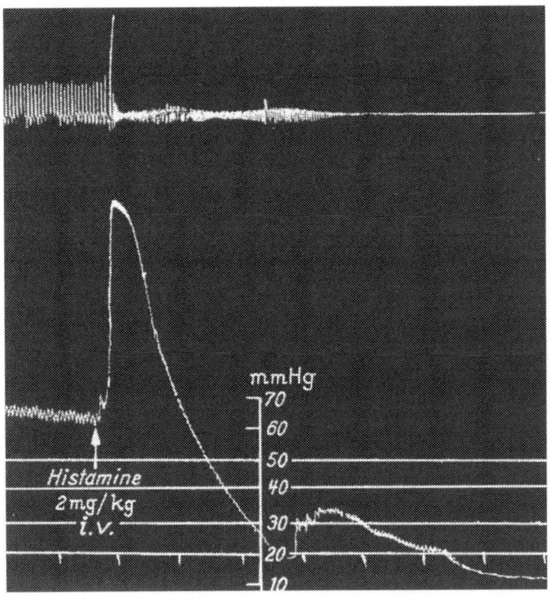

b

Fig. 5a and b. *Histamine shock in rabbits.* a, Rabbit, 1.5 kg, anesthetized with ether and prepared for recording respiration (upper tracing) and measurement of carotid blood pressure (lower tracing). Time in one-minute intervals (bottom line). At the arrow, histamine dihydrochloride in a sublethal dose (0.75 mg/kg), was rapidly injected by a jugular vein. Observe the sharp rise in blood pressure, two short periods of apnea followed by some bronchial obstruction. The irregularities in the blood pressure record during the hypertensive phase, correspond to extra-systoles. b, Rabbit, 1.3 kg, anesthetized with ether and prepared as above. At the arrow histamine in a lethal dose (2 mg/kg) was rapidly injected. Observe the sharp but transient rise of blood pressure which is followed by its fall to zero (original tracings)

One of the most outstanding changes is the marked constriction of the pulmonar artery and its ramifications, (Best and MacHenry, 1931; Woodbury and Hamilton, 1941) together with the constriction of the coronary vessels (Eichler and Mügge, 1931) which leads to the failure of the right ventricle. The vasoconstriction is not limited to the pulmonary artery but is largely a generalized phenomenon (Feldberg, 1927; Naranjo and Naranjo, 1958; Trendelenburg, 1961) which brings as a result an increase in the systemic blood pressure equivalent to 100 % or more of the normal value (fig. 5). The hypertensive phase lasts between one and two minutes, after which the pressure falls progressively to zero. The vasoconstriction is then replaced by a generalized dilatation of the vessels.

The respiratory alterations are less important and are similar to those observed in the dog and in the cat, a moderate obstruction of the bronchi of transitory nature is observed which generally does not produce emphysema, which if it appears is an exception and does so only in certain areas of the lung.

The changes in the abdominal viscera of smooth muscles are similar to those already described for other species.

D. Rat and mouse

These two species possess a natural tolerance to histamine (Rocha e Silva, 1955). Very high doses of histamine are required to produce toxic effects or death; and the toxic effects are very similar in the two species. When a lethal dose is given intravenously, death is produced within 3 minutes. With sublethal doses there is a short period of excitation after which there is an inhibition of the normal movements, bradypnea, bristling of the hair, micturition, defecation and diarrhea. When histamine is injected subcutaneously or intraperitoneally the symptoms are only of depressive nature. There is a slowing down of the movements, specially in rats, bristling of the hair and bradypnea with strong abdominal respiration. As the intoxication sets on, the equilibrium and the strength in the hind legs is impaired and the mice adopt an amphibian position, and finally the animals fall into collapse. Death is produced between 40 and 60 minutes after the injection. With sublethal doses, animals recover some 4 to 8 hours later.

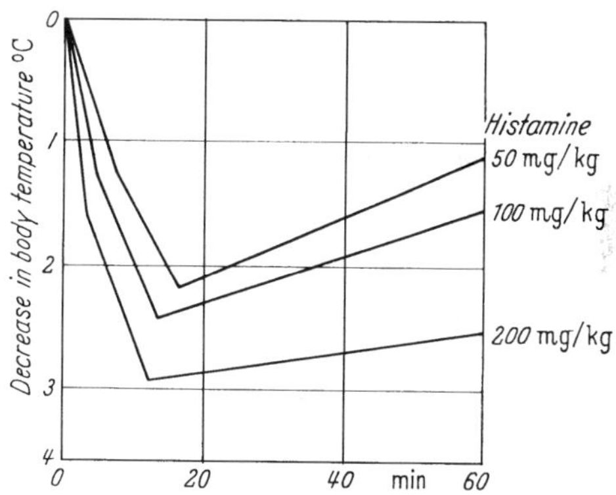

Fig. 6. *Effect of histamine on body temperature of mice.* Adult albino mice: rectal temperature was recorded after histamine diphosphate was injected subcutaneously. Each line is based on averages of 10 mice. Upper line, after Ambrus et al. 1952. Other lines, from unpublished data

A characteristic symptom in mice and rats is the fall in body temperature (fig. 6), being this an indication of the stage and degree of intoxication (Ambrus et al., 1952; Halpern and Briot, 1950; Halpern and Chmel, 1949). With sublethal doses the rectal temperature drops proportionally with the dose, 1 to 3° C, reaching the lowest level some 20 to 40 minutes after the injection. It rises again to the normal level, 1 to 3 hours later. When a lethal dose is administered, the temperature continues to fall gradually until the animal dies.

In spite of the metabolic alterations that are produced in the histamine intoxicated rat (Cordier and Cordier, 1955; Cordier and Peres, 1957) the sensitivity of the small intestine to epinephrine and acetylcholine or the mutual antagonism of these two drugs is not modified (CORDIER and DUVEAU, 1956).

E. Chicks

In experiments on chronic intoxication, when histamine is added to the food, the normal growth of chicks is impaired (SHIFRINE et al., 1959). The growth inhibition increases as the concentration of the histamine is increased (fig. 7). With concentrations below 0.2 %, no significant pathological changes are observed except a decrease of the growth rate and the total growth of chicks. When the concentration is above 0.5 % the animals show a slowing down of their normal activities, diarrhea, and loss of weight for a few days, after which the animals appear to adapt themselves to this kind of a diet. The general appearance of the animals improves, their appetite increases and they resume growth at approximately the same rate as the control chicks but with marked lag in the total growth.

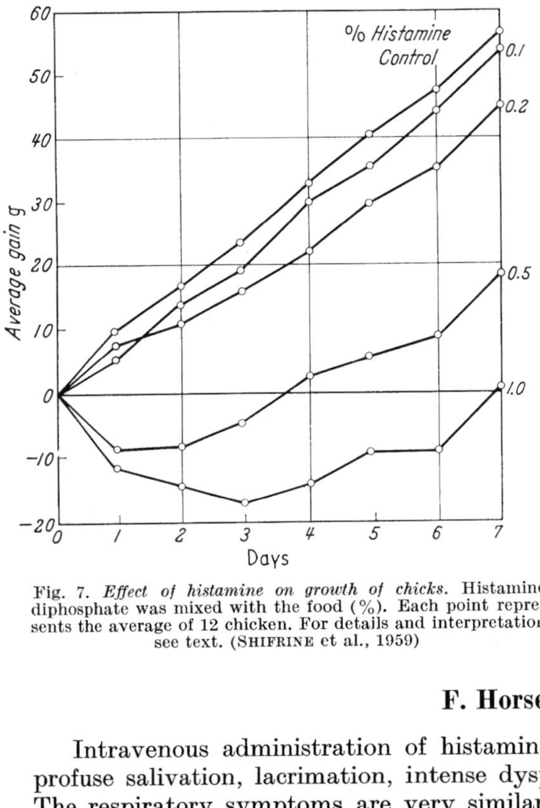

Fig. 7. *Effect of histamine on growth of chicks.* Histamine diphosphate was mixed with the food (%). Each point represents the average of 12 chicken. For details and interpretation see text. (SHIFRINE et al., 1959)

Poisoning of chick fed with spoiled foods, mainly spoiled fishes, would be explained by the formation of histamine due to microbial activity (GEIGER, 1955; KIMATA and KAWAI, 1953; SHIFRINE et al., 1959).

F. Horse

Intravenous administration of histamine to horses (JONES, 1957) produces profuse salivation, lacrimation, intense dyspnea, abdominal colic and diarrhea. The respiratory symptoms are very similar to those of an acute anaphylactic shock and, with the exception of coughing, to those characterizing acute alveolar emphysema.

G. Cow and sheep

Besides respiratory and circulatory changes, toxic doses of histamine may paralyze the rumen and inhibit eructation of gas (JONES, 1957). With doses of 2 to 5 mg/animal, injected intravenously in the cow (DOUGHERTY, 1942) an immediate though temporary ruminal paralysis is produced, which is followed by a longer period of depression. Subcutaneous injections of histamine are ineffective. Similar effects are produced in the sheep (CLARK, 1950), where the duration of ruminal atony has been shown to be proportional to the doses of histamine. The action of histamine, in both species, is exerted directly on the muscles of the rumen and reticulum. In spite of the paralysis of the rumen musculature, histamine causes hypermotility of the intestines, including the rectum.

H. Man

The fast intravenous injection of a small dose of histamine (0.25 to 0.5 mg of histamine diphosphate) produces in normal adults a violent pulsating headache with a sensation of craneal compression (HORTON, 1956; ROBINSON, 1958). The headache disappears within 5 to 10 minutes. During the first 5 minutes the face becomes flushed but later turns to paleness. Blood pressure changes little and transiently; in some patients, the systolic pressure rises some 10 mm and later falls some 10 to 15 mm below normal; in others there is only a fall of the systolic at the time that diastolic pressure tends to rise 10 to 15 mm. Simultaneously the cerebrospinal fluid pressure rises (PICKERING, 1933). Frequency of the pulse increases by 10 to 20 per minute. Almost all patients have anguish sensations, and some have nausea and even vomit and present diarrhea, along with sweating.

With higher doses, administered subcutaneously or intramuscularly (JONES, 1957; GOODMAN and GILMAN, 1955) there is a general vasodilation, with an increase of the cutaneous temperature, a precipitous fall in blood pressure, intense headache, visual disturbances, bronchospasm and dyspnea, a metallic taste, vomit and diarrhea.

An increase in the salivary, gastric and pancreatic secretions is also produced. In severe cases shock may occur.

II. Biochemical disturbances

A. Changes in proteinemia

It has been known for long time (DALE and LAIDLAW, 1919) that traumatic shock as well as histamine shock produces hypoproteinemia. This is due, in part, to the escape of plasma from the circulation as a result of the increased capillary permeability; but CORDIER and PERES (1957), after a critical examination of the problem have carried out in rats experiments which established an additional mechanism of said hypoproteinemia. Tables 1 and 2 show the most important results obtained by these authors.

Table 1. *Changes in proteinemia produced by toxic doses of histamine.* (CORDIER and PÉRÈS, 1957)

Doses of histamine mg/kg	Amino-nitrogen	Total proteins	Seroalbumins	Globulins	Ratio Alb./Glob.
	Concentration per 100 ml of serum[1]				
0	6.95	6.50	3.28	3.22	1.02
1.000	7.50	6.20	3.24	2.96	1.09
2.000	11.50	5.90	3.27	2.63	1.24
3.000	14.90	5.25	3.23	2.02	1.60
5.000	19.12	5.31	3.26	2.05	1.58

[1] Averages of 10 animals.

Table 2. *Changes in proteinemia during histamine intoxication.* (CORDIER and PÉRÈS, 1957)

Time elapsed after injection	Amino-nitrogen	Total proteins	Seroalbumins	Globulins	Ratio Alb./Glob.
	Concentration per 100 ml of serum[1]				
0	6.95	6.50	3.28	3.22	1.02
1 hour	8.70	6.30	3.27	3.03	1.08
3 hour	13.20	5.60	3.31	2.29	1.45
6 hour	19.12	5.31	3.26	2.05	1.58

[1] Averages of 10 animals.

One of the outstanding facts, during histamine shock is the increase in the aminoacid nitrogen, in amounts well above those corresponding to the amino-nitrogen of the histamine injected. There is a noticeable alteration in the albumin/globulin ratio, which is characterized by a decrease in the globulin fraction whereas the albumin fraction remains constant. The fall in globulin concentration is proportional to the histamine injected. It can be deduced that the increase in the plasma aminoacids and the hypoproteinemia takes place at the expense of the globulin fraction. It is to be noted that as the time progresses this change becomes more severe, until 6 hours after the injection. This protein disturbance would be explained as due to the anoxia. The catabolism of tissue proteins is increased whereas the synthesis is impaired. Aminoacids tend to accumulate in the blood as the liver becomes unable to perform deamination at a normal rate.

B. Disturbances in the glycogen phosphorolysis

Cordier and Cordier (1955), have found that when rats receive toxic doses of histamine (500 mg/kg subcutaneously every 20 minutes until a total dose of 5,000 mg/kg) the phosphorolysis of glycogen, *in vitro,* diminishes between 20 to 25 % both in liver and in muscle.

These authors esuggest that this biochemical change is due to intracellular disorders especially to those of enzymatic nature, brought about by the anoxia produced by histamine. In fact, histamine intoxication is characterized by a very complex anoxia:

a), anoxia by circulatory stasis due to hypotension, dilatation of the capillary system, alteration of the vascular endothelia and a progressive cardiac insuficiency;

b), anoxic anoxia, due to alterations in the alveolar capillaries and a constriction of the pulmonary veins followed by a decrease in hematosis, and

c), an anemic anoxia due to the loss of affinity of hemoglobin for oxygen.

A decrease in the rate of glycogen phosphorolysis similar to that observed during histamine intoxication, has been also described in cases of anoxia and asphyxia produced by other causes.

C. Changes in the blood sugar level and the epinephrine content of the adrenal glands

Satow (1938), re-examined the problem presented by toxic doses of histamine in changing the blood sugar level in man as well as in several laboratory species. Results of different authors appeared contradictory, but those obtained by Satow (1938) after a critical revision, seem to explain the existing contradictions. Satow found that after injecting, intravenously, into rabbits a dose of histamine of 0.4 to 0.5 mg/kg, in a very fast manner (5 to 20 seconds) a marked increase in the sugar level is observed which is followed by a fall beyond the normal level. If the same dose is administered slowly over a period of 1 to $1^1/_2$ minutes or subcutaneously, the only effect observed is hypoglycemia. These results have been confirmed later by Takita (1950) it being concluded that the glycemic changes do not depend only on the dose of histamine but also on the mode of administration and the rate at which it is given. Besides these facts, marked variations can be observed depending on the time elapsed between the administration of histamine and the time the blood is drawn for assay and whether or not the animal was anesthetized (Papacostas, et al., 1956).

La Barre (1927) and Ni (1926) found that if rabbits and guinea pigs were previously adrenalectomized or their adrenals denervated, histaminic hyperglycemia could not be produced. These results seem to point out that the hyperglycemia is due to a sudden release of endogenous epinephrine. As early as 1912, ELLIOT, showed that histamine administration, in the cat, produces a depletion of epinephrine of the adrenal medulla. Since then this phenomenon has been confirmed by direct (MALMEJAC et al., 1951; WADA et al., 1940) as well as by indirect methods (DALE, 1920; KELLAWAY and COWELL, 1922a). MALMEJAC et al. have further demonstrated that the epinephrine release by toxic doses of histamine, is first due to a fall in the blood pressure which produces a reflex stimulation by the way of the pressoceptors, so that if the adrenals are denervated this phenomenon is not produced. Secondly, the epinephrine release is due to a direct chemical stimulation of the medulla by the drug.

SUZUKI (1951), in experiments similar to those of SATOW (1938), designed to observe whether the rate of injection of histamine may alter the rate of epinephrine depletion from the adrenal medulla, found that as long as the drug is administered subcutaneously, depletion is produced, but if histamine is injected intravenously whether fast or slowly, no depletion is observed. It is well to note that SUZUKI sacrificed the animals in order to extract epinephrine from the adrenals, 30 minutes after the injection and that, within this time, it was possible that some new epinephrine could have been synthesized in the medulla.

III. Lethal doses

A. Relation of dose and lethal effect

As observed with many toxic agents, where the per cent mortalities are transformed into probits, a linear relationship is obtained with the logarithm of the doses.

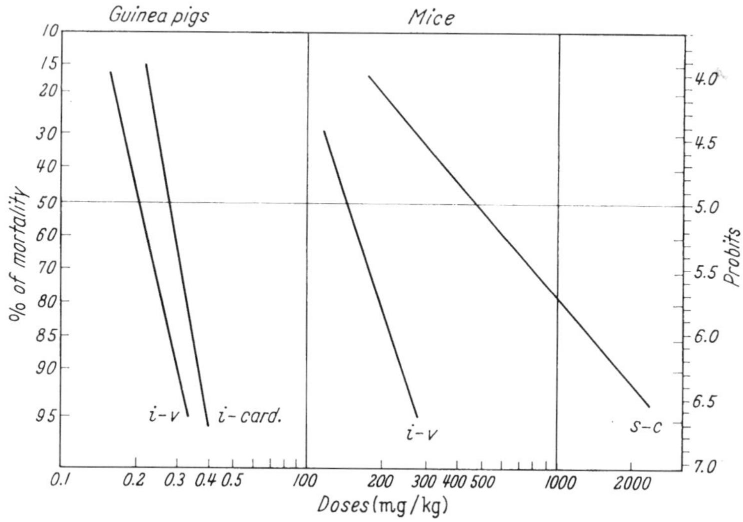

Fig. 8. *Relationship between histamine doses and per cent mortality.* Guinea pig: Regression line corresponding to intravenous administration, based on the data from NARANJO and NARANJO (1953b) and the one corresponding to intracardiac administrations, based on data from LEHMANN, (1948) Mice: Both regression lines based on data from AMBRUS et al. (1952). For details and interpretation consult text

When the drug is administered intravenously (fig. 8), the slope of the regression line is small for most species of animals. In fig. 8 it can be seen that the lines corresponding to guinea pigs and mice are practically parallel, also the line corresponding to the intracardiac administration of histamine to guinea pigs. In contrast when the drug is given subcutaneously, the slope of the regression is large, as can be seen in the same figure, where an experiment in mice has been used as an example. In these animals while the LD_{50}, subcutaneously, is only slightly above the value for the intravenous administration, the LD_{100} is 6 times greater than the value corresponding to the intravenous injection.

B. Lethal doses

Many authors have studied the lethal dose of histamine in different laboratory species, and it would be useless to list all the published data. In table 3 some of

Table 3. *Lethal doses of histamine in normal animals*

Species	Route of administ.	Type of lethal doses[1]	Dose mg/kg	Reference
Frog	s-c	LD	200—2300	FÜHNER (1932)
Mouse	s-c	LD_{100}	2300—2700	FÜHNER (1932)
		LD_{50}	230 P	AMBRUS et al. (1952)
	i-p	LD_{100}	2500	HALPERN and WOOD (1950)
		LD_{50}	2056 P	ANGELAKOS and LOEW (1957)
	i-v	LD_{100}	277 P	AMBRUS et al. (1952)
		LD_{50}	192 P	AMBRUS et al. (1952)
		LD_{50}	445 P	LISH et al. (1960)
Rat	s-c	MLD	1200	NOBLE and COLLIP (1941)
		LD_{100}	1300	HOUSSAY (1951)
		LD_{60}	1250	HOUSSAY (1951)
	i-p	MLD	1000	SCOTT (1927); WYMAN (1928)
		LD_{100}	1300	HOUSSAY (1951)
		LD_{50}	920	HOUSSAY (1951)
		LD_{50}	1781 P	ANGELAKOS and LOEW (1957)
	i-v	LD	500—700	CRIVELLARI (1926, 1927)
		LD_{100}	700	HOUSSAY (1951)
		LD_{50}	530	HOUSSAY (1951)
Guinea pig	s-c	LD	3,5—10	SCHMIDT und STÄHELIN (1929)
	i-p	LD	12—54	SCHMIDT und STÄHELIN (1929)
		LD_{50}	7	DOMENJOZ and JAQUES (1949)
	i-v	LD_{100}	0.6-b	HALPERN (1942)
		LD_{100}	1.10	ROTH and GOVIER (1958)
		LD_{100}	1.10 P	NARANJO and NARANJO (1953a)
		LD_{50}	0.60 P	NARANJO and NARANJO (1953b)
		LD_{50}	0.18 B	LANDS et al. (1949)
	i-card.	LD_{100}	0.4 B	LEHMANN (1948)
		LD_{50}	0.27 B	LEHMANN (1948)
	i-portal	LD_{50}	2.7 P	NARANJO and NARANJO (1953c)
	oral	MLD	100 B	DECOURT and PARROT (1947)
	i-gast.	LD_{100}	400 B	GABE (1952)
Rabbit	s-c	LD	12—15	SCHMIDT and STÄHELIN (1929)
	i-v	LD	0,6	OEHME (1913)
		MLD	1.2	OIKAWA (1931)
		LD	3.0	DECOURT and PARROT (1947)
		LD	3.5 C	REUSE (1948)
		LD_{100}	1.5 C	HALPERN (1947)
Dog	i-v	LD_{100}	10 C	HALPERN (1947)
Monkey	i-v	LD	50	FLURY (1925)
Cat	i-v	LD	10	DALE (1920)

Histamine as: B = free base; P = diphosphate; C = dihydrochloride.

[1] LD = Lethal dose (without additional specification); MLD = Minimal lethal dose; LD_{50}, LD_{60}, etc. = Lethal doses in 50%, 60%, etc. of animals.

the most representative data have been summarized: ANGELAKOS and LOEW (1957); AMBRUS, et al. (1952); CRIVELLARI (1927); DECOURT and PARROT (1947); DOMENJOZ and JAQUES (1949); GABE (1952); HALPERN (1947 a); HALPERN and WOOD (1950); HOUSSAY (1951); LANDS (1947, 1949); LEHMANN (1948); NARANJO and NARANJO (1953 a, b, c, d); NOBLE and COLLIP (1941); OIKAWA (1931); REUSE (1948); ROTH and GOVIER (1958). It can be observed in this table that certain discrepancies exist between the experimental values found by the different authors. In part, the discrepancy is due to the technique employed in the injection: speed of injection, concentration of drug, hour of the day, and the condition of the animal, whether it was fasted or not, etc.; and finally the difference may be only apparent, since the values, in some cases, correspond to histamine as the free base, whose molecular weight is 111.15, in others, to the dihydrochloride (m. w. = 184.08) or the diphosphate (m. w. = 307.15).

The relation between the LD_{50} or the LD_{100} and the route of the administration, as can be observed in table 3, varies according to the species. For instance, while in the mouse (AMBRUS et al., 1952) the LD_{50} when histamine is given subcutaneously, is only 1.2 times greater than when administered intravenously, in the rat it is approximately 2 times greater and in the guinea pig, 4 to 10 times. On the other hand, the difference between the oral (by means of a stomach tube, GABE, 1952) lethal dose and the intravenous is much greater than for most of the drugs. For example, the LD_{100} when histamine is given through a stomach tube in guinea pigs (GABE, 1952) is approximately 1,300 higher than the LD_{100} given intravenously, whereas if given intraportally or intrajugularly (NARANJO and NARANJO, 1953 b) the difference is only 4.5 times, which demonstrates that more than 99 % of the histamine taken up by the digestive system is destroyed in the gastrointestinal tract and of the part that is absorbed by the portal circulation, 80 % is further destroyed in the liver.

C. Lowering of the histamine toxicity: a) induced tolerance

AMBRUS et al. (1950, 1951 a, b) have demonstrated that daily administration of progressively higher doses of histamine for 3 or more weeks, develops a tolerance which permits the animal to receive lethal doses of the drug without suffering but slight toxic effects. In rats, these authors have been able to give 1,000 mg/kg subcutaneously, without even observing a drop in temperature which in these species is one of the signs of histamine intoxication. Guinea pigs in the same way are able to become resistant to histamine (ESSEX and HORTON, 1941), but in this species tolerance can be produced also by administering histamine through the respiratory system. AMBRUS et al., (1951 a) for instance, have subjected the animals to a histamine aerosol athmosphere, and after the appropriate treatment, the guinea pigs were able to inhale during 200 or more seconds the histamine aerosol without suffering shock, while normal animals that have not been previously exposed fall into mortal shock before 100 seconds of inhalation.

It is also possible to develop tolerance in an accelerated form if previously to the administration of lethal doses (one or more LD_{50}) of histamine an antihistamine is given (AMBRUS et al., 1951 a).

According to the results of AMBRUS et al., (1951 a), tolerance or histamine "resistance" is not due to an increased histaminase activity nor to any metabolic transformation of histamine into products with antihistamine activity but rather it is due to the fact that the tissues are able to accumulate the residual histamine in a bound nontoxic but protected form. Extracts of these tissues exhibit a higher histamine-like activity than extracts from tissues of nontolerant animals.

Although WELLS et al. (1941) have not been able to produce tolerance in dogs in reference to the gastric hypersecretion due to histamine, AMBRUS et al. (1951 b), using guinea pigs that were subjected to chronic treatment with increasing doses of histamine succeeded in producing this refractory stage in which a new dose of histamine did not elicit the gastric hypersecretory response and, in addition, in tolerant animals, development of gastric ulcers were not evident.

FABINYI and SZEBEHELYI (1949) and FEINBERG (1946) have extensively reviewed the problem of histamine tolerance both in laboratory animals as well as in humans.

b) Tachyphylaxis

By repeated doses of histamine, rabbits can be made insensitive. At the beginning this process is slow; but, finally, at a speedy supply of a dose of 5—10 mg of histamine, one succeeds easily to dispense the hundredfold of the lethal dose without harm. This procedure is accompanied by an acidosis and can be accelerated by adding acids (EICHLER and KILLIAN, 1931). The various organs loose their sensitiveness at different speed. First the coronary vessels are influenced, followed by the bronchial muscles then the branches of the pulmonary artery with the consequent decrease of the rise of the blood pressure in that artery, whereas the rise of the blood pressure in the great circular course shows the stiffest resistance (EICHLER and MÜGGE, 1931).

With cats tachyphylaxis can be produced as well. By chronic infusion the decrease of the blood pressure is constant, to lead after a certain time to death, partially due to oedema of the lungs. In this state epinephrine has a highly toxic effect. If the infusion is interrupted for a few minutes, its velocity can, after reinstalling the infusion, be raised without damage. In this way concentrations in the plasma are reached which are able to bring the intestine, previously inactivated through narcosis, to peristaltic movements (EICHLER, 1937).

D. Increase of histamine toxicity: "Sensitization"

Susceptibility of animals to the toxic effects of histamine can be increased by the administration of certain bacterial products (PARFENTJEV and GOODLINE, 1948).

LISH et al. (1960), found that the intravenous LD_{50} of histamine, in mice, greatly diminishes from 445 mg/kg to 24 mg/kg (histamine diphosphate) if the animals seven days prior to the histamine toxicity test are injected intraperitoneally with pertussis vaccine (approximately 3×10^9 *H. pertussis* cells). Likewise the administration of thyrotoxine "sensitizes" the animals to histamine. SPENCER and WEST (1961) found that in mice the LD_{50} of histamine decreased some 10-fold when animals were injected 2 mg/kg of thyrotoxine, 6 days in advance.

IV. Influence of the adrenal glands and the hypophysis on the toxicity of histamine

Since the investigations of DALE (1920) and KELLAWAY and COWELL (1922 b) it has been known that adrenalectomized animals become very sensitive to the toxic effects of histamine. The highest sensitivity in rats appears between 5 and 30 days after adrenalectomy (CRIVELLARI, 1926; HOUSSAY, 1951). The lethal dose of histamine, as can be seen in table 4, diminishes between 3 to 15 times depending on the mode of administration and the time elapsed after adrenalectomy (MARMORSTON-GOTTESMAN and GOTTESMAN, 1928; NOBLE and COLLIP, 1941; SCOTT, 1927; WYMAN, 1928).

This increase in sensitivity, in rats, persists for 5 or more months although it progressively diminishes as accessory adrenals develop.

The increased sensitivity to histamine varies quantitatively according to the species. BANTING and GAIRNS (1926) found that the adrenalectomized dogs die with doses 30 times smaller than those needed to produce death in normal animals, while HALPERN and WOOD (1950) found that adrenalectomized mice are 100 times more sensitive than the controls. On the other hand, in guinea pigs (GROSS, 1948),

Table 4. *Lethal doses of histamine in adrenalectomized or hypophysectomized rats*

Condition	Route of administ.	Type of LD	Doses μg/kg	References
Normal	s-c	LD	1200	WYMAN (1928)
Adrenalect. . . .	s-c	LD	500—600	WYMAN (1928)
Normal	i-p	LD	1000	SCOTT (1927)
Adrenalect. . . .	i-p	LD	100	SCOTT (1927)
Normal	i-v	LD	500—700	CRIVELLARI (1926)
Adrenalect. . . .	i-v	LD_{50}	40	CRIVELLARI (1926)
Normal	i-p	LD_{50}	1300 B	HOUSSAY (1951)
Adrenalect. . . .	i-p	LD_{50}	500 B	HOUSSAY (1951)
Normal	i-p	LD_{50}	920 B	HOUSSAY (1951)
Adrenalect. . . .	i-p	LD_{50}	70 B	HOUSSAY (1951)
Hypophysect.. . .	i-p	LD_{50}	670 B	HOUSSAY (1951)
Normal	i-v	LD_{100}	700 B	HOUSSAY (1951)
Adrenalect. . . .	i-v	LD_{100}	400 B	HOUSSAY (1951)
Normal	i-v	LD_{50}	500 B	HOUSSAY (1951)
Adrenalect. . . .	i-v	LD_{50}	70 B	HOUSSAY (1951)
Normal	s-c	LD_{100}	1400	NOBLE and COLLIP (1941)
Adrenalect. . . .	s-c	LD_{100}	500	NOBLE and COLLIP (1941)
Adrenalect. . . .	s-c	LD_{50}	440	NOBLE and COLLIP (1941)
Hypophysect.. . .	s-c	LD_{50}	530	NOBLE and COLLIP (1941)
Normal	i-p	LD_{100}	1400	PERLA (1935)
Adrenalect. . . .	i-p	LD_{50}	100	PERLA (1935)
Hypophysect.. . .	i-p	LD_{50}	400	PERLA (1935)

adrenalectomy produces only moderate increase in sensitivity and there are almost no changes in rabbits (HIRANO, 1939; OIKAWA, 1931). In this last species of animals the lethal dose, intravenously, diminishes only from 1.2 mg/kg to 0.9 mg/kg (OIKAWA, 1931).

The administration of epinephrine counteracts partially the effect of the adrenalectomy (INGLE, 1937; KELLAWAY and COWELL, 1922b). But a greater resistance to toxic doses of histamine has been obtained in adrenalectomized animals when they were previously injected cortical-adrenal extracts (KENDALL, 1941; MARMORSTON-GOTTESMAN and GOTTESMAN, 1928; PERLA and MARMORSTON-GOTTESMAN, 1941; WYMAN, 1928). Results even more consistent have been observed if instead of the extracts, the actual corticoids were given (HOUSSAY, 1951 and 1954; NOBLE and COLLIP, 1941). Results of different authors that have worked on this problem, show that the increased sensitivity in adrenalectomized animals, is due mainly to a lack of corticoids and secondly to a deficiency in epinephrine and norepinephrine, which are secondary to the extirpation of the adrenal glands.

LUCAS (1926), ROSE and BROWNE (1941) and others, found that after adrenalectomy the blood histamine level begins to rise as well as the histamine content of several tissues (WILSON, 1941). On the other hand, ROSE and BROWNE (1938) have demonstrated the capacity of blood and tissues of adrenalectomized animals to destroy the injected histamine, was markedly diminished. These results as well as those of KARADY et al. (1940) and CARLSTEN and WOOD (1950), show that one of the causes for the increased histamine sensitivity of adrenalectomized animals, is a fall in histaminase concentration, which rises again with the administration of cortical- adrenal extracts or corticoids (KARADY and et al., 1940). But a decrease in histaminase content probably has only a minor role since according to GADDUM (1956), SCHAYER (1956a, b; 1958), TABOR (1956) and ZELLER (1956) in most species the main metabolic pathway for histamine inactivation is not through oxidative deamination.

It is interesting to note that histamine tolerance attained in animals by the chronic administration of increasing doses of histamine, is maintained even after adrenalectomy. In fact these animals can withstand much higher doses than the control adrenalectomized animals (EICHLER and KILLIAN, 1931; KARADY, 1938); in addition, the survival ratio is also much higher than in the controls (MACKAY and CLARK, 1938).

Hypophysectomy also sensitizes animals to the toxic action of histamine, although in lesser degree than adrenalectomy. According to the results of HOUSSAY (1951), NOBLE and COLLIP (1941) and PERLA (1935), the lethal dose of histamine is between 3 and 5 times smaller in hypophysectomized rats. The administration of ACTH or corticoids antagonizes the sensitizing effect of hypophysectomy.

V. Histamine toxicity and antihistamines

According to what is described in other chapters of this book, antihistamines are capable of inhibiting almost all the effects of histamine, including the toxic one.

Table 5. *Histamine toxicity in animals previously treated with antihistamines*

Species	Antihistamine doses and route of administration		Histamine No. of LD_{50} and route adm.	References
	20 mg/kg, s-c, 20′ prior to histamine administ.		i-v	
Guinea pig	Pyranisamine (Neoantergan)		80	HALPERN (1947b)
Rabbit	Pyranisamine (Neoantergan)		30	
Dog	Pyranisamine (Neoantergan)		2—2,5	
Guinea pig	Promethazine (Phenergan)		1500—1600	
Rabbit	Promethazine (Phenergan)		400— 450	
Dog	Promethazine (Phenergan)		20	
Guinea pig	Synopen		300	DOMENJOZ and JAQUES (1949)
	Promethazine (Phenergan)		173	
	Pyranisamine (Neoantergan)		165	
	Diphenhydramine (Benadryl)		82	
	5 mg/kg, i-p, 30′ prior histamine adminst.		i-card.	
Guinea pig	Tripelennamine (Pyribenzamine)		22—30	LEHMANN (1948)
	Phenindamine (Thephorin)		15	
	Diphenhydramine (Benadryl)		6	
	Protective doses (PD_{50}) in μg/kg, i-v, 3′ prior histamine administ.		16 LD_{50}, i-v relative potency	
Guinea pig	Pyranisamine (Neoantergan)	9.4	100	NARANJO and NARANJO (1953c)
	Thiazinamium (Multergan)	10.5	89	
	Promethazine (Phenergan)	33.2	38	
	Thonzylamine (Neohetramine)	67.8	13	
	Methapyriline (Histadyl)	69.7	13	
	Prophenpyridamine (Trimeton)	97.0	9	
	Phenindamine (Thephorin)	101.7	9	

A very useful method in the evaluation of the antihistaminic activity of a compound consists in determining the number of LD_{50} of histamine that the animal can withstand if it has previously received a dose of an antihistamine.

As can be seen in table 5, the same dose of an antihistamine protects different species against a different number of LD_{50} (Halpern, 1947b). On the other hand considering only one species, protection varies according to the potency of the drug and the mode of administration, of both histamine and the antihistamine.

The potency of an antihistamine may vary according to the method of investigation and the parameter used to evaluate it, therefore it has only a relative value and should be considered cautiously. If the protective effect of pyranisamine is compared with that of promethazine (table 5), it is concluded that when a fixed dose of both antihistamines is injected to the animals and then the number of LD_{50} against which the animals are protected is determined, it is found that promethazine is some 20 times more effective. But if this experiment is reversed, this is if a fixed dose of histamine, for instance $16LD_{50}$ (Naranjo and Naranjo, 1953d) is chosen previously as the test dose and the experiment is designed to find the effective dose of the antihistamine necessary to protect 50 % of animals (ED_{50}), it results that pyranisamine is 3 times more effective than promethazine.

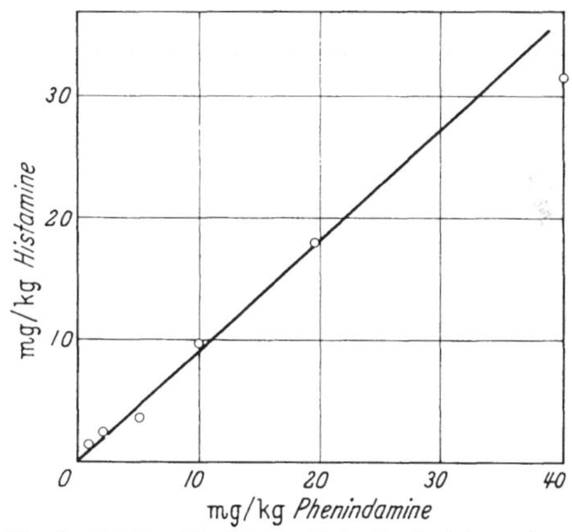

Fig. 9. *Relationship between histamine toxicity and an antihistamine: phenindamine.* Abscissa: phenindamine administered by intraperitoneal injection. Ordinate: Lethal dose of histamine (as free base), administered by intracardiac injection. [Lehmann 1948]

As the dose of an antihistamine increases, protection against histamine also increases. As can be seen in fig. 9 (Lehmann, 1948) a linear relationship exists between the dose of the antihistamine and the amount of histamine needed to produce the lethal effect. An exception to this general finding is observed in the rat and the mouse. In these two species pyranisamine and other antihistamines act synergistically with toxic doses of histamine given intravenously (Ambrus et al., 1952; Halpern, 1947), however they provide the animal with a slight protection if the lethal dose of histamine is given subcutaneously. According to Ambrus et al. (1952) and Deutsch and Loew (1954) some anthistamines proved of no protective value to mice against lethal doses of histamine, regardless of the route of administration.

VI. Histamine toxicity and sympathomimetic drugs

Since the classic investigations of Barger and Dale (1910b) the pharmacodynamic antagonism between epinephrine and histamine has been known.

Epinephrine, as many other sympathomimetic drugs, are capable of preventing the toxic and lethal effects of histamine, not only in adrenalectomized animals but in normals as well.

Guinea pigs subjected to the lethal effect of histamine aerosol can be protected by epinephrine and specially by isopropyl-arterenol (table 6) in a similar manner as the most active antihistamines do (Naranjo, 1954; Naranjo and Naranjo, 1953a, d). On the other hand, when histamine is administered subcutaneously or intravenously, sympathomimetic compounds confer only a very limited protection.

A large increase in the dose of isopropyl-arterenol, for example (fig. 10), produces only a slight increase in tolerance to lethal doses of histamine, in contrast to what happens with antihistamines. This fact is an indication that sympathomimetic amines selectively antagonize only certain effects of histamine particularly the

Table 6. *Median effective dose (ED_{50}) of some drugs against inhalatory histamine shock* (according to NARANJO, 1954).

Compound	ED_{50} mg/kg, s—c	Relative potency
Sympathomimetic drugs:		
Isopropyl-arterenol . .	0.023	100
Epinephrine	0.042	55
Phenyl-ephrine . . .	0.188	12
Norepinephrine . . .	0.356	6
Ephedrine	0.938	2
Antihistamines:		
Pyranisamine	0.043	55
Promethazine	0.356	12
Phenindamine	1.168	2

constriction of the bronchi which is so marked in guinea pigs. LANDS et al. (1947, 1950) have extensively studied the bronchodilator properties of the sympathomimetic amines and their capacity to antagonize histamine.

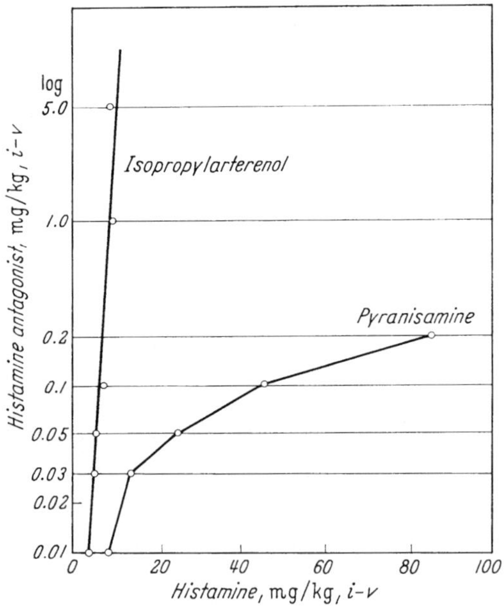

Fig. 10. *Correlation between lethal doses of histamine and protective doses of antagonists.* In the abscissa, the required doses of histamine to produce death in guinea pigs previously protected by a given dose of pyranisamine or isopropyl-arterenol. (NARANJO, 1954)

VII. Histamine toxicity and histaminase inhibitors

In contrast to the fast disappearance of exogenous histamine *in vivo* (ROSE and BROWNE, 1938), the *in vitro* inactivation in the presence of histaminase is extremely slow (BEST and MACHENRY, 1930). The studies of SCHAYER (1956a, b; 1958) and

SCHAYER et al. (1954) give evidence that histaminase plays a very important role in the overall catabolism of endogenous and exogenous histamine but only in a few species of animals, and particularly in the rat.

The works of ARUNLAKSHANA et al. (1954), LINDELL and WESTLING (1954) and MONGAR and SCHILD (1951), indirectly confirm the conclusions drawn by SCHAYER et al. (1954), since they have found that monoamine oxidase and diamine oxidase inhibitors potentiate certain pharmacological effects of histamine. Nevertheless the degree of potentiation is small, even though the effects have been studied in species and tissues that are considered highly susceptible to histamine.

Table 7. *Histamine toxicity (LD_{50}) in control and treated animals* (according to ANGELAKOS and LOEW, 1957).

Histaminase inhibitor	Dose mM/kg[1]	Histamine[2] LD_{50} mM/kg		Toxicity ratio A/B
		A normal	B treated	
Mouse				
Aminoguanidine	6.5	6.4	5.9	1.1[3]
Imidazole	6.0	6.4	2.8	2.3
Iproniazid	3.5	6.4	4.9	1.3
Semicarbazide	0.7	7.2	9.7	0.7
Isoniazid	0.55	6.4	5.9	1.1[3]
Stilbamidine	0.6	6.4	3.4	1.9[3]
Rat				
Aminoguanidine	8.5	5.0	4.2	1.2
Imidazole	5.0	5.2	0.4	13.0[3]
Iproniazid	1.5	5.1	4.5	1.1
Semicarbazide	1.15	5.6	5.4	1.0

[1] Dose in millimols (as free base) perkilog ram and equivalent to $^1/_2 LD_{50}$ of the respective compound.
[2] Histamine as diphosphate.
[3] Significantly different from 1.0.

ANGELAKOS and LOEW (1957) have investigated in rats and mice the influence that monoamine and diamine oxidase inhibitors have over the toxic and lethal effects of histamine. The main results obtained by ANGELAKOS and LOEW (1957) are depicted in table 7. With the exception of the imidazole, none of the other inhibitors produced a significant potentiation of the histamine toxicity. Imidazol reduced the lethal dose of histamine in rats but very little in mice, demonstrating a species selectivity.

From this report as well as from those mentioned above, that demonstrate that the major metabolic pathway for histamine inactivation is methylation, it can be deduced that although the inhibitors of histaminase can potentiate certain effects of histamine, selectively in certain species, the toxic and lethal effects specially in rats and mice, are not altered by most of the studied inhibitors and consequently it can be assumed that histaminase does not play an important role in the metabolic destruction of large amounts of exogenous histamine.

Literature

AMBRUS, J. L., C. M. AMBRUS and J. JACOB: Histamine desensitization in the guinea pig and the rat. Experientia (Basel) **6**, 272 (1950).
— — and J. W. E. HARRISON: Mode of action of histamine desensitization. Amer. J. Physiol. **167**, 268 (1951a).
— — — Effect of histamine desensitization on histamine induced gastric secretion of guinea pigs. Gastroenterology **18**, 249 (1951b).
— E. W. PACKMAN, G. V. ROSSI, C. M. AMBRUS and J. W. E. HARRISON: The antagonism and synergism of histamine and antihistamines in mice. J. Pharm. Pharmacol. **4**, 466 (1952).

ANGELAKOS, T. E., and E. R. LOEW: Histamine toxicity in mice and rats following treatment with histaminase inhibitors. J. Pharmacol. exp. Ther. **119**, 444 (1957).
ARUNLAKSHANA, O., J. L. MONGAR and H. O. SCHILD: Potentiation of pharmacological effects of histamine by histaminase inhibitors. J. Physiol. (Lond.) **123**, 32 (1954).
BANTING, F. G., and S. GAIRNS: Suprarenal insufficiency. Amer. J. Physiol. **77**, 100 (1926).
BARGER, G., and H. H. DALE: Beta-imidazol-ethyl-amine and other active principles of ergot. J. Chem. Soc. **97**, 2592 (1910a).
— — Chemical structure and sympathomimetic action of amines. J. Physiol. (Lond.) **41**, 19 (1910b).
BEST, C. H., and E. W. MACHENRY: The inactivation of histamine. J. Physiol. (Lond.) **70**, 349 (1930).
— — Histamine. Physiol. Rev. **11**, 371 (1931).
CARLSTEN, A., and D. R. WOOD: Restoration of normal lymph histaminase in adrenalectomized cats by adrenocortical extract. J. Physiol. (Lond.) **111**, 8 P (1950).
CLARK, R.: The paralytic action of histamine on the ruminal musculature. J. S. Afr. vet. med. Ass. **21**, 13 (1950).
CORDIER, D., et M. CORDIER: Troubles de la phosphorolyse du glycogène hépatique au cours de l'intoxication histaminique. J. Physiol. (Paris) **47**, 141 (1955).
—, et A. DUVEAU: Sensibilité à l'adrénaline et à l'acétylcholine de l'intestin grêle du rat intoxiqué par l'histamine. C. R. Soc. Biol. (Paris) **150**, 1954 (1956).
—, et G. PÉRÈS: Troubles de la protidémie au cours de l'intoxication histaminique. J. Physiol. (Paris) **49**, 107 (1957).
CRANE, J. T., S. LINDWAY and N. E. DAILEY: An attempt to prevent histamine induced ulcers in guinea pigs with Benadryl. Amer. J. Digest. Dis. **14**, 56 (1947).
CRIVELLARI, C. A.: Sensitivity of adrenalectomized rats to the action of some toxic substances. Rev. Soc. argent. Biol. **2**, 448 (1926).
— Sensibilité des rats décapsulés à l'égard de la nicotine, du cyanure, de l'acétylcholine et de l'histamine. C. R. Soc. Biol. (Paris) **96**, 223 (1927).
DALE, H. H.: Conditions which are conducive to the production of shock by histamine. Brit. J. exp. Path. **1**, 103 (1920).
—, and P. P. LAIDLAW: The physiological action of beta-iminazolyl-ethyl-amine. J. Physiol. (Lond.) **41**, 318 (1911).
— — Histamine shock. J. Physiol. (Lond.) **52**, 355 (1919).
DECOURT, M. J., et J. L. PARROT: Les bases physiologiques et physiopathologiques de la médication antihistaminique. Presse méd. **66**, 764 (1947). (Rapport au 26e Congrès Français de Médecine).
DELAUNOIS, A. L., R. KORDECKI, H. POLET and J. RYZEWSKI: Cardiac output, arterial blood pressure and pulmonary arterial pressure in histamine shock. Arch. int. Pharmacodyn. **120**, 114 (1959).
DEUTSCH, S., and E. R. LOEW: Failure of antihistamine drugs to antagonize lethal effects of histamine in mice. Fed. Proc. **13**, 348 (1954).
DOMENJOZ, R., u. R. JAQUES: Über Synopen, ein neues Antihistaminicum. Schweiz. med. Woch. **21**, 476 (1949).
DOUGHERTY, R. W.: A study of drugs affecting the motility of the bovine rumen. Cornell Vet. **32**, 269 (1942).
EICHLER, O.: Pharmakologie des Veritols. Naunyn-Schmiedeberg's Arch. exp. Path. Pharm. **187**, 433 (1937).
—, u. H. KILLIAN: Versuche zur Histaminwirkung am Kaninchen. Naunyn-Schmiedeberg's Arch. exp. Path. Pharmak. **159**, 606 (1931).
—, u. H. MÜGGE: Mechanismus der Histaminwirkung beim Kaninchen. Naunyn-Schmiedeberg's Arch. exp. Path. Pharm, **159**, 633 (1931).
ELLIOT, T. R.: The control of the suprarenal glands by the splachnic nerves. J. Physiol. (Lond.) **44**, 374 (1912).
ESSEX, H. E., and B. T. HORTON: Observations on development of resistance to histamine in the guinea pig. Proc. Mayo Clin. **16**, 603 (1941).
FABINYI, M., and J. SZEBEHELYI: The mechanism of desensitization with histamine. Acta allerg. (Kbh.) **2**, 233 (1949).
FEINBERG, S. M.: Histamine and antihistaminic agents; their experimental and therapeutic status. J. Amer. med. Ass. **132**, 702 (1946).
FELDBERG, W.: The action of histamine on the blood vessels of the rabbit. J. Physiol. (Lond.) **63**, 211 (1927).
— On some physiological aspects of histamine. J. Pharm. Pharmacol. **6**, 281 (1954).
—, and A. A. MILES: Regional variations of increased permeability of skin capillaries induced by histamine liberation and their relation to the histamine content of the skin. J. Physiol. (Lond.) **120**, 205 (1953).

FLURY, F.: In: Abderhalden's Handb. biol. Arbeitsmethoden. **4**, 7b, 1354 (1925).
FÜHNER, H.: Beiträge zur vergleichenden Pharmakologie; die giftigen und tödlichen Gaben einiger Substanzen für Frösche und Mäuse. Naunyn-Schmiedeberg's Arch. exp. Path. Pharmak. **166**, 437 (1932).
GABE, M.: Données histophysiologiques sur l'intoxication histaminique aiguë par voie gastrique. Arch. Mal. Appar. dig. **41**, 10 (1952).
GADDUM, J. H.: Histamine. Brit. med. J. **1948 I**, 867.
— The origin of histamine in the body. In: Histamine (Ciba Foundation Symposium), Little, Brown and Co. Publish. 285 (1956).
GEIGER, E.: Role of histamine in poisoning with spoiled fish. Science **121**, 865 (1955).
GOODMAN, L. S., and A. GILMAN: The pharmacological basis of therapeutics. 2nd. ed. New York, N. Y.: The Macmillan Co., Publ. 1955.
GRAHAM, J. D. P.: A comparison of some antihistamine substances. Brit. J. Pharmacol. **91**, 193 (1947).
GROSS, F.: Die Beeinflussung des Histaminschockes durch Desoxycorticosteron und Antihistaminica am nebennierenlosen Meerschweinchen. Helv. physiol. pharmacol. Acta **6**, 114 (1948).
HALPERN, B. N.: Les antihistaminiques de synthèse. Essai de chimiotherapie des états allergiques. Arch. int. Pharmacodyn. **68**, 339 (1942).
— Experimental research on a new series of chemical substances with powerful antihistaminic activity: the thiodiphenylamine derivatives. J. Allergy **18**, 263 (1947).
— Recherches sur une nouvelle série chimique de corps doués de propriétés antihistaminiques et anti-anaphylactiques: les dérivés de la thiodiphénylamine. Arch. int. Pharmacodyn. **74**, 314 (1947b).
— Sur le mécanisme d'action des antihistaminiques de synthèse. Presse méd. **65**, 949 (1949).
—, et M. BRIOT: Action des antihistaminiques de synthèse sur la température chez le rat normal et chez le rat surrénalectomisé. C. R. Soc. Biol. (Paris) **143**, 633 (1950).
—, et L. CHMEL: Etude de l'action de quelques antihistaminiques de synthèse sur la température du lapin. C. R. Soc. Biol. (Paris) **143**, 636 (1949).
—, and J. HAMBURGER: A new synthetic antihistamine substance derived from phenothiazine (Phenergan, 3.277 RP). Canad. med. Ass. J. **59**, 322 (1948).
—, et D. WOOD: Mise en évidence de l'action antitoxique d'un antihistaminique de synthèse vis-à-vis de l'histamine chez la souris par la surrénalectomie. C. R. Acad. Sci. (Paris) **230**, 138 (1950).
HAY, L. M., R. L. VARCO, C. F. CODE and O. H. WANGENSTEEN: The experimental production of gastric and duodenal ulcers in laboratory animals by the intramuscular injection of histamine in beeswax. Surg. Gynec. Obstet. **75**, 170 (1942).
HIRANO, T.: Non-importance of medulla in the susceptibility to histamine of suprarenalectomized rabbits. Tohoku J. exp. Med. **37**, 322 (1939).
HORTON, B. T.: Histamine cephalgia: differential diagnosis and treatment. Proc. Mayo Clin. **31**, 325 (1956).
HOUSSAY, R. H.: The adrenals in the hypoxia and the histamine intoxication. Buenos Aires: El Ateneo Publis. 1951.
— Protection par les corticostéroïdes ou la cortisone contre l'intoxication histaminique. C. R. Soc. Biol. (Paris) **148**, 907 (1954).
INGLE, J.: Resistance of the rat to histamine shock after destruction of the adrenal medulla. Amer. J. Physiol. **118**, 57 (1937).
JANCSO, M.: Histamine as a physiological activator of the reticuloendothelial system. Nature (Lond.) **160**, 227 (1947).
JONES, L. M.: Veterinary pharmacology and therapeutics. 2nd. Ed., The Iowa State College Press, 1957.
KAHLSON, G.: Histamine in normal physiology. Lancet **1960 I**, 67.
KARADY, S.: Changes in the total blood volume in histamine and surgical shock in normal rabbits and in those pretreated with histaminase. Amer. J. Physiol. **123**, 194 (1938).
— B. ROSE and J. S. L. BROWNE: Decrease of histaminase in tissue by adrenalectomy and its restoration by cortico-adrenal extracts. Amer. J. Physiol. **130**, 539 (1940).
KELLAWAY, C. H., and S. J. COWELL: The antagonism between histamine and adrenaline. J. Physiol. (Lond.) **56**, 20 (1922a).
— — On the concentration of the blood and the effects of histamine in adrenal insufficiency. J. Physiol. (Lond.) **57**, 82 (1922b).
KENDALL, E. C.: Hormones. Ann. Rev. Biochem. **10**, 298 (1941).
KIMATA, M., and A. KAWAI: Production of histamine by bacteria causing spoilage in fish. Bull. Res. Inst. Food Sci. Kyoto Univ. **13**, 29 (1953).
LA BARRE, J.: Sur les causes des variations de la glycémie au cours des chocs anaphylactique, histaminique et peptonique. Arch. int. Méd. exp. **3**, 42 (1927).

LANDS, A. M., J. O. HOPPE, O. H. SIEGMUND and F. P. LUDUENA: The pharmacological properties of three new antihistaminic drugs. J. Pharmacol. exp. Ther. **95**, 45 (1949).
— F. P. LUDUENA, J. I. GRANT and E. J. ANANENKO: The pharmacologic action of some analogs of 1-(3,4-dihydroxyphenyl)-2-amino-1-butanol (Ethylnorepinephrine). J. Pharmacol. exp. Ther. **99**, 45 (1950).
— V. L. NASH, H. M. MCCARTHY, H. R. GRANGER and B. L. DERTINGER: The pharmacology of N-alkyl homologues of epinephrine. J. Pharmacol. exp. Ther. **90**, 110 (1947).
LEHMANN, G.: Pharmacological properties of a new antihistaminic, 2-methyl-9-phenyl-2,3,4,9-tetrahydro-1-pyridindene (thephorin) and derivatives. J. Pharmacol. exp. Ther. **92**, 249 (1948).
—, and J. W. YOUNG: The antihistamine activity of diethylamino-ethyl-dihydroanthracen-carboxilate and other substances. J. Pharmacol. exp. Ther. **83**, 90 (1945).
LINDELL, S. E., and H. WESTLING: Potentiation of histamine effects by an antihistaminase. Acta physiol. scand. **32**, 230 (1954).
LISH, P. M., J. R. ALBERT, E. L. PETERS and L. E. ALIEN: Pharmacology of methdilazine (tacaryl). Arch. int. Pharmacodyn. **129**, 77 (1960).
LUCAS, G. H. W.: Blood and urine findings in desuprarenalized dogs. Amer. J. Physiol. **77**, 114 (1926).
MAC KAY, E. M., and W. G. CLARK: Effect of histamine pretreatment upon adrenalectomized rats. Proc. Soc. exp. Biol. (N. Y.) **39**, 56 (1938).
MALMÉJAC, J., A. GROSS et G. NEVERRE: Histamine et adrénalino-sécrétion. C. R. Soc. Biol. (Paris) **144**, 704 (1951).
MARMORSTON-GOTTESMAN, J., and J. GOTTESMAN: The use of histamine as a standard test for diminished resistance in suprarenalectomized rats. J. exp. Med. **47**, 503 (1928).
MONGAR, J. L., and H. O. SCHILD: Potentiation of action of histamine by semicarbazide. Nature (Lond.) **167**, 232 (1951).
NARANJO, P.: Bronchospasm and emphysema. An experimental study. Gaceta Méd. **6**, 200 (1951).
— Bronchodilator amines. Chemical structure and selectivity. Terapia **11**, 8 (1954).
— Protection of the experimental asthma by sympathomimetic and anticholinergic drugs. In: Proceedings of the IV Congress of Medicine, Vol. **I**, 457, Ed. Impta. Municipal Guayaquil (1953d).
—, and E. BANDA DE NARANJO: Hista-3 a new antihistamine combination. In: Proceedings of the IV Congress of Medicine, Vol. **I**, 432, Ed. Impta. Municipal, Guayaquil (1953a).
— — Inactivation of the antihistaminic drugs in the liver and in the gastrointestinal tract. J. Allergy **24**, 442 (1953b).
— — Studies of the combined action of some antihistaminc agents. Ann. Allergy **11**, 699 (1953c).
— — Pressor effect of histamine in the rabbit. J. Pharmacol. exp. Ther. **123**, 16 (1958).
— — Erworbene Antigentoleranz und Anaphylaxie. Allergie u. Asthma **7**, 259 (1961).
NI, T. G.: On the inverse change between the concentration of glucose and chloride in the blood. Amer. J. Physiol. **78**, 158 (1926).
NOBLE, R. L., and J. B. COLLIP: The response of normal, hypophysectomized and adrenalectomized rats to histamine administration. Amer. J. Physiol. **133**, 623 (1941).
OEHME, C.: Über die Wirkungsweise des Histamins. Naunyn-Schmiedeberg's Arch. exp. Path. Pharm. **72**, 76 (1913).
OIKAWA, K.: The susceptibility of doubly suprarenalectomized rabbits to nicotine, histamine ephedrine and typhoid vaccine. Tohoku J. exp. Med. **18**, 27 (1931).
PAPACOSTAS, C. A., P. MOZDEN and E. R. LOEW: Influence of histamine and histamine liberator, compound 48/80, on blood glucose of unanesthetized animals. Fed. Proc. **15**, 466 (1956).
PARFENTJEV, I. A., and M. A. GOODLINE: Histamine shock in mice sensitized with *Haemophilus pertussis* vaccine. J. Pharmacol. exp. Ther. **92**, 411 (1948).
PARROT, J. L., et J. REUSE: Rôle physiologique et physiopathologique de l'histamine. J. Physiol. (Paris) **46**, 99 (1954).
PERLA, D.: Effect of anterior hypophysis emulsion on natural resistance of hypophysectomized and normal rats to histamine poisoning. Proc. Soc. exp. Biol. (N. Y.) **33**, 121 (1935).
—, and J. MARMORSTON-GOTTESMAN: Natural resistance and clinical medicine. Boston: Little., Brown and Co. 1941.
PICKERING, G. W.: Observations on mechanism of headache produced by histamine. Clin. Sci. **1**, 77 (1933).
REUSE, J. J.: Histamine, antihistaminiques de synthèse et système circulatoire du Lapin. J. Physiol. (Paris) **40**, 289 (1948).
ROBINSON, B. W.: Histaminic cephalgia. Medicine **37**, 161 (1958).
ROCHA E SILVA, M.: Histamine, its role in anaphylaxis and allergy. Springfield, Ill.: Charles C. Thomas. Publish. 1955.

Rose, B., and J. S. L. Browne: The distribution and rate of disappearance of intravenously injected histamine in the rat. Amer. J. Physiol. **124**, 412 (1938).
— — The effect of adrenalectomy on the histamine content of the tissues of the rat. Amer. J. Physiol. **131**, 589 (1941).
Roth, F. E., and W. M. Govier: Comparative pharmacology of chlorpheniramine (chlortrimeton) and its optical isomers. J. Pharmacol. exp. Ther. **124**, 347 (1958).
Satow, J.: A measure to alter the glycaemic effect of histamine and peptone. Tohoku J. exp. Med. **32**, 239 (1938).
Schayer, R. W.: The origin and fate of histamine in the body. In: Histamine (Ciba Foundation Symposium), Little, Brown and Co. Publish., 183 (1956a).
— The origin of histamine in the body. In: Histamine (Ciba Foundation Symposium), Little, Brown and Co. Publish. 299 (1956b).
— Histamine metabolism. III. Congrès international d'allergologie, Paris, 377 (1958).
— Significance of induced synthesis of histamine in physiology and pathology. Chemotherapia **3**, 128 (1961).
— K. Y. T. Wu, and R. L. Smiley: Sources of urinary histamine in the rat. Amer. J. Physiol. **179**, 481 (1954).
Schmidt, G. W., u. A. Stähelin: Histaminempfindlichkeit und anaphylaktische Reaktionen. Z. Immun.-Forsch. **60**, 222 (1929).
Scott, W. J. M.: The effect of histamine in sublethal suprarenal insufficiency. Arch. Path. Lab. Med. **4**, 491 (1927).
Shifrine, M., L. E. Ousterhout, C. R. Grau and R. H. Vaughn: Toxicity to chicks of histamine formed during microbial spoilage of tuna. Appl. Microbiol. **7**, 45 (1959).
Spencer, P. S. J., and G. B. West: Sensitivity of the hyperthyroid and hypothyroid mouse to histamine and 5-hydroxytryptamine. Brit. J. Pharmacol. **17**, 137 (1961).
Stead, E. A., and J. V. Warren: The effect of injection of histamine into the brachial artery on the permeability of capillaries in the forearm and hand. J. Clin. Invest. **23**, 279 (1944).
Suzuki, T.: Adrenaline load of the suprarenal glands of rabbits in histamine poisoning. Tohoku J. exp. Med. **54**, 289 (1951).
Tabor, H.: The fate of histamine in the body. In: Histamine (Ciba Foundation Symposium), Boston: Little, Brown and Co. Publish. 318 (1956).
Takita, S.: Contribution to glycemic effect of histamine in dogs and rabbits. Tohoku J. exp. Med. **53**, 145 (1950).
Trendelenburg, U.: The pressor response of the cat to histamine and pilocarpine. J. Pharmacol. exp. Ther. **131**, 65 (1961).
Wada, M., F. Keizo, S. Hatiro, S. Huminchko and M. C. Li: The action of histamine upon the epinephrine secretion from the suprarenal gland in non-anaesthetized dogs. Tohoku J. exp. Med. **37**, 442 (1940).
Walpole, S. H., R. L. Varco, C. F. Code and O. H. Wangensteen: Production of gastric and duodenal ulcers in the cat by intramuscular implantation of histamine. Proc. Soc. exp. Biol. (N. Y.) **44**, 619 (1940).
Wells, J. A., J. S. Gray and C. A. Dragstedt: An investigation of the question of histamine tolerance. J. Allergy **13**, 77 (1941).
Wilson, A.: The effect of adrenalectomy on the blood histamine of rabbits. J. Physiol. (Lond.) **99**, 241 (1941).
Woodbury, R. A., and W. F. Hamilton: Effect of histamine on pulmonary blood pressure of various animals with and without anesthesia. J. Pharmacol. exp. Ther. **71**, 293 (1941).
Wyman, L. C.: Studies on suprarenal insufficiency. II. The relative importance of cortex and medulla in the susceptibility to histamine of suprarenalectomized rats. Amer. J. Physiol. **87**, 20 (1928).
Zeller, E. A.: The fate of histamine in the body, with particular reference to the enzymology of histamine oxidation. In: Histamine (Ciba Foundation Symposium), Boston, Little, Brown and Co. Publish., 339 (1956).

Section D. I

Action de l'histamine sur les muscles lisses

Par

Jean-Louis Parrot et Joseph Thouvenot

Avec 6 Figures

L'histamine fait contracter la plupart des muscles lisses de beaucoup d'espèces de Poissons, d'Oiseaux et de Mammifères; mais son action varie grandement selon l'espèce et selon l'organe.

Les muscles lisses du Chat et du Cobaye sont particulièrement sensibles; la grande sensibilité de l'iléon isolé de Cobaye, bien connue depuis 1916 grâce à Guggenheim et Löffler, est mise à profit pour le dosage biologique de l'histamine sur l'organe isolé. En revanche les muscles lisses du Rat et de la Souris sont particulièrement résistants à l'action de l'histamine; ceux du Chien et du Lapin occupent une position intermédiaire. Pour une espèce donnée, l'utérus et les bronches sont généralement les plus sensibles; la vessie, la vésicule biliaire et l'iris sont les plus résistants; et, entre ces extrêmes, se placent l'intestin et les artérioles.

C'est généralement l'effet que l'histamine exerce sur les muscles lisses qui donne le symptôme caractéristique de son action chez une espèce donnée. Ainsi les bronches chez le Cobaye constituent un test particulièrement sensible et l'on sait que la bronchoconstriction avec dyspnée expiratoire est le signe capital de l'intoxication histaminique aiguë chez cette espèce animale: c'est d'ailleurs l'obstruction bronchique avec asphyxie qui entraîne alors la mort du Cobaye et l'autopsie montre une distension emphysémateuse des poumons. Chez le Chien au contraire, les muscles lisses qui répondent d'une manière prédominante sont ceux du sphincter sus-hépatique; celui-ci par sa contraction détermine une stase dans la circulation porte et une hypotension dans le reste de la circulation sanguine. Chez le Lapin, ce sont les muscles lisses de la petite circulation qui donnent la réponse caractéristique: il y a constriction des artères pulmonaires d'où stase dans le coeur droit. Quant à l'Homme il peut réagir, selon les cas, par une crise de dyspnée expiratoire due à la réduction de la lumière bronchique ou par un collapsus cardio-vasculaire.

I. Action de l'histamine sur les bronches

L'effet bronchoconstricteur de l'histamine découvert par Dale et Laidlaw (1910) est l'un des plus généralement observés chez les diverses espèces animales; on l'obtient même chez la Grenouille, et déjà, à faible concentration (2 mg/l) (Carlson et Luckhardt, 1920); mais il est particulièrement net chez le Cobaye: chez cette espèce la dose liminaire (voie I. V.) peut descendre jusqu'à 1 μg/kg (Field et Drinker, 1930); chez le Chien, le bronchospasme histaminique est aussi très net après des doses de 0,2 à 0,3 mg/kg et il est généralement réversible; il est moins intense chez le Lapin et le Chat.

L'action bronchoconstrictrice de l'histamine peut entraîner d'importants effets secondaires qui résultent en somme d'une insuffisance de l'hématose: il y a chez le Lapin acidose gazeuse et stimulation du centre respiratoire; chez le Cobaye la broncho-constriction est beaucoup plus complète et il a été prouvé que, chez cette espèce, c'est par asphyxie que l'histamine entraîne la mort, du moins dans le cas d'intoxication aiguë; ainsi BURSTEIN (1946) a soumis le Cobaye à une respiration artificielle suffisamment intense pour rompre la résistance mécanique à la circulation de l'air et cet auteur a constaté qu'il devient alors possible d'injecter sans danger 30 doses mortelles. De même, lorsqu'une drogue protège le Cobaye contre une dose mortelle d'histamine c'est en s'opposant à l'action bronchoconstrictrice de cette substance, c'est ce qu'ont démontré BOVET et WALTHERT (1944).

Les techniques qui permettent d'enregistrer l'action de l'histamine sur les bronches, notamment chez le Cobaye, ont été très souvent appliquées à l'étude des antagonistes de l'histamine.

Ces techniques sont très diverses.

A. Bronchospasme par aérosol d'histamine

ALEXANDER, BECKE et HOLMES, dès 1926, puis KALLOS et PAGEL, onze ans plus tard (1937), avaient montré que l'inhalation d'histamine sous forme d'aérosol déclenche un syndrome dyspnéique chez le Cobaye, et ces auteurs ont engagé SCHAUMANN à utiliser ce test pour étudier diverses actions antagonistes. SCHAUMANN alors, à partir de 1940, a développé cette méthode en prenant comme test le retard apporté par une dose active de médicament à l'apparition du coma asphyxique.

Les aérosols d'histamine ont été maintes fois utilisés pour étudier ces antagonistes: on trouvera au chapitre correspondant le détail des diverses techniques; notons seulement ici que l'inhibition du bronchospasme provoqué par les aérosols d'histamine ne constitue pas chez le Cobaye un critère spécifique de l'activité antihistaminique; BOVET et BOVET-NITTI (1948), dans leur ouvrage classique, énumèrent, en particulier, six catégories de drogues qui, outre les antihistaminiques, peuvent lever ce spasme; mentionnons seulement l'atropine et certains spasmolytiques.

B. Enregistrement du spasme bronchique

Dès 1927 CORDIER et MAGNE avaient imaginé une technique sur le Cobaye dont le principe est le suivant: grâce à une canule trachéale l'air est insufflé sous pression constante; on enregistre alors la vitesse ou le volume de l'air qui pénètre dans la trachée à chaque inspiration passive; un bronchospasme diminue à la fois l'un et l'autre. STAUB (1939) a appliqué cette technique à l'étude des antagonistes de l'histamine.

Dans la technique de KONZETT et RÖSSLER (1940) c'est le volume total de l'air envoyé par la pompe qui est constant et l'on mesure la fraction de ce volume qui ne peut, à une pression donnée (8 à 12 cm d'eau), pénétrer dans la trachée. Un enregistreur de volume fournit un tracé continu. Au départ, le trop-plein de volume est règlé à quelques millilitres (4 à 6): qu'un spasme des bronches survienne et ce trop-plein augmente. C'est là un test très sensible. EMMELIN, KAHLSON et WICKSELL (1941) utilisent cette méthode pour évaluer l'histamine dans le plasma; ces auteurs peuvent déceler ainsi 0,5 μg d'histamine. L'enregistrement étant assuré par un manomètre à eau, HALPERN (1942) applique la même méthode à l'étude des antihistaminiques. BOVET et WALTHERT (1944), grâce à la technique de KONZETT et RÖSSLER, montrent chez le Cobaye que, à la suite de l'injection dans la veine jugulaire de 1 μg de mépyramine (néo-antergan) par kg, la sensibilité de l'animal à l'histamine diminue de 50 p. 100.

CHARLIER et VANDERMISSEN (1954) modifient cette méthode générale; l'appareil d'enregistrement est un tambour de Marey de grand diamètre; une fuite systématique limite la pression maximale de l'air; ces auteurs étudient le Chien anesthésié et enregistrent ainsi, grâce à une canule trachéale spéciale, les modifications du volume pulmonaire.

Collier, Holgate et coll. (1960), Collier et Shorley (1960) utilisent la méthode de Konzett et Rössler notamment pour comparer, sur le Cobaye, l'action de la bradykinine et de l'histamine. Holgate et Warner (1960) étudient de la même manière les antagonistes de l'histamine, de la 5-hydroxytryptamine et de l'acétylcholine.

Hansen et Zipf (1960) utilisent la méthode de Konzett et Rössler pour étudier les relations entre le tonus bronchique et les afférences vagales d'origine

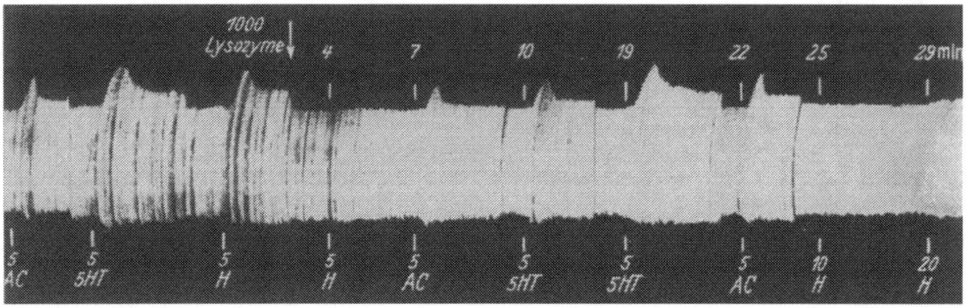

Fig. 1. Effet d'une préparation de lysozyme sur le bronchospasme provoqué sur un cobaye mâle de 500 g par du dichlorhydrate d'histamine (H), du chlorure d'acétylcholine (AC) et du sulfate double de 5-hydroxytryptamine et de créatinine. Dose en μg. Temps en min à partir de l'injection du lysozyme (Parrot et coll., 1962)

pulmonaire: il y a augmentation de ces afférences au moment du bronchospasme histaminique.

Parrot et coll. (1962) utilisent une variante de la méthode de Konzett et Rössler comportant une pression d'eau constante et un enregistrement par tambour de Marey (fig. 1).

Enfin D'Silva et Lewis (1961) déduisent la résistance bronchique à l'écoulement de l'air du diagramme de pression-volume. Ce dernier s'inscrit automatiquement sur l'écran de l'oscillographe selon la méthode générale de composition de deux variables périodiques (méthode des courbes de Lissajous). Cette méthode est assez analogue dans son principe à celle qui a été mise en oeuvre par Bargeton et coll. (1957) pour étudier la résistance bronchique.

Les résultats de D'Silva et Lewis concernant l'histamine indiquent qu'en réponse à cette substance les bronchioles se contractent jusqu'à 60 p. 100 de leur calibre normal; au-delà, elles se ferment soudainement et complètement. Ce calibre critique de fermeture peut être atteint chez le Cobaye, mais non chez le Lapin ou le Chat.

C. Pléthysmographie du poumon

Yonkman, Oppenheimer et coll. (1947), en utilisant la méthode de Jackson (1939), étudient, chez le Chien, la bronchoconstriction histaminique et l'action antagoniste de la pyribenzamine.

D. Moulage de l'arbre bronchique

Hanzlick (1925) réalise, après la mort de l'animal, un moule bronchique en injectant une solution acétonique de celluloïde dans la trachée. Le moule est ensuite dégagé après digestion des tissus. Chez le Cobaye, Bovet et Walthert (1944) ont étudié, grâce à cette méthode, le bronchospasme histaminique et sa prévention par les antihistaminiques.

E. Techniques in vitro

1. Perfusion du poumon (Sollmann et Oettingen, 1928)

On isole les poumons, on incise le parenchyme pulmonaire, et on perfuse l'ensemble par la trachée, l'histamine étant introduite dans le liquide de perfusion. Staub (1939), puis Yonkmann, Oppenheimer et coll. (1947) appliquent cette technique à l'étude de divers antihistaminiques, établissant ainsi la nature périphérique de l'effet protecteur.

2. Anneaux de trachée (Castillo et De Beer)

On prépare des anneaux bronchiques que l'on relie en chaînette. Cette technique a pu être appliquée aux bronches de l'Homme.

3. Trachée isolée (Fink et Akiyama, 1952)

La trachée d'un cobaye est isolée et maintenue en survie dans une solution physiologique. Le liquide qui la remplit est chassé, lorsqu'elle se contracte, dans un tube monté sur un levier; l'augmentation de poids abaisse alors le levier qui inscrit une ligne descendante. Légèrement modifiée, cette technique a été employée par Mariani (1960) pour comparer l'action de l'histamine à celle de la sérotonine.

II. Action de l'histamine sur la musculature lisse intestinale

L'intestin d'Oiseau et de Mammifère est en général très sensible à l'histamine, surtout dans sa partie distale: le coecum rectal isolé de Poulet a été proposé par Barsoum et Gaddum (1935). On lui préfère généralement l'iléon terminal isolé du Cobaye pour doser l'activité biologique de l'histamine.

Nous verrons que la réponse la plus constante des muscles lisses viscéraux à l'histamine est une contraction lente et durable, qui peut être accompagnée, chez certaines espèces (Lapin, Chat, Cheval), d'un accroissement de l'activité rythmique spontanée (Alexander, 1949; Ambache et Lessin, 1955).

Les fibres lisses intestinales réagissent très différemment à l'histamine selon l'espèce animale et cela dans tous les groupes zoologiques: ainsi, même chez les Poissons (Valette et Augereau, 1958), la répartition de la sensibilité de l'intestin à l'histamine est aussi variable que chez les Mammifères: parmi les Téléostéens, par exemple, on rencontre certaines espèces telles que le Brochet, dont la sensibilité de l'intestin à l'histamine est pratiquement comparable à celle du Cobaye. En revanche, les Sélaciens sont insensibles à cette substance.

Notre étude va porter plus particulièrement sur l'intestin grêle du Cobaye: c'est la préparation la plus sensible à l'histamine et elle a, pour cette raison, suscité divers travaux récents.

A. La technique d'étude de l'action de l'histamine sur l'iléon isolé du Cobaye

Un fragment d'iléon est prélevé sur un cobaye à jeun depuis 8 h environ, immédiatement après sacrifice de l'animal.

La technique la plus employée pour le dosage biologique de l'histamine dérive de celle de Magnus (1905): le fragment, long de 3 cm environ, est introduit dans une cuve thermostatique de faible capacité (de 2 à 15 ml). Une extrémité est fixée à la partie inférieure du récipient et sert de point fixe. L'autre est reliée par un fil à un myographe approprié.

De cette façon, seules s'inscrivent les contractions de la musculature longitudinale, lorsque le fragment n'est pas distendu de manière notable par le liquide que l'intestin sécrète dans sa lumière au cours de l'essai.

De nombreux dispositifs thermostatiques ont été réalisés. Citons celui de HARICHAUX et THOUVENOT (1960), de faible volume et de disposition commode.

Le liquide de survie est du type Tyrode qui peut, ou non, comporter du glucose (composition p. 1000 avec glucose: ClNa 8; ClK 0,2; Cl_2Ca 0,2; Cl_2Mg 0,1; PO_4HNa_2 0,05; CO_3HNa 1, glucose 1). Pour le dosage biologique, un simple barbotage d'air assure une oxygénation suffisante.

Le myographe isotonique s'avère le plus commode mais on doit s'assurer que la tension s'exerçant sur le fragment de l'intestin (1,5 à 2 g) est indépendante de la position du levier. SCHILD (1944) a proposé pour cela un système de compensation convenable. L'inscription peut être obtenue directement à partir du levier myographique muni d'une plume, mais, dans ce cas, les frottements de la plume d'inscription augmentent avec l'amplification.

Nous avons remarqué, en comparant les dispositifs, qu'au delà d'une amplification de 10 fois, les frottements peuvent perturber quelque peu les réponses de l'intestin. Aussi dans ce cas peut-on préférer l'emploi de dispositifs amplificateurs électroniques ou pneumatiques qui d'ailleurs introduisent de nouvelles difficultés d'étalonnage.

Dans ces conditions on obtient pour une concentration modérée d'histamine une contraction parfois précédée d'un bref relâchement.

B. Influence du glucose et de la température

La forme de la contraction dépend de la présence du glucose ainsi que de la température du bain.

1. Influence du glucose sur la contraction histaminique

En présence de glucose (10^{-3}) la contraction histaminique débute après un temps de latence de l'ordre 1,5 s et offre dans son ensemble un caractère soutenu. En fait on peut obtenir deux types de réponses (PARROT et THOUVENOT, 1956).

a) type simple: contraction soutenue avec ascension progressive en 35 à 40 s environ. Le raccourcissement peut se maintenir en présence d'histamine, pendant plusieurs minutes, dans les conditions isotoniques, sans relâchement spontané notable: c'est la réponse la plus constante. L'amplitude de la contraction soutenue dépend de la concentration du glucose dans le bain (de 0,25 à 5×10^{-3}), les autres conditions étant par ailleurs identiques.

b) type complexe: on l'observe fréquemment lorsque l'intestin est très sensible à l'histamine. Après une éventuelle chute initiale et très brève de la ligne de base (qui manque souvent), la contraction se développe en 2 temps (fig. 2): après une montée relativement rapide, le tracé dessine un premier sommet aigu au bout de 10 s environ. Après une phase intermédiaire de relâchement de 10 à 15 s, le tracé montre une nouvelle phase d'ascension plus lente, analogue à celle du type simple, et qui aboutit à la phase de plateau soutenue.

On retrouve, dans ce type complexe, la phase soutenue décrite plus haut; mais elle a été précédée d'une réponse d'un autre type, rapide et de courte durée. Cette réponse précoce est inconstante: elle s'observe dans $^1/_3$ à $^2/_3$ des cas selon la saison.

En l'absence de glucose, la première réponse, de type rapide, se manifeste sans changement notable d'amplitude; la deuxième phase, au contraire, n'est bien marquée que dans sa période d'ascension, elle perd ensuite tout caractère soutenu.

La contraction de type complexe est d'autant plus fréquente que l'organe est plus sensible à l'histamine. La sensibilité à l'histamine paraît dépendre:

1. de l'état digestif: l'iléon vide prélevé chez un animal à jeun depuis au moins 8 heures est plus sensible qu'en période digestive;

2. de la nutrition: la carence modérée en acide ascorbique et en facteur C_2 accroît notablement la sensibilité à l'histamine: le régime optimal qui permet d'obtenir ce résultat correspond à une ration de 25 à 35 g de chou par cobaye et par jour, complétée par du pain ou de l'avoine. La richesse du régime en calcium paraît être un facteur important (VALETTE et CALDERON, 1955).

3. de la saison et vraisemblablement de l'état endocrinien. Le minimum de sensibilité de l'iléon isolé de Cobaye (et de fréquence du caractère composite de sa

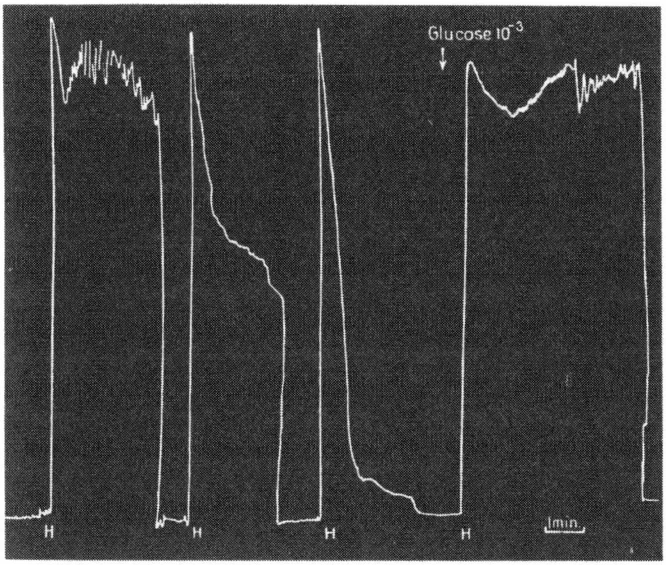

Fig. 2. Iléon de Cobaye (mâle 300 g); tension 2 g; amplification 15 fois. Tyrode sans glucose pour les 3 premiers essais. H: dichlorhydrate d'histamine $0,5 \times 10^{-7}$. Disparition progressive du second sommet. Restitution après addition de glucose (10^{-3}) (PARROT et THOUVENOT, 1956)

réponse à l'histamine) correspond aux mois de février à avril. Les animaux exposés au froid sont moins sensibles.

4. du sexe: le type de réponse composite est plus rarement obtenu chez les femelles, qui paraissent nettement moins sensibles que les mâles à l'histamine, surtout en période de gestation.

2. Influence de la température sur la contraction histaminique de l'iléon

Lorsqu'on obtient la double réponse de l'iléon de Cobaye à l'histamine, les deux composants de cette réponse contractile sont modifiés de manière différente sous l'effet des variations de température: grâce à un dispositif thermostatique spécial permettant de réaliser des variations rapides de la température du bain, on a pu constater que le premier composant fait en général défaut aux températures relativement basses (30° C), alors que l'amplitude du second n'est pas notablement modifiée par l'abaissement de température de 37° à 32°, les autres conditions étant par ailleurs identiques (THOUVENOT et HARICHAUX, 1959). A 35° C, ce même second composant apparaît même plus ample qu'à 37° C.

Ces observations s'accordent sur ce dernier point avec celles de ZADINA (1939), qui avait remarqué que l'amplitude globale de la contraction de l'iléon isolé de Cobaye à l'histamine est plus grande au voisinage de 32° C. Ainsi les deux composants de la contraction histaminique de cet organe sont différenciés par deux optimums thermiques différents, l'un situé à 37°—39° C pour le premier, l'autre à 32°—33° C pour le second.

C. Réponse des divers segments de l'intestin de Cobaye à l'histamine

Dans l'ensemble, la sensibilité du jéjunum à l'histamine est plus faible que celle de l'iléon; mais à condition de faire agir l'histamine à concentration suffisamment élevée (3×10^{-7} à 10^{-6}), on peut obtenir *in vitro* la double contraction de la musculature longitudinale de la partie orale ou moyenne du grêle (Parrot et Thouvenot, 1956).

Le côlon, au contraire, répond fréquemment à l'histamine par une double contraction (fig. 3) (Parrot et Thouvenot, 1956).

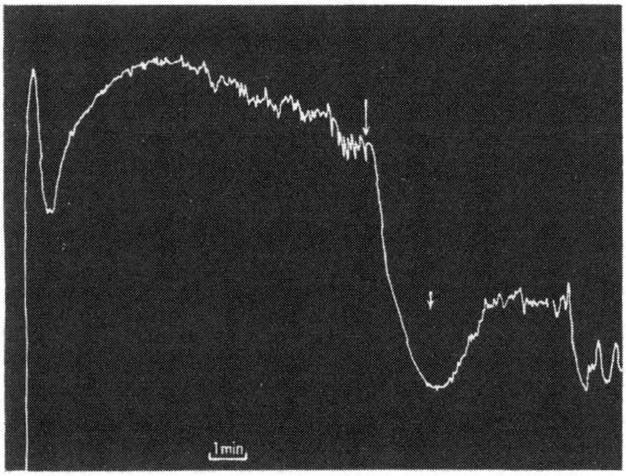

Fig. 3. Côlon gauche de Cobaye, 3 cm, sous tension de 4 g. Amplification 4,5 fois. Glucose 10^{-3}. Dichlorhydrate d'histamine 7×10^{-6}. Après un premier sommet aigu le tracé décrit une courbure dont on remarquera la grande lenteur: son sommet n'est atteint que 3 m 40 s après l'introduction de l'histamine. Activité tonique fortement déprimée par l'atropine (sulfate: 10^{-5} première flèche). Nouvelle addition d'histamine à la même concentration (seconde flèche): réponse de type lent et soutenu, d'ailleurs d'amplitude plus faible (Parrot et Thouvenot, 1956)

D. Caractéristiques mécaniques de la double réponse de l'intestin à l'histamine

A tension modérée (2 g environ), l'amplitude des deux composants peut être sensiblement égale et, dans ce cas, le travail développé (produit du raccourcissement par la tension) est sensiblement égal pour les deux composants. Mais si l'on fait intervenir la notion de temps, le composant initial rapide se révèle notablement plus puissant que le second. De plus, l'amplitude des deux composants est inégalement affectée par des variations de la tension initiale: soumis à des tensions élevées de 3 à 5 g, le premier composant est encore très ample alors que le second subit une réduction notable de son amplitude. Ainsi les deux composants contractiles s'opposent donc par leur inégale puissance (Parrot et Thouvenot, 1956).

Dans les conditions isométriques (Thouvenot et Harichaux, 1961*a*), la tension développée par le premier composant atteint 3 à 5 g en moins de 10 s. Le second correspond à une élévation de tension de 1 à 2 g par rapport au niveau de repos (0,8 à 1,2 g) et l'on observe alors dans ces conditions une chute lente et régulière de la tension, jusqu'au niveau de repos, en quelques minutes, malgré la présence de l'histamine.

Notons que l'excitabilité électrique de l'organe dépend elle aussi de la tension initiale (Thouvenot et Harichaux, 1961*b*).

E. Influence des conditions ioniques sur la double contraction de l'intestin de Cobaye à l'histamine

Dans leur travail original sur le dosage biologique de l'histamine, BARSOUM et GADDUM (1935) constatent diverses influences de la composition ionique sur la contraction du muscle lisse intestinal (cœcum rectal du Poulet). Ainsi l'ion potassium (2×10^{-6} et plus) renforce l'action de l'histamine dans des conditions où l'effet propre de l'ion K^+ est négligeable. Inversement, l'augmentation de la concentration du calcium réduit notablement la sensibilité de l'organe à l'histamine et peut agir en synergie avec les antihistaminiques (LECOMTE, 1950). Cependant ces influences ioniques n'affectent pas de la même manière les deux composants contractiles: l'amplitude du premier composant rapide dépend très étroitement de la concentration du milieu en potassium : elle s'accroît notablement lorsque la concentration du potassium augmente dans le milieu de survie, alors que l'amplitude du second composant soutenu ne subit guère de changements.

On peut obtenir des modifications analogues par augmentation relative du rapport K^+/Ca^{++} en réduisant la concentration du calcium du milieu. A l'opposé, toute réduction de ce rapport à un niveau convenable entraîne la disparition élective du premier composant sans affecter le second. Des perturbations plus profondes de la composition ionique entraînent une réduction de l'excitabilité globale du muscle lisse à divers stimulus de manière non spécifique. Ce point sera repris plus loin.

F. Relation concentration-action

L'étude de la relation quantitative entre la concentration de l'histamine et l'amplitude du raccourcissement a d'abord été poursuivie pour déterminer les conditions du dosage biologique de l'histamine (SCHILD, 1942; CHEN, ENSOR et CLARKE, 1948; PARROT, 1950; THOUVENOT, 1952).

De plus, elle a permis de mettre en évidence la dualité de la contraction histaminique de l'iléon, qui n'a été retrouvée sur les myogrammes qu'en présence de glucose au cours de recherches ultérieures (PARROT et THOUVENOT, 1952, 1956).

Lorsqu'on fait agir l'histamine sur l'iléon isolé de Cobaye, au cours d'essais répétés, on constate que l'amplitude de la contraction ne croît avec la concentration que dans d'étroites limites. Si l'on veut établir une relation précise entre l'action et la concentration de l'histamine sur une zone étendue, on doit:

1. tenir compte de conditions techniques particulières;
2. choisir un mode de représentation du diagramme concentration-action dans un système de coordonnées convenables.

1. Conditions techniques pour déterminer expérimentalement la relation concentration-action

Seule une préparation non distendue, prélevée sur un cobaye mâle de 300 g environ, soumis pendant 10 à 15 jours à un régime légèrement carencé en acide ascorbique et bien à jeun au moment du prélèvement conduit à de bons résultats.

1. On s'assure par des essais préliminaires que les réponses de l'organe isolé sont relativement constantes; ceci suppose en pratique: a) le choix d'une tension convenable avec un optimum voisin de 1,4 à 2 g environ selon la taille de l'intestin; b) la répétition des essais à intervalles rigoureusement constants, étant donné les fluctuations possibles de contractilité telles que nous pouvons les constater vis-à-vis de stimulus électriques, par exemple (THOUVENOT et PASSELEYGUE, 1962); c) le nombre de lavages de la préparation dans l'intervalle des essais doit être constant et effectué dans les mêmes conditions, car chaque lavage perturbe la répartition des ions au voisinage des structures excitables. Il est beaucoup plus difficile

d'obtenir une contractilité constante en présence de glucose; c'est pourquoi beaucoup d'auteurs suppriment le glucose du liquide de survie pour le dosage de l'histamine. Des appareils permettent d'effectuer automatiquement toutes les opérations de rinçage et d'addition d'histamine au bain grâce à des électro-vannes commandées par des circuits de temporisation (SCHILD, 1946).

Lorsque la longueur du fragment se maintient constante pendant sa phase de repos, on peut considérer que son excitabilité se maintient vraisemblablement aussi à une valeur stable. Si l'on constate l'ascension de la ligne de base, c'est-à-dire le raccourcissement progressif de la préparation, on peut s'attendre à voir l'excitabilité augmenter; l'essai doit alors être éliminé, et il faut reprendre l'expérience au cours d'une phase plus stable. Il est souvent utile de modifier légèrement la tension, puis de stimuler régulièrement l'organe par l'histamine jusqu'à obtention d'un nouvel état d'équilibre.

Tout raccourcissement spontané de la préparation correspond à un accroissement de contractilité. Ceci n'est vrai qu'en l'absence de toute contraction histaminique résiduelle. En effet il arrive fréquemment qu'à la suite d'une contraction intense et prolongée obtenue par une concentration élevée de l'histamine (dichlorhydrate 0,1 à 1×10^{-4}), la préparation devienne temporairement réfractaire à de nouvelles stimulations par l'histamine à plus faibles concentrations (CANTONI et EASTMAN, 1946).

2. Analyse des résultats et établissement du diagramme concentration-action

Lorsque le tracé réalisé en présence de glucose montre typiquement la double contraction pour certaines concentrations d'histamine, on peut vérifier dans la zone des faibles concentrations qu'un seul composant s'inscrit sur le myogramme; il s'agit le plus souvent du composant soutenu. Dans ces cas, l'autre composant de la contraction histaminique, qui s'inscrit habituellement sous forme de pointe, n'apparaît qu'aux concentrations plus élevées (PARROT et THOUVENOT, 1952). Pour établir le diagramme action-dose, il est nécessaire de rapporter l'amplitude de chaque contraction à celle de la contraction maximale: l'histamine, à cette concentration, détermine le raccourcissement maximal de la préparation par entrée en jeu de la totalité des éléments contractiles du muscle. Or, les concentrations élevées d'histamine provoquent une diminution de sensibilité pouvant persister pendant plusieurs minutes. D'où la nécessité d'espacer les essais pour les concentrations élevées d'histamine et de faire agir, dans l'intervalle des essais, du chlorure de potassium à dose convenable, de manière à hâter le retour de l'excitabilité à son niveau antérieur.

La hauteur de chaque contraction, mesurée à son sommet sur le tracé, peut être exprimée de manière relative en prenant pour la valeur 100 la hauteur de la contraction maximale. Ainsi exprimée, la hauteur relative de chaque contraction peut être portée en ordonnées et les diverses concentrations, en abscisses. Dans les coordonnées simples, le diagramme est alors représenté par une courbe sigmoïde très asymétrique. Une meilleure représentation est obtenue si on porte en abscisses non les concentrations d'histamine, mais leurs logarithmes: on sait en effet que les actions pharmacologiques sont proportionnelles au logarithme des concentrations du corps actif. Dans ces nouvelles coordonnées, le diagramme s'exprime fréquemment par une courbe sigmoïde symétrique: soixante-dix fois sur une étude de 106 diagrammes (PARROT et THOUVENOT, 1952; THOUVENOT, 1952).

Dans ces cas on peut considérer que dans la zone de 25 à 75 p. 100 de l'action maximale, le raccourcissement est sensiblement proportionnel au logarithme de la concentration d'histamine. La concentration correspondant au milieu de ce segment définit la concentration demi-maximale. Dans le cas le plus simple, un seul composant est représenté sur le myogramme. Un tel diagramme offre l'aspect d'une courbe en ogive de GALTON qui représente la distribution d'unités quantiques relativement indépendantes et normalement distribuées comme le serait la fréquence d'individus ayant succombé à l'action d'un toxique; c'est la distribution normale des statisticiens.

D'une manière générale un point du diagramme exprime, pour une abscisse donnée, le pourcentage d'unités quantiques qui ont répondu. Ces unités pourraient fort bien correspondre déjà à de petits groupements de fibres musculaires lisses, idée exprimée par BERTRAND, GAYET-HALLION et QUIVY (1951). Dans notre cas il fallait admettre à titre d'hypothèse que notre préparation musculaire lisse était composée d'unités contractiles suffisamment petites et nombreuses, indépendantes les unes des autres, normalement distribuées et dont la réponse unitaire est du type «tout ou rien». Si ce type de réponse est bien démontré pour la fibre musculaire striée, son existence est encore très discutée pour le muscle lisse viscéral. BOZLER (1927) admet l'organisation communautaire plutôt que l'indépendance absolue des unités en opposant ce type de muscle à celui du muscle lisse dit à unités multiples, type membrane nictitante du Chat, ce qui semble bien confirmé aujourd'hui (voir BÜLBRING, BURNSTOCK et HOLMAN, 1958).

Toutefois si les unités contractiles fournissent des réponses fluctuant de manière aléatoire autour d'une valeur moyenne et capables de s'additionner, l'on peut alors considérer notre préparation comme une population d'unités contractiles. Les premières unités recrutées sont les plus sensibles à l'histamine; les dernières, les moins sensibles.

Lorsqu'on porte chaque ordonnée sur une échelle probabilité, le diagramme peut être représenté plus simplement par une droite lorsque l'action de l'histamine est simple en présence d'antihistaminiques par exemple (CHEN, ENSOR et CLARKE, 1948). On utilise pour cela les propriétés de l'écart réduit utilisé par GADDUM (1933) ou les probits de BLISS (1934) qui en dérivent.

Un autre système d'ordonnées du type «logistique» permet aussi d'obtenir un diagramme pratiquement linéaire: il consiste à prendre pour ordonnée l'expression log (r/100-r), où r est le raccourcissement relatif rapporté au raccourcissement maximal pris pour valeur 100 (THOUVENOT, 1952).

Dans une étude de 166 diagrammes construits dans le système de coordonnées log-probit (raccourcissement relatif exprimé sous forme de probits en ordonnées, et logarithme des concentrations d'histamine exprimées en abscisses), PARROT et THOUVENOT (1952) ont obtenu dans 34 p. 100 des cas un certain type de diagramme complexe où l'on reconnaît deux parties (fig. 4): un segment de droite, correspondant aux faibles doses, prolongé vers les doses plus élevées par un segment curviligne où la pente croît assez régulièrement jusqu'au voisinage de la dose maximale.

Dès la constatation de ce type de diagramme complexe, l'interprétation suivante a été formulée (PARROT, 1950): pour les faibles concentrations, l'action de l'histamine est simple et correspond au segment de droite initial, mais, aux concentrations plus élevées, l'action résulte de l'addition de deux mécanismes différents mettant en jeu les effecteurs musculaires disponibles.

Une construction graphique permet en effet d'individualiser les deux diagrammes simples dont l'addition rend compte du diagramme complexe.

Grâce à ce système de coordonnées probabilité-logarithme l'action simple de l'histamine sur le muscle lisse est représentée par un diagramme concentration-action linéaire. On peut alors définir la concentration d'histamine correspondant à la moitié de l'action maximale, celle qui met en jeu 50 p. 100 des effecteurs (tableau 1). Il est difficile naturellement de situer avec précision les concentrations correspondant au seuil ou à l'action maximale. Mais le tableau 1 indique les concentrations de dichlorhydrate d'histamine correspondant à 16 et 84 p. 100 de l'action maximale, ce qui permet de définir la pente du diagramme.

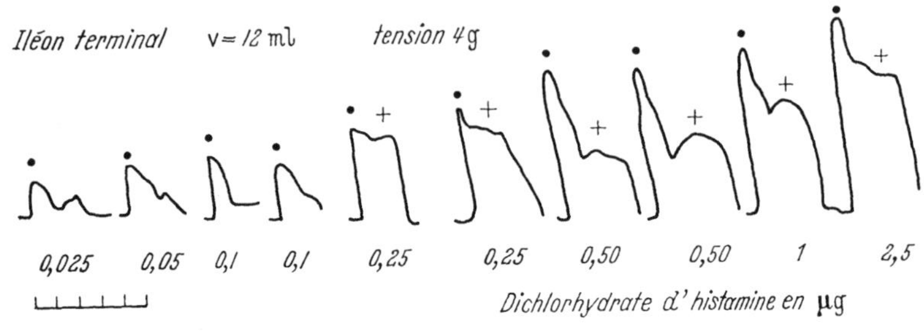

a

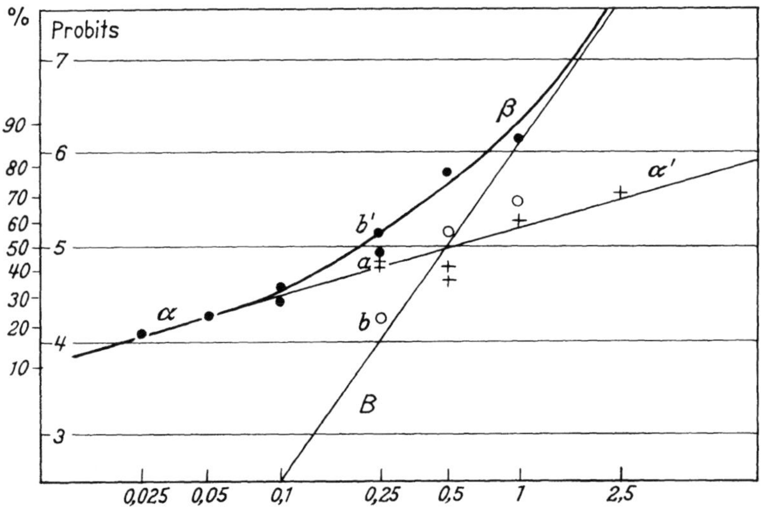

b

Fig. 4. En haut, myogramme isotonique; iléon terminal de Cobaye. L'échelle des temps est indiquée en fractions de 30 s. Les points et les croix indiquent les instants où l'amplitude a été mesurée. En bas, diagramme correspondant. Les doses sont représentées sur une échelle logarithmique. Les amplitudes des contractions sont représentées en pourcentage de la contraction maximale. Les points et les croix correspondent aux mesures fournies par le myogramme. On a utilisé pour les ordonnées une échelle dite de probabilité. Les amplitudes initiales, indiquées par des points, dessinent un diagramme complexe $\alpha\,\beta$; mais une droite $\alpha\,\alpha'$ fournit une représentation satisfaisante de l'un des composants; l'autre composant fournit une autre droite B. (Parrot et Thouvenot, 1952)

Lorsque le diagramme répond au type complexe, l'analyse fondée sur l'addition de deux composants permet de définir les deux droites qui leur correspondent (tableau 1).

La confrontation des diagrammes et des myogrammes complexes fait apparaître qu'un même composant du diagramme correspond à un même composant du myogramme à condition toutefois que les deux réponses phasiques et toniques soient relativement bien séparées dans le temps.

Ainsi ces recherches montrent la double possibilité d'action de l'histamine sur l'intestin.

Tableau 1. *Action de l'histamine sur l'iléon isolé du cobaye caractéristique du diagramme action-dose. Concentrations moyennes exprimées en µg de dichlorhydrate d'histamine par centimètre cube.* (Les chiffres entre parenthèses indiquent les limites entre lesquelles 68 pour cent des résultats se placent; ils sont fournis par le calcul de l'écart-type sur le logarithme des doses)

Type de diagr.	Nb. de diagr.		Concentration correspondant à la contraction représentant 16 pour 100 de l'action maximale[1]	Concentration correspondant à la contraction demi-maximale	Concentration correspondant à la contraction représentant 84 pour 100 de l'action maximale[1]
Rectil.	70		0,033 (0,027—0,040)	0,110 (0,104—0,113)	0,354 (0,29—0,43)
Composite	36	α	0,037 (0,035—0,040)	0,38 (0,31—0,47)	3,90 (3,7—4,1)
		β	0,096 (0,035—0,26)	0,17 (0,072—0,40)	0,30 (0,11—0,81)

[1] Ces valeurs ont été obtenues en partant de l'écart-type sur le logarithme des doses. Celui-ci est évalué en fonction de la pente de la droite correspondante obtenue dans le système logarithme-probabilité (droite unique ou droites α et β suivant le cas); cet écart-type, qui caractérise le groupement des unités contractiles mises en jeu, est inversement proportionnel à la pente. (D'après PARROT et THOUVENOT, 1952).

Une même dualité se retrouve à propos de l'antagonisme histamine-antihistaminique pour lequel SEGRE et FALCO (1952) trouvent avec la mépyramine (néo-antergan) deux types de récepteurs: un type d'antagonisme s'exerce à faible concentration de mépyramine, l'autre à concentration plus élevée. PARROT et THOUVENOT (1957*b*) ont constaté avec ce même antihistaminique à faible concentration (10^{-12}) la disparition élective de la réponse nerveuse, comme si l'antihistaminique se fixait plus facilement sur les structures nerveuses du plexus myentérique que sur les structures musculaires.

G. Mécanisme d'action de l'histamine sur le muscle lisse viscéral

1. Essais de dissociation de la part nerveuse et musculaire directe de l'action de l'histamine

Le muscle lisse intestinal est en étroite relation avec le plexus nerveux myentérique d'AUERBACH; celui-ci est situé entre les deux couches musculaires, et son automatisme résiste à l'énervation extrinsèque (LANGLEY). Aussi l'activation du muscle lisse par l'histamine pourrait-elle résulter d'une action s'exerçant soit directement soit par l'intermédiaire du système nerveux ganglionnaire intrinsèque. AMBACHE (1946) puis J. LÉVY et MICHEL-BER (1953) se sont efforcés de définir expérimentalement les critères de l'action musculaire directe ou de l'action musculaire indirecte que certains agents pharmacologiques peuvent exercer par le jeu des neurones ganglionnaires.

Ces neurones peuvent être inactivés expérimentalement par trois méthodes: le traitement par le froid, l'emploi des ganglioplégiques et enfin l'énervation par des toxines spécifiques: toxine botulinique (AMBACHE et LESSIN, 1955).

2. L'action musculaire directe

a) Mise en évidence

En fait les conclusions sur le mode d'action direct ou indirect de l'histamine se sont dégagées progressivement de résultats expérimentaux parfois contradictoires. C'est ainsi qu' AMBACHE (1946) observe, après traitement de l'intestin par le froid, la perte de sa réactivité vis-à-vis de l'histamine, ainsi que des chlorures de potassium ou de baryum; l'action de l'histamine déprimée dans ces expériences pourrait correspondre au composant d'origine nerveuse. En revanche l'action musculaire directe de l'acétylcholine et l'effet de la stimulation électrique persistent. Un autre critère de l'action indirecte de l'histamine est, selon AMBACHE, l'aptitude de cette amine, comme de l'ion Ba^{++}, à stimuler la synthèse de l'acétylcholine. FELDBERG (1950) montre cependant que la synthèse de l'acétylcholine par l'intestin peut être active dans un tissu qui est dépourvu d'éléments nerveux ou dans lequel ceux-ci sont rendus inactifs.

De leur côté, EMMELIN et FELDBERG (1947) observent que l'action de l'histamine est réduite comme d'ailleurs celles de l'acétylcholine et de la pilocarpine sous l'effet de la nicotine. Toutefois l'exclusion fonctionnelle des éléments nerveux du plexus d'AUERBACH par la nicotine s'est heurtée à des difficultés. Cette substance, en effet, s'est montrée, elle aussi, capable d'action secondaire musculaire dépressive, surtout lorsqu'elle vient d'être introduite dans le bain; c'est ainsi que, sous son effet, l'action de l'histamine sur l'intestin est réduite temporairement, et il en est de même des réponses à de faibles concentrations d'acétylcholine, de pilocarpine, de 2268 F (AMBACHE, 1949); or ce sont des agents qui exercent une action musculaire prédominante. En revanche on assiste fréquemment, après élimination de la nicotine par lavages, à un rebondissement des effets de l'histamine (FELDBERG, 1951; PARROT et THOUVENOT, 1957b).

Certains corps à action nicotinique plus spécifique à concentration dépressive (iodure de phénoxycholine: $2,6 \times 10^{-6}$; mono et dibromophénylcholine: 8×10^{-7} à 8×10^{-6}) n'ont pas modifié le composant soutenu de l'action de l'histamine; or à ces concentrations la réponse précoce à l'histamine est complètement supprimée, de même que l'action répétée de ces mêmes corps à concentration stimulante; ceci peut être interprété comme la preuve de l'interruption de la transmission au niveau des synapses du plexus d'AUERBACH (PARROT et THOUVENOT, 1957b).

L'emploi des ganglioplégiques tels que l'hexaméthonium a permis de constater que la principale action de l'histamine résiste au bloquage ganglionnaire; celui-ci est contrôlé par l'emploi de nicotiniques stimulants, nicotine, chlorure de potassium dont l'action disparaît (FELDBERG, 1951). Dans ces expériences de FELDBERG, l'iléon de Cobaye était aussi maintenu en présence de glucose (10^{-3}) et la réponse de l'organe correspondait vraisemblablement au type soutenu à l'état pur.

Ce fait a été confirmé par PARROT et THOUVENOT (1954) au cours d'expériences comportant un contact limité à quelques minutes avec le bromure d'hexaméthonium (10^{-5}): dans ces conditions la disparition du composant précoce fait contraste avec la persistance de l'action directe de l'histamine sur la fibre lisse.

Cette phase soutenue de la réponse à l'histamine résiste de plus à l'action d'agents dépresseurs de la conduction nerveuse (cocaïne, procaïne) qui font au contraire disparaître le composant précoce et inconstant (PARROT et THOUVENOT, 1957b); la phase soutenue peut même se trouver renforcée en présence de cocaïne comme le signale FELDBERG (1950).

Ainsi la comparaison des modifications pharmacologiques des composants précoce et tardif suggère bien l'opposition des mécanismes d'action: l'action soutenue de l'histamine apparaît ainsi comme une action musculaire directe, insensible à l'action d'agents pharmacologiques aux concentrations capables de déprimer électivement la réponse précoce.

L'atropine (sulfate $0,5 \times 10^{-7}$ à 10^{-5}) ne modifie pas non plus la réponse soutenue de l'intestin à l'histamine. Ainsi la réponse lente et soutenue apparaît comme la principale action de l'histamine qui n'engage que la fibre lisse; et cette action est différente de celle qu'exerce l'acétylcholine dans son action musculaire directe.

b) *Nature de l'action directe de l'histamine*

α) La spécificité des récepteurs musculaires à l'histamine. Il semble d'après l'étude de l'antagonisme histamine-antihistaminiques que les récepteurs du muscle lisse à l'histamine soient distincts de ceux sur lesquels agissent la 5-hydroxytryptamine et l'acétylcholine dans leurs actions musculaires directes; les antihistaminiques les plus spécifiques, la mépyramine par exemple aux concentrations pour lesquelles l'action de l'histamine est électivement déprimée (10^{-9} à 10^{-12}), ne modifient pas notablement la réponse à ces autres agents[1]; d'autre part lorsque l'atropine bloque l'action musculaire directe de l'acétylcholine, on n'observe aucune modification significative du composant soutenu de la contraction histaminique.

On met depuis longtemps cette propriété en application pour le dosage de l'histamine dans des extraits contenant par ailleurs des corps, dont l'action est voisine de celle de l'acétylcholine, et souvent plus stables que cette dernière substance: tel est le facteur étudié par PARROT et RICHET (1943) dans certains échantillons de sang humain.

β) Histamine et polarisation membranaire. Un autre point concerne le mécanisme de l'excitation musculaire. Les électrophysiologistes ont bien montré la relation qui existe entre les mécanismes de polarisation membranaire et l'excitation; ce fait est bien démontré pour le nerf et le muscle strié (HUXLEY, 1957) et paraît l'être pour le muscle lisse (BÜLBRING, 1955). Le muscle intestinal s'apparente aux tissus autorythmiques par l'instabilité de la polarisation membranaire dont le fonctionnement rappelle un peu celui du tissu nodal.

Lorsque, à la suite d'une décharge, la cellule musculaire se repolarise, cette repolarisation ne se maintient pas à niveau stable; la polarisation décroît ensuite jusqu'au point de déclenchement du potentiel d'action propagé (BÜLBRING, 1957): cette décroissance spontanée et rapide du potentiel de membrane se révèle sur les enregistrements électriques sous forme d'un prépotentiel. Ceux-ci peuvent persister en présence d'atropine, alors que les potentiels de pointe rapides disparaissent (BURNSTOCK, 1958).

Tout agent capable de faire décroître la polarisation augmente l'excitabilité: tel est le cas de l'histamine comme de l'acétylcholine; au contraire, une substance capable de favoriser la polarisation de la membrane diminue l'excitabilité; tel est le cas de l'adrénaline dans certaines conditions (BÜLBRING, 1957, BÜLBRING et BURNSTOCK, 1960).

On connaît les nombreux travaux qui ont récemment démontré l'origine métabolique de la polarisation membranaire (CIER, 1961): celle-ci n'est que la conséquence de l'inégale répartition des ions de part et d'autre des membranes cellulaires. Cette répartition ionique est, on le sait, déterminée par les transferts actifs métaboliques. La cellule au repos concentre le potassium à l'intérieur, et rejette activement le sodium (processus dit de la «pompe à sodium» de HODGKIN et HUXLEY, 1952). Il existe une relation linéaire assez étroite entre la valeur du potentiel de repos (de 50 à 70 mV) et le logarithme de la concentration du milieu extracellulaire en potassium. L'histamine fait croître de manière importante la fuite du potassium de l'intestin. Cet effet disparaît en présence d'un antihistaminique tel que la mépyramine (PARROT, THOUVENOT et LONGUEVALLE, 1953). Cette libération du potassium sous l'effet de l'histamine a été confirmée par MACMILLAN et VANE (1956), et BORN et BÜLBRING (1956).

γ) Potentiels d'action du muscle lisse et effet de l'histamine. Les potentiels d'action spontanés du muscle lisse intestinal sont aussi très particuliers: leur amplitude,

[1] Toutefois on a signalé une action secondaire anti-5-hydroxytryptamine de la mépyramine, relativement faible.

de l'ordre de 60 mV, est assez variable, contrairement à celle des potentiels d'action des muscles striés, qui est de l'ordre de 120 mV. Lorsque les potentiels d'action du muscle lisse se répètent sous forme de salves, leur amplitude est d'autant plus faible que la fréquence est plus élevée. Quoi qu'il en soit, la tension développée par le muscle lisse, dans des conditions isométriques, est en relation avec la fréquence des potentiels rapides (fig. 5) (Bülbring, 1955, 1961). Cependant la polarisation du muscle lisse n'est pas dominée par le jeu des variations de concentration en potassium de manière aussi étroite que pour le muscle strié: si l'on compare la composition ionique du muscle lisse à celle du muscle strié, on constate

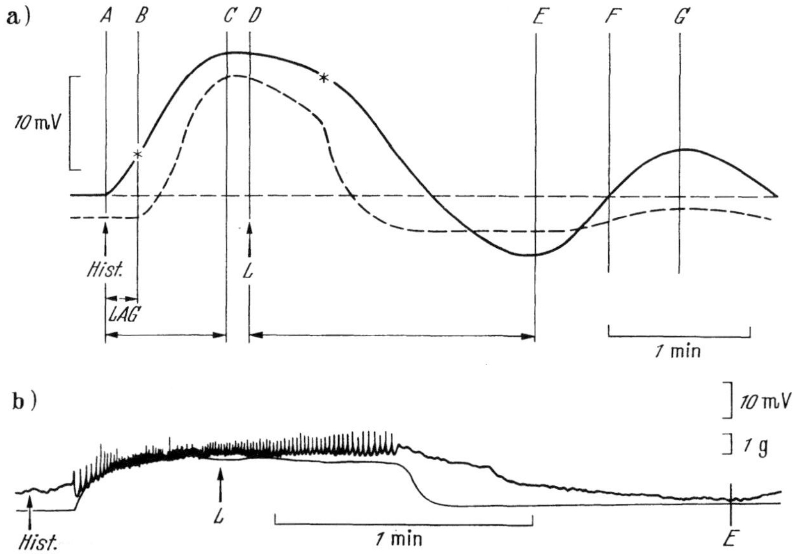

Fig. 5. (a) Diagramme représentant la suite des phénomènes consécutifs à l'administration d'une substance qui stimule le muscle lisse. Ligne continue: potentiel de membrane; ligne interrompue: tension (en g) AB = „LAG": temps de latence; en B: début des potentiels d'action et accroissement de la tension. C: réponses électrique et mécanique maximales; D: lavage; DEFG: fluctuations oscillatoires de la polarisation modifiant parallèlement l'excitabilité. (b) Enregistrement des variations électriques (tracé supérieur) et des variations de tension (tracé inférieur) produites par l'histamine à 10^{-7}. (Bülbring et Burnstock, 1960)

que le milieu intracellulaire du premier renferme moins de potassium (environ 105 mEq) et davantage de sodium (environ 64 mEq) que le muscle strié (K^+: 155 mEq; Na^+: 12 mEq; v. Burnstock, Holman et Prosser, 1963). Il est possible que l'excitabilité du muscle lisse et sa sensibilité à l'histamine ne dépendent pas uniquement des variations de concentration en potassium de part et d'autre de la membrane. C'est ainsi que la réduction de moitié de la concentration du sodium d'une solution de Krebs rétablit la sensibilité à l'histamine de l'utérus de Cobaye qui avait été déprimée par un antihistaminique (McDowall et Soliman, 1954).

Une préparation musculaire lisse plus pure est représentée par le *taenia coli* du Cobaye: sa réponse à l'histamine est précédée et accompagnée de potentiels d'action, mais ceux-ci ressemblent davantage aux potentiels locaux des muscles d'Arthropodes, survenant au cours de la phase de dépolarisation soutenue, qu'aux potentiels quantiques de la fibre striée (Bülbring, 1955).

δ) Possibilité d'une action plus directe de l'histamine sur les éléments contractiles indépendante des phénomènes d'excitation électrique. La stimulation électrique de l'intestin, qui suscite si facilement des contractions de type rapide, ne provoque pas les contractions lentes et soutenues comparables à celles qu'on obtient si aisément avec l'histamine, quels que soient les paramètres ou les conditions techniques (Parrot et Thouvenot, 1957a). Ceci peut suggérer que l'histamine pourrait agir sur l'élément contractile de la fibre lisse, indépendamment des processus d'excitation qui résultent du bloquage des transferts ioniques au niveau de la membrane. La stimulation électrique ne fait d'ailleurs jouer que ces derniers mécanismes. On connaît dans d'autres domaines des exemples d'une dissociation analogue entre l'excitabilité électrique et la sensibilité aux agents chimiques: la membrane nictitante du Chat, peu excitable à la stimulation électrique, surtout lorsqu'elle est énervée, est en revanche très sensible, comme on le sait, à l'adrénaline (Eccles et Magladery, 1937); dans le même ordre d'idée rappelons l'existence dans le système nerveux central de certaines formations plus sensibles aux agents chimiques qu'aux agents électriques (Grundfest et Schedlowski, 1957).

Il apparaît raisonnable d'admettre que les organites contractiles de la fibre musculaire lisse puissent être mis en jeu de deux manières: soit indirectement par la chaîne des processus membranaires, soit directement par couplage plus direct avec les processus chimiques qui aboutissent à la contraction des myofibrilles.

Cette conception peut être appuyée sur des expériences qui montrent les possibilités du découplage entre l'activité électrique et les phénomènes mécaniques: le 2—4 dinitrophénol, par exemple, fait croître la fréquence des potentiels d'action du muscle lisse ainsi que la fuite du potassium; cependant la force contractile décroît (Bülbring, 1957; Bülbring et Lüllmann, 1957). Il en est de même pour d'autres inhibiteurs du métabolisme (Axelsson, Bueding et Bülbring, 1959). On connaît, depuis les travaux de Bacq (1939) et de ses collaborateurs, l'efficacité de diverses substances, dont la vératrine, et ses principaux alcaloïdes (cévadine, vératridine, etc.), pour augmenter l'action dépolarisante de l'ion potassium. Or Parrot et Thouvenot (1953, 1957b) ont observé que ces substances modifient peu la phase soutenue de la réponse à l'histamine, contrairement à la phase précoce et inconstante de cette réponse.

Ces corps vératriniques retentissent vraisemblablement sur les mécanismes qui assurent la polarisation membranaire, de même que certains glucosides cardiotoniques (Dunham et Glynn, 1961). La phase soutenue de la contraction histaminique pourrait être dans certaines conditions relativement indépendante des phénomènes de polarisation membranaire.

De plus le refroidissement conjugué à la suppression du glucose conduit au renforcement paradoxal de l'activité électrique et, comme nous l'avons vu, à la disparition de toute contraction de caractère soutenu en réponse à l'histamine. Enfin la dissociation entre les phénomènes mécaniques et électriques du muscle lisse peut être encore obtenue grâce à l'emploi de milieux dépourvus d'ions Na (l'isotonie est alors assurée par du ClLi, ou par de l'hydrazine ou encore par de la choline); dans ces cas toute activité mécanique disparaît alors que persiste l'activité électrique (Burnstock et Straub, 1958).

Inversement on peut citer d'après le travail d'Evans, Schild et Thesleff (1958) des cas où l'activité mécanique du muscle lisse persistait malgré la disparition de toute activité électrique: ainsi la caféïne peut faire croître le tonus du muscle lisse sans variation du potentiel de membrane.

Dans ce même travail, ces auteurs rapportent qu'un muscle lisse, tel que celui de l'amnios de Poulet, complètement dépolarisé par séjour dans une solution riche en K^+ mais complètement dépourvue de Na^+, devient totalement inexcitable au courant électrique, mais reste encore parfaitement capable de répondre à l'histamine ainsi qu'à l'acétylcholine, la 5-hydroxytryptamine et l'ocytocine.

Aussi entrevoyons-nous deux possibilités pour l'action musculaire directe de l'histamine, une action excitante par dépolarisation et une action plus directe sur le métabolisme lié à la contraction; celle-ci serait encore différente de celle qu'exercent l'acétylcholine et la 5-hydroxytryptamine, en raison de la spécificité relative des antagonistes pharmacologiques.

H. Mécanisme de la contraction histaminique précoce

1. Son existence

Si l'action musculaire directe est la principale action de l'histamine sur la fibre lisse intestinale, l'analyse du diagramme concentration-action d'abord (Parrot, 1950), puis du myogramme obtenu en présence du glucose (Parrot et Thouvenot, 1952, 1956) nous a révélé que l'histamine peut provoquer assez fréquemment une contraction précoce puissante, mais de courte durée: celle-ci interfère assez fréquemment avec la phase soutenue, de sorte que bien souvent elle est peu apparente sur les tracés myographiques et qu'elle échappe à beaucoup d'auteurs travaillant sur ce test biologique, l'iléon de Cobaye.

Lorsque cette réponse précoce est assez bien différenciée sur le myogramme, on peut constater que de nombreuses interventions expérimentales la modifient électivement.

Plusieurs faits plaident en faveur d'un mécanisme ganglionnaire pour cette action précoce de l'histamine.

C'est ainsi que le bloquage ganglionnaire obtenu par l'hexaméthonium ou des nicotiniques dans leur action dépressive (bromophénylcholine et phénoxycholine) supprime électivement ce composant précoce, le composant tardif, nous le savons, n'étant pas modifié (Parrot et Thouvenot, 1954, 1957). On peut de plus constater sa disparition sous l'effet d'un refroidissement modéré (Parrot et Thouvenot, 1957b; Thouvenot et Harichaux, 1959) et sous l'effet de la fatigue; sa labilité et son inconstance ont été constatées dès le début de ces recherches (Parrot et Thouvenot, 1952).

De plus, la procaïne et la cocaïne font disparaître cet effet précoce de l'histamine (Parrot et Thouvenot, 1957 b), fait à rapprocher des constatations de Frommel, Favre et Vallette (1947) concernant déjà la dépression de l'action de l'histamine sur l'iléon de Cobaye, sans que ces auteurs aient dissocié les deux composants.

D'ailleurs l'accroissement rapide de la concentration du potassium dans le bain à un niveau donné ($2{,}5 \times 10^{-4}$, par exemple) peut provoquer une réponse phasique en tout point analogue au premier composant de l'action de l'histamine. Feldberg (1951) a montré, grâce à l'emploi de l'hexaméthonium alors récemment découvert, l'action excitoganglionnaire de l'ion K^+ dans les conditions de concentration utilisées.

De plus l'action «phasique» de l'ion K^+ subit les mêmes modifications pharmacologiques que le composant précoce de l'action de l'histamine: renforcement par la vératrine et ses alcaloïdes ainsi que par le sulfocyanure de sodium (Parrot et Thouvenot, 1953, 1957b).

L'interprétation de ces diverses expériences conduit à supposer que l'histamine agit en amont de la chaîne nerveuse qui met en jeu le neurone cholinergique effecteur: l'hexaméthonium par exemple ne se comporte pas comme un agent compétitif de l'histamine, mais bien de l'acétylcholine libérée par excitation du neurone préganglionnaire. La commande de la fibre musculaire sous l'effet de ce mécanisme nerveux paraît bien être cholinergique; l'atropine supprime électivement cette action de l'histamine, l'ésérine (sulfate: 10^{-10} et 10^{-9}) la renforce (Parrot et Thouvenot, 1957b).

Ce type de contraction phasique est d'ailleurs analogue à celle que provoquent les agents nicotiniques stimulants ainsi que l'ion potassium.

On a pu obtenir ce même type de réponse phasique au moyen de la stimulation électrique itérative appliquée concentriquement à l'intestin sous distension modérée (Paton, 1955; Parrot et Thouvenot, 1957a).

2. Signification du mécanisme nerveux déclenché par l'action pharmacologique de l'histamine

L'histamine, dans sa phase précoce, peut susciter l'excitation des neurones préganglionnaires et mettre en jeu artificiellement un mécanisme nerveux cholinergique; celui-ci est alors capable de déterminer un type de réponse phasique qui doit bien correspondre à un mécanisme physiologique élémentaire de la motricité intestinale.

Ce problème a été abordé grâce à l'enregistrement des contractions longitudinales de deux zones orale et aborale d'un long fragment d'intestin; la technique permet de dissocier, parmi les diverses activités contractiles, celles qui restent localisées de celles qui sont capables de se propager dans le sens oral-aboral (THOUVENOT, 1957; THOUVENOT et HARICHAUX, 1961a, b et c).

Dans ces conditions il est possible de retrouver la double action de l'histamine et de constater que la distension de l'intestin favorise l'apparition du composant rapide; la distension réalisée, de l'ordre de 0,2 à 0,5 cm d'eau, est inférieure à celle qui provoque le déclenchement du péristaltisme; cette distension infraliminaire peut faire apparaître le composant phasique de l'action de l'histamine alors que l'action initiale de l'histamine est simple et de type soutenu[1].

De plus on a pu constater la propagation sous forme d'onde contractile du composant phasique à la vitesse de 4 à 16 cm/s (fig. 6); cette vitesse est du même ordre de grandeur que celle que ces auteurs ont obtenue dans leurs essais de péristaltisme *in vitro*. Il existe d'ailleurs une réelle analogie mécanique entre la réponse phasique à l'histamine et la phase d'évacuation du péristaltisme telle que l'a décrite TRENDELENBURG (1917). Cette phase d'évacuation consiste en une réponse des deux couches circulaires et longitudinales en opposition ou en concordance de phase selon les cas (TRENDELENBURG, 1917; KOSTERLITZ et coll., 1956; THOUVENOT

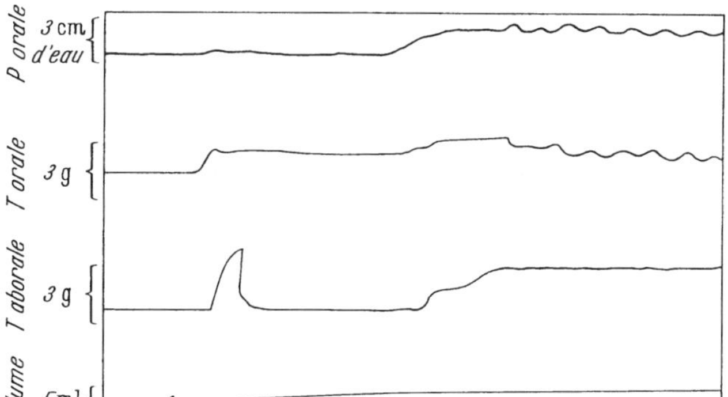

Fig. 6. Action péristaltogène de l'histamine dans son action précoce sur l'iléon isolé de Cobaye (longueur totale du fragment étudié 38 cm). *De haut en bas:* 1° pression intra-intestinale de la zone orale; 2° tension des fibres longitudinales de la zone orale sur une longueur de 4 cm; 3° tension des fibres longitudinales de la zone aborale terminale dans les mêmes conditions; 4° volume débité par l'anse. L'histamine (50 µg), déposée dans la partie orale de la cuve (signal en surimpression sur la ligne de débit), suscite la réponse orale diphasique; le composant précoce se propage en 1,9 s à la zone aborale, provoquant l'onde péristaltique à l'état pur. Elle s'accompagne d'un début d'évacuation. Ultérieurement la distension de 3 cm d'eau de l'extrémité orale provoque le péristaltisme oral, dont la propagation n'est plus observée sur la zone aborale. Temps: 5 s, température 37° C. Volume total du bain: 40 ml (celui-ci est irrigué dans le sens antipéristaltique). (THOUVENOT et HARICHAUX, 1961)

[1] L'action soutenue de l'histamine peut perturber la phase préparatoire du péristaltisme (KOSTERLITZ et ROBINSON, 1957) mais ne supprime pas son déclenchement (THOUVENOT et HARICHAUX, 1961) (v. fig. 6).

et HARICHAUX, 1961); elle met en jeu le plexus nerveux d'AUERBACH. L'hexaméthonium bloque électivement ce type de réponse (KOSTERLITZ et ROBINSON, 1957).

On peut alors se demander si le composant précoce de l'action de l'histamine ne résulterait pas de l'intervention de facteurs mécaniques locaux.

Il est possible que la seule action musculaire de l'histamine modifie l'état des récepteurs de distension à l'origine du réflexe péristaltique tels qu'ils ont été étudiés récemment par GINZEL (1959); cette hypothèse expliquerait que le déclenchement de la réponse phasique résulte de la sommation du stimulus distension et du stimulus histamine dans les conditions du péristaltisme *in vitro*. Ainsi se pose de nouveau le problème des interactions des facteurs mécaniques dans l'étude des actions pharmacologiques, problème sur lequel TRENDELENBURG (1917) avait déjà attiré l'attention.

Cette hypothèse permet d'expliquer la mise en jeu d'un arc nerveux comportant plusieurs neurones dont certains sont cholinergiques et dont la signification fonctionnelle est liée habituellement à l'activité propulsive de l'intestin.

Conclusion

L'histamine fait contracter la plupart des muscles lisses chez de nombreuses espèces de Poissons, d'Oiseaux et de Mammifères.

C'est souvent la sensibilité de telle ou telle musculature lisse qui caractérise chez une espèce donnée les signes de l'intoxication aiguë. Ainsi la broncho-constriction du Cobaye exposé aux aérosols d'histamine entraîne une mort rapide.

La broncho-constriction est à la base de certaines techniques de dosage biologique. Il est aussi possible d'étudier l'effet directement sur des préparations isolées d'«anneaux bronchiques». L'accroissement de la résistance bronchique a pu aussi être étudié récemment à partir des relations pression-débit ventilatoire.

L'action que l'histamine exerce sur la fibre lisse intestinale est plus complexe, car elle est étroitement liée au fonctionnement du plexus myentérique. Elle peut être étudiée chez le Cobaye, qui est l'espèce la plus sensible à l'histamine: l'iléon isolé est utilisé depuis longtemps pour le dosage biologique. L'histamine suscite à certaines concentrations une double réponse contractile de cette préparation: une réponse précoce, rapide, puissante, mais non soutenue, suivie d'une réponse lente et moins ample; l'amplitude et la durée de cette dernière dépend de la concentration du glucose dans le bain d'organe. Ces deux types de réponse peuvent expliquer la complexité du diagramme qui représente l'action contractile en fonction de la concentration de l'histamine: l'addition de deux composants élémentaires rend compte de la courbe complexe que l'on obtient en coordonnées probit-logarithme; on sait que ces coordonnées permettent généralement de représenter par une ligne droite les actions pharmacologiques, simples, qui s'exercent sur une population d'effecteurs musculaires indépendants les uns des autres, normalement distribués et réagissant de manière quantique.

Des deux composants, celui qui est lent et tardif représente l'action constante de l'histamine sur la fibre lisse; celle-ci résiste à l'atropine, aux bloquants ganglionnaires, aux modifications ioniques et à celles de la perméabilité membranaire. Il s'agit d'une action directe que l'histamine exerce sur la fibre lisse, et qui est distincte de celle qu'exerce l'acétylcholine ou la 5-hydroxytryptamine.

Il est possible que cette action soutenue dépende peu des phénomènes d'excitation membranaire qui sont à l'origine des manifestations électriques, bien qu'une action dépolarisante de l'histamine ait été décrite et bien étudiée.

Quant à la contraction puissante et précoce que suscite fréquemment l'histamine, elle est supprimée électivement par bloquage ganglionnaire: elle résulte de l'intervention de neurones cholinergiques. Ce type de réponse peut être identifié à la composante longitudinale du mouvement péristaltique qui met en jeu le plexus myentérique; il est intéressant de constater que l'histamine peut la déclencher.

Bibliographie

ALEXANDER, F.: The action of some humoral agents on the horse intestine. Quart. J. exp. Physiol. **35**, 11—24 (1949).

ALEXANDER, H. L., W. G. BECKE, and J. A. HOLMES: Reactions of sensitized guinea pigs to inhaled antigens. J. Immunol. **11**, 175—189 (1926).

AMBACHE, N.: Interaction of drugs and the effect of cooling on the isolated mammalian intestine. J. Physiol. (Lond.) **104**, 266—287 (1946).

— The nicotinic action of substances supposed to be purely smooth-muscle stimulating (a) effects of α, β ethylal-γ-trimethyl-ammonium-propanediol (2268 F) upon skeletal muscle and ganglion cells. J. Physiol. (Lond.) **110**, 145—163 (1949).

—, and A. W. LESSIN: Classification of intestinomotor drugs by means of type D botulinum toxin. J. Physiol. (Lond.) **127**, 449—478 (1955).

AXELSSON, J., E. BUEDING, and E. BÜLBRING: The action of adrenaline on phosphorylase activity and membrane potential of smooth muscle. J. Physiol. (Lond.) **148**, 62—63 P (1959).

BACQ, Z. M.: Ions et corps vératriniques. Arch. int. Pharmacodyn. **63**, 59—87 (1939).

BARGETON, D., G. BARRÈS, R. LEFEBVRE DES NOETTES et P. GAUGE. Mesure de la résistance des voies aériennes de l'homme dans la respiration normale. J. Physiol. (Paris) **49**, 37—40 (1957).

BARSOUM, G. S., and J. H. GADDUM: The pharmacological estimation of adenosine and histamine in blood. J. Physiol. (Lond.) **85**, 1 (1935).

BERTRAND, I., TH. GAYET-HALLION et D. QUIVY: Existence de groupements fonctionnels de la musculature de l'intestin révélée par l'analyse de variance. C. R. Acad. Sci. (Paris) **232**, 1157 (1951).

BLISS, C. I.: The method of "probits". Science **74**, 38—39 et 408—409 (1934).

BORN, G. V. R., and E. BÜLBRING: The movement of potassium between smooth muscle and the surrounding fluid. J. Physiol. (Lond.) **131**, 690—703 (1956).

BOVET, D., et F. BOVET-NITTI: Structure et activité pharmacodynamique des médicaments du système nerveux végétatif. 1 vol. 849 p. Bâle-New-York: S. Karger 1948.

—, et F. WALTHERT: Structure chimique et activité pharmacodynamique des antihistaminiques de synthèse. Ann. pharm. franç. **2** (suppl. n° 4), 1—43 (1944).

BOZLER, E.: Über die Tätigkeit der einzelnen glatten Muskelfaser bei der Kontraktion. Z. vergl. Physiol. **6**, 361—377 (1927).

BÜLBRING, E.: Correlation between membrane potential, spike discharge and tension in smooth muscle. J. Physiol. (Lond.) **128**, 220—221 (1955).

— Humoral transmitters and smooth muscle. Brit. med. Bull. **13**, (3), 172—180 (1957).

— Die Physiologie des glatten Muskels. Pflügers Arch. ges. Physiol. **273**, 1—17 (1961).

—, and G. BURNSTOCK: Membrane potential changes associated with tachyphylaxis and potentiation of the response to stimulating drugs in smooth muscle. Brit. J. Pharmacol. **15**, 611—624 (1960).

— —, and M. E. HOLMAN: Excitation and conduction in the smooth muscle of the isolated taenia coli of the guinea-pig. J. Physiol. (Lond.) **192**, 420—437 (1958).

—, and H. LÜLLMANN: The effect of metabolic inhibitors on the electrical and mechanical activity of the smooth muscle of the guinea-pig's taenia coli. J. Physiol. (Lond.) **136**, 310—323 (1957).

BURNSTOCK, G.: The action of adrenaline on excitability and membrane potential in the taenia coli of the guinea-pig and the effect of D.N.P. on this action and on the action of acetylcholine. J. Physiol. (Lond.) **143**, 183—194 (1958).

—, M. E. HOLMAN, and C. L. PROSSER: Electrophysiology of smooth muscle. Physiol. Rev. **43**, 482—527 (1963).

—, and R. W. STRAUB: A method for studying the effects of ions and drugs on the resting and action potentials in smooth muscle with external electrodes. J. Physiol. (Lond.) **140**, 156—167 (1958).

BURSTEIN, M.: Recherches sur la physiologie des muscles brouchiques. Thèse Doct. Sci. Paris 96 p 1946.

CANTONI, G. L., and G. EASTMAN: On the response of the intestine to smooth muscle stimulants. J. Pharmacol. exp. Ther. **87**, 392—399 (1946).

Carlson, A. J., and A. B. Luckhardt: Studies on the visceral sensory nervous system. I. Lung automatism and lung reflexes in the frog. Amer. J. Physiol. **54**, 55—95 (1920).

Castillo, J. del, et E. J. de Beer: Cité d'après Bacq et coll. Pharmacodynamie biochimique, 1 vol. 1227 p. Voir p. 234. Paris: Masson éd. 1961.

Charlier, R., et L. Vandermissen: Une méthode simple d'enregistrement des modifications du volume pulmonaire chez le chien anesthésié. Arch. int. Physiol. **62**, 433—444 (1954).

Chen, G., Ch. R. Ensor, and I. G. Clarke: The biological assay of histamine and diphenhydramine hydrochloride (benadryl hydrochloride). J. Pharmacol. exp. Ther. **92**, 90—97 (1948).

Cier, J. F.: Les facteurs métaboliques et hormonaux de la répartition intra et extracellulaire du sodium et du potassium. J. Physiol. (Paris) **53**, 3—74 (1961).

Collier, H. O. J., J. A. Holgate, M. Schachter and P. G. Shorley: The bronchoconstrictor action of bradykinin in the guinea-pig. Brit. J. Pharmacol. **15**, 290—297 (1960).

—, and P. G. Shorley: Analgesic antipyretic drugs as antagonists of bradykinin. Brit. J. Pharmacol. **15**, 601—610 (1960).

Cordier, D., et H. Magne: Physiologie des muscles bronchiques du Cobaye. Ann. Physiol. Physicochim. biol. **3**, 486—488 (1927).

Dale, H. H., and P. P. Laidlaw: The physiological action of β-iminazolylethylamine. J. Physiol. (Lond.) **41**, 318—344 (1910).

Dunham, E. T., and I.M. Glynn: Adenosine triphosphatase activity and the active movements of alkali metal ions. J. Physiol. (Lond.) **156**, 274—293 (1961).

Eccles, J. C., and J. W. Magladery: Responses of denervated smooth muscle. J. Physiol. (Lond.) **89**, 45—46 P (1937).

Emmelin, N., and W. Feldberg: The smooth muscle contracting effects of various substances supposed to act on nervous structures in the intestinal wall. J. Physiol. (Lond.) **106**, 482—502 (1947).

— G. Kahlson, and F. Wicksell: Histamine in plasma and methods of its estimation. Acta physiol. scand. **2**, (2), 123—142 (1941).

Evans, D. H. L., H. O. Schild, and S. Thesleff: Effects of drugs on depolarized plain muscle. J. Physiol. (Lond.) **143**, 474—485 (1958).

Feldberg, W.: A discussion on the action of local hormone. On the origin and function of acetylcholine in the intestinal wall. Proc. roy. Soc. B **137**, 285—292 (1950).

— Effects of ganglion-blocking substances on the small intestine. J. Physiol. (Lond.) **113**, 484—505 (1951).

Field, M. E., and C. K. Drinker: The action of histamine on the bronchioles and pulmonary vessels of the guinea-pig. Amer. J. Physiol. **93**, 138—145 (1930).

Fink, L. D., and J. Akiyama: Response of excised guinea-pig tracheal muscle to morphine and meperidine. Arch. int. Pharmacodyn. **91**, 322—329 (1952).

Frommel, E. M., M. Favre et F. Vallette: L'action antiacétylcholine et antihistaminique des anesthésiques locaux (cocaïne, novocaïne, percaïne) étudiée à l'aérosol et par les méthodes de la contraction de l'iléon de Cobaye. Arch. int. Pharmacodyn. **73**, 355—366 (1947).

Gaddum, J. H.: Reports on biological standards. III. Methods of biological assay depending on a quantal response. Special Report 183 Med. Research Council Lond. **46** P. (1933).

Ginzel, K. G.: Investigations concerning the initiation of the peristaltic reflex in the guinea-pig ileum. J. Physiol. (Lond.) **148**, 75—76 P (1959).

Grundfest, H., and I. Schedlowski: Electrochemistry in biology and medicine. Voir page 141. New York: John Wiley and Sons 1957.

Guggenheim, M., u. W. Loeffler: Biologischer Nachweis proteinogener Amine in Organextrakten und Körperflüssigkeiten. Biochem. Z. **72**, 303 (1916).

Halpern, B. N.: Les antihistaminiques de synthèse. Essais de chimiothérapie des états allergiques. Arch. int. Pharmacodyn. **68**, 339—408 (1942).

Hansen, K., u. H. F. Zipf: Beziehungen zwischen Bronchotonus und Lungen-Vagusafferenzen und ihre pharmakologische Beeinflussung. Naunyn-Schmiedeberg's Arch. exp. Path. Pharmak. **240**, 253—274 (1960).

Hanzlik, P. J.: Demonstration of bronchial constriction and compression from physical and other causes. Amer. J. Physiol. **71**, 558—569 (1925).

Harichaux, P., et J. Thouvenot: Un nouveau dispositif thermostatique pour organes isolés. Rev. méd. Tours **1**, 292—296 (1960).

Hodgkin, A. L., and A. F. Huxley: Currents carried by sodium and potassium ions through the membrane of the giant axon of Loligo. J. Physiol. (Lond.) **116**, 449—472 (1952).

Holgate, J. A., and B. T. Warner: Evaluation of antagonists of histamine, 5-hydroxytryptamine and acetylcholine in the guinea-pig. Brit. J. Pharmacol. **15**, 561—566 (1960).

Huxley, A. F.: Muscle structure and theories of contraction. Recent advances in biophysics **7**, 257—318. London: Pergamon Press 1957.

Jackson, D. E.: Experimental Pharmacology 2nd ed. St.-Louis: Mosby 1939.

KALLOS, P., u. W. PAGEL: Experimentelle Untersuchungen über Asthma bronchiale. Acta med. scand. **91**, 292—305 (1937).
KONZETT, H., u. R. RÖSSLER: Versuchsanordnung zu Untersuchungen an der Bronchialmuskulatur. Naunyn-Schmiedeberg's Arch. exp. Path. Pharmak. **195**, 71—74 (1940).
KOSTERLITZ, H. W., V. W. PIRIE, and J. A. ROBINSON: The mechanism of the peristaltic reflex in the isolated guinea-pig ileum. J. Physiol. (Lond.) **133**, 681—694 (1956).
—, and J. A. ROBINSON: Inhibition of the peristaltic reflex of the isolated guinea-pig ileum. J. Physiol. (Lond.) **136**, 249—262 (1957).
LECOMTE, J.: Antihistaminiques de synthèse et ions potassium. Arch. int. Pharmacodyn. **82**, 360 (1950).
LEVY, J., et E. MICHEL-BER: Mécanisme de l'action de divers excitoganglionnaires et intestin isolé de rongeurs. J. Physiol. (Paris) **45**, 687—722 (1953).
MACMILLAN, W. H., and J. R. VANE: The effects of histamine on the plasma potassium levels of cats. J. Pharmacol. exp. Ther. **118**, 182—192 (1956).
MCDOWALL, R. J. S., and A. A. I. SOLIMAN: A mode of drug action. Lancet **1954 I**, 1166—1167.
MAGNUS, R.: Versuche am überlebenden Dünndarm von Säugetieren. Pflügers Arch. ges. Physiol. **108**, 1 (1905).
MARIANI, L.: Attività associata dell'istamina e della serotonina sulla muscolatura bronchiale della cavia. Atti Accad. med. lombarda **15**, (2) 165—170 (1960).
PARROT, J.-L.: Action de l'histamine sur l'iléon isolé de Cobaye. Analyse du diagramme action-dose. J. Physiol. (Paris) **42**, 697—699 (1950).
— G. NICOT, C. LABORDE et P. CANU: Action antihistaminique du lysozyme. J. Physiol. (Paris) **54**, 739—748 (1962).
—, et G. RICHET: Sur une substance vasodilatatrice présente dans certains extraits de sang et d'exsudat. C. R. Acad. Sci. (Paris) **217**, 580 (1943).
—, et J. THOUVENOT: Action de l'histamine sur l'iléon isolé de Cobaye; double réaction des fibres longitudinales. Schweiz. med. Wschr. **40**, 1014—1018 (1952).
— — Dualité d'action de l'histamine sur l'iléon isolé de Cobaye. Augmentation de l'une des réponses par deux substances (vératrine et sulfocyanure de sodium) qui renforcent l'action du potassium. C. R. Soc. Biol. (Paris) **147**, 1199 (1953).
— — Influence de l'hexaméthonium sur la contraction histaminique de l'iléon isolé de Cobaye. J. Physiol. (Paris) **46**, 496—498 (1954).
— — Sur la contraction du muscle lisse intestinal. Sa dualité fonctionnelle chez le Cobaye. J. Physiol. (Paris) **48**, 33—47 (1956).
— — Double mécanisme contractile de l'intestin isolé de Cobaye. Essai d'analyse par stimulation électrique coaxiale. J. Physiol. (Paris) **49**, 329—332 (1957a)
— — Dualité d'action de l'histamine sur l'iléon isolé de Cobaye. Essai d'analyse pharmacologique. J. Physiol. (Paris) **49**, 1149—1170 (1957b).
— — et S. LONGUEVALLE: Libération de potassium par les organes isolés du Cobaye. Action de l'histamine et de l'un de ses antagonistes de synthèse. J. Physiol. (Paris) **45**, 215—218 (1953).
PATON, W. D. M.: The response of the guinea-pig ileum to electrical stimulation by coaxial electrodes. J. Physiol. (Lond.) **127**, 40 P (1955).
SCHAUMANN, O.: Über eine neue Klasse von Verbindungen mit spasmolytischer und zentralanalgetischer Wirksamkeit unter besonderer Berücksichtigung des 1-Methyl-4-phenyl-piperidin-4-carbonsäure-äthylesters (Dolantin). Naunyn-Schmiedeberg's Arch. exp. Path. Pharmak. **196**, 109—136 (1940).
SCHILD, H. O.: Method of conducting a biological assay on a preparation giving repeated graded response illustrated by the estimation of histamine. J. Physiol. (Lond.) **101**, 115—130 (1942).
— An approximately linear and isotonic frontal writing lever. J. Physiol. (Lond.) **103**, 11 P. (1944).
— Automatic apparatus for pharmacological assay on isolated preparations. Brit. J. Pharmacol. **1**, 135—138 (1946).
SEGRE, G., ed E. M. FALCO: Studi quantitativi sull'antagonismo. IV. Istamina e neoantergan sull'ileo di cavia. Boll. Soc. ital. Biol. sper. **28**, 1370—1372 (1952).
D'SILVA, J. L., and A. F. LEWIS: The measurement of bronchoconstriction in vivo. J. Physiol. (Lond.) **157**, 611—622 (1961).
SOLLMANN, T., and W. F. OETTINGEN: Bronchial perfusion of isolated lung as method for studying pharmacologic reactions of bronchiolar muscle. Proc. Soc. exp. Biol. (N. Y.) **25**, 692—695 (1928).
STAUB, A. M.: Recherches sur quelques bases synthétiques antagonistes de l'histamine. Ann. Inst. Pasteur **63**, 400—436 et 485—524 (1939).
THOUVENOT, J.: Etude critique du dosage biologique de l'histamine. Thèse méd. Paris, 57 p. R. Vezin Edit. (1952).

THOUVENOT, J.: Un dispositif permettant l'étude *in vitro* du péristaltisme de l'intestin de petit Mammifère. J. Physiol. (Paris) **49**, 429—431 (1957).

—, et P. HARICHAUX: Sur les composants neurogène et myogène de la contraction longitudinale de l'intestin isolé de Cobaye. Essai de dissociation par variation de températures. C. R. Soc. Biol. (Paris) **153**, 2074—2077 (1959).

— — Sur le péristaltisme intestinal: ses interactions avec l'histamine sur le jéjuno-iléon isolé de Cobaye. C. R. Soc. Biol. (Paris) **155**, 608—611 (1961 a).

— — Sur le déclenchement du péristaltisme. Etude *in vitro* sur le jéjuno-iléon isolé de Cobaye. C. R. Soc. Biol. (Paris) **155**, 1681—1685 (1961 b).

— — Fonction propulsive de l'intestin. Rôle des fibres longitudinales. Etude sur le jéjuno-iléon isolé de Cobaye. Rev. méd. Tours **2** (n° 18), 621—639 (1961 c).

—, et D. PASSELEYGUE: Variations cycliques d'excitabilité du muscle lisse longitudinal de l'intestin grêle chez le Cobaye. C. R. Soc. Biol. (Paris) **156**, 1138 (1962).

TRENDELENBURG, P.: Physiologische und pharmakologische Versuche über die Dünndarmperistaltik. Naunyn-Schmiedeberg's Arch. exp. Path. Pharmak. **81**, 55—129 (1917).

VALETTE, G., et P. AUGEREAU: Réactivité des muscles lisses des Poissons à l'histamine et à d'autres agents contracturants (5-hydroxytryptamine, acétylcholine et chlorure de baryum). J. Physiol. (Paris) **50**, 1067—1074 (1958).

—, et C. E. CALDERON: Effets de la teneur du régime alimentaire en calcium sur la sensibilité du Cobaye à l'histamine. C. R. Acad. Sci. (Paris) **241**, 1620 (1955).

YONKMAN, F. F., E. OPPENHEIMER, B. R. RENNICK, and T. A. PELLE: Pharmacodynamic studies of a new antihistaminic agent, pyribenzamine; effects on smooth muscle of guinea-pig and dog lung. J. Pharmacol. exp. Ther. **89**, 31—41 (1947).

ZADINA, R.: Influence de la température sur la contraction histaminique de l'intestin du Cobaye. C. R. Soc. Biol. (Paris) **132**, 283—31 (1939).

Section D, II

Action of Histamine on the Smooth Muscle

(On the nature of the receptors for histamine in the guinea pig ileum)

By

M. ROCHA E SILVA

With 7 Figures

A. Parameter of affinity drug-receptor *(pKn)*

In the discussion about the mechanism by which histamine acts upon smooth muscle, PARROT and THOUVENOT (see Preceeding Part of this Section) confined themselves to one view of the phenomenon by assuming a random distribution of contractile units which would respond according to the rules of "all or none" processes. A similar approach, but with different connotations is to assume that for each successful hit at the drug receptor, a quantum of "free energy" should be released. In such a case, the intensity of the response registered by an isotonic and frontal lever, should be proportional to the number of receptors interacting with the agonist. This assumption is the basis to derive CLARK's equation relating the intensity of the effect (y) to the dose or concentration (x) of the agonist

$$y = \frac{K_c x}{1 + K_c x} \text{ or } y = \frac{x}{K_n + x} \; if \; K_n = \frac{1}{K_c} \tag{1}$$

In these equations K_c (Clark's constant) is a constant of affinity and its reciprocal $K_n = \frac{1}{K_c}$, a constant of dissociation. We have taken the reciprocal of the logarithm of K_n

$$pK_n = -\log K_n = \log K_c$$

as a "parameter of affinity" drug-receptor, since by thermodynamic considerations the free energy (or free enthalpy) of formation of the complex [HR] is linearly related to the value of pK_n

$$-\Delta G = \text{RT} \ln K_n \quad \text{or} \quad \Delta G = 2.3 \text{ RT } pK_n \tag{2}$$

Clark's equation can be deduced by considerations similar to those of derivation of the Michaelis-Menten equation in which K_M plays a similar role as K_n in our equations. If we assume that a concentration [H] of the agonist (histamine) acts upon a random population of receptors [R] it will produce a reversible combination [HR], according to the reaction:

$$[\text{H}] + [\text{R}] \underset{K_n}{\overset{K_c}{\rightleftarrows}} [\text{HR}] \quad K_c = \frac{1}{K_n} = \frac{[\text{AR}]}{[\text{A}][\text{R}]} \tag{3}$$

At equilibrium, the value of the constant K_n can be measured and the amount of free energy given by equation 2.

It is easy to verify that Clark's equation can be put in the logarithmic form:

$$p(x) = pK_n - \log \frac{y}{1-y} \tag{4}$$

where x represents the concentration of the agonist in g/ml and y the response in percentages of the maximum ($y_m = 1.00$). When $y = 0.50$ (or 50% of the maximum), the above equation is reduced to

$$p(x_{50}) = pK_n$$

i.e. the parameter of affinity (pK_n) can be measured numerically by the reciprocal of the logarithm of the concentration (px_{50}) of the agonist producing 50% of the maximum effect. This relationship has been widely verified by the experiment (Rocha e Silva, 1959, 1961).

The logarithmic form (4) of Clark's equation is interesting because it emphasizes the analogy existing between the equilibrium "drug-receptors" and the five other equilibria known to biochemists and listed by Dixon (1953). On the other hand, the deduction that the constant pK_n is numerically identical with the reciprocal of the logarithm of the concentration which gives 50% of the maximal response might provide a method of determination of the value of pK_n, similar to

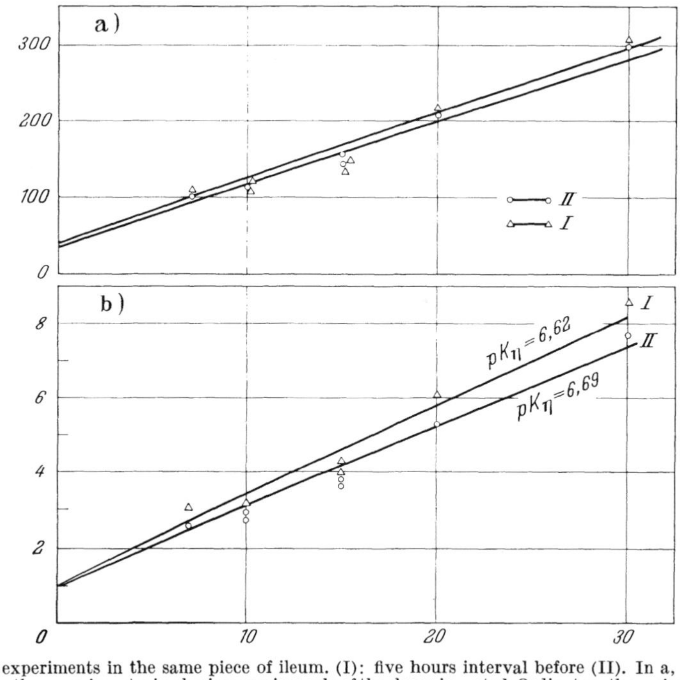

Fig. 1. Two experiments in the same piece of ileum. (I): five hours interval before (II). In a, the lines obtained directly from the experiments; in abscissae reciprocals of the doses in μg/ml. Ordinates: the reciprocal of the effects. In b, the same lines reduced to their normalized forms, with intercept 1 and effects indicated as reciprocals of the percentage of the maximum ($\times 10^{-2}$). (According to Rocha e Silva, 1960)

that utilized in the determination of the Michaelis-Menten constant, as the concentration of the substrate which corresponds to a half of the maximum initial velocity of the enzymatic reaction.

It is, however, easier to deduce the value of K_n and therefore the value of the parameter of affinity (pK_n) by utilizing the method well known to biochemists by the name Lineweaver-Burk's invertion. In fact, Clark's equation can be put into the "normalized form":

$$\frac{1}{y} = \frac{K_n}{x} + 1 \quad \text{or} \quad \frac{1}{y} = K_n \left(\frac{1}{x}\right) + 1 \tag{5}$$

It is easy to see that if any agonist follows Clark's equation a linear relationship should be found between the reciprocals of the responses $\left(\frac{1}{y}\right)$ and the reciprocals of the doses or concentrations $\left(\frac{1}{x}\right)$ of the agonist. In that form, we avoid the obvious difficulty of measuring directly the maximal contraction ($y_m = 1$) in Clark's equation. Though feasible under certain conditions, the direct measurement of the maximal response by adding a great excess of the agonist to the bath containing the muscle strip, is a procedure bound to present unsurmountable difficulties. By utilizing the inverted form of Clark's equation, however, the value of the maximal response can be derived from milder responses given by *physiological concentrations* of the agonist, avoiding the need to measure the shortening of the muscle in presence of a large excess of the agonist. It is easy to see that if the double reciprocal plot is a straight line, the reciprocal of the maximal response can be graphically measured, as the intercept of the line with the axis of the ordinates, as indicated in Fig. 1.

Table 1 gives a complete description of the calculation of pK_n in an experiment with the guinea pig ileum in Tyrode bicarbonate, at pH = 8.3.

Table 1. *Calculation of the constant pK_n from the experimental data* (according to ROCHA E SILVA, 1960)

x (µg/ml)	y (mm height)	$\frac{1}{y}$	y % (10^{-2})	$\frac{1}{y\ \%}$	$\frac{1}{x \cdot 10^{-6}}$	Slope $K_n \cdot 10^8$
0.100	89	112	0.31	3.22	10.0	22.0
0.066	66	151	0.23	4.35	15.1	22.0
0.050	47	213	0.16	6.25	20.0	26.0
0.033	33	303	0.11	8.69	30.3	25.0
0.066	68	147	0.24	4.17	15.1	21.0
0.100	85	118	0.30	3.33	10.0	23.0
0.133	95	105	0.33	3.03	7.5	27.0

Calc. $y_m = 285$ $1/y_m = 35$

$K_n = 23.7 \cdot 10^{-8}$

$pK_n = 6.62$

$K_c = 4.2 \cdot 10^6$

Legend: The reciprocal of the maximum response ($1/y_m$) is derived graphically as the intercept of the line with the axis of ordinates ($1/y$) using the reciprocals of the experimental data. This example is selected to indicate that the value of the maximum response (y_m) can be far out of the range of the direct measurements, and obtained by extrapolation. In terms of percentage of the maximum, a height of 95 mm in the registered response, is only 35% of that maximum. The standard error of the mean slope calculated over the experimental data did not exceed the 3% level.

B. Definition of pharmacological receptors

Table 2 gives a survey of the experimental data utilized in the determination of Clark's constant ($K_c = 1/K_n$) and its logarithm ($\log K_c = pK_n$), referred to g/ml of histamine and responses in percentages of the maximum (= 1.00). The values of pK_n are given in w/v and could be transformed to molar values, by subtracting log 11.0 = 1.05, from the numerical values given in Table 2.

Table 2. *Parameters of the line for calculation of Clark's constant (K_c) and the index pK_n* (according to ROCHA E SILVA, 1959)

Exp. N°	Range of concentr. of histamine (μg/ml) $x10^{-3}$	Number of doses in 4 replicates each.	$1/y_{max}$	y_{max} (mm)	Slope K (aver.)	Slope $K_n x 10^9$	$K_c = 1/K_n$ $x 10^{-9}$	log K_c (pK_n)
I	2.4—15.0	5	30	330	0.96	60.0	0.017	7.23
	2.4—15.0	6	30	330	0.89	60.8	0.016	7.20
II	10.0—30.0	4	125	80	1.19	19.2	0.052	7.72
	5.0—30.0	4	125	80	1.29	23.2	0.043	7.63
III	2.0—15.0	4	50	200	0.40	16.2	0.061	7.78
IV	5.0—20.0	3	50	200	1.27	50.4	0.020	7.30
V	5.0—30.0	4	100	100	0.74	14.8	0.067	7.83
	5.0—30.0	4	100	100	0.74	14.8	0.067	7.83
VI	20.0—60.0	4	70	142	3.15	89.0	0.011	7.04
VII	10.0—40.0	4	50	200	1.68	70.0	0.014	7.14
	10.0—40.0	4	50	200	1.41	51.0	0.020	7.30
VIII	4.0—20.0	4	50	200	1.06	43.0	0.023	7.36
IX	5.0—10.0	3	40	250	0.85	43.0	0.023	7.36
	5.0—10.0	3	40	250	0.74	38.6	0.026	7.41
X	12.0—40.0	5	25	400	2.10	170.4	0.006	6.78
	6.0—20.0	3	25	400	1.53	124.0	0.008	6.90
XI	3.0—10.0	6	50	200	0.41	16.5	0.060	7.78
XII	7.0—15.0	5	35	285	0.67	38.0	0.026	7.41

The slope K refers to the experimental line; the slope K_n refers to the "normalized" line, with intercept $1/y = 1$; the constant K_c is Clark's constant, calculated from a concentration of the agonist (g/ml) in the smooth muscle chamber and the responses in fractions of the maximum (= 1.00). The log K_c is an absolute measure of the affinity of the agonist (histamine) for the receptors, in the conditions of the assay, $pK_n = \log K_c$.

It is easy to see (Table 2) that the values of the maximum responses are usually out of the range of a direct measurement upon the muscle strip. In fact, it is rather undesirable that such a measurement should be obtained by any direct means. The graphical method outlined above permits a deduction of what should be called the *total number of receptors* available. In the deduction of Clark's equation, the assumption is made that any response (y) actually *measures* the number of receptors successfully hit or occupied at the concentration of the agonist producing such a response. Therefore, the maximum response, or the reciprocal of the intercept of the line with the ordinates, in the double reciprocal plot ($y_m = 1/\text{intercept}$), will obviously measure the number of receptors *available*. In most cases, this datum would be unobtainable by direct means, since large amounts of the agonist should be added to the bath, and still the maximum shortening might not be attained owing to the bulk of the reacting structure (something similar to the co-volume in real gases). However, by using the inversion of Clark's equation, a reproducible constant value can be obtained which could theoretically be taken as the maximal number of available receptors. It is irrelevant to know whether this value indicates the *total* number of receptors present in the strip utilized, or if there are other receptors which are not attainable at any concentration of the agonist. From the linearity of the double reciprocal plot, we can assume that a certain "population of receptors" is taking part in the production of the response, at a "physiological range" of concentrations of the agonist. The fact that by adding an antagonist to the bath, the same sequence of responses can be obtained with higher levels of concentrations of the agonist, is no argument against the above assumption, but in favor of it, since the role of the antagonist is obviously to decrease the probability of a successful hit of the molecules of the agonist, as some of the "available" receptors are knocked out by the antagonist.

Whatever be the idea one has of the intimate nature of such "working units" or receptors, one might assume that the number of receptors which combine with the agonist is linearly related to the intensity of the response obtained. In a kind of axiomatic way, one might define "receptors" by the linear relation between intensity (y) and number (n) of receptors occupied:

$$y = \alpha n . \tag{6}$$

The question that arises from this assumption is to know whether it might constitute a useful definition of receptors. In my opinion, this is the only useful definition of receptors, since it brings forth the idea of the receptor as a "gadget" holding an "energetic unit" to be released by a successful hit of the agonist molecule. The only limitation to this statement is the method utilized to measure the intensity (y) of the effect. If the intensity is registered directly or through an isotonic and frontal lever, one can fairly assume that the response (y) is proportional to the number of energetic units mobilized by a combination of the receptor with the agonist, according to equation 3. As the method described above allows the calculation of an equilibrium constant (K_c) or its reciprocal (K_n), according to the law of the independency of the enthalpies of formation of any compounds in heterogeneous systems, one might tentatively calculate the free energy (or enthalpy) involved in the formation of the [RH] complex.

C. Free energy of formation of the complex drug-receptors

By thermodynamical considerations, if we assume that the reaction between n_1 mols of the agonist with n_2 "mols of receptors" generates n_3 "mols of the complex drug-receptor," according to the reaction.

$$n_1 \mathrm{H} + n_2 \mathrm{R} \rightleftarrows n_3 [\mathrm{HR}]$$

the net variation of free enthalpy will be given by the expression

$$- \Delta G = n_3 \Delta\mu_3 - n_1 \Delta\mu_1 - n_2 \Delta\mu_2 \tag{7}$$

where μ_i is the so-called "chemical potential" at constant temperature, pressure and constancy of any other concentration of the components of the system (n_j constituents):

$$\mu_i = \left(\frac{\partial G}{\partial n_i}\right) T,\ P,\ n_j$$

and since

$$\Delta\mu_i = \mathrm{RT}\, \Delta \ln x_i$$

where x_i represents the molar concentrations of the reagents, the relation (7) becomes:

$$- \Delta G = \mathrm{RT}\, [n_3 \ln x_3 - n_1 \ln x_1 - n_2 \ln x_2]$$

where n_i represents the stoechiometric coefficients of the reaction. The expression under brackets is no less than $\ln K_c = - \ln K_n$ and therefore

$$\Delta G = \mathrm{RT} \ln K_n$$

where R = 1.987 cal/deg/mol and T = 310.10°K (37°C).

If we take pK_n (g/ml) equal to 6.78 to 7.83, the values of pK_n (molar) will range from 5.73 to 6.78 and

$$- \Delta G = - 1.987 \times 310.1 \times 2.302 \times \begin{cases} 5.73 = 7.86 \text{ kcal/mol.} \\ 6.78 = 9.38 \text{ kcal/mol.} \end{cases}$$

Therefore, the values of "free energy" of formation of the complex [HR], in the case of histamine, fall between the range of 7.86 to 9.38 kcal/mol.

It might be a coincidence, though a remarkable one, that the "free energy" of formation of the complex [AR] approaches the accepted values for a high energy phosphate bond.

This coincidence might induce one to complete the microconfiguration of the "histamine receptor" assuming that for each successful hit, a high energy phosphate bond ($\sim P$) would be released to produce the mechanical work of contraction ($-\Delta W$) and again by thermodynamic considerations this value ($-\Delta W$) should be numerically inferior to the maximum attainable in a reversible process ($-\Delta G$). In part we have verified that the mechanical work obtainable in such conditions never exceeds 20 to 30% of the theoretical value ΔG (molar) of the assumed maximum "free energy" released.

$$-\Delta W = 0.20 \text{ to } 0.30\,(\Delta G)$$

Fig. 2 gives a pictorial view of the "histamine receptor" as arising from the above considerations.

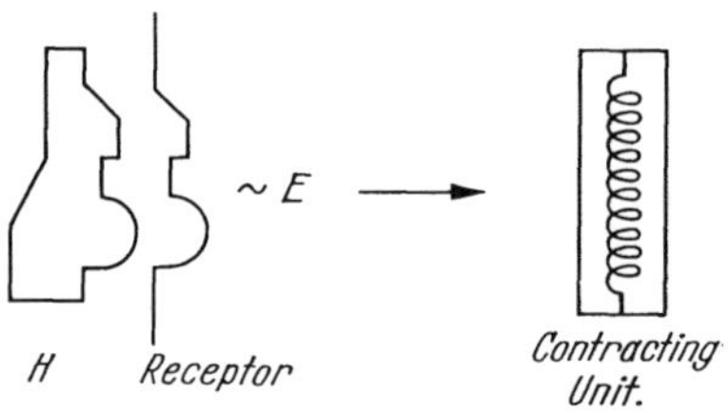

Fig. 2. Possible representation of the histamine receptor, built up for the release of an "energetic unit" ($\sim E$) when the molecule of the agonist (H) approaches the complementary pattern of its exposed configuration

D. Influence of pH on the equilibrium drug-receptor

In order to have a more definite insight into the structure of the histamine receptors, the influence of pH on the values of the parameter of affinity pK_n was studied. According to a well known theory by DIXON (1953) a sharp bend in the curve representing the plot of pK_n versus pH would indicate the pK of an ionizable group either of the receptor or of the drug. The two pKs of histamine

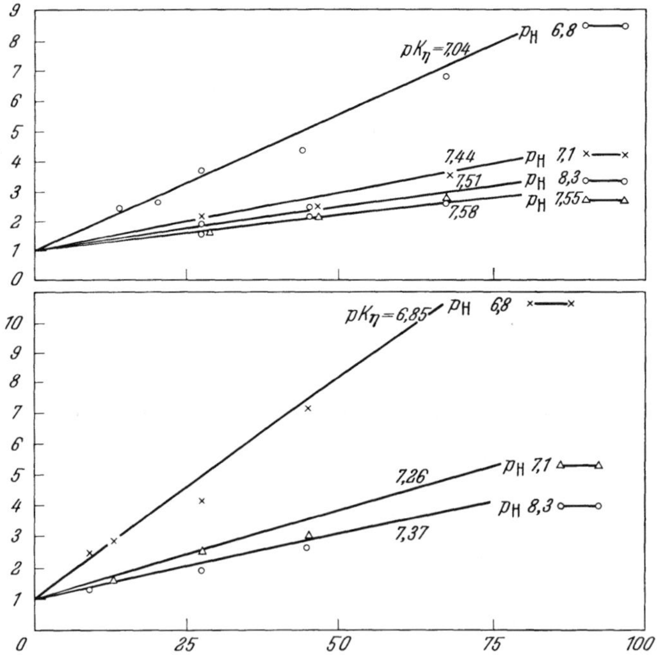

Fig. 3a. Double reciprocal plots of 6 experiments to show variation of pK_n, in function of pH. It can be seen that the values of pK_n (slope of the line) are not significantly different between pH 8.3 to pH 7.1, but as the pH falls to 6.8, there is a sharp increase in the slope of the line. (According to ROCHA E SILVA, 1960)

are known: 5.9 and 9.7 according to LEVY (1935). Therefore, in the useful range of pHs from 8.3 to 6.7, the pKs of histamine are probably not interfering in the results. A sharp change in the value of pK_n around pH 6.8 to 7.1, as observed in our experiments (ROCHA E SILVA, 1960, 1961) and presented in Fig. 3a, b, would most likely depend upon the pK of an active group of the receptor.

To avoid any influence of the histaminolytic enzyme (histaminase) present in the preparation, all experiments were done in presence of 2×10^{-6} concentration of aminoguanidine, and to avoid variations of pH due to changes in concentration of CO_2, instead of the usual bicarbonate buffer, a maleate buffer was employed. For this purpose, two solutions were prepared: A) maleic acid 23.8 g + 8 g NaOH per liter and B) 0.2 M NaOH solution. A fixed volume (50 ml) of solution A was added to increasing quantities of sol. B to raise the pH, and the final volume was adjusted to 200 ml. From this mixture, 50 ml were added to 950 ml of Tyrode solution (without bicarbonate, but still containing phosphate). A final adjustment of pH was done before or during the experiment. Although the maleate buffer is more efficient at pH below 7.0 (COLOWICK and KAPLAN, 1954) the presence of phosphate and the fact that above 7.0 the effect of pH was negligible upon the value of pK_n, in some experiments the maleate buffer was utilized over the entire range of pH from 8.3 to 6.6.

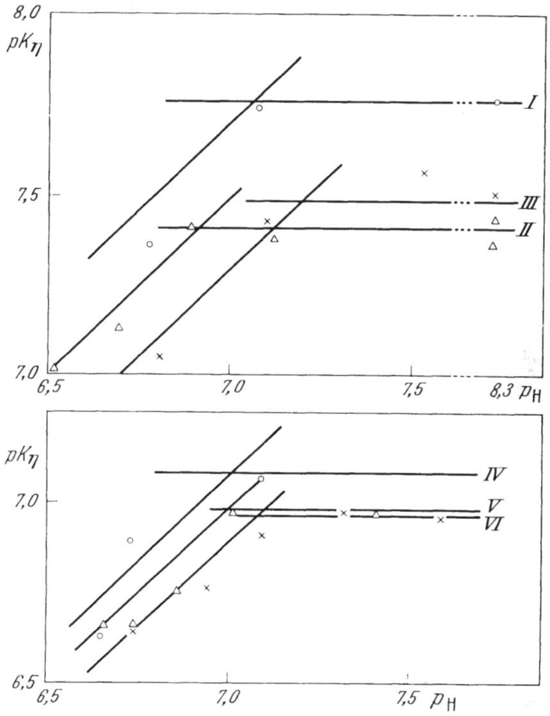

Fig. 3b. Variation of the "affinity" constant pK_n in function of pH of the external fluid, in 6 different experiments. It can be seen that between 8.3 to 7.1 no substantial alterations in the slope of the line could be detected but as the pH drops below 7.0 a sharp bend of the line takes place. If the two lines (slope 0 and slope + 1) are drawn, the intersection lies between 6.9 and 7.0 in all experiments (According to ROCHA E SILVA, 1960)

Fig. 3b presents the variation of the values of pK_n with pH in six experiments with histamine upon the guinea pig ileum. Over a large interval, from 8.3 to 7.1 the variations in the values of pK_n are small and comparable to those obtained upon the same piece of intestine, under constant pH at different time intervals. One might assume a "0-slope" line correlating the values of pK_n to those of pH over that range of variation. As the pH falls to 7.0 or 6.9, the lines show an abrupt change in slope, with a downward bend, tending to + 1 values. If the two lines are plotted as in Fig. 3b, the intersection could indicate an abrupt change of ionization of an active grouping of the receptor. The corresponding value of pH would measure the pK of the active center. Analysing the different lines in Fig. 3b, it is seen that in all cases, the intersections of the lines fall between 6.8 to 7.1, and therefore the pK of the active center of the receptor will be in that range, nearer the lower than the upper limits.

In fact, from the double reciprocal plots presented in Fig. 3a, it is reasonable to assume that hydrogen ions compete with histamine in its interaction with the receptors (increase in slope without change of intercept) and therefore one might assume that the log of the concentration of hydrogen ions (– pH) which duplicates the slope of the double reciprocal plot can measure the constant of ionization of the active center of the receptor (pK). In the case presented in Fig. 3b, the value of $pK = 6.8$, since $pA_2 = 6.8$ (= – pH). Similar confirmatory results have been presented by ARIËNS and SIMONIS (1963).

E. Probable presence of an imidazol ring in the receptors for histamine

As for the nature of this ionizable group in the receptors for histamine in the guinea pig ileum, with a pK around 6.8 to 7.1 we have assumed that it belongs to the imidazol ring of a histidyl radical (ROCHA E SILVA, 1960). It is well known that imidazol has a pK in that range of pH (MASSEY, 1953; BARNARD and STEIN, 1958) and it seems reasonable to speculate around the possibility of an imidazol ring being one of the active centers in the receptors for histamine in the guinea pig ileum. Actually it has been stated that the imidazol ring is about the only group known in proteins having a pK in that region. According to data in BARNARD and STEIN (1958), the pK of tertiary imidazol is 7.03; for histidyl-histidine it is 6.80 and for anserine (β-alanyl-N-methyl-histidine) it is 7.08. Therefore the identification of the active center, revealed in our experiments, with an imidazol ring, though not the only possibility, is by far the most probable.

It remains to see whether the presence of an imidazol ring in the histamine receptors might introduce some conceptual simplifications to afford a comprehensive theory on the mechanism by which the "gadget" represented by the receptor, would start the energetic changes to initiate the muscle contraction.

F. The receptor as an energetic gadget

Any theory on the nature of a pharmacological receptor should provide a hint to understand the dynamic aspects of the interaction of the agonist with the effector system. The receptor should be considered primarily a "gadget" to release an energetic metabolite to act upon the reacting structure. In the case of histamine acting upon the guinea pig ileum, the theory should account for the two fundamental implications:

a) that the equilibrium drug-receptors obeys the law of mass action; and

b) that there is a linear relationship between the intensity of the effect and the number of receptors hit or occupied by the molecule of the agonist.

As shown before, these two implications are contained in the deduction of Clark's equation as shown in the beginning of this paper, and well confirmed by the linearity of the double reciprocal plot (ROCHA E SILVA, 1959, 1960). The linearity of the double reciprocal plot, as regards the actions of histamine and acetylcholine upon the guinea pig ileum, was recently confirmed by GODFRAIND and GODFRAIND-DE BECKER (1960).

The simplest way to conform to both postulates would be to assume that the trigger "unit," or receptor, presents a bond holding some energetic metabolite, as for instance a high energy phosphate bond ($\sim P$). The release of $\sim P$, as a consequence of the collision of one molecule of histamine with the receptor, would contribute with a quantitative factor, the energy contained in $\sim P$ to start the contraction. The response observed would be linearly related to the number of $\sim P$ units set free by the agonist.

The imidazol is conveniently fit to provide for such a mechanism. In the imidazol ring, we have to consider the "pyrrol" and the "pyridine" nitrogen. The first one is a center of positive charge and its hydrogen can be replaced by other groups as acetyl (Ac) or phosphoryl ($\sim P$).

Though never isolated from biological structures, N. phosphoryl-imidazols have been chemically prepared (BARNARD and STEIN, 1958; RATHLEV and ROSENBERG, 1956). The pyridine nitrogen, on the contrary, is a locus of negative charges ready to fix a "proton" or to form hydrogen bonding with complementary structures.

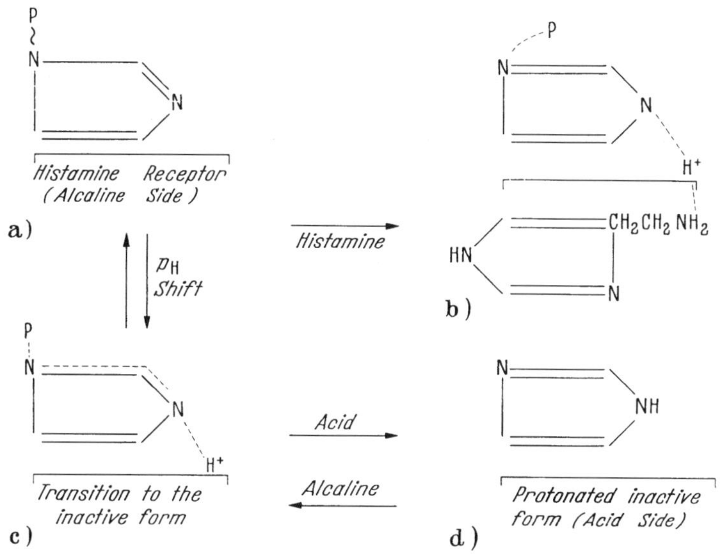

Fig. 4. Schematic representation of the receptor for histamine in different conditions of pH. a, resting condition at pH above 7.0. At b, interaction of a histamine molecule with formation of a hydrogen bond with the imidazol ring of the receptor. c, activated form of the receptor, when the pH is shifted from a higher to lower values; this form is understood as a transition to the inactive state (d), when the gadget is completely discharged of its energetic metabolite $\sim P$. (According to ROCHA E SILVA, 1961)

Fig. 4 attempts to show the changes undergone by the imidazol ring presumably present in the receptors for histamine. The maximum efficiency of the gadget would be in the alkaline side (Fig. 4, a). If the pH is shifted to lower values, the imidazol center might undergo a transitory "activation" in which the effect of the agonist might be potentiated. This "activated" state, represented by the dots in Fig. 4 c, could be invariably observed, in our experiments, when the pH was shifted to the acid side and before any decrease in sensitivity or affinity occurred; the ileum responds to the same small or large doses of histamine with increasing intensity before it falls to equilibrium levels.

G. Histamine as a proton carrier

At the conditions of pH of the tissue, it has been suggested by NIEMANN and HAYS (1942) that histamine behaves as an univalent cation (Fig. 5) forming a

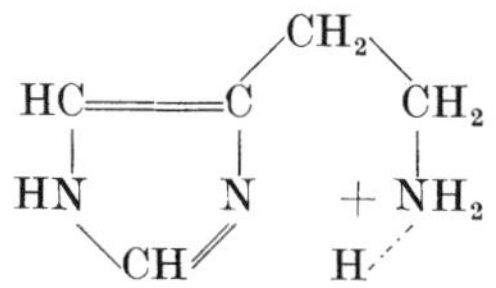

Fig. 5. Ionized form of histamine under physiological conditions.

chelate structure with a hydrogen bond between the lateral chain and the pyridine nitrogen in the imidazol ring. Therefore, histamine might contribute as a proton carrier to start the changes in the imidazol nucleus characteristic of the transformation leading to the discharge of the "gadget."

By examining a number of compounds with histamine-like activity, LEE and JONES (1949) reached the conclusion that intramolecular hydrogen bonding between the side chain and the ring is one of the requisites for a histamine-like activity. Other peculiarities of the ring are necessary. Methylation in position (2) will not affect the activity, although methylation in position (5) in the ring, will reduce the activity to 1/300 as shown first by ALLES, WISEGARVER and SHULL (1943).

H. The second anchorage group for histamine

It has been admitted for long time that histamine has another anchorage group and ACKERMANN (1939), on the basis of the inhibition by arginine, histidine and guanidine derivatives, postulated that this second group should be the =NH imine group of the imidazol ring of histamine. If an excess of either arginine or histidine is previously added to the perfusing bath, histamine would have no chance to combine with the occupied receptors to produce its characteristic stimulating effect. In 1944, in confirmation to this theory we have observed (ROCHA E SILVA, 1944) that compounds of histamine with aminoacids, which by themselves are inactive pharmacologically, display an inhibitory effect upon histamine of the same order of magnitude as histidine itself or of benzoyl-1. arginine amide, which, among the derivatives of arginine showed a maximum of anti-histamine effect.

This theory, therefore, suggested that the histamine molecule has two poles by which it could affect the receptors, a "haptophore" one, represented by the imine radical situated in the imidazol ring, having only anchoring capacity, and the "toxophore" group represented by the free amine radical in the lateral chain. This provided a clear cut demonstration of the hypothesis emitted by CLARK (1937) that a drug must have at least two anchorage groups, one inactive by itself, and the other indispensable for its pharmacological activity. In the case of histidine, and histamine compounds with aminoacids, the toxophore group ($-NH_2$) is blocked by a neighboring $-COOH$ radical or combined with it, but the haptophore group (=NH) would be free to hold the inhibitor to the anchorage of histamine to its receptors.

I. A comprehensive view on the structure of the receptors for histamine in the guinea pig

To comply with the idea of a histidyl radical in the receptor for histamine, and conciliate it with the idea of two anchorage points for histamine, we have to complete the picture of the receptor by assuming that the anchorage group for the imine (=NH) radical is at a distance to the left in the scheme of Fig. 6, that might fit the dimensions of the agonist. The simplest assumption is to admit that the second anchorage group is provided by a peptide bond $-CO-NH-$ to the left of the imidazol ring in the scheme of Fig. 6. The polar carbonyl =C=O might form a transitory bond with the imine =NH of the imidazol ring of histamine. The possibility of this model to fit the histamine molecule has been also suggested by using a Hirschfelder model as indicated in Fig. 7a and b.

A few points should be discussed in connection with this scheme. LEE and JONES (1949) have assayed a compound isomer of histamine, with the $-NH-$ group in position of carbon (5) and found it completely inactive. Its isosteric similar, having –S– in that position (5), on the contrary, was highly active with 1/3 of the activity of histamine itself. However, when the –S– group was in the position of the –NH— imine group (position 1) the compound was found to have only 1/50 of the activity of histamine.

It is understandable that a –S– in position (1) will face the negative pole (carbonyl radical) of the peptide bond, although in position (5) it might contribute to the anchorage of histamine since it will face the positive side of the peptide bond.

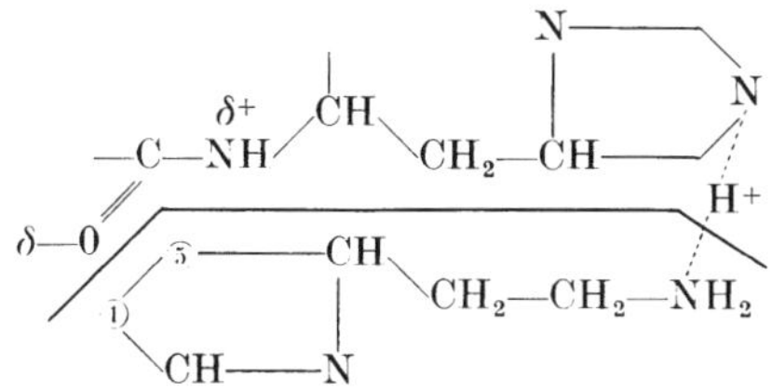

Positions	①	—NH—	—CH—	—S—	—CH—
	⑤	—CH—	—NH—	—CH—	—S—
Compound		Histamine	XIII	V	IV
Activities		1	0	0.02	0.3

Fig. 6. Schematic representation of the receptor for histamine in the ileum of the guinea pig. The compounds numbered are those assayed by Lee and Jones (1949). (According to Rocha e Silva, 1961)

The opposite would be true for the imine –NH– radical which in position (5) would face the positive pole of the peptide bond. The compounds described by Lee and Jones (1949) are indicated in Fig. 6.

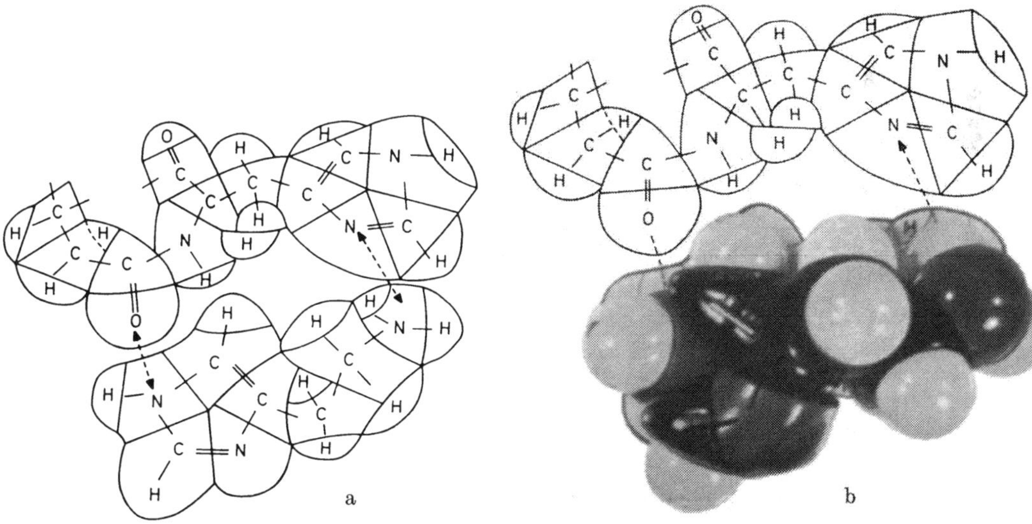

Fig. 7a and b. a) A histamine molecule represented as a projection of its atom model, faces the hypothetical scheme of its receptor, represented as a histidyl residue of a peptide chain. b) Atom model of the histamine molecule facing the receptor in the ileum of the guinea pig. The transitory bonds are represented by the dotted arrows pointing to the active groups at the receptor and at the histamine molecule. (According to Rocha e Silva, 1961)

J. A fit for bound histamine

The experiments described above refer to the transient equilibrium between histamine and its receptors in the smooth muscle, but it would be tempting to speculate further on the possibility that a similar frame might hold histamine tightly bound to the protein molecules in its normal storage sites in other structures, such as the mast cells, or rabbit's platelets. In 1953, in a private discussion of the subject, LINDERSTROM-LANG had suggested that bound histamine might simply depend upon a "fit" to the molecule to be retained in place by secondary valence forces of hydrogen bondings.

We know now that histamine can be released by the following procedures: a) organic solvents or heat denaturation, or by any other means of denaturing proteins; b) by proteolytic enzymes as trypsin, or by chymotrypsin; c) by ammonia, the most efficient agent to release histamine; d) by basic compounds such as amines, diamines, as well as by alkaloids as D. tubocurarine, strychnine, atropine and so forth and by the synthetic polymer 48/80.

Fig. 6 provides a possible "fit" for bound histamine, in the aminoacid chain of proteins. It is obvious that in that connection, arginine might take the place of the histidine moiety since there is a remarkable similarity of structure between bound histidine or bound arginine, as indicated in BARNARD and STEIN (1958). In that case, the four possibilities for the release of histamine might receive a simple explanation, since ammonia or basic compounds might break the hydrogen bonding between the side chain of histamine and the imidazol ring of the receptor, or viceversa; also the specificity of trypsin would be satisfied, if the breaking of a peptide bond involving a basic aminoacid disrupts the whole frame, and finally any denaturation of the proteins might break down the weak bonds holding histamine to its receptors, as by heating or the action of organic solvents.

Recently, a phosphorylation procedure has been postulated as a possible step in the release of histamine by the antigen-antibody (MOUSSATCHÉ and PROUVOST-DANON, 1958) reaction or, in the rat, by the releaser 48/80 (ROTHSCHILD et al., 1961). The scheme of Fig. 4 might suggest an obvious explanation for the release of histamine by a simple phosphorylation of the imidazol, or of an arginine group possibly present in its receptors, since the entrance of a $\sim P$ radical might contribute to weaken the hydrogen bonding with the lateral chain of histamine, in a way opposite to that which has been postulated for the release of the contracting energy in the receptor of the smooth muscle, as shown in Fig. 4.

All these possibilities are, of course, purely speculative.

References

ACKERMANN, D.: Zur Kenntnis des Histamins und seiner Beziehung zur Anaphylaxie. Naturwissenschaften **27**, 515 (1939).

ALLES, G. A., B. B. WISEGARVER, and M. A. SHULL: Comparative physiological actions of some "imidazolyl-4-alkylamines." J. Pharmacol. exp. Ther. **77**, 54 (1943).

ARIËNS, E. J., and A. M. SIMONIS: pH and drug action. Arch. int. Pharmacodyn. **141**, 309 (1963).

BARNARD, E. A., and W. D. STEIN: The roles of imidazole in biological systems. Advanc. Enzymol. **20**, 51 (1958).

CLARK, A. J.: General Pharmacology. In: HEFFTERS Handb. exptl. Pharmakol. IV. Berlin: Julius Springer 1937.

COLOWICK, S. P., and N. O. KAPLAN: In: Methods in Enzymology, I. New York: Academic Press Inc. 1954.

DIXON, M.: The effect of pH on the affinities of enzymes for substrates and inhibitors. Biochem. J. **55**, 161 (1953).

GODFRAIND, T., et A. GODFRAIND-DE BECKER: Antagonisme du Cu^{++}, du Zn^{++}, du Fe^{++} vis-à-vis de l'histamine et de l'acétylcholine. Arch. int. Pharmacodyn. **126**, 96 (1960).

LEE, H. M., and R. G. JONES: The histamine activity of some β-aminoethyl heterocyclic compounds. J. Pharmacol. exp. Ther. **95**, 71 (1949).

LEVY, M.: A note on the titration constants of imidazole derivatives. J. biol. Chem. **109**, 361 (1935).

MASSEY, V.: Studies on fumarase. 4. The effects of inhibitors on fumarase activity. Biochem. J. **55**, 172 (1953).

MOUSSATCHÉ, H., and A. PROUVOST-DANON: Influence of oxidative phosphorylation inhibitors on the histamine release in the anaphylactic reaction *in vitro*. Experientia (Basel) **14**, 414 (1958).

NIEMANN, C., and J. R. HAYS: Relation between structure and histamine-like activity. J. Amer. chem. Soc. **64**, 2288 (1942).

RATHLEV, T., and T. ROSENBERG: Non-enzymic formation and rupture to nitrogen linkages in phosphoramido derivatives. Arch. Biochem. **65**, 319 (1956).

ROCHA E SILVA, M.: Inhibition of histamine effects by compounds of histamine, histidine and arginine. J. Pharmacol. exp. Ther. **80**, 399 (1944).

— Concerning the theory of receptors in pharmacology. A rational method of estimation of pA_x. Arch. int. Pharmacodyn. **117**, 74 (1959).

— Influence of pH on the interaction of histamine with its receptors in the guinea pig ileum. Arch. int. Pharmacodyn. **128**, 355 (1960).

— On the nature of the receptors for histamine. Chemotherapia **3**, 544 (1961).

ROTHSCHILD, A. M., I. VUGMAN, and M. ROCHA E SILVA: Metabolic studies on the release of histamine by compound 48/80 in the rat diaphragm. Biochem. Pharmacol. **7**, 248 (1961).

Section E

Action of Histamine upon the Circulatory Apparatus

By

M. ROCHA E SILVA

With 19 Figures

I. Mechanism of histamine shock. Historical survey

The complexity of the effects of histamine upon the circulatory apparatus might explain what was called, in earlier times, the "histamine paradox". When injected intravenously in cats and dogs, histamine produced a sharp fall in arterial blood pressure, though when perfused through isolated tissues or organs, not infrequently, a pure vaso-constrictor effect with decline in outflow was observed. This constrictor effect upon isolated perfused organs was particularly seen in cats (DALE and RICHARDS, 1918). With improvement in the conditions of the perfusion experiments, and especially when dogs or monkeys were utilized as donors of the biological structure to be perfused, a vasodilation with increase in volume of the perfused limb and its venous outflow was observed (BURN and DALE, 1926). However, in rabbits and rats the main effect of histamine, when injected into the perfusing cannula, was a sharp decrease in outflow, in spite of the fact that when the amine was injected intravenously in the intact rat, a consistent fall in blood pressure could be observed. Even in the rabbit, under special conditions of anesthesia, histamine produced a fall of arterial blood pressure (FELDBERG, 1927). Therefore, the paradox persists and can be understood only through an extensive analysis of the mode of action of histamine upon the cardio-vascular system.

The circulatory effects of histamine depend upon so many factors varying from animal to animal that it is convenient to present a general description of the differences before embarking on a detailed study of the histamine effects in each animal species. One can broadly admit that the effects of histamine depend mainly upon three factors:

a) action upon the smooth muscle coats of the arterioles and venules;
b) a generalized capillary vaso-dilation with increased capillary permeability, and
c) alterations in the dynamics of the heart, with changes in rhythm, increased or decreased contractility with dilation or constriction of the coronary bed.

To these, so to speak, primary effects, one can add the release of catechol amines from the adrenal glands and, probably also, from other stores in the tissues (as for instance the heart) and the terminals of the sympathetic nervous system. This effect will compensate in part for the long lasting fall in B. P. produced by large doses of histamine (secondary rise) and therefore will change the pattern of the histamine shock (DALE, 1920b; BURN and DALE, 1926; SZCZYGIELSKI, 1932; EICHLER and KILLIAN, 1931; WENT and VARGA, 1952; SLATER and DRESEL, 1952; ROBINSON and JOCHIM, 1960; TRENDELENBURG, 1961; and many others). The subject will be treated in a different Section of this Chapter (see Effects of histamine on the autonomous nervous system).

The interplay of such diverse effects, combined with the fact that different species react differently to the intravenous injection of histamine, might explain a great deal of the "histamine paradox". On the other hand, the calling into play of such diverse and, up to a certain point, contradictory effects would lend support to no single theory on the mechanism of production of the shock by large amounts of histamine. In that connection, and mainly from a historical point of view, one might recall a few major conceptions which have been proposed to explain the precipitous fall in blood pressure provoked by a single large injection of histamine.

A. The Mautner and Pick theory

The Mautner and Pick theory attributed the fall in blood pressure to a predominantly constricting action of histamine upon certain "strategic points" in the circulatory apparatus with relative thickness of the smooth muscle layers in the arteriolar or venular walls. This theory, which derived mainly from experiments of perfusion of the dog's liver, had a profound influence on the studies about the mechanism of peptone and anaphylactic shock in this species (MAUTNER and PICK, 1915, 1922, 1929). According to the theory, the circulatory apparatus presented two main strategic points which might be influenced by the action of histamine or by conditions conducive to spasm of smooth muscles, as in the above mentioned kinds of shock. In the dog, there was predominance of the so-called *Lebersperre* to produce stasis in the splanchnic area, though in other species, as the cat and the rabbit, the spasm occurred in the lung vessels. When the shock agents were perfused through the isolated liver of the dog, a considerable decrease in flow was observed, contrasting with the increase observed in other organs of the same species.

The decrease in flow of the perfused liver was understood to depend upon the presence in the supra-hepatic veins of a thick layer of smooth muscle forming a kind of throttling valve near the orifices into the inferior vena cava.

The anatomical basis for this conception was presented first by AREY and SIMONDS (1920) who stated: "*Histological examination of the hepatic veins of the dog reveals a relatively enormous amount of smooth muscle in the wall, thus demonstrating an adequate anatomical basis for impeded vascular flow would spasm occur.*" SIMONDS (1923) has also investigated 22 different species and found the hepatic veins of the dog the richest in smooth muscle fibers. POPPER (1931) described the fibers in the hepatic veins as a thick layer arranged in longitudinal columns, such that when these columns are contracted (as in the liver fixed under the action of histamine) they caused projection of the intima into the lumen, so that the latter appeared star-shaped in section and was almost obliterated. According to BAUER et al. (1932) the muscle fibers near the orifices of the hepatic veins were continuous with the smooth muscle fibers of the caval vein, without any evidence of a true sphincter with transversally disposed fibers.

A more systematic approach to the problem was presented by AREY (1941) after examining the liver of 30 mammalian species. Only 3, the dog, the racoon and the seal (all carnivora), showed peculiar arrangements of smooth muscles in the larger veins, and rings or spirals in the smaller tributaries to the hepatic veins. In the racoon the muscle was mainly distributed in spaced rings. In the seal, the rings were incomplete or branched with slanting connections giving the semblance of a spiral. In the dog, the arrangement varied from an imperfect spiral, through a loose, perfect spiral to a ring (the latter appeared mainly in the largest vessels). Reviewing the literature on the anatomy of the hepatic veins, SNYDER (1942) described those structures appearing in the liver of the dog and the seal: "*In the hepatic vein and venules of dogs and amphibious mammals, the smooth muscle cells are not arranged in continuous sheets as in ordinary veins, but grouped into slender spirally arranged bands, and especially where the hepatic venules empty into the thoracic vein, the band becomes thickened and quite annular, so as to provide a sphincter.*"

In more recent times, ELIAS and BENGELSDORF (1952) confirmed the existence of such sphincters in the dog's liver and also in the carp. See also MAUTNER (1955).

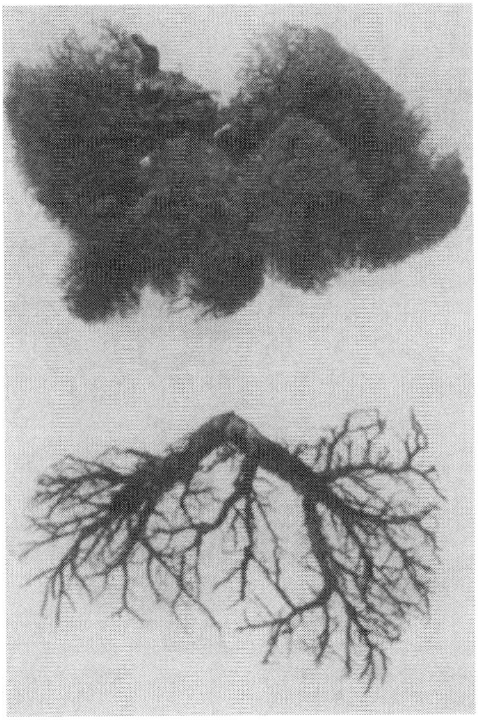

Fig. 1. *A* (upper). Cast of hepatic veins of a control dog. *B* (lower). Cast of the hepatic veins after an injection of an extract of Ascaris suum. This cast was indistinguishable from those made after anaphylactic or histamine shock had been induced ($^1/_2$ natural size) (According to THOMAS and ESSEX, 1949)

The existence of these sphincters in the liver of the dog regulating the outflow of blood through the suprahepatic veins and contributing to liver stasis, "should spasm occur," was also demonstrated by THOMAS and ESSEX (1949) by the aid of a technique allowing visualization of spasm of the small vessels of the liver in conditions of shock by *Ascaris* extracts, histamine, anoxia and anaphylactic shock. By injecting a plastic material (vinyl acetate) into the hepatic artery, the portal vein and, in retrograde manner, into the hepatic veins, THOMAS and ESSEX (1949) made casts of the hepatic circulation in normal animals and animals submitted to a variety of shocks. Especially in the dog, the small veins of the liver were shown to be powerfully contracted (Fig. 1).

Another approach to the question of localization of the sphincters in the subsidiary branches of the hepatic veins, was by use of the technique described by KNISELY (1936, 1938) of transillumination of living structures for microscope study. Evidences were presented that there was contractile tissue, which could be stimulated by histamine, near the openings of the sinusoids into the intralobular veins (see BURN, 1948) as indicated in Fig. 2. Following constriction, the sinusoids filled with blood coming from the portal veins and the hepatic artery, but the escape into the hepatic veins was prevented or impaired.

Any attempt to apply these views to the cat met with failure because, according to DALE and RICHARDS (1918) and BAUER et al. (1932), there was nothing in the liver of the cat to suggest a similar structure which might explain a fall in blood pressure when histamine was given. By measuring the time elapsing from the injection of the amine to the moment when the blood pressure started to fall, the shortest interval corresponded to the intra-arterial injection (in the aorta) and the longest to the injection into the portal vein (DALE and RICHARDS, 1918). Furthermore, if the liver was removed from the circulation, the fall in blood pressure following the intravenous injection of histamine was of about the same intensity as when the experiment was done in the intact animal. According to McDowall (1923) and Feldberg and Schilf (1930) the main accumulation of smooth muscle in the cat would occur in the pulmonary artery, since histamine produced a sharp rise in pulmonary artery pressure when injected intravenously, as shown first by Dale and Laidlaw (1910). Nonetheless, by utilizing the technique of making a cast of the liver circulation, Thomas and Essex (1949) mentioned that the cat also showed some constriction of the hepatic veins under the action of *Ascaris* extracts or histamine, though rabbits and rats did not present any reaction of the hepatic veins under comparable conditions. The reaction of cats, however, was considerably less than that among dogs.

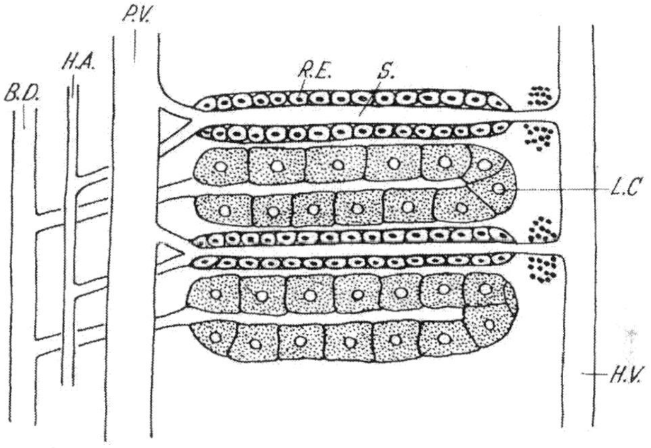

Fig. 2. Diagram of arrangement of blood-supply in the liver suggested by Knisely. *P.V.* portal vein from which blood goes through the sinusoids to the intralobular vein *H.V.* and so to the hepatic vein. The reticulo-endothelial cells, *R.E.*, line the sinusoids *S.* Liver cells, *L.C.*, disposed around the first part of the smallest bile-ducts *B.D.* Histamine causes swelling of the liver in the dog by constricting muscle around the openings of the collecting venules into the hepatic vein (According to Burn, 1948)

In the rabbit, Coca (1919) had shown an enormous thickness of smooth muscle in the branches of the pulmonary artery which contracted powerfully during anaphylaxis (Airila, 1914; Coca, 1919; Drinker and Bronfenbrenner, 1924) or under the action of histamine (Feldberg, 1927; Rocha e Silva, 1940a).

In favor of the theory of "strategic points" in the circulatory apparatus, one might mention the peculiar pattern of histamine shock in some species of animals. In the dog, the predominance of stasis in the liver and in the portal region, with only discrete or slight participation of the pulmonary circulation, and in the cat, the smaller participation of the liver in the mechanism of fall of blood pressure, with a definite rise in the pressure of the pulmonary artery, might fit nicely into that scheme. Even the case of the guinea pig, where the main symptom of histamine shock depended upon the thickness of the smooth muscle coats of the bronchioli fitted into that scheme of "strategic points" since it was assumed that the subsequent slow fall in arterial blood pressure was caused in part by the emphysema consequent to bronchioli constriction (Auer and Lewis, 1910). Also the rabbit, though reacting to histamine as a rule by a rise in blood pressure, showed a definite constriction of the pulmonary artery bed under the influence of histamine.

The main weakness of the conception of "strategic points" is the great emphasis upon constriction of smooth muscles to explain the circulatory effects of histamine. Other factors, as we are going to show, are as much or even more important to account for the steep fall of blood pressure in animals when large doses of histamine are given intravenously. Even in the dog, removal of the liver by an Eck fistula did not abolish completely, but only reduced, the magnitude of the fall in systemic blood pressure. By injecting small doses of histamine into the jugular vein, Feldberg, Schilf and Zernick (1928) were able to show a pressure fall in systemic circulation and in the portal vein, though if the same doses were injected directly into a branch of the portal vein, a smaller effect was seen upon the systemic pressure, in spite of the fact that the pressure in the portal vein increased conspicuously (Fig. 3, 4). From these experiments, the German workers concluded: "*daß die Gefäße des großen Kreislaufs empfindlicher gegen Histamin sind als die Lebergefäße*" (FELDBERG and SCHILF, 1930).

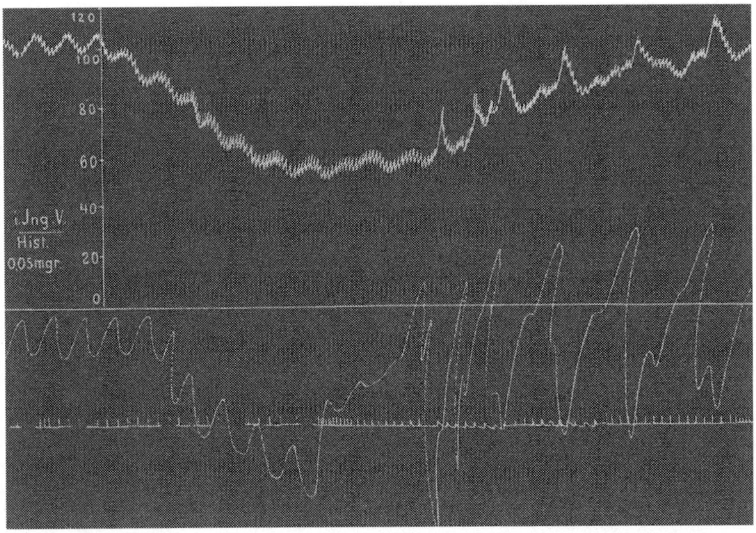

Fig. 3. Dog. Intrajugular injection of 0.05 mg of histamine. Upper tracing, arterial blood pressure; lower tracing, pressure in the portal vein. (According to FELDBERG, SCHILF and ZERNICK, 1928)

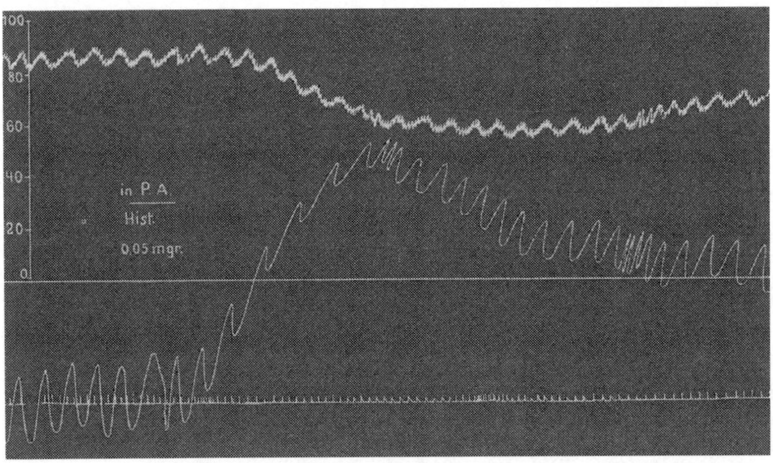

Fig. 4. Continuation of tracings of Fig. 3. Intraportal injection of 0.05 mg of histamine. The return of blood pressure is slower than seen in Fig. 3. (According to FELDBERG, SCHILF and ZERNICK, 1928)

By making plethysmographic records immediately following the intraarterial injection of 1 mg of histamine into the hind limb of a dog, RANSON et al. (1923) demonstrated an increase in the limb volume, independent of the integrity of the local nerve supply, and thus indicated that, on the one hand, the liver could not be the only factor in histamine shock, and on the other hand, that the effects are peripheral. A decreased viscosity of the blood, induced by histamine, was described by WAUD (1928), who invoked this effect to explain, in part, the fall in blood pressure.

We have to remark that the liver might play a larger role if the constriction of the sinusoid or supra-hepatic sphincters were of such an intensity to entrap a significant proportion of the circulating blood in the portal region reducing the venous return by stasis in the abdominal vessels. In fact, this can be achieved with large doses of histamine, but the diffusibility of this substance is such that its effects are not very lasting and are never as persistent as those obtained with peptone, *Ascaris* extracts and anaphylactic shock, in which conditions the symptomatology is dominated by the liver with enormous stasis in the portal region, as described in another chapter of this book. (See Chapter 3, Section D: Release of Histamine in Anaphylaxis.) That the obliteration of the hepatic circulation should have a great significance in the genesis of such kinds of shock has been shown in the experiments by SIMONDS and BRANDES (1927), who interrupted the circulation in the supra-hepatic veins by tying a rubber tubing around the vessels just below the diaphragm and above the dome of the liver obliterating the orifices into the caval vein. Concomitant with a shock-like fall in arterial blood pressure, the liver increased in size as a consequence of this mechanical *Lebersperre.* After removal of the ligature, the blood pressure rapidly rose to higher levels than the initial one (Fig. 5). But, even so, this mechanical obstruction did not reproduce the exact situation obtained when the liver stasis is produced by a discharge of histamine as in anaphylactic shock, since the presence of the released amine produces further endothelial damage with extravasation of plasma and stagnation of blood in the vessels subsidiary to the portal vein.

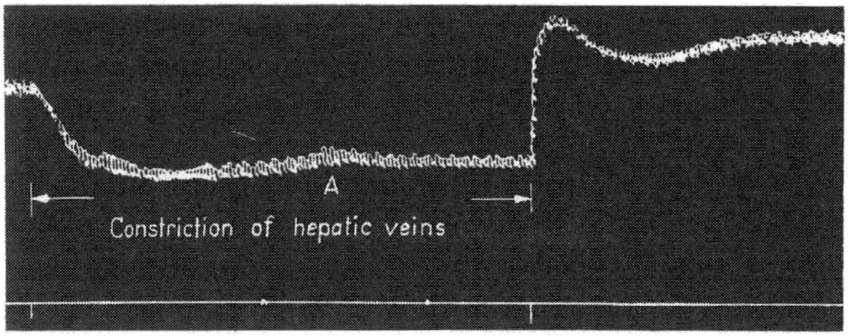

Fig. 5. Effect of constriction of the hepatic vein of a dog on the arterial blood pressure. Duration of constriction (between the arrows) was 1.5 min. The small increase (*A*) of the blood pressure was due to a slight release of the ligature (According to SIMONDS and BRANDES, 1927)

B. Inchley's theory

Inchley's theory constituted an interesting complement to the MAUTNER and PICK conception by assuming that the fall in blood pressure produced by histamine could arise from a generalized constriction of the venous system (INCHLEY, 1923, 1926) with stasis in the whole capillary bed and decreased venous return to the heart. The advantage of Inchley's conception was to explain a little further the "histamine paradox", since a generalized venous constriction might account for a fall in blood pressure *in vivo* and at the same time, explain the reduction in outflow from perfused organs other than the liver or the lungs (which are covered by the strategic points theory). However, the main weakness of Inchley's conception was to reduce to a single factor such a complex phenomenon, histamine shock. According to this theory the vasodilation produced by histamine upon the capillary bed would be mainly secondary to a partial obliteration of the circulation in the venous system.

The experiments by INCHLEY (1926) were done in pigs and cats, and the higher sensitivity of isolated pieces of veins, when compared with strips of arterioles, to the stimulating action of histamine appeared to be conclusive evidence about the locus of action of the latter. In a series of perfusion experiments, INCHLEY (1926) showed that the decrease in flow occurred mainly where segments of veins were introduced into the perfusion circuit, although perfusion of the arterial system, including the capillary network, did not present the decrease of flow seen in the intact organs. This relative insensitivity of the cat's arterial system to the action of histamine confirmed some experiments performed earlier by DALE and RICHARDS (1918), who perfused the arterioles after cutting through the mesentery close to the wall of the intestine and measured the flow of blood dripping from the ends of the severed small arteries. A discrete but distinct decrease in flow volume was observed with histamine, though acetylcholine and amyl nitrite produced a conspicuous increase in flow indicating arteriolar vasodilation.

Data accumulated in the literature are sometimes against, sometimes in favor of Inchley's views. Direct observations of the ear vessels of the cat indicated a generalized dilation of the small veins (HOOKER, 1920). In the omentum of the cat, RICH (1921) showed a general dilation of veins and capillaries following histamine shock. Later on, FLEISCH (1931) obtained variable results, depending upon the concentration of histamine in perfusion experiments of the veins of cats and dogs. With high histamine concentrations up to 1:1 milion, a strong venous constriction was observed, while with lower concentrations (from 10^{-6} to 10^{-9}) the constriction was preceeded by a short dilation. In the range of 10^{-7} to 10^{-9}, in 70–80% of the cases, histamine produced a pure dilation: *Diese dilatorische Wirkung des Histamins auf die Venen liefert einen weiteren Baustein für das Verständnis des Histaminschocks. Die Venenerweiterung, die sich mit der Capillarerschlaffung assoziert, begünstigt das Liegenbleiben des Blutes in der Peripherie, was zur Ursache des venösen Rückflusses und damit zum Kreislaufschock durch Histamin führt* (FLEISCH, 1931). A description of the many-sided effects of histamine upon the venous and arterial system was presented by MATEEFF and SCHNEIDER (1935). In modern times, HADDY (1960) described the increased pressure of the small veins in the dog's foreleg concluding that "low concentrations of histamine raise small venous pressure by arteriolar dilation, that higher concentrations raise it both by arteriolar dilation and venous constriction, and that the venous constriction results both from direct and indirect (blocked by a sympatholytic agent) actions of histamine." HADDY (1960) also concluded that histamine edema may be adequately explained by elevation of capillary hydrostatic pressure. In one point, however, the findings of HADDY diverge from those of INCHLEY in that the increased venous pressure is accompanied by arteriolar dilation. HADDY's work is going to be presented in a more detailed way in the second part of this Section.

C. Dale's theory (capillary vasodilation)

INCHLEY's conception was in conflict with the demonstration by DALE and RICHARDS (1918), DALE and LAIDLAW (1919) and BURN and DALE (1926) who showed that under certain experimental conditions, especially in the dog and in the monkey, histamine induced considerable vasodilation when injected through a perfused limb. Even in the cat under careful perfusion conditions, histamine in small doses produced an increase in flow, followed by a period of insensitivity (tachyphylaxis), during which the perfused leg failed to respond to the same dose of histamine. This situation was interpreted as due to a loss of tone of the small vessels, especially capillaries, under the action of such minute doses of histamine. If, however, a small dose of adrenaline (1:5 million) was added to the perfusing fluid, the preparation responded again to the same dose of histamine (BURN and DALE, 1926). In subsequent experiments, comparing the effect of other drugs, such as acetylcholine, amyl nitrite and adrenaline itself, using an improved method of perfusion, DALE and RICHARDS (1927) regularly produced a vasodilation by histamine in the cat without the addition of adrenaline. The previous failure to show a regular dilating effect of histamine, was attributed to the improper conditions of the perfusion experiments, leading to an irreversible loss of the capillary tone. If the conditions of the perfusion were improved by maintaining a high level of tone in the capillary bed, histamine regularly produced, even in cats, the same vasodilation that it produced in dogs and monkeys: "*For no reason which we could analyse we now for the first time found it possible, in many artificial perfusions of a cat's limb with plain defibrinated blood, without any addition of adrenaline or other vaso-tonic agent, to observe the development of a vascular tone as distributed that histamine would reproduce the vasodilation characteristic of its action in vivo. The "paradox" thus disappeared; but we did not know why. Of course, (Richards and I) speculated on the possibility that this tone was produced by a normal, though minimal content of adrenaline in the shed blood.*" (DALE, 1953, pg. 411).

To HEMINGWAY and McDOWALL (1926) the tone of the capillary bed was maintained to a great extent by the H^+ ion concentration of the perfusing fluid. An increase in alkalinity from 7.4 to 7.6 increased the tone and the reactivity to the vasodilating action of histamine, and the opposite was observed by reducing the inflow pH to lower levels. When the capillary tone had disappeared in the course of an experiment, the addition of N/100 NaOH or $NaHCO_3$ to the perfusing fluid restored it, rendering the system more reactive to the vasodilating effect of histamine, though the effect of the addition of a strong base disappeared after a short interval of time. Therefore, the conclusion was drawn that the loss of tone, observed after a long perfusion through isolated organs, could be mainly caused by formation of lactic acid, CO_2 and other metabolites.

Concomitant with the stasis in the capillary bed, produced by the intravenous injection of histamine in the cat (which might explain, according to DALE and co-workers, the precipitous fall in blood pressure occurring in cats and dogs) a generalized leakage of plasma took place, with increased hematocrit volume and a parallel rise in the hemoglobin value and red-cell count, as indicated in Table 1 (DALE and LAIDLAW, 1919).

Table 1. *Parallelism between the changes in hemoglobin value, corpuscular volume, by hematocrit and red-cell count in cats* (according to DALE and LAIDLAW, 1919)

Hemoglobinometer			Hematocrit			Red cells per c.mm ($\times 10^{-3}$)		
Normal	Shock	Ratio	Normal	Shock	Ratio	Normal	Shock	Ratio
74	98	1.32	30	40	1.33	8,344	11,360	1.36

Direct measurements of plasma showing a reduction of the circulating fluid could be taken as a direct demonstration that the numerical changes in circulating red cells were due to leakage of plasma and consequent hemoconcentration, secondary to increased capillary permeability produced by histamine (DALE and LAIDLAW, 1919).

The attempt to apply such views to the explanation of traumatic shock in which participation of histamine was an obvious possibility, was presented by DALE et al. (1919) and DALE (1923). This view is not generally accepted (WIGGERS, 1950).

The increase in red cell count and hemoconcentration was many times confirmed in subsequent years in the cat and the dog (KELLAWAY and COWELL, 1923; HASHIMOTO, 1925–1926; SMITH, 1928; FLATOW, 1929; FLATOW and HÜTTEL, 1930; DOMENECH-ALSINA, 1933; and others) and in other species (FELDBERG and SCHILF, 1930). By estimating blood volume with the dye T-1824, in the unanesthetized dog, SILVER et al. (1944) studied the effect of a single intravenous injection of histamine (1.5 mg/kg). Hematocrit values were also determined. Within 2 minutes after the injection of histamine, a sharp increase in the hematocrit values and fall in plasma volume concomitant with a sharp decrease in circulating dye concentration, indicated a rapid passage of plasma and dye through the capillary walls which were rendered more permeable by the action of histamine. The same experiment repeated in the anesthetized dog showed the appearance of dye in the lymph collected in the thoracic and cervical duct (Fig. 6).

By the subcutaneous route, however, the effects of histamine on cats and dogs were different from those obtained by the intravenous route. Though the hematocrit rose conspicuously after the subcutaneous injection of 3 to 12 mg of histamine base per kilo, the rate of escape of the dye T-1824 did not appear to increase significantly (DEYRUP, 1944). The increase in the hematocrit reading could not be ascribed to contraction of the spleen, since it occurred also regularly in dogs submitted to a previous splenectomy. However, the persistance of the initial plasma volume remained unexplained and attributed by DEYRUP to the way of introduction of the base (subcutaneously) and the fact that the animals were unanesthetized. Actually, when two etherized cats were injected intravenously with histamine, DEYRUP (1944) could confirm DALE and LAIDLAW's findings.

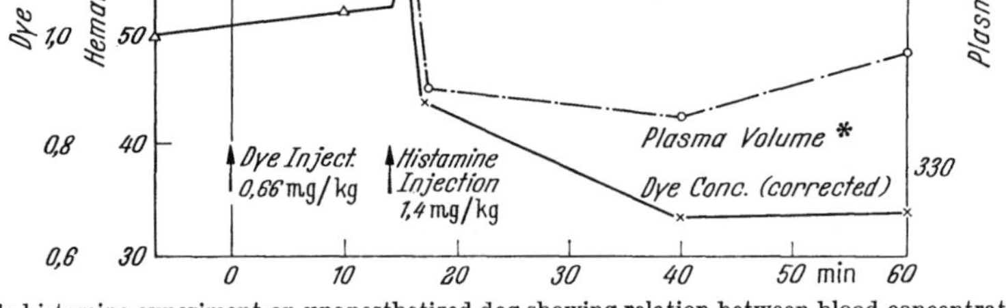

Fig. 6. Single histamine experiment on unanesthetized dog showing relation between blood concentration changes and disappearance curve of the dye (According to SILVER et al., 1944)

Though the parallelism between hemoconcentration and the intensity of shock is not complete (NEUWELT et al. 1941), a situation similar to that seen in histamine shock only infrequently can be obtained with other vasodilator agents, such as amyl nitrite and acetylcholine (DALE and LAIDLAW, 1919). On the other hand, in conditions in which histamine-like poisons appeared to be released, as in anaphylactic and peptone shock, hemoconcentration with similar characteristics could be observed (MOON, 1938, 1940).

That the increased number of red cells per cmm could be accounted for by a leakage of plasma through the capillary walls was also suggested by experiments by FLATOW and HÜTTEL (1930). They were unable to find reticulocytes in the circulation of animals submitted to shock, and only an occasional erythroblast could be detected under similar conditions. The possibility of the spleen discharging its depots of erythrocytes into the circulation was also excluded, since in splenectomized cats, the increase in the number of red cells after histamine, was not significantly different from that occurring in normal cats (DALE and LAIDLAW, 1919; BARCROFT and FELDBERG, 1930). Again, as regards the effect of histamine upon the number of erythrocytes and hemoglobin values, the rabbit behaved in an anomalous way, showing a decrease rather than an increase, following the subcutaneous injection of large doses of histamine (UNDERHILL and ROTH, 1922; FLATOW, 1929; FELDBERG and SCHILF, 1930, pg. 362).

It appeared, therefore, that the conception by DALE (1920, 1923) that histamine produced a shock-like condition by a generalized dilation of the capillary bed followed by leakage of plasma through the endothelial walls made more permeable through the direct action of the amine, acquired a broad experimental basis in subsequent years.

Nevertheless, the relative importance of the vasoconstrictor effects of histamine upon arterioles and venules and the dilating effect upon capillaries varied from one species to another, and these variations might explain some facets of the "histamine paradox". In cats and dogs, under normal conditions, it appeared evident that a predominance of the capillary dilation over the spasmogenic action of histamine upon arterioles and veins was a major contributing factor in the production of the fall in blood pressure regularly observed in *carnivora*. The rabbit, however, presented a condition in which the equilibrium between the two tendencies could be shifted in either direction, according to the anesthesia under which the experiments were done (FELDBERG, 1927). By direct observation of the denervated ear vessels, the injection of 0.03 to 0.05 mg of histamine in the normal ear of a rabbit induced constriction of the central artery with an almost simultaneous increase in the number of visible venules and dilation of the previously visible ones: "*In some instances the arterial constriction was severe and the general reddening and venous filling correspondingly small; in others the arterial constriction was slight, and the general dilator effect very pronounced*" (FELDBERG, 1927). This was in agreement with previous observation by LEWIS and MARVIN (1927) which showed hyperemia in the rabbit ear following a skin puncture through a drop of a 1:10,000 solution of histamine. However, the contention by FELDBERG (1927) that the nature and degree of anesthesia might explain the different reactions of the rabbit toward histamine was challenged by DIXON and HOYLE (1930).

For many years, histamine was the only endogenous agent with capillary activity which had been proved beyond doubt. Acetylcholine and other vasodilating substances, such as amyl nitrite, or adenosine and adenyl compounds, acting mainly upon the arterial system or the heart, did not reproduce the shock-like picture shown by histamine, with plasma leakage through increased capillary permeability. We knew that many irritating substances induced an increase of capillary permeability, as revealed by the passage of blue dye from the circulation to the subcutaneous spaces, but this effect could be caused by a release of histamine, as will be discussed in another section of this Chapter (see Part III: *Action of histamine upon the capillaries*).

Now we know that a number of polypeptides, such as bradykinin, angiotensin and substance-P can act upon the capillary wall, increasing its permeability

(Feldberg, 1956; Spector, 1958; Lewis, 1961; Schachter, 1961; Frimmer, 1961). They can, therefore, be called upon to explain many facets of the shocks produced by anaphylaxis, bacterial toxins, trauma or hemorrhage, when a simple release of histamine does not explain all symptoms observed. These problems will be discussed in another chapter of this book.

D. Cardiac failure

In spite of the fact that the previous observations by Dale and Laidlaw (1910,1919) had attributed a minor role to the heart in the genesis of the histamine shock, Rühl (1929, 1930) brought forward the question of damage to the heart as one of the causes of the fall in blood pressure induced by histamine. According to Rühl, the right heart appeared less damaged than the left one, and its alterations could be accounted for by the increased resistance in the pulmonary circulation (in cats and rabbits) or by stasis in the venous system (in the dog). Therefore, attention was directed mainly toward the behavior of the left heart, since any increase in pressure in the left cavities, especially the left auricle, concomitant with a steep fall in systemic B. P. would indicate, according to Rühl, an acute insufficiency of the heart muscle. This effect, and also an increase in volume of the whole heart, was observed not only *in vivo* (cats) but also in heart-lung preparations (dogs). The increase in pressure in the left auricle was considerably more conspicuous than that registered in the right one (Fig. 7).

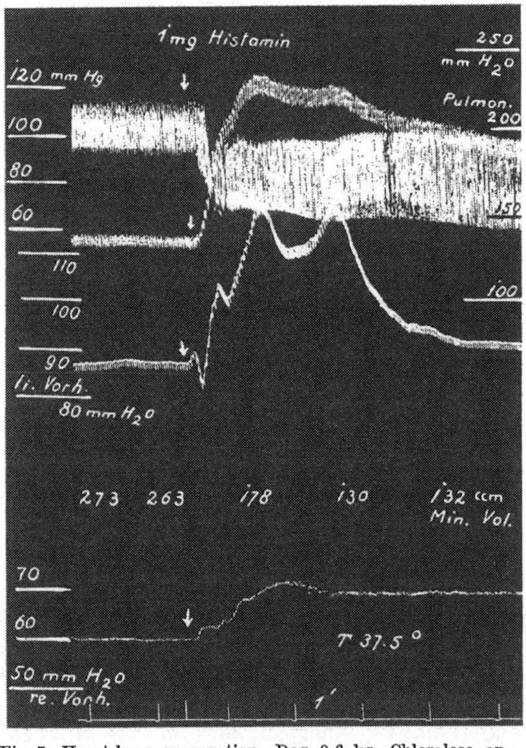

Fig. 7. Heart-lung preparation. Dog 9.6 kg. Chloralose anesthesia. Arterial resistance (80 mm Hg). Pulmonary artery pressure, pressures in the left and right auricles. The large oscillations indicate the systemic minute volume. At the arrow: injection of 1 mg of histamine. (According to Rühl, 1929)

From his experiments on the heart-lung preparation, Rühl concluded: "*that the severe insufficiency of the left ventricle should come in the foreground.*" The same conclusion was drawn by Klisiecki and Holobut (1937) in experiments in the intact dog.

A similar increase in the pressure in the left heart with decreased cardiac output was described by Rössler (1930) in experiments of heart-lung preparations in the dog. Papaverine counteracted these effects, though when pitressin was given before histamine, the latter corrected the heart insufficiency produced by the pituitary hormone, apparently by counteracting the coronary vasoconstriction induced by pitressin (Rössler, 1930).

Cardiac arrhythmias were found in heart-lung preparations by Rühl (1929) and in the intact animal by Feldberg and Schilf (1930) with large doses of histamine. Besides trivial alterations in the frequency or amplitude of the beats, extrasystoles were observed (RÜHL, 1929) and electrocardiographic changes persisted, even after section of the vagus (HASHIMOTO, 1925), with an increased P. R. interval, suggesting a direct effect of histamine upon the auriculo-ventricular bundle with partial or total block.

DIXON and HOYLE (1930) also suggested damage of the heart to explain the fall of B. P. in the right auricle and pulmonary artery in the dog after the injection of 0.5 to 2.0 mg of histamine intravenously. However, the main cause for the incomplete filling of the right heart was ascribed to *Lebersperre* in agreement with the MAUTNER and PICK theory. In the cat, with doses ranging from 0.5 to 1.0 mg i. v., a sharp increase in the pulmonary artery pressure was observed. This could not be accounted for by heart damage nor by arteriolar constriction. The explanation, according to DIXON and HOYLE, might reside in the coronary vasodilation which is a common finding in cats under the influence of histamine. By increasing coronary flow, a considerable amount of blood would be short-circuited from the left to the right heart, thus explaining the increase in the circulatory volume of the lung observed in cats. The increase in pulmonary artery pressure as observed in rabbits could only be due to arteriolar constriction since in this animal species histamine produces coronary constriction and a decrease in lung volume follows the injection of histamine. On the other hand, the indication by DIXON and HOYLE of a vasoconstrictor effect of histamine upon the coronary bed in the intact dog has not been confirmed by others as we are going to discuss in a later paragraph. With the heart-lung preparation in the dog, MÜLLER et al. (1932) were unable to find diastolic heart dilation when small doses (up to 0.1 mg) of histamine were injected, but even the damage observed after larger doses (above 0.5 mg) was not seen if these doses were given after repeated administrations of small doses (< 0.1 mg) of histamine. These observations agreed with the findings described by FELDBERG and SCHILF (1930) that the symptoms obtained with large doses of histamine did not appear or were short-lived when preceeded by treatment with small doses.

ETTINGER et al. (1936) gave histamine for as long as 266 days to dogs by intravenous infusion of a 1:10,000 solution at the rate of 2 to 4 ml per 90 minutes. These amounts were enough to double or triple the heart rate. *Post mortem* examination revealed no evidence of degenerative changes in the coronary arteries or myocardium. In acute experiments, giving high doses of histamine to dogs, cats, rabbits, and guinea pigs, KIRCH (1933) observed a dilation of the right ventricle, of the type he had classified as "*tonogene Dilatation*", but no permanent damage to the heart: "*Eine Herzinsuffizienz durch Histamin* (RÜHL) *ist für meine hier mitgeteilten Untersuchungen sicher abzulehnen*". The increase in tone of the right ventricle according to Kirch could be attributed to the venous stasis in the lung causing a compensatory heart dilation of the tonic type. Therefore, instead of failing, the heart would be reacting against the increased resistance to flow in the pulmonary circulation.

The effect of small doses of histamine upon the cardiac output has been highly controversial. EPPINGER and SCHÜRMEYER (1928) described marked reduction. This agrees with findings of BLALOCK and LEVY (1937). However, JOHNSON and BLALOCK (1931) found no change or an increase of cardiac output in anesthetized dogs following subcutaneous injection of small doses of histamine. With large subcutaneous doses (10 mg per kg), in the unanesthetized dog, histamine produced a marked reduction in cardiac output, with drops in the A-V O_2 differential and O_2 consumption, with increased peripheral resistance (DEYRUP and ROOT, 1947).

In a fresh approach to the problem, DELAUNOIS et al. (1959) used thermistors (DELAUNOIS, 1961) to register the cardiac output in the anesthetized dog and observed a sharp increase in output following the intravenous infusion of 250 to 300 μg of histamine per kg of body weight, concomitant with a profound fall in arterial blood pressure to 50 to 80% of the original levels. Parallel to the arterial blood pressure fall, a slight increase in the pulmonary artery pressure occurred, which persisted for the duration of the arterial B. P. fall. From these experiments it was concluded: "*that the arterial blood pressure fall in the histamine shock has its primary cause in the dilation of the peripheral vessels and not in a decrease of the cardiac output due to heart failure,*" (DELAUNOIS et al., 1959).

In 25 patients receiving intravenous infusions of histamine there was no evidence of anginal pains, signs of coronary constriction, or of permanent heart damage (PETERS and HORTON, 1944 a).

From this analysis of the literature, we have to conclude that the heart plays only a subsidiary role in the genesis of histamine shock. Rather, the genesis of histamine shock is mainly caused by a generalized dilation of capillaries and small vessels, increased smooth muscle tone at strategic points in the venous system and pulmonary circulation with secondary peripheral stasis (largely in the splanchnic area), decreased venous return, slowing of the lung circulation, insufficient filling of the left heart, and reduction of effective circulating volume. The picture can vary from species to species, as we are going to see in the next section of this chapter, but in all cases the alterations observed in the heart *in situ* can be ascribed mainly to one or the other alterations in the peripheral circulation. When saline is infused into an animal under histamine shock, with rapid increase in the circulation volume, the heart resumes its normal function (DALE and LAIDLAW, 1910; RICH, 1921).

These conclusions were strengthened by the observation of the effects of histamine directly upon the isolated heart, presented below.

E. Effects on the isolated mammalian heart

Upon the isolated mammalian heart perfused by LANGENDORFF's technique, the effects of small doses of histamine varied considerably from species to species as far as sensitivity was concerned, but in general there was an increase in the frequency and amplitude of the beat (DALE and LAIDLAW, 1910; RABE, 1912; ROTHLIN, 1920; VIOTTI, 1924; GUNN, 1926; STAUB and GRASSMANN, 1930, and others, as indicated in Table 3). The differences in sensitivity of the different species were considerable, as the cat's heart was shown to be 5 times less sensitive than the rabbit's heart (GUNN, 1926). A slight increase in heart tonus, before the usual acceleration of rhythm and increased amplitude, was observed by ROTHLIN (1920). The effects even in the same preparation depended upon the dose. VIOTTI (1924) demonstrated, by the use of the rabbit heart, that the smallest concentrations (10^{-7}) increased the frequency without any effect upon the amplitude, while higher concentrations (8×10^{-7}) invariably decreased the frequency and increased the amplitude, with reduction of the volume of fluid passing through the heart; with the guinea pig heart, concentrations of the order of 2.5×10^{-7} produced increased amplitude and frequency, with sharp reduction of the volume of perfusion fluid, though concentrations of the order of 10^{-5} caused marked increase in amplitude with diminution of frequency, with a late reduction in the volume of fluid. VIOTTI concluded that the highest and lowest concentrations of histamine provoked increased frequency and eventually an increase in amplitude, though intermediate doses did produce a decrease in both frequency and amplitude. The inhibitory effects of histamine upon the isolated hearts of the rabbit and guinea pig were blocked by atropine (VIOTTI, 1924). Similar results were obtained in the rabbit by GUNN (1926) and STAUB and GRASSMANN (1930). With high doses, especially when the heart was perfused with Ringer-Locke solution, heart block and extra-systoles were obtained (EINIS, 1913; GUNN, 1926). ANDRUS and WILCOX (1939) compared the effects of histamine and anaphylaxis upon the isolated guinea pig heart and observed an increase in heart rate, arrhythmias and coronary vasoconstriction. Atropine antagonized the effects of histamine on the coronary bed, but was without effect upon the alterations of rhythm. A release of histamine from the isolated heart of sensitized guinea pigs was demonstrated by FEIGEN et al. (1960), who also indicated the perfect similarity between the effects of histamine and those of the antigen in this animal species, as shown in Table 2.

The effects of histamine upon the mammalian heart were strikingly similar to those produced by sympathomimetic amines, as far as the changes in rhythm were concerned (ROCHA e SILVA, 1946). Because histamine could discharge catechol amines from the adrenals and possibly also from any stores of chromaffin tissue in the body, it has been a strong possibility that it might act upon the heart by releasing these amines, since the heart contains stocks of nor-adrenaline and adrenaline (GOODALL, 1951; TRUEX, 1950 and others) which might be mobilized by histamine. In accordance with this view, WENT et al. (1952) showed a blockade of the effects of histamine upon the heart by a treatment with ergotamine. One difficulty in this view was the fact that upon the coronary bed, in some species, as the guinea pig and the rabbit, histamine produced vasoconstriction. However, if histamine was given first to the perfused guinea pig heart a subsequent injection of adrenaline further constricted the coronary bed (ROCHA e SILVA, 1946). The problem has been reinvestigated recently by MANNAIONI (1960) and TRENDELENBURG (1960) by using dichloroisoproterenol (DCI) which has been shown by MORAN and PERKINS (1958) to block the effects of catechol amines upon the heart. This reagent had only a small effect upon the alterations of rhythm provoked by histamine, indicating that histamine acts to a greater extent by a direct action upon the myocardium and not through the β-receptors of adrenaline. A further discussion of this problem is presented by VON EULER, in another section of this chapter (see: *Relationship between histamine and the autonomous nervous system.*)

Upon the isolated auricle of the rabbit and the guinea pig, histamine, in moderate doses, invariably produced increased amplitude and acceleration of the rhythm (DEWS and GRAHAM, 1946; PENNA et al. 1959; HOLTZ, 1960 and FEIGEN et al. 1960), as in the whole perfused heart. In *in vivo* experiments or in

Table 2. *Effects of ovalbumin and histamine on the sensitized guinea pig heart* (according to FEIGEN, 1960)

	Control ± S.E.	Challenge ± S.E.	Per cent change
	*Reactions to ovalbumin**		
Heart rate (beats/min)	206.8 ±13.19	256.6 ±16.10	+ 24.1
Amplitude (mm)	26.4 ± 2.10	56.3 ± 5.03	+113.1
Coronary flow (ml/g/min)	6.48 ± 0.72	3.36 ± 0.48	— 48.1
	*Reactions to histamine***		
Heart rate (beats/min)	184.5 ±13.69	215.8 ±18.43	+ 17.0
Amplitude (mm)	15.6 ± 2.58	34.3 ± 4.44	+120.0
Coronary flow (ml/g/min)	2.50 ± 0.41	1.92 ± 0.42	— 23.2

* Reaction to 1 mg of ovalbumin.

** Reactions to 0.25 ml of 10^{-3} M histamine.

heart-lung preparations, in all animal species, including man, histamine produced acceleration and increased amplitude of the beat, as indicated in Table 3.

Upon the coronary circulation, histamine produced dilation or constriction depending upon the species of animal studied or the conditions of the experiment. In cats and dogs, and possibly in man, histamine produced, as a rule, a dilation

Table 3. *Cardio-vascular alterations produced by histamine on the systemic and pulmonary circulation*

Strategic points	Species	Effects observed	Influence on B.P.	References
Venous system	Cat	Constriction ++	↓↓	1, 40, 59, 75, 104
	Cat	Dilation		48, 91
	Cat	No effect	0	85
	Dog	Constriction ++	↓↓	32, 40, 44, 53
	Pig	Constriction ++	↓↓	59
	Rabbit	Constriction +++	↓↓↓	38, 47, 115
	Human	Constriction		
Pulmonary artery	Cat	Constriction +++	↓↓↓	1, 17, 20, 25, 41, 42, 70, 72, 85, 99
	Dog	Constriction +	↓	22, 25, 49, 67, 77, 82, 99, 129
	Rabbit	Constriction +++	↓↓↓	6, 10, 17, 25, 81, 92, 98, 105, 129, 130
	G. pig	Constriction +	↓	45
Supra-hepatic veins	Cat	No effect	0	7, 39, 41, 51, 78, 103
	Dog	Constriction +++	↓↓↓	5, 7, 26, 37, 42, 44, 56, 73, 78, 112
	Cat	Relaxation (passive)	↑	7, 78
	Cat	Constriction ++	0	112
	Monkey	No effect	0	43, 78
	Rabbit	No effect	0	43, 78, 112
	G. pig	No effect	0	43, 78
Arterial system	Cat	Constriction +	↑	21, 50, 75, 103, 108, 51
	Dog	Dilation	↓	8, 13, 21, 51, 100, 111
	Pig	Constriction +	↑	59, 107
	Rabbit	Constriction +++	↑↑↑	47, 56, 108, 115
Capillary bed				
A) Vaso-motor effects	Cat	Dilation	↓	8, 13, 20, 21, 91, 99
	Dog	Dilation	↓	13, 20, 21, 56, 98, 99
	Monkey	Dilation	↓	13, 99
	Rabbit	Depending on tone	↑↓	43, 56, 58, 69, 81
	Human	Flushing of face, peripheral vaso-dilation		15, 29, 30, 54, 88, 119, 121
B) Increased permeability	Several	+ Hemoconcentration		2, 21, 32, 43, 67, 71, 110, 131 84, 106, 111
		Blueing of the skin area		11, 16, 79, 90, 93, 94
	Human	Wheal formation (skin)		29, 30, 68
Blood volume	Dog	No change or slow fall		23
	(in vivo)	Reduction		14, 32
Brain vessels	Cat	Dilation		59, 126
	Dog	Dilation		62, 66, 102, 118
	Human	Dilation		102
	Rabbit	Constriction		101
	Monkey	Dilation		27
Kidney vessels	Cat	Constriction		50, 74
	Dog	Constriction		74
Blood cells				
A) Red cells (Hematocrit)	Dog	Reduction		57
	Dog	Increased		23, 46, 111
	Cat	Increased		20
	G. pig	Increased		46
B) W. B. C.	Monkey, human	Leukocytosis		80
	Human	No change		28

Table 3 (continuation). *Cardio-vascular alterations produced by histamine on the heart and coronary circulation*

Locus of action or effects	Conditions of the experiments	Animal species	Effects observed	References
Cardiac output	In vivo or HLP	Dog	Reduction ++	12, 23, 24, 25, 32
		Dog	No change	60
		Dog	Increase	22, 75
		Cat	Increase	20
		Human	Increase	35, 121
Right ventricle	In vivo or HLP	Rabbit	Increase +++	34, 63
		Dog	Increase +	34, 63
		Cat	Dilation ++	17, 20, 34, 63
		Dog	Decrease	95, 99
Left auricle (Pressure)	In vivo or HLP	Dog	Increase	95, 99
		Cat	Increase	99
		Cat	No effect	70
Rhythm	In vivo	Human	Tachycardia	9, 54, 55, 119, 120, 121, 122
		Dog	Tachycardia	23, 34
		Cat	Tachycardia	64
		Cat	Bradycardia	20
	HLP	Dog	Tachycardia	83
	In vitro (Langendorff's)	Several (cat, dog, g. pig, rabbit)	Positive ino- and chronotropic effects	31, 36, 52, 86, 89, 97, 109, 113, 114, 116, 117, 123, 124, 125, 128
Arrhythmias	HLP	Dog	Extra-systoles (alt. ECG)	55, 99
	In vivo	Dog	Extra-systoles	43, 65
	In vivo	Human	Alt. ECG	55, 87, 121, 122
Coronary circulation	In vitro	Cat	Vaso-dilation	19, 52, 57, 83, 96
		Dog	Vaso-dilation	52, 83
		G. pig	Constriction	3, 36, 52, 117, 127, 128
		Rabbit	Constriction	19, 20, 52, 96, 109
	In vivo	Dog	Dilation	33, 56
	HLP	Dog	Dilation	76, 83, 99
		Human	Dilation	4
Myocardial damage	In vivo or HLP	Dog		99
Papillary muscle	In vitro	Cat	Neg. inotropic effect	18

1. Abe (1920)
2. Abramson and Engel (1938)
3. Andrus and Wilcox (1939)
4. Anrep (1936)
5. Baer and Rössler (1926/27)
6. Barbour (1912/13)
7. Bauer et al. (1932)
8. Bauer and Richards (1928)
9. Benson and Horton (1945)
10. Best and McHenry (1931)
11. Bier and Rocha e Silva (1939)
12. Blalock and Levy (1937)
13. Burn and Dale (1926)
14. Butler et al. (1931)
15. Carrier (1922)
16. Chappell et al. (1952)
17. Cloetta and Anderes (1914)
18. Cobbin and Thorp (1959)
19. Cruickshank and Subba Rau (1927)
20. Dale and Laidlaw (1910)
21. Dale and Richards (1918)
22. Delaunois et al. (1959)
23. Deyrup (1944)
24. Deyrup and Root (1947)
25. Dixon and Hoyle (1930)
26. Donnet et al. (1946)
27. Dumke and Schmidt (1943)
28. Dzsinich and Gallé (1939)
29. Ebbecke (1917)
30. Ebbecke (1923)
31. Einis (1913)
32. Eppinger and Schürmeyer (1928)
33. Essex et al. (1940)
34. Ettinger et al. (1936)
35. Euler and Liljestrand (1929)
36. Feigen et al. (1960)
37. Feldberg (cit. in 43)
38. Feldberg (1927)
39. Feldberg (1929)
40. Feldberg et al. (cit. in 43)
41. Feldberg and Kellaway (1937a)
42. Feldberg and Kellaway (1937b)
43. Feldberg and Schilf (1930)
44. Feldberg et al. (1928)
45. Field and Drinker (1930)
46. Flatow (1929)
47. Fleckenstein (1952)
48. Fleisch (1931)
49. Fühner and Starling (1913)
50. Ganter and Schretzenmayr (1929)

51. GANTER and SCHRETZENMAYR (1930)
52. GUNN (1926)
53. HADDY (1960)
54. HARMER and HARRIS (1926)
55. HASHIMOTO (cit. in 43)
56. HOCHREIN and MEIER (1930)
57. HUEPER and ICHNIOWSKI (1943)
58. HUNT (1917; cit. in 43)
59. INCHLEY (1926)
60. JOHNSON and BLALOCK (1931)
61. KELLAWAY and COWELL (1923)
62. KELLER (1930)
63. KIRCH (1933)
64. KISCH (1929)
65. KLISIECKI and HOLOBUT (1937)
66. KOOPMANS (1939)
67. LAMSON et al. (1923)
68. LAMSON (1929)
69. LEWIS and MARVIN (1927)
70. LUISADA (1928)
71. MCCARRELL and DRINKER (1941)
72. MCDOWALL (1923)
73. MANWARING et al. (1923)
74. MARIMOTO (1928)
75. MATEEFF and SCHNEIDER (1935)
76. MATSUMOTO (cit. in 43)
77. MAUTNER and PICK (1915)
78. MAUTNER and PICK (1929)
79. MILES and MILES (1952)
80. MOON et al. (1935)
81. MOREL and MAROIS (1949)
82. MÜLLER et al. (1932)
83. NARAYANA (1933)
84. NEUWELT et al. (1941)
85. OSAWA (1930)
86. PENNA et al. (1959)
87. PETERS and HORTON (1944b)
88. PICKERING and HESS (1933)
89. RABE (1912)
90. RAMSDELL (1928)
91. RICH (1921)
92. ROCHA E SILVA (1940a)
93. ROCHA E SILVA and BIER (1939)
94. ROCHA E SILVA and DRAGSTEDT (1941)
95. RÖSSLER (1930)
96. RÖSSLER and PASCUAL (1932)
97. ROTHLIN (1920)
98. ROTHLIN and GUNDLACH (1921)
99. RÜHL (1930)
100. SCHILF (1927)
101. SCHMIDT and HENDRIX (1937)
102. SCHNEIDER and SCHNEIDER (1934)
103. SCHRETZENMAYR (1934)
104. SHARPEY-SCHAFER (1961)
105. SHARPEY-SCHAFER and MACDONALD (1926)
106. SILVER et al. (1944)
107. SMITH (1951)
108. SOLLMANN and GILBERT (1938)
109. STAUB and GRASSMANN (1930)
110. STEAD and WARREN (1944)
111. SZABÓ and MAGYAR (1961)
112. THOMAS and ESSEX (1949)
113. TRIBE-OPPENHEIMER (1929)
114. TRIPOD et al. (1951)
115. VALLERY-RADOT (1937)
116. VAUGHAN-WILLIAMS (1961)
117. VIOTTI (1924)
118. VIRNO et al. (1956)
119. WAKIM et al. (1949)
120. WEISS et al. (1929a)
121. WEISS et al. (1929b)
122. WEISS et al. (1932)
123. WENT et al. (1954)
124. WENT and LISSÁK (1935)
125. WENT and MARTIN (1939)
126. WHITE (1961)
127. WILCOX and ANDRUS (1938)
128. WILCOX and SEEGAL (1942)
129. WOODBURY (1946)
130. WOODBURY and HAMILTON (1941)
131. WYMAN and SUDEN (1930)

of the coronary vessels (GUNN, 1926; CRUICKSHANK and SUBBA RAU, 1927; MATSUMOTO, 1930; RÜHL, 1929; NARAYANA, 1933; ANREP, 1936; HOCHREIN and MEIER, 1930 and others, indicated in Table 3). In the guinea pig and rabbit there were consistent evidences that histamine produced, as a rule, a vasoconstriction of the coronary bed (DALE and LAIDLAW, 1910; GUNN, 1926; VIOTTI, 1924; WILCOX and ANDRUS, 1938 and others, see Table 3). Under conditions of ventricular fibrillation, VANREMOORTERE et al. (1951) observed a coronary vasodilation in the isolated heart of the rabbit. In the unanesthetized dog, using a permanent Stromuhr technique, ESSEX et al. (1940) demonstrated a considerable increase in coronary flow from 155 to 239% of the normal after the injection of 0.1 to 0.5 mg of histamine. Though this result was in accordance with other data from the literature, the technique was critized by ECKENHOFF et al. (1947) and the results questioned.

II. Cardiovascular effects of histamine in different species and in humans

From the above survey of the mechanism of production of shock by histamine, it became obvious that no single theory could explain the main symptom of fall in B.P. Nevertheless, the idea of "strategic points" in its broader meaning including besides smooth muscles, other sectors directly affected by histamine, as the heart and the capillary bed, still is the best frame of reference for a theoretical background of the mechanism of histamine shock.

This view has oriented the collection of data for Table 3 which summarizes the work done on the cardiovascular effects of histamine. We see, in another Chapter (*Release of histamine in anaphylaxis*), that the idea of "strategic points" still is the more comprehensive one to account for species differences in the symptomatology of anaphylactic and related shocks. With this idea it becomes understandable why these shocks have a common pattern, similar to that produced by histamine, in spite of the fact that their mechanisms are complex and are by no means strictly dependent upon a release of histamine. This group comprises shocks produced by bacterial toxins, animal venoms, peptone and proteolytic enzymes, and a number of anaphylactoid reactions produced by a variety of inorganic and organic poisons. These problems will be dealt with in another chapter.

In the first section of this sub-chapter we have followed the analytical method to disentangle all possible aspects of the action of histamine upon the cardiovascular system. Now we are going to integrate this fragmentary knowledge by describing the main symptoms occurring after administration of histamine in the different species of animals.

A. Cats and dogs

The intravenous administration of large doses of histamine in the cat and the dog produces a steep fall in systemic blood pressure followed, in a second stage, by incomplete recovery and renewed fall leading to death. In the cat, the first

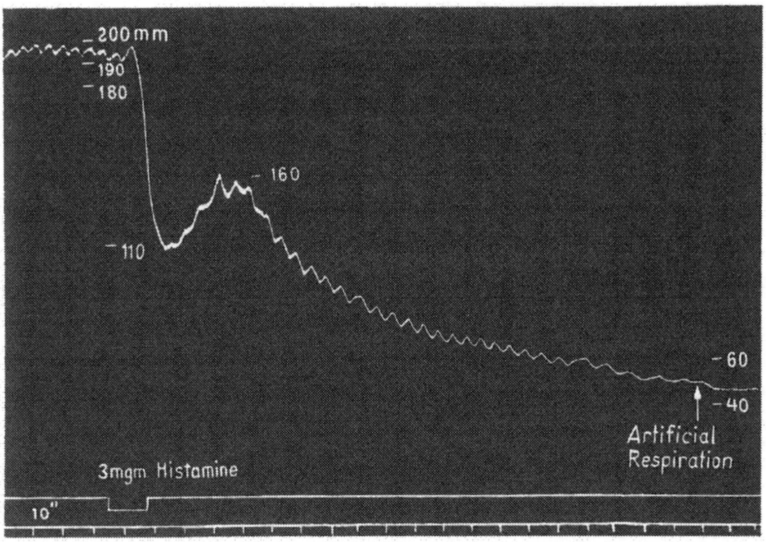

Fig. 8. Cat, ether anesthesia. Action of 3 mg of histamine on blood pressure: primary fall, secondary recovery, and third main fall of pressure (According to DALE and LAIDLAW, 1919)

phase is the result of a violent spasm in the pulmonary artery, dilation of the right heart and stasis in the venous system. The second phase, during which a partial recovery takes place, depends upon constriction of large arteries, and also on the discharge of catechol amines (see Chapter 2, Section H: *Relationship of histamine with the autonomous nervous system*). The third phase, in which the blood pressure falls slowly and irreversibly, can be interpreted as dependent upon the generalized dilation of smaller vessels and increased capillary permeability. Fig. 8 gives an idea of the succession of phenomena in the triphasic shock produced by histamine in the anesthetized cat (DALE and LAIDLAW, 1919).

In the dog, the three phases described by SMITH (1928) can be explained in a similar way, differing in that the effect of histamine upon the pulmonary circulation is not predominant and could not account for the initial fall of systemic

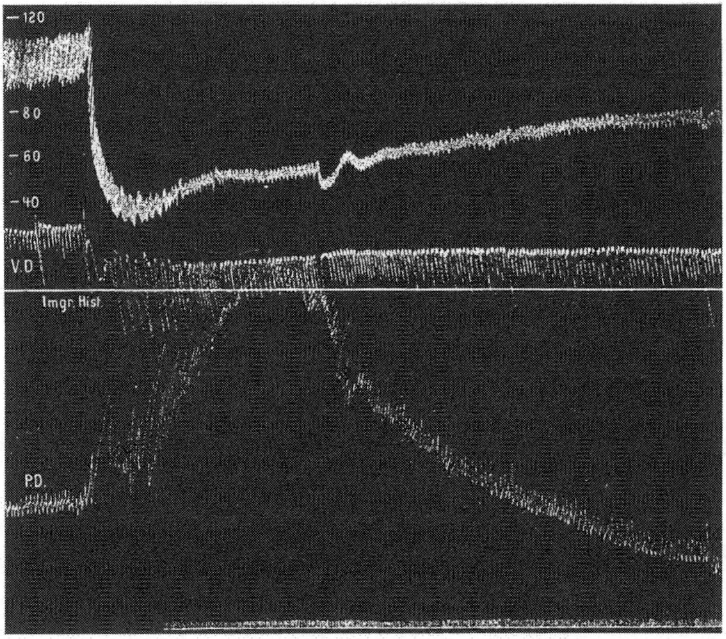

Fig. 9. Dog under chloralose anesthesia. Effect of the injection of 1 mg histamine upon the carotid blood pressure (upper tracing), the venous pressure (*VD*) and the pressure in the portal vein (*PD*). (According to FELDBERG et al., 1928)

pressure. The role played by the pulmonary artery in the cat is taken over by the vessels of the liver (*Lebersperre*) in the dog. Fig. 9 indicates this correlation between fall in carotid blood pressure and increase in pressure in the portal vein of a dog receiving 1 mg of histamine (FELDBERG et al. 1928).

Microscopic observations of the action of histamine on small vessels of cats anesthetized with pentobarbital were presented by LEE (1957). In the skin and skeletal muscle, when applied topically, histamine dilated the small arteries with calibers less than 107 μ in diameter. However, upon the vessels of the mesentery and intestine (over 52 μ diameter) no dilating effect was observed. When histamine was applied locally or given intravenously (above 80 μg/kg) the intestinal and mesenteric small veins (above 200 μ in diameter) showed localized constrictions. Histamine, given intravenously or applied topically, reversed the arteriolar constriction produced by a continuous infusion of epinephrine. The effects on the vessels were less marked. According to LEE (1957) the mechanism of histamine hypotension in cats would depend upon the balance of all these effects and of the doses employed, the higher the histamine dosage, the greater would be the importance of venous constriction.

With the aid of plethysmographic methods, also in the cat, FELIX (1960) admitted a central component to the increased flow through the inferior mesenteric and femoral veins when histamine was infused intravenously (first phase of shock). Morphine and synthetic analgesics, as well as barbiturates, reduced considerably, or reverted the fall in blood pressure provoked by histamine.

By a simultaneous record of the pressures in the brachial artery, in a small arterial branch and in a small vein of the dog's foreleg, under normal conditions or by using a pump to maintain blood flow to the paw, HADDY (1960) showed that a continuous infusion of increasing concentrations of histamine consistently produced fall in the arteriolar pressure and rise in the small veins. Edema became

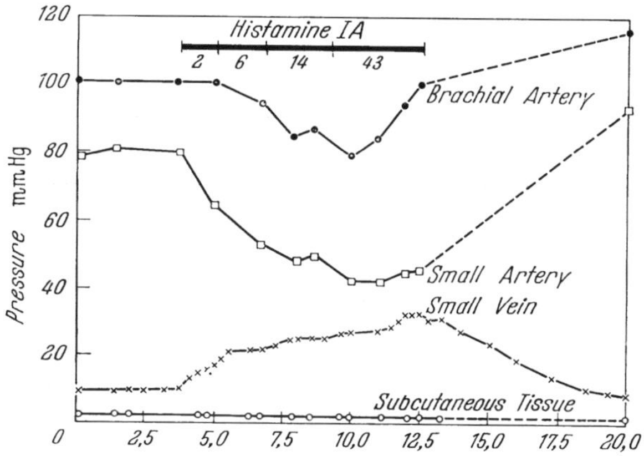

Fig. 10. Effect of histamine infused intra-arterially at low and moderate rates upon foreleg vascular and interstitial pressures. Numbers refer to μg/min histamine base administered into the brachial artery (According to HADDY 1960)

apparent when venous pressure in the small vessels exceeded 26 mm Hg for 7 or more minutes. If the blood flow was kept constant (by the aid of a pumping device), low rates of histamine infusion did not produce appreciable changes in the small vein pressure; if the rate of infusion was increased to an average value of 30 μg/min, coinciding with a fall in the aortic blood pressure, there was a definite increase in the pressure in the small veins, in spite of the fact that the blood flow was kept constant by the pumping device. Section of all nerves to the foreleg, during or before the administration of histamine did not change the rise in the pressure of the small veins. However, the injection of the sympatholytic agent phentolamine (regitine) did prevent the change produced by histamine in one experimental dog and sharply reduced it in another one. Figs. 10 and 11 from HADDY (1960) give an idea of the course of the phenomena by infusion of histamine without (Fig. 10) and with (Fig. 11) control of the blood flow rate.

From these and previous experiments (HADDY, 1958,60) it was concluded that histamine at low rate infusion raises the pressure in the small veins by arteriolar dilation, since that effect is not seen if the blood flow is kept constant. At high rates of infusion, above 30 μg/min, the venous constriction results from a direct action, but also through the release of catecholamines since a sympatholytic agent reduced it (HADDY, 1960). According to HADDY, histamine edema may be adequately explained by the increase in capillary hydrostatic pressure. This conclusion, however, is difficult to accept in view of the evidences that increased permeability produced by histamine and noxious agents appears to be an active phenomenon, being induced in constricted vessels (WILHELM, 1962). Histamine hypotension in the dog might result both from a decrease in peripheral resistance and a decrease in venous return plus edema formation subsequent to arteriolar dilation and venous constriction. In the dog as in the cat, the last phase of the phenomenon might depend upon widening of the capillaries and leakage of plasma through the capillary walls rendered more permeable by the action of histamine (see also Szabó and Magyar, 1961).

By measuring the O_2 content and pH of blood taken from the femoral artery, femoral and portal veins, in dogs, Kowalewski and Wisniewski (1962) have shown a marked fall in both parameters in all samples taken during shock by intravenous injection of 5 mg/kg of histamine. The pattern of the changes corresponded to one observed in anoxia and acidosis which follows stagnation of blood in the splanchnic area.

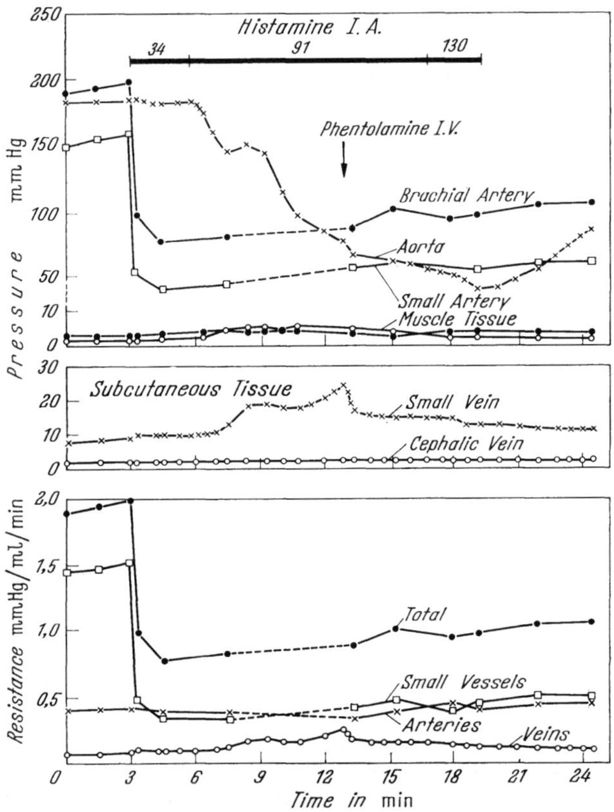

Fig. 11. Effect of histamine infused intra-arterially at high rates upon aortic pressure, foreleg pressures and foreleg resistances with brachial artery blood flow held constant at 100 ml/min. Numbers refer to μg/min histamine base administered into brachial artery. *Arrow* indicates injection of 2.5 mg phentolamine methanesulfonate into hindleg vein (According to Haddy, 1960)

A finer analysis of the effect of histamine upon the terminal vessels of the dog's leg was reported by Piiper and Schürmeyer (1955) by measuring total blood flow and the permeation of the arterio-venous (A-V) anastomoses, with the aid of microscopic wax spherules (19 to 38 μ diameter) injected intraarterially. The increase in total blood flow and concomitant reduction in the number of spherules which could be recovered at the venous side, were taken as an indication that the main effect of histamine is to increase the caliber of capillaries and small vessels, closing (actively or passively) the A-V shunts. After reduction of both total and A-V flow by a previous injection of adrenaline, histamine sharply increased (104.5%) total blood flow, though affecting very slightly the A-V anastomoses permeation to the wax spherules. These results agree with previous findings by SCHROEDER (1952), and constitute additional evidence of the direct action of histamine upon capillaries and small vessels (of caliber less than 19 μ diameter).

From the previous discussion (Part I) one can conclude that histamine, given acutely or chronically to dogs and cats, does not produce any lasting damage to the heart and that the changes observed in this organ, *in vivo* or *in vitro*, are rather trivial or dependent upon the conditions in other sectors of the circulatory system. The concept of an acute heart insufficiency as proposed by RÜHL (1929) and KLISIECKI and HOLOBUT (1937) has not been accepted by the majority of workers in that field (MÜLLER et al. 1932; ETTINGER, HALL and LANG, 1936; KIRCH, 1933, and others), and has been disproved by experiments with the isolated mammalian heart in which histamine produced positive inotropic and chronotropic effects and only occasional auriculo-ventricular blocks and arrhythmias when the doses were too large.

B. Rabbits

In the unanesthetized rabbit of medium size, the injection of 2 mg of histamine produced prostration and difficult respiration; the cardiac beats became intermittent and feeble, but the animal survived. If a second dose of 2 mg was given before the effects of the first subsided, all the symptoms were aggravated and some of the animals died after a few minutes. At necropsy, the heart was seen to be dilated with dark blood, as a consequence of the increased pressure in the pulmonary circulation (DALE and LAIDLAW, 1910). If the rabbit was anesthetized with ether, the effect of histamine was predominantly hypertensive (ACKERMANN and KUTSCHER, 1910; DALE and LAIDLAW, 1910; and others). Under chloralose, or in the first stages of anesthesia by urethane, histamine was hypotensive (FELDBERG, 1927). These differences were attributed to differences in the tonus of the capillaries, which was maintained high under chloralose but impaired under ether and in the last stage of urethane anesthesia. Here, as in the cat, the constrictor effect of histamine upon the pulmonary artery of the rabbit (ROCHA E SILVA, 1940 a), luxuriantly provided with smooth muscle (COCA, 1919), with stasis in the right heart and in the whole venous system, accounted for the main pattern of shock when a fall in blood pressure occurred. Decreased venous return forced the capillaries to dilate, provoking stasis in the abdominal organs. We have analysed (ROCHA e SILVA, 1940 a) the importance of the pulmonary artery trunk in the rabbit for the regulation of blood pressure. By mechanically constricting and releasing the pulmonary artery trunk by loose ligature, a state of permanent low blood pressure was obtained, simulating shock. Under these conditions of persistent loss of capillary tone, if histamine was injected, a powerful vasopressor effect was observed, as shown in Fig. 12.

In the sensitized rabbit submitted to this kind of mechanical shock, the antigen produced a pure vasopressor effect (ROCHA E SILVA, 1940 a).

It is, however, to be mentioned that EICHLER and KILLIAN (1931) described a rise in blood pressure, when histamine was given to unanesthetized rabbits.

MOREL and MAROIS (1949) studied the action of histamine upon the cardiovascular system of the rabbit using radioactive ${}^{24}_{11}Na$. The method consisted in the injection of radioactive sodium in different phases of a reaction produced by the intravenous administration of 0.1 to 0.5 mg/kg of histamine with timed observations of the Na concentration in arterial blood. Compared with the controls, histamine induced: a) delay in the appearance of radiosodium in the arterial blood, indicating slow flow and decreased cardiac output; b) a much higher maximum concentration of ${}^{24}_{11}Na$, indicating reduction of the circulatory volume and c) an abrupt fall of the concentration of radiosodium coinciding with the moment the blood pressure started to fall. This late effect would indicate expansion of the circulatory volume caused by capillary dilation and regression of the arterial spasm. By direct observation, MOREL and MAROIS (1949) described the acute effects of histamine in the rabbit as caused by a rapid rise in the pressure of the

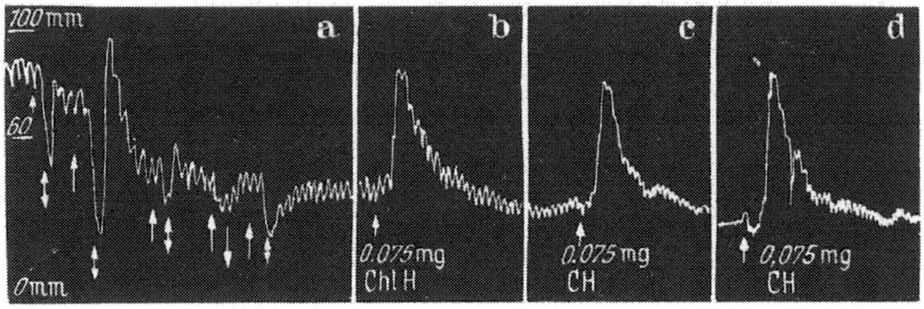

Fig. 12. Normal rabbit. Section *a*, at the arrows, mechanical constriction and release of the pulmonary arterial trunk. Sections *b*, *c*, and *d*, pressor action produced by three successive injections of 0.075 mg of histamine dihydrochloride (According to ROCHA E SILVA, 1940 a)

pulmonary artery concomitant with a rise in systemic blood pressure, and a late generalized dilation of the capillary bed coinciding with decrease in blood flow and stagnation in the peripheral system.

These experiments, as those by FELDBERG (1927) and ourselves (1940 a), have stressed the importance of a balance between the vasopressor effect of histamine and the vasodepressor one due to constriction of the pulmonary bed and generalized dilation of the smaller vessels of the rabbit. The situation here was different from that seen in cats and dogs, in which the secondary rise in blood pressure following large doses of histamine could be mainly ascribed to a discharge of adrenaline from the adrenals. In a recent analysis of the mechanism of rise of blood pressure in rabbits, NARANJO and NARANJO (1958) demonstrated that the pressor effect was neither abolished by adrenalectomy, nor diminished or reversed by sympatholytic agents (regitine-HCl) or ganglionic blocking agents (hexamethonium, pendiomide) nor increased by cocaine. Fig. 13, from NARANJO and NARANJO (1958), gives an idea of the contrast of the pressor effects produced by histamine and adrenaline toward the reagents utilized.

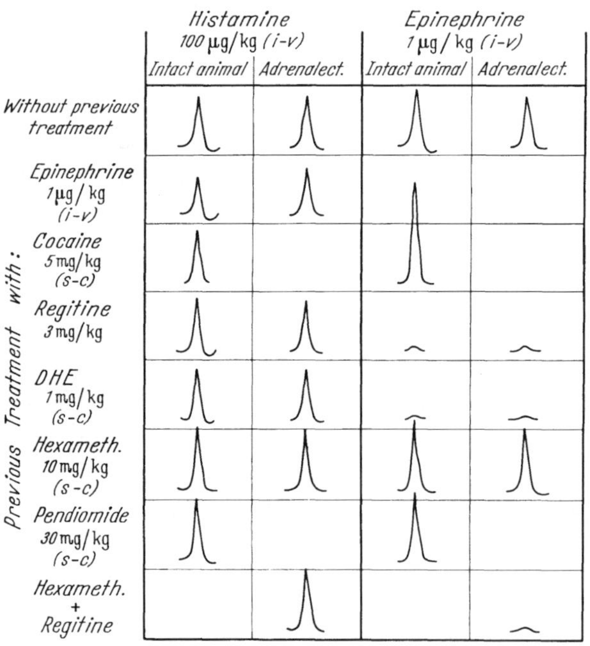

Fig. 13. Pressor effects of histamine and epinephrine after various drugs before and after adrenalectomy (According to NARANJO and NARANJO, 1958)

In this connection, it is interesting to recall that VALLERY-RADOT (1937,49) by roentgenologic observations, concluded that histamine contracted the arteriolar and venous systems of the rabbit. Since capillary dilation in rabbits was as conspicuous as that seen in *carnivora*, it is understandable that some times (under ether anesthesia) a pure hypertensive effect predominated. It is also interesting to recall that injection of an anti-histaminic agent in the rabbit reversed the pressor into a depressor effect (STAUB, 1939) or potentiated the vasodilating effect of histamine (RAMANAMANJARY, 1944). It is conceivable that the anti-histaminic abolished the stimulating effect of histamine upon the arterial system, especially that on larger vessels and accentuated the vasodilator action due to capillary stasis, since anti-histaminics are more effective in preventing the action of histamine upon smooth muscles than upon capillaries.

C. Rats and mice

As other species are considered, such as rats and mice, the analysis of the shock produced by histamine does not lead to any clear cut definition of "strategic points" in the circulatory apparatus.

One reason for this lack of "shock organ" in rats and mice might be the absence of a thickness of smooth muscle in the hepatic or lung vessels, as it occurs in dogs, cats, and rabbits. Another reason might be the insensitivity of such structures to the action of histamine, since we know that in general the smooth muscles of rats and mice are insensitive or even refractory to the action of histamine. These species might depend mainly upon a generalized vascular dilation in response to a dose of histamine. If that is so, the capillary bed in mice is probably largely insensitive to histamine when compared to other species, even to rats.

In the rat, histamine regularly produced a fall in arterial blood pressure (FELDBERG and SCHILF, 1930; WENT and MARTIN, 1939). In a recent approach to the problem, LECOMTE (1961) obtained a sharp hypotensive effect with extremely small doses of histamine given intravenously. Small fractions of a microgram per 100 g of body weight were enough to produce distinct falls in arterial blood pressure in the normal rat. The effect increased regularly with doses up to 10 μg/100 g. Above these levels a secondary rise probably caused by a discharge of catechol amines from the adrenals, took place and could be potentiated by a previous treatment of the rat with guanethidine (0.5 mg/100 g). This drug is known to increase the effect of catechol amines in the rat. Adrenalectomy supressed this secondary rise and rendered more effective the injection of moderately large doses of histamine. A physiological antagonism between histamine and adrenaline in relation to vascular effects was also described (LECOMTE, 1961). The acute hypotensive effect of histamine in the normal or adrenalectomized rat was not affected by ACTH or by hydrocortisone. Large doses of hydrocortisone or desoxycorticosterone acetate (5 mg/100 g) had a moderate, but probably not significant, effect in correcting the vascular changes induced by histamine in the adrenalectomized rat (LECOMTE, 1961).

As far as mortality is concerned, the rat could be made much more sensitive to histamine by removal of the adrenals (CRIVELLARI, 1927; MARMORSTON-GOTTESMAN and GOTTESMAN, 1928; WYMAN and SUDEN, 1930; MARMORSTON-GOTTESMAN and PERLA, 1931; INGLE, 1937; NOBLE and COLLIP, 1941; LECOMTE, 1961).

This increase in sensitivity has been ascribed to a decrease in histaminase after removal of the adrenals, as shown by ROSE and BROWNE, 1938; ROSE and KARADY, 1939; CARLSTEN and WOOD, 1951; and others. Concomitantly, there also occurred an increase in the histamine content of the small intestine and stomach, and a smaller increase in the liver and the lung (ROSE and BROWNE, 1941). The total body histamine was found to increase by 30% in the adrenalectomized rat (MARSHALL, 1943). It seems, however, difficult to correlate these changes of histamine and histaminase in the adrenalectomized animal with its increased sensitivity to the toxic action of histamine. It seems unlikely that a 10 fold increase in toxicity of histamine might depend upon a decreased rate of destruction, as we know that even a complete blockade of histaminase in the tissues will increase only slightly the effects of histamine. Not even the increase in tissue histamine could be correlated to a drop in histaminase content. Newly bound histamine comes exclusively from decarboxylated histidine, and, therefore, would not be increased by simple preservation of circulating free histamine. (See other Sections of this book.)

Most of the experiments showing the influence of adrenalectomy on the sensitivity of rats to histamine were chronic experiments and a large part of the effects observed should be ascribed to a lack of adreno-cortical hormones. In chronic experiments, the sensitivity to histamine returned to normal after administration of cortico-adrenal extracts (MARMORSTON-GOTTESMAN and PERLA, 1931). Likewise, the increased histaminase in adrenalectomized cats could be reduced to normal by adreno-cortical extracts and not by adrenaline (CARLSTEN and WOOD, 1951).

However, since adrenaline is a physiological antagonist of histamine in many of the latter's actions on the circulatory system, it was natural to think of catechol amines as a factor in the increased (histamine) sensitivity of adrenalectomized animals. This possibility would more likely play a role in acute experiments where adrenalectomy is performed a short time before the injection of histamine, as in the experiments by DALE and RICHARDS (1918), DALE (1920 b) and BURN and DALE (1926), which showed increased sensitivity of cats after extirpation of the adrenals. A fresh attack to the problem has been presented by LECOMTE (1961), showing protection by adrenaline against the shock produced by histamine in adrenalectomized rats. However, since the protective effect of the adrenals extends to such a great variety of toxic agents (alkaloids, glycosides, animal venoms and bacterial toxins, proteolytic enzymes and so forth), it would be difficult to think of catechol amines as the sole agents in the protection of animals against histamine (INGLE, 1937; NOBLE and COLLIP, 1941; HALPERN et al. 1952; HOUSSAY, 1955).

The problem of increased sensitivity of animals after extirpation of the adrenals has, of course, strong impact upon the problem of the mechanism of stress. When administered to animals, histamine provokes manifestations which are typical of the so-called "Alarm Reaction" (SELYE, 1936,37,51,56 - for a definition of stress on cardiovascular diseases, see SELYE, 1961), causing inhibition of growth, adrenal hypertrophy, thymus-lymphatic atrophy, eosinopenia, and above all, a depletion of the ascorbic acid content of the adrenal glands (FORTIER, 1952). The discharge of ascorbic acid provoked by histamine is indirect through stimulation of the pituitary gland, since hypophysectomy abolished such an effect. The effect upon the hypophysis with release of ACTH appears to be a direct one and not through a release of adrenaline, since in adrenal-demedullated rats the effect could still be observed (GORDON, 1950). The discharge of ascorbic acid from the adrenals provoked by a small dose of histamine was extremely rapid and not prevented by a previous injection of cortico-adrenal extracts or cortisone. However, a possible role of histamine as a mediator for pituitary activation during exposure to stressful stimuli has been denied by GUILLEMIN and FORTIER (1953) and GUILLEMIN (1955).

A new approach to the relationship between histamine and stress has been presented by SCHAYER (1961), who observed an increase in histidine decarboxylase after local trauma or application of bacterial endotoxins. This problem, however, will be discussed in another chapter of this book (*Metabolism of Histamine*, Chapter 4, Section D). A more detailed discussion of the problem of stress is out of the scope of this book and reference is made to the Annual Reports on Stress (SELYE, 1951 and subsequents years) and the Symposium on the Mechanism of Inflammation (1953).

Mice are extremely insensitive to histamine. It is even doubtful whether the large amounts of histamine needed to kill mice do that by a simple peripheral collapse. Mice tolerate as much as 750 mg of histamine per kg body weight (MAYER, 1950). Instead of becoming more resistant to histamine by previous treatment with anti-histaminics, these drugs sensitize mice to the lethal effect of histamine (MAYER and BROUSSEAU, 1946; HALPERN, 1947). Anaphylaxis in mice, however, was not influenced by pyribenzamine (MAYER, 1950) nor by phenergan (HALPERN and WOOD, 1950). Whatever the cause of death, mice became more sensitive to histamine and to anaphylaxis by a previous treatment with *Haemophilus (Bordetella) pertussis* vaccine (WEISER et al. 1941; PITTMAN., 1951; KIND, 1953,58; KIND and GADSDEN, 1953; PARFENTJEV and GOODLINE, 1948; HALPERN and ROUX, 1949; MALKIEL and HARGIS, 1952a, b; MALKIEL et al. 1953; SOLOTOROWSKY and WINSTEN, 1953; PITTMAN and GERMUTH, 1954; PARFENTJEV, 1955; MUÑOZ and SCHUCHARDT, 1953,54; MUÑOZ et al. 1958). It appeared that *H. pertussis* vaccine induced changes in mice similar to those produced by adrenalectomy, since cortisone and other adrenal steroids protected *H. pertussis* - treated mice from fatal anaphylaxis, histamine and serotonin (KIND, 1954; MUÑOZ and SCHUCHARDT, 1954; SOLOTOROWSKY and WINSTEN, 1954). Adrenalectomized mice, like *Pertussis* - treated animals, became more sensitive to histamine (HALPERN et al. 1952; MUÑOZ and SCHUCHARDT, 1953,54) and to anaphylaxis (WEISER et al. 1941). However, increased susceptibility of mice to histamine could be observed in animals with normal adrenal glands or function (KIND and GADSDEN, 1953; MALKIEL, 1956; KIND, 1958).

Rats, like mice, could be made more sensitive to histamine and anaphylaxis by a previous treatment with *Haemophilus (Bordetella) pertussis* vaccine (MALKIEL and HARGIS, 1952c; MOTA, 1958; CODE et al. 1961). The significance of these findings will be discussed in another chapter of this book (see MOTA, Chapter 3, Section F).

D. Man

In humans, histamine given by intravenous infusion produced a peripheral vasodilator effect (WEISS et al. 1929, a, b, 32; DUFF and WHELAN, 1954; ELLIOTT et al. 1960; FOX et al. 1961), increased cardiac output (WEISS et al. 1932), dilation of the brain vessels (PICKERING, 1933; SICUTERI et al. 1957), irregularities in the heart rate (WEISS et al. 1932; PETERS and HORTON, 1944a; BENSON and HORTON, 1945), and a special type of cephalalgia (HORTON, 1944,55).

When injected by slow infusion in man, histamine produced a rise in O_2 consumption and an increase in the minute volume of the heart (EULER and LILJESTRAND, 1929). The increase in basal metabolism was roughly proportional to the amount of the drug injected (PETERS et al. 1945). When the flow of histamine was stopped the effects on basal metabolism also ceased. When the histamine infusion was increased in rate, a gradually increasing vasodilation spread over the thorax, abdomen and upper extremities. Vasodilation "was more marked in blonds and red-heads than in brunets" (PETERS and HORTON, 1944b; PETERS et al. 1945).

This gradient of vasomotor effects of histamine in the peripheral vessels was also seen by WAKIM et al. (1949) and others who have injected histamine by slow intravenous infusion. A similar gradient was described with bradykinin (KONZETT, personal communication) and, in normal individuals, with alcohol and typhoid vaccine (HORTON et al. 1936) or by warming up the skin (PICKERING and HESS, 1933). The maximum degree of vasodilation occurred in the face and the fingers, spreading to the lower extremities as the concentration of histamine or other vasodilators increased. Regardless of the vasodilator used, the rise in surface temperature appeared first in the face, then in the fingers, and later in the toes. Contrariwise, when vasoconstriction occurred it was greater in the toes than in the fingers. Even when histamine was given into the leg veins, the increase in blood flow was greater in the upper parts of the body (WAKIM et al. 1949).

WEISS, ROBB and ELLIS (1932) found the minimum effective dose of histamine, by intravenous infusion, in man to be 0.003 mg per min. Increasing doses of histamine failed to produce any lowering of the systolic arterial blood pressure, but the diastolic B.P. showed a tendency to fall. The most characteristic effect of histamine was vasodilation of the venules with cyanotic flush independent of the vasodilator effects on arterioles. The intravenous infusion of 0.02 to 0.03 mg of histamine base per minute, produced an increase in cardiac output (to about 20 % above the control) and reduction of the stroke volume. HARMER and HARRIS (1926) found a slight fall when infusing 0.05 mg of histamine per minute intravenously, but could not detect any increase in peripheral blood flow by using plethysmography of the whole limb.

With the aid of venous occlusion plethysmography with a compensatory spirometer recorder, as described by BERRY et al. (1948), and histamine infusion, WAKIM et al. (1949) observed peripheral vasodilation appearing in the order described by PETERS et al. (1945): face → neck → thorax → arms → lower extremities. The histamine solution (1:250,000 diphosphate) was given at a rate of 0.004 to 0.024 mg per minute. There was a definite increase in skin temperature and in heart rate with slight decrease in diastolic blood pressure. The blood flow in the lower extremities increased in proportion to the dosage, reaching 244 % of the control value in the left arm, 120 % in the right arm and 76 % and 18 % respectively in the left and right legs. All symptoms subsided shortly after cessation of the infusion.

Large differences in sensitivity of patients to the intravenous infusion of histamine were registered by KARADY (1934). A group of patients (200) receiving 0.005 mg histamine were classified into four types: I. those which reacted with a 25 to 30 mm Hg fall in B.P. within 15 to 30 seconds of the injection; II. those who showed after a fall of 10-60 mm Hg, a rise of 40-120 mm Hg; III. those who only showed slight changes in B.P.; and IV. those who after a small fall (10 mm) showed a small increase (10 mm Hg). The significance of these results is difficult to assess since histamine was given in a single injection and the effects were registered at a later period.

Changes in ECG. Electrocardiographic changes among patients, receiving histamine have been described since SCHENK (1921) reported ventricular extrasystoles and marked arrhythmias after subcutaneous injections of large doses of histamine. WEISS et al. (1929 a) detected a rapidly vanishing inversion of the T wave (in Lead II) and WEISS et al. (1932), by continuous intravenous administration of histamine, reported depression of all the complexes of the normal ECG with infusion rates as low as 0.004 mg per minute. When a single intravenous injection was given, depression of the T wave, with acceleration of the heart was observed. When the rate of infusion was increased, the T wave became inverted.

PETERS and HORTON (1944 a) studied the effects of an intravenous infusion of histamine, (up to a total of 2.75 mg of histamine diphosphate = 1 mg of base) at the rate of 0.0017 to 0.044 mg of base per minute, upon the electrocardiogram in 25 patients. The predominant effect of histamine seemed to be on the T wave. Depression to the isoelectric level was observed in all cases and complete inversion in 14 cases. The extent of loss of T wave voltage was roughly parallel to the rate of administration. The cardiac rate was increased in the average, from 68 beats per minute to 94. Impairment of the A-V conduction was seen in only one case, in all other cases there was decrease of the P-R interval. Premature ventricular contraction was observed in four cases when the rate of infusion was high. From these experiments, PETERS and HORTON (1944 a) drew the following conclusion: "*No clinical or electrocardiographic evidence of permanent cardiac damage was observed in any of the twenty-five patients. No anginal distress or definite symptoms of coronary insufficiency were observed.*"

Capillary dilation. By applying histamine to the base of a finger nail (1:10,000 to 1:1,000 solution) CARRIER (1922) observed widening of the capillaries and acceleration of the capillary flow. A controlled study of the action of histamine on the capillary permeability by injections into the brachial artery showed an increase in hematocrit reading and hemoglobin concentration with a rise in protein concentration (STEAD and WARREN 1944). Application of histamine by iontophoresis to human skin induced escape of lymph, as observed by ABRAMSON and ENGEL (1938) and ABRAMSON and GETTNER (1941). A comparative study of the cutaneous effects of histamine, and other vasodilating drugs was presented by DUNÉR and PERNOW (1952) and HERXHEIMER and SCHACHTER (1959). With the aid of injected sodium fluorescein, the action was re-studied by MÖLLER and RORSMAN (1958), as well as the effect of 5-HT which appears to act in man by releasing small amounts of histamine (MÖLLER and RORSMAN, 1959). The problem will be re-studied in a later subsection of this chapter.

A review of the effects of histamine in man as well as its possible significance in physiological and pathological conditions is presented by DUNÉR and PERNOW (1960). The reactions of human capillaries to the intracutaneous injection of histamine will be discussed in another part of this Section (see *Effects on Capillary Permeability*). Some specific problems of metabolism of histamine in man are treated in another section of this book by LINDELL and WESTLING (See: *Metabolism of histamine in man*) Chapter 4, Section F, and the participation of *Histamine in allergy*, by SERAFINI (Chapter 5, Section D).

III. Action of histamine upon the capillaries

The analysis of the mechanism of histamine shock as presented in Part I of this Section, led invariably to the conclusion that one of the most predominant features of this and the so-called anaphylactoid shocks produced by peptone, *Ascaris* extracts, bacterial toxins, and so forth, is a generalized dilation of the small vessels, including capillaries, with extravasation of plasma into the interstitial space. The proofs for this have been of three categories:

a) hemoconcentration revealed by the hematocrit values which rise conspicuously following the injection of a large dose of histamine;

b) passage of a dye through the capillary walls, which appears in increased amounts in the lymph draining special organs, such as the liver of the dog;

c) observations of the local changes produced upon the skin capillaries, either directly (as in the human skin where histamine and other noxious agents produce a typical pattern, the so-called "triple response") or by the aid of an intravenously injected dye, such as trypan, Evans, Pontamine or Geigy blue, or colloidal suspensions such as silver or mercury sulphide, which will accumulate in the skin area around the site of the histamine injection.

In the large majority of papers utilizing this last technique one or the other of the blue dyes were utilized. Hence this test will be called "blue test", and its positive reaction, "blueing of the skin" (see Table 3). For a critical review of such methods, see SPECTOR (1958) and WILHELM (1962).

When dealing with the shock provoked by a chemical, the first concern is to determine whether the action upon the capillaries is direct, due to the pharmacologic effects of the substance upon the endothelial lining, or indirect, as a consequence of the fall in blood pressure and stagnation of blood in areas luxuriantly provided with capillaries. It is commonly assumed that the capillary endothelium is sensitive to changes in physiologic conditions, such as pH, oxygen tension, CO_2 and other products of metabolic activity, though common metabolic products never show vaso-dilating properties comparable to those elicited by tissue hormones such as histamine, acetylcholine or bradykinin (FLEISCH and SIBUL, 1933; HILTON, 1962). It is also doubtful whether changes in pH might attain the levels needed to produce capillary atony (KROGH, 1929). It is, however, known that under the influence of many noxious agents, the endothelium loses its normal tonus and becomes abnormally permeable to plasma. Anoxia is one of the most important factors leading to this loss of tone, though we still do not know the final mechanism of the vaso-dilation following circulatory occlusion, for instance (see discussion at the end of this Section). Impairment of the general circulation by heart failure, obstruction in the venous system (as occurring in many kinds of anaphylactoid reactions), by constriction of the hepatic veins (in the dog and possibly also in the cat) and/or of the pulmonary artery leading to stasis in the whole venous system, or direct constriction of the large veins, will lead to stagnation in the capillary bed impeding the exchange of metabolic products which tend to accumulate in the area submitted to stasis. It is possible that under many circumstances, activation of tissue hormones (as bradykinin for instance) which act upon the capillary wall, might be a predominant factor.

The first coherent doctrine about filtration through the capillary walls, was proposed by STARLING (1895-96; 1909) who established a definite relationship between hydrostatic pressure, colloidosmotic pressure and leakage of fluid into the interstitial space. This theory had a tremendous impact upon all studies of mechanism by which the capillaries become permeable to plasma proteins. Direct measurements on the capillaries of the mesentery of the frog, led to a quantitative confirmation of Starling's theory, since the fluid movement across the capillary wall was proportional to the difference between the hydrostatic capillary pressure and the colloidosmotic pressure in plasma (LANDIS, 1927). It is to be noted, however, that in Starling's mind, the capillary endothelium should be considered as an inert filtering membrane. The present conception of increased vascular permeability in injury or under the action of mediators (histamine, serotonin, polypeptides, proteases) postulates opening up the channels across the endothelial membrane, allowing the passage of the blood constituents and the consequent edema formation, in conditions of isobarism (not only osmotic but also hydrostatic) between plasma and interstitial fluid.

It is, however, true that a simple mechanical obstruction of pressing on the venous side of the capillary wall with a glass rod will increase capillary permeability, as shown many years ago by LANDIS (1927-34) and KROGH (1929).

This effect can have practical implications in the formation of all kinds of edemas and, especially of the pulmonary edema, which develops when the pressure in the left auricle rises above 50 mm Hg and causes extravasation of fluid through the lung capillaries. Other factors will, of course, contribute to the extravasation of plasma in acute pulmonary edema (Gray and Field, 1961) and local mediators released at the site of injury would certainly play a role.

The immediate consequence of any endothelium injury is the extravasation of plasma leading to a local or generalized hemo-concentration, with increase in number of red cells per cubic millimeter. This has been proved to occur with great regularity in histamine shock, though there are discrepant opinions about the parallelism between the intensity of these effects and the severity of shock as measured by the most typical signs, for instance the fall in blood pressure. On the other hand, when the capillaries become atonic with an increased capacity, a general insufficiency of the circulation tends to aggravate stasis, and therefore, to force more fluid across the capillary walls and further dilate the capillaries. This vicious circle (Moon, 1940) could explain the third phase of shock, in which, after the exhaustion of the organism in trying to overcome the peripheral collapse, a secondary fall in arterial blood pressure takes place leading to death, in spite of the fact that the causal agent (injected or released histamine) no longer can be detected in the circulating blood. This possibility should be kept in mind when interpreting data obtained in the intact animal under histamine or anaphylactic and peptone shock.

A. Direct methods to measure increased vascular permeability

Apparently, the third method, that is, observing the local changes of the capillary network, either directly or by the use of a microscope or by any of the methods described utilizing blue dyes or particulate matter, such as colloidal silver or mercury sulphide or India ink, is less vulnerable to the above criticism, when histamine or other pure active materials, such as serotonin or polypeptides, are locally injected. However, when other agents, such as inflammatogens or irritating materials, are injected locally, the staining of the skin area could not by itself indicate that the material acts directly upon the capillary endothelium, since a release of histamine, serotonin, bradykinin, or other endogenous active materials could explain a positive blue test. Therefore, extreme caution should be taken in concluding that an agent is active on capillaries on the basis of such a local skin test. Intradermal injections of hypertonic solutions can produce a positive blue test. According to Zweifach (1955) the local introduction of hypertonic solution (NaCl, glucose, sucrose, albumin) will result in a shrinkage of the endothelial elements with increased loss of fluid and, eventually, extravasation of red cells. Most organic solvents will give a blue color, some of them, as for instance alcohol, xylene and chloroform, by simply rubbing on the outer surface of the skin (Rigdon, 1940,42; Jancsó, 1961).

More elaborate methods using isotopic labelled compounds have been developed, by using iodinated (I^{131}) serum proteins (Aschheim and Zweifach, 1961; Spector, 1956), colloidal gold Au ^{198} (Frimmer, 1961), with results comparable to those obtained with the blue dyes, though refinements in the technique are made possible through the inherent advantages of measuring radioactivity instead of confining the observation to the naked eye by measuring diameters of the areas stained with the blue dyes. Especially, studies on the rate of passage of materials from the blood stream to the interstitial spaces, are made possible by the aid of isotopic techniques. Fig. 14, from Frimmer (1961) gives a picture of the course of the phenomenon of increased capillary permeability to the colloidal gold (Au^{198}) under the influence of locally injected bradykinin, and Fig. 15 shows the relative potencies of bradykinin, histamine and acetylcholine, to increase the rate of filtration of colloidal gold through the capillary walls of the rabbit's skin. In these experiments, serotonin had no effect or a rather decreasing one upon the capillary permeability. This fact confirmed one quoted by WILHELM (1962) that serotonin is completely inactive in the rabbit's and guinea pig's skin.

There is now a complete agreement that bradykinin is by far the most active material to increase capillary permeability in all species studied, followed by histamine. Serotonin is only effective in rats and mice.

The combined use of fine colloidal solutions (blue dyes, colloidal gold, iodinated proteins), and suspensions of coarse particles (India ink, silver and mercury sulphide, etc.) permits

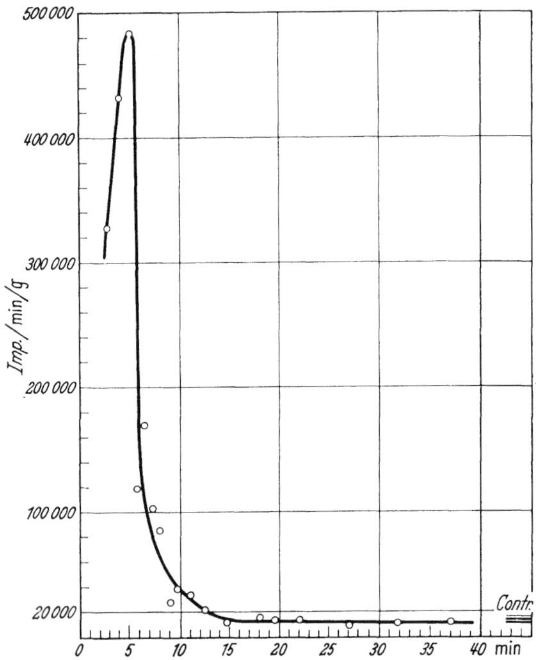

Fig. 14

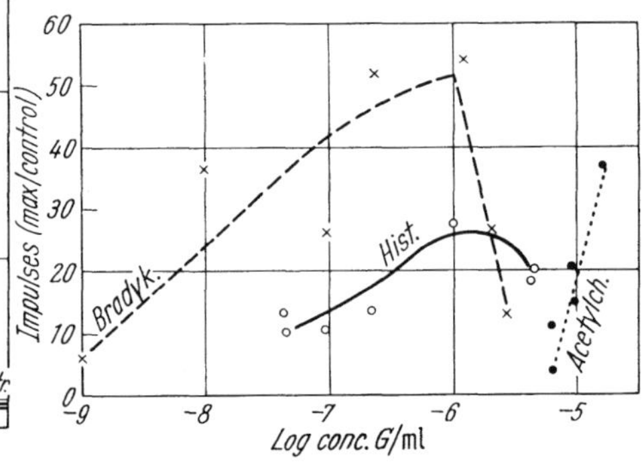

Fig. 15

Fig. 14. Time curve of changes in capillary permeability to colloidal gold (Au^{198}) in the rabbit skin capillaries under the action of 0.01 μg of bradykinin

Fig. 15. Relative potencies of bradykinin, histamine and acetylcholine as related to increase of capillary permeability to colloidal gold (Au^{198}) in the rabbit skin capillaries (calculated from data by FRIMMER, 1961)

a sharp visualization of two aspects of the problem of vascular permeability i. e. increased filtration through diffusion of dissolved materials or transport by ferrying of particles along channels across the endothelial cells or the periendothelial space, as we are going to discuss later on in this Section. For deciding some of the morphological aspects of this phenomenon, the observations with the electron microscope have been of invaluable aid.

B. Mechanism of increased capillary permeability

It would be beyond the scope of this Section, to follow in minute detail the history of our present conception of the mechanism by which capillaries and small vessels (venules) become more permeable to protein molecules, large particles and blood cells (red cells, platelets and phagocytes). The old idea of the existence of *stomata* as virtual windows in the intercellular spaces, presented first by ARNOLD (1875,76), was strongly supported by experiments by LANDIS (1927-34) and KROGH (1929) showing increased permeability by simple dilation due to mechanical obstruction of the small veins serving the region. The simplest way to explain such a phenomenon was the idea that the capillary wall is provided with permanent windows (*stomata*) that could be widened by mechanical stretching. ZWEIFACH

(1937,40) demonstrated that these *stomata* become numerous and visible in the dilated capillaries, and CHAMBERS and ZWEIFACH (1940,47) pointed to the endothelial pericellular cement as a possible locus where capillary permeability could be influenced by mechanical stretching or by poisoning with drugs, such as histamine or histamine liberators. This idea of preformed and normally collapsed holes in the capillary wall dominated the picture for many years. The endothelial cell was thought to be a passive barrier permitting the diffusion of O_2, CO_2 and other metabolites through the capillary walls and allowing plasma and lipid insoluble substances to cross through pores and channels. This view was theoretically worked up by PAPPENHEIMER (1952) and RENKIN and PAPPENHEIMER (1957) who predicted the existence of channels of about 30 Å of radius occupying 0.2 % of the capillary surface. The presence of such pores in the surface of the endothelial cells was challenged by direct observation with the electron microscope by BENNETT (1956), BENNETT et al. (1959) and ALKSNE (1959) who were unable to find any such permanent holes in the normal capillary wall. However, the old conception of the *stomata* was recently revived by MAJNO and PALADE (1961) on the basis of light and electron microscope observations. According to MAJNO and PALADE (1961), such gaps, known as *stomata* would open between endothelial cells of somewhat larger vessels than capillaries (venules), permitting the leakage of plasma proteins, colloidal suspensions, platelets and red cells, when histamine or serotonin was injected locally in the cremaster muscle of the rat.

In opposition to the common belief, MAJNO et al. (1961) localized in the smaller veins of 20 to 30 micra diameter, the sites of maximum leakage of carbon or mercuric sulphide particles, when histamine or serotonin was injected. The vessels with diameter inferior to 7 micra were almost completely free of carbon particles (India ink injected intravenously). Leaks developed with great regularity in vessels about twice this diameter and were found in venules as large as 75 to 80 micra diameter.

Fig. 16 a, from MAJNO et al. (1961) is a striking demonstration that under the influence of serotonin (or histamine), the leakage of intravenously injected carbon particles (India ink) can only be observed through vessels which correspond to a limited segment (from 20 to 80 μ diameter) of the venular system with exclusion of the abundant capillary network which can be visualized in the same Fig. 16 (b) by the intraarterial injection of a thick suspension of India ink in gelatin.

These experiments raised the interesting question of defining with exactitude what is meant by "capillary". The smallest vessels (3-4 micra diameter) with a single endothelial layer, protected only by a basement membrane, would obviously be the "capillary proper". In this case, according to MAJNO et al. (1961), neither histamine nor serotonin would act upon capillaries, since these vessels appeared tightly closed against leakage of colloidal or carbon particles. Nevertheless, in view of the great similarity between the structure of capillaries and that of small veins up to 50 micra diameter in that both are lined with endothelial cells and do not contain smooth muscle fibers, "*if one were to base the definition of capillary on the absence of smooth musculature, the diameter of the capillaries would reach at least 50 micra*" (MAJNO et al. 1961). I am of the opinion that this broader definition of a capillary vessel is more likely to satisfy the mental requirements of a non-morphologically oriented mind. Therefore, we can hold the statement that "histamine increases capillary permeability" with the possible admonition that its locus of action resides in the endothelial lining of vessels above 7 micra diameter, a morphological finesse probably above the usual physiological or pharmacological standards. The main problem at issue, is to determine whether the particles or large molecules have to find their way through the endothelial cytoplasm, as indicated by ALKSNE (1959), or if there are preformed or newly formed windows between the endothelial cells which would allow plasma and colloidal particles to pass across the walls of the vessels to reach the intercellular space.

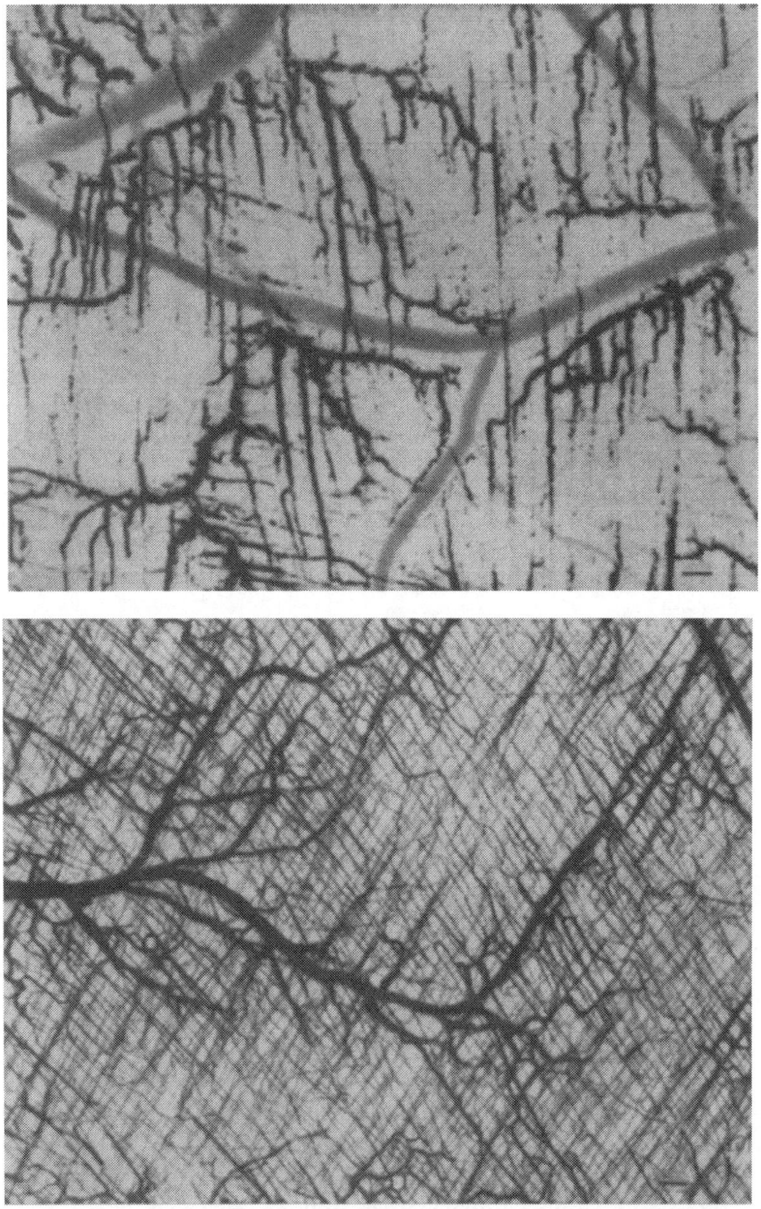

a

b

Fig. 16. Rat cremaster muscle. (a) Typical example of vascular labeling, induced by serotonin. Scale 100 micra. (b) Entire vascular system injected with a mixture of carbon and gelatin. This preparation shows a large number of very fine vessels (capillaries, in the strictest sense) superimposed in different planes. By comparing with photograph (a) it becomes obvious that the great majority of these fine vessels are not blackened by the method of vascular labeling. Scale 100 micra (According to MAJNO, PALADE and SCHOEFL, 1961)

In order to understand the whole problem, we have to go back to early experiments by JANCSÓ (1942,47) which showed that slight damage to the skin or intracutaneous injection of histamine stimulated the reticulo-endothelial-system (RES) to engulf India ink particles injected intravenously. On direct observation of the skin areas treated with histamine, the endothelial cells of the capillary (venular) walls were found to be engorged with the carbon particles picked up from the circulating blood. Likewise, in experiments of liver perfusion, JANCSÓ demonstrated the enhanced activity of Kupffer cells in capturing the granules of India Ink, when histamine was present in the perfusing fluid. This effect of histamine, stimulating phagocytosis by liver cells when added to the perfusing fluid, was confirmed in the rat by KEWITZ and MORGAN (1954), who attributed this effect to the slowing down of the liver circulation, but not to a direct stimulating effect of histamine upon the Kupffer cells. This "granulopectic" activity of histamine was again described by TÖRÖ (1942) and by BIOZZI, MENÉ and OVARY (1948,49) in the skin and reviewed recently by JANCSÓ (1961). In order to study the effect of histamine or histamine-liberating substances, BIOZZI et al. (1948) developed in the rat a technique of injecting the test substances (0.01 ml) intradermally followed immediately by intravenous India Ink (10 % in 1 % saline solution of gelatin). After two hours, the animal was killed and the reaction in the inner face of the skin was observed directly or under the microscope, after it was rendered diaphanous with xylene. After the injection of histamine or histamine-liberating substances, the endothelial cells of the capillaries around the site of injection were engorged with black granules, indicating an abnormally increased phagocytic activity of these cells. More recently, JANCSÓ and JANCSÓ-GABOR (1960) have described a new method for the visualization of inflammatory reactions in the tissues of rats by injecting into the blood stream a 1 % solution of colloidal silver in 5 % glucose solution. Around the area of a local inflammation, a large quantity of silver was seen to be bound by the tissue and formed colored coatings along the internal surface of the smallest veins. In confirmation to JANCSÓ's views, MATOLTSY and MATOLTSY (1951) observed under the light microscope that in sections of the skin treated with histamine among animals which received suspension of India Ink and were sacrified 24 hours later, most of the carbon particles were inside the cells of the capillary wall.

These observations were made under the light microscope, and it seems now that what appeared as engulfed particles were depots of the India Ink in the peri-endothelial space, retained by the basal membrane from going through to the interstitial spaces. The particles that succeeded to get through the *stomata* might, of course, be taken up by phagocytes in the connective tissue. This more conservative point of view, confirming the classical conception of the presence of *stomata* in the venous side of the capillary bed is born out from experiments with the electron microscope (MAJNO and PALADE, 1961; PETERSON and GOOD, 1962). The passage of thorotrast intravenously injected through the wall of small veins at sites of the guinea pig skin submitted to passive cutaneous anaphylaxis, was also studied by PETERSON and GOOD (1962). Though under the light microscope the particles seemed to be engulfed by the endothelial cells, with good resolution at higher magnifications, however, the thorotrast was always found to be outside the cells, along channels (*stomata?*) through the intercellular spaces (PETERSON and GOOD, 1962), thus excluding granulopexy as a mechanism of passage of particulate matter from the lumen of the capillary to the connective tissue.

PALADE (1953,60) was the first to describe the structure of capillaries as revealed by the electron microscope. On the luminal surface of the endothelial cells there are indentations of the limiting membrane known as *caveolae intracellulares* that can also appear in the external surface of the cells. Inside the cytoplasm, there appear vesicles which are usually 500 to 700 Å in diameter. This system would normally constitute a transporting system for fluid or suspended colloidal particles from the lumen to the interstitial space across the endothelial wall. Minute droplets of plasma would be engulfed into the *caveolae* and incorporated into the cytoplasmic vesicles; the vesicle is ferried across the cytoplasm

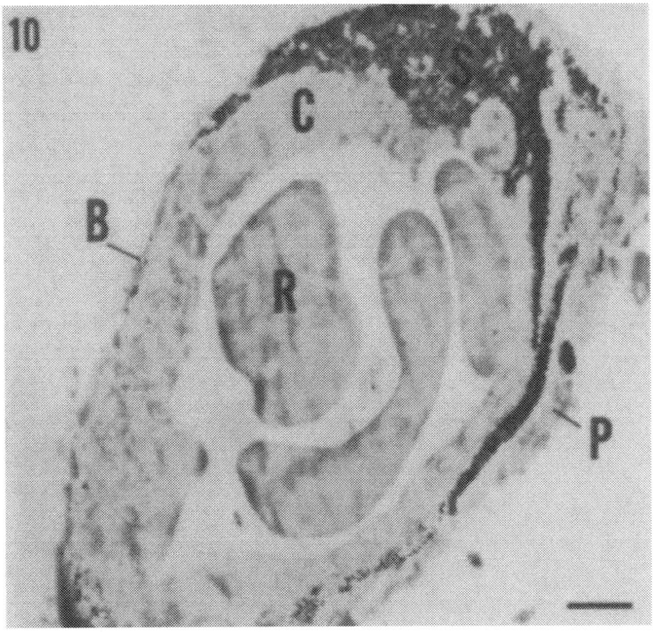

Fig. 17. Electron micrograph of a capillary from an area of skin treated with histamine and fixed 20 min. after injection of colloidal HgS. Note the considerable quantity of HgS (*S*) which has crossed the endothelial cell during the 20 min. interval. Many particles have accumulated between the basement membrane (*B*), or periendothelial cell (*P*), and the external surface of the endothelial cell (*C*). A few particles of HgS are seen in the endothelial cytoplasm, most of them within definite membrane-lined vesicles. × 13,000 (According to ALKSNE, 1959)

and discharged on the external surface under the basement membrane. According to Palade, the selective permeability of capillaries would reside in this basement membrane. Therefore, the capillary-active substances, such as histamine, serotonin or bradykinin, might act predominantly upon this basement membrane. Similar observations were described by ALKSNE (1959), who used a 8% solution in distilled water of colloidal mercuric sulphide (HgS) with particles from 50 to 250 Å in diameter. A solution of histamine was applied topically to the shaved back of mice and five minutes later, 0.15 ml of the colloidal mercury sulphide solution was injected via the tail vein. Skin samples were taken at intervals of time following the fixation for electron microscopy *in situ* by intradermal injection of a 1 per cent osmium tetroxide in veronal acetate buffer. The skin was immediately excised in 1 mm blocks and immersed in the fixative for an additional 30 minutes, then dehydrated with alcohol and embedded in methacrylate. Fig. 17 shows the electron micrograph of a capillary from an area of skin treated with histamine and fixed 20 minutes after the injection of the colloidal HgS. It is interesting to note that a considerable quantity of HgS particles has crossed the endothelial cell through infoldings or fenestrations through the endothelial cytoplasm (ALKSNE, 1959).

Though quite impressive, the pictures presented by ALKSNE (1959) are somehow at variance with the later description by MAJNO and PALADE (1961), MAJNO et al. (1961), and PALADE (1961) who examined the small blood vessels in the cremaster muscle of the rat, after topical application of histamine, serotonin or bradykinin. They could find no alterations in the vesicles of the endothelial

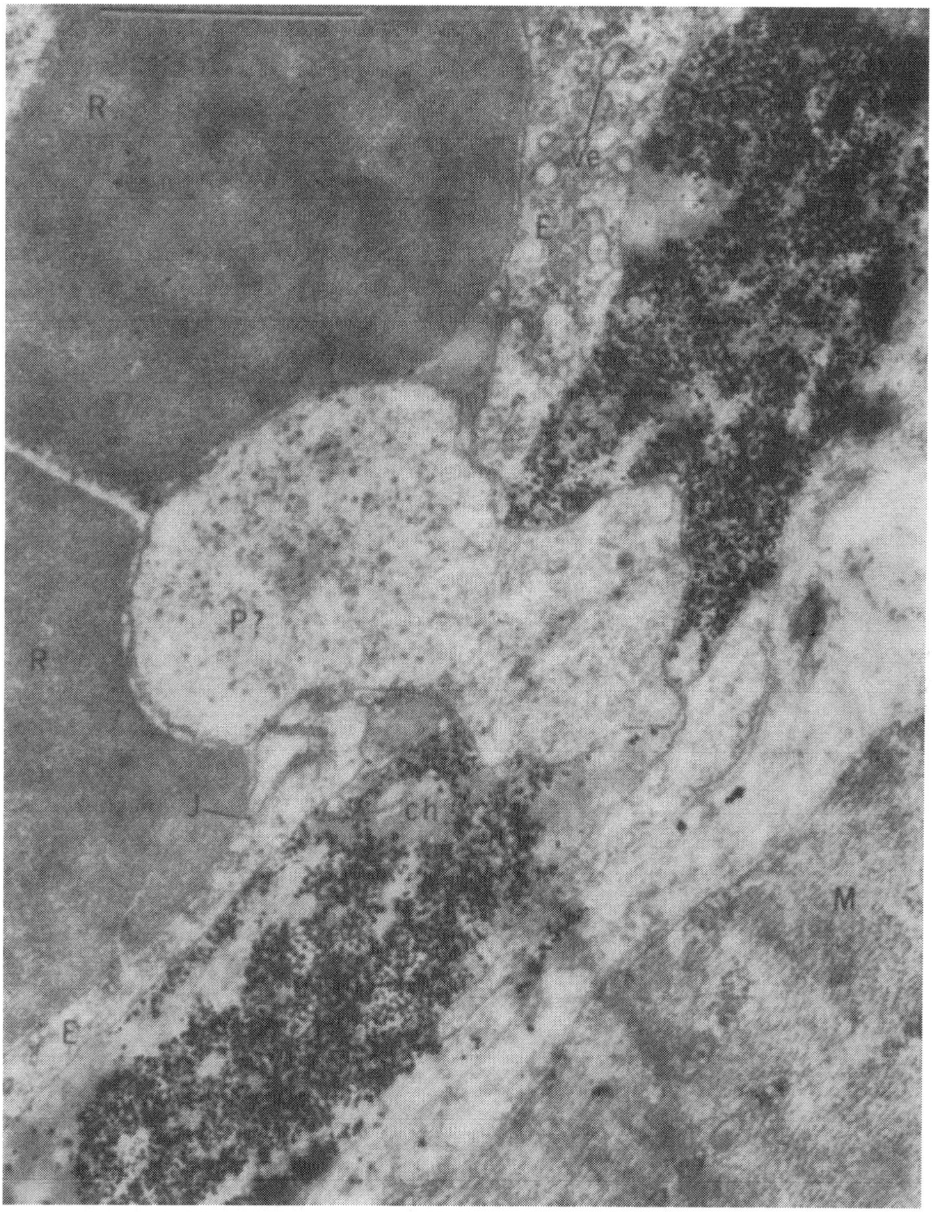

Fig. 18. Electron micrograph of a leaking vessel after a local injection of serotonin and i.v. injection of HgS. In the center, a portion of a cell (possibly a platelet) engaged inside an endothelial gap, in the neighbourhood of an intracellular junction (J). The vascular wall is thickened by a large accumulation of the injected particles. In the endothelial cell (E) only one particle can be spotted in the intracellular vessels (Ve). Magnification 39,000 ×. (According to MAJNO and PALADE, 1961)

cytoplasm and no holes through the cytoplasm, only discontinuities in the walls of some of the minute vessels at the junctions of the endothelial cells. These structures, which were reminiscent of the *stomata* described by earlier workers, let through not only plasma, but also fine particles of HgS and blood platelets. A dramatic contrast between ALKSNE's (1959) picture and MAJNO and PALADE's (1961) is demonstrated in Figs. 17 and 18.

The plasma apparently clotted outside the endothelial cells, with the formation of fibrin threads, and the particles, as well as the blood platelets were held by the basement membrane. In a review of the subject, FLOREY (1961) described experiments with carbon particles (colloidal) injected into the blood stream after inflicting a local trauma to the skin (FLOREY et al. 1959). The carbon particles, after escaping from the lumen, became entrapped for a time between the cells and the periendothelial tissues. The conclusion was reached that: "*in normal vessels transport of fluid may be principally through the substance of the endothelial cells but in pathological conditions there may be an actual solution of continuity of the vessel wall, probably at the cell junctions*".

The mention of a fibrin depot in connection with the transport mechanism across the capillary wall is interesting in view of the fact, described by JANCSÓ (1961) and JANCSÓ and JANCSÓ-GABOR (1960) that anticoagulants, as liquoid, germanin and other synthetic anticoagulants, exert a strikingly protective effect upon the enhancement of capillary permeability produced by a variety of agents. Along this line, one might mention the observations by COPLEY and TSULUCA (1961) of the inhibition of the increased capillary permeability by histamine and bradykinin, when the animal was prepared by a local and intravenous injection of fibrinolysin.

It has not been proved, however, that histamine only acts by a direct poisoning effect upon the capillary walls, and not in part at least by increasing hydrostatic pressure in the venous side of the capillary bed. When injected locally, histamine increases the small vein and reduces the arteriolar blood pressure. The total gradient across small vessels increases by as much as 50 mm Hg (HADDY, 1960). This would be already enough to produce stasis in the venous side of the capillary bed, facilitating the opening up of *stomata*, as seen at the electron microscope. Even when injected intradermally, histamine increases the pressure in the venous end of the capillaries to levels of 39 mm Hg, as measured by LANDIS (1930) by direct micropuncture in the histamine flare: "These findings indicate that a primary change in the permeability of the capillary membrane need not be postulated to account for the edema" (HADDY, 1960). It is doubtful, however, whether such vaso-motor mechanism might hold to explain increased capillary permeability in inflammation or by other agents, such as proteases (trypsin, kininogenins) or bradykinin and related polypeptides.

C. Increased capillary permeability in inflammation

With the above discussion as background, we can rapidly review the arguments in favor or against the participation of histamine in the phenomenon of increased capillary permeability produced by noxious agents.

The origins of the blue tests to indicate increased capillary permeability are found in the work by MACCARDY and EVANS (1912), WINTERNITZ and HIRSCHFELDER (1913) and LEWIS (1916) who have shown that a dye, such as trypan blue or trypan red, injected intravenously accumulated in the area of inflammation, no matter the site or the nature of the agent causing the inflammation. Using a similar procedure, McClellan and Goodpasture (1923—24) showed the accumulation of trypan blue in herpetic lesions of the rabbit brain, and Okuneff (1924) showed a similar accumulation of several dyes in the skin areas submitted to local burns. Kusuetzowsky (1924) demonstrated a similar phenomenon by local application of irritating agents, such as heat and mustard oil. A first attempt to correlate release of histamine with a positive trypan blue test was undertaken by Ramsdell (1928), who compared the effects of histamine and of the local injection of an antigen in areas of the skin of sensitized rabbits and guinea pigs.

On the basis of such preliminary experiments, Menkin (1938,39) made extensive use of this technique to study increased capillary permeability in inflammation, e.g. using trypan blue as the revealing dye and the shaved abdominal skin of the rabbit as test object. The method was further utilized by Menkin to isolate a principle-"leukotaxine" — which reproduced two of the basic features of inflammation: increased capillary permeability as revealed by the trypan blue test, and leukotactic attraction when given subcutaneously or introduced in small tubes inside the peritoneal cavity of rabbits.

According to Menkin (1939,1940) leukotaxine could be sharply distinguished from histamine by its lack of activity upon the guinea pig ileum and also by the fact that histamine was unable to attract leukocytes when injected subcutaneously or tested under comparable conditions in the rabbit's peritoneal cavity. Another major difference between histamine and leukotaxine, according to Menkin (1939), was the sharp distinction between the reactions produced by these agents upon the rabbit's skin under conditions of the so-called trypan blue test. Although leukotaxine produced a homogenous spot, histamine, when given in large doses (1 mg or higher), developed a central whitish area surrounded by a pale blue halo. In a series of papers, Bier and Rocha e Silva (1939) and Rocha e Silva and Bier (1939) presented a strong criticism of the evidence presented by Menkin in characterizing leukotaxine. Firstly, the exudates collected from the rabbit's peritoneal cavity were heavily contaminated with histamine and under this circumstance, the capillary permeability effect could be sharply separated from the leukotactic effect of the exudates. They confirmed that histamine was unable to attract leukocytes when introduced into the rabbit's peritoneal cavity under conditions in which the inflammatory exudates were strongly active (Rocha e Silva and Bier, 1939). Furthermore, the contention by Menkin that histamine was unable to reproduce the homogenous blue spot when injected intracutaneously was completely disproved: the blue halo surrounding the whitish area, described by Menkin as characteristic of histamine, was shown to be due to the large concentration of histamine used in his experiments. When given in concentrations below 1:100,000, histamine induced a homogenous blue spot similar to that obtained by inflammatory exudates and by leukotaxine.

On the other hand, when inflammatory agents such as chloroform, xylene, etc, were applied to the skin, they induced a cutaneous reaction similar to that produced by higher concentrations of histamine (Bier and Rocha e Silva, 1939; Rocha e Silva and Dragstedt, 1941). As the trypan blue test is a highly unspecific one, and since rabbit's skin contains histamine in amounts which might account for a positive reaction in the case of its release, the hypothesis was advanced that leukotaxine induced the increased capillary permeability either by containing histamine or by releasing it from the rabbit's skin. Actually, it was shown that any material known to release histamine would give a positive trypan blue test (Rocha e Silva and Dragstedt, 1941). Snake venoms (*Crotalus t. terrificus*), bee venom, staphyloccocal toxin, Bactoprotone and Bactopeptone, proteolytic enzymes also produced a positive trypan blue test. Contrariwise, insulin, heparin and acetylcholine did not produce a positive trypan blue test. The capacity of histamine to produce a positive trypan blue test in rats was described by HECHTER (1943) and became a common finding since then (see other sections of this Book).

By that time, histamine was the only endogenous principle, the capillary activity of which had been accurately determined. However, looking in perspective now, we can assume that other materials, especially polypeptides might be playing a role in the phenomenon described by MENKIN (1938). Using paper chromatography, SPECTOR (1951) obtained from peptic digests of fibrin several polypeptide fractions with an average chain length of 8 to 18 amino acid residues, displaying the basic properties of "leukotaxine": increasing capillary permeability and attracting leukocytes. SPECTOR was able to separate a fraction that continued to induce leukocytic migration being, however, inactive upon capillary permeability. Anti-histaminics (anthisan = neoantergan) blocked the increased capillary permeability induced by peptic digests of fibrin in the rabbit skin, though having no effect upon the leukocytic migration induced by the same material.

Furthermore, a sharp distinction between time of the increased vascular permeability to colloidal dyes and the migration of leukocytes, could be achieved after application of histamine or of mild injury (by rubbing xylene or applying heat) to the rat's or rabbit's skin (RIGDON, 1940,41,42; SPECTOR and WILLOUGHBY, 1959). According to SPECTOR and WILLOUGHBY (1959) after an initial phase in which histamine and other short living mediators might participate, characterized by increased capillary permeability and edema formation, a second phase would coincide with more chronic alterations of the connective tissues with alteration of leukocytes, possibly induced by the chemotactic effect of a released mediator. These results agree with earlier findings showing that histamine has by itself no leukotactic effect, and that there are endogenous materials which might attract leukocytes without affecting the vascular permeability to blue dyes.

In 1952, MILES and MILES submitted the blue test to a careful experimental analysis, comparing the effects of histamine with those produced by leukotaxine and a powerful histamine releaser, the basic compound 48/80. Though not quite conclusive, the experiments by MILES and MILES suggested that leukotaxine might act upon capillaries by releasing histamine. The differences found could be ascribed to the fact that the effects of the histamine released *in loco* are not identical with those of injected histamine, since similar differences were obtained with the basic releaser (48/80). A partial or total inhibition of leukotaxine prepared by the method of CULLUMBINE and RYDON (1946) was observed in the rat and the guinea pig by treating the animals with neoantergan (DEKANSKI, 1949; MILES and MILES, 1952). The fact that CULLUMBINE (1947) could not detect any inhibitory effect of leukotaxine by anti-histaminics was aptly explained by MILES and MILES (1952): "*Leukotaxine in the skin can have a very shallow dosage-response slope, so that as much as a 10-fold drop in potency might diminish the diameter of the lesion by as little as 2 mm. Unless the neutralization test is made at several dose-levels in several animals, a genuine though small neutralization effect might well be missed. The relative insusceptibility of leukotaxine to neoantergan may well be determined by factors responsible for the similar behaviour of 48/80 and other liberators.*"

The experiments by MILES and MILES (1952) differed from ours and MENKIN'S because they made use of guinea pigs instead of rabbits. We know how much animal species can differ toward the effect of histamine releasers and irritating substances. For instance, in the rat, and possibly in mice, serotonin is a powerful capillary-active agent (ROWLEY and BENDITT, 1956; MAJNO and PALADE, 1961), though in the rabbit, it rather decreases capillary permeability (FRIMMER, 1961). As the rat's skin is extremely rich in histamine, the possibility of serotonin acting by a local release of histamine has been suggested (SPARROW and WILHELM, 1957). A similar suggestion of a release of histamine by serotonin to explain its effects upon human skin has been advanced by MÖLLER and RORSMAN (1959). A release of histamine in the rat's skin was again suggested to explain the localization of the edema produced by egg white in the rat's paw and nose, apparently the sites containing the highest concentrations of histamine (FELDBERG and MILES, 1953; FELDBERG and TALESNIK, 1953). This problem is being discussed in another Section of this book, Chapter 3, Section E.

To correlate the release of histamine with the vascular changes which are typical of inflammatory reactions, we have to consider the recent findings by SEVITT (1958) showing an early and delayed phases of the increased capillary permeability produced by burning of the skin. After applying to the guinea pig skin a temperature of 60° C for 5 to 6 seconds, an immediate mild response was followed in 30 to 60 minutes by a second stronger response. A similar phenomenon was also observed by applying other noxious agents, such as xylene, U.V. light and bacterial toxins (see WILHELM, 1962), or by gentler heating to 54° to 58° C in the rat's (SPECTOR and WILLOUGHBY, 1958,59) and the rabbit's (WILHELM, 1962) skin. With bacterial toxins, such as the α-toxin of *Cl. oedematiens*, the delayed reaction can last for many hours or days (ELDER and MILES, 1957; WILHELM, 1962). The antihistaminics were found to interfere only in the few minutes after injury, diminishing, to a certain extent, the early reaction, but having no effect upon the later phases of the increased capillary permeability (WILHELM, 1962). These findings have been adduced against participation of histamine in more than the earliest phases of the inflammatory process, and definitely support the belief that the continuous activation of the enzymatic releaser of some ever present capillary active agent, should be earnestly considered. Among these factors we have to think first of proteases which might act as kininogenins (such as plasmin or plasma kallikrein) and the globulin permeability factor described by MILES and WILHELM (1955,60) obtained by simply diluting the plasma of most species of animals and humans.

An entirely new approach to the problem of mediators of the increased capillary (venular) permeability in inflammation is now in full swing with the observation that synthetic or pure bradykinin is 10 to 100 times more active, on a weight basis, than histamine in producing increased capillary permeability (BHOOLA et al. 1960; ELLIOTT et al. 1960; KONZETT and STÜRMER, 1960; SCHACHTER, 1961; FRIMMER, 1961; WILHELM, 1962, and many others). The effects of bradykinin upon capillaries apparently extend to all animal species utilized when tested with blue dyes. The spot produced in the skin is of the homogenous type, no matter what the concentration utilized. As bradykinin seems to be released through an endogenous enzymatic process (activation of proteases) its participation in inflammatory processes becomes a great possibility. At least in one form of edema, obtained in the rat's paw by gentle heating (44–45° C), a release of bradykinin seems to play a role, to the exclusion of histamine or serotonin (ROCHA E SILVA and ANTONIO, 1960). Releasers of bradykinin (kininogenins) such as kallikrein or trypsin, might act mainly by their intermediary product upon the skin capillaries. As early as 1940, the demonstration was made that kallikrein produces a positive trypan blue test, in spite of the fact that all attempts to show a release of histamine with such a material failed (ROCHA E SILVA, 1940b). This fact has been confirmed and extended by BHOOLA et al. (1960), SCHACHTER (1961) and FRIMMER (1961). Now we know that kallikrein acts indirectly on the skin capillaries mainly through the product(s) originated by its action upon plasma proteins, as bradykinin or kallidin (1. lysyl-bradykinin). The capillary active factor obtained by diluting plasma globulins, the

"Globulin PF" factor of MILES and WILHELM (1955) is probably a kinin forming enzyme (WILHELM, 1962).

A pertinent question is whether MENKIN's leukotaxine might have been a forerunner of bradykinin. To this question, we can answer "no". Though bradykinin might have appeared in some of MENKIN's experiments, it was fairly well demonstrated that leukotaxine was completely inactive upon the guinea pig ileum. On the other hand, the methods utilized by MENKIN to extract leukotaxine would be unsuitable for the isolation of bradykinin.

D. Histamine and the triple response in the human skin

The first observations on the effect of histamine upon the human skin were by EPPINGER (1913), SOLLMANN and PILCHER (1917) followed by EBBECKE (1917,23) and SCHENK (1921), who have described the typical wheal obtained by intradermal injection of histamine. However, the accurate description of this reaction was given by LEWIS and GRANT (1924) and LEWIS (1927) with the elegant technique of pricking the skin through a drop of a histamine solution, observing the reaction under variable experimental conditions. The name of "triple response" was then proposed to define a triad of reactions involving: a) the local capillaries; b) small arteries and venules around the injected area and c) the local sensory nerve endings. The vasodilation, depending upon the integrity of the sensory nerve supply, according to LEWIS (1927), would have the same origin as the well known antidromic vasodilation studied by BAYLISS (1901,02), in dogs. As the vasodilation by antidromic stimulation of sensory fibers occurs after a latency of 2 to 8 seconds, the contention was held that a vasodilating metabolite is released (LANGLEY, 1923; FELDBERG, 1926). The possibility of histamine or a histamine-like material being released under these circumstances was advanced by LEWIS (1927) and LEWIS and MARVIN (1926–27,27).

The triad of responses depicting the effect of histamine upon human skin are: a) the red point at the site of puncture, representing the immediate effect upon the vessels of the skin directly reached by the drug; b) the flush or erythema which develops 30 to 45 seconds after the initial aggression, produced by the reflex vasodilation of the small vessels of the skin in a large area around the point of attack, and is completely abolished by anesthetizing the skin with cocaine or by degeneration of the sensory fibers, as it occurs in certain forms of leprosy; c) the wheal or edema that develops as a consequence of this increased permeability of the capillaries, this wheal being due to the extravasation of plasma through the walls of the capillaries along the lymphatics of the skin (formation of pseudopodes).

According to LEWIS (1927), the erythema (phase b) around the point of injection, extending over an area of 3 to 5 cm^2 is the consequence of an axon reflex along dichotomized sensory nerve fibers around the point of attack. When injected intradermally, histamine would stimulate the sensory nerve endings and through a reflex, involving no cellular or synaptic connections, would determine dilation of the smaller vessels of the skin closely connected with the other endings of the dichotomized fibers (axon reflex). Therefore, in LEWIS' explanation, the erythema originates as a consequence of the antidromic stimulation of the sensory nerve endings of the skin. But, in LEWIS' mind the connection between antidromic vasodilation and histamine effect was more than one of a fortuitous overlapping of actions upon the same anatomical structures. According to LEWIS, histamine would be a necessary link in the phenomenon of antidromic vasodilation. When the peripheral ends of sensory nerves are stimulated, histamine would be released at the extremities in direct contact with the skin cells and this liberated histamine could then stimulate the dermal endings of dichotomized fibers, producing vasodilation by an axon reflex.

In 1931, DALE and GADDUM completed this scheme suggesting that the erythema might be due to a release of acetylcholine at the other end of the axon reflex. The scheme presented by DALE and GADDUM (1931) would complete LEWIS' scheme (Fig. 19).

In 1937, 38 WYBAUW demonstrated the liberation of acetylcholine by stimulation of the posterior roots of lumbar nerves, in the cat, thus giving experimental support to DALE's scheme. Nevertheless, the difficulties of a cholinergic mediation in the antidromic vasodilation, and, therefore, of a similar mechanism to explain

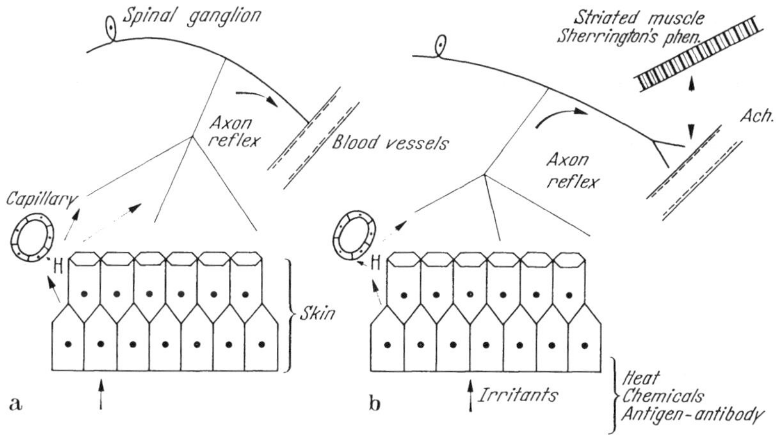

Fig. 19. Scheme of the probable mechanism of the triple response induced in the skin by the action of irritants (↓). (*A*) Lewis' scheme. (*B*) Dale's scheme. The histamine liberated from the skin cells will produce a direct effect upon the capillaries and through an axon reflex a dilatation of the small arteries around the site of its release (According to ROCHA E SILVA, 1955)

the erythema produced by histamine, have been stressed ever since. Though antihistaminics can block the effect of histamine when applied locally (HALEY and HARRIS, 1949) they have no effect upon the antidromic vasodilation (PARROT and LEFÈBVRE, 1943; PARROT, 1954). This would not constitute a serious argument against participation of histamine in this phenomenon, as the hyperemia produced by antidromic impulses is not the direct effect of the released histamine, but of the supposed cholinergic mediator at the other end of the axon reflex. However, it is the nature of this mediator itself that is far from settled. Atropine was unable to block the antidromic vasodilation and eserine rather decreased the reaction (HOLTON and PERRY, 1951). Other endogenous vasodilating materials such as ATP, polypeptides and so forth have been suggested as possible mediators of the phenomenon (HOLTON and HOLTON, 1952, 53; HILTON and LEWIS, 1957; HOLTON, 1959; LEWIS, 1961 and others). The question, however, remains unsettled whether histamine released at one end of the sensorial skin fibers might act as a reinforcing agent to explain antidromic vasodilation, in view of some suggestive evidence of the existence of histaminergic nerve fibers (UNGAR, 1937; KWIATKOWSKI, 1943; EULER and ASTRÖM, 1948, and IBRAHIM et al. 1951). For a discussion of the problem, see GADDUM (1952) and the corresponding section of this book (Chapter 5, Section A).

E. Reactive hyperemia

Also highly controversial is the participation of endogenous histamine in the so-called "reactive hyperemia" which occurs in tissues previously rendered ischemic by occlusion of the artery or the veins for a long time interval. The most plausible theory to explain this phenomenon assumed formation or release of a vasodilating mediator during the period of vascular obstruction to cause relaxation of capillaries and arterioles. The previous suggestion by ANREP that histamine might be such a mediator was supported by LEWIS and GRANT (1924) and LEWIS (1927) by assuming that under abnormal conditions of anoxia a histamine-like substance (H-substance) might be released to account for the vascular effects. PHEMISTER and HANDY (1927—28) though accepting the explanation of the release of a vasodilating endogenous material as the cause of the hyperemia observed after re-injecting blood submitted to varying degrees of trauma, by shaking and hemolysis outside of the body, did not accept *in totum* the idea that histamine might be the mediator.

The difficulty of a histamine mediation was also stressed by EICHLER (1930) on the basis that its effects are blocked or diminished at low pHs or at high CO_2-pressure, conditions prevailing in the genesis of the phenomenon of the reactive hyperemia. We might add now that release of histamine is also hindered or decreased in the absence of molecular O_2 in *in vitro* experiments (see other sections of this book) and at any rate a spontaneous release of histamine is unlike to occur as a consequence of blood stasis or increased anoxemia of the tissues.

The histamine hypothesis, however, received considerable support from experiments performed in Cairo. BARSOUM and GADDUM (1935) working in dogs found that the histamine equivalent of venous blood collected from a hind limb during reactive hyperemia increases above normal, reaching a maximum immediately after release from obstruction. Even without complete arrest of the circulation an increase in venous blood histamine could be obtained by ANREP and BARSOUM (1935). These results were confirmed in man by BARSOUM and SMIRK (1936) who have obtained a 2-to 4-fold increase of plasma histamine after a 10—20 minute obstruction of the circulation of the arm. These experiments were extended and again confirmed by ANREP et al. (1944) showing increases in plasma histamine after occlusion with a sphygmomanometer inflated above the systolic pressure for 10 to 20 minutes. The increases were especially marked when the subject was submitted to muscular exercise with the occluded arm. A critical point stressed by ANREP et al. (1944) was the moment to take the last sample before the release of the occluding cuff. This detail of technique would explain the negative results by KWIATKOWSKI (1941) who collected the last sample *after* the release of the cuff. Working on the rabbit, BILLINGS and MAEGRAITH (1938) claimed that after the release of the clamp at the hind limbs of rabbits, not only histamine but also a substance with the properties of adenosine, could be found in the venous blood emerging from the ischemic limb. The contribution of histamine to the production of the phenomenon in rabbits could not be great, according to KWIATKOWSKI (1941), since the rabbit reacts to histamine with an increase in blood pressure, under conditions of anesthesia allowing the observation of the fall in blood pressure consequent to the release of the circulation in the ischemic area. But even in cats, receiving a large dose of cysteine intravenously, the typical fall due to reactive hyperemia would appear, in conditions in which the vasodilating effect of histamine was no longer detectable, as cysteine is endowed of some antihistaminic activity. Furthermore, in the dog, EMMELIN et al. (1941 a) were unable to find any increase of the histamine content in the venous blood coming from an ischemic limb, after release of the ligature, even when the abdominal aorta was clamped for 10 to 20 minutes. Similar negative experiments were also done in cats and guinea pigs.

It is true that the impossibility of detecting increase of free histamine in the blood would not completely invalidate the idea that histamine might be the mediator, as it is known (ROSE, 1940; EMMELIN et al. 1941 b) that histamine, when injected intravenously, can produce marked symptoms without there being detectable increased amounts by the most sensitive methods. However, using anti-histaminics, such as diphenhydramine (benadryl), EMMELIN and EMMELIN (1947) showed that reactive hyperemia produced in the cat by unclamping the iliac artery is not affected by a previous injection of 10 mg/kg of benadryl, while the vasodilation produced by the injection of histamine was fully prevented by the anti-histaminic. Similarly, FOLKOW, HAEGER and KAHLSON (1948) observed that the sensitivity of the small vessels of cats to histamine and to the fall in blood pressure after release of the clamp in the iliac artery (reactive hyperemia) did not run parallel. Furthermore, if the vessels were rendered less sensitive or insensitive to histamine by a previous treatment with anti-histaminics and/or by a previous treatment with large doses of histamine, the hyperemia was observed with undiminished intensity, after unclamping the vessel. As adenosinetriphosphate (ATP) did produce a vasodilator effect in doses of the order of $0.1-0.2$ μg when injected intra-arterially in the hind limb of the cat, it was suggested as an obvious possible mediator in reactive hyperemia (FOLKOW et al. 1948).

The similar and possibly related phenomenon of vasodilation following a tetanus of striated muscle, has been extensively analysed from a similar standpoint. Acetylcholine and histamine have been ruled out as possible mediators, since neither atropine nor anti-histaminics have any inhibitory effect (HILTON, 1953,59). Seventy intermediary products were investigated for vasodilator activity by FLEISCH and SIBUL (1933) and FLEISCH and WEGER (1937). Most of them had very small activity when compared with acetylcholine and ATP. This last metabolite could not be found in perfusates collected from the connective tissue in association with the tetanized muscle (HILTON, 1962). It was shown by HILTON (1959,62) that section of the sciatic nerve, but not sympathectomy or posterior root ganglionectomy will diminish or abolish the responses. Therefore, the possibility of participation of a network of fibrils extending over arteries, arterioles and capillaries to conduct at slow speed (10 cm/sec) a vaso-dilating stimulus arising from the contracting muscle along the vascular walls, was postulated by HILTON (1959,62), with a possible participation of vasodilating polypeptides (bradykinin, kallidin) released at distance from the arteriolar walls.

The evidences presented by ANREP et al. (1936) of the release of enormous amounts of histamine (up to 2.0 to 40.6 μg/min) by the cardiac muscle, when the blood was taken from a coronary vein in a heart-lung-preparation, were not confirmed by CODE et al. (1938). More recently, DUNÉR and PERNOW (1958) found a significant increase in blood histamine in healthy individuals submitted to strenuous work. However, the final decision whether this increased histamine was bound to the increased leukocytes or was free and physiologically active in plasma to cause vasodilation, was left open.

A comparative analysis of the effects of intra-arterially injected bradykinin and the changes observed in the circulation of the finger after prolonged ischemia (reactive hyperemia) led BURCH and DE PASQUALE (1962) to conclude: "*The precise similarity of the digital vascular responses during reactive hyperemia and after the injection of bradykinin suggests that reactive hyperemia may be due to the release of bradykinin*".

References

ABE, K.: Cit. in FELDBERG und SCHILF (1930). Tohoku J. exp. Med. **1**, 389 (1920).

ABRAMSON, H. A., and M. ENGEL: Skin reactions; effect of allergic and histamine wheals on rate of absorption of dyes and blood from human cutis. J. invest. Derm. **1**, 65 (1938).

—, and H. GETTNER: Skin reactions; lymphatic escape following electrophoresis of histamine and epinephrine. J. invest. Derm. **4**, 243 (1941).

ACKERMANN, D., u. F. KUTSCHER: Untersuchungen über die physiologische Wirkung einer Secalebase und des Imidazoläthylamins. Z. Biol. **54**, 387 (1910).

AIRILA, Y.: Über die Ursache der tödlichen Blutdrucksenkung im akuten anaphylaktischen Schock beim Kaninchen. Skand. Arch. Physiol. **31**, 388 (1914).

ALKSNE, I. F.: The passage of colloidal particles across the dermal capillary wall under the influence of histamine. Quart. J. exp. Physiol. **44**, 51 (1959).

ANDRUS, E. C., and H. B. WILCOX: Effects of anaphylaxis upon coronary arteries in the isolated heart. J. exp. Med. **69**, 545 (1939).

ANREP, G. V.: Lane Medical Lectures: Studies in cardiovascular regulation. Stanford Univ. Press, vol. 3 (1936).

—, and G. S. BARSOUM: Appearance of histamine in the venous blood during muscular contraction. J. Physiol. (Lond.) **85**, 409 (1935).

— — S. SALAMA and Z. SOUIDAN: Liberation of histamine during reactive hyperaemia and muscle contraction in man. J. Physiol. (Lond.) **103**, 297 (1944).

— — and M. TALAAT: Liberation of histamine by the heart muscle. J. Physiol. (Lond.) **86**, 431 (1936).

AREY, L. B.: Throttling veins in the livers of certain mammals. Anat. Rec. **81**, 21 (1941).

—, and J. P. SIMONDS: The relation of the smooth muscle in the hepatic veins to shock phenomena. Anat. Rec. **18**, 219 (1920).

ARNOLD, J.: Über das Verhalten der Wandungen der Blutgefäße bei der Emigration weißer Blutkörper. Virchows Arch. path. Anat. **62**, 487 (1875).

— Über die Kittsubstanz der Endothelien. Virchows Arch. path. Anat. **66**, 77 (1876).

ASCHHEIM, E., and B. W. ZWEIFACH: Kinetics of blood protein leakage in inflammation. Circulat. Res. **9**, 349 (1961).

AUER, J., and P. A. LEWIS: The physiology of the immediate reaction of anaphylaxis in the guinea-pig. J. exp. Med. **12**, 151 (1910).

BAER, R., u. R. RÖSSLER: Über die Bedeutung der Leber für die Blutverteilung; Durchströmungsversuche an überlebender Hundeleber. Wien. klin. Wschr. **39**, 1033 (1926).

— — Beiträge zur Pharmakologie der Lebergefäße. Über die Abhängigkeit der Histaminwirkung von der Durchströmungsrichtung (Versuche an isoliert durchströmter Hundeleber). Naunyn-Schmiedeberg's Arch. exp. Path. Pharmak. **119**, 204 (1927).

BARBOUR, H. G.: Note on the action of histamine upon surviving arteries. J. Pharmacol. exp. Ther. **4**, 245 (1912—1913).

BARCROFT, J., and W. FELDBERG: Cit. in FELDBERG und SCHILF (1930).

BARSOUM, G. S., and J. H. GADDUM: The liberation of histamine during reactive hyperaemia. J. Physiol. (Lond.) **85**, 13P (1935).

—, and F. H. SMIRK: Observations on histamine yielding substance in plasma and red cells of normal human subjects and of patients with congestive heart failure. Clin. Sci. **2**, 353 (1936).

BAUER, W., H. H. DALE, L. T. POULSSON and D. W. RICHARDS: The control of circulation through the liver. J. Physiol. (Lond.) **74**, 343 (1932).

—, and D.W. RICHARDS JR.: A vaso-dilator action of acetates. J. Physiol. (Lond.) **66**, 371 (1928).

BAYLISS, W. M.: On the origin from the spinal cord of the vasodilator fibers of the hind limb and on the nature of these fibers. J. Physiol. (Lond.) **26**, 173 (1901).

— Further researches on antidromic nerve impulses. J. Physiol. (Lond.) **28**, 276 (1902).

BENNETT, H. S.: The concepts of membrane flow and membrane vesiculation as mechanisms for active transport and ion pumping. J. biophys. biochem. Cytol. **2**, suppl. 99 (1956).

— J. H. LUFT and J. C. HAMPTON: Morphological classification of vertebrate blood capillaries. Amer. J. Physiol. **196**, 381 (1959).

BENSON, A. J., and B. T. HORTON: Effects on continuous intravenous administration of histamine on the blood pressure and pulse rate in cases of multiple sclerosis. Proc. Mayo Clin. **20**, 113 (1945).

BERRY, M. R., E. J. BALDES, H. E. ESSEX and K. G. WAKIM: Compensating plethismokymograph for measuring blood flow in human extremities. J. Lab. clin. Med. **33**, 101 (1948).

BEST, C. H., and E. W. MCHENRY: Histamine. Physiol. Rev. **11**, 371 (1931).

BHOOLA, K. D., J. D. CALLE and M. SCHACHTER: The effect of bradykinin, serum kallikrein and other endogenous substances on capillary permeability. J. Physiol. (Lond.) **152**, 75 (1960).

BIER, O. G., u. M. ROCHA E SILVA: Untersuchungen über Entzündungen. I. und III. Virchows Arch. path. Anat. **303**, 325 u. 343 (1939).

BILLINGS, F. T., and B. G. MAEGRAITH: Chemical changes in tissues following obstruction of blood supply. Quart. J. exp. Physiol. **27**, 249 (1938).

BIOZZI, G., G. MENÉ et Z. OVARY: L'histamine et la granulopexie de l'endothélium vasculaire. Rev. Immunol. (Paris) **12**, 320 (1948).

— — — Ricerche sui rapporti tra istamina e granuloplessia dell'endotelio vascolare. I. e II. Sperimentale **99**, 341, 352 (1949).

BLALOCK, A., and S. E. LEVY: Partition of venous return during shock and after histamine. Amer. J. Physiol. **118**, 734 (1937).

Burch, G. E., and N. P. De Pasquale: Bradykinin, digital flow, and the arteriovenous anastomoses. Circulat. Res. **10**, 105 (1962).

Burn, J. H.: The Background of Therapeutics. London, New York, Toronto: Oxford Univ. Press 1948.

—, and H. H. Dale: The vaso-dilator action of histamine and its physiological significance. J. Physiol. (Lond.) **61**, 185 (1926).

Butler, V., J. W. Beard and A. Blalock: Experimental Shock. XI. A study of the alterations in the volume of blood and in the water content of blood and of muscle that are produced by histamine. Arch. Surg. **23**, 848 (1931).

Carlsten, A., and D. R. Wood: Increased lymph histaminase in adrenalectomized cats and its restoration by adrenocortical extract but not by adrenaline. J. Physiol. (Lond.) **112**, 142 (1951).

Carrier, E. B.: Studies on the physiology of capillaries. V. The reaction of the human skin capillaries to drugs and other stimuli. Amer. J. Physiol. **61**, 528 (1922).

Chambers, R., and B. W. Zweifach: Capillary endothelial cement in relation to permeability. J. cell. comp. Physiol. **15**, 255 (1940).

— — Intercellular cement and capillary permeability. Physiol. Rev. **27**, 436 (1947).

Chappell, J. W., R. H. Ebert and W. R. Barclay: Effects of cortisone (adrenocortical preparation) on cutaneous histamine response of rabbits using Evans blue dye as indicator. J. Lab. clin. Med. **39**, 896 (1952).

Cloetta, M., u. A. Anderes: Besitzen die Lungen Vasomotoren? Naunyn-Schmiedeberg's Arch. exp. Path. Pharmak. **76**, 124 (1914).

Cobbin, L. B., and R. H. Thorp: The cardioactive principle in spleen. Brit. J. Pharmacol. **14**, 392 (1959).

Coca, A. F.: The mechanism of the anaphylaxis reaction in the rabbit. J. Immunol. **4**, 219 (1919).

Code, C. F., C. Lowatt-Evans and R. A. Gregory: Blood histamine and cardiac activity. J. Physiol. (Lond.) **92**, 344 (1938).

— D. T. Cody, M. Hurn, J. C. Kennedy and M. J. Strickland: The simultaneous release of histamine and a histamine destroying factor during anaphylaxis in rats. J. Physiol. (Lond.) **156**, 207 (1961).

Copley, A. L., and V. Tsuluca: The antibradykinin action of fibrinolysin, etc. In: Symposium on Bradykinin, 1st International Pharmacological Meeting, Stockholm (1961). Biochem. Pharmacol. **10**, 67 (1962).

Crivellari, C. A.: Sensitiveness of adrenalectomized rats to certain toxin substances. Amer. J. Physiol. **81**, 414 (1927).

Cruickshank, E. W. H., and A. Subba Rau: Reactions of isolated systemic and coronary arteries. J. Physiol. (Lond.) **64**, 65 (1927).

Cullumbine, H.: Leukotaxine and histamine. Nature (Lond.) **159**, 841 (1947).

—, and H. N. Rydon: A study of the formation, properties and partial purification of leukotaxine. Brit. J. exp. Path. **27**, 33 (1946).

Dale, H. H.: The Herter Lectures. I. Capillary poisons and shock. II. Anaphylaxis. III. Chemical structure and physiological action. Bull. Johns Hopk. Hosp. **31**, 257, 310, 373 (1920a).

— Conditions which are conducive to the production of shock by histamine. Brit. J. exp. Path. **1**, 103 (1920b).

— The activity of the capillary blood vessels, and its relationship to certain forms of toxaemia. Brit. med. J. **1**, 959, 1006 (1923).

— Adventures in Physiology with Excursions into Autopharmacology. London: Pergamon Press 1953.

—, and J. H. Gaddum: Reactions of denervated voluntary muscle and their bearing on the mode of action of parasympathetic and related nerves. J. Physiol. (Lond.) **70**, 109 (1931).

—, and P. P. Laidlaw: The physiological action of β-iminazolylethylamine. J. Physiol. (Lond.) **41**, 318 (1910).

— — Histamine shock. J. Physiol. (Lond.) **52**, 355 (1919).

— — and A. N. Richards: The action of histamine: its bearing on traumatic toxaemia as a factor in shock. In: Spec. Rep. Ser. med. Res. Coun. (Lond.) **26**, 8 (1919).

—, and A. N. Richards: The vasodilator action of histamine and of some other substances. J. Physiol. (Lond.) **52**, 110 (1918).

— — The depressor (vaso-dilator) action of adrenaline. J. Physiol. (Lond.) **62**, 397 (1927).

Dekanski, J.: The effect of protein hydrolysates (leukotaxine) on skin-histamine in cats. J. Physiol. (Lond.) **108**, 233 (1949).

Delaunois, A. L.: Continuous measurement of blood flow and cardiac output by means of a cournand catheter equipped with thermistors. Arch. int. Pharmacodyn. **134**, 245 (1961).

— R. Kordecki, H. Polet and J. Ryzewski: Cardiac output arterial blood pressure and pulmonary arterial pressure in histamine shock. Arch. int. Pharmacodyn. **120**, 114 (1959).

DEWS, P. B., and J. D. P. GRAHAM: The antihistamine substance 2786 R. P. Brit. J. Pharmacol. **1**, 278 (1946).
DEYRUP, I. J.: Circulatory changes following the subcutaneous injection of histamine in dogs. Amer. J. Physiol. **142**, 158 (1944).
—, and W. S. ROOT: The effect of subcutaneous histamine injection on the cardiac output of the unanesthetized dog. Amer. J. Physiol. **148**, 134 (1947).
DIXON, W. E., and J. C. HOYLE: Studies in pulmonary circulation; action of histamine. J. Physiol. (Lond.) **70**, 1 (1930).
DOMENECH-ALSINA, F.: Studies on histamine hypotension. J. Physiol. (Lond.) **78**, 54 (1933).
DONNET, V., M. LÉANDRI et P. ZWIRN: Effets de l'histamine sur la pression artérielle pulmonaire. C. R. Soc. Biol. (Paris) **140**, 619 (1946).
DRINKER, C. K., and J. BRONFENBRENNER: The pulmonary circulation in anaphylactic shock. J. Immunol. **9**, 387 (1924).
DUFF, F., and R. F. WHELAN: Effects of antihistamine substances on the response to histamine of the human forearm. Brit. J. Pharmacol. **9**, 413 (1954).
DUMKE, P. R., and C. F. SCHMIDT: Quantitative measurements of cerebral blood flow in macaque monkey. Amer. J. Physiol. **138**, 421 (1943).
DUNÉR, H., and B. PERNOW: Cutaneous reactions produced by local administration of acetylcholine, acetyl-β-methylcholine (methacholine), piperidine and histamine. Acta Physiol. scand. **25**, 38 (1952).
— — Histamine and leukocytes in blood during muscular work in man. Scand. J. clin. Lab. Invest. **10**, 394 (1958).
— — Histamine in man under physiological and pathological conditions. Acta med. scand. **168**, 307 (1960).
DZSINICH, A., u. T. GALLÉ: Zum Wirkungsmechanismus des Histamins. Z. klin. Med. **135**, 669 (1939).
EBBECKE, V.: Die lokale vasomotorische Reaktion (L. V. R.) der Haut und der inneren Organe. Pflügers Arch. ges. Physiol. **169**, 1 (1917).
— Capillarerweiterung, Urticaria und Schock. Klin. Wschr. **2**, 1725 (1923).
ECKENHOFF, J. E., J. H. HAFKENSCHIEL and C. M. LANDMESSER: The coronary circulation in the dog. Amer. J. Physiol. **148**, 582 (1947).
EICHLER, O.: Zur Pharmakologie der Hofmeisterschen Reihe. Habilitationsvortrag (1930).
—, u. H. KILLIAN: Versuche zur Histaminwirkung am Kaninchen. Naunyn-Schmiedeberg's Arch. exp. Path. Pharmak. **159**, 606 (1931).
EINIS, W.: Über die Wirkung des Pituitrins und β-Imidazoläthylamins (Histamins) auf die Herzaktion. Versuche am isolierten Frosch- und Säugetierherzen. Biochem. Z. **52**, 96(1913).
ELDER, J. M., and A. A. MILES: The action of lethal toxins of gas-gangrene clostridia on capillary permeability. J. Pathol. Bact. **74**, 133 (1957).
ELIAS, H., and H. BENGELSDORF: The structure of the liver of vertebrates. Acta anat. (Basel) **14**, 297 (1952).
ELLIOTT, D. F., E. W. HORTON and G. P. LEWIS: Actions of pure bradykinin. J. Physiol. (Lond.) **153**, 473 (1960).
EMMELIN, K., and N. EMMELIN: Histamine and reactive hyperaemia. Acta physiol. scand. **14**, 16 (1947).
EMMELIN, N., G. KAHLSON and F. WICKSELL: Blood histamine in reactive hyperaemia and in muscle tetanus. Acta physiol. scand. **2**, 110 (1941a).
— — — Histamine in plasma and methods of its estimation. Acta physiol. scand. **2**, 123 (1941b).
EPPINGER, H.: Über eine eigentümliche Hautreaktion hervorgerufen durch Ergamin. Wien. med. Wschr. **63**, 1414 (1913).
—, u. A. SCHÜRMEYER: Über den Kollaps und analoge Zustände. Klin. Wschr. **7**, 777 (1928).
ESSEX, H. E., R. G. E. WEGRIA, J. F. HERRICK and F. C. MANN: The effects of certain drugs on the coronary blood flow of the trained dog. Amer. Heart J. **19**, 554 (1940).
ETTINGER, G. H., G. E. HALL and J. LANG: The effect of repeated injections of histamine in the dog; on the heart and blood vessels. Canad. med. Ass. J. **35**, 184 (1936).
EULER, U. S. v., and A. ASTRÖM: Liberation of histamine and sympathin by stimulation of isolated splenic nerves from cattle. Acta physiol. scand. **16**, 97 (1948).
—, u. G. LILJESTRAND: Die Wirkung von Adrenalin, Sympathol, Tyramin, Ephetonin und Histamin auf Gaswechsel und Kreislauf beim Menschen. Skand. Arch. Physiol. **55**, 1 (1929). See also J. Physiol. (Lond.) **65**, 22P (1928).
FEIGEN, G. A., E. M. VAUGHAN-WILLIAMS, J. K. PETERSON and C. B. NIELSEN: Histamine release and intracell potentials during anaphylaxis in the isolated heart. Circulat. Res. **8**, 713 (1960).
FELDBERG, W.: The peripheral innervation of the vessels of the external ear of the rabbit. J. Physiol. (Lond.) **61**, 518 (1926).

FELDBERG, W.: The action of histamine on the blood vessels of the rabbit. J. Physiol. (Lond.) **63**, 211 (1927).
— Das Verhalten des Pfortaderdruckes nach Injektion von Histamin und Pepton in den Kreislauf der Katze. Naunyn-Schmiedeberg's Arch. exp. Path. Pharmak. **140**, 156 (1929).
— The role of mediators in the inflammatory tissue response. Int. Arch. Allergy **8**, 15 (1956).
— G. KATZ u. E. SCHILF: Cit. in FELDBERG and SCHILF (1930).
—, and C. H. KELLAWAY: The circulatory and pulmonary effects of the venom of the Australian Copperhead (Denisonia superba). Aust. J. exp. Biol. med. Sci. **15**, 81 (1937a).
— — Circulatory effects of the venom of the Indian cobra (Naia naia) on dogs. Aust. J. exp. Biol. med. Sci. **15**, 441 (1937b).
—, and A. A. MILES: Regional variations of increased permeability of skin capillaries by a histamine liberator and their relation to the histamine content of the skin. J. Physiol. (Lond.) **120**, 205 (1953).
—, u. E. SCHILF: Histamin. Seine Pharmakologie und Bedeutung für die Humoralphysiologie. Berlin: Springer 1930.
— — u. H. ZERNIK: Das Verhalten des Pfortaderdruckes nach Injektion von Histamin und Pepton in den Kreislauf des Hundes. Pflügers Arch. ges. Physiol. **220**, 738 (1928).
—, and J. TALESNIK: Reduction of tissue histamine by compound 48/80. J. Physiol. (Lond.) **120**, 550 (1953).
FELIX, W.: Histaminwirkung auf Blutdruck und Durchblutung des Mesenteria und des Femoralisgebietes unter abnormen Kreislaufverhältnissen. Naunyn-Schmiedeberg's Arch. exp. Path. Pharmak. **238**, 101 (1960).
FIELD, M. E., and C. K. DRINKER: Action of histamine on bronchioles and pulmonary vessels of the guinea pig. Amer. J. Physiol. **93**, 138 (1930).
FLATOW, E. M.: Die Wirkung des Histaminschocks auf das Blutbild. II. Tagung d. Deut. Physiol. Gesellschaft in Kiel. Ber. ges. Physiol. **50**, 301 (1929).
FLATOW, E., u. H. HÜTTEL: Cit. in FELDBERG und SCHILF (1930).
FLECKENSTEIN, A.: A quantitative study of antagonists of adrenaline on the vessels of the rabbit's ear. Brit. J. Pharmacol. **7**, 553 (1952).
FLEISCH, A.: Die Wirkung von Histamin, Acetylcholin und Adrenalin auf die Venen. Pflügers Arch. ges. Physiol. **228**, 351 (1931).
—, u. I. SIBUL: Über nutritive Kreislaufregulierung. II. Die Wirkung von p_H, intermediären Stoffwechselprodukten und anderen biochemischen Verbindungen. Pflügers Arch. ges. Physiol. **231**, 787 (1933).
—, u. P. WEGER: Über eine gefäßerweiternde Substanz der Erythrocyten. Pflügers Arch. ges. Physiol. **239**, 476 (1937).
FLOREY, H.: Anniversary address. Proc. roy. Soc. Med. **155**, 314 (1961).
—, J. C. F. POOLE and G. A. MEEK: Endothelial cells and "cement" lines. J. Pathol. Bact. **77**, 625 (1959).
FOLKOW, B., K. HAEGER and G. KAHLSON: Observations on reactive hyperaemia as related to histamine, on drugs antagonizing vasodilatation induced by histamine and on vasodilator properties of adenosine triphosphate. Acta physiol. scand. **15**, 264 (1948).
FORTIER, C.: Facteurs humoraux et nerveux de la réponse hypophysosurrénalienne au stress. Acta neuroveg. (Wien) **5**, 55 (1952).
FOX, R. H., R. GOLDSMITH, D. J. KIDD and G. P. LEWIS: Bradykinin as a vaso-dilator in man. J. Physiol. (Lond.) **157**, 589 (1961).
FRIMMER, M.: Beeinflussung der Durchlässigkeit von Blut-Capillaren der Kaninchenhaut für Makromoleküle durch einige biogene, gefäßaktive Substanzen. Naunyn-Schmiedeberg's Arch. exp. Path. Pharmak. **242**, 390 (1961).
FÜHNER, H., and E. H. STARLING: Experiments on the pulmonary circulation. J. Physiol. (Lond.) **46**, 286 (1913).
GADDUM, J. H.: Beiträge zum Histaminproblem. Acta neuroveg. (Wien) **4**, 268 (1952).
GANTER, G., u. A. SCHRETZENMAYR: Über die Wirkung des Histamins auf die Nierengefäße. Naunyn-Schmiedeberg's Arch. exp. Path. Pharmak. **147**, 123 (1929).
— — Über die Wirkung des Histamins auf den Kreislauf der Katze. Naunyn-Schmiedeberg's Arch. exp. Path. Pharmak. **147**, 128 (1929).
— — Über den Mechanismus der Histaminwirkung beim Hunde. Naunyn-Schmiedeberg's Arch. exp. Path. Pharmak. **151**, 49 (1930).
GOODALL, M.: Studies of adrenaline and noradrenaline in mammalian heart and suprarenals. Acta physiol. scand. **24**, Suppl. 85, 1 (1951).
GORDON, M. L.: An immediate response of the demedullated adrenal gland to stress. Endocrinology **47**, 13 (1950).
GRAY, F. D., and A. S. FIELD: Fluid interchange at the pulmonary capillary wall in lung edema. Yale J. Biol. Med. **34**, 75 (1961).

GUILLEMIN, R.: A re-evaluation of acetylcholine, adrenaline, nor-adrenaline and histamine as possible mediators of the pituitary adrenocorticotrophic activation by stress. Endocrinology **56**, 248 (1955).
—, and C. FORTIER: Role of histamine in the hypothalamohypophyseal response to stress. Trans. N. Y. Acad. Sci. **15**, 138 (1953).
GUNN, J. A.: The action of histamine on the heart and coronary vessels. J. Pharmacol. exp. Ther. **29**, 325 (1926).
HADDY, F. J.: Effect of histamine upon large and small vessels of dog forelimb. Circulation **18**, 732 (1958).
— Effect of histamine on small and large vessel pressure in the dog foreleg. Amer. J. Physiol. **198**, 161 (1960).
HALEY, T. J., and D. H. HARRIS: Effect of topically applied antihistaminic drugs on mammalian capillary bed. J. Pharmacol. exp. Ther. **95**, 293 (1949).
HALPERN, B. N.: Experimental research on new series of chemical substances with powerful antihistaminic activity; thiodiphenylamine derivatives. J. Allergy **18**, 263 (1947).
— B. BENACERRAF and M. BRIOT: Potentiation by adrenaline (epinephrine) of protective effect of cortisone (adrenocortical preparation) on histamine toxicity in adrenalectomized mice. Proc. Soc. exp. Biol. (N. Y.) **79**, 37 (1952).
— — — Roles of cortisone, desoxycorticosterone (adrenocortical preparation) and adrenaline (epinephrine) in protecting adrenalectomized animals against hemorrhagic, traumatic and histamine shock. Brit. J. Pharmacol. **7**, 287 (1952).
—, et J. ROUX: Interférence entre l'immunisation par l'Hémophilus pertussis et l'intoxication histaminique. C. R. Soc. Biol. (Paris) **143**, 923 (1949).
—, and D. R. WOOD: The action of promethazine (phenergan) in protecting mice against death to histamine. Brit. J. Pharmacol. **5**, 510 (1950).
HARMER, I. M., and K. E. HARRIS: Observations on the vascular reactions in man in response to histamine. Heart **13**, 381 (1926).
HASHIMOTO, H.: Transient change in the auriculoventricular condition following the injection of histamine. Arch. intern. Med. **35**, 609 (1925).
— Blood chemistry in acute histamine intoxication. J. Pharmacol. exp. Ther. **25**, 381 (1925—1926).
HECHTER, O.: Effect of histamine upon capillary permeability in the skin and muscle of normal and adrenalectomized rats. Endocrinology **32**, 135 (1943).
HEMINGWAY, A., and R. J. S. MCDOWALL: On the survival of striped mammalian muscles. J. Physiol. (Lond.) **61**, 6 (1926).
— — The chemical regulation of capillary tone. J. Physiol. (Lond.) **62**, 166 (1926).
HERXHEIMER, A., and M. SCHACHTER: Wheal and flare in human skin produced by histamine and other substances. Nature (Lond.) **183**, 1501 (1959).
HILTON, S. M.: Experiments on the post-contraction hyperaemia of skeletal muscle. J. Physiol. (Lond.) **120**, 230 (1953).
— A peripheral arterial conducting mechanism underlying dilatation of the femoral artery and concerned in functional vasodilatation in skeletal muscle. J. Physiol. (Lond.) **149**, 93 (1959).
— Local mechanisms regulating peripheral blood flow. Physiol. Rev. **42**, Suppl. 5, 265 (1962).
—, and G. P. LEWIS: Functional vasodilatation in the submandibular salivary gland. Brit. med. Bull. **13**, 189 (1957).
HOCHREIN, M., u. R. MEIER: Über den Mechanismus der Blutdrucksenkung durch Histamin. Naunyn-Schmiedeberg's Arch. exp. Path. Pharmak. **153**, 309 (1930).
HOLTON, F. A., and P. HOLTON: Vasodilator activity of spinal roots. J. Physiol. (Lond.) **118**, 310 (1952).
— — The possibility that ATP is a transmitter at sensory nerve endings. J. Physiol. (Lond.) **119**, 50 P (1953).
HOLTON, P.: The liberation of adenosine triphosphate on antidromic stimulation of sensory nerves. J. Physiol. (Lond.) **145**, 494 (1959).
—, and W. L. M. PERRY: On the transmitter responsible for antidromic vaso-dilatation in the rabbit's ear. J. Physiol. (Lond.) **114**, 240 (1951).
HOLTZ, P.: Über die Wirkung von Cholinestern und biogenen Aminen am isolierten Vorhof des Herzens. Acta neuroveg. (Wien) **21**, 445 (1960).
HOOKER, D. R.: The functional activity of the capillaries and venules. Amer. J. Physiol. **54**, 30 (1920).
HORTON, B. T.: Head and face pain. Collected Papers Mayo Clin. Mayo Found. **36**, 520 (1944).
— Histaminic cephalalgia: differential diagnosis and treatment. Collected Papers Mayo Clin. Mayo Found. **47**, 384 (1955).
— M. R. GRACE and A. W. ADSON: Observations on some differences in the vasomotor reactions of the hands and feet. Proc. Mayo Clin. **11**, 433 (1936).

HOUSSAY, R. H.: Sensibilité vis-à-vis de l'histamine des rats à surrénales accessoires ou démédullisés. C. R. Soc. Biol. (Paris) **149**, 1664 (1955).
HUEPER, W. C., and C. T. ICHNIOWSKI: Hematic and organic reaction in standardized and graded histamine shock in dogs. J. Pharmacol. exp. Ther. **78**, 127 (1943).
HUNT, R.: (1917). Cit. in FELDBERG und SCHILF (1930).
IBRAHIM, F. D., G. STELLA and M. TALAAT: The mechanism of antidromic vasodilatation. Quart. J. exp. Physiol. **36**, 189 (1951).
INCHLEY, O.: The action of histamine on the veins. Brit. med. J. **1**, 679 (1923).
— Histamine shock. J. Physiol. (Lond.) **61**, 282 (1926).
INGLE, D.: Resistance of the rat to histamine shock after destruction of the adrenal medulla. Amer. J. Physiol. **118**, 57 (1937).
JANCSÓ, N.: (1942). Cit. in JANCSÓ (1961).
— Histamine as a physiological activator of the reticulo-endothelial system. Nature (Lond.) **160**, 227 (1947).
— Inflammation and the inflammatory mechanisms. J. Pharm. Pharmacol. **13**, 577 (1961).
—, u. A. JANCSÓ-GABOR: Wirkung von Anticoagulantien auf entzündliche Gewebsreaktionen. Naunyn-Schmiedeberg's Arch. exp. Path. Pharmak. **238**, 83 (1960).
JOHNSON, G. S., and A. BLALOCK: Experimental shock. XII. Study of the effects of hemorrhage, of trauma to muscles, of trauma to intestine, of burns and of histamine on the cardiac output and on blood pressure of dogs. Arch. Surg. **23**, 855 (1931).
KARADY, S.: Histaminempfindlichkeit. Wien. klin. Wschr. **1**, 622 (1934).
KELLAWAY, C. H., and S. J. COWELL: On the concentration of the blood and the effects of histamine in adrenal insufficiency. J. Physiol. (Lond.) **57**, 82 (1923).
KELLER, C. J.: Untersuchungen über die Gehirndurchblutung; gibt es eine Autonomie der Gehirngefäße. Naunyn-Schmiedeberg's Arch. exp. Path. Pharmak. **154**, 357 (1930).
KEWITZ, H., u. K. MORGAN: Über die Bedeutung des Histamins für die Phagocytose von Tuschepartikelchen durch Endothelien. Naunyn-Schmiedeberg's Arch. exp. Path. Pharmak. **223**, 399 (1954).
KIND, L. S.: The altered reactivity of mice after immunization with Hemophilus pertussis vaccine. J. Immunol. **70**, 411 (1953).
— Inhibition of histamine death in pertussis-inoculated mice by cortisone and neoantergan. J. Allergy **24**, 52 (1953).
— Antagonism of cortisone to body temperature reducing effect of histamine. Proc. Soc. exp. biol. (N. Y.) **85**, 371 (1954).
— The altered reactivity of mice after inoculation with Bordetella pertussis vaccine. Bact. Rev. **22**, 173 (1958).
—, and R. H. GADSDEN: Adrenal function tests in mice sensitized to histamine with Hemophilus pertussis vaccine. Proc. Soc. exp. biol. (N. Y.) **84**, 373 (1953).
KIRCH, E.: Über tierexperimentelle Erzeugung von tonogener Dilatation und Hypertrophie des rechten Herzens durch hochdosierte Histamininjektionen. Naunyn-Schmiedeberg's Arch. exp. Path. Pharmak. **171**, 691 (1933).
KISCH, F.: Tierexperimentelle Untersuchungen über den Einfluß des Histamins auf die Zirkulationsgröße. Z. ges. exp. Med. **66**, 799 (1929).
KLISIECKI, A., u. W. HOLOBUT: Die linke Herzkammer als Herdsitz des Histaminschocks. Naunyn-Schmiedeberg's Arch. exp. Path. Pharmak. **186**, 57 (1937).
KNISELY, M. H.: A method of illuminating living structures for microscopic study. Anat. Rec. **64**, 499 (1936).
— An improved fused quartz living tissue illuminator. Anat. Rec. **71**, 503 (1938).
KONZETT, H., and E. STÜRMER: Biological activity of synthetic polypeptides with bradykinin-like properties. Brit. J. Pharmacol. **15**, 544 (1960).
KOOPMANS, S.: Functions of blood vessels in brain; effect of some narcotics, hormones and drugs. Arch. néerl. Physiol. **24**, 250 (1939).
KOWALEWSKI, K., and C. WISNIEWSKI: Oxygen content and pH of arterial, venous and portal blood in dogs after histamine. Proc. Soc. exp. biol. (N. Y.) **109**, 161 (1962).
KROGH, A.: Anatomy and physiology of the capillaries. New Haven, Conn.: Yale Univ. Press 1929.
KUSUETZOWSKY, N.: Über den Einfluß lokaler Reize auf den Prozeß der Vitalfärbung. Z. ges. exp. Med. **44**, 646 (1924).
KWIATKOWSKI, H.: Observations on the relation of histamine to reactive hyperaemia. J. Physiol. (Lond.) **100**, 147 (1941).
— Histamine in nervous tissue. J. Physiol. (Lond.) **102**, 32 (1943).
LAMSON, P. D., A. F. ABT, C. A. OOTHUISEN and S. M. ROSENTHAL: The influence of arterial blood supply to the liver on hemoglobin concentration in certain acute conditions. J. Pharmacol. exp. Ther. **21**, 401 (1923).
LAMSON, R. W.: Skin reactions to pollen and to histamine. Proc. Soc. exp. biol. (N. Y.) **26**, 611 (1929).

LANDIS, E. M.: Micro-injection studies of capillary permeability. I. Factors in the production of capillary stasis. Amer. J. Physiol. **81**, 124 (1927).
— Micro-injection studies of capillary blood pressure in human skin. Heart **15**, 209 (1930).
— Micro-injection studies of capillary blood pressure in Raynaud's disease. Heart **15**, 247 (1930).
— Capillary pressure and capillary permeability. Physiol. Rev. **14**, 404 (1934).
LANGLEY, J. N.: Antidromic action. I. J. Physiol. (Lond.) **57**, 428 (1923).
— Antidromic action. II. Stimulation of the peripheral nerves of the cat's hind foot. J. Physiol. (Lond.) **58**, 49 (1923).
LECOMTE, J.: Sur les facteurs surrénaliens qui conditionnent la résistance du rat intoxiqué par l'histamine. Arch. int. Physiol. Biochem. **69**, 563 (1961).
LEE, J. S.: Microscopic observations on the action of histamine on small blood vessels. Amer. J. Physiol. **190**, 503 (1957).
LEWIS, G. P.: Pharmacological actions and functions of bradykinin. In: Symposium on Bradykinin 1st International Pharmacological Meeting (1961). Biochem. Pharmacol. **10**, 29 (1962).
LEWIS, P. A.: The distribution of trypan red to the tissues and vessels of the eye as influenced by congestion and early infection. J. exp. Med. **23**, 669 (1916).
LEWIS, T.: The blood vessels of the human skin and their responses. London: Shaw & Sons, Ltd., 1927.
—, and R. T. GRANT: Vascular reactions of the skin to injury. II. The liberation of a histamine-like substance in injured skin: the underlying cause of factitious urticaria and of wheals produced by burning, and observations upon the nervous control of certain skin reactions. Heart **11**, 209 (1924).
—, and H. M. MARVIN: Herpes Zoster and antidromic impulses. J. Physiol. (Lond.) **62**, 19 (1926—1927).
— — Observations relating to vasodilatation arising from antidromic impulses, to herpes zoster and trophic effects. Heart **14**, 27 (1927).
LUISADA, A.: Neuere Untersuchungen über die Wirkung des Morphins auf Blutgefäße. besonders der Lungengefäße. Naunyn-Schmiedeberg's Arch. exp. Path. Pharmak. **132**, 296 (1928).
MAC CARDY, J. I., und H. M. EVANS: Experimentelle Läsionen des Centralnervensystems, untersucht mit Hilfe der vitalen Färbung. Berl. klin. Wschr. **49**, 1695 (1912).
MCCARREL, J. D., and C. K. DRINKER: Cervical lymph production during histamine shock in the dog. Amer. J. Physiol. **133**, 64 (1941).
MCCLELLAN, R. H., and E. W. GOODPASTURE: A method of demonstrating experimental cross lesions of the central nervous system. J. med. Res. **44**, 20 (1923—1924).
MCDOWALL, R. J. S.: On the nature of histamine action. J. Physiol. (Lond.) **57**, 146 (1923).
MAJNO, G., and G. E. PALADE: Studies on inflammation. I. Effect of histamine and serotonin on vascular permeability. An electron microscopic study. J. biophys. biochem. Cytol. **11**, 571 (1961).
— — and G. I. SCHOEFL: Studies on inflammation. II. The site of action of histamine and serotonin along the vascular tree. A topographic study. J. biophys. biochem. Cytol. **11**, 607 (1961).
MALKIEL, S.: Anaphylactic shock in mouse vaccinated with Hemophilus pertussis; studies on adrenal gland. J. Allergy **27**, 445 (1956).
—, and B. J. HARGIS: Anaphylactic shock in the Pertussis-vaccinated mouse. J. Allergy **23**, 352 (1952a).
— — Anaphylactic shock in the Pertussis-vaccinated mouse. Proc. Soc. exp. Biol. (N. Y.) **80**, 122 (1952b).
— — Histamine sensitivity and anaphylaxis in the Pertussis-vaccinated rat. Proc. Soc. exp. Biol. (N. Y.) **81**, 689 (1952c).
— — and S. M. FEINBERG: Anaphylactic shock in the mouse vaccinated with Hemophilus Pertussis. III. Antigens, antibody, and passive transfer studies. J. Immunol. **71**, 311 (1953).
MANNAIONI, P. F.: Interaction between histamine and dichloroisoproterenol, hexamethonium, pempidine and diphenhydramine in normal and reserpine treated heart preparations. Brit. J. Pharmacol. **15**, 500 (1960).
MANWARING, W. H., R. E. MONACO, and H. D. MARINO: Hepatic reactions in anaphylaxis. VI. Histamine reactions in isolated canine tissues. J. Immunol. **8**, 217 (1923).
MARIMOTO, M.: Über die Wirkung von Histamin auf die Nierengefäße. Naunyn-Schmiedeberg's Arch. exp. Path. Pharmak. **135**, 194 (1928).
MARMORSTON-GOTTESMAN, J., and J. GOTTESMAN: The use of histamine as a standard test for diminished resistance in suprarenalectomized rats. J. exp. Med. **47**, 503 (1928).
—, and D. PERLA: Effect of injections of cortin on resistance of suprarenalectomized rats to large amounts of histamine. Proc. Soc. exp. Biol. (N. Y.) **28**, 1022 (1931).
MARSHALL, P. B.: The influence of adrenal cortical deficiency on the histamine content of rat tissues. J. Physiol. (Lond.) **102**, 180 (1943).

Mateeff, D., u. M. Schneider: Analyse der peripheren Kreislaufswirkungen des Histamins. Pflügers Arch. ges. Physiol. **236**, 606 (1935).
Matoltsy, A. G., and M. Matoltsy: The action of histamine and antihistaminic substance on the endothelial cells of the small capillaries of the skin. J. Pharmacol. exp. Ther. **102**, 237 (1951).
Matsumoto, Y.: Cit. in Feldberg und Schilf (1930).
Mautner, H.: The role of veins in the circulation. Arch. Pediatr. **72**, 387 (1955).
—, u. E. P. Pick: Über die durch „Schockgifte" erzeugten Zirkulationsstörungen. Münch. med. Wschr. **62**, 1141 (1915).
— — Über die durch „Schockgifte" erzeugten Zirkulationsstörungen. II. Das Verhalten der überlebenden Leber. Biochem. Z. **127**, 72 (1922).
— — Über die durch „Schockgifte" erzeugten Zirkulationsstörungen. III. Der Einfluß der Leber auf Blutdruck und Schlagvolumen. Naunyn-Schmiedeberg's Arch. exp. Path. Pharmak. **142**, 271 (1929).
Mayer, R. L.: The activity of pyribenzamine and related compounds with special reference to their mode of action. Ann. N. Y. Acad. Sci. **50**, 1127 (1950).
—, and D. Brousseau: Anti-histaminic substances in histamine poisoning and anaphylaxis in mice. Proc. Soc. exp. Biol. (N. Y.) **63**, 187 (1946).
Menkin, V.: Studies on Inflammation. XIV. Isolation of the factor concerned with increased capillary permeability in injury. J. exp. Med. **67**, 129 (1938).
— Studies on Inflammation. XVI. On the formation of a chemotactic substance by enzymatic action. J. exp. Med. **67**, 153 (1938).
— A note on the differences between histamine and leukotaxine. Proc. Soc. exp. Biol. (N. Y.) **40**, 103 (1939).
— Dynamics of Inflammation. New York: McMillan Co. 1940.
Miles, A. A., and E. M. Miles: Vascular reaction to histamine, histamine liberator (compound 48/80, phenylethylamine compounds) and leukotaxine in skin of guinea pigs. J. Physiol. (Lond.) **118**, 228 (1952).
—, and D. L. Wilhelm: Enzyme-like globulins from serum reproducing the vascular phenomena of inflammation. An activable permeability factor and its inhibitor in guinea pig serum. J. exp. Pathol. **36**, 71 (1955).
— — The activation of endogenous substances inducing pathological increases of capillary permeability. 51. Biochem. Response to Injury, Symposium, Semmering, Austria, 1958 (Publ. 1960).
Möller, H., and H. Rorsman: Studies on vascular permeability factors with sodium fluorescein. I. The effect of intracutaneously injected histamine, human serum and its protein fractions in normal individuals. Acta derm.-venereol. (Stockh.) **38**, 233 (1958).
— — Studies on vascular permeability factors with sodium fluorescein. III. The effect in man of intracutaneously injected 5-hydroxytryptamine. Acta derm-venereol. (Stockh.) **39**, 12 (1959).
Moon, V. H.: Shock and Related Capillary Phenomena. Oxford, Med. Publications, New York 1938.
— Circulatory failure of capillary origin. J. Amer. med. Ass. **114**, 1312 (1940).
— M. M. Lieber, and P. J. Kennedy: Histamine and leukocytosis. Arch. Path. **20**, 1209 (1935).
Moran, N. C., and M. E. Perkins: Adrenergic blockade of the mammalian heart by a dichloro-analogue of isoproterenol. J. Pharmacol. exp. Ther. **124**, 223 (1958).
Morel, F. E., et M. Marois: Actions de l'histamine sur le système vasculaire du lapin étudiées au moyen du radiosodium. C. R. Soc. Biol. (Paris) **143**, 464 (1949).
Mota, I.: Mast cell and histamine in rat anaphylaxis. The effect of Hemophilus pertussis. Nature (Lond.) **182**, 1021 (1958).
Müller, E. A., H. Salomon u. G. Zuelzer: Die Wirkung von Histamin auf Herz und Lungen. Naunyn-Schmiedeberg's Arch. exp. Path. Pharmak. **164**, 441 (1932).
Muñoz, J., and L. F. Schuchardt: Studies on the sensitivity of mice to histamine following injections of Hemophilus pertussis. J. Allergy **24**, 330 (1953).
— — Sensitivity to histamine of adrenalectomized mice from different strains. J. Allergy **25**, 125 (1954).
— —, and W. F. Verwey: Anaphylaxis in Hemophilus pertussis, treated mice. I. Passive anaphylaxis with heterologous rabbit antibody. J. Immunol. **80**, 77 (1958).
Naranjo, P., and E. B. Naranjo: Pressor effect of histamine in the rabbit. J. Pharmacol. exp. Ther. **123**, 16 (1958).
Narayana, B.: Vaso-constricteurs et vaso-dilateurs coronaires. C. R. Soc. Biol. (Paris) **114**, 550 (1933).
Neuwelt, F., S. O. Levinson and H. Necheles: Studies on shock. III. Variability of the shock syndrome in toxic drug shock. Surgery **9**, 503 (1941).
Noble, R., and J. Collip: The response of normal, hypophysectomized and adrenalectomized rats to histamine administration. Amer. J. Physiol. **133**, 623 (1941).

OKUNEFF, N.: Über den Einfluß lokaler thermischer Reize auf die Abwanderung eines intravenös injizierten kolloidalen Farbstoffs aus dem Blut. Virchows Arch. path. Anat. **204**, 261 (1924).
OSAWA, Y.: Die Durchblutung der Katzenlunge nach Histamin. Naunyn-Schmiedeberg's Arch. exp. Path. Pharmak. **156**, 309 (1930).
— Die Bedeutung der lungengefäßverengernden Wirkung des Histamins für Blutdruck und Venendruck der Katze. Naunyn-Schmiedeberg's Arch. exp. Path. Pharmak. **156**, 323 (1930).
PALADE, G. E.: Fine structure of blood capillaries. J. appl. Physiol. **24**, 1429 (1953).
— Transport in quanta across the blood capillaries. Anat. Rec. **136**, 254 (1960).
— Blood capillaries of the heart and other organs. Circulation **24**, 368 (1961).
PAPPENHEIMER, J. R.: Capillary permeability deductions concerning the number and dimensions of ultramicroscopic openings in the capillary wall. Ann. N. Y. Acad. Sci. **55**, 465 (1952).
PARFENTJEV, I. A.: Anaphylaxis and histamine shock in mice. Proc. Soc. exp. Biol. (N. Y.) **89**, 297 (1955).
—, and M. A. GOODLINE: Histamine shock in mice sensitized with Hemophilus pertussis vaccine. J. Pharmacol. exp. Ther. **92**, 411 (1948).
PARROT, J. L.: The place of histamine in neurohumoral transmission. Pharmacol. Rev. **6**, 119 (1954).
—, et J. LEFÈBVRE: Analyse de la triple réaction cutanée au moyen d'un antagoniste de l'histamine. C. R. Soc. Biol. (Paris) **137**, 316 (1943).
PENNA, M., A. ILLANES, M. UBILLA, and S. MUJICA: Effect of histamine and of the anaphylactic reaction on isolated atria. Circulat. Res. **7**, 521 (1959).
PETERS, G. A., and B. T. HORTON: Continuous intravenous administration of histamine: effect on the electrocardiogram and serum potassium. Amer. Heart J. **27**, 845 (1944a).
— — Effect of continuous intravenous administration of histamine on basal metabolism of human beings. Proc. Centr. Soc. Clin. Res. **17**, 65 (1944b).
— —, and W. M. BOOTHBY: Effect of continuous intravenous administration on basal metabolism in human beings. J. clin. Invest. **24**, 611 (1945).
— — — The effect of continuous intravenous administration of histamine on basal metabolism in human beings. Coll. Pap. Mayo Clin. Mayo Found. **37**, 778 (1945).
PETERSON, R. D. A., and R. A. GOOD: Morphology of vascular permeability. Lab. Invest. **11**, 507 (1962).
PHEMISTER, D. B., and J. HANDY: Vascular properties of traumatized and laked blood. J. Physiol. (Lond.) **61**, 155 (1927—1928).
PICKERING, G. W.: Observations on mechanism of headache produced by histamine. Clin. Sci. **1**, 77 (1933).
—, and W. HESS: Vasodilatation in hands and feet in response to warming the body. Clin. Sci. **1**, 213 (1933).
PIIPER, J., u. E. SCHÜRMEYER: Über den Einfluß von Doryl und Histamin auf die arteriovenösen Anastomosen in der Hundeextremität. Pflügers Arch. ges. Physiol. **261**, 234 (1955).
PITTMAN, M.: Sensitivity of mice to histamine during respiratory infection by Hemophilus pertussis. Proc. Soc. exp. Biol. (N. Y.) **77**, 70 (1951).
—, and F. G. GERMUTH: Some quantitative aspects of passive anaphylaxis in pertussis-vaccinated mice. Proc. Soc. exp. Biol. (N. Y.) **87**, 425 (1954).
POPPER, H.: Über Drosselvorrichtungen an Lebervenen. Klin. Wschr. **10**, 2129 (1931).
RABE, F.: Die Reaktion der Kranzgefäße auf Arzneimittel. Z. exp. Path. Ther. **11**, 175 (1912).
RAMANAMANJARY, W.: Action des antihistaminiques sur les effects tensionnels de l'histamine chez le lapin. C. R. Soc. Biol. **138**, 480 (1944).
RAMSDELL, S. G.: The use of trypan blue to demonstrate the immediate skin reaction in rabbits and guinea pigs. J. Immunol. **15**, 305 (1928).
RANSON, S. W., L. R. FAUBION, and C. J. ROSS: Vasodilator mechanisms. IV. The intra-arterial injection of histamine. Amer. J. Physiol. **64**, 311 (1923).
RENKIN, E. M., and J. R. PAPPENHEIMER: Wasserdurchlässigkeit und Permeabilität der Capillarwände. Ergebn. Physiol. **49**, 59 (1957).
RICH, A. R.: Condition of the capillaries in histamine shock. J. exp. Med. **33**, 287 (1921).
RIGDON, R. H.: Capillary permeability in areas of inflammation produced by xylene. Arch. Surg. **41**, 101 (1940).
— Observations on effect of histamine phosphate on capillary permeability and inflammation. J. Lab. clin. Med. **27**, 1554 (1941—1942).
ROBINSON, R. L., and K. E. JOCHIM: Histamine and anaphylaxis on adrenal medullary secretion in dogs. Amer. J. Physiol. **199**, 429 (1960).
ROCHA E SILVA, M.: Anaphylaxis in the rabbit. J. Immunol. **38**, 333 (1940a).
— Kallikrein and histamine. Nature (Lond.) **145**, 591 (1940b).
— Histamina e Anafilaxia. Sao Paulo: Edigraf Ltda. 1946.
— Histamine. Its Role in Anaphylaxis and Allergy. Springfield, Ill.: Charles C. Thomas 1955.
—, and A. ANTONIO: Release of bradykinin and the mechanism of production of a "thermic edema (45° C)" in the rat's paw. Med. exp. (Basel) **3**, 371 (1960).

ROCHA E SILVA, M., u. O. G. BIER: Untersuchungen über Entzündungen. II. Virchows Arch. path. Anat. **303**, 337 (1939).
—, and C. A. DRAGSTEDT: Observations on the trypan blue capillary permeability test in rabbits. J. Pharmacol. exp. Ther. **73**, 405 (1941).
ROSE, B.: Production of symptoms by subcutaneous injection of histamine without increase of the blood histamine. Science **92**, 454 (1940).
—, and J. S. L. BROWNE: Distribution and rate of disappearance of intravenously injected histamine in rat. Amer. J. Physiol. **124**, 412 (1938).
— — The effect of adrenalectomy on the histamine content of the tissues of the rat. Amer. J. Physiol. **131**, 589 (1941).
—, and S. KARADY: Histamine metabolism in the adrenalectomized rat. Amer. J. Physiol. **126**, P 614 (1939).
RÖSSLER, R.: Über experimentelle Herzschädigung durch Koronargefäßverengerung und ihre Beeinflussung durch Pharmaka. Naunyn-Schmiedeberg's Arch. exp. Path. Pharmak. **153**, 1 (1930).
—, and W. PASCUAL: The coronary circulation in the isolated perfused heart. J. Physiol. (Lond.) **74**, 1 (1932).
ROTHLIN, E.: Über die Einwirkung des Milzextraktes (Lienins) auf die Tätigkeit des Froschherzens in situ und des isolierten Säugetierherzens. Pflügers Arch. ges. Physiol. **185**, 111 (1920).
—, et R. GUNDLACH: Étude expérimentale de l'influence de l'histamine sur la sécrétion gastrique. Arch. int. Physiol. **17**, 59 (1921).
ROWLEY, D. A., and E. P. BENDITT: 5-hydroxytryptamine and histamine as mediators of the vascular injury produced by agents which damage mast cells in rats. J. exp. Med. **103**, 399 (1956).
RÜHL, A.: Über Herzinsuffizienz durch Histamin. Naunyn-Schmiedeberg's Arch. exp. Pathol. Pharmak. **145**, 255 (1929).
— Über Gefäßinsuffizienz. Naunyn-Schmiedeberg's Arch. exp. Path. Pharmak. **148**, 24 (1930).
SCHACHTER, M.: Bradykinin and other capillary active factors. In: Symposium on Bradykinin, 1st Int. Pharmacological Meeting (1961). Biochem. Pharmacol. **10**, 87 (1962).
SCHAYER, R. W.: Significance of induced synthesis of histamine in physiology and pathology. Chemotherapia **3**, 128 (1961).
SCHENK, P.: Über die Wirkungsweise des β-imidazoläthylamins (Histamin) auf den menschlichen Organismus. Naunyn-Schmiedeberg's Arch. exp. Path. Pharmak. **89**, 332 (1921).
SCHILF, E.: Über die Wirkung von Atropin und Histamin (nach vorhergehender Atropingabe) auf die Gefäße des Hundes. Naunyn-Schmiedeberg's Arch. exp. Path. Pharmak. **126**, 37 (1927).
SCHMIDT, C. F., and J. P. HENDRIX: Cit. in VIRNO (1956). Ass. Res. nerv. Dis. Proc. **18**, 229 (1937).
SCHNEIDER, M., u. D. SCHNEIDER: Untersuchungen über die Regulierung der Gehirndurchblutung. I. Mitt. Naunyn-Schmiedeberg's Arch. exp. Path. Pharmak. **175**, 606 (1934).
— — Untersuchungen über die Regulierung der Gehirndurchblutung. II. Mitt. Einwirkung verschiedener Pharmaka auf die Gehirndurchblutung. Naunyn-Schmiedeberg's Arch. exp. Path. Pharmak. **175**, 640 (1934).
SCHRETZENMAYR, A.: Über die regulatorische Bedeutung der großen Arterien. II. Adenosinphosphorsäure, Histamin, Padutin und Tonephin. Naunyn-Schmiedeberg's Arch. exp. Path. Pharmak. **176**, 160 (1934).
SCHRÖDER, W.: Zit. in PIIPER u. E. SCHÜMEYER (1955). Verh. dtsch. Ges. Kreisl.-Forsch. **18**, 289 (1952).
SELYE, H.: The alarm reaction. Can. med. Ass. J. **34**, 706 (1936).
— The significance of the adrenal glands for adaptation. Arch. int. Pharmacodyn. **55**, 431 (1937).
— First Annual Report on Stress. Montreal: Acta Inc., Med. Publ. 1951.
— The stress of life. New York: McGraw Hill 1956.
— Stress and cardiovascular disease. Wld-Wide Abstr. gen. Med. **4**, 8 (1961).
SEVITT, S.: Early and delayed edema and increase in capillary permeability after burns of the skin. J. Path. Bact. **75**, 27 (1958).
SHARPEY-SCHAFER, E. P.: Venous tone. Brit. med. J. **1961 II**, 1589.
—, and A. D. MAC DONALD: The actions of extracts of the posterior lobe of the pituitary body on the pulmonary circulation. Quart. J. exp. Physiol. **16**, 251 (1926).
SICUTERI, F., M. FICINI, R. MONFARDINI e M. RICCI: Cefalea sperimentale da istamina; studi sulle modificazioni sfigmiche del circolo esocranico nel soggetto normale. Settim. med. **45**, 21 (1957).
SILVER, A., I. E. STECK, and C. I. REED: A study of the effects of vitamin D on capillary permeability by the use of the dye T-1824. J. Lab. clin. Med. **29**, 48 (1944).

SIMONDS, J. P.: A study of the simultaneous changes in blood pressure in the carotid artery and jugular and portal veins in anaphylactic and peptone shock in the dog. Amer. J. Physiol. **65**, 512 (1923).
—, and W. W. BRANDES: Anaphylactic shock and mechanical destruction of the hepatic veins in the dog. J. Immunol. **13**, 1 (1927).
SLATER, I. H., and P. E. DRESEL: The pressor effect of histamine after autonomic ganglionic blockade. J. Pharmacol. exp. Ther. **105**, 101 (1952).
SMITH, D. J.: *In vitro* action of cortisone on vasoconstriction due to histamine. Proc. Soc. exp. Biol. (N. Y.) **77**, 534 (1951).
SMITH, M. I.: Studies on experimental shock with special reference to its treatment. J. Pharmacol. exp. Ther. **32**, 465 (1928).
SNYDER, C. D.: Recent advances in knowledge of the liver. Physiol. Rev. **22**, 54 (1942).
SOLLMANN, T., and A. J. GILBERT: Reaction of carotid arteries of small animals. J. Pharmacol. exp. Ther. **62**, 236 (1938).
—, and J. D. PILCHER: Endermic reaction. J. Pharmacol. exp. Ther. **9**, 309 (1917).
SOLOTOROVSKY, M., and S. WINSTEN: Anaphylaxis in mouse produced with crystalline bovine albumin. J. Immunol. **71**, 296 (1953).
— — Inhibition of fatal anaphylactic shock in mouse with cortisone. J. Immunol. **72**, 177 (1954).
SPARROW, E. M., and P. L. WILHELM: Species differences in susceptibility to capillary permeability factors; histamine, 5-HT and compound 48/80. J. Physiol. (Lond.) **135**, 51 (1957).
SPECTOR, W. G.: The role of some higher peptides in inflammation. J. Path. Bact. **63**, 93 (1951).
— Mediation of altered capillary permeability in acute inflammation. J. Path. Bact. **72**, 367 (1956).
— Substances which affect capillary permeability. Pharmacol. Rev. **10**, 475 (1958).
—, and D. A. WILLOUGHBY: Experimental suppression of increased capillary permeability in thermal burns in rats. Nature (Lond.) **182**, 949 (1958).
— — Experimental suppression of the acute inflammatory changes of thermal injury. J. Path. Bact. **78**, 14 (1959).
STARLING, E. H.: On the absorption of fluids from the connective tissue spaces. J. Physiol. (Lond.) **19**, 312 (1895—1896).
— The fluids of the body. Chicago: Univ. Chicago Press 1909.
STAUB, A. M.: Recherches sur quelques bases synthétiques antagonistes de l'histamine. I. Ann. Inst. Pasteur **63**, 400 (1939).
STAUB, H., u. W. GRASSMANN: Über die Wirkungsgrenze einiger Gifte am isolierten Säugetierherzen. Naunyn-Schmiedeberg's Arch. exp. Path. Pharmak. **154**, 317 (1930).
STEAD, E. A., and J. V. WARREN: The effect of the injection of histamine into the brachial artery on the permeability of capillaries of the forearm and hand. J. clin. Invest. **23**, 279 (1944).
Symposium on The Mechanism of Inflammation. Edit. G. JASMIN and A. ROBERT. Montreal: Acta Inc., Medical Publishers 1953.
SZABÓ, G., u. S. MAGYAR: Die Wirkung der Sympathicusblockade im Histaminschock. Z. ges. exp. Med. **135**, 193 (1961).
SZCZYGIELSKI, J.: Die adrenalinabsondernde Wirkung des Histamins und ihre Beeinflussung durch Nikotin. Naunyn-Schmiedeberg's Arch. exp. Path. Pharmak. **166**, 319 (1932).
THOMAS, W. D., and H. E. ESSEX: Observations on hepatic venous circulation with special reference to the sphyncteric mechanism. Amer. J. Physiol. **158**, 303 (1949).
TÖRÖ, J.: (1942). Cit. in JANCSÓ (1961).
TRENDELENBURG, U.: The action of histamine and 5-hydroxytryptamine on isolated mammalian atria. J. Pharmacol. exp. Ther. **130**, 450 (1960).
— The pressor response of the cat to histamine and pilocarpine. J. Pharmacol. exp. Ther. **131**, 65 (1961).
TRIBE-OPPENHEIMER, E.: Studies on the so-called heart hormone. Amer. J. Physiol. **90**, 656 (1929).
TRIPOD, J., E. WIRZ et R. MEIER: Influence de l'histamine sur l'activité cardiaque du chat. Arch. int. Pharmacodyn. **88**, 51 (1951).
TRUEX, R. E.: Chromaffin tissue of the sympathetic ganglia and heart. Anat. Rec. **108**, 687 (1950).
UNDERHILL, F. P., and S. C. ROTH: The influence of water deprivation, pilocarpin, and histamine upon changes in blood concentration in the rabbit. J. biol. Chem. **54**, 607 (1922).
UNGAR, G.: Les substances histaminiques et la transmission chimique de l'influx nerveux. Paris: Hermann et Cie., Éditeurs 1937.
VALLERY-RADOT, P.: L'anaphylaxie humaine et expérimentale. Paris: Masson et Cie. 1937.
— Précis des Maladies Allergiques 18. Paris: Flammarion 1949.
VANREMOORTERE, E., H. MAZZELLA et J. LECOMTE: Action de l'histamine sur le débit coronarien du coeur isolé du lapin, en fibrillation ventriculaire. Arch. int. Physiol. **59**, 471 (1951).

Vaughan-Williams, E. M.: The action of quinidine, acetylcholine and anaphylaxis interpreted from simultaneous and intracellular potentials in the heart. In: The Scientific Basis of Medicine. Ann. Rev. University of London. The Athlone Press 302 (1961).

Viotti, C.: Action de l'histamine sur le coeur et importance de l'atropine à cet égard. C. R. Soc. Biol. (Paris) **91**, 1085 (1924).

Virno, M., S. B. Gertner, and D. Bovet: Action of histamine on the jugular venous pressure and cerebral circulation of the dog. Effects of antihistaminic drugs (pyrilamine and chlorpheniramine) and a histamine liberating agent (48/80 B. W.). J. Pharmacol. exp. Ther. **118**, 63 (1956).

Wakim, K. G., G. A. Peters, J. C. Terrier, and B. T. Horton: Effects of intravenously administered histamine on peripheral circulation in man. J. Lab. clin. Med. **34**, 380 (1949).

Waud, R. A.: Viscosity of the blood in histamine shock. Amer. J. Physiol. **84**, 563 (1928).

Weiser, R. S., O. J. Golub. and D. M. Hamre: Studies on anaphylaxis in the mouse J. infect. Dis. **68**, 97 (1941).

Weiss, S., L. B. Ellis, and G. P. Robb: Bodily responses in man during the continuous intravenous administration of histamine. Amer. J. Physiol. **90**, 551 (1929a).

— G. P. Robb, and H. L. Blumgart: The velocity of blood flow in health and disease as measured by the effect of histamine on the minute vessels. Amer. Heart J. **4**, 664 (1929b).

— —, and L. B. Ellis: The systemic effects of histamine in man; with special reference to the responses of the cardiovascular system. Arch. intern. Med. **49**, 360 (1932).

Went, I., u. E. Varga: Experimentelle Untersuchungen über die chemische Gegenregulation des Blutdruckes. Acta physiol. Acad. Sci. hung. **3**, 377 (1952).

— — E. Szücs u. O. Fehér: Eine Analyse der sympathomimetischen Wirkung des Histamins an isolierten Säugetierherzpräparaten. Acta physiol. Acad. Sci. hung. **5**, 121 (1954).

Went, S., u. K. Lissak: Histamin und Proteinwirkung am normalen und sensibilisierten Meerschweinchenherz. Naunyn-Schmiedeberg's Arch. exp. Path. Pharmak. **179**, 609 (1935).

—, u. J. Martin: Über die Schockresistenz der weißen Ratte. Naunyn-Schmiedeberg's Arch. exp. Path. Pharmak. **191**, 545 (1939).

— E. Varga, E. Szücs u. O. Fehér: Über eine „sympathomimetische" Wirkung des Histamins. Naunyn-Schmiedeberg's Arch. exp. Pharmak. **215**, 129 (1952).

White, T.: Some effects of histamine and two histamine metabolites on the cat's brain. J. Physiol. (Lond.) **159**, 198 (1961).

Wiggers, C. J.: Physiology of Shock. New York: The Commonwealth Fund. 1950.

Wilcox, H. B., and E. C. Andrus: Anaphylaxis in the isolated heart. J. exp. Med. **67**, 169 (1938).

—, and B. C. Seegal: Influence of an ethylenediamine derivative on histamine intoxication and anaphylactic shock in the intact guinea pig and the isolated guinea pig heart. J. Immunol. **44**, 219 (1942).

Wilhelm, D. L.: The mediators of increased vascular permeability in inflammation. Pharmacol. Rev. **14**, 251 (1962).

Winternitz, M. C., and A. D. Hirschfelder: Studies upon experimental pneumonia in rabbits. J. exp. Med. **17**, 657 (1913).

Woodbury, R. A.: Influence of epinephrine and atropine on pulmonary pressor action of histamine. J. Pharmacol. exp. Ther. **86**, 78 (1946).

—, and W. F. Hamilton: Effect of histamine on pulmonary blood pressure of various animals with and without anesthesia. J. Pharmacol. exp. Ther. **71**, 293 (1941).

Wybauw, L.: Transmission humorale de la vaso-dilatation provoquée par l'excitation du bout périphérique des racines postérieures lombaires chez le chat. C. R. Soc. Biol. (Paris) **123**, 524 (1937).

— Contribution à l'étude du rôle vaso-moteur et trophique des nerfs sensitifs. Arch. int. Physiol. **46**, 293 (1938).

Wyman, L. C., and C. T. Suden: The blood volume of the rat in suprarenal insufficiency, anaphylactic shock and histamine shock. Amer. J. Physiol. **93**, 700 (1930).

Zweifach, B. W.: Structure and reactions of small blood vessels in amphibia. Amer. J. Anat. **60**, 473 (1937).

— The structural basis of permeability and other functions of blood capillaries. Cold Spr. Harb. Symp. quant. Biol. **8**, 216 (1940).

— Structural makeup of the capillary wall. Ann. N. Y. Acad. Sci. **61**, 670 (1955).

Section F

Action of Histamine upon Salivary Glands

By

NILS EMMELIN

I. Flow of saliva caused by histamine

The early papers on the pharmacology of histamine describe salivary secretion as a characteristic effect of this drug (DALE and LAIDLAW, 1910; BARGER and DALE, 1910; ACKERMANN and KUTSCHER, 1910; FRÖHLICH and PICK, 1913). Intravenous injection of 2—10 mg histamine was found to cause a profuse secretion in unanaesthetized cats, and in anaesthetized cats and dogs histamine was observed to evoke a flow of saliva from the cannulated submaxillary duct.

Generally, it may be stated that secretion of saliva is not one of the more conspicuous effects of histamine. Fairly large doses of histamine are required to cause a flow of saliva, compared with those needed to produce effects on the blood pressure, on smooth muscle or on the gastric glands, and with repeated injections the secretory responses of the salivary glands often diminish or disappear. In some experiments no secretion is seen even after the first injection. MARGARET MACKAY (1927) could demonstrate a flow of saliva in less than 50 per cent of cats in chloralose anaesthesia when histamine was given intravenously, intramuscularly or subcutaneously, and similar results were obtained in dogs. GIBBS and MCCLANAHAN (1937), administering the drug in close arterial injection to the submaxillary gland of cats under dial could produce a flow of saliva in two thirds of the cases. This irregularity seems in part to be due to the fact that anaesthetics suppress the secretory responses of the salivary glands to histamine. In decerebrated cats M. MACKAY found histamine regularly to produce secretion of saliva. Similarly, CORNIL and MALMÉJAC (1938) observed a more pronounced secretion in curarized dogs than in dogs anaesthetized with chloralose. According to STAVRAKY (1931), morphine followed by light ether anaesthesia is favourable when studying effects of histamine on salivary glands of dogs, whereas YONKMAN, CHESS, MATHIESON and HANSEN (1946) recommend urethane or this drug combined with dial for experiments on cats.

A further reason for the variable results obtained with histamine on the salivary glands may be that the comparatively large doses necessary cause profound effects on the circulation, thus interfering with the flow of blood through the glands; the picture may in addition be complicated by release of catechol amines from the adrenals, as discussed below.

In spite of numerous investigations, our knowledge of the mechanism by which histamine is able to elicit salivation is inadequate. This is no doubt in part due to the fact that the responses are so irregular and decrease with repeated injections. Several different points of attack have been demonstrated. It may well be that a flow of saliva observed in an experiment is the result of more than one type of action of histamine. The contributions of different actions may vary with the species, the mode of administration of the drug, the dose and, if an anaesthetic is used, the compound chosen. The type of gland investigated is, likewise, of importance. For instance, the submaxillary gland of most cats, contrary to the parotid of that species, has a well developed sympathetic innervation through which secretory effects may be mediated.

Most experiments on histamine and salivary secretion have been carried out on the submaxillary gland of cats and dogs. Some observations have been made on the parotid gland of the dog (STAVRAKY, 1931). No experiments on the effect of histamine on the sublingual gland, or on the small glands of the oral mucosa, have been described. Secretion of saliva in humans following administration of histamine has been reported (GOMPERTZ and COHEN, 1929; CORNIL, 1938) but not referred to a specified salivary gland; this applies to monkeys also (BERTHELOT and BERTRAND, 1912).

Under physiological conditions the salivary glands are activated reflexly, parasympathetic secretory fibres serving as the efferent link of the reflex arc. Experimentally, secretion can be evoked from some glands by stimulation of sympathetic fibres; the significance of this nerve supply is little understood. The same glands respond to injected adrenaline (or noradrenaline) and under exceptional circumstances catechol amines released from the adrenal medulla may cause a flow of saliva. Apart from this, no hormonal mechanism resulting in salivary secretion is known. This brief summary suggests the following possibilities when considering the mode of action of histamine on the salivary glands.

A. Reflex actions

In human beings the subcutaneous injection of 2 mg histamine was found to give rise to a salty taste after about three minutes (SCHENK, 1921). When 0.001 mg histamine was injected quickly intravenously the subjects experienced a sensation in the tongue described as salty, metallic or electric (WEISS, ROBB and BLUMGART, 1929). If this sensation is accompanied by a flow of saliva has not been investigated.

Secretion observed in dogs after intracarotid injection of histamine was by CORNIL and MALMÉJAC (1938) in part attributed to a reflex elicited from the carotid sinus. Whether such an effect was thought to be mediated via the salivary nuclei or involved a fall in blood pressure and a liberation of catechol amines was not discussed.

B. Central actions

POPIELSKI (1920) injected 0.03 mg histamine per kg intravenously in dogs under chloralose and observed a secretion of saliva. When the chorda tympani was cut and a second injection given, no flow of saliva was seen. From this finding he concluded that the point of action of histamine in eliciting salivary secretion is central. Later investigators have found the response to be reduced but not abolished by acute denervation of the salivary gland (e. g. STAVRAKY, 1931). In this connection the fact that the secretory effects of repeated doses tend to decline has to be borne in mind. It seems advisable to study the effect of a single dose of histamine when one gland is acutely denervated and the contralateral one intact. In such experiments M. MACKAY (1927) saw no difference between the responses of the two glands. Histamine was given intravenously, and the experiments suggest that under such conditions a central effect can play a minor role only. Different results may be obtained if histamine is given through the carotid artery; CORNIL and MALMÉJAC (1938) then saw a more pronounced secretion from the innervated than from the denervated gland. The secretory effect was greatly reduced by ligation of the internal carotid artery and therefore thought to be mainly of central origin, although an action on the carotid sinus was assumed to contribute to some extent.

That histamine is able to evoke a flow of saliva by virtue of a central action is apparent from the investigations of FELDBERG and SHERWOOD (1954). Among the effects of histamine (150–200 μg), injected intraventricularly in unanaesthetized cats through a permanent cannula, salivation is mentioned. Such an effect seems to be more difficult to elicit in monkeys; LIGHT and BYSSHE (1933) found no salivary secretion after intraventricular injection of as much as 10 mg histamine. It should be noted, however, that no secretion was obtained after intravenous or subcutaneous injection of 2 mg in these animals. BERTHELOT and BERTRAND (1912), who were able to elicit salivary secretion in monkeys by intravenous injection of histamine, used considerably larger doses, 8–45 mg in small animals.

It is obviously possible to evoke a secretion of saliva through a central mechanism at least in dogs and cats. Whether the central stimulation results in impulses in the secretory parasympathetic or sympathetic nerves or a release of catechol amines from the adrenals has not been investigated. In the experiments of FELDBERG and SHERWOOD (1954) the intraventricular injection of histamine was followed by relaxation of the nictitating membrane. The flow of saliva observed could therefore not be due to catechol amines in the blood, for doses of these substance causing salivary secretion should certainly strongly contract the membrane. There was apparently no general discharge of impulses in the sympathetic nerves. Very likely the secretory effect was mediated by way of the parasympathetic path.

C. Ganglionic actions

Histamine has been shown to stimulate sympathetic ganglion cells in cats through an action different from that of nicotine-like substances (TRENDELENBURG, 1959). With regard to salivary secretion this possible mode of action has not been studied. The doses required to stimulate the ganglion are fairly large (TRENDELENBURG, 1954) but not larger than those used to evoke secretion of saliva. When secretion was obtained with histamine in "denervated" glands, a ganglionic point of attack was not excluded, for these glands were not "denervated" in the restricted sense of the word but "decentralized", both sympathetic and parasympathetic ganglia being left intact. The analysis could be carried out on parotid glands in which both types of secretory fibres can be cut postganglionically. If pharmacological tools are used in such experiments it should be kept in mind that the ganglion-stimulating action of histamine is not abolished by drugs acting through competitive blocking. The ganglionic effect of histamine is selectively abolished by antihistaminic agents. It is interesting in this connection that pyribenzamine has been found to abolish the secretory effect of histamine (YONKMAN, CHESS, MATHIESON and HANSEN, 1946). This was apparently a specific histamine antagonism, for the secretory effects of chorda stimulation or pilocarpine were not annulled; some antihistamines, e. g. benadryl, have an atropine-like action on the salivary glands (ANDERSON and EMMELIN, 1947).

D. Actions directly on the salivary glands

A peripheral effect of histamine on the gland is well demonstrated in experiments in which the drug is given by close arterial injection. Doses of 1–100 μg administered in this way into the cat's submaxillary gland often produce a marked secretion (GIBBS and MCCLANAHAN, 1937). Such an effect is generally assumed to be exerted to a great extent on the glandular cells, although a ganglionic action has not been excluded, the submaxillary gland containing numerous parasympathetic ganglion cells. Another way of producing a local effect in the gland is to inject drugs backwards through the salivary duct. In such an experiment on a dog, 3–300 μg histamine produced no flow of saliva from the submaxillary gland (Emmelin, Muren and Strömblad, 1954); in view of the great individual variations in susceptibility of the salivary glands to histamine this experiment ought to be repeated on a series of animals.

According to M. MacKay (1927, 1930), Osborne (1928), Babkin (1929) and Stavraky (1931) histamine has a dual action on the salivary gland (apart from its vascular effect). It has a motor effect, expelling saliva present in the duct system, and it has a "true secretory" effect on the gland cells.

Arguments in favour of the existence of a contractile effect of histamine on the gland are of the following type. Plethysmographically it can be shown that histamine causes a marked and long lasting diminution of the submaxillary gland, preceded by a short and small increase in size (Babkin and MacKay, 1931). When histamine is injected several times the number of drops falling from a cannula in a salivary duct decreases quickly; if fluid is blown back into the gland through the cannula a subsequent dose of histamine causes a large effect (MacKay, 1927; Stavraky, 1931). Instead of by forcing fluid backwards, the ducts can be filled by stimulation of the chorda; afterwards histamine will produce a marked flow of saliva. This effect is obtained even if the time interval between the chorda stimulation and the injection of histamine is long enough to allow the excitability of the gland cells, raised by nerve stimulation, to return to its pre-stimulation level (see below). The fact that the response to histamine depends on the amount of saliva present in the ducts can no doubt to some extent explain the common finding that the flow decreases with repeated doses. Babkin and MacKay (1931) excluded the possibility that this mechanical effect of histamine could be of vascular origin and inferred that it is due to a contraction of myoepithelial cells. These can be activated by sympathetic fibres also, and this effect is abolished by ergotamine. Histamine, however, retains its motor effect and is therefore supposed to act directly on the myoepithelial cells. The motor effect of histamine does not seem to be abolished by atropine either (Babkin, 1929; MacKay, 1930; Stavraky, 1931).

Salivation caused by histamine cannot be entirely explained as due to a motor effect. This is apparent already from the fact that the amount of saliva obtained is often much larger than that which can be present in the ducts. The experiments of Gibbs and McClanahan (1937) clearly show that in many cats considerable quantities of saliva can be discharged from the submaxillary gland when histamine is injected intraarterially and that in some cases there is no decline in the responses to repeated doses. These responses are ascribed to a "true secretory" effect of histamine. This effect is abolished by atropine (Dale and Laidlaw, 1910; Gibbs and McClanahan, 1937; Yonkman, Chess, Mathieson and Hansen, 1946). It may therefore be classified as muscarinic. Dale and Laidlaw (1910) compared it with that of pilocarpine and pointed out that both drugs contain an imidazol ring. It may be worth mentioning that salivary secretion, abolished by atropine, can be obtained with two other imidazole derivates, privine (Yonkman, Rennick and Schwerma, 1945) and priscol (Hermann and Vial, 1942; Chess and Yonkman, 1946; Roch-Besser, 1950).

Gibbs and McClanahan (1937) call in question whether the secretory effect of histamine can be considered muscarine-like. They observed that the effect can be increased by eserine and further that histamine can potentiate the effect of chorda stimulation but not that of intraarterially injected acetylcholine. Assuming histamine nevertheless to possess a real muscarinic effect these findings could tentatively be interpreted as follows. Eserine causes accumulation of acetylcholine, constantly leaking from the postganglionic parasympathetic endings (for discussion see EMMELIN, 1960). This acetylcholine, in subthreshold or superthreshold amount, adds its effect to that of histamine, increasing the secretory response. The potentiation of the chorda effect by a previous injection of histamine could be due to a raised excitability of the gland cells caused by the secretory agent histamine and persisting for a short time period. This should in other words be an example of a "true augmented secretion" in LANGLEY's sense. If so it would be reasonable to expect histamine to increase the effect of injected acetylcholine also, but that did not occur; it may be that the dose of acetylcholine quickly injected was sufficient to cause a maximal response.

The effect on the submaxillary gland of histamine, like that of most other secretory agents, can be increased by previous denervation (EMMELIN, unpublished observation). In that way it is often easier to show that the amount of saliva delivered by the gland on injection of histamine is so large that it cannot be due wholly to a motor effect of the drug. Another mode of increasing the responses to histamine has been used by earlier investigators (MACKAY, 1927, 1930; STAVRAKY, 1931). Before the administration of histamine the chorda has been stimulated; histamine has been given as soon as the flow due to nerve stimulation has ceased. An "augmented secretion" is thereby obtained which in part is due to the fact that the ducts are filled with saliva to be expelled by the activated myoepithelial cells and partly is a "true augmented secretion".

In this connection the interaction between pilocarpine and histamine on the salivary glands ought to be mentioned. Several investigators have remarked that secretion caused by pilocarpine is reduced by the injection of histamine. Such an effect was observed in cats under chloralose anaesthesia by M. MACKAY (1927) and in unanaesthetized dogs with a salivary fistula by KLEITMAN (1930) and VINEBERG and BABKIN (1931). These findings can probably be explained in the following way. The glands were secreting at a maximal or nearly maximal rate under the influence of pilocarpine, and their blood vessels were maximally dilated. Normally histamine dilates the vessels of the salivary glands but under these conditions the sole effect of histamine was to reduce the flow of blood through the glands owing to the fall in arterial pressure. It is well known that a gland secreting near its maximum is very sensitive to a reduced flow of blood and quickly responds with a diminished rate of secretion. This interpretation is supported by the fact that very large doses of pilocarpine were given (for instance 7 mg in the experiments of VINEBERG and BABKIN) and by the following statement (MACKAY, 1927): "It is interesting to note that in a few instances with cats, histamine produced an acceleration of the pilocarpine secretion, but this was observed when the effect of pilocarpine was wearing off. Different results were obtained in the dog, histamine usually giving an acceleration and an inhibition only after large doses of pilocarpine." When the doses of pilocarpine were moderate, the effects of the two drugs were obviously additive, as could be expected.

The action of atropine on salivary secretion deserves some further comments. Some investigators have found that the effect of histamine on the glands cannot be completely abolished by atropine (OSBORNE, 1928; STAVRAKY, 1931); this seems to apply particularly to the parotid gland. This could be interpreted to mean that the action of histamine on the salivary gland cells differs from that of, say, acetylcholine in the same way as it is supposed to do in the gastric glands. If so, histamine should be the only agent known with a real "direct" effect on the gland cells (with the possible exception of some nitrogen mustards; see EMMELIN, 1961). Before such a far-reaching conclusion is accepted the following possibilities ought to be considered:

α) the effect remaining after atropine may be a purely motor one on the myoepithelial cells,
β) it may be mediated via the sympathetic innervation, or
γ) due to catechol amines released from the adrenal medulla.

E. Actions via the adrenal medulla

As is well known, histamine may liberate catechol amines from the adrenals. Since these substances, and particularly adrenaline, can evoke a flow of saliva from some glands, for instance the submaxillary and sublingual glands of the cat and the parotid gland of the rabbit, the possibility has to be considered that salivary secretion observed after injection of histamine can be indirect and due to adrenaline. If so, the effect ought to remain after the acute denervation of the salivary glands but to be abolished by sympatholytic agents. The adrenaline liberating effect of histamine, injected into the arteries of the adrenals, is abolished by antihistamine compounds, and this effect is specific; the action of acetylcholine, potassium or bile salts on the adrenals is not affected (EMMELIN and MUREN, 1949). Secretion of saliva caused by histamine acting on the adrenals therefore can be supposed to be abolished by histamine antagonists, just as the secretory effect exerted directly on the salivary gland.

A complicating factor is that there seems to be some kind of antagonism between histamine and adrenaline in the effects on the salivary glands (FRÖHLICH and PICK, 1913; MACKAY, 1929). There is even experimental evidence to show that the secretory responses to histamine may be increased by adrenalectomy (MACKAY, 1929). These interesting observations seem to deserve further analysis.

II. Secretory effects mediated by histamine

Curarine is known to cause a flow of saliva, mainly of central origin. It has, however, a peripheral action also, for a small dose injected into the artery of the submaxillary gland causes salivation, as seen already by CLAUDE BERNARD (1864). Flow of saliva can also be observed when the gland is perfused with a solution containing curarine. The possibility that this effect is due to histamine, released by curarine, has been considered but regarded as unlikely since fairly large doses of histamine have to be added to the perfusion fluid in order to elicit an even scanty secretion (EMMELIN and MUREN, 1950). Recently, however, some evidence has been given to show that curarine is able to release histamine in the submaxillary gland in amounts sufficient to cause a flow of saliva (ELWELL, 1960). It would be interesting to know if other histamine liberators have a secretory effect on the salivary glands.

There is no reason to assign to histamine a role as a mediator in salivary secretion under physiological conditions. The fact that some of the histamine antagonists suppress secretion of saliva (ANDERSON and EMMELIN, 1947; MCDONALD, 1953) cannot be used as an argument in favour of such a view. The effect is unspecific and no doubt due to a central action and in some instances to an atropine-like effect of the drugs.

III. Effect on the composition of saliva

The only investigation dealing with the composition of saliva secreted after injection of histamine is that by STAVRAKY (1931). He found the saliva richer in organic matter but with a lower ash content than saliva secreted in response to stimulation of the chorda tympani.

IV. Excretion of histamine in saliva

Kamenowa (1930) found no histamine in saliva and Ungar and Pocoulé (1937) significant amounts in some cases only, but some investigators demonstrate considerable quantities (Gibertini, 1942; Sanders, 1955). At least some of this histamine may not have been excreted by the gland but originate from leucocytes. The fact that saliva contains kallikrein which may contract the guinea-pig ileum in the presence of protein and lower the blood pressure should be kept in mind if the effect of saliva is studied on these test objects without extraction procedures inactivating the kallikrein.

V. Vascular effects of histamine in the glands

Histamine increases the flow of blood through the submaxillary gland (Fröhlich and Pick, 1913; MacKay, 1927, 1928). When histamine causes secretion, a reactive vasodilatation is to be expected. In addition, however, histamine no doubt has a powerful direct vasodilator action in the gland, for it causes a pronounced increase in the blood flow. The vasodilator action is in fact so marked that after an intravenous injection the blood flow is augmented in spite of the lowered blood pressure.

References

Ackermann, D., u. F. Kutscher: Untersuchungen über die physiologische Wirkung einer Secalebase und des Imidazolyläthylamins. Z. Biol. **54**, 387—394 (1910).
Anderson, D. J., and N. Emmelin: The action of β-dimethylaminoethyl benzhydryl ether hydrochloride on salivary secretion. Acta physiol. scand. **13**, 72—74 (1947).
Babkin, B. P.: Innervation of the salivary glands. Amer. J. Physiol. **90**, 271 (1929).
—, and Margaret E. MacKay: Concerning the motor mechanism of the salivary glands. Amer. J. Physiol. **91**, 370—376 (1931).
Barger, G., u. H. H. Dale: Die physiologische Wirkung einer Secalebase und deren Identifizierung als Imidazolyläthylamin. Zbl. Physiol. **24**, 886—889 (1910).
Bernard, C.: Du role des actions réflexes paralysantes dans le phénomène des sécrétions. J. Anat. (Paris) **1**, 507—513 (1864).
Berthelot, A., et D.-M. M.Bertrand: Contribution à l'étude de la toxicité de la β-imidazoléthyl-amine. C. R. Acad. Sci. (Paris) **55**, 360—362 (1912).
Chess, Dorothy, and F. F. Yonkman: Adrenolytic and sympatholytic actions of Priscol (benzyl-imidazoline). Proc. Soc. exp. Biol. (N. Y.) **61**, 127—130 (1946).
Cornil, quoted by Cornil and Malméjac.
Cornil, L., et J. Malméjac: Sur la sécrétion salivaire sous-maxillaire provoquée par l'histamine. C. R. Soc. Biol. (Paris) **129**, 680—681 (1938).
Dale, H. H., and P. P. Laidlaw: The physiological action of β-imidazolethylamine. J. Physiol. (Lond.) **41**, 318—344 (1910—1911).
Elwell, L. H.: Effects of d-tubocurarine on the submandibular salivary gland. Amer. J. Physiol. **198**, 621—624 (1960).
Emmelin, N.: Is there a leakage of acetylcholine from postganglionic parasympathetic nerve endings? Nature (London) **185**, 297—298 (1960).
— 1961. In: Burgen, A. S. V., and N. G. Emmelin: Physiology of the Salivary Glands. Monographs of the Physiological Society. London: Arnold 1961.
—, and A. Muren: Effects of antihistamine compounds on the adrenaline liberation from the suprarenals. Acta physiol. scand. **17**, 345—355 (1949).
— — Acetylcholine release at parasympathetic synapses. Acta physiol. scand. **20**, 13—32 (1950).
— — and R. Strömblad: Secretory and vascular effects of various drugs injected into the submaxillary duct. Acta physiol. scand. **32**, 325—338 (1954).
Feldberg, W., and S. L. Sherwood: Injections of drugs into the lateral ventricle of the cat. J. Physiol. (Lond.) **123**, 148—167 (1954).
Fröhlich, A., u. E. P. Pick: Die Folgen der Vergiftung durch Adrenalin, Histamin, Pituitrin, Pepton, sowie der anaphylaktischen Vergiftung in bezug auf das vegetative Nervensystem. Naunyn-Schmiedeberg's Arch. exp. Path. Pharmak. **71**, 23—61 (1913).

Gibbs, O. S., and H. H. McClanahan: The effect of histamine on salivary secretion. J. Pharmacol. exp. Ther. **61**, 218—229 (1937).
Gibertini, G.: Il contenuto in istamina nella saliva, nel succo gastrico, nella bile. Boll. Soc. ital. biol. sper. **17**, 360—361 (1942).
Gompertz, L. M., and W. Cohen: The effect of smaller doses of histamine in stimulating human gastric secretion. Amer. J. med. Sci. **177**, 59—64 (1929).
Hermann, H., et J. Vial: Sur quelques actions pharmacodynamiques du 2-benzyl-imidazoline (C. 3259). C. R. Soc. Biol. (Paris) **136**, 803—805 (1942).
Kamenowa 1930. In: Feldberg, W., u. E. Schilf: Histamin. Seine pharmakologische Bedeutung für die humorale Physiologie. Berlin: Springer 1930.
Kleitman, N.: Effect of histamine upon the salivary flow induced by pilocarpine in dogs. Proc. Soc. exp. Biol. (N. Y.) **28**, 134—135 (1930—1931).
Light, R. U., and S. M. Bysshe: The administration of drugs into the cerebral ventricles of monkeys: pituitrin, certain pituitary fractions, pitressin, pitocin, histamine, acetylcholine and pilocarpine. J. Pharmacol. exp. Ther. **47**, 17—36 (1933).
MacKay, Margaret E.: Histamine and salivary secretion. Amer. J. Physiol. **82**, 546—556 (1927).
— The vascular reaction of the pilocarpinized submaxillary gland to histamine. J. Pharmacol. exp. Ther. **32**, 147—159 (1928).
— Histamine and adrenaline in relation to the salivary secretion. J. Pharmacol. exp. Ther. **37**, 349—358 (1929).
— Further data concerning the histamine salivary secretion. Amer. J. Physiol. **91**, 123—131 (1930).
McDonald, R. E.: The effect of antihistamine drugs on salivary flow and viscosity. J. dent. Res. **32**, 224—226 (1953).
Osborne, W. A.: Low blood pressure and secretory activity. Austral. J. exp. Biol. med. Sci. **5**, 171—172 (1928).
Popielski, L.: β-Imidazolyläthylamin und die Organextrakte. Naunyn-Schmiedeberg's Arch. exp. Path. Pharmak. **178**, 214—236 (1920).
Roch-Besser, B.: La benzyl-imidazoline (Priscol). Helv. med. acta Suppl. **27**, 1—175 (1950).
Sanders, S. G.: Chemical determination of histamine content of oral tissues and saliva. J. oral Surg. **13**, 193—199 (1955).
Schenk, P.: Über die Wirkungsweise des β-Imidazolyläthylamins (Histamin) auf den menschlichen Organismus. Naunyn-Schmiedeberg's Arch. exp. Path. Pharmak. **89**, 332—339 (1921).
Stavraky, G.: The response of the submaxillary and parotid glands of the dog to histamine. J. Pharmacol. exp. Ther. **43**, 265—275 (1931).
Trendelenburg, U.: The action of histamine and pilocarpine on the superior cervical ganglion and the adrenal glands of the cat. Brit. J. Pharmacol. **9**, 481—487 (1954).
— Non-nicotinic ganglion-stimulating substances. Fed. Proc. **18**, 1001—1005 (1959).
Ungar, G., et A. Pocoulé: Sur les voies d'élimination de l'histamine et son absence dans les urines normales. C. R. Soc. Biol. (Paris) **124**, 1204—1206 (1937).
Vineberg, A. M., and B. P. Babkin: Histamine and pilocarpin in relation to the gastric secretion. Amer. J. Physiol. **97**, 69—73 (1931).
Weiss, S., G. P. Robb and H. L. Blumgart: The velocity of blood flow in health and disease as measured by the effect of histamine on the minute vessels. Amer. Heart. J. **4**, 664—691 (1929).
Yonkman, F. F., Dorothy Chess, D. Mathieson and N. Hansen: Pharmacodynamic studies of a new antihistamine agent, N'-pyridyl-N'-benzyl-N-dimethylethylene diamine HCl, pyribenzamine HCl. J. Pharmacol. exp. Ther. **87**, 256—264 (1946).
— B. Rennick and H. L. Schwerma: Pharmacologic studies of a new vasoconstrictor: 2-naphthyl-(1')-methyl-imidazoline hydrochloride (privine or naphazoline). J. Pharmacol. exp. Ther. **84**, 197—202 (1945).

Section G

Effect of Histamine on Gastric Secretion

By

A. C. Ivy and W. H. Bachrach

With 6 Figures

I. Introduction

The powerful effect of histamine as a stimulant of gastric secretion was discovered by Popielski and by Keeton, Luckhardt and Koch in 1919—1920 in experiments on dogs. A similar action in humans was demonstrated (Carnot et al., 1922) soon thereafter, and it was subsequently shown that histamine stimulates gastric secretion in all species adequately tested, including the groundhog (Marmota monax) (Friedman and Armour, 1936), the rhesus monkey (Schnedorf and Ivy, 1937), the pigeon (Friedman, 1939; Ojha, 1960), the chicken (Friedman, 1939), the cat (Bjorkman et al., 1943), the mouse (Davenport and Chavre, 1950), the tortoise (testudo graeca) (Wright and Trethewie, 1956), the lizard (teliqua nigrolutea and tachysaurus rugosus) (Davenport and Chavre, 1950), the rat (Kyle and Welbourn, 1956; Lane, 1957), the guinea pig (Marks, 1957), and the wild boar (sus scrofa) (Gill et al., 1960).

II. Route of administration

Popielski (1920) and Keeton et al. (1920) elicited the histamine response in dogs after subcutaneous, but not after oral or intravenous administration; Rothlin and Gundlach (1921—1922) reported the same experience. Later investigations proved however, that with proper dosage, a secretory response to histamine could be obtained by both the oral (Ivy et al., 1923) and intravenous (Gutkowski, 1924; Ivy and Javois, 1924—1925) as well as by the subcutaneous routes.

III. Characteristics of the secretory response

A. Hydrochloric acid

The most extensively studied aspect of the gastric secretory response to histamine is the secretion of HCl.

Histamine is an extremely potent stimulus to the acid-forming cell. Popielski (1920) noted acid concentrations in the dog as high as 166 "units". Assuming a "unit" to be equal to one milliequivalent per liter, the observed acidity was at or close to the peak capacity of the parietal cell.

Following an average dose (of the order of 0.5 mg of histamine base) subcutaneously in the human, the volume and acidity of the gastric juice begins to rise above the basal level after a latent period of up to 15 min, averaging about 7 min, followed by a rapid climb in volume to a level of 3 or 4 times the basal, usually within the first half hour. The secretion returns to the basal level in the next 30 to 60 min, the total duration of the response usually amounting to about an hour[1].

The rise in acid concentration is somewhat more gradual than that of the volume, and the duration of response somewhat longer, so that the curve of total acid output shows a slower downslope relative to the volume. A typical curve illustrating the gastric secretory response, taken from the work of Lim et al. (1923), is shown in Fig. 1.

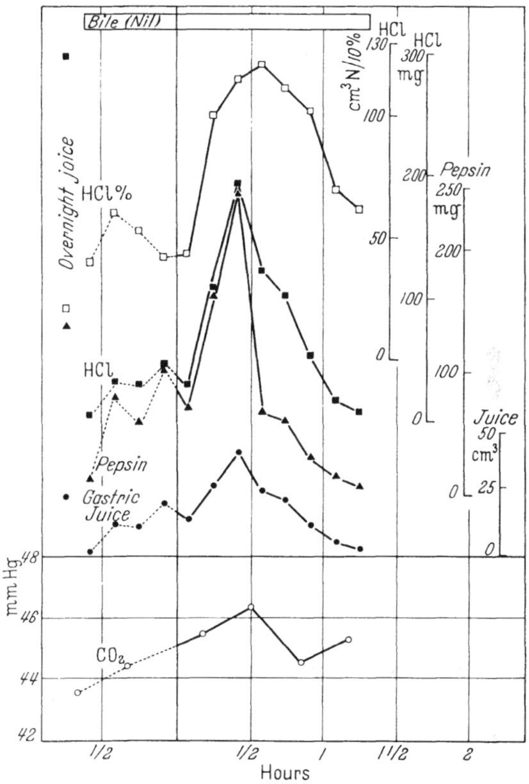

Fig. 1. Gastric and alveolar CO_2 analyses. Histamine was injected at the time indicated by the vertical line. Subject L. T. (Lim et al., 1923)

1. Dose-response relationship of acid secretion to histamine

a) Oral route

Ivy et al. (1923) and Ivy and Javois (1924–1925) found in the dog, that 50 mg of histamine dihydrochloride orally, was approximately a threshold dose, while 150mg provoked a secretion equivalent to that following a meat meal. In the human, 200 mg of the dihydrochloride orally produced a definite secretion without side effects. It has been reported recently (Chirico and Falchi, 1960) that oral administration of histamine hydrochloride in dose of 1.5 mg caused an increased acidity in most of the human subjects tested, but the data are inadequate to support this conclusion. (For further information see p. 831 and 845, Chapter 5, Section B, this volume).

b) Subcutaneous route

α) Rat. Komarov et al. (1944) had difficulty demonstrating a secretory effect even with "very large doses" (exceeding 0.9 mg of histamine dihydrochloride/100 g/bd. wt.) and Friedman (1953) concluded that histamine had little, if any, effect in the rat because doses of 3.5 to 5.5 mg/kg were required to obtain a measurable increase in acidity. Kyle and Welbourn (1956) obtained a 50% increase in the volume and hydrogen ion concentration of the gastric contents in pylorus-ligated rats with doses of 9 to 18 mg of histamine/kg/bd. wt. No toxicity was observed with these doses. The range of variation in the results reported may be appreciated further from the data of Roe and Dyer (1939) and Dyer and Roe (1941) on the one hand, in whose work 0.24 mg histamine disphosphate/kg/bd. wt. over a 2 hr period yielded an increase of acidity but not of volume, and those of Bovet and Walthert (1944), who obtained a 50-fold increase in volume during a

[1] In man after removing the gastric residuum of the fasting stomach, the aspiration should be either continuous or conducted every 10 min as a control for 30 min before injecting histamine. In the dog two 30 min control periods should precede the injection.

1.5-hr period after an injection of 50 mg/kg. In view of these marked discrepancies and the differences in experimental design which appeared responsible for them, LANE (1957) and LANE et al. (1957) undertook an investigation of the dose-response relationship to histamine in chronic gastric fistula rats. Preliminary observations indicated a threshold dose of 0.1 mg histamine disphosphate in a 350 g rat, or 0.0363 mg of the base every 10 min, or 3.63 µg/rat/min subcutaneously. On a kilogram basis, the threshold dose is 10.37 µg/kg/min. With progressively increasing doses, the percentage increase in output of HCl in milligrams for the hour after histamine, as compared with the hour before, varied with the dose as follows (Fig. 2): 0.25 mg, 63%; 0.5 mg, 94%; 1.0 mg, 171%; 2.0 mg, 233%; 3.0 mg, 220%; 4 mg, 136%. Toxic effects become evident when the 2.0 mg dose is exceeded. It is of interest that the total dose for consistent stimulation in the rat is the same as for the human, the dog and the cat.

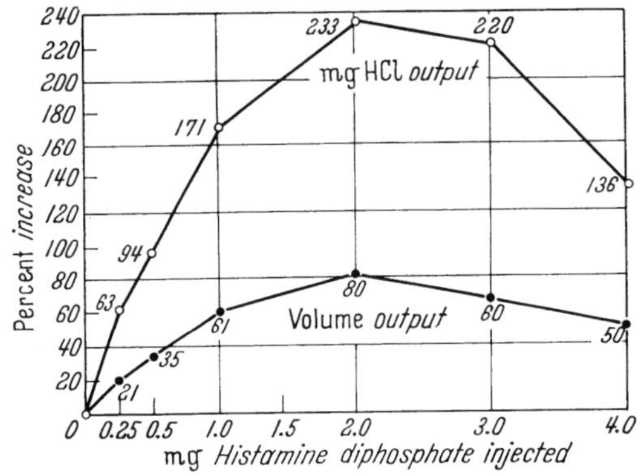

Fig. 2. Average response of 7 chronic gastric fistula rats to various doses of histamine diphosphate, a dose above 2 mg subcutaneously being "toxic". Percentage represents the increment over the control divided by the control. (LANE and IVY, 1957)

β) **Dog.** The first dose-response data were those of POPIELSKI (1920). With a dose of 32 mg (of the hydrochloride), acid secretion started in 10 min, reached a volume peak in 45–60 min and an acidity peak (166 mEq/l) in 3 hrs, returning to the basal level after 5 hrs and 45 min; the total volume was 938 ml. With 3.2 mg the secretion

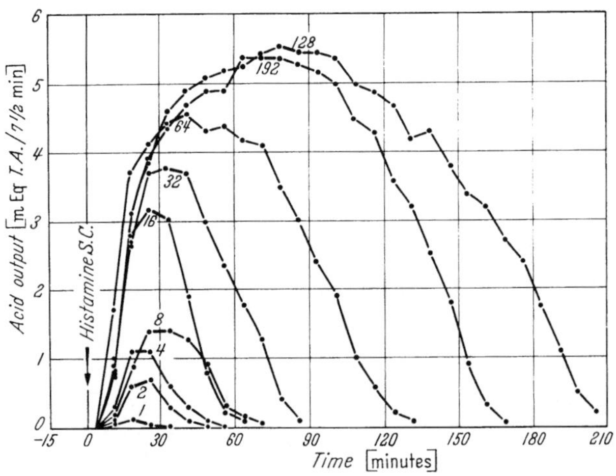

Fig. 3. Acid secretory responses to graded doses of histamine administered subcutaneously (*dog 5*). *Heavy line* in each curve connects the two $7^1/_2$ min outputs used in calculating the 15-min plateau rate of acid output; the corresponding numeral is the dose in arbitrary units (1 U = 1.85 µg/kg s.c.). (MARKS et al., 1958)

lasted 2 hrs and 15 min with an acidity reaching 164 mEq/l and a volume half that of the preceding dose. 0.32 mg evoked a secretion lasting 45 min and yielding some 90 ml; the acidity was not stated.

In both intact dogs and in vagotomized total-stomach-pouch dogs receiving histamine subcutaneously every 10 min, HANSON et al. (1948) found the average minimal effective dose to be 0.03 μg/kg/min and the maximal effective dose 0.75 μg/kg/min. At the maximal dose the average output of HCl was 11.6 mEq/hr in the pouch dogs and 9.8 mEq/hr in the intact animals. Employing the same dose schedule in anesthetized dogs, MARKS et al. (1958) reported a minimal effective dose of something less than 0.04 μg/kg/min and an average maximal effective dose of 1.9 μg/kg/min; at this dose the average output of HCl was 17.3 mEq/hr. In further experiments, MARKS and his associates (1960) examined the dose-response relationships of *single* subcutaneous doses in gastric-fistula dogs. In the one dog in which it was studied in greater detail, the minimal effective dose was 1.8 μg/kg. In this animal, the response to graded doses illustrates (Fig. 3) the progressive increase in both intensity and duration of secretory response with increasing doses.

γ) Human. Starting with 0.01 mg/kg as a "body-weight dose", KAY (1953) was able to determine the dose-response relationship of successive multiples of this dose by pre-treating the subjects with correspondingly increasing amounts of an antihistamine preparation. He found that the HCl output increased in response to increasing amounts of histamine up to 4 body-weight doses (i. e., 0.04 mg/kg in a single subcutaneous injection), with no significant increase above that amount, up to 12 body-weight doses (Fig. 4).

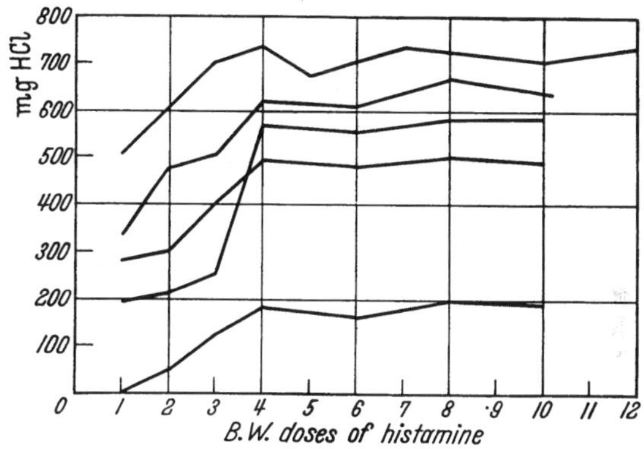

Fig. 4. Dose-response curves in five normal subjects. (KAY, 1953)

The "inhibitory" effect of a supraoptimal dose of histamine occurs in the rat, dog and human.

c) Intravenous route

α) Cat. According to WOOD (1948) the infusion of 2 to 3 μg of histamine per kilo per minute causes a submaximal secretion in most cats. In cats under chloralose anesthesia, 15 mg histamine per minute produced between 1 and 4 ml of gastric secretion per minute (THOMPSON and VANE, 1953). IVY (1958) found the threshold dose in anesthetized cats to range from 0.005 to 0.01 μg/kg/min, the average was 0.015 when given over a period of 20 min.

β) Dog. IVY and JAVOIS (1924/1925) showed that histamine was effective when given intravenously, provided the dose was properly adjusted. A decided secretory response, without peripheral vasodilatation, occurred in a Pavlov pouch dog on intravenous infusion of histamine dihydrochloride at a rate of 1 μg/kg/min. EMMELIN et al. (1941) were able to observe a secretory response with 0.5 μg/kg/min, while a dose one-tenth that amount produced a secretory response in the hands of ÖBRINK (1946), who found that the maximal effective dose was of the order of 1.7 μg/kg/min. A dose-response curve derived from these and the intervening values led ÖBRINK to conclude that there was no threshold dose of histamine.

HANSON et al. (1948) thoroughly investigated this problem in a series of dogs with and without the vagi sectioned. In both groups the average minimal effective dose of histamine base was 0.045 μg/kg/min. The average maximal effective dose was, paradoxically, higher for the intact dogs (2.6 μg/kg/min) than for the pouch dogs (1.3 μg/kg/min). The average maximal output of HCl was 12 mEq/hr for both groups. Among 4 dogs, MARKS et al. (1960) observed a maximal effective dose of 2.4 μg/kg/min in two, and 1.6 μg/kg/min in two. The maximal output of HCl in mEq/15 min varied from 5.4 in a dog weighing 9.1 kg to 10.8 in one weighing 28.2 kg.

γ) Human. PETERS and HORTON (1940) observed a significant secretion of HCl on infusion of histamine in a dilution of 1 to 250,000 at a rate of 0.7 to 2 cc/min, which, for a 70 kg subject would be 0.04 to 0.12 μg/kg/min. McELIN and HORTON (1946) obtained a rise in gastric acidity in one subject with an approximate dose of 0.03 μg/kg/min.

HANSON et al. (1948) obtained an average of 0.004 μg/kg/min for the minimal effective dose with a range of 0.001 to 0.016 μg. No consistent correlation was observed between the secretory threshold and side reactions such as flushing, headache and in skin temperature. (It should be kept in mind that swallowing and keeping a tube in the stomach causes flushing, sweating and a headache in some human subjects; also fasting alone.) The maximal effective dose was not established; gastric secretion was still increasing in one subject at a level of 0.18 μg/kg/min and in another subject the maximal secretion may have been reached at a dose of 0.33 μg/kg/min, where the HCl output was 34 mEq/hr.

NORDGREN (1958) reported maximal secretion with a dose of 20 μg/kg/hr, which approximates 0.33 μg/kg/min. The findings of ADAM et al. (1954a, b) agree with those of HANSON et al. (1948) in that they found threshold rates in 3 healthy subjects of 0.004, 0.009 and 0.013 μg/kg/min, respectively; they were able to relate the dose to the response up to doses of 0.117, 0.114 and 0.094 μg/kg/min in the respective subjects. Their observations indicated that the subjective effects of histamine infusions up to a rate of 0.03 μg/kg/min were indistinguishable from those of the control saline solution.

2. Duration of the acid secretory response to continued histamine stimulation

Numerous data are available to indicate that the acid production stimulated by histamine continues unabated as long as the stimulus continues to be applied, provided toxicity and dehydration are avoided. For example, CODE and VARCO (1942) incorporated doses of 15 to 50 mg of histamine in beeswax to provide for slow absorption from subcutaneous depots. In dogs receiving such injections, the secretion of gastric juice began during the first 15 min, reached its maximum during the first 10 hrs and continued for 24 or more hours at an acid concentration of approximately 150 mEq/l.

AMBRUS and his co-workers (1951a, b, 1953) claim to have demonstrated a progressive decrease in both the histamine response and the interdigestive secretion, in rats and guinea pigs treated with increasing doses of histamine. They attribute the effect to either a "desensitization" or to an exhaustion of the parietal cells. WELLS et al. (1941) found that tachyphylaxis and desensitization, as measured by the gastric secretory response, could not be produced in dogs. In these animals, and in rats (LANE et al., 1957) the histamine response persists as long as nutrition and hydration are preserved. However, IVY and JAVOIS (1924—1925) and others have remarked, but not established, that after repeated stimulation of a pouch with histamine it may be more refractory to other stimuli.

3. Reproducibility of the acid response

NYMAN (1943) used the double tube technique to determine the 60-minute gastric secretory response to a subcutaneous injection of 0.1 mg/10 kg body weight, in each of 8 human subjects on two occasions 24 to 48 hrs apart. He reported a difference of less than 5% between values for the two tests, in most cases not exceeding 10% in any subject. These figures are for the volume; no values are given for the concentration of HCl. MARKS (personal communication) finds a close correspondence in the maximal acid output, as obtained by the "augmented histamine" test of KAY (1953) (see Appendix) in repeated tests on the same individuals. However, the experience of most observers coincides with that reported (to select a couple of examples from a literature too extensive to cite in detail) by ENGELBACH and BROWN, in 1933, and by PALMER et al., in 1940, who found decided unexplained variations in both the volume and acid response to histamine in the same individuals on different days. We have observed this to be true in the rat, dog, monkey and man[1]. In dogs the response from day to day in the same dog may vary as much as ± 25%. Some dogs will vary no more than ± 10%. (See Appendix.)

4. Relation of acid output to number of parietal cells

RAGINS et al. (1957) and MARKS and his associates (1958, 1960) and CARD and MARKS (1960) have supplied experimental support for the reasonable assumption, that the amount of acid formation resulting from the administration of the maximal effective dose of histamine, is a function of the amount of acid-secreting tissue, or "parietal cell mass". The only challenge to this idea to be found in the literature is that of GREGORY (1958) who found that, after a portocaval shunt in denervated gastric pouch dogs, the maximal secretory response to histamine was more than doubled. It must be kept in mind, however, that the pouch was denervated; perhaps its blood flow was increased by the operation.

B. Pepsin

α) Human. Without exception every report of experiments in the human shows that histamine increases the output but not necessarily the concentration of gastric pepsin[2] (CARNOT et al., 1922; LIM et al., 1923; MATHESON and AMMON, 1923; RACHON and WALAWSKI, 1928; POLLAND and BLOOMFIELD, 1929; AUSTIN and GAMMON, 1931; POLLAND, 1932; HELMER et al., 1932; MEIENBERG and BROWN, 1933; BLAKELY and WILKINSON, 1933; BLOOMFIELD and POLLAND, 1933; OSTERBERG et al., 1937; RIVERS and VAN ZANT, 1937–1938; TOBY, 1937a, b; CARNOT, 1939; LEHMANN et al., 1946; ASHFORD et al., 1949; HUNT, 1950; MERTEN and FETSCHER, 1956; FRIEDMAN et al., 1957; HIRSCHOWITZ et al., 1959; PIPER, 1960). Nevertheless, for many years a difference in the interpretation of methods and results has existed on whether histamine actually stimulates pepsin secretion; and some responsible investigators are certain that it does not. For example, MARKS et al. (1960), in their work on maximal acid response to histamine in the dog, defined a true histamine response "as one in which the *pepsin concentration*, at the height of a secretory response, fell to a level not measurable with the Mett method." He illustrated the results of an experiment in which the highest level of acid secretion, occurring in the 90 to 120 min period after the subcutaneous injection of a large dose of histamine,"was not considered to be due to the histamine alone since it was associated with an increase in pepsin secretion."

The basic question is: Does the evidence justify this conviction that pepsin secretion is not evoked by histamine in the dog?

[1] When making a study of the effect of some procedure on the response of an animal's or man's stomach to histamine, at least 10 tests on each individual should be done and the significance of the difference between two means should be mathematically determined. In the case of dogs, we now select them for an experiment on the basis of their consistency in response to histamine or a test-meal.

[2] Uropepsin excretion is not increased after histamine, according to FLORKIEWICZ (1960).

β) Dog. In 1921/1922, ROTHLIN and GUNDLACH, apparently the first to study the pepsin response to histamine in dogs, found that the enzyme secretion was not significantly augmented; but in view of our present knowledge they came to the paradoxical conclusion that histamine has a parasympathomimetic effect on the stomach. LIM and LIU, in 1926, reported that the canine stomach continued to secrete both acid and pepsin for as long as histamine was administered. There followed a series of reports[1] from BABKIN's laboratory, showing that during histamine stimulation the *pepsin concentration* of the gastric juice first rises, then falls until, at the height of the acid response, the pepsin content of the secretion is reduced to, or near, zero. The conclusion of these investigators was that the initial increase in pepsin concentration represents a washing out of preformed pepsin by the acid secretion, and that histamine stimulates the chief cells little, if at all. It was also reported (ALLEY, 1935) that histamine inhibits the secretion of pepsin. Histological examination of the gastric mucosa, (BOWIE and VINEBERG, 1935) after repeated subcutaneous administration of histamine, showed no diminution in the pepsinogen granules in the chief cells, as occurs after vagal stimulation. The histamine juice was contrasted with the secretion in response to pilocarpine, which was decidedly concentrated in enzymes, a fact with which every investigator agrees.

Failure of histamine to stimulate pepsin secretion in dogs was reported also by GILMAN and COWGILL (1931) and by LINDE (1950). GOODMAN (1938), on the other hand, interpreted the results of his single and double histamine experiments as showing that histamine definitely stimulated pepsin secretion.

In attempting to evaluate the foregoing evidence, BUCHER and IVY (1941), BUCHER et al. (1941) and BUCHER (1949) formed the opinion that the disagreement was the result of inadequacies in the experimental design. In their experiments, histamine appeared to stimulate pepsin secretion (BUCHER and IVY, 1941) and continued to do so over long periods of time and after high doses of histamine (BUCHER et al., 1941). They could not attribute the sustained output of pepsin, though low in concentration and total output, to a washing out process, and they could not find any evidence that histamine in "non-toxic" amounts inhibited the secretion of pepsin. ABRAMS and BROOKS (1960) and PIPER (1960) also observed a continued output of pepsin, though low in concentration and total output, in histamine stimulated canine gastric juice. Using the plasma pepsinogen as an index of gastric pepsin secretion, KOWALEWSKI and his associates (1955/1956) reported an increase following histamine administration.

γ) Cat. The finding of BJORKMAN et al. (1943) that histamine does not stimulate the secretion of pepsin in the cat was not confirmed by BUCHER (1949).

δ) Rat. The zymogen content of peptic cells was gradually depleted by daily subcutaneous injection of histamine (CAMBEL and SGOURIS, 1952), and a histamine-liberator evoked increased plasma pepsinogen (KOWALEWSKI, 1960) in rats.

ε) Other species. KOWALEWSKI (1954,1 957) observed an increase in gastric pepsin, and in plasma and urine pepsinogen in guinea pigs receiving large doses of histamine. Pepsin secretion appeared to be stimulated by histamine in the chicken but not in the pigeon (FRIEDMAN, 1939) or the groundhog (FRIEDMAN and ARMOUR, 1936).

C. Mucus

In the experiments of KOMAROV et al. (1949), histamine did not increase, and in large doses appeared to depress, the secretion of mucus in dogs. KOWALEWSKI

[1] BABKIN, 1930; WEBSTER, 1931; VINEBERG and BABKIN, 1931; BOWIE and VINEBERG, 1935; ALLEY, 1935; TOBY, 1936.

and SILBERMANN (1958) and KOWALEWSKI and WILLIAMS (1958) interpreted the rate of uptake of labelled sulfate by the gastric mucosa as an index of mucus formation, and with this technique obtained evidence suggesting mucus stimulation by histamine in dogs (KOWALEWSKI and SILBERMANN, 1958), and guinea pigs (KOWALEWSKI and WILLIAMS, 1958). BANCHE et al. (1955) reported an increased secretion of mucoprotein in the human. This matter obviously requires further investigation.

IV. Histamine tests of gastric secretory function

A. Single histamine test

The method of performing the single histamine test on a human subject is illustrated in Figure 1. The same design is generally used in animals. The dose of histamine is generally 0.1 mg/10 kg bd. wt. (B. W. dose) of histamine acid phosphate or histamine dihydrochloride. When 0.1 mg of the phosphate is used, only 0.033 mg of the base is being given; when 0.1 mg of the dihydrochloride is used, then 0.066 mg of the base is being used (RIVERS and VAN ZANT, 1937/1938).

B. The double histamine test

This consists in emptying the stomach of its 12-hour fasting residuum and withdrawing out the contents every 10 min during a period of 30 min as a control, and then injecting the standard dose of histamine decided on (generally 0.1 mg base/10 kg of body weight) and withdrawing the gastric contents every 10 min for 1.5 or 2.0 hrs, and then repeating the injection of histamine (WELLS et al., 1941; RIVERS and VAN ZANT, 1937/1938).

C. The augmented histamine test

The results of this test provide two items of information, namely, the "Basal Secretion in mEq or mg of HCl" and an expression of the maximal parietal cell activity. The test is performed as follows (KAY, 1953):

1. The test is preceded by a 12 hr fast.

2. A No. 9 stomach tube is introduced into the stomach and the fasting juice aspirated by means of a 50 ml syringe. It is essential to alter the position both of the tube and of the patient until the tip of the tube reaches the most dependent part of the stomach and permits aspiration of the residual pool of fluid. This position of the tube is now maintained by fixing it to the side of the face and by insisting that the patient does not alter his position until completion of the test. This will usually mean that he will lie comfortably on his left side.

3. The spontaneously secreted gastric juice is now collected for a period of 45 min and the basal secretion expressed in milligrams of HCl produced in this time interval.

4. 4 ml of mepyramine is now given by intramuscular injection.

5. The gastric juice is aspirated for the next 30 min and is discarded.

6. A subcutaneous injection of 0.1 mg/10 kg of body weight of histamine acid phosphate is now made.

7. The histamine-provoked secretion is continuously aspirated and the volume secreted in the half-hour from 15–45 min after injection is measured and its titratable free HCl estimated. The weight of HCl produced in this 30-minute period is the figure expressing the maximum parietal cell response.

This test of gastric secretion has certain advantages over other gastric-function tests. It is simple to do and lasts only two hours. The systemic effects following the administration of a large dose of histamine are prevented and the main subjective sensation is the drowsiness due to the antihistamine.

The pharmacology or toxicology of histamine in peptic ulcer production will not be considered here (Ivy et al., 1951).

References

Abrams, R., and F. P. Brooks: Intravenous histamine and gastric pepsin in the unanesthetized dog. Proc. Soc. exp. Biol. (N. Y.) **104**, 278 (1960).

Adam, H. M., W. I. Card, M. J. Riddell, M. Roberts and J. A. Strong: The effect of intravenous infusions of histamine on the urinary histamine and on gastric secretion in man. Brit. J. Pharmacol. **9**, 62 (1954a).

— — — — — and B. Woolf: Dose-response curves for the effect of histamine on acid gastric secretion in man. Brit. J. Pharmacol. **9**, 329 (1954b).

Alley, A.: The inhibitory effect of histamine on gastric secretion. Amer. J. dig. Dis. **1**, 787 (1935).

Ambrus, J. L., C. M. Ambrus and J. W. E. Harrison: Effect of histamine desensitization on histamine induced gastric secretion on guinea pigs. Gastroenterology **18**, 249 (1951a).

— — — Gastric acid secretion and gastric ulcer formation of rats and guinea pigs. Amer. J. Physiol. **173**, 95 (1953).

Ambrus, J., C. Ambrus et J. Jacob: Contribution à l'étude de la désensibilisation histaminique chez le rat et chez le cobaye. Arch. int. Pharmacodyn. **86**, 350 (1951b).

Ashford, C. A., H. Heller and G. A. Smart: Effect of antihistamine substances on gastric secretion in man. Brit. J. Pharmacol. **4**, 157 (1949).

Austin, J. H., and G. D. Gammon: Gastric secretion after histamine: Sodium and potassium content and pepsin estimation. J. clin. Invest **10**, 287 (1931).

Babkin, B. P.: The value of histamine as a test of gastric secretion from a physiological point of view. Canad. med. Ass. J. **23**, 268 (1930).

Banche, M., E. Fama e F. Presti: Ricerche comparative sulla secrezione gastrica parietale e non parietale; raffronto fra secrezione parietale e secrezione mucoproteinica dopo stimulo meccanico da sondino e istaminico. Minerva gastroent. **1**, 21 (1955).

Bjorkman, G., A. Norden and B. Uvnäs: Histamine and peptic secretion. Acta physiol. scand. **6**, 108 (1943).

Blakely, A. P. L., and J. F. Wilkinson: The influence of histamine and pilocarpine on the human gastric secretion. Brit. J. exp. Path. **14**, 349 (1933).

Bloomfield, A. L., and W. S. Polland: Gastric Anacidity; Its Relation to Disease. New York: MacMillan Co. 1933.

Bovet, D., et F. Walthert: Structure chimique et activité pharmacodynamique des anti-histaminiques de synthèse. Ann. pharm. franç. Suppl. 2, No. 4, Sept.-Dec. (1944).

Bowie, D. J., and A. W. Vineberg: The selective action of histamine and the effect of prolonged vagal stimulation on the cells of gastric glands in the dog. Quart. J. exp. Physiol. **25**, 247 (1935).

Bucher, G. R.: Further studies on the pepsin content of histamine stimulated gastric juice. Fed. Proc. **8**, 18 (1949).

—, and A. C. Ivy: The inherent inadequacies of the double histamine test for studies on pepsin secretion. Amer. J. Physiol. **132**, 654 (1941).

— — and J. S. Gray: Is histamine able to maintain an augmented pepsin response comparable to that of pilocarpine? Amer. J. Physiol. **132**, 698 (1941).

Cambel, P., and J. T. Sgouris: Pathologic changes in the gastric mucosa of the rat after histamine administration. Amer. J. Path. **28**, 1079 (1952).

Card, W. I., and I. N. Marks: The relationship between the acid output of the stomach following maximal histamine stimulation and the parietal cell mass. Clin. Sci. **19**, 147 (1960).

Carnot, P.: Sur trois tests de la sécrétion gastrique (test du repas fictif; test de l'alcool; test de l'histamine). Monde méd. **49**, 713 (1939).

— W. Koskowski et E. Libert: Action de l'histamine sur les sucs digestifs chez l'homme. C. R. Soc. Biol. (Paris) **86**, 670 (1922).

Chirico, G., and F. Falchi: Therapeutic importance of the gastro-secretory effect of small doses of orally administered histamine. Arch. Sci. med. **110**, 215 (1960).

Code, C. F., and R. L. Varco: Prolonged action of histamine. Amer. J. Physiol. **137**, 225 (1942).

Davenport, H. W., and V. J. Chavre: Conditions affecting acid secretion by mouse stomachs *in vitro*. Gastroenterology **15**, 467 (1950).

Dyer, H. M., and J. H. Roe: The relation of nutrition to gastric function. III. The effect of vitamin B_1 deficiency. Amer. J. dig. Dis. **8**, 329 (1941).

Emmelin, N., G. Kahlson and F. Wicksell: Histamine in plasma and methods of its estimation. Acta physiol. scand. **2**, 123 (1941).

ENGELBACH, F., and C. L. BROWN: Variations in the volume and in the acid content of gastric secretion of normal individuals following stimulation by histamine. Ann. intern. Med. **6**, 1560 (1933).

FLORKIEWICZ, H.: Effect of histamine on the uropepsin level. Pol. Tyg. lek. **15**, 1713 (1960).

FRIEDMAN, M. H. F.: Gastric secretion in birds. J. cell. comp. Physiol. **13**, 219 (1939).

— Histamine ineffective in the rat as a gastric secretory stimulant. Proc. Soc. exp. Biol. (N. Y.) **54**, 42 (1953).

—, and J. D. ARMOUR: Gastric secretion in the groundhog (Marmota Monax) during hibernation. J. cell. comp. Physiol. 8, 201 (1936).

FRIEDMAN, E., I. POLINER and H. M. SPIRO: Effect of histamine on gastric peptic secretion in man. New Engl. J. Med. **257**, 901 (1957).

GILL, J. H., H. HOFFMANNOVWA and R. PIEKARZ: Wplyw Histaminy Na Przebieg Procesow Trawienno-Wydzielniczych Wzolad ku Dzik (Sus Scrofica L.). Digestive capacity of the salivary glands, pancreas and duodenum and the size of the digestive system in boars (Sus scrofica L.). Acta physiol. pol. **11**, 707 (1960).

GILMAN, A., and G. R. COWGILL: The effect of histamine upon the secretion of gastric pepsin. Amer. J. Physiol. **97**, 124 (1931).

GOODMAN, L. S.: Peptagogic action of choline esters, pilocarpine, histamine, food and alcohol on canine isolated gastric pouches. J. Pharmacol. exp. Ther. **63**, 11 (1938).

GREGORY, R. A.: Gastric secretory responses after portal venous ligation. J. Physiol. (Lond.) **144**, 123 (1958).

GUTOWSKI, B.: Sécrétion du suc gastrique sous l'influence de l'histamine introduite directement dans la circulation du sang. C. R. Soc. Biol. (Paris) **91**, 1346 (1924).

HANSON, M. E., M. I. GROSSMAN and A. C. IVY: Histamine and gastric secretion. Amer. J. Physiol. **153**, 242 (1948).

HELMER, O. M., P. J. FOUTS and L. G. ZERFAS: Gastrointestinal studies. I. Gastric juice in pernicious anemia. J. clin. Invest **11**, 1129 (1932).

HIRSCHOWITZ, B. I., J. L. LONDON and H. M. POLLARD: Histamine stimulation of gastric pepsin secretion in man. Gastroenterology **32**, 85 (1959).

HUNT, J. N.: An interpretation of the histamine test of gastric secretion. Gastroenterology **16**, 231 (1950).

IVY, A. C.: Proof that histamine is a gastric secretory hormone. Proceedings of the World Congress of Gastroenterology, p. 102, 1958.

— W. H. BACHRACH and M. I. GROSSMAN: "Peptic Ulcer". Philadelphia: Blakiston & Co. 1951.

—, and A. J. JAVOIS: Contributions to the physiology of gastric secretion. VI. The stimulation of gastric secretion by amines and other substances. Amer. J. Physiol. **71**, 604 (1924—1925).

—, and K. W. LIEPINS: Effect of 1,2,4-triazole ethylamine on gastric secretion. Amer. J. Physiol. **198**, 614 (1960).

— T. M. LIN, E. K. IVY and E. KARVINEN: Effect of histaminase inhibitors on gastric secretion. Amer. J. Physiol. **186**, 239 (1956).

— — and G. LANGBERG: Gastric secretory response to various amounts of food. Amer. J. Physiol. **188**, 71 (1957).

— G. B. MCILVAIN and A. J. JAVOIS: The stimulation of gastric secretion by histamine. Science 58, 286 (1923).

KAY, A. W.: Effect of large doses of histamine on gastric secretion of HCl. An augmented histamine test. Brit. med. J. **2**, 77 (1953).

KEETON, R. W., A. B. LUCKHARDT and F. C. KOCH: Gastrin studies. III. The response of the stomach mucosa of various animals to gastrin bodies. Amer. J. Physiol. **51**, 454 (1920). Gastrin studies: IV. The response of the stomach mucosa to food and gastrin bodies as influenced by atropin. Amer. J. Physiol. **51**, 469 (1920).

KOMAROV, S. A., H. SHAY, M. REYPORT and S. S. FELS: Some observations on gastric secretion in normal rats. Gastroenterology **3**, 406 (1944).

— — and H. SIPLET: Secretion of gastric mucin in response to sham-feeding and histamine stimulation. Amer. J. Physiol. **158**, 194 (1949).

KOWALEWSKI, K.: Uropepsin and plasma pepsinogen after injection of histamine dihydrochloride in doses provoking acute gastric ulcers in guinea pigs. Canad. J. Biochem. **32**, 553 (1954).

— Effect of histamine on gastric pepsinogen, pepsin secretion, and blood pepsinogen in guinea pigs. Canad. J. Biochem. **35**, 729 (1957).

— Effect of compound 48/80 on plasma pepsinogen in rats. Surg. Forum **11**, 345 (1960).

— H. A. HYDE and S. T. NORVELL JR.: Effect of ACTH and histamine on plasma pepsinogen in normal, hypophysectomized, thyroidectomized and adrenalectomized dogs. Surg. Forum **6**, 316 (1955).

— S. T. NORVELL JR. and W. C. MCKENZIE: The gastric endocrine and exocrine response to histamine in dogs and effect of passage of blood through the gastric and hepatic vessels on its pepsinogen content. Canad. J. Biochem. **34**, 244 (1956).

Kowalewski, K., and O. Silbermann: Effect of histamine on the excretion of radiosulphur by the gastric pouch in dogs. Arch. int. Pharmacodyn. **117**, 197 (1958).

—, and H. T. G. Williams: Observations on the uptake of radiosulphate by the gastric tissue and gastric secretion in histamine-treated guinea pigs. Canad. J. Biochem. **36**, 847 (1958).

Kyle, J., and R. B. Welbourn: The effect of histamine on gastric secretion and ulceration in the pylorus-ligated rat. Gastroenterology **30**, 593 (1956).

Lane, Ardelle: The dose-response relationship to histamine in the chronic gastric fistula rat. Fed. Proc. **16**, 77 (1957).

Lane, A., A. C. Ivy and E. K. Ivy: Response of the chronic gastric fistula rat to histamine. Amer. J. Physiol. **190**, 221 (1957).

Lehmann, H., F. P. Kayser and J. W. Simpson: Secretion of pepsin in achlorhydric human subjects after injection of histamine. Nature (Lond.) **157**, 194 (1946).

Lim, R. K. S., u. A. C. Liu: Ermüdung der Magensekretion. Pflüger's Arch. ges. Physiol. **211**, 647 (1926).

— A. R. Matheson and W. Schlapp: Observations on the human gastroduodenal secretions with special reference to the action of histamine. Quart. J. exp. Physiol. **13**, 361 (1923).

Linde, S.: Studies on the stimulation mechanism of gastric secretion. Acta physiol. scand. **21**, Supplement 74 (1950).

McElin, T. W., and B. T. Horton: Clinical observations on the use of Benadryl: Its effect on histamine induced gastric acidity in man. Gastroenterology **7**, 100 (1946).

Marks, I. N.: Personal communication.

— The effect of prolonged histamine stimulation on the parietal cell population and the secretory function of the guinea-pig stomach. Quart. J. exp. Physiol. **42**, 180 (1957).

— S. A. Komarov and H. Shay: Acid secretory responses to histamine and the parietal cell mass in the dog. Amer. J. Physiol. **195**, 528 (1958).

— — — Maximal acid secretory response to histamine and its relation to parietal cell mass in the dog. Amer. J. Physiol. **199**, 579 (1960).

Matheson, A. R., and S. E. Ammon: Observations on the effect of histamine on the human gastric secretion. Lancet **1923I**, 482.

Meienberg, L. J., and C. L. Brown: The effect of pilocarpine on the volume, free and combined-acid, total chlorides and pepsin of gastric secretion; and a comparison with the effects of histamine stimulation. Ann. intern. Med. **7**, 762 (1933).

Merten, R., u. W. Fetscher: Beziehungen zwischen Gesamtausscheidung und Konzentration von freier Salzsäure, Pepsin und Kathepsin in der Basalsekretion, nach Histamin und Insulin. Z. ges. exp. Med. **127**, 133 (1956).

Nordgren, B.: Aspects of gastric acid secretion in man. Acta med. scand. **161**, 221 (1958).

Nyman, E.: On the reproducibility of human gastric secretion after subcutaneous injections of histamine. Acta med. scand. **113**, 416 (1943).

Öbrink, K. J.: Some relations in gastric stimulation by intravenous injection of histamine. Acta physiol. scand. **12**, 213 (1946)

Ojha, K. N.: A new method of studying the effects of drugs on gastric secretory response to histamine in pigeons. Indian J. med. Sci. **14**, 426 (1960).

Osterberg, A. E., F. R. Van Zant, W. C. Alvarez and A. B. Rivers: Studies of pepsin in human gastric juice. III. Physiologic aspects. Amer. J. dig. Dis. **3**, 35 (1937).

Palmer, W. L., J. B. Kirsner and P. B. Nutter: Spontaneous variations in gastric secretion in response to histamine stimulation. Amer. J. dig. Dis. **7**, 427 (1940).

Peters, G. A., and B. T. Horton: The effect of intravenous administration of histamine on gastric acids in man. Proc. Mayo Clin. **15**, 545 (1940).

Piper, D. W.: The effect of histamine on pepsin secretion. Amer. J. dig. Dis. **5**, 880 (1960).

Polland, W. S.: Stimulation of gastric pepsin by histamine. J. clin. Invest. **11**, 449 (1932).

—, and A. L. Bloomfield: Quantitative measurements of pepsin in gastric juice before and after histamine stimulation. J. clin. Invest **7**, 57 (1929).

Popielski, L.: β-Imidazolyläthylamin und die Organextrakte. Erster Teil. β-Imidazolyläthylamin als mächtiger Erreger der Magendrüsen. Pflüger's Arch. ges. Physiol. **178**, 214 (1920).

Rachon, K., et J. Walawski: Influence de l'histamine sur la sécrétion du suc gastrique dans un cas de fistule gastrique permanente. C. R. Soc. Biol. (Paris) **98**, 383 (1928).

Ragins, H., S. O. Evans, L. R. Dragstedt II, S. P. Rigler and L. R. Dragstedt: Quantitative studies on the effect of gastric resection on secretion of gastric juices. Arch. Surg. **74**, 266 (1957).

Rivers, A. B., and F. R. Van Zant: A study of peptic activity by means of the double histamine test. Amer. J. dig. Dis. **4**, 304 (1937—1938).

Roe, J. H., and H. M. Dyer: Relation of nutrition to gastric function. I. An experimental method. Proc. Soc. exp. Biol. (N. Y.) **41**, 603 (1939).

Rothlin, E., et R. Gundlach: Étude experimental de l'influence de l'histamine sur la sécrétion gastrique. Arch. int. Physiol. **17**, 59 (1921—1922).

Schnedorf, J. G., and A. C. Ivy: The incidence and permanence of unexplained gastric anacidity in the rhesus monkey after histamine and mecholyl, with hematologic studies. Amer. J. dig. Dis. **4**, 429 (1937).

Thompson, J. E., and J. R. Vane: Gastric secretion induced by histamine and its relationship to the rate of blood flow. J. Physiol. (Lond.) **121**, 433 (1953).

Toby, C. G.: Effect of different types of stimuli on the composition of the gastric juice. Quart. J. exp. Physiol. **26**, 45 (1936).

— The composition of human gastric juice secreted in response to histamine administration. Amer. J. dig. Dis. **3**, 896 (1937a).

— Does histamine stimulate the secretory activity of the peptic cells in man? Amer. J. dig. Dis. **3**, 902 (1937b).

Vineberg, A. M., and B. P. Babkin: Histamine and pilocarpin in relation to the gastric secretion. Amer. J. Physiol. **97**, 69 (1931).

Webster, D. R.: Changes in composition of gastric juice under different stimuli. Roy. Soc. Can. **25**, (Sec. V) 213 (1931).

Wells, J. A., J. S. Gray and C. A. Dragstedt: An investigation of the question of histamine tolerance. J. Allergy **13**, 77 (1941).

Wood, D. R.: The effect of gastric secretion of different rates of histamine infusion and of "Neoantergan". Brit. J. Pharmacol. **3**, 231 (1948).

Wright, R. D., and E. R. Trethewie: Histamine of the reptilian stomach and lung. Nature (Lond.) **178**, 546 (1956).

Appendix

Some observations regarding methodology

The following information is provided because it pertains to the methodology of the use of dogs with gastric pouches for various pharmacological purposes. This cannot be discussed completely because of the question of space. Original articles should be consulted for various types of experimental designs. Unfortunately the older investigators did qualitative experiments with very few exceptions. Even many – too many – modern investigators do not perform enough tests to render their conclusions quantitative. And, we believe that this fault is the cause of many discrepancies in the literature.

A. "Basal state" is important before applying stimulus

This has been studied by Ivy et al. (1957). By "basal state" is meant that the pouch should be secreting no "free acid" (pH 4.5) to Topfer's reagent. If a dog is fed the daily ration at 3:00 or 4:00 p.m., the pouch, as a rule, will secrete no juice containing free acid 14 to 16 hrs later. This also applies to most human subjects, but there are numerous exceptions which can only be taken care of by statistical reasoning with proper control data.

In Table 1, two Heidenhain pouch and one transplanted pouch (Ivy) dogs were used. They were fed a small meal 4 hrs apart. When the response to the first meal had returned to almost basal but "free acid" was still present in the secretion, the second meal was fed. It will be noted that the average response, in from 9 to 10 tests on each dog, is greater after the second meal. The daily data on Dog 2 are provided to show the variations which occur in output from day to day under ideal conditions of feeding and control.

B. Size of meal

The importance of the size of the meal is indicated in Table 2 and Fig. 5.

Quantitative gastric secretory work is very time consuming. The rate of the work can be speeded by using a small team of dogs every day. It is possible to collect a basal control secretion from 7:00 to 8:00 a.m., feed a meal consisting of the daily ration at 8:00 a.m., and by 6:00 p.m. the response to the meal is practically concluded. This can be done every day. Or, if a drug is to be used in an experiment,

Table 1. *Response to a double test-meal of 100 g of mixed food with 200 cc H_2O given twice 4 hr apart* (Ivy et al. 1957)

Response to first meal		Response to second meal	
Total vol.	Total HCl	Total vol.	Total HCl
cc	mg	cc	mg
Dog 2			
36.3	147.9	30.5	149.0
38.8	159.4	55.0	206.7
32.7	128.8	41.9	161.8
36.9	113.1	38.2	151.0
33.2	130.5	55.5	243.2
34.0	139.8	42.4	176.1
34.7	139.9	43.3	145.6
42.8	170.8	53.5	217.8
46.8	202.1	50.6	211.2
Average response in the three dogs			
Dog 2			
37.5	141.8	48.5	195.3
Dog 1			
32.8	108.6	43.7	144.8
Dog 3			
15.0	20.2	22.1	30.1

Dogs 1 and *2* had a Heidenhain pouch; *dog 3* had a transplanted pouch. Ave. of 9 to 10 tests

Table 2. *Ratio of volume and acid output to meals of various sizes in two Heidenhain pouch (dogs 1 and 2) and in one transplanted pouch (dog 3).* (Ivy et al., 1957)

Size meal, gm	Dog 1 (H)				Dog 2 (H)				Dog 3 (T)			
	Vol. output		Acid output		Vol. output		Acid output		Vol. output		Acid output	
	cc	Ratio vol/ meal, gm	mg	Ratio mg/ meal, gm	cc	Ratio vol/ meal, gm	mg	Ratio mg/ meal, gm	cc	Ratio mg/ meal, gm	mg	Ratio mg/ meal, gm
100	33	0.328	118	1.18	38	0.380	142	1.42	15	0.150	20	0.200
300	146	0.488	609	2.03	100	0.333	422	1.40	60	0.200	240	0.800[1]
400	165	0.410	750	1.87								
450	215	0.433	960	2.10					92	0.204[1]	395	0.877[1]
600	262	0.436	1205	2.01	184	0.306	845	1.41				
900	413	0.460	2037	2.27	114	0.350	1464	1.60	125	0.140	530	0.590
Av. 300 to 900 incl.		0.448		2.06		0.342		1.46				
Conc. of acid, mg/cc, av. 300—900	2.06 / 0.448 = 4.60 mg/cc				1.46 / 0.342 = 4.25 mg/cc				0.839[1] / 0.202[1] = 4.15 mg/cc			

[1] Only the data for the linear part of the sigmoid curve are averaged. The averages represent from 8 to 12 trials on the same dog.

the basal control can be collected from 7:00 to 8:00 or to 9:00 a.m.,and the drug given at 8:00 or 9:00 a.m. The response to a drug usually is over by 3:00 p.m. The daily ration can be fed at 3:00 p.m. In this way a test can be performed on each dog daily. Pouch dogs work much better on a routine daily or 6 times a week schedule. When not used, the feeding routine should be followed. *It is important to guard against coprophagia.*

The quality of the meal is very important, as is well known. Meat or liver in the daily ration is important for a copious response to a meal. Canned food may be used but some dogs tire of such food unless some fresh meat is stirred into the meat or ration.

C. Dose response curve to a standard meal

IVY et al. (1957) determined the dose-response curve in two Heidenhain and one transplanted pouch (IVY) dogs to meals of various sizes. Figure 5 shows the total curve in response to meals. Figure 6 shows the curve of response to sham feeding, the output of HCl being zero, and then the response to small amounts of food.

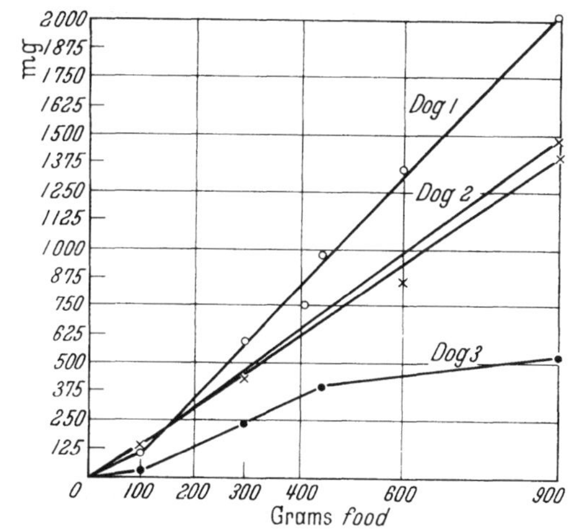

Fig. 5. Average output of HCl in mg secreted in response to meals of different sizes. (IVY et al., 1957)

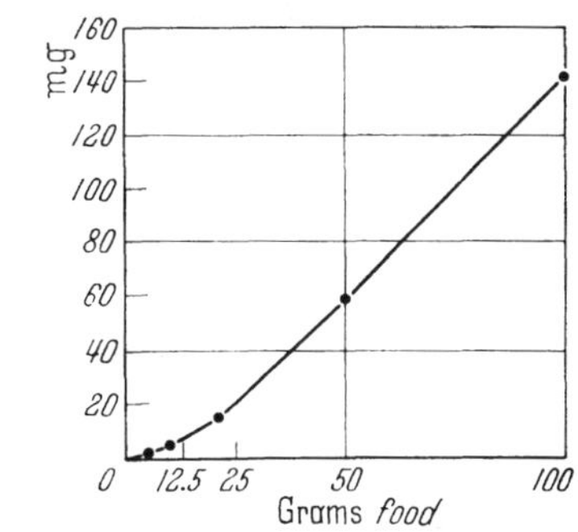

Fig. 6. Output of HCl in mg in a Heidenhain pouch dog when sham fed (0 mg) and then fed 12.5, 25, 50 and 100 mg, of food in 50 cc of water. (IVY et al., 1957)

It should be noted that the secretion of the transplanted pouch dog leveled out after a meal of 400 gm, but that of the two Heidenhain pouch dogs did not. This may be explained by pointing out that the capacity of the transplanted pouch to secrete was reached after the 400 gm meal; whereas this was not true of the large Heidenhain pouches which these two dogs had. The capacity of the two Heidenhain pouches could not be tested because the dogs would not eat more than 900 gm. That is, their appetite was satiated, and the dogs were not fed by stomach tube because being "stuffed" or fed by a tube might inhibit secretion. Therefore, the capacity of their Heidenhain pouch to secrete in response to a meal was greater than could be measured because of limits in appetite and the development of satiety. This suggests that in the presence of a normal average appetite the capacity of the stomach to secrete is not tested. But, when histamine is used, the maximum secretory capacity can be tested because appetite is not involved. When histamine is used a sigmoid curve or a limited capacity to secrete is found (HANSON et al., 1948).

In Table 3, it will be observed how gastric pouch dogs were used to determine the histamine equivalent dose of 1,2,4-triazole. In line 4 of the table 0.5 mg of histamine di-HCl caused an output of 53 $\pm$ 9 mg HCl in Dog Le and 59 $\pm$ 10 in Dog Bu. In line 11 0.7 mg of the Triazole di-HCl produced 49 $\pm$ 7 in Dog Le and 64 $\pm$ 16 in Dog Bu. 0.7 mg di-HCl is the approximate Triazole equivalent of 0.5 mg

Table 3. *Augmentation of 1,2,4-triazole by aminoguanidine (histaminase inhibitor) when aminoguanidine is given in dose of 6 mg/kg body weight* (Ivy and Liepins 1960)

Li-ne	Procedure*	Dog Le			Dog Bu		
		No tests	HCl, mg	Significance	No tests	HCl, mg	Significance
1	Saline injection hourly for 5 hr	5	5		5	2	
2	4 mg/kg of aminoguanidine (AG) alone hourly for 5 hr	10	5		10	3	
3	Same as 2; 6 mg/kg/hr AG	8	8.6		9	5	
4	0.5 mg histamine di-HCl single dose alone	12	53±9		10	59±10	
5	Same as 4; plus 4 mg/kg AG/hr	10	56±11	4 vs. 5 = n.s.[2]	10	88±11	4 vs. 5 = $P < 0.01$
6	Same as 4; plus 6 mg/kg AG/hr	10	68±10	4 vs. 6 = $P < 0.001$	10	91±14	4 vs. 6 = $P < 0.001$
7	0.5 mg triazole di-HCl alone	22	31±4		22	31±4	
8	Same as 7; plus 4 mg/kg AG/hr	10	38±10	7 vs. 8 = n.s.	10	42±11	7 vs. 8 = n.s.
9	0.65 mg triazole di-HCl alone	10	42±8		10	43±6	
10	Same as 9; plus 6 mg/kg AG/hr	10	87±14	9 vs. 10 = $P < 0.001$	10	66±10	9 vs. 10 = $P < 0.001$
11	0.7 mg triazole di-HCl alone	19	49±7		19	64±16	
12	Same as 9; plus 6 mg/kg AG/hr	15	87±8	11 vs. 12 = $P < 0.001$	15	74±17	11 vs 12 = n.s.
13	0.075 mg triazole di-HCl alone	10	68±9	Mean = 71.5±12	10	75±15	

[1] All injections subcutaneous. [2] n.s. = not significant.

histamine di-HCl. When the output of Dog Le (53 mg) and of Dog Bu (59 mg) in response to 0.5 mg of histamine are averaged, the result is 56 mg. When the responses to 0.7 mg of the Triazole in the two dogs are averaged, the result is 56 mg (line 11, Table 3, 49 + 64 = 113 ÷ 2 = 56 mg). In Table 3 it will be noted that in each test, when aminoguanidine was given subcutaneously in 4 to 6 mg/kg doses hourly for 5 hr along with a single injection of either histamine or triazole, the output of HCl was augmented but not to a statistically significant extent in all cases.

Since in such a study, the tests extend over a period of months, the consistency of the response of the pouch to the same stimulus must be checked. An illustration is given for two dogs in Table 4.

Table 4. *Consistency of response to 0.5 and 0.7 mg 3-β-Aminoethyl-1,2,4-Triazole dihydrochloride* (Ivy and Liepins 1960)

Dog	Dose, mg	No. Tests	HCl output, mg				
			Control 1 hr	Hours after injection			
				1st hr	2nd hr	3rd hr	Total
Le	0.5	12 in April	0.3	22.8	7.6	2.3	32.7
	0.5	10 in July	0.3	17.6	10.7	2.1	30.4
Mean			0.3	20.2	9.1	2.2	31.5±4
Bu	0.5	13 in April	0.3	20.2	9.0	2.3	31.5
	0.5	10 in July	0.3	20.3	10.2	1.7	32.2
Mean			0.3	20.2	9.6	2.0	31.8±4
Le	0.7	10 in August	0.25	27.3	15.0	3.3	45.6
	0.7	9 in Nov.	0.22	35.2	12.5	3.4	51.1
Mean			0.23	31.2	13.8	3.3	48.8±7
Bu	0.7	10 in August	0.27	44.0	17.1	4.5	65.6
	0.7	9 in Nov.	0.15	42.0	16.0	3.6	61.6
Mean			0.21	43.0	16.6	4.0	63.6±16

More detailed data on the consistency of a response to the same meal is provided in Table 5. The consistency is less than in the case of a drug like histamine or 1,2,4-Triazole ethylamine.

Comment: It should be obvious that in making any comparative studies, using gastric secretion as an indicator, the experiment should be designed according to statistical reasoning and all differences in averages checked statistically for significance of differences due to random sampling.

Table 5. *Augmenting effect of a threshold dose of aminoguanidine given intravenously on gastric secretory response to a 100-g test-meal* (Ivy et al. 1956)

Test No.	Controls: No Aminoguanidine		Test No.	Treated: Aminoguanidine		
	Vol.[1] output	HCl[1] output		Amount inject.	Vol.[1] output	HCl[1] output
	cc	mg		mg/kg	cc	mg
A. Dog 1, Heidenhain pouch[2]						
1	32.4	87	1	8	73.8	249
2	20.0	55	2	10	52.5	224
3	48.1	182	3	12	53.6	230
4	50.3	216	4	20	56.9	257
5	42.7	170	5	20	69.7	313
6	23.9	67	6	20	89.5	446
7	28.7	91	7	20	79.8	384
8	30.4	100	8	20	52.0	224
9	28.9	111	9	20	50.2	210
10	52.4	190	10	20	54.5	221
11	37.8	158				
12	23.0	90				
13	37.5	129				
14	20.0	46				
15	22.9	73				
16	25.4	69				
17	19.7	60				
Av.	32.0	111	Av.	(10)[3]	64.0	276
B. Dog 2, Heidenhain pouch[4]						
1	26.9	101	1	20	43.7	182
2	36.1	133	2	20	45.6	198
3	28.6	97	3	20	61.0	277
4	48.7	144	4	20	49.4	211
5	36.7	88	5	20	68.0	278
6	27.3	107	6	20	48.9	201
7	30.6	128				
8	32.0	86				
9	19.9	70				
10	17.9	70				
11	24.1	94				
Av.	30.0	101	Av.	(6)	53.0	225
C. Dog 3, Ivy transplanted pouch[5]						
1	20.0	48	a	3	21.8	49
2	11.2	16	b	3	10.6	12
3	18.6	41	c	6	13.8	26
4	11.8	26	d	10	19.7	40
5	9.6	12	Av.		16.4	32
6	12.2	16				
7	16.4	27				
8	20.6	19	1	20	29.6	96
9	19.2	36	2	20	28.8	87
10	15.9	18	3	20	49.4	177
11	21.8	49	4	20	30.5	85
12	10.6	22	5	20	29.0	100
13	13.8	12	6	20	42.6	166
14	19.7	40				
15	15.2	21				
Av.	15.8	26	Av.	(6)	35.0	120

[1] Volume and HCl output is for a 4-hr period, the latter being calculated from the free acid.

[2] 20 mg of aminoguanidine given alone produced only 8.3 mg of HCl in 4 hr; therefore the augmentation is striking.

[3] The differences are highly significant.

[4] 20 mg/kg of aminoguanidine alone produced an average of 2.7 mg of HCl in a 4-hr period. The augmentation is striking. The t for the difference in volume output was 5.047, and for the difference in HCl output was 7.67, both being definitely significant.

[5] 20 mg of aminoguanidine given alone produced 16.7 mg in a 4-hr period. The augmentation is striking. The t value for the differences in volume output is 11.65, and for the difference in HCl output is 11.55, both being highly significant. Note that 3—10 mg/kg which were subthreshold did not augment the response to the meal; compare 15.8 cc the control average with 16.4 cc the test average.

Section H

Relationship Between Histamine and the Autonomous Nervous System

By

U. S. v. Euler

With 6 figures

I. Effect of histamine on the functional activity of the adrenosympathetic system

A. Effects on the adrenal medullary cells

A stimulating effect of histamine on the adrenal medulla was first observed by Burn and Dale (1926), causing a liberation of catecholamines which exert their characteristic effects on the blood pressure of the cat. This effect was confirmed by Szczygielski (1932) who noted a high sensitivity of the adrenal medulla towards histamine and also found that the effects of small doses of histamine could be abolished by nicotine. This inhibitory effect of nicotine has later been explained by its depolarizing action on the chromaffin cells. The histamine effect on the chromaffin cells is a direct one as shown by Siehe (1934) who demonstrated that it persisted after denervation of the adrenal medulla.

There is good evidence that the major part of the rise in blood pressure observed after histamine is due to a liberation of medullary amines, although the effect may be reinforced by the stimulating and potentiating effect of histamine on sympathetic ganglion cells (Trendelenburg 1954, 1955, 1957a).

Burn and Dale (1926) as well as Root (1951) and Slater and Dresel (1952) found that the rise in blood pressure after histamine was abolished by anti-adrenaline substances, indicating that the effect was due to catecholamines. The first-named authors also directly showed that the effect was due to a liberation of pressor substances from the adrenal medulla. However, both Root (1951) and Slater and Dresel (1952) observed that histamine exerted some pressor effect even after removal of the adrenal glands, suggesting that it stimulated also some other structures, thereby liberating pressor substances. The possible implications of these findings will be discussed in more details below.

The histamine actions on the adrenal medullary cells have been analyzed to a certain extent by Trendelenburg (1954, 1955). When administered in the central end of the coeliac artery 0.13—3.5 μg histamine caused a rise in blood pressure of 15—50 mm Hg (Trendelenburg 1954). Desensitization phenomena were observed if the intervals between injections were shorter than 10 minutes. Further Trendelenburg (1955) showed that while intravenous histamine in a dose of 20 μg usually caused a secondary rise of blood pressure in the spinal cat as a sign of catecholamine liberation from the adrenal medulla, this effect occurred only occasionally in the cat under chloralose. However, after a dose of 2 mg hexamethonium SLATER and DRESEL (1952) observed that the secondary rise was a regularly occurring phenomenon also in the cat under chloralose anaesthesia. This effect is explained by the potentiating effect of hexamethonium on the pressor response to both adrenaline and noradrenaline. After repeated doses of hexamethonium, 2—120 mg intravenously, the effects of noradrenaline and even more of adrenaline increased considerably. A striking increase of the secondary rise in blood pressure following an intravenous injection of 20 μg histamine was also noted after hexamethonium. As shown in Fig. 1, taken from TRENDELENBURG's paper (1955), the response to noradrenaline is increased by some 100 per cent while the secondary rise after histamine is increased nearly 10 times after the

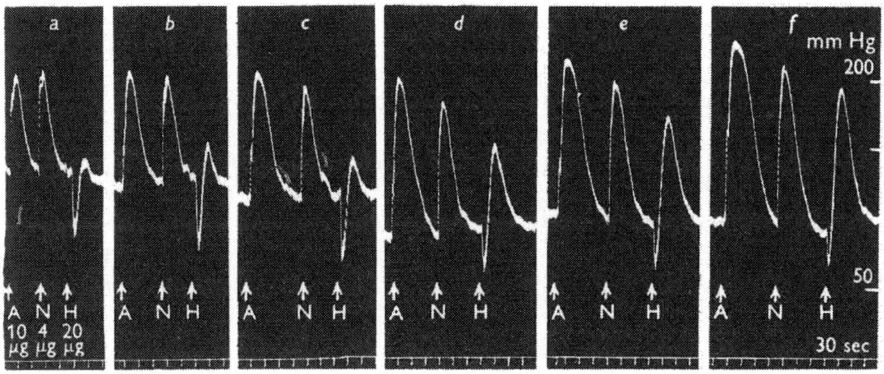

Fig. 1. Cat, chloralose, arterial blood pressure. A = intravenous injection of 10 μg adrenaline, N = that of 4 μg noradrenaline, H = that of 20 μg histamine. Responses of the blood pressure before (a) and after hexamethonium 2 mg (b), 6 mg (c), 18 mg (d), 54 mg (e) and 120 mg (f) injected intravenously. (After TRENDELENBURG, 1955)

largest dose of hexamethonium. It is hardly likely that such a large potentiation is due only to the increased peripheral sensitivity and is more suggestive of some other additional effect, possibly an increased liberation. This finding also indicates that hexamethonium does not prevent the stimulating effect of histamine on the chromaffin cells which, thus, is a direct one, and possibly analogous to that observed on the ganglion cells (TRENDELENBURG 1954).

While cocaine blocks the action of histamine on the superior cervical ganglion it does not interfere with the release of catecholamines from the adrenal medulla (TRENDELENBURG 1954). Thus after cocaine, which potentiates the action of the catecholamines, the blood pressure rise caused by histamine is increased.

Nicotine in large doses, on the other hand, prevents the liberation of catecholamines from the adrenal medulla by histamine, and consequently prevents the secondary rise in blood pressure (TRENDELENBURG 1955). After recovery, however, which may occur after a relatively short time (10 min.), a second series of nicotine injections failed to block the releasing effect of histamine. A failure of nicotine to block the releasing effect of histamine from the adrenal medulla was also observed after a dose of hexamethonium sufficient to block the pressor effect of nicotine itself. This refractoriness of the chromaffin cells towards the blocking effect of repeated doses of nicotine has been interpreted as a blocking without depolarization (TRENDELENBURG 1955). Thus PATON and PERRY (1953) observed that the block of the superior cervical ganglion caused by 0.2 mg nicotine given by close arterial injection had a longer duration than the depolarization of the ganglion cells. A second injection still produces a block but hardly any depolarization. If the same mechanism holds true for the chromaffin cells of the adrenal medulla, the recovery of the catecholamine-releasing effect of histamine suggests that the cells, although blocked against neural stimuli and nicotine itself, still react to the direct action of histamine. This interpretation implies (1) that depolarization prevents the catecholamine-releasing effect of histamine and (2) that the pressor response observed with histamine after a second treatment with nicotine is due to released catecholamines.

After small doses of nicotine (0.5—1 mg/kg) the effect of intravenous doses of histamine (5—10 μg/kg in the cat) are moderately increased (TRENDELENBURG 1961). A "sensitization" of this kind was not observed after tetramethylammonium, which causes ganglionic block by pure depolarization (PATON and PERRY 1953).

TRENDELENBURG (1955) also states that, in order to obtain constant blood pressure response after an intravenous dose of histamine, the injections had to be spaced with an interval of 5—10 min.

A release of catecholamines from the adrenal medulla may also be demonstrated by direct analysis of the secretion in the adrenal venous blood. Experiments of this kind have been reported by WADA et al. (1940) on the dog. With a dose of 1 mg/kg the hypersecretion lasted for 40 minutes with a maximum rate of 0.4 μg/kg/min. and a total extra secretion of 10 μg/kg.

WOODS et al. (1956) found no increase in plasma catecholamines after intra-aortic injection of histamine. A slight increase of "epinephrine-like material" was noted, however, by MANGER et al. (1957) after intravenous administration of 1 mg of histamine. DE SCHAEPDRYVER (1959) found increased catecholamine secretion in the adrenal vein in dogs. In experiments on dogs ROBINSON and JOCHIM (1960) also found a marked increase in the catecholamine secretion into the adrenal venous blood, reaching a maximum within the first 6—8 minutes and then rapidly decreasing in the next few minutes. Recovery to normal secretion was attained 20—30 minutes after the injection, depending on the dose of histamine (1—5 mg). In adreno-jugular cross-circulation experiments the maximal response to histamine was noted in less than 2 minutes after the injection. In most animals the increase in adrenaline was slightly greater than that of noradrenaline as also noted by DE SCHAEPDRYVER (1959).

Moderate increases in the excretion of catecholamines in urine after subcutaneous injections of histamine in man have been observed by EULER and LUFT (unpublished observations) presumably as a result of a releasing effect chiefly on the adrenal medulla.

In the experiments of TRENDELENBURG (1955) intravenous doses of 20 μg histamine generally caused a small or moderate secondary rise in blood pressure of the cat under chloralose anaesthesia. This small effect is in marked contrast to the large effects of small doses observed by EULER (1946) in the cat under chloralose, pretreated with ergotamine and cocaine. In these cases extracts of various organs were given, however. Judging from the amounts of extracts administered it can be concluded that doses of histamine of approximately 1 μg released a similar amount of catecholamines. Whether the simultaneous occurrence of other substances in the extract have contributed to the large effects observed cannot be stated at present.

The release of catecholamines from the cat adrenal medulla caused by histamine is abolished by antihistamine drugs (EMMELIN and MUREN 1949).

Further studies of the nature of the pressor effect of histamine and its dependence on catecholamine release from various sources have been induced by the availability of a series of new drugs known to affect the biosynthesis, storage, and release of catecholamines.

Choline 2,6-xylylether bromide (TM 10) is known to prevent the liberation of noradrenaline from adrenergic nerve endings (EXLEY 1957). After injection of this substance in a dose of 10 mg/kg in the cat the pressor effect of histamine was unaltered in normal preparations but abolished in the adrenalectomized animal (TRENDELENBURG 1961). This is in accord with the observation that TM 10 does not prevent the release of catecholamines from the adrenal medulla.

Pretreatment of the cat with reserpine in doses which reduce or abolish the response to sympathetic nerve stimulation (3 mg/kg 24 and 48 hours before experiment) caused a diminished or abolished blood pressure response to histamine (TRENDELENBURG 1961). This effect is of interest since reserpine in this dose usually does not deplete the catecholamine content of the adrenal in the cat completely (KRONEBERG and SCHÜMANN 1957). The result suggests that reserpine causes some kind of block of the chromaffin cells rendering them less sensitive to the direct stimulating effect of histamine. It should also be recalled that the sensitivity to released catecholamines is increased after reserpine.

After injections of histamine in the rat, HÖKFELT (1951) noticed marked changes in the catecholamine content of various organs in regard to amount as well as to proportions of the amines. 3 hours after a dose of 0.5 mg/kg histamine in the rat he observed that noradrenaline had disappeared in the suprarenals whereas adrenaline had increased by 50 per cent.

SUZUKI (1951) observed a fall in the adrenaline content of the adrenals in rabbits after injection of histamine.

B. Effect of histamine on extra-adrenal chromaffin cells

In the experiments of TRENDELENBURG (1955) it was shown that adrenalectomy greatly reduced the secondary rise in blood pressure in the cat after histamine, but did not abolish it. Similar observations had previously been made by SLATER and DRESEL (1952) who also noticed that the remaining effect was abolished by cocaine. It was also annulled by nicotine. Since these drugs abolish the stimulating effect of histamine on sympathetic ganglia, it has been concluded (TRENDELENBURG 1955) that the residual effect of histamine on the blood pressure of the adrenalectomized cat was due to an action on the ganglia. The possibility of an action of histamine on extra-adrenal chromaffin cells should be taken into consideration, however, since there is increasing evidence that such cells are widely spread in the organism, even though relatively few in number. A dose of 20 μg histamine intravenously would hardly suffice to cause the secondary rise observed in adrenalectomized cats by ganglionic stimulation in view of the statement (TRENDELENBURG 1954) that the doses of histamine required to cause ganglionic stimulation are of the order of 50 μg. Furthermore, hexamethonium in doses up to 20 mg does not influence the ganglionic response to histamine (TRENDELENBURG 1954, 1955) while it increases the blood pressure response to histamine in the adrenalectomized cat (TRENDELENBURG 1955) which speaks in favour of an effect on chromaffin cells.

Histamine exerts a stimulating action also on chromaffin tumour cells (ROTH and KVALE 1945). The release of catecholamines from the tumour cells has been utilized as a diagnostic test in suspected cases of phaeochromocytoma.

Tentative evidence for a stimulating effect of histamine on chromaffin cells in organs have been obtained in some instances. Thus it has been known for a long time that histamine stimulates the isolated heart of the rabbit and the cat (DALE and LAIDLAW 1910, VIOTTI 1924, GUNN 1926, STAUB and GRASSMANN 1930, TRIPOD,

WIRZ and MEIER 1951), of the guinea-pig (WENT and LISSÁK 1935, PENNA et al. 1959, HOLTZ 1960) and of the rat and frog (WENT et al. 1952). It also stimulates the isolated auricle of the rabbit (DEWS and GRAHAM 1946).

This effect might be interpreted either as a direct effect of histamine on myocardial receptors or possibly as secondary to a release of catecholamines (TRUEX 1950, KOTTEGODA 1953, WENT et al. 1954). Although there is some evidence that histamine acts directly on the myocardium it does not seem to be

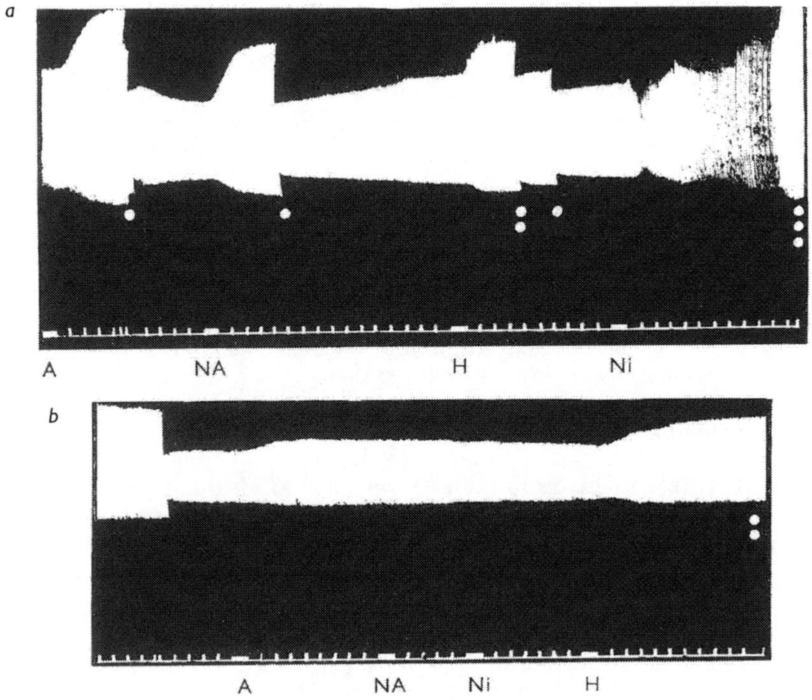

Fig. 2. Dichloroisoproterenol 1×10^{-4} prevents the effects of the catecholamines and nicotine in guinea-pig isolated auricles; the effect of histamine is still present. (a) The effect of adrenaline 1×10^{-7} (A), noradrenaline 1×10^{-7} (NA), nicotine 5×10^{-5} (Ni), and histamine 1×10^{-6} (H). (b) The effect of the same substances 60 min. after treatment with dichloroisoproterenol. Upper tracing: height of contraction. Lower tracing: time, 10 sec. The washings are indicated by the white dots. (After MANNAIONI, 1960).

entirely excluded that it may cause an effect by stimulating the release of catecholamines from chromaffin cells for instance, or possibly from adrenergic neurons.

Isolated auricles, brought to a standstill by reserpine, are activated by histamine as well as by adrenaline and noradrenaline, but not by nicotine (GIOTTI 1954, PEPEU, MASI and GIOTTI 1959).

MANNAIONI (1960) has reinvestigated the problem of histamine action on the heart with the use of dichloroisoproterenol (DCI) which was introduced by POWELL and SLATER (1958) and shown to be a specific antagonist of the catecholamines on the heart (MORAN and PERKINS 1958). He found that while DCI (10 μg/ml for 30 min) practically annulled the effect of adrenaline and noradrenaline in doses of 1 μg/ml on the isolated auricles of the guinea-pig, it did not suppress the action of histamine. From the tracings it can be seen, however, that even after DCI adrenaline may have a slight action on the contraction and that the effect of histamine is greatly reduced (Fig. 2). After pretreatment with reserpine and DCI the effect of adrenaline was very much reduced while the average effect of histamine on contraction height was hardly affected. After DCI the effect of histamine on the heart rate was markedly diminished, however.

The ganglionic blocking agents hexamethonium (100 μg/ml) and pempidine (0.1 μg/ml) acting for 30 minutes did not alter the effect of histamine on isolated guinea-pig auricles pretreated with reserpine. After 90 minutes exposure to the ganglionic blocking agents histamine had lost its action, however.

According to WENT et al. (1952) the stimulating effect of histamine on the isolated heart is abolished by ergotamine. Moreover WENT et al. (1954) have reported that, after stimulation of the isolated heart with histamine, substances inhibiting smooth muscle appear in the perfusate.

It is not at present possible to decide with complete certainty whether the stimulant action of histamine on the isolated heart is due to a release of catecholamines or not. The heart contains chromaffin cells which might be stimulated by histamine like those in the adrenal medulla.

If hexamethonium by itself causes a release of catecholamines from chromaffin cells, which may be considered as an explanation of its potentiating effect on the effect of histamine on the blood pressure, this might explain why it prevents the effect of histamine on the isolated heart after having acted for 90 minutes. It appears less likely that this treatment should abolish direct action of histamine on the myocardium.

The persisting effect of histamine after reserpine does not exclude the possibility of a release of catecholamines from chromaffin cells in the heart, since these have been found to be more resistent to the depleting effect of reserpine than the nerve stores.

As to the abolishment after DCI of the action of adrenaline, but not of histamine, this result obviously seems to be better explained by assuming a direct action of histamine on the myocardium. However, in these two systems, the conditions for an antagonism are not strictly comparable, since an action of exogenous adrenaline might well be antagonized by DCI in a different way from that of catecholamines released intramurally from chromaffin cells. MANNAIONI (1960) also considers the possibility that histamine may act through the release of stimulating substances which are not antagonized by DCI.

Should more conclusive evidence be obtained for an action of histamine on the heart through liberation of catecholamines, or possibly of other compounds, the actions of histamine on a variety of other organs will have to be reconsidered, since chromaffin cells in all probability are present in most organs.

Thus an effect of this kind may be partly responsible for the contraction of vessels in the rabbit ear caused by histamine.

Another effect of histamine which may be partly attributed to the release of catecholamines is the antagonistic action against depolarizing neuromyal blocking agents. SCHENK and ANDERSON (1958) have demonstrated that histamine, when administered by close arterial injection, is capable of antagonizing a neuromyal block caused by depolarizing agents such as decamethonium or succinylcholine (Fig. 3). This effect is similar to that exerted by adrenaline (PATON and ZAIMIS 1950) but since the effect is not altered by adrenalectomy, SCHENK and ANDERSON conclude that the histamine effect is not due to adrenaline. The possibility of a local release of adrenaline from chromaffin cells in this case as in the several others where the effects of histamine closely mimick those of adrenaline should not be overlooked, however.

MacMillan (1955) observed that close arterial injection of histamine caused a small tetanic contraction in the chronically denervated cat tibialis but not in the normal muscle.

Whether histamine will also cause a release of dopamine from the specific cells containing this substance (Falck, Hillarp and Torp 1959, Coupland and Heath 1961) is at present unknown.

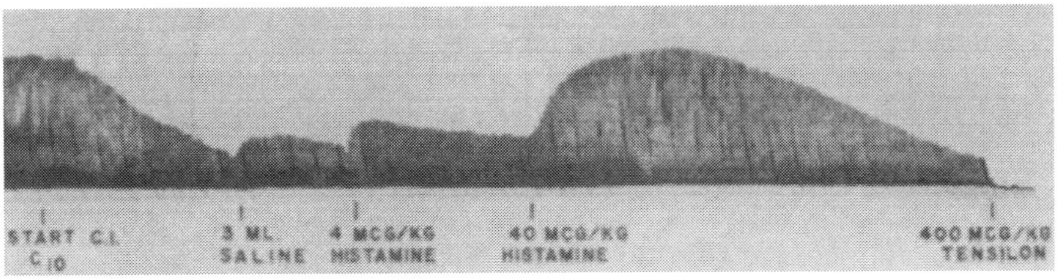

Fig. 3. Record of contractions of cat tibialis anticus muscle, showing antagonistic effect of intraarterial histamine in doses of 4 and 40 μg/kgm. on decamethonium (C_{10}) block maintained by constant infusion. Intraarterial saline injection produced minimal reversal. Tensilon antagonism indicates maintained depolarization at conclusion of experiment. (After Schenk und Anderson 1958)

C. Effects on sympathetic ganglion cells

Burn and Trendelenburg (1954) observed on some occasions that the innervated nictitating membrane of the cat gave a stronger response to histamine than the denervated preparation, and also that a response was obtained even after adrenalectomy. Since it could be shown in other experiments that no reaction occurred upon injections of histamine in the perfused head, it seemed possible that the effect observed was on the superior cervical ganglion. Previous experiments by Feldberg and Vartiainen (1935) failed to reveal a stimulating effect of histamine on the isolated perfused ganglion but in Konzett's study (1952) 4 out of 22 preparations responded with stimulation.

Trendelenburg (1954) observed a stimulating effect of histamine on the superior cervical ganglion after intravenous injection in doses above 50 μg. The denervated membrane did not respond after adrenalectomy, the effect thus being due to liberation of catecholamines from the gland. The innervated membrane contracted upon injection of histamine even in the adrenalectomized animal, however.

Using intraarterial injections into the lingual artery, responses were obtained with histamine (as hydrochloride) in doses of 2—55 μg. Desensitization occurred after intravenous as well as intraarterial injections and the recovery was fairly slow, requiring from 5 to 30 min.

An interesting difference was noticed between the stimulating effect of histamine and those of acetylcholine or nicotine, the former requiring a considerably longer time to develop. Unspecific stimulation and direct actions on the membrane could be excluded, and actions mediated by adrenaline from the adrenals as well. Removal of the ganglion or cutting of the postganglionic fibres abolished the histamine effect. Adrenaline in a small dose caused contraction of the nictitating membrane when injected through the lingual artery without occlusion of the external carotid artery, while histamine caused the effect only when this artery was occluded.

All these observations combined prove that the contraction of the nictitating membrane produced by histamine in the cat is mediated through the superior cervical ganglion. This conclusion has been further corroborated by pharmacological analysis in which a number of "autonomic" drugs have been used.

Hexamethonium in doses up to 20 mg had no effect on the ganglionic response to histamine, although it abolished, as expected, the effect of preganglionic stimulation and of acetylcholine.

A series of nicotine injections (0.5—10 mg) sufficient to block the effect of stimulation on the blood pressure also blocked the effect of histamine on the ganglion. After recovery some 30—60 min later the response to histamine was sometimes more marked than before nicotine.

Cocaine administered in doses of 0.5 mg intravenously, which have no effect on the response to submaximal preganglionic stimulation, was found to reduce considerably the effect of histamine on the nictitating membrane. A dose of 20 mg cocaine intramuscularly prevented the response to 2 μg histamine intraarterially for more than 4 hours (TRENDELENBURG 1954).

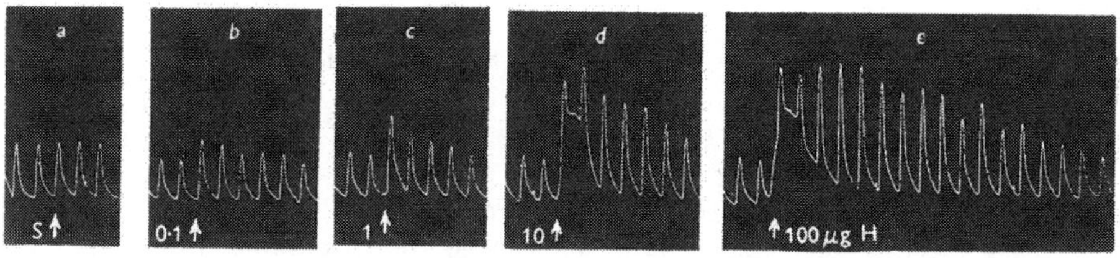

Fig. 4. Cat, chloralose, adrenals removed. Normal nictitating membrane. Submaximal stimulation of preganglionic fibres 2/min for 5 sec each. Injections of 0.2 ml. saline (*S*) in (a), and of 0.1 μg histamine in (b), 1 μg in (c), 10 μg in (d) and 100 μg histamine in (e). (After TRENDELENBURG, 1955)

Atropine in doses up to 2 mg had no effect on the ganglionic response to histamine, while mepyramine in sufficiently large doses (0.15 mg) blocked the effects of histamine.

Morphine antagonized the stimulant effect of histamine on the superior cervical ganglion and is also said to diminish the release of transmitter from adrenergic nerve endings (TRENDELENBURG 1957c). In doses of 1 mg/kg intravenously it did not affect the pressor response to histamine in the normal cat but diminished the response after adrenalectomy (TRENDELENBURG 1961).

Histamine is also able to potentiate the action of nicotine-like substances on the perfused superior cervical ganglion (KONZETT 1952). In doses which are not large enough to stimulate the ganglion (1 μg), histamine also exerts a potentiating action on the response of the nictitating membrane to submaximal preganglionic stimulation. This potentiating effect increased with increasing doses of histamine intraarterially (Fig. 4). While the minimal dose of histamine for stimulation of the ganglion was between 2 and 20 μg by the intraarterial route, 0.01 to 0.1 μg was required for the potentiating action. The potentiating effect was abolished by mepyramine but not influenced by atropine. Hexamethonium, nicotine and cocaine abolished this effect of histamine.

The effect of intraarterial injections of histamine is predominantly on the ganglion cells, as indicated by the finding that when pre- and postganglionic fibres of the superior cervical ganglion were stimulated intermittently with submaximal stimuli, only the effects of preganglionic stimulation on the contraction height of the nictitating membrane were potentiated (TRENDELENBURG 1957a).

An attempt has been made to analyse the effect of histamine on the ganglion cells by recording postganglionic action potentials after stimulation of preganglionic fibres. It was shown by ECCLES (1935) that the cervical sympathetic chain contains two groups of fibres, conducting with 15—22 and 7—14 m/sec respectively. These groups were named S_1 and S_2. A close correlation between the contraction height of the nictitating membrane and the amplitude of action potentials of the S_1 fibres was found. Action potentials of the S_2 group were only found when the stimulation strength was further increased, and when the response of the nictitating membrane was already maximal. After cutting the postganglionic fibres, there was a close correlation between the corresponding group of pre- and postganglionic action potentials. The findings of ECCLES (1935) have been confirmed by TRENDELENBURG (1957a) in that the S_1-impulses in the preganglionic fibres were conducted through the postganglionic S_1-fibres causing contraction of the nictitating membrane on stimulation. The S_2-fibres, on the other hand, do not carry fibres to the nictitating membrane. The impulses travelling in the S_2-fibres were, however, potentiated by histamine. It has been concluded (TRENDELENBURG 1957a) that histamine also potentiates the impulses conducted in the S_1-fibres although direct evidence for this has not been produced.

D. Effects of histamine on sympathetic centers

The biological actions of histamine observed after its injection into the blood supply to the superior cervical ganglion differ depending on whether the central connections of the ganglion are intact or not. After section of the preganglionic fibres, any actions observed have been regarded as purely ganglionic ones, while the effects observed in preparations with intact preganglionic fibres have been interpreted as partly due to actions on the sympathetic centers.

If cocaine is administered intravenously in doses of 2.5 mg or more, causing hypersensitivity to adrenaline and noradrenaline, the response of the nictitating membrane to intraarterial injections of histamine is unchanged or increased, in contrast to the effect of small doses of cocaine, 0.1—1 mg, which antagonize the stimulant effect of histamine on the ganglion (TRENDELENBURG 1957b). These results suggest that the effect observed with histamine after the larger dose of cocaine is not due to a direct action on the ganglion, but rather due to nerve impulses reaching the sensitized ganglions from a point central to the ganglion, presumably from sympathetic centers. The effects of histamine in preparations subjected to the larger doses of cocaine disappeared after sectioning of the preganglionic nerve fibres to the ganglion.

The assumption that the observed effect of histamine was due to a central stimulation acting on a sensitized nictitating membrane was supported by the finding that while intravenous histamine (15 μg) as well as noradrenaline (1 μg) had no effect on the membrane when the central connections were left intact, both injections caused contraction of the membrane 30 minutes after 8 mg/kg cocaine, i. e. when full sensitization had occurred. After section of the preganglionic fibres the contraction caused by histamine was abolished (Fig. 5). The same effect was produced by injections of a ganglion blocker, hexamethonium, in a dose of 10 mg intravenously.

The possibility of tonic impulses through the superior cervical ganglion being the cause of the contraction through the potentiating effect of histamine could be ruled out since this effect is abolished by cocaine (TRENDELENBURG 1957b).

The centrally stimulating effect of histamine just described is not observed if the interval between successive histamine injections is too short (10 min) while it is regularly observed at intervals of 20 min. This observation makes it unlikely that the effect was due to circulatory changes affecting secondarily the sympathetic centers.

The observed action of histamine was reduced by section of the spinal cord at the level of the second vertebra which suggested that histamine acts also on sympathetic centers in the spinal cord.

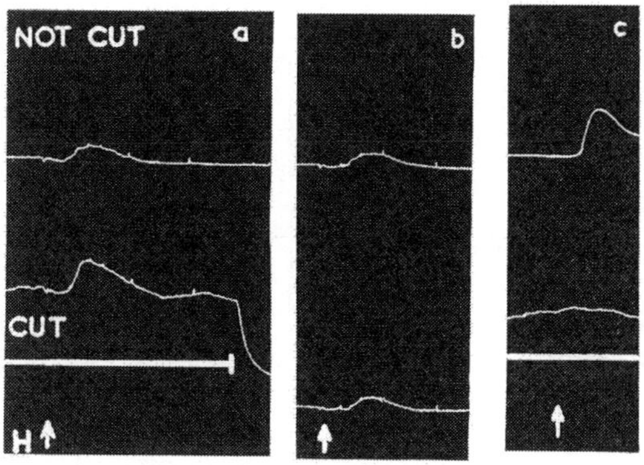

Fig. 5. Cat under chloralose, 3.3 kg, adrenals removed. Normal nictitating membrane with its central connections intact (upper trace) and other side, with its preganglionic fibers cut (lower trace). Intravenous injections of 50 μg histamine at arrow. In (a) and (c) submaximal preganglionic stimulation of one side (lower trace), as indicated by solid line. No stimulation in (b). Intramuscular injection of 8 mg/kg cocaine 30 min before (c). (After TRENDELENBURG, 1957b)

II. Presence of histamine in autonomic nerves

Histamine has been observed to occur in autonomous nerves in a variety of animals. Although there is no proportionality between the histamine content and the amounts of the adrenergic transmitter in sympathetic nerves these nerves seem to be particularly rich in histamine. This makes it possible and even probable that the occurrence of histamine is in some way functionally or morphogenetically connected with the postsynaptic adrenergic neurons. Even if the adrenergic neuron itself should prove to contain no histamine, the observed relationships between histamine and sympathetic nerves seem to be close enough to make desirable a presentation of the available data in this context.

A. Histamine content of autonomic nerves

Quantitative data on the occurrence of histamine in nerves are available from a number of studies beginning with KWIATKOWSKI (1943). Using bioassay technique he showed that most peripheral nerves in rats, guinea-pigs, rabbits, cats, dogs, monkeys and man contained histamine. Sensory nerves were generally found to contain more histamine than motor nerves, whereas the spinal roots and spinal cord were almost free from histamine. The presence of histamine in nerves was also reported by KOSHTOJANZ, RIVKINA and MITROPOLITANSKAYA (1945), WERLE and WEICKEN (1949), RIVKINA (1947) and WERLE and PALM (1950). In 1948 EULER reported remarkably high contents of histamine in bovine adrenergic nerves. Thus the splenic nerves were found to contain some 100 μg histamine per g of fresh tissue. These findings were further extended by EULER (1949) and by WERLE and WEICKEN (1949), who reported high amounts in sympathetic nerves and ganglia and also in other autonomous nerves. In Table 1 the average figures from the data of EULER (1949), EULER and PURKHOLD (1951b) and of WERLE and PALM (1950) from nervous tissue of man, dog, cow, and sheep, are presented.

Table 1. *Average histamine content of nervous tissue from man, dog, cow, and sheep (μg/g histamine dihydrochloride)*

Nerve	Man	Dog	Cow		Sheep
	WERLE and PALM (1950)	WERLE and PALM (1950)	WERLE and PALM (1950)	EULER (1949)	EULER and PURKHOLD (1951b)
Splenic	—	16	64	98	13
Symp. gangl.	—	—	61	93	—
Symp. trunk	6	8	31	93	3.5
Sup. mesent. gangl.	—	19	—	—	—
Mesenteric	—	—	—	78	7.5
Hepatic	—	13	—	—	7
Splanchnic	7	13	49	(65)	4.7
Coeliac gangl.	—	—	—	(60)	—
Stellate gangl.	8	8	80	(33)	—
Sup. cervical gangl.	10	—	50	29	5.5
Phrenic	—	6	—	28	—
Vagus	6	16	18	24	2.4
Vagus gangl.	—	11	(37)	—	—
Intercostal	3	7	10	22	—
Sciatic	—	9	—	17	0.3
Spinal gangl.	6	—	46	12	—
Optic	—	—	—	8.5	—
Dorsal roots	0.5	—	2.2	4—11	—
Ventral roots	0.4	—	2.2	5—9	—
Spinal cord	0.05	0.3	0.5	1.4	—
Entire brain	—	—	—	0.1—1	—

Figures within brackets refer to single determinations.

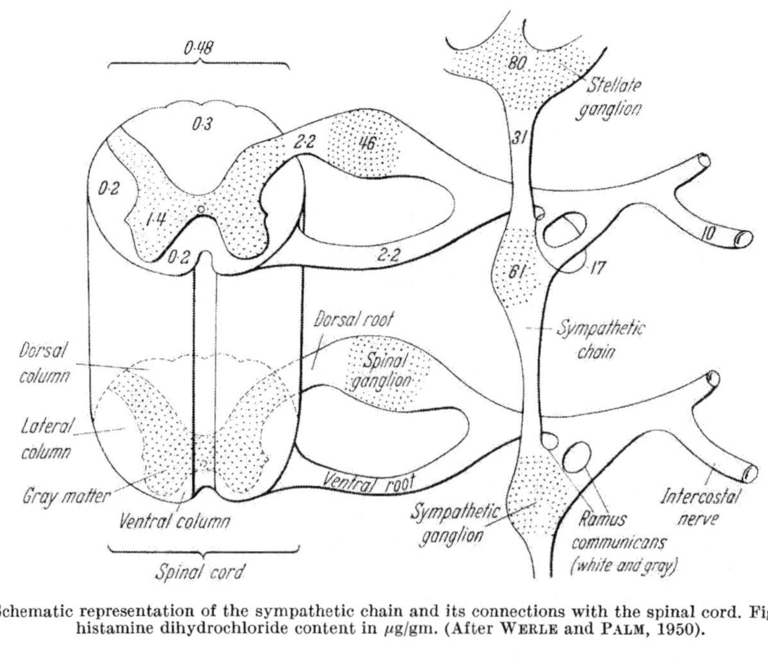

Fig. 6. Schematic representation of the sympathetic chain and its connections with the spinal cord. Figures give histamine dihydrochloride content in μg/gm. (After WERLE and PALM, 1950).

The Table shows that the highest figures are found, as a rule, in sympathetic nerves and ganglia although variations are observed, not only between different species by the same authors, but also in the same kind of nerves by different investigators. The original data also reveal a fairly large scatter of the values.

As noticed by KWIATKOWSKI (1943) the histamine content of the central nervous system is generally very low. Higher histamine values were found in the cervical and thoracal spinal roots than in lumbosacral roots, as well as higher figures in the dorsal roots (EULER 1949, WERLE and PALM 1950) (Fig. 6).

B. Histamine-noradrenaline ratio in autonomic nerves

A comparison of the histamine and noradrenaline contents of various nerves reveals that the ratio varies widely, as shown in Table 2.

According to WERLE and WEICKEN (1949) the histamine is probably present in the nerve fibrils and not in the nerve sheath or glia. The lack of a constant relationship between the histamine and noradrenaline contents of various nerves led, however, EULER (1949) to question the probability that histamine should appear solely as an ingredient in postganglionic adrenergic fibres. Furthermore the distribution of histamine in parasympathetic and in sensory nerves and the low amounts in the spinal cord makes it unlikely that histamine is bound to the axons. Analysis of homogenates from bovine splenic nerves showed that histamine occurred in the supernatant from the centrifuged homogenate but not in the storage granules which only contained catecholamines (EULER and HILLARP 1956, EULER 1958).

Table 2. *Average histamine and noradrenaline content of bovine nervous tissue*

	Histamine	Noradrenaline	Ratio Nor/Hi
Splenic	98	15	1:7
Mesenteric . . .	78	2.3	1:34
Splanchnic . . .	65	0.4	1:160
Carotid nerve . .	60	0.8	1:75
Saphenous . . .	34	0.5	1:68
Vagus (neck) . .	24	0.1	1:240

The results of histamine analyses in guinea-pig nerves at different intervals after nerve section also make it highly improbable that histamine should be an action substance in the neuron proper. Thus WERLE and WEICKEN (1949) did not observe any consistent change in the histamine content of the sciatic nerve up to a fortnight after nerve section. Also after section of the lumbar sympathetic trunk the histamine content in the sciatic nerve was unchanged in cats (KWIATKOWSKI 1943) and in dogs (WERLE and PALM 1950).

Section of the sympathetic nerves to an organ causes a rapid disappearance of its noradrenaline content (CANNON and LISSÁK 1939, GOODALL 1951, EULER and PURKHOLD 1951a). After section of the sympathetic nerves to various organs EULER and PURKHOLD (1951b) observed no change in histamine content in the submaxillary and parotid glands, and in the kidney and the liver of sheep. A loss of histamine was found only in the spleen and in lymph glands. From this it may be inferred that the histamine in most organs is not derived from the nerves as it is the case for noradrenaline. FELDBERG (1951), likewise, observed no histamine loss in the rabbit's ear after sectioning the nerves to the ear.

Since the nerve loses its conductivity within 72 hours after sectioning and also most of its content of chemical transmitters within this time, it is hard to believe that the histamine could be present in the neuron itself.

The results suggest that the histamine found in nerves may be present outside the neuron. The most likely assumption seems at present to be that the histamine occurs in mast cells located in the nerve connective tissue and perhaps associated with the vascular supply. There is at present no fact directly supporting the belief that it should occur in the neurons. Likewise nothing speaks against its occurrence in specific cells outside the neurons. On the other hand the peculiar fact still remains to be explained that peripheral nerves rich in adrenergic nerve fibres are also rich in histamine. Assuming that histamine is present in mast cells the question arises whether these have any relationship to the adrenergic nervous system. Such a connection could be based on a morphogenetical kinship between mast cells and chromaffin cells or their homologues, the postsynaptic adrenergic neurons. It should also be recalled that the dopamine cells, discovered by FALCK et al. (1959) are considered to be closely related to the mast cells (COUPLAND and HEATH 1961).

WERLE and WEICKEN (1949) studied the uptake of histamine in sections of stellate ganglia and found that histamine was either taken up or released depending on the histamine concentration in the bath. No "active" uptake was observed. These authors also found a decreased histamine content in nerves taken from animals which had been stored in the cold room in the slaughter house.

The release of histamine from isolated bovine splenic nerves reported by EULER and ÅSTRÖM (1948) need not be regarded as contradictory to the belief expressed by the present author that the histamine is, at least chiefly, located extraaxonally in the nerves. It might well be the case that nerve stimulation can affect histamine-containing cells present in the vicinity of the axons, thus causing a release. The normal mechanism of release of heparin and histamine (and 5-hydroxytryptamine) from mast cells is still obscure. The histamine release from isolated nerves described by EULER and ÅSTRÖM might therefore be an artifact. Some differences between the release of noradrenaline and histamine from isolated bovine splenic nerves were also noted by these authors. Thus noradrenaline was usually detected only during the first stimulations of a quite fresh nerve, whereas histamine effects as a rule could be elicited as a result of stimulation even after a few hours.

GISCAFRE, TANTURI and VAN ARMAN (1952) observed a release of histamine in the surrounding fluid following electrical stimulation of freshly excised sympathetic trunks from man.

The presence of histamine derivatives and of enzymes capable of splitting such compounds have been studied by WERLE and PALM (1952), who found small amounts of acetylhistamine in the stellate ganglion.

III. Histamine release by adrenaline

It has been claimed by several authors that adrenaline can liberate histamine in the body (EICHLER and BARFUSS 1940, STAUB 1946, KOCH and SZERB 1950, WENT and VARGA 1952). According to CSALAY, HORVÁTH and LUDÁNY (1955) splanchnic stimulation can cause increased histamine content of the blood. The same effect was observed after stimulation of the cut central end of the sciatic nerve in the dog but only when the adrenals were left intact (BORNEMISZA et al. 1955). MONGAR and WHELAN (1953), on the other hand, found no change in the histamine concentration of the blood after infusion of adrenaline 10 and 20 μg/min in man. Intra-arterial infusion of adrenaline was also ineffective in this respect.

According to LAMBERT and ROSENTHAL (1943) splanchnic nerve stimulation increases the histamine content of the skin in the dog.

References

BORNEMISZA, GY., L. CSALAY, G. HORVÁTH u. G. LUDÁNY: Die Wirkung des Schmerzreizes auf den Histamingehalt des Blutplasmas. Acta med. Acad. Sci. hung. **8**, 187—192 (1955).

BURN, J. H., and H. H. DALE: The vaso-dilator action of histamine, and its physiological significance. J. Physiol. (Lond.) **61**, 185—214 (1926).

—, and U. TRENDELENBURG: The hypersensitivity of the denervated nictitating membrane to various substances. Brit. J. Pharmacol. **9**, 202—209 (1954).

CANNON, W. B., and K. LISSÁK: Evidence for adrenaline in adrenergic neurones. Amer. J. Physiol. **125**, 765—777 (1939)

COUPLAND, R. E., and I. D. HEATH: Chromaffin cells, mast cells and melanin. II. The chromaffin cells of the liver capsule and gut in ungulates. J. Endocr. **22**, 71—76 (1961).

CSALAY, L., G. HORVÁTH u. G. LUDÁNY: Untersuchungen über die Adrenalin-Histamin-Gegenregulation. Acta physiol. Acad. Sci. hung. **8**, 109—118 (1955).

DALE, H. H., and P. P. LAIDLAW: The physiological action of iminazolylethylamine. J. Physiol. (Lond.) **41**, 318—344 (1910).

DEWS, P. B., and J. D. P. GRAHAM: The antihistamine substance 2786 R.P. Brit. J. Pharmacol. **1**, 278—286 (1946).

ECCLES, J. C.: The action potential of the superior cervical ganglion. J. Physiol. (Lond.) **85**, 179—206 (1935).

EICHLER, O., u. F. BARFUSS: Untersuchungen über den Histamingehalt des Blutes bei Infusion von Adrenalin und Histamin. Naunyn-Schmiedeberg's Arch. exp. Path. Pharmak. **195**, 245—257 (1940).

EMMELIN, N., and A. MUREN: Effects of antihistamine compounds on the adrenaline liberation from the suprarenals. Acta physiol. scand. **17**, 345—355 (1949).

EULER, U. S. v.: A specific sympathomimetic ergone in adrenergic nerve fibres (sympathin) and its relation to adrenaline and noradrenaline. Acta physiol. scand. **12**, 73—97 (1946).

— Sympathin, histamine and acetylcholine in mammalian nerves. J. Physiol. (Lond.) **107**, 10P—11P (1948).

— Histamine as a specific constituent of certain autonomic nerve fibres. Acta physiol. scand. **19**, 85—93 (1949).

— The presence of the adrenergic neurotransmitter in intraaxonal structures. Acta physiol. scand. **43**, 155—166 (1958).

—, and N. Å. HILLARP: Evidence for the presence of noradrenaline in submicroscopic structures of adrenergic axons. Nature (Lond.) **177**, 44—45 (1956).

—, and A. PURKHOLD: Effect of sympathetic denervation on the noradrenaline and adrenaline content of the spleen, kidney, and salivary glands in the sheep. Acta physiol. scand. **24**, 212—217 (1951a).

— — Histamine in organs and its relation to the sympathetic nerve supply. Acta physiol. scand. **24**, 218—224 (1951b).

—, and A. ÅSTRÖM: Liberation of histamine and sympathin by stimulation of isolated splenic nerves from cattle. Acta physiol. scand. **16**, 97—104 (1948).

EXLEY, K. A.: The blocking action of choline 2:6-xylyl ether bromide on adrenergic nerves. Brit. J. Pharmacol. **12**, 297—305 (1957).

FALCK, B., N.-Å. HILLARP and A. TORP: Some observations on the histology and histochemistry of the chromaffin cells probably storing dopamine. J. Histochem. Cytochem. **7**, 323—328 (1959).

FELDBERG, W.: Personal communication (1951).

—, and A. VARTIAINEN: Further observations on the physiology and pharmacology of a sympathetic ganglion. J. Physiol. (Lond.) **83**, 103—128 (1935).

GIOTTI, A.: Interaction of nicotine and eserine, ephedrine, atropine, hexamethonium, and adrenaline in isolated guinea-pig auricles. Brit. J. Pharmacol. **9**, 15—23 (1954).

GISCAFRE, L., C. TANTURI e C. G. VAN ARMAN: Aumento de la histamina en la sangre por la inyección de sympatol, usando la acidez gástrica como indicador. Día méd. **24**, 1427 (1952).

GOODALL, McC.: Studies of adrenaline and noradrenaline in mammalian heart and suprarenals. Acta physiol. scand. **24**, Suppl. 85 (1951).

GUNN, J. A.: The action of histamine on the heart and coronary vessels. J. Pharmacol. exp. Ther. **29**, 325—337 (1926).

HÖKFELT, B.: Noradrenaline and adrenaline in mammalian tissues. Distribution under normal and pathological conditions with special reference to the endocrine system. Acta physiol. scand. **25**, Suppl. 92 (1951).

HOLTZ, P.: Über die Wirkung von Cholinestern und biogenen Aminen am isolierten Vorhof des Herzens. Acta Neuroveg. **21**, 445—460 (1960).

KOCH, J., and J. SZERB: Liberation of histamine by adrenaline from isolated lung. Arch. int. pharmacodyn. **81**, 91—98 (1950).

KONZETT, H.: The effect of histamine on an isolated sympathetic ganglion. J. Mt. Sinai Hosp. **19**, 149—153 (1952).
KOSHTOJANZ, CH. S., D. E. RIVKINA and R. L. MITROPOLITANSKAYA: System histamine-histidine decarboxylase-histaminase in the nerve tissue of homiothermal animals subjected to different conditions. C. r. Acad. Sci. U.R.SS. **49**, 381 (1945).
KOTTEGODA, S. R.: Stimulation of isolated rabbit auricles by substances which stimulate ganglia. Brit. J. Pharmacol. **8**, 83—86 (1953).
KRONEBERG, G., u. H. J. SCHÜMANN: Die Wirkung des Reserpins auf den Hormongehalt des Nebennierenmarks. Naunyn-Schmiedeberg's Arch. exp. Path. Pharmak. **231**, 349—360 (1957).
KWIATKOWSKI, H.: Histamine in nervous tissue. J. Physiol. (Lond.) **102**, 32—41 (1943).
LAMBERT, E., and S. R. ROSENTHAL: Study of skin histamine (with some results of splanchnic nerve stimulation). Proc. Soc. exp. Biol. (N.Y.) **52**, 302 (1943).
MACMILLAN, W. H.: Effects of histamine on skeletal muscle. J. Pharmacol. exp. Ther. **113**, 35 (1955).
MANGER, W. M., B. E. SCHWARZ, C. W. BAARS, K. G. WAKIM, J. L. BOLLMAN, M. C. PETERSEN and J. BERKSON: Epinephrine and arterenol (norepinephrine) in mental disease. Arch. Neurol. Psychiat. (Chic.) **78**, 396—412 (1957).
MANNAIONI, P. F.: Interaction between histamine and dichloroisoproterenol, hexamethonium, pempidine, and diphenhydramine, in normal and reserpine-treated heart preparations. Brit. J. Pharmacol. **15**, 500—505 (1960).
MONGAR, J. L., and R. F. WHELAN: Histamine release by adrenaline and D-tubocurarine in the human subject. J. Physiol. (Lond.) **120**, 146—154 (1953).
MORAN, N. C., and M. E. PERKINS: Adrenergic blockade of the mammalian heart by a dichloro analogue of isoproterenol. J. Pharmacol. exp. Ther. **124**, 223—237 (1958).
PATON, W. D. M., and W. L. M. PERRY: The relationship between depolarization and block in the cats superior cervical ganglion. J. Physiol. (Lond.) **119**, 43—57 (1953).
—, and E. J. ZAIMIS: Actions and clinical assessment of drugs which produce neuromuscular block. Lancet **1950 II**, 568—570.
PENNA, M., A. ILLANES, M. UBILLA and S. MUJICA: Effect of histamine and of the anaphylactic reaction on isolated guinea-pig atria. Circulat. Res. **7**, 521—526 (1959).
PEPEU, G., R. MASI and A. GIOTTI: Nicotine-like actions of ephedrine on isolated guinea-pig auricles. Arch. int. pharmacodyn. **119**, 334—344 (1959).
POWELL, C. E., and I. H. SLATER: Blocking of inhibitory adrenergic receptors by a dichloro analog of isoproterenol. J. Pharmacol. exp. Ther. **122**, 480—488 (1958).
RIVKINA, D. E.: Comparative examinations of the acetylcholine contents and the system histidinedecarboxilase-histaminase of nerves in irritation. Bjull. eksp. biol. med. **24**, 53—57 (1947).
ROBINSON, R. L., and K. E. JOCHIM: Histamine and anaphylaxis on adrenal medullary secretion in dogs. Amer. J. Physiol. **199**, 429—432 (1960).
ROOT, M.: Certain aspects of the vasopressor action of pilocarpine. J. Pharmacol. exp. Ther. **101**, 125—131 (1951).
ROTH, G. M., and W. F. KVALE: A tentative test for pheochromocytoma. Amer. J. med. Sci. **210**, 653—660 (1945).
SCHAEPDRYVER, A. F. DE: Physio-pharmacological effects on suprarenal secretion of adrenaline and noradrenaline in dogs. Arch. int. pharmacodyn. **121**, 222—253 (1959).
SCHENK, E. A., and E. G. ANDERSON: The effect of histamine on neuromyal blocking agents. J. Pharmacol. exp. Ther. **122**, 234—238 (1958).
SIEHE, H. J.: Die Reaktion des denervierten Nebennierenmarkes auf humorale Sekretionsreize. Arch. ges. Physiol. **234**, 204—209 (1934).
SLATER, I. H., and P. E. DRESEL: The pressor effect of histamine after autonomic ganglionic blockade. J. Pharmacol. exp. Ther. **105**, 101—107 (1952).
STAUB, H.: Mechanism of action of adrenaline. Schweiz. med. Wschr. **76**, 818 (1946).
—, u. W. GRASSMANN: Über die Wirkungsgrenze einiger Gifte am isolierten Säugetierherzen. Naunyn-Schmiedeberg's Arch. exp. Path. Pharmak. **154**, 317—341 (1930).
SUZUKI, T.: Adrenaline load of suprarenal glands of rabbits in histamine poisoning. Tohoku J. exp. Med. **54**, 289—293 (1951).
SZCZYGIELSKI, J.: Die adrenalinabsondernde Wirkung des Histamins und ihre Beeinflussung durch Nikotin. Naunyn-Schmiedeberg's Arch. exp. Path. Pharmak. **166**, 319—332 (1932).
TRENDELENBURG, U.: The action of histamine and pilocarpine on the superior cervical ganglion and the adrenal glands of the cat. Brit. J. Pharmacol. **9**, 481—487 (1954).
— The potentiation of ganglionic transmission by histamine and pilocarpine. J. Physiol. (Lond.) **129**, 337—351 (1955).
— The action of histamine, pilocarpine and 5-hydroxytryptamine on transmission through the superior cervical ganglion. J. Physiol. (Lond.) **135**, 66—72 (1957a).

TRENDLENBURG, U.: Stimulation of sympathetic centers by histamine. Circulat. Res. **5**, 105—110 (1957b).

— The action of morphine on the superior cervical ganglion and on the nictitating membrane of the cat. Brit. J. Pharmacol. **12**, 79—85 (1957c).

— The pressor response of the cat to histamine and pilocarpine. J. Pharmacol. exp. Ther. **131**, 65—72 (1961).

TRIPOD, J., E. WIRZ et R. MEIER: Influence de l'histamine sur l'activité cardiaque du chat. Arch. int. pharmacodyn. **88**, 51—62 (1951).

TRUEX, R. E.: Chromaffin tissue of the sympathetic ganglia and heart. Anat. Rec. **108**, 687—693 (1950).

VIOTTI, C.: Action de l'histamine sur le coeur et importance de l'atropine à cet égard. (Action of histamine on heart and action of atropin in this respect.) C. R. Soc. Biol. (Paris) **91**, 1085—1088 (1924).

WADA, M., K. FUZII, H. SIBUTA and H. SAKURAI: The action of histamine upon the epinephrine secretion from the suprarenal gland in non-anaesthetized dogs. Tohoku J. exp. Med. **37**, 442—465 (1940).

WENT, I., u. E. VARGA: Experimentelle Untersuchungen über die chemische Gegenregulation des Blutdruckes. Acta physiol. Acad. Sci. hung. **3**, 377—393 (1952).

— — E. SZÜCS u. O. FEHÉR: Eine Analyse der sympathomimetischen Wirkung des Histamins an isolierten Säugetierherzpräparaten. Acta physiol. Acad. Sci. hung. **5**, 121—130 (1954).

WENT, S., u. K. LISSÁK: Histamin und Proteinwirkung am normalen und sensibilisierten Meerschweinchenherz. Naunyn-Schmiedeberg's Arch. exp. Path. Pharmak. **179**, 609—615 (1935).

— E. VARGA, E. SZÜCS u. O. FEHÉR: Über eine sympathomimetische Wirkung des Histamins. Naunyn-Schmiedeberg's Arch. exp. Path. Pharmak. **215**, 129—132 (1952).

WERLE, E., u. D. PALM: Histamin in Nerven II. Biochem. Z. **320**, 322—334 (1950).

— — Histamin in Nerven. III. Biochem. Z. **323**, 255—264 (1952).

—, u. G. WEICKEN: Über das Vorkommen von Histamin in Nerven. Biochem. Z. **319**, 457—462 (1949).

WOODS, E. F., J. A. RICHARDSON, A. K. RICHARDSON and R. F. BOZEMAN: Plasma concentrations of epinephrine and arterenol following the actions of various agents on the adrenals. J. Pharmacol. exp. Ther. **116**, 351—355 (1956).

Chapter 3

Release of Histamine

Section A

Release of Histamine by Animal Venoms and Bacterial Toxins

By

W. T. BERALDO and W. DIAS DA SILVA

With 12 Figures

I. Introduction

The problem of release of histamine by animal venoms and bacterial toxins was born out from earlier experiments described by BRUCE (1910) in which he claimed that the reddening and swelling that follow the instillation of mustard oil into the conjunctival sac of the rabbit are dependent upon the integrity of the conjunctival nerves. STEVENSON and REID (1915) repeated BRUCE's experiments and could not reproduce his findings. GROLL (1922), HIRSCHFELDER (1924), NAKAMURA and TAKAHASHI (1924), TANNENBERG and DEGENER (1925), HANZLIK (1926), TAINTER and REICHERT (1928) using several local anesthetics were unanimous in their findings that the chemosis produced by mustard oil in the anesthetized eye is not appreciably different from the opposite non-anesthetized control.

LEWIS (1927) has found that in the human skin the inflammatory reaction consists of three distinct phases: an initial reddening followed by the wheal and finally by the appearance of a flare. He postulated that the stimulus elicits the signs of inflammation not directly, but indirectly when the cells are injured by any kind of noxious agent releasing a histamine-like substance (H-substance). Since then experimental evidence in support of this view has been obtained in anaphylaxis and other kinds of cell injury (see corresponding Sections of this Chapter).

As the acute effects of snake venoms resemble those of histamine and anaphylaxis and as such venoms are considered general cytolytic poisons (KELLAWAY, 1929; ESSEX and MARKOWITZ, 1930 a, b), KELLAWAY and LE MESSURIER (1936) tried to demonstrate that this similarity might probably be due to the liberation of histamine by venoms. Though in a first attempt to demonstrate this fact KELLAWAY and LE MESSURIER (1936) failed, FELDBERG and KELLAWAY (1937 a) however, were able to show a histamine release from the perfused guinea-pig and cat lungs by several kinds of snake venoms.

Many other animal venoms and bacterial toxins have been intensively investigated, as far as their ability in producing cell damage and histamine release are concerned. *In vivo*, the aggression by such noxious agents produces local and general symptoms. Pain, erythema, swelling and urticarial eruptions occur frequently. Symptoms of systemic intoxication revealed by repeated vomiting, defecation, urination and circulatory collapse are observed. Gastrointestinal congestion and hemorrhage in dogs and pulmonary emphysema in the guinea-pig were found very often at necropsy. *In vitro*, cell injury has been usually evaluated by the capacity of the noxious agent of releasing histamine and protein from perfused organs.

Besides histamine many other pharmacologically active substances can be released when tissue is injured. As shown by WATERS et al. (1938) heparin is released from dog's liver during anaphylactic and peptone shock. FELDBERG and KELLAWAY (1937 b) found in experiments on perfused guinea-pig lungs that the perfusate, after the injection of bee venom caused not only a rapid contraction due to histamine but sometimes also a delayed and slow contraction of the isolated ileum of the guinea-pig. Similar effect was also observed on the perfused lungs and liver of dogs and monkeys with cobra venom (FELDBERG and KELLAWAY, 1938 a). Slow reacting substances (SRS) have been also found when tissue is damaged by other kinds of injury such as those produced by *Clostridium welchii*, Type D toxin (KELLAWAY et al. 1940) and trypsin (TRETHEWIE, 1942). The appearance of SRS frequently coincides with the release of histamine.

Adenyl compounds are also released when tissues are injured (TRETHEWIE, 1942; KELLAWAY et al. 1940). The role played by SRS and adenyl compounds in the biochemical and pharmacological mechanism of cell injury is still unknown.

The term SRS, as currently used, means a slow type of contraction of the guinea-pig ileum produced by perfusates of isolated organs or tissue extracts after contact with the venoms. Up to now, at least three active substances have been isolated which probably share some of the properties of SRS. Bradykinin, a basic polyptide released from blood by snake venoms and trypsin (ROCHA e SILVA et al. 1949) appears in the blood during anaphylactic and peptone shock in dogs (BERALDO, 1950). SRS-A, seems to be an acidic substance with a certain though not predominant lipid-solubility, found in perfusates from shocked human asthmatic lung and shocked isolated guinea-pig lungs (BROCKLEHURST, 1956). SRS-C is an unsaturated fatty acid derived from lecithin, first observed by FELDBERG and KELLAWAY (1937b, 1938a), and FELDBERG et al. (1938) during an investigation on the mode of action of bee and cobra venoms and further studied by VOGT (1956). The subject was recently reviewed by VOGT (1958).

Finally, serotonin (5-hydroytryptamine) whose role in the anaphylactic and anaphylactoid reaction of the rat, the mouse and the rabbit has been recently discussed (See corresponding Section of this Chapter).

As already mentioned concomitantly with the release of active substances, a certain degree of tissue damage was observed, as shown by morphologic alterations of perfused organs and the presence of protein in the perfusates (FELDBERG and KELLAWAY, 1938a). Using adequate histological techniques it has been possible to demonstrate that characteristic cell damage confined to certain types of cells takes place. Clumping and disintegration of leucocytes and platelets were observed in dogs liver after the injection of trypsin, peptone *Ascaris* extract and the specific antigen (ROCHA E SILVA and TEIXEIRA, 1946; ROCHA E SILVA et al. 1946; ROCHA E SILVA, 1946). Histologic alterations of liver mast cells in the dog were observed by WILANDER (1938) in peptone shock and by JAQUES and WATERS (1941) in anaphylactic shock. These findings supported the conclusion that the heparin present in the blood during anaphylactic and peptone shock originates from the liver mast cells. Similar histologic alterations of the mast cells not only in the dog, but also in other species, were related to the liberation of histamine and serotonin (RILEY, 1953; MOTA et al. 1953; BHATTACHARYA and LEWIS, 1956). Morphologic alterations of the enterochromaffin cell were recently demonstrated by GERSHON and ROSS (1962) in the anaphylactic shock in mice. These alterations are consistent with the participation of serotonin in the mechanism of anaphylactic shock in these animals.

Among the active substances found when tissue is damaged, histamine has been the most extensively investigated. The present Section deals mainly with the histamine release by animal venoms and bacterial toxins.

II. Methods usually employed to demonstrate histamine release

Until recently, the ways by which histamine could be mobilized from tissue stores were relatively few. However, the field has been extraordinarily extended after the work of ALAM et al. (1939), ROCHA E SILVA and SCHILD (1949), MACINTOSH and PATON (1949) which started a new line of research on histamine release.

The methods commonly used for the study of the release of histamine can be divided into three general items consisting of:

A. *In vivo*, experiments.
B. Experiments using isolated organs and tissues.
C. Experiments in which isolated cells and intracellular particles are used.

A. In vivo, experiments

1. Increase of histamine in blood, lymph, urine and peritoneal fluid

A simple method consists of an intravenous injection of the releaser followed by taking blood or lymph samples at suitable time intervals.

Using this method DRAGSTEDT and GEBAUER-FUELNEGG (1932), GEBAUER-FUELNEGG and DRAGSTEDT (1932) demonstrated, for the first time, an increase of blood and lymph histamine in dogs after the injection of the specific antigen. A similar method permitted MACINTOSH and PATON (1949) to discover certain organic bases which release histamine. These authors studying the effect of licheniformin, an antibiotic polypeptide extracted from *Bacillus licheniformis*, found a characteristic lowering of the cat's arterial blood pressure. It was the correct analysis of a very small diference between the depressor effect of histamine and that of licheniformin which led to the discovery of a new class of histamine liberators. With histamine the fall started within a few seconds, with licheniformin, a histamine releaser, there was a delay of 20 to 25 seconds between injection and appearance of the depressor effect (Fig. 1). MONGAR and WHELAN (1953) investigated the histamine releasing activity of adrenaline and D-tubocurarine in man injecting the drugs into the brachial artery and estimating the histamine released in the venous blood collected from an anticubital vein of the same arm. Adrenaline did not produce any rise in histamine level and the injection of D-tubocurarine resulted in over 20-fold increases in plasma histamine. The method presents inconveniences owing to technical difficulties inherent to experiments performed in human beings.

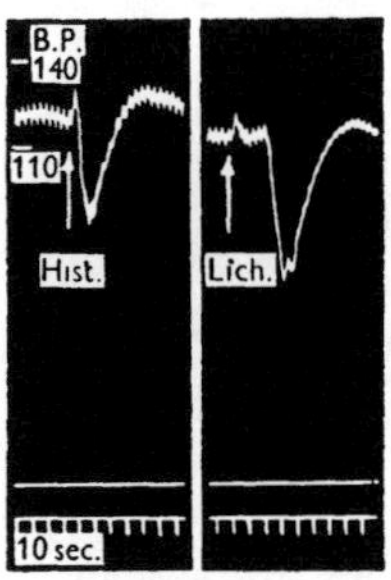

Fig. 1. Cat, chloralose: blood pressure. Hist., injection of 0.2 μg/kg of histamine. Lich., injection of 0.95 mg/kg of licheniformin hydrochloride

Another method using intact animals was described by FAWCETT (1954). This method consists of injecting the histamine releaser, dissolved in large volume of Tyrode solution, into the peritoneal cavity of the rat. Fifteen to twenty minutes after injection, samples of the peritoneal fluid were withdrawn and assayed for histamine and histologic examination of the mast cells. This is a very convenient method to study simultaneously histamine release and the alterations in the morphology of the mast cells.

Wilson (1954), on the basis of previous experiments by Anrep et al. (1944), developed a method for studying histamine release, using the urinary excretion of histamine in the rat. This method gives a quantitative measure of the way in which the animal reacts to the histamine releaser and permits the comparison of the effects of different liberators under the same experimental conditions and provides the means of investigating histamine metabolism and the factors which influence it.

2. Increase of HCl gastric secretion

Determination of free HCl in gastric secretion is a very sensitive method for detecting a gradual release of histamine for long periods of time. Using this method, Tinel and Ungar (1935) demonstrated an increase of gastric acid secretion by heating to 50°C the hind paw of the cat. This increased acid secretion was attributed to the histamine release. Feldberg and Holmes (1941) using this method were able to demonstrate histamine release during decerebrate rigidity, stimulation of motor nerves and after injection of curarine.

3. Increase of capillary permeability

The first demonstration of the increase of capillary permeability producing a wheal, was presented by Ebbecke (1923) showing that if trypan blue (a colloidal dye) was injected into the blood stream, it appeared in the area of the wheal. Since, normally, the vessel walls retain the dye confining it to the blood stream, Ebbecke's experiment was a clear demonstration of increased vascular permeability in the area of the wheal. The simple production of a wheal by intradermal injection of morphine was reported by Pilcher and Sollmann (1924). Since then, the method has been used by many investigators to test histamine-releasing

Table 1. *Histamine content of various regions of skin of guinea-pigs weighing 400—600 g*

Site	Histamine in μg/g skin							Mean values (abdominal skin taken as unity)
	Expt. 1	Expt. 2	Expt. 3	Expt. 4	Expt. 5	Expt. 6	Expt. 7	
Ear margin	—	—	—	18.5	14.0	14.7	14.0	5.9
Ear base	—	—	—	12.5	10.3	13.0	12.0	4.6
Submental	15.5	—	17.2	12.0	11.2	13.3	10.5	4.5
Areola of nipples	15.5	—	14.2	—	—	—	11.3	3.7
Lids	11.0	—	8.9	11.5	10.0	—	—	3.7
Bristle area	13.0	—	11.5	7.3	10.5	—	—	3.6
Anal margin	—	—	—	6.0	—	8.7	11.7	3.1
Paws; forelegs	—	—	—	7.0	5.8	11.4	5.9	2.9
Paws; hind-legs	—	—	—	6.8	5.6	8.0	4.3	2.7
Vertex	10.0	9.2	8.9	8.0	5.8	—	—	2.6
Lips and nose	11.0	—	11.5	6.0	—	7.2	6.6	2.6
Cheek	—	—	—	5.0	—	7.6	8.5	2.4
Fore-leg	—	—	—	5.0	6.2	6.7	—	2.4
Scrotum	5.0	—	—	—	—	6.5	—	1.7
Abdomen	4.0	4.0	3.8	2.4	2.1	3.0	3.2	1.0
Calf	—	—	—	—	2.0	4.0	2.5	1.0
Back (middle lumbar)	3.0	3.8	4.2	2.4	1.5	2.6	2.2	0.9
Thigh	—	—	—	—	1.2	2.9	1.5	0.7

activity of several compounds (MacIntosh and Paton, 1949; Bain, et al. 1949; Collier and Macauley, 1952). Using this method Feldberg and Miles (1953) found that the regional pattern of blueing was related to the histamine content of the skin. (Figs. 2, 3 and Table 1)

Other applications of this method to show release of histamine under varying experimental conditions will be presented in other parts of this Section.

B. Isolated organs and tissues

1. Perfusion of isolated organs and tissues

The method consists of irrigating organs or fragments of tissues through their vascular system with Ringer, Locke, Tyrode or Jalon solutions to which the histamine releaser is added. Defibrinated and

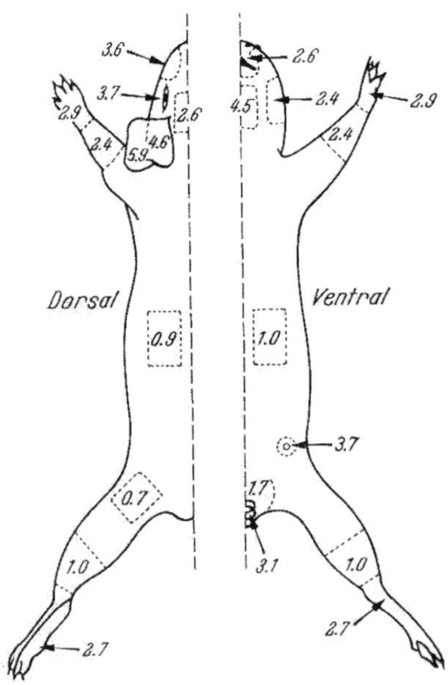

Fig. 2

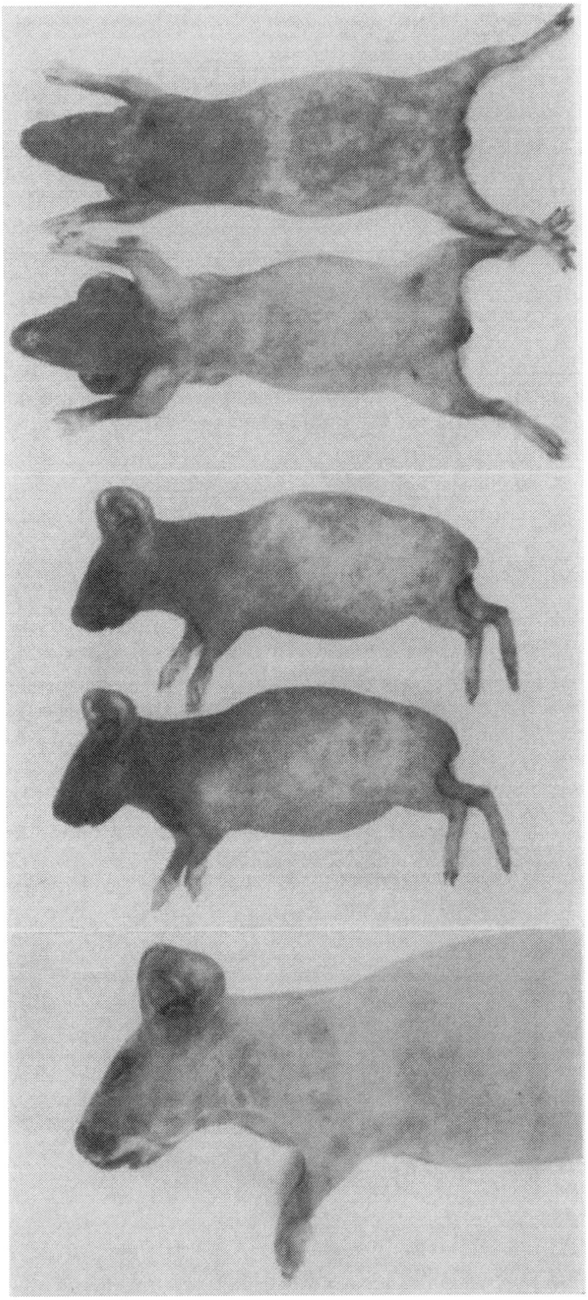

Fig. 3

Fig. 2. Distribution of histamine in various regions of guinea-pig's skin. The figures are those given in the last column of Table 1 and represent mean values for each region, the abdominal skin being taken as unity

Fig. 3. Blueing of the skin after intravenous injection of 48/80 into three guinea-pigs with pontamine blue in their circulation. Animals A and B were killed after full blueing had developed and depilated. Guinea-pig C was killed before the blueing was complete to show the early blueing round the lips, nose, eyes and ears. The depilation of this animal is incomplete; the white areas round the mouth and along the base of the jaw are remnants of hair whole blood has also been used. The pressure, temperature, oxygen supply are controlled, according to the purpose of the experiment.

By perfusing the sensitized guinea-pig lung BARTOSCH et al. (1932) presented conclusive evidence relating a liberation of histamine to the contact of the antigen with sensitized tissues. This method consisted of perfusing guinea-pig lungs from the pulmonary artery with Tyrode solution and collecting the venous outflow for assay from a cannula tied into the left auricle. The antigen was injected into the arterial perfusion cannula. For the preparation of the guinea-pig lungs the animal was killed by a blow on the head. The trachea and lungs were exposed, a cannula tied into the trachea and the pericardium opened. The lower half of the animal was cut away proximal to the diaphragm; cannulae were quickly tied

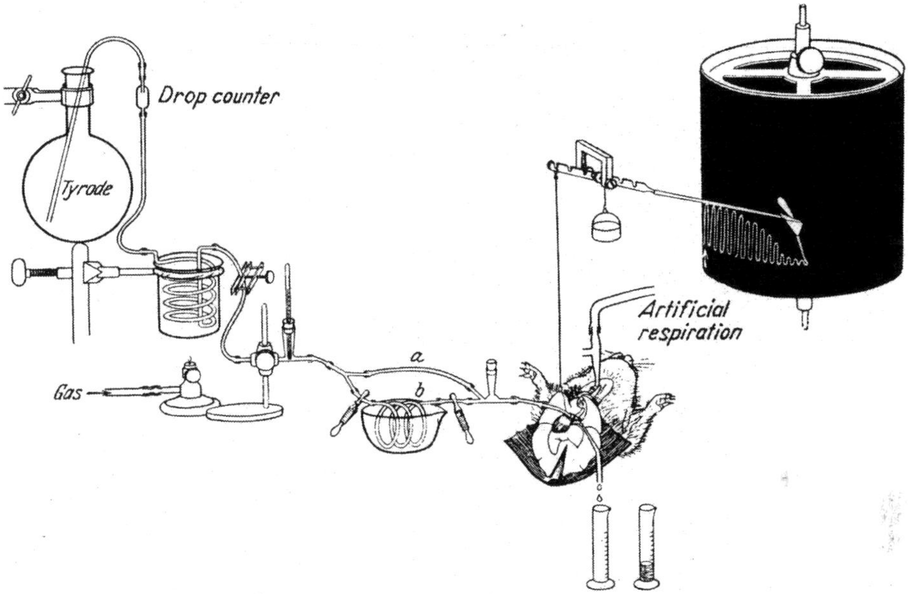

Fig. 4. Perfusion of sensitized isolated guinea-pig lungs. Effect of the antigen on the inflation of air into the lungs

into the pulmonary artery and left auricle, perfusion was started and the aorta tied. The lungs were ventilated rhythmically 9-14 times per min. from a positive pressure pump. The presence of histamine in perfusates was estimated on the guinea-pig ileum and on the cat blood pressure (Figs. 4 and 5).

Since blood was not used, the cellular theory of anaphylaxis received an important support from this experiment. Perfusion of lungs of other species (dog, cat and monkey) has also been used (FELDBERG and KELLAWAY, 1937b, 1938a) to demonstrate liberation of histamine by snake venoms.

Perfusion of the isolated liver is another method used to demonstrate histamine release. FELDBERG and KELLAWAY (1937b, 1938a) were able to show histamine release from dog's liver by perfusing the organ with cobra venom. The perfusion is performed inserting a cannula into the portal vein. The cannula makes connection with a reservoir containing Tyrode solution. The hepatic artery is clamped. The animal is bled through a cannula inserted into the carotid artery. After ligation of the rami to the portal vein distal to the cannula, the left and central lobes of the liver are tied off and excised. The organ is transferred to an appropriate warm chamber from which the perfusates are collected. Injections of the histamine releaser are made into rubber tubing connecting the cannula with the perfusing system.

Perfusing the isolated sensitized dog's liver with Tyrode solution or defibrinated blood to which the antigen or *Ascaris* extracts were added, ROCHA E SILVA and GRAÑA (1946b) were unable to obtain histamine release from this organ. SCROGGIE and JAQUES (1949), perfused sensitized liver, *in situ*, as follows: the inferior vena cava in the thorax was clamped. The abdominal aorta and inferior vena cava were ligated above the level of the kidneys but below the superior mesenteric artery. During the experiment the dog was perfused with blood through a cannula

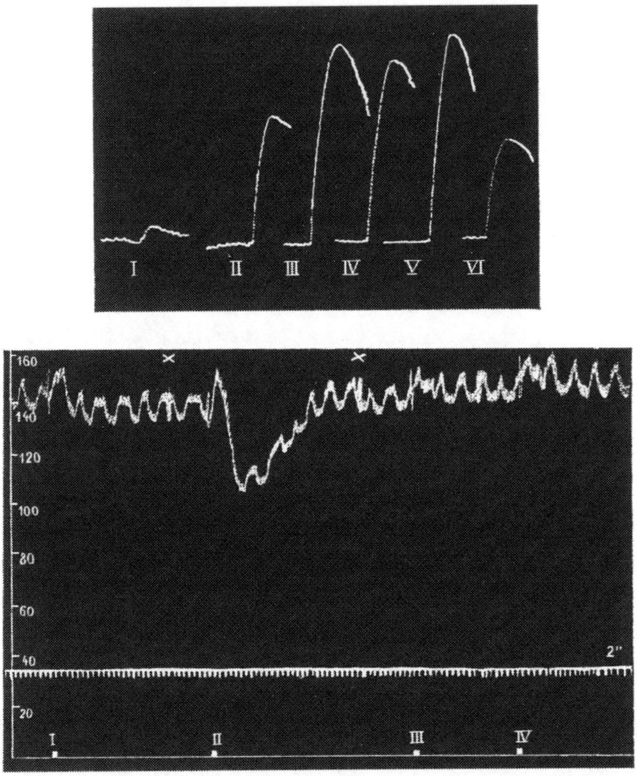

Fig. 5. Assays of perfusates on the guinea-pig ileum and on the cat blood pressure

inserted into the brachial vein. The antigen was injected into the portal vein. Blood samples were collected for histamine and heparin assays from the clamped inferior vena cava below the diaphragm. Using this preparation the Canadian authors were able to demonstrate release of significant amounts of histamine and heparin from the dog's liver.

These experiments show that the blood, although not absolutely essential to the anaphylactic reaction, must in some way contribute to the reaction. The discrepancy observed in the experiments above, when dog's liver is perfused, showed that different results can be obtained when different conditions of perfusion are employed. Blood proved to be definitely superior to Tyrode solution as a perfusing fluid, maintaining the tissues in good physiological conditions for the reaction leading to the release of histamine.

The perfusion of the cat's skin flap was shown to be one of the most sensitive preparations for detecting histamine release (FELDBERG and PATON, 1951). An area of skin from the right hindleg, supplied by the saphenous artery was perfused with Locke solution. The skin was cut by two incisions right round the leg, one about 4-6 cm above the knee joint, the other about 2 cm above the ankle. The two incisions were joined by a further incision along the lateral aspect of the leg. The saphenous vein was tied and cut, at the border of lower circular incision. The skin was then dissected off from the underlying structures, starting from the longitudinal incision and working from both sides to the center where the saphenous artery and vein enter and leave it. The saphenous artery and vein up to the femoral vessels were carefully isolated. The femoral artery below the origin of the saphenous was ligated and cut. A cannula, connected with a reservoir by means of a rubber tubing, was inserted into the femoral artery above the saphenous. Another cannula was tied into the femoral vein above the saphenous vein, for the collection of the venous effluent. The entirely isolated patch of skin was transferred to a warmed paraffin bath. Injections of the histamine liberators were made through the rubber tubing which connects the cannula with the reservoir.

By using this preparation FELDBERG and SCHACHTER (1952) showed the release of histamine from the skin of the cat by horse serum without previous sensitization of the animal. This was a direct demonstration of the release of histamine in a non-sensitized animal by a foreign protein.

Perfusion of the gastrocnemius muscle has also been used to demonstrate histamine release (FELDBERG and PATON, 1951). The isolated muscle was perfused through a cannula inserted into its artery and the venous effluent collected from a cannula tied into its vein. All branches of the popliteal vessels not supplying the gastrocnemius muscle were ligated and cut. The histamine liberators were injected through the artery cannula after the venous effluent had become free of blood and control samples had been collected.

Using perfused hind quarters (muscle and skin) of the rat FELDBERG and MONGAR (1954) studied comparatively the liberation of histamine by compound 48/80 and octylamine. For the perfusion of the hind quarters a cannula was inserted into the lower abdominal aorta and the venous outflow collected from a cannula in the vena cava. A mass ligature was firmly tied around the body proximal to the cannulation sites and the upper half of the animal cut off.

Perfusion of the isolated rabbit's ear was used by SCHACHTER (1953) to study histamine release by antigen and by 48/80. The entire ear was removed after cutting away excess fur and clipped on to a sloping square piece of glass. A needle cannula connected with the perfusion system was inserted into the central artery of the ear. The perfusates were run along the margin of the supporting glass plate and were collected as they dropped. The histamine releasers were injected through a rubber tubing into the central artery.

More recently, UVNÄS (1955) reported a method for the study of histamine liberation from the isolated paw of the cat. The tibial or the radial artery was cannulated with plastic tubing connected with the perfusion system. The perfusates oozed from the cut surface and were collected in a plastic disc which drained into a test tube. Using this method HÖGBERG et al. (1956) studied histamine release by *Ascaris* and jelly-fish extracts.

2. Sliced and minced tissues

UNGAR and PARROT (1936) were the first to demonstrate the histamine release in anaphylaxis using tissue slices. These authors suspended the isolated ileum of a normal guinea-pig in Tyrode solution containing lung slices from a sensitized guinea-pig. The addition of the specific antigen produced a contraction of the ileum which was due to the histamine released from the lung slices. A modification of this method was introduced by SCHILD (1937, 1939), allowing the study of the release of histamine on a quantitative basis. More recently MONGAR and SCHILD (1953) improved the method, using samples of lung tissues obtained

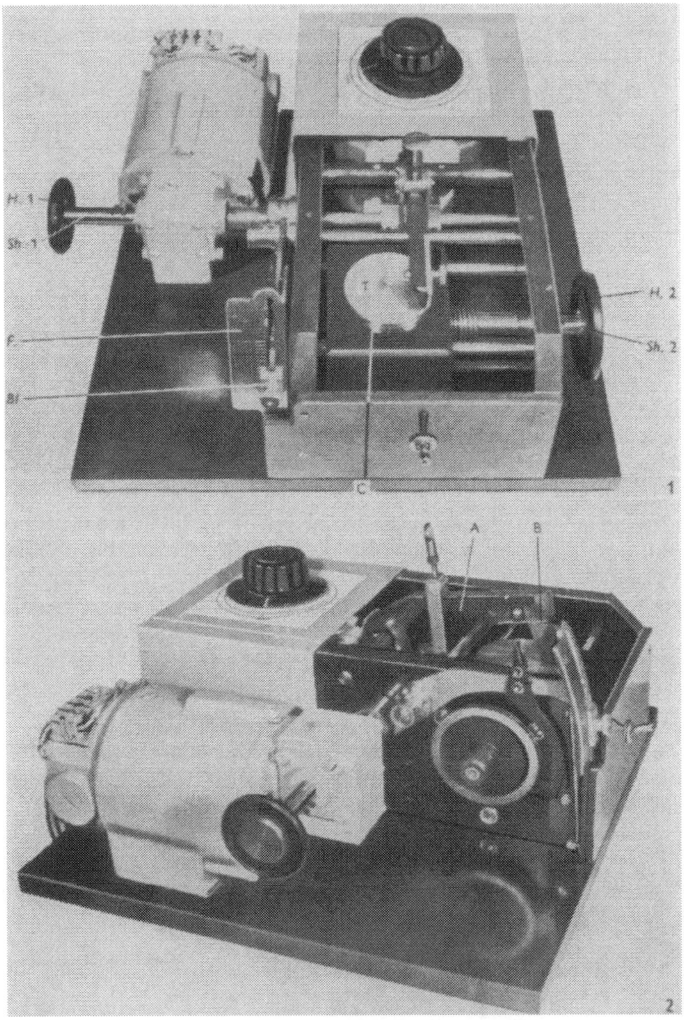

Fig. 6. The chopper. *A*, cutting-arm carrying blade *B*; *H* 1, handwheel on shaft *Sh* 1 which also carries the two cams; *H* 2, handwheel on shaft *Sh* 2 which also carries the leadscrew. *T*, cutting table on the carriage *C* which is moved by the leadscrew. *Bl*, adjustable block whose position in the frame *F* conditions the thickness of section cut

with a MCILWAIN tissue chopper (MCILWAIN and BUDDLE, 1953). This apparatus (Fig. 6) gives tissue slices of uniform size and in good physiological conditions for *in vitro* experiments. Tissue samples so obtained were then incubated at 37°C, for 15min. with the nutrient fluid containing the histamine releaser.

Fragments of other tissues than rat diaphragm and the skin are also frequently used. The technique using sliced and minced tissues has the advantage of standardization of all conditions for histamine release, which has permitted the study of the enzymatic processes involved in the mechanism of histamine release. (See other Sections of this Chapter).

C. Isolated cells and intracellular particles

1. Isolated cells

As first shown by KATZ (1940) when the antigen is added to sensitized rabbit's blood, there is a shift of histamine from the formed elements to plasma. Heparinized blood collected from a sensitized rabbit was incubated at 37°C for a certain interval of time with antigen, *in vitro*. After centrifugation the histamine content of the plasma was found to increase as compared with the control. These findings have been confirmed as far as the antigen is concerned and extended to histamine releasers (ROSE and BROWNE, 1940; KATZ and COHEN, 1941; DRAGSTEDT and ROCHA E SILVA, 1941; GOTZL and DRAGSTEDT, 1942; MCINTIRE et al. 1951; HAINING, 1956).

The striking positive correlation observed between mast cell number and histamine content as found in many tissues by RILEY and WEST (1952) suggested that mast cells are containers of histamine. WILANDER (1938), JAQUES and WATERS (1941) observed alteration of mast cell in conditions in which heparin and histamine liberation occurred. RILEY (1952) and MOTA et al. (1953) called attention to the fact that histamine releasers disrupt mast cells, thus supporting the hypothesis that histamine arises from mast cells. Further progress along this line was accumulated after development of a technique which permitted separation of normal mast cells from other cellular elements and tissue fluids. The method is based on differential centrifugation of rat's peritoneal fluid (PADAWER and GORDON, 1955). With this technique a fraction containing about 75% of mast cells was obtained. MOTA and DIAS DA SILVA (1960) presented results showing that washed isolated mast cells taken from sensitized animals still disrupt when in contact with the specific antigen. Release of histamine and 5-hydroxytryptamine from washed cells of the peritoneal fluid of rats by organic bases was reported by GARCIA-AROCHA (1961). These experiments demonstrated that the presence of other cellular elements or tissular fluid are not necessary for mast cell disruption and histamine release.

2. Intracellular particles

According to TRETHEWIE (1938) histamine is still retained in fragments of tissue when they are divided into small particles. By perfusing the dog's liver FELDBERG and KELLAWAY (1938b) found that the perfusate, obtained after an intraportal injection of staphylococcal toxin, contained cellular debris rich in histamine. COPENHAVER et al. (1953), by means of differential centrifugation of the dog's liver homogenate, pointed out that the mitochondrial fraction contained the major portion of the histamine present in the whole homogenate. However, MOTA et al. (1954) demonstrated that the mitochondrial fraction of the dog's liver was highly contaminated with mast cell granules. It is therefore probable that the higher histamine concentration of that fraction, as found by COPENHAVER et al. (1953), might be due, at least in part, to its contamination with mast cell granules. Besides the liver, other tissues have been used. MOTA et al. (1954) were able to release histamine from isolated rat mast cell granules by heating or contact with compound 48/80. MONGAR and SCHILD (1956) have shown that histamine can be released from intracellular particles of the guinea-pig lung by organic bases. When specific antigen was used, however, histamine release was not observed. The authors concluded that the cell disintegration interrupted a process required for the histamine release in anaphylaxis.

After being released the histamine can be estimated by the usual methods utilizing biological structures or by chemical means, as extensively described in another Chapter of this Book. See also a discussion of such methods by the American group of the Histamine-Club, edited by UNGAR (1961).

III. Release of histamine by animal venoms

Animal venoms are toxic substances secreted by a special glandular tissue and excreted by an appropriated injector apparatus, generally causing lesion when in contact with animal tissues. This Sub-chapter will deal also with toxic substances extracted from the animal body which, when injected into experimental animals or human beings, cause toxic manifestations.

The nature of the animal venoms is extremely complex. Its chemical composition varies according to the species and within the same species, regional differences are also observed. Usually, they are complex enzymatic mixtures containing proteases, lecithinases and hyaluronidase-like enzymes. These agents destroy or digest the tissues and pharmacologically active substances are set free by gross cell damage. Moreover, the venoms themselves may contain active substances such as histamine, 5-hydroxytryptamine (serotonin), bradykinin-like factors, adenyl compounds which may be responsible for, at least, part of their action.

It seemed to us convenient to study the problem of the release of histamine by venoms, following the order of structural complexity of the organisms of the venomous animals.

A. Coelenterata

It was in the Coelenterata that the problem concerned with the histamine release by animal venoms started. GOSSE (1860), for the first time, obtained cutaneous reactions by the local application of anemone tentacles. It was as a consequence of a study on the toxicity of the stinging tentacles of the *Physalia* and *Actinia* that PORTIER and RICHET on the 15th of February 1902 discovered anaphylaxis. From a crude extract of *Actinia* tentacles those investigators obtained three pharmacologically active fractions presenting distinct effects when injected intravenously in dogs. They termed these fractions thalassine, congestine and hypnotoxin, which produced severe and generalized pruritus, pulmonary oedema and sedation, respectively. The chemical nature of these fractions is so far unknown. As far as the pharmacological activity of these fractions is concerned, it should be reviewed in the light of the modern methods of chemical separation. Thalassine, the pruritogenic fraction can be obtained as a stable, dry powder by repeated alcoholic extraction.

JAQUES and SCHACHTER (1954a) demonstrated the release of histamine from perfused cat's skin and whole animal by thalassine. These investigators also showed in the plasma of the injected animals, a substance which produced a delayed slow contraction of the guinea-pig ileum. Thalassine preparations had no effect on the isolated guinea-pig ileum, even in high concentrations. The thalassine preparations so far obtained are rather crude. After the intravenous injection of 10mg/kg in the intact cat a prolonged fall in arterial blood pressure was observed. The fall in blood pressure was regularly delayed for approximately 30 seconds following the injection. This delay is characteristic of substances whose main circulatory depressor action is due to the release of histamine (MACINTOSH and PATON, 1949). It was not demonstrated, however, whether thalassine is a genuine active principle or is dependent on the action of the peptone present in the extracts.

Another Coelenterate which has engaged the attention of biologists and physiologists is the jelly-fish (*Cyanea capillata*). Contact with its tentacles causes burning sensation, itching, pain, redness of the skin and oedema. UVNÄS (1960) demonstrated that extracts obtained from the tentacles contained no histamine, but presented a rather high histamine releasing activity on the cat skin and the perfused cat's paw. The principle was heat stable and soluble in hot absolute alcohol. The histamine-releasing action showed temperature and pH dependence. It was blocked by some enzyme inhibitors (DNP, ninhydrin, etc). The action of the *Cyanea* principle on human skin, however, was not studied.

B. Platyhelminthes

The spontaneous rupture of *Taenia echinococcus* cysts has been reported to cause severe urticaria. Intravenous injection of the fluid of cysts into the rabbit or the guinea-pig killed the animal within a few hours (MOURSON and SCHLAGDENHAUFFEN, 1882 and HUMPHREY, 1887). DEBOVE (1888) induced experimental urticaria after the injection of hydatid fluid in two patients.

MESSINEO and CALAMIDA (1902) investigating the toxicity of an aqueous extract of *Taenia* in the rabbit, guinea-pig and dog, verified that the intravenous injection of an aqueous extract of *Taenia* produced convulsions, paresis of the hind leg and lowering of temperature. The animals recovered completely after 24 hours. MINGAZZINI (1901) found that the extracts of the intestinal worm were very toxic for dogs, guinea-pigs and rabbits. VAULLEGEARD (1901) isolated two different toxic substances from Cestodes and Nematodes, one soluble in alcohol with a curare-like action and the other which was precipitated by alcohol was supposed to act directly on the central nervous system.

The toxicity of the fluid of cysts of *Echinococcus granulosa* has been repeatedly reported (DESSY and MAROTTA, 1912). PARISOT and SIMONIN (1920) and GIUSTI and HUG (1923) have shown that hydatid fluid produced severe to fatal shock when injected intravenously into dogs, cats, guinea-pigs and rabbits. In the dog the symptoms were somewhat similar to those of anaphylactic shock, since there was a fall of carotid blood pressure with tachyphylaxis, leukopenia and incoagulability of the blood. In man, accidents produced by the rupture of hydatid cysts have been reported in several instances (DEW, 1928; LOZANO, 1934). Those accidents were usually attributed to phenomena of sensitization. The rupture of the cysts would bring the system into contact with substances to which the organism had been progressively sensitized and anaphylactic accidents would follow combination of the antigen with the respective antibodies.

GRAÑA et al. (1943) have shown an increase of the histamine content of the blood following injection of hydatid fluid into the veins of dogs and assumed a certain relationship between the release of histamine from the tissues and the fall of carotid blood pressure, which is a constant symptom following the injection of hydatid fluid. ROCHA E SILVA and GRAÑA (1945), reexamining the problem of the histamine release in the dog by the injection of hydatid fluid, found rather a decrease of the total blood histamine. Only in the late stages there was, occasionally, a small increase of the histamine in the venous blood, which occurred frequently when the carotid blood pressure was returning to normal. That a release of histamine accompanies the shock seems to be very probable from data obtained by estimation of the concentrations of histamine in pieces of liver taken before and after injection of hydatid fluid. In four of six animals there was a definite decrease in the histamine content of the liver; however, there was no parallelism between the decrease of the concentration of histamine in the liver and the intensity of the shock. Perfusion of the dog's liver with hydatid fluid did not lead to any appreciable release of histamine. All these facts point to the conclusion that the release of histamine is not seriously concerned with the production of shock in dogs following the injection of hydatid fluid. On the other hand, in no case has there been any indication of the release of slowly reacting substances. The authors discussed the possibility of an unidentified substance as a mediator of the shock produced by hydatid fluid.

C. Nematoda

LINSTROW (1896) had the opportunity to verify that a substance obtained from *Ascaris* produced conjunctivitis and chemosis. CATTANEO (1903) injecting guinea-pigs, intraperitoneally, with a liquid which had been in contact with *Ascaris* observed that the animal showed unrest, paresis and death after 3 to 17 hours. CHANSON (1906) reported that patients infested with *Ascaris* presented conjunctivitis, coryza or laryngitis. SHINAMURA and FUJI (1917) isolated from *Ascaris lumbricoides* an "albumose-peptone" which they designated as "askaron", a very toxic substance for dogs. In 1939 MACHEBOUEF and MANDOUL showed that deproteinized extracts from *Ascaris megalocephala*, when injected intravenously into guinea-pigs, produced a reaction reminiscent of anaphylaxis. BIER (1939) showed that *Ascaris lumbricoides* contained a substance very active in producing an anaphylaxis-like shock in guinea-pigs. ROCHA E SILVA and GRAÑA (1946a, b), using a deproteinized and dialysed extract from *Ascaris lumbricoides*, were able to produce fatal shocks in dogs and guinea-pigs. Further purification of this material led them to identify the active fraction as a proteose of high molecular weight. NAKAJIMA (1954), after heating to 80°C an aqueous extract of *Ascaris lumbricoides*, purified it by alcohol precipitation and obtained an active fraction containing nitrogen and phosphorus. HÖGBERG et al. (1956), precipitating *Ascaris* extracts in alcohol followed by passage through an Amberlite IRC-50 (XE-64) column, obtained an active fraction which released histamine from the perfused paw of the cat.

OLIVER-GONZALEZ and KOPPISCH (1958) studied the effects produced by the injection of substances extracted from tissues of *Ascaris lumbricoides* in the dog, guinea-pig and the mouse. They reported anaphylactoid reactions in the dog. The main pathological findings were congestion of the liver and intestinal veins. Marked decrease in leukocytes, platelets and incoagulability of the blood were also described. The results of these experiments agree with those previously reported by ROCHA E SILVA et al. (1946). OLIVER-GONZALEZ and KOPPISCH (1958) suggested that the autoagglutination of the erythrocytes may have an important role in the effect of *Ascaris* extracts in the dog. The α_2-isoagglutinins would be present in the blood of the animal and A_2-isoagglutinogen-like factor in the *Ascaris* extract. Guinea-pigs and mice, on the other hand, exhibited no symptoms after injection with each *Ascaris* tissue extracts.

Recently, GAZZINELLI et al. (1961) showed that the active fraction of *Ascaris lumbricoides* was a complex substance containing carbohydrate and protein. BERALDO et al. (1961) showed that intravenous injection of a purified fraction produced in the guinea-pig a fatal anaphylaxis-like reaction. These experiments confirm those described by previous investigators. Moreover, the perfusion of the guinea-pig lungs with purified *Ascaris* fractions led to a release of histamine which ranged from 0.9 to 5.8 μg. These results agree with those obtained by BARTOSCH et al. (1932) in guinea-pig lungs perfused with the specific antigen.

The alterations of mast cells produced by purified *Ascaris* fractions were very similar to those induced by anaphylatoxin (MOTA, 1959) or the specific antigen in the sensitized guinea-pig (MOTA and VUGMAN, 1956).

The experiments with the isolated ileum of the guinea-pig (Fig. 7) showed that *Ascaris* fractions were able to produce a strong contraction of this organ, indistinguishable from that induced by anaphylaxis (SCHULTZ, 1910 a, b; DALE, 1913) or by anaphylatoxin (ROTHSCHILD and ROCHA E SILVA, 1954).

MONGAR and SCHILD (1957) showed that previous heating of the sensitized guinea-pig's ileum abolishes the anaphylactic contraction. MOTA (1959) observed that this treatment did not modify the contraction produced by anaphylatoxin.

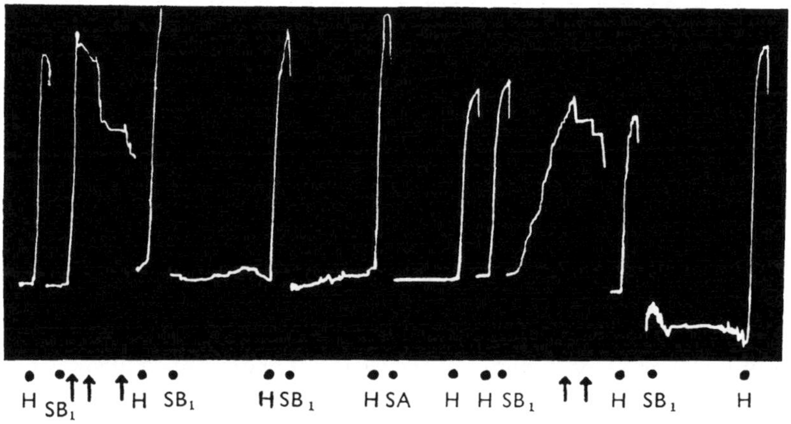

Fig. 7. Guinea-pig ileum suspended in 10 ml. Tyrode solution: H = 0.05 μg histamine. SB_1 = 130 μg *Ascaris* fraction. SA = 10 ml spleen extract precipitate (50% ammonium sulphate saturation) dissolved in distilled water and dialysed against saline, allowed to remain in the bath for 2 hr. The arrows indicate washings with Tyrode solution. The substances were added to the bath at 2 min intervals

Furthermore desensitization to anaphylatoxin did not interfere with the anaphylactic response. Previous heating of the ileum to 45° C abolishes the contraction produced by *Ascaris* fraction. The desensitization by anaphylatoxin, on the other hand, has no effect on the contraction. These experiments excluded the participation of the anaphylatoxin and suggested an antigen-antibody reaction in the mechanism of this contraction.

This problem was further studied by sensitization of ilea by spleen extract *in vitro*. It was observed that a 50% saturation ammonium sulphate precipitate obtained from spleen extract retains the ability of sensitizing the ileum. The possibility of spontaneous or non-specific resensitization, in the absence of sensitizing spleen extract, was excluded by experiments of spleen extract from guinea-pigs with ilea insensitive to the *Ascaris* fractions. These experiments supported the view that we were dealing with a passive sensitization by antibodies present in spleen extract. Fig. 7 shows one of these experiments. These results do not imply that spleen extracts are richer in antibodies than serum, for in the experiments presented above no comparative study was undertaken.

Those guinea-pigs in which the intravenous injections of the *Ascaris* fractions did not cause any effect also showed no mast cell damage. In such guinea-pigs the ilea proved insensitive to the *Ascaris* fractions and the release of histamine from the lungs did not occur.

In vitro experiments (DIAS DA SILVA et al. 1961) showed that purified fractions of *Ascaris* extracts released histamine from slices of guinea-pig lung and produced mast cells degranulation in the mesentery. Both processes were inhibited by the inhibitors of anaphylaxis. On the basis of the experiments described by GAZZINELLI et al. (1961), BERALDO et al. (1961) and DIAS DA SILVA et al. (1961) it is suggested that all effects produced by *Ascaris* extracts on the guinea-pig depend on a natural sensitization of the animals to the antigens likely present in the *Ascaris lumbricoides*.

DIAMANT (1961) claimed that injections of *Ascaris* extracts caused negligible histamine release, as compared with the controls. Degranulated mast cells were in no case observed in the guinea-pig mesentery after intraperitoneal injection of the *Ascaris* extract. Guinea-pigs, therefore, are considered by the author not to be susceptible to the effect of the *Ascaris* extract in the concentrations used. These results agree with those previously reported by OLIVER-GONZALEZ and KOPPISH (1958). Both the results presented by DIAMANT (1961) and OLIVER-GONZALEZ and KOPPISH (1958) disagree with those reported by other authors. DIAMANT (1961), however, presented results obtained from experiments performed in 3 guinea-pigs, injected intraperitoneally, one of them being used as control animal. As far as the results presented by OLIVER-GONZALEZ and KOPPISCH (1958) are concerned, a plausible explanation for their findings is the difference in the method of extraction used, since they extracted the material at pH 8.9, whereas the majority of authors extracted it with an acid solution.

HÖGBERG et al. (1956) compared the 48/80 and *Ascaris* extract histamine-releasing ability on the perfused paw of the cat. They found that the *Ascaris* extracts are five time less active than compound 48/80.

UVNÄS et al. (1960), on the basis of the influence of pH, ionic milieu, temperature and enzyme inhibitors on the mast-cell disruption caused by *Ascaris suis* extract in the rat, believe that the disruption depends on the activation of an enzymatic process producing lysis of the mast cell membrane. The hypothetical enzyme was not isolated, but indirect evidence pointed to an enzyme identical with, or related to phospholipase A.

An interesting question which arises from the discussion on the release of histamine by *Ascaris* extracts is to know whether an antigen-antibody reaction is also involved in other species as it was strongly suggested in the guinea-pig.

D. Mollusca

The cephalopod octopods have attracted the attention of biologists and physiologists since many years ago. Their salivary glands have been the object of many investigations, where enzymes and a great deal of pharmacologically active substances have been found.

The venomous properties of the posterior gland secretion were suggested by the early experiments described by BELLESME (1879) on the paralytic effect of the secretion in the crab. However, it had no effect on the rat and rabbit (LIVON and BRIOT, 1905). More recently, the function of the salivary gland of these animals has been extensively studied and a great number of pharmacologically active amines, amine oxidases and other enzymes were found in the gland. For reference see the papers by HARTMAN et al. (1960) and CLARK et al. (1960).

UNGAR and PARROT (1937) demonstrated the presence of histamine in several tissues of the *Octopus vulgaris*. They found considerable amounts of histamine in the nervous tissue.

We were not able to find in the literature any reference on the release of histamine by tissue extracts or secretions of the cephalopods.

E. Arthropoda

1. Arachnida

a) Scorpionidea

The scorpion uses its venom as defence against its enemies.

JOYEUX-LAFFUIE (1882) divides the action of the scorpion venom into two phases. The first is characterized by violent contractions of the skeletal muscles resembling the contractions produced by strychnine. The second phase of the intoxication is recognized as a generalized depression which kills the animal by asphyxia. BERT (1865) and JOYEUX-LAFFUIE (1882) also described a curare-like action of the venom. WILSON (1904), on the other hand, admitted a direct action on the muscle. This author also observed hypersecretion of saliva, lachrymation and increase in the blood pressure followed by a decrease after the injection of the venom. The local action of the scorpion venom is characterized by violent pain, swelling and tissue hemorrhage.

BELLESME (1871/72) described a hemolytic action of the scorpion venom for the blood of certain species (fishes, amphibia and birds) but it had no hemolytic action on mammalian blood (SANARELLI, 1889).

CALMETTE (1895a) was able to kill mice with 0.05 mg and rabbits with 0.5 mg *Scorpio afer* venom.

Experimental and clinical observations reported from Egypt (BERT, 1865), Algiers (GUYON, 1865), Mexico (ALTAMIRANO, 1899), Argentina (HOUSSAY, 1919) and Brazil (MAGALHÃES, 1928) suggest that the pharmacological actions of venoms from a great variety of scorpions are very similar. These actions have been extensively studied by DEL POZO et al. (1944) and DEL POZO (1956).

Recently, DINIZ and GONÇALVES (1956) submitted to a pharmacological analysis the action of Brazilian scorpion venoms on smooth muscle. They showed that scorpion venom produced a sustained and strong contraction of the guinea-pig's gut which is not inhibited by antihistaminics. The action of venom upon smooth muscles is similar in many ways to the action of serotonin.

DINIZ and GONÇALVES (1960) injecting the whole venom (100 μg) into the abdominal skin of the rat verified an increase of vascular permeability (capillaries) to Evans blue dye. Phenergan (4 mg/kg) administered intravenously 30 min. before the venom, inhibited the oedema and the extravasation of the dye. Although some of its actions suggest a possible release of histamine by the scorpion venom, a direct histamine-releasing activity has not yet been demonstrated.

To clarify this point, perfusions of isolated guinea-pig lungs and rat hind quarters were performed in our laboratory.

The scorpion venom was obtained by electric stimulation of the distal coils of the tail and collecting it in a watch glass. It was dried and kept in the refrigerator. The venom was weighed and dissolved in 2 ml saline immediately before use. Its histamine-releasing property was tested on the perfused guinea-pig lungs and on the perfused hind quarters of the rat. The guinea-pigs were anaesthetized with pentobarbitone sodium, intraperitoneally, the lungs perfused through the pulmonary artery with Tyrode solution, and the venous outflow collected from the left ventricle, according to the method described by BARTOSCH et al. (1932). The rats were similarly anaesthetized and the hind quarters perfused through the lower abdominal aorta and the venous outflow collected from the vena cava, as described by FELDBERG and MONGAR (1954). After washing the preparations, freed of blood as completely as possible, three perfusate samples were collected as controls. The perfusion was then stopped and 2 ml saline, containing the scorpion venom, were injected through the cannula inserted into the pulmonary artery or into the lower abdominal aorta. The injected solution was allowed to remain in contact with the tissues. Five minutes later the perfusion was continued until only traces of histamine could be detected in the perfusates, which were assayed for histamine on the atropinized guinea-pig ileum. All values of histamine are referred to as the base.

As can be seen from Table 2 scorpion venom releases small amounts of histamine, both from guinea-pig lungs and from hind quarters of the rat.

Table 2. *Histamine release from perfused guinea-pig lungs and hind quarters of the rat by scorpion venom (Tityus bahiensis)*

	No.	mg scorpion venom injected	Total of histamine released in μg
Guinea-pig lungs	1	630	0
	2	430	1.6
	3	440	1.0
Rat hind quarters	1	6.8	1.8
	2	220	0
	3	8.8	2.3

b) *Araneida*

Bordas (1901a, b, 1905) described local symptoms produced by the spider bite. It is very painful, chiefly during the first hours. There is always some swelling, redness at the site of the bite. Local necrotizing effects, generalized hemolytic and hemorrhagic manifestations have also been reported.

The black widow spider (*Latrodectus mactans*) bite was responsible for 55 fatalities in the United States during the period from 1726 to 1943 (Thorp and Woodson, 1945).

In human beings *Phoneutria fera* venom is very painful and besides the local reaction it produces alteration of the pulse, cardiac and visual disturbances. Blindness has been recorded. Fever, sweating, kidney disorders are included among the systemic symptoms of poisoning. Venoms of the Brazilian spiders, *Lycosa raptoria* and *Ctenus nigriventer* (Phoneutria), show proteolytic activity. This enzyme is similar in action to trypsin extracted from beef pancreas (Kaiser, 1953). The venoms contain considerable amounts of a hyaluronidase-like substance (Pantlitschko and Kaiser, 1951).

Antihistamines have been given as part of the treatment of spider bite poisoning, partly on the supposition that allergic sensitization to venom proteins may be present, but this is still to be demonstrated.

Diniz (1962) demonstrated by paper chromatography and pharmacological tests the presence of histamine and 5-hydroxytryptamine (serotonin) in spider venoms (*Lycosa erythrognata* and *Phoneutria fera*). Histamine was found in enormous concentration (14 to 19 mg/g of venom). The greatest amount of histamine found so far was in the wasp venom (17 mg/g) (Jaques and Schachter, 1954b). Such an enormous amount of histamine must play an important rôle in the appearance of symptoms caused by spider bites.

2. Insecta

a) *Lepidoptera*

Urticating caterpillars have been studied by Ihering (1914), Foot (1922) and Gaminara (1928). Estable et al. (1945) extracted from the *Megalopyge urens* venom a globulin with necrotizing, hemolytic and immunological properties. The local and systemic reactions following contact or injection of caterpillar extracts would depend on liberation of active agents from tissues or on the presence of active agents in the extract or to both. No experiments have been done to decide this question.

VALLE et al. (1954) studying the pharmacological properties of crude extracts from setae of urticating caterpillars verified the presence of conspicuous amounts of histamine in the pinetree-like spines of caterpillars, belonging to the genus *Dirphia*. These authors also studied the genus *Megalopyge*. In *Megalopyge* the histamine content was found to be very low. Acetylcholine was not detected in both cases. VALETTE and HUIDOBRO (1957) were not able to demonstrate the presence of histamine in extracts from setae of *Thaumetopoea pityocampa*, however they showed that the extracts release histamine from skin and diaphragm of guinea pig and from rabbit blood.

Dermatitis caused by venomous moths and butterflies has also been reported (LEGER and MOUZELS, 1918; BOYÉ, 1932; TISSEUIL, 1935; ALLARD and ALLARD, 1958). Recently, GUSMÃO et al. (1961) described an epidemic dermatitis produced by lepidoptera of the genus *Hylesia* in Brazil, presenting epidemiological and experimental data which showed that the cutaneous manifestations are essentially of an irritative nature. Although no special studies concerned with this reaction have been reported, it seems reasonable to presume the participation of a release of histamine in the mechanism of such a reaction.

b) *Coleoptera*

GOELDI (1902) observed that certain species of coleoptera in Amazonia (Brazil) when put into contact with the skin produced a strong cutaneous reaction. PIRAJÁ DA SILVA (1912) showed that *Paederus columbianus* produced severe dermatitis in man. PICKEL (1940) admits approximately 200 species of coleoptera which when in contact with the skin cause severe dematitis characterized by intense burning pain, reddening, swelling, itching and inflammation. Conjunctivitis can also be observed when the lesion occurs in the eyes. In Africa the syndrome is known as Nairobi's eye.

Recently, MAGALHÃES (1960) reproduced experimentally in guinea-pigs the inflammatory lesions produced by *Paederus columbianus*.

Although so far no attempt has been made to demonstrate the liberation of histamine by *coleoptera* the general symptoms observed in man and experimentally in animals suggest that it may occur.

c) *Hymenoptera*

Usually the result of bee and wasp sting is the immediate sensation of pain at the point of the sting, followed by erythema, swelling and urticaria. Frequently the patients suffer severe symptoms after a single sting. They often become nauseated and vomit, and at times develop mild respiratory distress, cramps in the muscles of the extremities. Itching and oedema are most distressing and irritating. If the sting is in the region of the mouth glottis oedema can take place.

LANGER (1896, 1899) injecting bee venom in dogs observed appearance of neurological symptoms (clonus, trismus, nystagmus and opisthotonos). Respiratory paralysis and generalized hemorrhages in the gastrointestinal tract, pancreas and kidney were also observed. The *in vitro* hemolytic action of the bee venom gives an experimental support for LANGER's findings *in vivo*.

FELDBERG and KELLAWAY (1937b) were able to demonstrate the liberation of histamine from perfused lungs of guinea-pig by bee venom. The total output after the injection of five stings corresponded to between 65 and 75% of the lung histamine. Besides histamine a slowly contracting substance (SRS) was also found in perfusates.

NEUMANN et al. (1953) described two hemolysing principles in bee venom.

JAQUES and SCHACHTER (1954b) demonstrated that wasp venom contained three active smooth muscle stimulating agents: histamine, 5-hydroxytryptamine and a highly potent substance similar to bradykinin. The average concentration of histamine in the dried venom was approximately 16 to 20 mg/g. Such huge amounts of histamine will contribute to the pain and oedema which follow a wasp sting. The concentrations of 5-hydroxytryptamine were of the order of 0.32 mg/g. This concentration would also be greater than the pain producing threshold concentration for human skin (ARMSTRONG et al., 1953). JAQUES and SCHACHTER (1954b) also reported that wasp venom occasionally releases histamine from isolated perfused cat skin. The amount released ranged from 3.2 to 15.4 μg.

In addition to the direct effect of the active substances contained in the venoms, a sensitization to antigens present in bee and wasp venoms has been frequently reported (CATOLA, 1928; LUDWIG, 1934; PEÇANHA and OLIVEIRA LIMA, 1954).

As the histamine-releasing mechanism by these and snake venoms are intimately connected, both processes will be discussed with more detail later on.

F. Chordata

1. Pisces

In 1888 MOSSO reported that the serum of the European moray eel, *Gymnothorax helena* contained a substance which, when injected into certain mammals, resulted in hemolysis, decreased sensitivity to pain, hypersalivation, respiratory distress, clonic convulsion, paralysis and death. The toxin was inactivated by gastric enzymes and presented hemolytic properties. Reviews of the toxic properties of moray eel serum have been given by PHISALIX (1922) and PAWLOWSKY (1927). For other references see the paper by HALSTEAD (1956).

Certain species as stonefish (*Synanceja verrucosa*) when it stings the animal produces extreme pain, ischemia and oedema. Systemic effects include weakness, sweating, respiratory distress and convulsions; death may occur. DUHIG and JONES (1928) and GAIL and RAGEAU (1956) have described the effect of the venom in animals; in addition, a hemolytic action has been reported (DUHIG, 1929).

The systemic effect of the stonefish venom was recently investigated in the rabbit by SAUNDERS (1959). The author found that 7.7 μg to 11 μg/kg of the venom protein produced fall in arterial blood pressure and alteration in the respiratory rate.

Although no experiment to demonstrate a histamine release by these venoms has been so far carried out, the hemolytic action of fish venoms and their effects on the blood pressure may suggest that it might occur.

2. Reptilia

Snake venoms are complex mixtures of toxic proteins, many of which possess enzymatic properties. The symptoms observed in experimental animals injected with venom or in man when bitten by snakes are produced by the combined action of all the toxic principles contained therein.

CALMETTE (1895a, b) working on preparations of anticobra serum, was the first to start this line of investigation. As far as the physiological action of snake venom is concerned, MITCHELL (1861) and MITCHELL and REICHERT (1886), studying *Crotalus horridus* and *Crotalus atrox* venoms demonstrated their hypotensive action on mammals. ARTHUS (1921) called attention to the similarity between symptoms caused by *Crotalus adamanteus, Vipera russellii* and *Vipera aspis* venoms and anaphylactic shock.

KELLAWAY (1929) showed that Australian elapines have a powerful stimulant action upon the *in vitro* plain muscles (guinea-pig, rat and rabbit uterus), of a type which does not appear to have been described previously either for snake venoms or for any other substance. The effect of venoms resembles closely the anaphylactic response of the sensitized plain muscle. When the muscle has responded to one venom it will not respond to the same or any other venom of the group, but its reaction to other stimuli is unaffected. Having been once thoroughly desensitized to the venom it does not recover its sensitiveness. The reaction has a latent period of the same order as that of the anaphylactic response of sensitized plain muscle. The venoms also cause contraction of the isolated uterus of the rat. Since histamine produces relaxation of this preparation, the contraction of the guinea-pig and the rabbit uterus are probably not wholly due to a histamine release. The very close similarity which exists between the action of snake venom and the anaphylactic reaction, raised the question whether a hypothetical stimulant substance produced by contact of the sensitized uterus with its specific antigen was identical with the stimulant substance present in the snake venoms. That this is not the case is shown by the fact that the sensitized guinea-pig uterus still gives the typical anaphylactic response after it has become tachyphylactic to the snake venom. Conversely after desensitization with the specific antigen the muscle still reacts with the snake venom.

ESSEX and MARKOWITZ (1930a, b, c, d, e) in a series of papers on the physiologic action of the venoms from the rattlesnakes *Crotalus horridus* and *Crotalus atrox* described the action of intravenous injection on the blood pressure of dogs, rabbits and guinea-pigs. In each case, there is a remarkably sharp, profound drop in blood pressure to a shock level. The analysis of the mechanism of this fall in blood pressure showed that it was probably peripheral in nature. The authors also found a striking similarity of the results of their experiments with venoms with those following injection of the specific antigen into a sensitized animal. In the course of these studies they described a toxic action of th evenoms on the heart and the skeletal muscle. On the isolated guinea-pig uterus, the venoms caused strong contraction, which according to the American investigators differed from the anaphylactic response by its longer latent period and by the fact that desensitization required repeated doses of the venom. The isolated intestine of the rat relaxed when the venom was added to the perfusing bath.

In view of the analogies and differences already mentioned among the effect of snake venoms, anaphylactic reaction and histamine (KELLAWAY, 1929; ESSEX and MARKOWITZ, 1930a, b) an impetuous rush to demonstrate the release of histamine by snake venoms was undertaken by a group of Australian investigators.

The first attempt to demonstrate the histamine release by snake venoms was not successful (KELLAWAY and LE MESSURIER, 1936). FELDBERG and KELLAWAY (1937a) pursuing this line of enquiry in experiments on the perfused lungs of the guinea-pig and the cat showed that histamine was liberated by the three venoms examined (*Denisonia superba, Naia naia* and *Crotalus atrox*). With increasing doses of the venom of *Denisonia superba* up to 10 mg the lung became almost completely depleted of its histamine (Fig. 8).

Denisonia superba was the most active venom in releasing histamine and that of *Crotalus atrox* the least active. On the guinea-pig gut, all of them caused contraction with a latent period of some seconds, followed by desensitization.

As far as the mechanism of histamine release by snake venoms is concerned, FELDBERG and KELLAWAY (1938a) put forward the theory that the venom causes the formation in the tissues of lysocithin-like substances which might represent an intermediate step in the liberation of histamine by snake and bee venoms. The authors went further, admitting that this mechanism is not confined to the action of haemolytic poisons but plays a role in other conditions of general cell injury in which histamine is released, such as antigen-antibody reaction, peptone, etc. Working with a preparation of lysocithin, FELDBERG and KELLAWAY (1938a) demonstrated the liberation of histamine from perfused liver of the dog and monkey. In the intact animal (cat and dog) it caused a steep fall of systemic arterial blood pressure which in the cat was associated with a rise of pressure in the pulmonary artery and in the dog with a rise of pressure in the portal vein. A positive correlation was found by TRETHEWIE (1939) between the hemolytic activity of venoms and their capacity to liberate histamine.

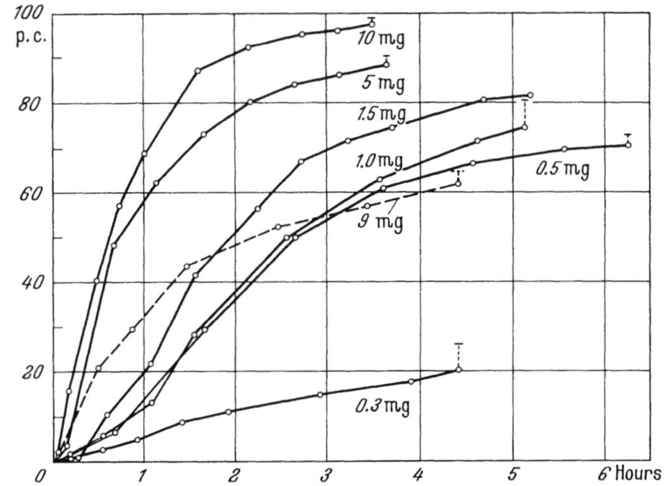

Fig. 8. Histamine output from perfused guinea-pig lungs produced by various doses of venoms. The continuous curves are for copperhead and the dotted curve is for cobra venom

Apart from the presence of histamine in the perfusates collected from organs perfused with snake venom FELDBERG and KELLAWAY (1938a) found a substance which caused slow delayed contraction of the guinea-pig gut. Many effects of snake venoms which cannot be reproduced by histamine may perhaps be explained by the action of the slowly contracting substance.

Recently, a renewed interest on the lysocithin has arisen from the investigation by UVNÄS and colleagues (1958) who claimed that a lytic enzymatic process hydrolysing the lipoprotein phospholipids of mast cell membrane occurs during the release of histamine by histamine releasers and in antigen-antibody reactions. The experimental basis for this view resides in the fact that lecithinase A is the only enzyme among 25 tested which is capable of disrupting mast cells in the rat mesentery. These findings agree with the lysolecithin theory presented previously by FELDBERG and KELLAWAY (1938a).

It is a known fact that some snake venoms possess strong proteolytic activity which, at least in part, is responsible for their toxic activity. As has been shown by ROCHA E SILVA and ANDRADE (1943) proteolytic enzymes release histamine. The histamine releasing properties of snake venoms might well be connected also with the proteolytic activity of venoms beside the presence of lecithinase A, as was already discussed. Figs. 9 and 10 show the histamine release by snake venom (*Bothrops atrox*), which presents a strong proteolytic activity.

DUTTA and NARAYANAN (1952) demonstrated that cobra (*Naia naia*) venom is a potent liberator of histamine from rat diaphragm, *in vitro*. After incubation of the muscle with 100 μg/ml of the venom, for 75 min., the preparation was completely depleted of its histamine. The participation of proteolytic enzymes in the histamine release by cobra venom cannot be ruled out, for the existence of more than one protease in this venom was suggested by RAO and RAO (1956).

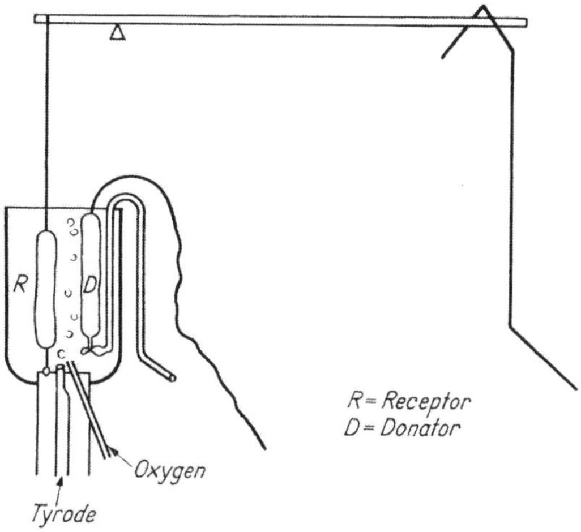

Fig. 9. Diagram showing the experiment to demonstrate the release of gut stimulating principles from a fresh piece of gut "donator" to a desensitized piece of the same guinea pig gut "receptor". In Fig. 10, a tracing obtained in one experiment performed with the venom of *Bothrops atrox*.

Although the histamine releasing properties of snake venoms have been demonstrated by several authors, we do not know of any effort to isolate from the venoms the histamine releasing fraction. More recently, however, MOURA GONÇALVES and ROCHA E SILVA (1958), using crotamine, a basic protein isolated from the Brazilian rattlesnake (MOURA GONÇALVES and VIEIRA, 1950), reported the first experiments on histamine release by a purified fraction from venoms.

Besides histamine, snake venoms release bradykinin (ROCHA E SILVA et al. 1949), adenyl compounds (KELLAWAY and TRETHEWIE, 1940), adrenaline (FELDBERG, 1940). REID and JENKINS (1948) have shown that the injection of the cobra

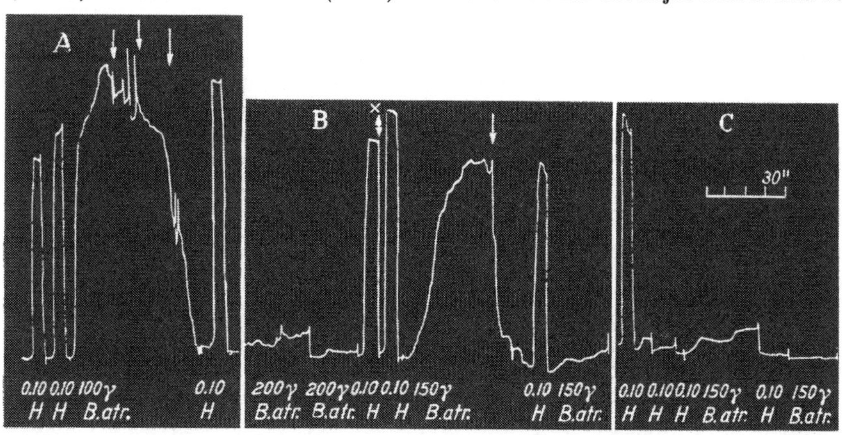

Fig. 10. A typical experiment with the set up of Fig. 9. A) Contraction of the "receptor" with 100 μg of the venom of *Bothrops atrox;* *B*) after desensitization of the "receptor" to 200 μg of the venom, a piece of "donator" was introduced in the chamber at the signal (×) and 150 μg of the same venom added; a second addition of the same venom did not elicit any further contraction (exhaustion of the "donator"); *C*) a fresh piece of gut "donator" was introduced in the bath containing 0.3 ml of a 1:500,000 solution of pyribenzamine: only a slight or no effect was induced by the addition of 150 μg of the venom of *Bothrops atrox*.

venom releases renin from the kidney. These numerous activities of the venoms explain the variety of symptoms caused by snake bite and make the nature of this subject extremely complex.

3. Mammalia

The existence of venomous animals among mammals is exceptional. Only one species in Australia (*Ornithorhynchus paradoxus*), the male of which carries its poison device at the hind legs, was described (Flury, 1930). The animal is a mixture of bird and mammal, a paradoxical animal. The action of the venom in man is limited to a local action such as oedema and swelling. Hunting dogs when hurt and inoculated by the venom died (Fonseca, 1949).

A toxic substance from the salivary glands of an American mammal, the short-tailed shrew (*Blarina brevicauda*), was reported by Pearson (1942). The bite of the shrew is able to incapacitate, but not to kill, a mouse. Upon parenteral injection, a submaxillary gland extract produced a local inflammatory reaction, hypotension, bradycardia and respiratory difficulties. Ellis and Krayer (1955) isolated a toxin from the submaxillary gland of the shrew and determined the LD 50 of the purified toxin in mice. The toxin appeared to be of a proteic nature. Although some of the actions of the toxin on the blood pressure, on peripheral vessels, on the suprarenal medulla and on isolated smooth muscle preparations resemble the corresponding actions of histamine, the final demonstration of histamine release from tissues treated with this shrew toxin has not been carried out.

IV. Release of histamine by bacterial toxins

Bacterial toxins are toxic substances possessing antigenic properties and usually classified into exotoxin and endotoxin. The exotoxins in general are proteins excreted into the culture media, relatively unstable (inactivated by heating at 60° C, storage or ultraviolet light). They produce effects which are highly specific for certain tissues such as heart muscle, nerves and adrenals. The endotoxins, on the other hand, are liberated only after disintegration of the microorganism (gram-negative), being polysaccharide-protein-lipid complexes, containing phosphorus. In contrast to the exotoxins, they are relatively stable to heating, storage and ultraviolet light. The endotoxins are variously known as Boivin antigen, Boivin glucolipid toxins, Shwartzman-active toxins and bacterial pyrogens.

Dale in a note appended to a paper by Robertson (1919), on the basis of a few experiments, suggested that the toxin of *Cl. septique* has a pressor effect and a direct action on the heart of the rabbit. Buttle and Trevan (1928), studying the action of *Vibrion septique* and *B. welchii* toxin, on isolated rabbit's uterus and intestine demonstrated that the action of the toxin was specific, for the effects of both the *septique* and *Welch* toxins are prevented by mixing the toxin with the specific antisera.

Liberation of histamine from perfused guinea-pig and cat lungs by staphylococcal toxin was demonstrated by Feldberg and Keogh (1937). The histamine output amounted to between 4 and 15 % of the cat lung histamine.

Kellaway et al. (1941) in a more extensive study on the pharmacological effects of the *Cl. septique* toxins verified that the injection of the toxin in doses of 20 and 60 mg into the pulmonary artery caused release of histamine from the isolated perfused lungs of the guinea-pig. This effect is not wholly specific because neutralized toxin (toxin and antitoxin) in similar dosage still causes histamine release, though in smaller amounts.

Kellaway et al. (1940, 1941 a, b) in a series of papers in which they studied tissue damage caused by various types of *Cl. welchii* toxin demonstrated the release of considerable amounts of histamine, from perfused lungs of the cat by type D toxin (Fig. 11). Type A *Cl. welchii* toxin, on the other hand, failed to cause the liberation of histamine, nevertheless it caused definite injury to cells as indicated by the hemolysis test, release of coagulable protein and adenyl compounds. The difference between the toxins of *Cl. welchii* A and D in respect to their ability to liberate histamine must be regarded as qualitative rather than quantitative, the capacity to liberate histamine being a property of the non-hemolytic ε constituent (GLENNY et al. 1933), of which the D toxin used was almost wholly composed, whereas the hemolytic α fraction (corresponding to A toxin) fails to do so. Finally, the toxins of *Cl. welchii* type B and C showed different qualitative pharmacological actions. Type B toxin caused liberation of histamine from the perfused lungs of the cat but failed to release it from the perfused lungs of the guinea-pig, whereas type C toxin caused the release of a slowly reacting muscle stimulant from both preparations.

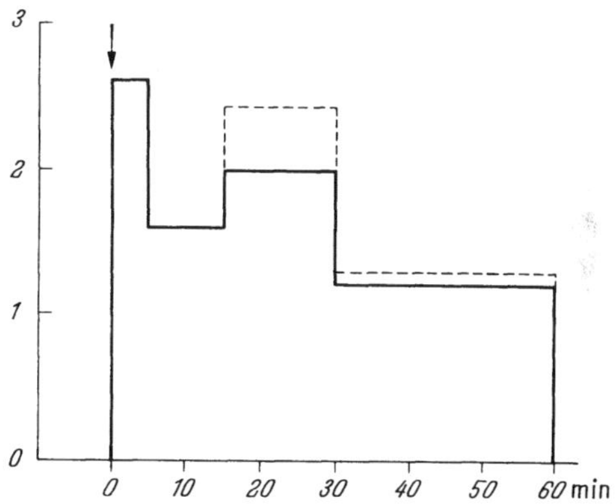

Fig. 11. Output of histamine from the perfused lung of the cat. At the arrow 50 mg toxin. Ordinates, histamine in γ per minute; abscissae, time in minute

RILEY (1958) and HABERMANN (1959) reported that α-toxin from *Cl. welchii* caused alterations in mast cells and that this toxin was identical or intimately related to phospholipase C. FREDHOLM et al. (1960), on the other hand, investigating the nature of this mast cell alterating factor, observed that such a factor was similar to phospholipase A and not to phospholipase C. It was also demonstrated that the mast cell alterating factor was present even in sterile culture medium, for it did not increase after the growth of *Cl. welchii*. These observations agree with those described by KELLAWAY and TRETHEWIE (1941a) which showed that the toxin of *Cl. welchii* type A, which contains phospholipase C (MACFARLANE and KNIGHT, 1941) failed to cause release of histamine.

As early as 1909, ANDERSON and ROSENAU recognized certain analogies between the physiologic changes produced by endotoxin and by anaphylaxis. They predicted at that time that further studies of anaphylaxis would offer an explanation for the poisonous nature of endotoxin.

The local vascular effects of endotoxins have been extensively studied in animals, particularly with reference to the Shwartzman reaction (KARSNER and MORITZ, 1934; THOMAS and GOOD, 1952; THOMAS, 1954). KUN (1947) studying the effect of meningococcal endotoxin on histamine content of blood and tissues of rabbit found that the blood histamine level fell in the first 5 minutes after the injection of the endotoxin. It remained well below the level found in control animals, until death. These findings are parallel to those reported by ROSE and WEIL (1939) who have shown that during anaphylactic shock in the rabbit there is a marked decrease in the blood histamine, in contrast to the increased amounts that are found in the dog and the guinea-pig.

In the course of a series of investigations on the circulatory effects of endotoxins from gram-negative bacteria, WEIL et al. (1955, 56) and MACLEAN and WEIL (1956), in dogs and cats, observed a sharp fall in arterial blood pressure, rise in portal vein pressure and a fall in systemic venous pressure.

WEIL and SPINK (1957) made a comparative study between shock due to endotoxin (*B. melitensis, E. coli, S. typhosa* and *S. marcescens*) with anaphylactic shock, in the dog. They found great similarities, as far as hemodynamics is concerned. However, two important points of difference were noted between the shocks caused by endotoxin and anaphylaxis. No change in blood coagulability occurred after endotoxin and this is in contrast to the liberation of heparin in anaphylaxis in dogs. The authors also found a sharp rise and rapid fall of blood histamine following the injection of endotoxin. The explosive liberation of histamine was closely related to the onset of hypotension and rise in portal vein pressure (fig. 12).

Kuida et al. (1958) studying the effect of endotoxin from *E. coli* bacteria on pulmonary vessels of the dog and the cat found an increase in the pulmonary artery pressure. The authors suggested that the effect may not be produced

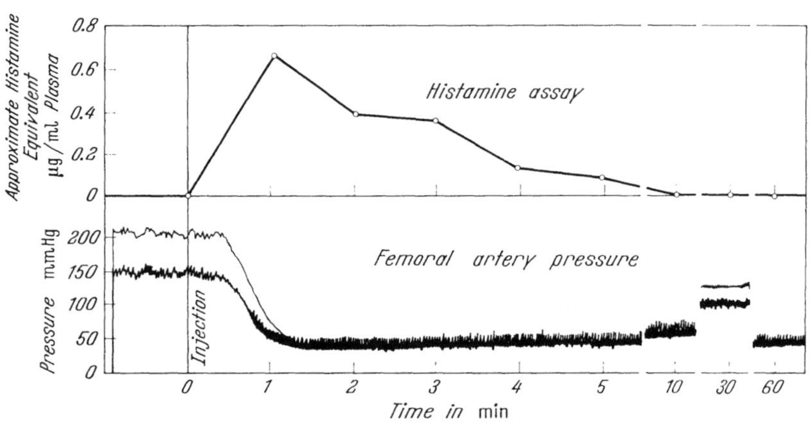

Fig. 12. Relationship of the amount of histamine-like substance in inferior vena cava blood of the dog to the arterial pressure following injection of crude *E. coli* endotoxin

directly by the endotoxin upon the smooth muscle, but rather through the release of an active agent or agents in the blood, for when blood is replaced by dextran or gelatin solution, endotoxin does not produce its effect on the isolated lung preparation. The authors discarded the possibility of histamine being involved in the mechanism of the effect of endotoxin on pulmonary vessels, as injected histamine failed to elicit the response in conditions in which endotoxin still produced significant changes in the vascular resistance. This does not definitely rule out the participation of histamine, for if histamine is released close to the receptor sites in the tissue, the amounts of extrinsic histamine which must be added from the outside to produce a response are considerably higher. Recently, Hinshaw et al. (1961) verified that lethal doses of *E. coli* endotoxin given to anesthetized dogs caused hypotension with simultaneous increase of blood histamine, histamine-histidine ratio and circulating hematocrit readings. The authors emphasized the role of histamine in the endotoxin shock and suggested the possible conversion of histidine into histamine following the endotoxin administration.

These results are in conflict with those obtained by Rothschild and Corrado (1962) who were unable to show any significant increase of blood histamine in dogs submitted to severe shocks with *E. coli* endotoxin, even when the blood was collected directly from hepatic veins by catheterization through a jugular vein, in spite of the fact that the liver reacted to the toxin with appreciable increase in volume. These negative results contrasted with the easiness with which histamine increases were detected in peptone and anaphylactic shocks. The differences in histamine contents of pieces of liver taken before and after the injection of the toxin did not warrant the idea that histamine might be an important factor in the genesis of endotoxin shock in the dog.

Another group of toxic substances, produced by microorganisms in culture medium during growth, releases histamine from animal tissues. Among these substances, dextrans and polymyxins have been extensively investigated.

Dextran, a polymer of glucose, formed by the action of microorganisms, (Genera *Leuconostoc*) when injected in the rat produces an anaphylactoid reaction (VOORHEES et al. 1951). This reaction was inhibited by antihistaminics and corticoides (MORRISON et al. 1951). HALPERN and BRIOT (1952) showed that dextran released histamine from rat skin, in *in vitro* experiments. GOTH et al. (1957) demonstrated that the alloxan diabetic rat failed to show the characteristic oedema and elevated plasma histamine produced by dextran. Recently, ADAMKIEWICZ and ADAMKIEWICZ (1960) demonstrated that rats simultaneously injected with dextran and glucose did not show anaphylactoid reaction. DIAS da SILVA, et al. (1962) studying the mechanism of the anaphylactoid reaction produced by dextran and the inhibitory effect of alloxan diabetes on this reaction, found that alloxan diabetic rats failed to show the skin reaction produced by dextran. These authors also showed that dextran produces disruption of mast cells which occurred, simultaneously, with a histamine release. Both these processes are inhibited by glucose and other related carbohydrates. As far as the inhibition of the effect of dextran by glucose is concerned a competitive mechanism was suggested. Using inhibitors of anaphylaxis (Ca^{++}-lack, previous heating at 45° C, 2,4-dinitrophenol, sodium iodoacetate and N-ethylmaleimide) it was verified that the release of histamine by dextran showed steps similar to those observed in anaphylaxis.

Finally, among the substances formed by microorganisms which present histamine releasing properties are included several antibiotics. Licheniformin, a polypeptide extracted from *Bacillus licheniformis* by CALLOW et al. (1947), is a potent histamine releaser (MACINTOSH and PATON, 1949).

Polymyxins are a group of polypeptides produced by many strains of a widely distributed soil organism, *Bacillus polymyxa*. According to the strains of *Bacillus polymyxa* several polymyxins were isolated: polymyxin A, B, C, D and E. They present antibiotic activity (AINSWORTH et al. 1947; BENEDICT and LANGLYKKE, 1947; STANSLY et al. 1947). Some of the side-effects of polymyxins B and E in man and experimental animals might be due to the release of histamine. SWIFT and BUSHBY (1953) observed that injection of a histamine-free polymyxin in man produced a typical histamine "triple response". The release of histamine by polymyxins B and E was demonstrated by BUSHBY and GREEN (1955). Subcutaneously, in rats, they are about as active as 48/80 in releasing histamine from skin and in causing disruption of the mast cells. Intravenously in dogs they cause increase in blood histamine.

NORTON and BEER (1955) studying the effects of a series of antibiotics (Polymyxin, Aureomycin, Bacitracin, Penicillin and Achromycin) on rat mast cells, *in vitro*, found that polymyxin B was the most active of the antibiotics tested. The action of the drug was related to its concentration.

References

ADAMKIEWICZ, V. W., and L. M. ADAMKIEWICZ: Glucose and the dextran anaphylactoid inflammation. Amer. J. Physiol. **198**, 51 (1960).

AINSWORTH, G. C., A. M. BROWN, and G. BROWNLEE: "Aerosporin", an antibiotic produced by Bacillus aerosporus Greer. Nature (Lond.) **160**, 263 (1947).

ALAM, M., G. V. ANREP, G. S. BARSOUM, M. TALAAT, and E. WIENINGER: Liberation of histamine from the skeletal muscle by curare. J. Physiol. (Lond.) **95**, 148 (1939).

ALLARD, H. F., and H. A. ALLARD: Venomous moths and butterflies. J. Wash. Acad. Sci. **48**, 18 (1958).
ALTAMIRANO, F.: Algunas observaciones fisiologicas sobre los efectos de la ponzona del alacran de jojutla. Mem. soc. cient. Antonio Alzate **14**, 327 (1899).
ANDERSON, J. F., and M. J. ROSENAU: Anaphylaxis. Arch. intern. Med. **3**, 519 (1909).
ANREP, G. V., M. S. AYADI, G. S. BARSOUM, J. R. SMITH, and M. M. TALAAT: The excretion of histamine in urine. J. Physiol. (Lond.) **103**, 155 (1944).
ARMSTRONG, D., R. M. L. DRY, C. A. KEELE, and J. W. MARKHAM: Observations on chemical excitants of cutaneous pain in man. J. Physiol. (Lond.) **120**, 326 (1953).
ARTHUS, M.: De l'anaphylaxie à l'immunité. Paris: Masson 1921.
BAIN, W. A., J. L. BROADBENT, and R. P. WARIN: Comparison of anthisan (Mepyramine maleate) and phenergan, as histamine antagonists. Lancet **1949** II, 47.
BARTOSCH, R., W. FELDBERG u. E. NAGEL: Das Freiwerden eines histaminähnlichen Stoffes bei der Anaphylaxie des Meerschweinchens. Pflügers Arch. ges. Physiol. **230**, 129 (1932).
BELLESME, J.: Essai sur le venin de scorpion. Rev. Magazin Zool. **23**, 150 (1871/72).
— Recherches sur la digestion chez les mollusques céphalopodes. C. R. Acad. Sci. (Paris) **138**, 428 (1879).
BENEDICT, R. G., and A. F. LANGLYKKE: Antibiotic activity of Bacillus polymyxa. J. Bact. **54**, 24 (1947).
BERALDO, W. T.: Formation of bradykinin in anaphylactic and peptone shock. Amer. J. Physiol. **163**, 283 (1950).
— W. DIAS DA SILVA, and J. PUDLES: Antigenic properties of purified fractions from Ascaris lumbricoides var. suum on naturally sensitized guinea-pig. Brit. J. Pharmacol. **17**, 236 (1961).
BERT, P.: Contribution a l'étude des venins (venin de scorpion). C. R. Soc. Biol. (Paris) **17**, 136 (1865).
BHATTACHARYA, B. K., and G. P. LEWIS: The release of 5-hydroxytryptamine by histamine liberators. Brit. J. Pharmacol. **11**, 202 (1956).
BIER, O., cited by M. ROCHA E SILVA: Histamina e Anafilaxia. São Paulo: Edigraf 1946.
BORDAS, L.: Recherches sur les glandes venimeuses du Latrodectus 13-guttatus Rossi. Associat. franc. pour l'Avanc. des Sci. Congrès d'Ajaccio, 8. Sept. (1901a).
— Recherches sur les effets des piqures de Lactrodectus 13-guttatus Rossi ou Malmignatte. C. R. Soc. Biol. (Paris) **133**, 953 (1901b).
— Recherches anatomiques, histologiques et physiologiques sur glandes venimeuses ou glandes des chélicères des Malmignattes (Lactrodectus 13-guttatus Rossi). Ann. Sci. nat. Zool. **79**, 147 (1905).
BOYÉ, R.: La papillonite guyanaise. Bull. Soc. Path. exot. **25**, 1099 (1932).
BROCKLEHURST, W. E.: Ciba Foundation Symposium on Histamine. A slow reacting substance in anaphylaxis "SRS-A". London: Churchill Ltd. 1956.
BRUCE, A. N.: Über die Beziehung der sensiblen Nervenendigungen zum Entzündungsvorgang. Naunyn-Schmiedeberg's Arch. exp. Path. Pharmak. **113**, 424 (1910).
BUSHBY, S. R. M., and A. F. GREEN: The release of histamine by polymyxin B and polymyxin E. Brit. J. Pharmacol. **10**, 215 (1955).
BUTTLE, G. A. H., and J. W. TREVAN: The action of Vibrion septique and B. welchii toxin on isolated organs. Brit. J. exp. Path. **9**, 182 (1928).
CALLOW, R. K., R. E. GLOVER, P. D. A. HART, and G. M. HILLS: Licheniformin, antibiotic substance from Bacillus licheniformis active against Mycobacterium tuberculosis. Brit. J. exp. Path. **28**, 418 (1947).
CALMETTE, A.: Contribution à l'étude des venins, des toxines et des sérums antitoxiques. III. Venin des Scorpions. Ann. Inst. Pasteur **9**, 53 (1895a).
— Contributions a l'étude des venins, des toxines et des sérums antitoxiques. Ann. Inst. Pasteur **9**, 225 (1895b).
CATOLA, G.: Crises vaso-motrices céphaliques et ménieriformes par venin d'abeille. Rev. neurol. **35**, 260 (1928).
CATTANEO, C.: Nota preventiva sulla tossicità degli Ascaridi. Associazione medico-chirurgica di Parma. Zit. nach Biochem. Zbl. (1903).
CHANSON, V.: Contribution à l'étude des accidents produits par les Ascarides. C.R. Soc. Biol. (Paris) **48**, 38 (1906).
CLARK, W. G., W. J. HARTMAN, R. A. LIEBHOLD, A. L. JORDON, and S. D. CYR: Some aspects of the biochemical pharmacology of the octopus. Proc. W. Pharmacol. Soc. **3**, 106 (1960).
COLLIER, H. O. J., and B. MACAULEY: The pharmacological properties of "laudolissin" — A long — action curarizing agent. Brit. J. Pharmacol. **7**, 378 (1952).
COPENHAVER, J. H., M. E. NAGLER, and A. GOTH: The intracellular distribution of histamine. J. Pharmacol. exp. Ther. **109**, 401 (1953).
DALE, H. H.: The anaphylactic reaction of plain muscle in the guinea-pig. J. Pharmacol. exp. Ther. **4**, 167 (1913).

Debove, M.: De l'intoxication hydatique. Bull. Soc. Med. Hôp. Paris **5**, 113 (1888).
del Pozo, E. C.: Mechanism of pharmacological actions of scorpion venoms. In: Venoms. Ed. E. E. Buckley and N. Porges. Washington, D. C. Amer. Ass. Advanc. Sci. (1956).
— L. G. Anguiano y J. Gonzalez: Acciones del veneno de alacran sobre el sistema vasomotor. Rev. Inst. Salubr. Enferm. trop. (Mex.) **5**, 227 (1944).
Dessy, S., y R. A. Marotta: Toxicidad del liquido del quiste hidático. Rev. Soc. Med. Arg. **20**, 373 (1912).
Dew, H. R.: Hydatid disease; its pathology, diagnosis and treatment. Sidney: Aust. Med. Publ. Co. Ltd. 1928.
Dias da Silva, W., W. T. Beraldo, and J. Pudles: Histamine release and mast cell damage induced by purified fraction from Ascaris lumbricoides, in vitro. Effect of inhibitors of anaphylaxis. Acta physiol. lat.-amer. **11**, 264 (1961).
— A. D. L. Fernandes, and W. T. Beraldo: Inhibitory effects of carbohydrates on histamine release and mast cell disruption by dextran. Brit. J. Pharmacol. **19**, 405 (1962).
Diamant, B.: Histamine release elicited by extracts from Ascaris suis. Influence of oxygen lack and glucose. Acta physiol. scand. **52**, 8 (1961).
Diniz, C. R.: Chromatographic separation of smooth muscle active substances from spider venoms. Acta physiol. lat.-amer. (in press) (1962).
—, and J. M. Gonçalves: Some chemical and pharmacological properties of Brazilian scorpion venoms. In: Venoms, Ed. E. E. Buckley and N. Porges. Washington, D. C. Amer. Ass. Advanc. Sci. (1956).
— — Separation of biologically active components from scorpion venoms by zone electrophoresis. Biochim. biophys. Acta **41**, 470 (1960).
Dragstedt, C. A., and E. Gebauer-Fuelnegg: Studies in anaphylaxis. I. The appearance of a physiologically active substance during anaphylactic shock. Amer. J. Physiol. **102**, 512 (1932).
—, and M. Rocha e Silva: Effect of trypsin upon blood histamine of rabbits. Proc. Soc. exp. Biol. (N. Y.) **47**, 420 (1941).
Duhig, J. V.: Nature of venom of "Synanceja horrida" (stonefish). Z. Immun.-Forsch. **62**, 185 (1929).
—, and G. Jones: The venom apparatus of the stone fish (Synanceja horrida). Mem. Queensland Museum **9**, 136 (1928).
Dutta, N. K., and K. G. A. Narayanan: Release of histamine from rat diaphragm by cobra venom. Nature (Lond.) **168**, 1064 (1952).
Ebbecke, U.: Capillarerweiterung, Urticaria und Schock. Klin. Wschr. **2**, 1725 (1923).
Ellis, S., and O. Krayer: Properties of a toxin from the salivary gland of the shrew, Blarina brevicauda. J. Pharmacol. exp. Ther. **114**, 127 (1955).
Essex, H. E., and J. Markowitz: The physiologic action of rattlesnake venom (crotalin). I. Effect on blood pressure: symptoms and post-mortem observations. Amer. J. Physiol. **92**, 317 (1930a).
— — II. The effect of crotalin on surviving organs. Amer. J. Physiol. **92**, 329 (1930b).
— — III. The influence of crotalin on blood, in vitro and in vivo. Amer. J. Physiol. **92**, 335 (1930c).
— — IV. The effect on lower forms of life. Amer. J. Physiol. **92**, 342 (1930d).
— — Some experiments on immunity to crotalin. Amer. J. Physiol. **92**, 345 (1930e).
Estable, C., P. Ferreira-Berruti y M. I. Ardao: Contribucion al conocimiento de la toxina de Megalopyge urens y de su acción farmacodinámica. Arch. Soc. Biol. Montevideo **12**, 186 (1945).
Fawcett, D. W.: Cytological and pharmacological observations on the release of histamine by mast cells. J. exp. Med. **100**, 217 (1954).
Feldberg, W.: The action of bee venom, cobra venom and lysolecithin on the adrenal medulla. J. Physiol. (Lond.) **99**, 104 (1940).
— H. F. Holden, and C. H. Kellaway: The formation of lysocithin and of a muscle-stimulating substance by snake venoms. J. Physiol. (Lond.) **94**, 232 (1938).
—, and B. Holmes: The effect of muscular contraction and of curarine on acid gastric secretion in cats. J. Physiol. (Lond.) **99**, 3 P (1941).
—, and C. H. Kellaway: Liberation of histamine from the perfused lung by snake venoms. J. Physiol. (Lond.) **90**, 257 (1937a).
— — Liberation of histamine from the perfused lung of the guinea-pig by bee venom. J. Physiol. (Lond.) **91**, 2 P (1937b).
— — Liberation of histamine and formation of lysocithin-like substances by cobra venom. J. Physiol. (Lond.) **94**, 187 (1938a).
— — Liberation of histamine by staphylococcal toxin and mercuric chloride. Aust. J. exp. Biol. med. Sci. **16**, 249 (1938b).
—, and W. V. Keogh: Liberation of histamine from the perfused lung by staphylococcal toxin. J. Physiol. (Lond.) **90**, 280 (1937).

FELDBERG, W., and A. A. MILES: Regional variations of increased permeability of skin capillaries induced by histamine liberator and their relation to histamine content of skin. J. Physiol. (Lond.) **120**, 205 (1953).
—, and J. L. MONGAR: Comparison of histamine release of compound 48/80 and octylamine in perfused tissues. Brit. J. Pharmacol. **9**, 197 (1954).
—, and W. D. M. PATON: Release of histamine from skin and muscle in the cat by opium alkaloids and other histamine liberators. J. Physiol. (Lond.) **114**, 490 (1951).
—, and M. SCHACHTER: Histamine release by horse serum from skin of the sensitized dog and non-sensitized cat. J. Physiol. (Lond.) **118**, 124 (1952).
FLURY, F.: Handbuch der normalen und pathologischen Physiologie. Berlin: Springer 1930.
FOOT, N. C.: Pathology of the dermatitis caused by Megalopyge opercularis, a Texan caterpillar. J. exp. Med. **35**, 737 (1922).
FONSECA, F.: Animais Peçonhentos. São Paulo (Brazil), Emp. Graf. Revistas dos Tribunais, Ltda. (1949).
FREDHOLM, B., B. HÖGBERG, and B. UVNÄS: Role of phospholipase A and C in mast cell degranulation induced by non-purified Clostridium welchii toxin. Biochem. Pharmacol. **5**, 39 (1960).
GAIL, R., et J. RAGEAU: Premières observations sur un poisson marin venimeux de la nouvelle-calédenie: La synancée (Synanceia verruces Bloch). Bull. Soc. Path. exot. **49**, 846 (1956).
GAMINARA, A.: Le venin de la larve de Megalopyge urens. Bull. Soc. Path. exot. **21**, 656 (1928).
GARCIA-AROCHA, H.: Release of histamine and 5-hydroxytryptamine from cells of the peritoneal fluid of rats. Canad. J. Biochem. Physiol. **39**, 395 (1961).
GAZZINELLI, G., M. M. GUIA, A. G. G. NEVES, J. PUDLES, W. T. BERALDO, and W. DIAS DA SILVA: Purification of the toxic fractions from Ascaris lumbricoides and their effect on the guinea-pig. Nature (Lond.) **190**, 813 (1961).
GEBAUER-FUELNEGG, E., and C. A. DRAGSTEDT: Studies in anaphylaxis. II. The nature of a physiologically active substance appearing during anaphylactic shock. Amer. J. Physiol. **102**, 520 (1932).
GERSHON, M. D., and L. L. ROSS: Studies on the relationship of 5-hydroxytryptamine and the enterochromaffin cell to anaphylactic shock in mice. J. exp. Med. **115**, 367 (1962).
GIUSTI, L. et E. HUG: Propriétés pharmacodynamiques du liquide hydatique. C. R. Soc. Biol. (Paris) **88**, 344 (1923).
GLENNY, A. T., M. BARR, M. LLEWELLYN-JONES, T. DALLING, and H. E. ROSS: Multiple toxins produced by some organisms of Cl. welchii group. J. Path. Bact. **37**, 53 (1933).
GOELDI (1902): Quoted by FONSECA, F.: Animais peçonhentos. São Paulo (Brazil), Emp. Graf. Revistas dos Tribunais. Ltda. (1949).
GOSSE, P. H.: A history of the British Sea Anemones. London: Ray Society 1860.
GOTH, A., W. L. NASH, M. NAGLER and J. HOLMAN: Inhibition of histamine release in experimental diabetes. Amer. J. Physiol. **191**, 25 (1957).
GOTZL, F. R., and C. A. DRAGSTEDT: Peptone shock in rabbits. J. Pharmacol. exp. Ther. **74**, 33 (1942).
GRÃNA, A., P. RECARTE, and E. BALEA: La histaminemia en la alergia hidatidica. Medicina (Madr.) **3**, 198 (1943).
GROLL, H.: Die Entzündung in ihren Beziehungen zum nervösen Apparat. (Eine experimentelle Studie). Beitr. Path. Anat. **70**, 20 (1922).
GUSMÃO, H. H., O. P. FORATTINI e A. ROTBERG: Dermatite provocada por lepidópteros do gênero Hylesia. Rev. Inst. Med. trop. S. Paulo **3**, 114 (1961).
GUYON, M.: Sur les accidents produits sur les animaux a sang chaud, mammifères et oiseaux, par le venin des scorpions. C. R. Soc. Biol. (Paris) **60**, 16 (1865).
HABERMANN, E.: Gewinnung und pharmakologische Bedeutung einiger Komponenten des Giftes des Gasbranderregers (clostridium Welchii Typ A). Naunyn-Schmiedeberg's Arch. exp. Path. Pharmak. **236**, 274 (1959).
HAINING, C. G.: Activation of rabbit serum protease by dextran sulphate. Brit. J. Pharmacol. **11**, 107 (1956).
HALPERN, B. N., et M. BRIOT: Liberation d'histamine par la peau du rat sous l'effet du contact avec le dextran, in vitro. C. R. Soc. Biol. (Paris) **146**, 1552 (1952).
HALSTEAD, B. W.: Animal phyla known to contain poisonous marine animals. Venoms, Washington D. C. Amer. Ass. Advanc. Sci. (1956).
HANZLIK, P. J.: Nerve mechanisms in production and treatment of certain edemas, and role of adrenals in preventive effects of certain drugs. Calif. west. Med. **24**, 33 (1926).
HARTMAN, W. J., W. G. CLARK, S. D. CYR, A. L. JORDON, and R. A. LIEBHOLD: Pharmacologically active amines and their biogenesis in the octopus. Ann. N. Y. Acad. Sci. **90**, 637 (1960).
HINSHAW, L. B., M. M. JORDAN, and J. A. VICK: Mechanism of histamine release in endotoxin shock. Amer. J. Physiol. **200**, 987 (1961).

HIRSCHFELDER, A. D.: Studies upon vascular and capillary phenomena and supposed axon reflexes concerned in development of edema in mustard oil conjunctivitis, together with effects of vasodilator drugs, local anesthetics and vital stains. Amer. J. Physiol. **70**, 507 (1924).

HÖGBERG, B., G. THUFVESSON, and B. UVNÄS: Histamine liberation produced in the perfused paw of the cat by 48/80 and extracts from jelly-fish (Cyanea capillata) and eelworm (Ascaris lumbricoides) from swine. Acta physiol. scand. **38**, 135 (1956).

HOUSSAY, B. A.: Action physiologique du venin des scorpions (Buthus quinquestriatus et Tityus bähiensis). J. Physiol. Path. gén. **18**, 305 (1919).

HUMPHREY, L.: An inquiry into the severe symptoms occasionally following puncture of hydatid cysts of the liver. Lancet **1887 I**, 120.

IHERING, R. VON: Estudo biológico das lagartas urticantes ou tatoranas. An. Paul. Med. Cirurgia **3**, 129 (1914).

JAQUES, L. B., and E. T. WATERS: The identity and origin of the anticoagulant of anaphylactic shock in the dog. J. Physiol. (Lond.) **99**, 454 (1941).

JAQUES, R., and M. SCHACHTER: A sea anemone extract (thalassine) which liberates histamine and a slow contracting substance. Brit. J. Pharmacol. **9**, 49 (1954a).

— — The presence of histamine, 5-hydroxytryptamine and a potent slow contracting substance in wasp venom. Brit. J. Pharmacol. **9**, 53 (1954b).

JOYEUX-LAFFUIE, J.: Sur l'appareil venimeux et le venin du scorpion. C. R. Soc. Biol. (Paris) **95**, 866 (1882).

KAISER, E.: The enzymatic activity of spider venom. Mem. inst. Butantan. **25**, 35 (1953).

KARSNER, H. T., and A. R. MORITZ: Pathologic histology of the Shwartzman phenomenon with interpretative comments. J. exp. Med. **60**, 37 (1934).

KATZ, G.: Histamine release from blood cells in anaphylaxis in vitro. Science **91**, 221 (1940).

—, and S. COHEN: Experimental evidence for histamine release in allergy. J. Amer. med. Ass. **117**, 1782 (1941).

KELLAWAY, C. H.: The action of Australian snake venoms on plain muscle. Brit. J. exp. Path. **10**, 281 (1929).

—, and D. H. LE MESSURIER: Vaso-depressant action of venom of Australian copperhead (Denisonia superba). Aust. J. exp. Biol. med. Sci. **14**, 57 (1936).

— G. REID, and E. R. TRETHEWIE: Circulatory and other effects of the toxin of Cl. septique. Aust. J. exp. Biol. med. Sci. **19**, 297 (1941).

—, and E. R. TRETHEWIE: Liberation of adenyl compounds from perfused organs by cobra venom: Aust. J. exp. Biol. med. Sci. **18**, 63 (1940).

— — Tissue injury by the toxin of Cl. welchii type A. Aust. J. exp. Biol. med. Sci. **19**, 17 (1941a).

— — The injury of tissue cells and the liberation of pharmacologically active substances by the toxins of Cl. welchii types B. and C. Aust. J. exp. Biol. med. Sci. **19**, 77 (1941b).

— —, and W. TURNER: The liberation of histamine and of adenyl compounds by the toxin of Cl. welchii type D. Aust. J. exp. Biol. med. Sci. **18**, 253 (1940).

KUIDA, H., L. B. HINSHAW, R. P. GILBERT, and M. B. VISSCHER: Effect of gram-negative endotoxin on pulmonary circulation. Amer. J. Physiol. **192**, 335 (1958).

KUN, E.: Effect of meningococcal endotoxin on histamine content of blood and tissues of rabbit. Proc. Soc. exp. Biol. (N. Y.) **66**, 197 (1947).

LANGER, J.: Über das Gift unserer Honigbiene. Naunyn-Schmiedeberg's Arch. exp. Pharm. Pathol. **38**, 381 (1896).

— Abschwächung und Zerstörung des Bienengiftes. Arch. int. Pharmak. **6**, 181 (1899).

LEGER, M., et P. MOUZELS: Dermatose prurigineuse déterminée par des papillons saturnidae du genre Hylesia. Bull. Soc. Path. exot. **11**, 104 (1918).

LEWIS, T.: The blood vessels of the human skin and their responses. London: Shaw and Sons Ltd. 1927.

LINSTROW, O.: Über den Giftgehalt der Helminthen. Intern. Mschr. Anat. Physiol. **13**, 188 (1896).

LIVON, C., et A. BRIOT: Le suc salivaire des céphalopodes est un poison nerveux pour les crustacés. C. R. Soc. Biol. (Paris) **58**, 878 (1905).

LOZANO Y MONZÓN, R.: Chascos y peligros de la hidatidosis; el "schock" anafilatico mortal. Arch. int. Hidatid. **1**, 95 (1934).

LUDWIG, O.: Anaphylaktischer Schock durch Insektenstich. Münch. med. Wschr. **18**, 1564 (1934).

MACHEBOUEF, M., et R. MANDOUL: À propos de la toxité des extraits d'Ascaris. C. R. Soc. Biol. (Paris) **130**, 1032 (1939).

MACFARLANE, M. G., and B. C. J. G. KNIGHT: The biochemistry of bacterial toxins. I. The lecithinase activity of Cl. welchii toxins. Biochem. J. **35**, 884 (1941).

MACINTOSH, F. C., and W. D. M. PATON: The liberation of histamine by certain organic bases. J. Physiol. (Lond.) **109**, 190 (1949).

MacLean, L. D., and M. H. Weil: Hypotension (shock) produced by Escherichia coli endotoxin. Circulat. Res. 4, 456 (1956).
Magalhães, O.: Contribuição para o conhecimento da intoxicação pelo veneno dos escorpiões. Mem. Inst. Osw. Cruz. 21, 5 (1928).
— Estudos sôbre os coleópteros vesicantes. Brasil-med. n°s. 10 a 13, 11 (1960).
McIlwain, H., and H. L. Buddle: Techniques in tissue metabolism. I. A mechanical chopper. Biochem. J. 53, 412 (1953).
McIntire, F., L. W. Roth, and M. Sproull: Histamine release in rabbit blood by simple molecules; inhibition and reaction rate studies. Amer. J. Physiol. 167, 233 (1951).
Messineo, E., u. D. Calamida: Über das Gift der Tänien. Anal. in Arch. ital. Biol. 38, 490 (1902).
Mingazzini, P.: Sull'esistenza di una secrezione emessa dalla superficie del corpo dei cestodi adulti. Atti Acad. Lincei Roma 10, 307 (1901).
Mitchell, S. W.: Physiology and toxicology of the venom of the rattlesnake Smithson. Contrib. 12, 1 (1861).
—, and E. T. Reichert: Researches upon the venoms of poisonous serpents. Smithson. Contrib. 26, 1 (1886).
Mongar, J. L., and H. O. Schild: Quantitative measurement of the histamine-releasing activity of a series of monoalkylamines using minced guinea-pig lung. Brit. J. Pharmacol. 8, 103 (1953).
— — Effect of antigen and organic bases on intracellular histamine in guinea-pig lung. J. Physiol. (Lond.) 131, 207 (1956).
— — Effect of temperature on the anaphylactic reaction. J. Physiol. (Lond.) 135, 320 (1957).
—, and R. F. Whelan: Histamine release by adrenaline and D-tubocurarine in the human subject. J. Physiol. (Lond.) 120, 146 (1953).
Morrison, J. L., A. P. Richardson, and W. L. Bloom: The effects of antihistaminic agents on the reaction of the rat to dextran. Arch. int. Pharmacodyn. 88, 98 (1951).
Mosso, A.: Un venin dans le sang des Murénides. Arch. ital. biol. 10, 139 (1888).
Mota, I.: The mechanism of action of anaphylatoxin. Its effect on guinea-pig mast cells. Immunology 2, 403 (1959).
— W. T. Beraldo, A. G. Ferri, and L. C. U. Junqueira: Intracellular distribution of histamine. Nature (Lond.) 174, 698 (1954).
— —, and L. C. U. Junqueira: Protamine-like property of compound 48/80 and stilbamidine and their action on mast cells. Proc. Soc. exp. Biol. (N. Y.) 83, 455 (1953).
—, and W. Dias da Silva: Antigen-induced damage to isolated sensitized mast cells. Nature (Lond.) 186, 245 (1960).
—, and I. Vugman: Effects of anaphylactic shock and compound 48/80 on the mast cells of the guinea-pig lung. Nature (Lond.) 177, 427 (1956).
Moura Gonçalves, J., e M. Rocha e Silva: Fator de permeabilidade capilar no veneno de Crotalus terrificus crotaminicus. Ciênc. e Cultura 10, 163 (1958).
—, e L. G. Vieira: Estudos sôbre venenos de serpentes brasileiras. I. Analise eletroforética. Acad. Bras. Ciências 22, 141 (1950).
Mourson, J., et F. Schlagdenhauffen: Nouvelles recherches chimiques et physiologiques sur quelques liquides organiques (Eau des oursins, eau des kystes hydatiques et des cysticerques, liquide amniotique). C. R. Acad. Sci. (Paris) 95, 791 (1882).
Nakajima, M.: Biochemical studies on the nature of ascaris toxin. Yokohama med. Bull. 5, 10 (1954).
Nakamura, M., and H. Takahashi: Sensory nerve terminals and inflammation from skin irritants. Tohoku J. exp. Med. 5, 288 (1924).
Neumann, W., E. Habermann, and H. Hansen: Differentiation of two hemolytic factors in the bee's venom. Naunyn-Schmiedeberg's Arch. exp. Path. Pharmak. 217, 130 (1953).
Norton, S., and E. J. de Beer: Effect of some antibiotics on rat mast cells in vitro. Arch. int. Pharmacodyn. 102 352 (1955).
Oliver-Gonzalez, J., and E. Koppisch: Immunological and pathological phenomena related to substances from tissues of Ascaris lumbricoides. Rice Inst. Pamphlet 45, 141 (1958).
Padawer, J., and A. S. Gordon: Isolation of mast cells from other cellular elements of rat peritoneal fluid. Proc. Soc. exp. Biol. (N. Y.) 88, 29 (1955).
Pantlitschko, M., u. E. Kaiser: Untersuchungen über Aktivierung und Hemmung der Hyaluronidase. Biochem. Z. 322, 137 (1951).
Parisot, J., et P. Simonin: Action du liquide hydatique sur les appareils circulatoire et respiratoire. C. R. Soc. Biol. (Paris) 83, 149 (1920).
Pawlowsky, E. N.: Gifttiere und ihre Giftigkeit. Jena: Gustav Fischer 1927.
Pearson, O. P.: On the cause and nature of a poisonous action produced by the bite of a shrew (Blarina brevicauda). J. Mammal. 23, 159 (1942).
Peçanha, J., e A. Oliveira Lima: Alergia aos antígenos de abelhas e de vespas. Hospital 46, 341 (1954).

PHISALIX, M.: Poissons Toxicophores. Animaux Venimeux et Venins. Paris: Masson et Cie. (1922).
PICKEL, B.: Uma dermatite purulenta causada por potós em São Paulo. Arch. Biol. **24**, 153 (1940).
PILCHER, J. D., and T. SOLLMANN: Skin-reaction to morphine. Arch. int. Med. **33**, 516 (1924).
PIRAJÁ DA SILVA, M.: Paederus colombianus est vesicant. Arch. Parasitol. **15**, 431 (1912).
PORTIER, P., et C. RICHET: De l'action anaphylactique de certain venins. C. R. Soc. Biol. (Paris) **54**, 170 (1902).
RAO, S. S., and S. S. RAO: Proteases of cobra (Naja, naja) venom. In: Venoms. Ed. E. E. BUCKLEY and N. PORGES Washington, D. C. Amer. Ass. Advanc. Sci. (1956).
REID, G., and H. A. JENKINS: The liberation of renin from the kidney by tissue injury with cobra venom. Aust. J. exp. Biol. med. Sci. **26**, 215 (1948).
RILEY, J. F.: Proc. Scot. Soc. exp. Med. Dundee Meeting, 9. Feb. 1952. Cit. in: RILEY, J. F. The riddle of mast cell. Lancet **1954 I**, 241.
— The effects of histamine liberators on the mast cells of the rat. J. Path. Bact. **65**, 471 (1953).
— The mechanism of histamine release from mast cells. J. Pharm. Pharmacol. **10**, 271 (1958).
—, and G. B. WEST: Histamine in tissue mast cells. J. Physiol. (Lond.) **117**, 72 P (1952).
ROBERTSON, M.: Serological groupings of vibrion septique and their relation to the production of toxin. J. Path. Bact. **23**, 153 (1919).
ROCHA E SILVA, M.: Histamina e anafilaxia em suas relações com patogenia das doenças alérgicas. São Paulo: Edigraf 1946.
—, and S. O. ANDRADE: Histamine and proteolytic enzymes. Liberation of histamine by papain. J. biol. Chem. **149**, 9 (1943).
— W. T. BERALDO, and G. ROSENFELD: Bradykinin, a hypotensive and smooth muscle stimulating factor released from plasma globulin by snake venoms and by trypsin. Amer. J. Physiol. **156**, 261 (1949).
—, and A. GRAÑA: Shock produced in dogs by hydatid fluid. Amer. J. Physiol. **143**, 306 (1945).
— — Anaphylaxis-like reactions produced by Ascaris extracts: I. The changes in the histamine content and the coagulability of the blood in guinea-pigs and dogs. Arch. Surg. **52**, 523 (1946a).
— — Anaphylaxis-like reactions produced by Ascaris extracts. II. The mechanism of the shock induced in dogs. Arch. Surg. **52**, 713 (1946b).
— —, and S. O. ANDRADE: Anaphylaxis-like reactions produced by Ascaris extracts. Arch. Surg. **53**, 199 (1946).
—, and H. O. SCHILD: The release of histamine by D-tubocurarine from the isolated diaphragm of the rat. J. Physiol. (Lond.) **109**, 448 (1949).
—, and R. M. TEIXEIRA: Role played by leucocytes, platelets and plasma trypsin in peptone shock in the dog. Proc. Soc. exp. Biol. (N. Y.) **61**, 376 (1946).
ROSE, B., and J. S. L. BROWNE: Changes in the blood histamine in shock. Proc. Soc. exp. Biol. (N. Y.) **44**, 182 (1940).
—, and P. WEIL: Blood histamine in the rabbit during anaphylactic shock. Proc. Soc. exp. Biol. (N. Y.) **42**, 494 (1939).
ROTHSCHILD, A., and A. CORRADO: (Personal communication) (1962).
—, and M. ROCHA E SILVA: Activation of a histamine releasing agent (anaphylatoxin) in normal rat plasma. Brit. J. exp. Path. **35**, 507 (1954).
SANARELLI, G.: Über Blutkörperchenveränderungen bei Skorpionenstich. Zbl. klin. Med. **10**, 153 (1889).
SAUNDERS, P. R.: Venom of the stonefish Synanceja verrucosa. Science **129**, 272 (1959).
SCHACHTER, M.: Anaphylaxis and histamine release in the rabbit. Brit. J. Pharmacol. **8**, 412 (1953).
SCHILD, H. O.: Release of histamine-like substance in anaphylactic shock from various organs of the guinea-pig. J. Physiol. (Lond.) **90**, 34 P (1937).
— Histamine release in anaphylactic shock from various tissues of the guinea-pig. J. Physiol. (Lond.) **95**, 393 (1939).
SCHULTZ, W. H.: Physiological studies in anaphylaxis. I. The reaction of the smooth muscle of the guinea-pig sensitized with horse serum. J. Pharmacol. exp. Ther. **1**, 549 (1910a).
— Physiological studies in anaphylaxis. II. Reaction of smooth muscle from guinea-pig rendered tolerant to large doses of serum. J. Pharmacol. exp. Ther. **2**, 221 (1910b).
SCROGGIE, A. E., and L. B. JAQUES: The release of histamine and heparin by antigen from the isolated perfused liver of the sensitized dog. J. Immunol. **62**, 103 (1949).
SHINAMURA, T., and N. J. FUJI: J. coll. Agric. **4**, 189 (1917), (cited by ESSEX, H. E., J. MARKOWITZ, and F. C. MANN). Physiologic responses and immune reactions to extracts of certain intestinal parasites. Amer. J. Physiol. **98**, 18 (1931).
STANSLY, P. G., R. G. SHEPHERD, and H. J. WHITE: Polymyxin: a new chemotherapeutic agent. Bull. Johns Hopk. Hosp. **81**, 43 (1947).

STEVENSON, N., and M. R. REID: The relation of the sensory nerves to inflammation. Bull. Johns Hopk. Hosp. **26**, 21 (1915).

SWIFT, P. N., and S. R. M. BUSHBY. Clinical aspects of toxicity of polymyxins A, B and E. Lancet **1953 I**, 110.

TAINTER, M. L., and F. L. REICHERT: Alleged mechanisms of local nerves in causation and in treatment of edema caused by irritants. Arch. Path. **6**, 872 (1928).

TANNENBERG, J., u. M. DEGENER: Experimentelle Untersuchungen über lokale Kreislaufstörungen. Die Leukocytenabwanderung und die Diapedese der roten Blutkörperchen. Frankf. Z. Path. **31**, 351 (1925).

THOMAS, L.: The physiological disturbances produced by endotoxins. Ann. Rev. Physiol. **16**, 467 (1954).

—, and R. A. GOOD: Studies on the generalized Shwartzman reaction. I. General observations concerning the phenomenon. J. exp. Med. **96**, 605 (1952).

THORP, R. W., and W. D. WOODSON: The black widow: America's most poisonous spider. Chapel Hill: Univ. of North Carolina Press 1945.

TINEL, J., et G. UNGAR: Vasodilatation et libération locale de substances histaminiques. C. R. Soc. Biol. (Paris) **118**, 1148 (1935).

TISSEUIL, J.: Contribution à l'étude de la papillonite guyanaise. Bull. Soc. Path. exot. **28**, 719 (1935).

TRETHEWIE, E. R.: Experiments on problem of "free" and "bound" histamine and acetylcholine. Aust. J. exp. Biol. med. Sci. **16**, 225 (1938).

— Comparison of haemolysis and liberation of histamine by two Australian snake venoms. Aust. J. exp. Biol. med. Sci. **17**, 145 (1939).

— Injury by trypsin. Aust. J. exp. Biol. med. Sci. **20**, 49 (1942).

UNGAR, G.: (Editor): Les méthodes employées pour l'étude du metabolisme et de la liberation de l'histamine. J. Physiol. (Paris) **53**, 847 (1961).

—, et J. L. PARROT: Recherches sur le choc anaphylactique in vitro. Mise en liberté d'une substance active par le poumon isolé du cobaye sensibilisé. C. R. Soc. Biol. (Paris) **123**, 676 (1936).

— — Sur la présence de substance histaminiques dans les tissus des invertébrés marins. C. R. Soc. Biol. (Paris) **126**, 1156 (1937).

UVNÄS, B.: Histamine and histamine liberators. Nord. Med. **53**, 770 (1955).

— The mechanism of histamine liberation. J. Pharm. Pharmacol. **10**, 1 (1958).

— Mechanism of action of a histamine-liberating principle in jelly-fish (Cyanea capillata). Ann. N. Y. Acad. Sci. **90**, 751 (1960).

— B. DIAMANT, B. HÖGBERG, and I. L. THON: Mechanism of mast-cell disruption induced by a principle extracted from Ascaris suis. Amer. J. Physiol. **199**, 575 (1960).

VALETTE, G., et H. HUIDOBRO: Pouvoir histaminolibérateur de la chenille processionnaire du pin — Thaumetopoea pityocampa, Schiff. Arch. int. Pharmacodyn. **109**, 344 (1957).

VALLE, J. R., Z. P. PICARELLI, and J. L. PRADO: Histamine content and pharmacological properties of crude extracts from setae of urticating caterpillars. Arch. int. Pharmacodyn. **98**, 324 (1954).

VAULLEGEARD, A.: Etude expérimentale et critique sur l'action des helminthes. I. Cestodes et Nematodes. Bull. Soc. Linné, Normand. Caen. **4**, 84 (1901).

VOGT, W.: Pharmacologically active substances formed in egg yolk by cobra venom. J. Physiol. (Lond.) **136**, 131 (1956).

— Naturally occurring lipid-soluble acids of pharmacological interest. Pharmacol. Rev. **10**, 407 (1958).

VOORHEES, A. B., H. J. BAKER, and E. J. PULASKI: Reactions of albino rats to injections of dextran. Proc. Soc. exp. Biol. (N. Y.) **76**, 254 (1951).

WATERS, E. T., J. MARKOWITZ, and L. B. JAQUES: Anaphylaxis in the liverless dog. Science **87**, 582 (1938).

WEIL, M. H., L. D. MAC LEAN, M. B. VISSCHER, and W. W. SPINK: Investigations on the role of the central nervous system in shock produced by endotoxin from gram-negative microorganism. J. Lab. clin. Med. **46**, 962 (1955).

— — — — Studies on the circulatory changes in the dog produced by endotoxin from gram-negative microorganisms. J. clin. Invest. **35**, 1191 (1956).

—, and W. W. SPINK: A comparison of shock due to endotoxin with anaphylactic shock. J. Lab. clin. Med. **50**, 501 (1957).

WILANDER, O.: Studien über Heparin. Skand. Arch. Physiol. **81**, Suppl. 15 (1938).

WILSON, C. W. M.: Factors influencing the urinary excretion of histamine in the rat. J. Physiol. (Lond.) **126**, 141 (1954).

WILSON, W. H.: The physiological action of scorpion venom. J. Physiol. (Lond.) **31**, 48 (1904).

Section B

Release of Histamine by Noxious Physical Agents, Organic Compounds and by Metals

By

Itamar Vugman

With 3 Figures

The similarity between the reaction of the blood vessels of human skin to intradermal injection of histamine and to several kinds of injury, – mechanical, thermal and electrical as well as by some chemical agents – led Lewis (1927) to suggest that the skin response to trauma is due to the release of histamine.

I. Release of histamine by physical stimulation

A. Radiant energy

1. Thermal injury

A few years after the report of Lewis (1927), Bennet and Drury (1931) made the first demonstration that histamine is actually released from tissues by the action of heat, showing that when a perfused rabbit's heart is burnt, a substance resembling histamine is liberated and can be detected in the perfusate. From dog's grinded liver extracts, heating increased the histamine yield from two to six times as compared to the yield from unheated extracts; heating the sediment obtained by centrifuging the liver extracts brought large amounts of histamine into solution (Trethewie, 1938).

The release of histamine by heat and some other kinds of stimuli has been carefully studied and reported in several papers by Rosenthal and co-workers. They have used split thicknesses of skin obtained from human beings and experimental animals secured with the cut surface inward at one end of glass cylinders. After immersing the skin in hot water, or after mechanical or electrical stimulation, it was found that histamine diffused into the Ringer-Locke solution contained inside the glass cylinder (Rosenthal and Minard, 1939). Using this method, Rosenthal, et al. (1957) found a direct relationship between the amount of histamine liberated from dog's skin and the temperature of burning. Detectable amounts of histamine were released after fifteen seconds of burning at 96° C and 85° C, after forty-five seconds at 75° C, and after two minutes at 55° C. Only trace amounts of histamine were released after exposure to 47° C. Quite surprisingly, burning for five minutes at 85° C or 96° C released consistently less histamine than at 65° C and 75° C. In order to make feasible the collection of larger amounts of material and to extend the time of collection of perfusates, Rosenthal et al. (1960) made use of the air pocket method described by Selye (1954). In this method, 30 ml of air are injected into the back of an anesthetized rat, between the skin and underlying tissues. The skin of the dome-shaped pocket formed is subjected to scalding and the histamine released is that diffusing into the solution injected into the pocket. Confirming their previous results, ROSENTHAL et al. (1960) found that burning the skin of the pocket at 96° C released less histamine than heating at 60° C.

Through the air pocket method, ROCHA E SILVA and ROSENTHAL (1961), besides confirming the liberation of histamine by scalding, studied the relationship between the fluid injected into the air pocket and the release of histamine by heat. Washing the air pocket of unburned rats with distilled water released histamine while no histamine could be detected when Tyrode's solution was introduced. On the other hand, Tyrode solution wash enabled a greater amount of histamine to be released by burning as compared to that occurring in the presence of distilled water, despite the histamine liberating action of the latter (Table 1).

Table 1. *Estimations of histamine in samples of fluid from air pockets*

Time of collection after burn (min)	Rat No. 1 control unburned, wash with distilled water (μg/5 ml)	Rat No. 2 burned 15 sec at 96° C, wash with distilled water (μg/5 ml)	Rat No. 3 burned 15 sec at 96° C, wash with tyrode's solution (μg/5 ml)	Rat No. 4 control unburned, wash with tyrode's solution (μg/5 ml)	Rat No. 5 burned 15 sec at 96° C, wash with tyrode's solution (μg/5 ml)
5	12.35	19.00	70.00	0	50.0 (5 min)
15	12.35	26.25	50.00	0	37.5 (10 min)
30	7.00	19.80	50.00	0	25.0 (20 min)
60	3.60	19.00	53.00	0	25.0 (30 min)
120	3.75	26.25	33.00	0	19.0 (40 min)
220—240	3.25	19.00	33.00	0	15.0 (50 min)
					12.5 (60 min)
Totals	42.30	129.30	289.00	0	184.0 (60 min)

The schedule of time for collection of the wash fluids was the same for rats 1, 2, 3, and 4; in rat 5 more washings were done in the first hour after burn and the experiment finished after that time. Five ml of fluid were injected into the pocket at each interval noted and allowed to remain there for 2 minutes after gentle shaking. (According to ROCHA E SILVA and ROSENTHAL, 1961).

The action of heat in releasing histamine from isolated tissues has been studied by MONGAR and SCHILD (1957) who worked with slices of guinea pig lung incubated for twenty-four minutes at several temperatures. Under these conditions, histamine release induced by heat began to occur at 55° C, and at 65° C as much as eighty-five per cent of the histamine contained in the tissue was released. By the method of "coaxial perfusion" ROCHA E SILVA and ANTONIO (1960) have been able to show that when paws of rats were heated at temperatures from 37° to 57° C the release of detectable amounts of histamine occurred only at 57° C.

Although ROSENTHAL et al. (1957), MONGAR and SCHILD (1957) and ROCHA E SILVA and ANTONIO (1960) found that release of histamine began at 55° C, the release of small amounts of histamine at temperatures ranging from 37° C to 50° C was described by KELLAWAY and RAWLINSON (1944), where six to seven per cent of the total histamine content of the guinea pig lung was released during a six hour perfusion. Such small amounts of histamine do not seem to have been released by the action of heat but are due to spontaneous release, since similar amounts of histamine (two to four per cent) were released from isolated rat diaphragm incubated during forty minutes at 36° C and 45° C (VUGMAN, 1961); also the same histamine content was found in symmetrical pieces of rat skin after heating at 37° C and 45° C during thirty minutes (ANTONIO, 1961).

In the rabbit, the action of heat apparently leads to an increase in the skin histamine content. Loos (1931) found that by immersing a rabbit's ear in hot water, its histamine content increased eight times as compared to that of the control, the unheated ear of the same animal. HILDEBRANDT (1940) also found that the histamine content of the skin of the trunk of rabbits began to increase three hours after being heated at temperatures just above 40° C, reaching a maximum of five hundred per cent four to twelve hours later. Such increases, however, seem to be due to capillary dilatation and blood stasis caused by heat, thus inducing an apparently heightened histamine content of the skin since rabbit blood is very rich in histamine.

Heat-induced increases in tissue histamine content, probably not due to blood histamine, were reported by KISIMA (1938) and by DEKANSKI (1945, 47). KISIMA found that cutaneous burns in dogs increased the histamine content of all tissues studied as well as that of the blood. This increase was due to formation of histamine in the skin, since removal of the burned skin prevented the increase in the histamine

Table 2. *Individual results of series 1. Histamine equivalents (μg) for normal (N) mice and mice exposed to 60° for 30 sec. Extracts prepared chemically* (according to DEKANSKI, 1945)

Time after burning	Skin	Stomach and intestines	Rest of body	Excreta[1]	Total (including excreta when obtained)
(*N*)	110	10	72	—	192
	146	11	81	—	238
	172	6	45	—	223
	137	13	62	—	212
1—4 min	164	10	70	—	244
	164	8	72	—	244
	140	7	82	—	229
	205	7	61	—	273
5—10 min	230	17	185	—	432
	282	14	91	—	387
	260	17	125	—	402
	223	11	113	—	347
	227	13	90	—	330
1 hr	282	13	78	0.11	373
	294	15	154	—	463
	288	10	125	—	423
	378	9	115	0.08	502
3 hr	253	11	88	—	352
	302	6	157	0.15	465
	264	18	125	—	407
	231	14	76	0.25	321
5 hr	281	10	73	0.8	364
	225	3	182	0.2	410
	230	14	166	1,2	411
	233	16	100	1.1	350

[1] Faeces only, no urine excreted.
(*N*) = neither anaesthetized, nor immersed in water, nor burned.

content of blood and tissues. In the blood there was an initial rise in the histamine level within six to twelve hours after the injury, reaching its maximum forty-eight to ninety-six hours later. After two to three days this high level gradually decreased toward normal values. DEKANSKI (1945) found that plunging mice into hot water at 60° C for ten to thirty seconds increased the total histamine content of the animals. This increase occurred mainly in the skin, the total amount of histamine being almost doubled in ten minutes and reached its maximum value within one hour or less. Surviving mice excreted the excess histamine mostly in the urine during the next forty-eight hours. As there was an increase in the total histamine of the body, these changes could not have been due to transference of histamine from one part of the body to another, but to production of new histamine due to some physical or chemical change in the skin itself (Tables 2, 3).

Table 3. *Individual results of series 2. Histamine equivalents (µg) for control (C) mice and mice exposed to 60° C for 10 sec. Extracts prepared chemically* (according to DEKANSKI, 1945)

Time after burning or immersion hr	Skin	Stomach and intestines	Rest of body	Excreta	Total (including excreta)
5	242	7	72	—	321
	215	12	90	17	334
	305	8	78	0.9[1]	392
	215	13	85	75	388
12	267	10	86	2[1]	365
	245	9	105	2.8[1]	362
	230	12	74	20	336
	228	13	70	40	357
(*C*)	132	8	45	1	181
24	264	7	62	20	353
	268	9	54	20	351
	281	6	75	1[1]	362
	220	8	95	40	363
(*C*)	110	5	35	1.3	157
48	210	10	50	60	330
	176	6	50	100	332
	267	8	40	180	495
	226	8	60	144	437
(*C*)	146	5	34	3	188

[1] Faeces only, no urine excreted.
(*C*) = anaesthetized and immersed in water at room temperature.

Burning outlined patches of skin of cats also led to similar results (DEKANSKI, 1947). While control pieces of skin averaged 10.5 µg per outlined area, burning at 60° C for sixty seconds increased to 22.6 µg the histamine extractable from equivalent areas. Maximum increase was found to occur at three hours after burning, but five hours later the histamine content of the skin was still higher than that of controls. Heating at 80° C for sixty seconds or at 140° C for fifteen seconds reduced the histamine content of the skin.

The formation of histamine by the action of heat as described by KISIMA and DEKANSKI has not been confirmed by BALLANI et al. (1959b). According to their report, mice immersed in hot water at 60° C for ten seconds, ten minutes, two and twenty-four hours after the burning did not show any alteration in histamine values in the tissues studied (whole skin, subcutaneous tissue, outer skin, spleen and lungs). Mast cells observed in subcutaneous tissue spreads and mesentery were disrupted suggesting that there should have been histamine release caused by the burning. In another paper, BALLANI et al. (1959a) again found no increase in histamine content of tissues of mice and rats also heated in hot water at 60° C for ten seconds. Twenty-four hours after the burning there actually occurred a moderate lowering of the histamine content of the skin along with mast cell degranulation and rupture. An increase of fifty per cent in the histamine content of the whole skin occurred only nineteen to twenty-one days after burning and of one hundred and fifty per cent later on. This increase in the histamine content has not been followed by a significant proliferation of mast cells in subcutaneous tissue. Results similar to those of BALLANI's et al. were described by SANYAL (1962). Heating of rats and mice under the same conditions led again to a fall in the histamine content of the skin accompanied by mast cell alterations soon after the heat treatment. A delayed rise in the skin histamine content occurring earlier in the rat and later in the mouse was also observed; in the rat this increase began on the seventh day and in the mouse on the 14th day after the heating.

Our own experiments on heating mice in a water bath at 60° C also do not suggest any alteration in skin histamine content as caused by such heating. No significant difference was found between the skin histamine content of control mice and that of the skin of mice one hour after being heated for ten, fifteen or thirty seconds at 60° C (Table 4). Also the histamine content of the ears of mice taken before heating was strictly comparable to that of the ears taken after heating the animals.

Table 4. *Histamine content of the skin of mice heated at 60° C*

	Controls	10 sec	15 sec	30 sec
	57.0	180.0	178.0	138.4
	91.0	106.0	93.0	100.0
	83.0	94.0	106.2	111.0
	125.0	100.0	94.0	100.0
	111.0	140.0	106.2	66.8
	75.0	70.0		84.5
	85.0	106.8		52.0
	113.0	100.0		120.0
	89.0			
	89.0			
Average	91.8	102.1	115.5	96.6

The mice were heated at 60° C for the time indicated, the skin has been taken out one hour later and the histamine extracted by grinding in 0.1 N HCl and boiling. Values are given as μg of histamine (base). No statistical difference has been found between the different treatments and controls.

Ever since the demonstration that the effects of a large dose of histamine resemble the shock-like picture sometimes observed in burned patients, the possibility that histamine might be liberated in these conditions has been considered. Much work has been done trying to demonstrate such causal relationship. Most of the first trials were very indirect, remained unconfirmed, and only after the description by BARSOUM and GADDUM (1935) of the first reliable method for extraction of histamine from the blood did a better approach to the problem become possible. Subsequent to the description of this method, the influence of cutaneous burns on the blood histamine level of burned patients or under experimental conditions began to be studied. The assay of the histamine content of blood in physiological and pathological conditions had then become feasible. Quite naturally, soon after reporting their method, BARSOUM and GADDUM (1936) described the alterations occurring in the blood histamine level of nine patients suffering from extensive cutaneous burns. In these patients, the blood histamine content rose to at least four times its normal level on the fourth and sixth days, maintained at high values and slowly settled again to its normal level. There appeared to be a direct relationship between the area of burns and the magnitude and duration of the rise in the blood histamine content. The next year, CODE and MACDONALD (1937) reported another case of a patient with severe burns. In this patient, on the day after the burn the blood histamine content was well within normal values, rose considerably on the twelfth day, then gradually subsided but did not reach normal levels until two months later. While BARSOUM and GADDUM and CODE and MACDONALD had not reached their patients immediately after the injury, ROSE and BROWNE (1942) were able to assay the blood histamine content of three burned patients one hour after the burning. An increase in the blood histamine content was then found. In the days following the trauma, in these patients as well as in four other cases, the blood histamine content followed the clinical picture of the other patients: there was a fall in the blood histamine when their condition became worse and a return to normal or higher than normal values with their clinical improvement. ROSE and BROWNE have not observed the slow increase in the blood histamine content as reported in the previous papers.

More recently, BIRKE et al. (1958) have followed the blood histamine alterations occurring in several burned patients. They have found markedly elevated blood histamine levels one to three hours after the injury. Urinary excretion of histamine was also high during the first twenty-four hours. Both high histamine blood level and urinary excretion of the amine subsided rapidly afterwards: four days later they were found to be comparable to control values. Notwithstanding the great individual variation, some correlation between the severity of the injury and initial excretion of histamine seemed to exist. In another paper, DUNÉR et al. (1961) also found a significantly higher urinary histamine excretion in three burned patients during the first day after trauma. This high histamine excretion returned to normal values on the third day.

Experimental work has been done by BEHRMANN et al. (1946), who followed the blood histamine alterations in fourteen dogs receiving third degree burns over fifty to sixty per cent of their body surface. Twenty-four to forty-eight hours later the blood histamine level had risen to two and a half times the average normal figure with a maximum increase of approximately five times about the fourth day. After the sixth to seventh day the blood histamine level gradually decreased toward normal in the succeeding days. Unfortunately, in this paper, no mention is made on the blood histamine levels immediately after the injury. Another experimental evidence is presented by UNGAR and BOLGERT (1938), who have shown that the inhalation of water steam by guinea pigs and dogs increases the histamine content of blood and kills the animals.

Since histamine is released by heat, when anti-histamine drugs were developed their use in the treatment of local burns and shock induced by burning seemed indicated. The protection afforded and the prevention of symptoms would suggest a participation of the released histamine in the symptomatology observed. Such reasoning led GUNNAR and WEEKS (1949) to induce a burn shock in rabbits by immersing them in hot water after a pre-treatment with large doses of intravenously injected tripelennamine. No differences in the severity, delay of onset or inhibition of progression of shock were noted between treated and untreated animals. On localized burns, however, PELLERAT et al. (1950) described a partial protection afforded to the injured part of the skin of rats and guinea pigs by local pre-treatment with two per cent promethazine. Similar results were not obtained by SEVITT (1949) who was unable to find any protection afforded by the anti-histamines: Benadryl, Antistin and Anthisan to skin burns of different degrees of severity. The symptoms observed after burn included erythema, presence of capillary permeability changes, stagnation or stasis in the dermal blood supply, edema formation, followed by the clinical course of the burns. In man also, two circular burns inflicted on anesthetized skin of the arm (60° C for fifteen seconds) developed in the same manner whether Antistin had been previously taken or not (SEVITT et al. 1952).

The role played by locally released histamine in the development of burns was carefully studied by SPECTOR and WILLOUGHBY (1958, 1959b). They have inflicted standard burns of two different intensities in the skin of rats, and capillary permeability changes as evidenced by leakage of intravenously injected Trypan blue and edema formation were observed. In the less severe burns increased capillary permeability developed only after a latent period, whereas after severe burns this vascular change began immediately. The initial phase of the delayed increase in capillary permeability was suppressed by small systemic doses of mepyramine and, less consistently, by prior depletion of body histamine. After burns of greater intensity the immediate increase of capillary permeability was unaffected by these treatments. These results suggest that in rats increased capillary permeability following burns of moderate severity is initiated by release of histamine and then maintained by other endogenous mechanisms. According to WILHELM and MASON (1958) mild heat treatment of the skin of guinea pigs is followed by vascular permeability changes similar to those described by SPECTOR and WILLOUGHBY. They have also been able to inhibit with anti-histamines the initial and short-lived increase in capillary permeability, but again the delayed and more prolonged response was unaffected. Some participation of histamine in the development of burns is also indicated by FERLUGA and STERN (1960) who have shown that the depletion of body histamine by a histamine liberator partially protects rats from third degree burns covering up to fifty per cent of the skin area. When the third degree burns did not exceed twenty-five per cent of the body surface the burned rats behaved in the same manner as the controls. When second degree burns were inflicted in the skin of guinea pigs in regions with either a high or low histamine content, they were of lower intensity in the region poor in histamine. The same pattern was followed when the histamine content of rat skin was artificially decreased.

It seems clear then that above a certain temperature heat releases histamine from tissues as shown by the histamine appearing in the perfusates of burned isolated organs and by the increase in the blood histamine content of patients and animals appearing shortly after the burning. However the delayed alterations in blood histamine content reported in the literature do not seem to be related to release of histamine from the injured tissues caused directly by the burning. Most probably causes secondary to the trauma influence these blood histamine alterations. On the other hand, only a small part of the symptoms appearing after local burns and probably none of those observed in shock state due to burning seem to be caused by the histamine released by thermal injury.

2. Injury by heat-producing radiations

The demonstration of histamine release by types of radiant energy which act through heat production has also been made. Thus, KELLAWAY et al. (1938) have shown that after exposure of a perfused dog lung to infra-red and to visible light a small amount of histamine appears in the perfusate. Short-waves and diathermy, according to HILDEBRANDT (1938, 1940), also may release histamine as shown by the increased histamine content of the blood of dogs submitted to these irradiations, while in cats exposed to short-waves the skin histamine content fell two hours after exposure. Using the air pocket method, ROCHA E SILVA and ROSENTHAL (1961) found a good parallelism between the histamine released when the skin was scalded at 96° C for fifteen seconds or burned with an infra-red lamp for two minutes.

3. Ultra-violet light

Ultra-violet light induced skin changes such as erythema followed by edema were long thought to be due to histamine release, since they resemble those caused by the injection of histamine into the skin. The early demonstration by ELLINGER (1928) that histamine was formed in a histidine solution after ultra-violet irradiation seemed to lend support to this contention. But although histamine formation from irradiated histidine solutions was confirmed (ELLINGER, 1934; HOLTZ, 1934), and notwithstanding KAWAGUCHI's report (1930) of an increased histamine content of the guinea pig skin after exposure to sun light or to ultra-violet light, no increase of histamine content of the skin seems really to occur after ultra-violet irradiation. ELLINGER himself was unable to find any changes in the histamine content of the guinea pig skin (1928) of pig skin (1930) after ultra-violet exposure, and KAWAGUCHI's results do not seem to have been supported by other experimental evidences. It seems, on the contrary, that ultra-violet light lowers the histamine content by releasing it from tissues as it was shown by the work of TARRAS-WAHLBERG (1937a). Cats and rabbits were submitted to ultra-violet irradiation, and at different times after exposure, the histamine content of the irradiated skin was compared to that of symetrical non-irradiated pieces of skin taken from the same animal. Since symmetrical pieces of skin contain an equivalent histamine content, the frequent difficulties in the interpretation of experimental results arising from the high individual variation and from differences in histamine content between the several regions of the skin of one and same animal were avoided. The results of TARRAS-WAHLBERG's experiments show that after ultra-violet irradiation the histamine content of the cat skin clearly fell below control values in a few hours and three days later it still was low. In the rabbit, the histamine content of the exposed skin increased in the first two days, falling in the third and fourth days. TARRAS-WAHLBERG suggests that the different results obtained in the cat and rabbit could be explained by the hyperemia and edema appearing after irradiation. In the cat there is a ratio of two thousand to one between the histamine content of the skin and that of the blood, while in the rabbit this ratio is two to one. On a weight basis, hyperemic and edematous rabbit skin would then have an increased histamine content, even if some of the histamine it originally contained had been lost subsequent to the injury. The same would not happen in the cat skin where a similar weight increase could even cause an apparent lowering of the content in the skin in spite of no histamine being actually lost. Figures 1 and 2 show such a relationship between histamine content and skin weight.

The histamine releasing action of ultra-violet light has been confirmed by KELLAWAY et al. (1938). Perfused isolated dog lung upon being irradiated by ultra-violet light during half to one hour liberated small but measurable amounts of histamine found in the perfusate, the lung surface having been kept moist and cool during the experiment so as to avoid histamine release by heat injury.

In the subsequent analysis of the role played by histamine in the vascular response of the skin to ultra-violet irradiation different experimental approaches were tried, mainly indirect ones. Most results have cast doubts on histamine being the substance responsible for the vascular alterations or even being released during the process. Contrasting to skin alterations induced when histamine is released, ABRAMSON (1940) noticed that the borders of the wheal formed after ultraviolet irradiation always initially coincide with the exposed area and that pseudopods never formed. By reverse electrophoresis of histamine he was also unable to isolate a whealing substance from the irradiated skin. Results also suggesting no participation of histamine in this process are those of PARTINGTON (1954) who found that lowering the histamine content of the skin by intradermal injection of histamine liberators (pethidine, 500 or 5,000 μg; compound 48/80, 100 or 500 μg) in man either four hours or immediately before irradiation did not alter the subsequent development of erythema, while, as shown by MACINTOSH and PATON (1949) a second injection of a histamine liberator produces either no response or one that is much reduced. Furthermore the histamine content of human skin, as indicated by the erythema response to intradermal injection of compound 48/80, seemed not to be affected after ultra-violet exposure (PARTINGTON, 1954). Similarly, the

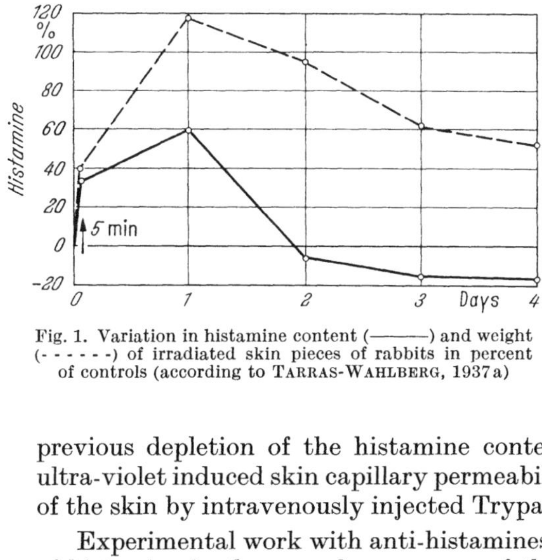

Fig. 1. Variation in histamine content (———) and weight (- - - - - -) of irradiated skin pieces of rabbits in percent of controls (according to TARRAS-WAHLBERG, 1937a)

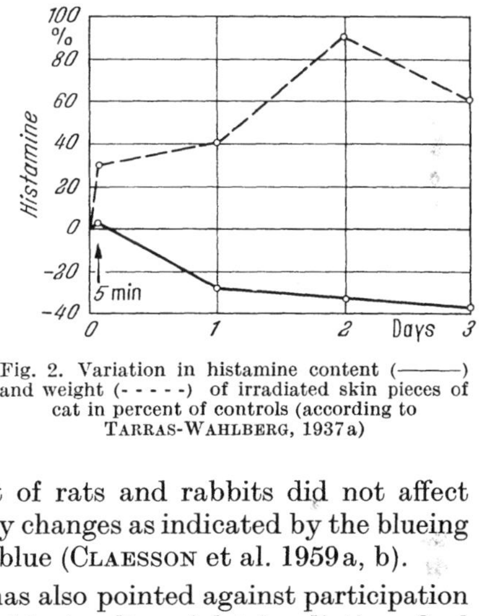

Fig. 2. Variation in histamine content (———) and weight (- - - - -) of irradiated skin pieces of cat in percent of controls (according to TARRAS-WAHLBERG, 1937a)

previous depletion of the histamine content of rats and rabbits did not affect ultra-violet induced skin capillary permeability changes as indicated by the blueing of the skin by intravenously injected Trypan blue (CLAESSON et al. 1959a, b).

Experimental work with anti-histamines has also pointed against participation of histamine in the vascular response of the skin to ultra-violet irradiation. Oral pre-treatment with mepyramine reduced in man the red reaction of the skin to injected histamine but not that produced by ultra-violet light, and also did not prevent the blueing by intravenously injected Trypan blue of the ultra-violet irradiated area of the skin of the rabbit (PARTINGTON, 1954). Anti-histamines also were not effective against cutaneous erythema induced in human skin by exposure to ultra-violet light; of three drugs tested, phenindamine, promethazine and chlorcyclizine, only the last one has raised significantly the erythema threshold (ROSS, 1951). In rats, this erythema reaction could be decreased by injection of methotrimepazine, an anti-histamine which also has anti-5-hydroxytryptamine activity (CLAESSON et al., 1959a).

Prevention of ultra-violet erythema by local aplication of some anti-histamines can be due to the absorption of the erythema producing wave-lengths by the drugs. This was clearly demonstrated by KLINE and BAER (1948) who prevented the ultra-violet induced erythema by interposing between the skin and the ultra-violet source a five per cent pyribenzamine solution contained in a quartz cup; direct anti-histamine effects of pyribenzamine having been thus excluded. KALZ and BOWER (1950) confirmed this observation by showing that the previous iontophoretic application of pyrilamine and pyribenzamine to the skin markedly reduced the erythema caused by ultra-violet irradiation, pyrilamine being twice as potent as pyribenzamine. Their application after the exposure was of no effect. The erythema caused by different wave-length radiations (ultra-soft roentgen rays) was not regularly influenced by such drugs.

4. X-Rays and β-radiations

X-ray induced alterations in histamine content of tissues are usually delayed, although differing appreciably according to the organ and to the animal species.

EISEN et al. (1956) described the changes in the histamine content of rat tissues induced by X-rays. It was shown that after total body dorsal x-irradiation of 605 r the histamine content of the skin fell on the fifth post-irradiation day, reaching a minimum value on the tenth day. In the following days it increased slightly. In the pyloric portion of the stomach the histamine content began to decrease during the first twenty-four hours after total-body irradiation of 1025 r and reached its minimum value on the fifth day. Later on it increased slightly but it was still significantly below the control values fifteen days after irradiation. In the jejunum three hours after irradiation the histamine content began to diminish and on the fifth post-irradiation day it had already fallen to its minimum value. The irradiation of the abdominal skin with high x-ray doses (1000 and 2000 r) produced a greater fall in the skin histamine value, but the effects followed the same time pattern as after a 605 r dose. The changes in the histamine content of the different tissues following total-body irradiation are shown in Fig. 3. Whereas the histamine content of the stomach wall and skin decreased to about sixty per cent, that of the jejunum fell to seven and half per cent of the normal value. The figure also shows that the changes in the skin occur considerably later than those in the stomach and jejunum.

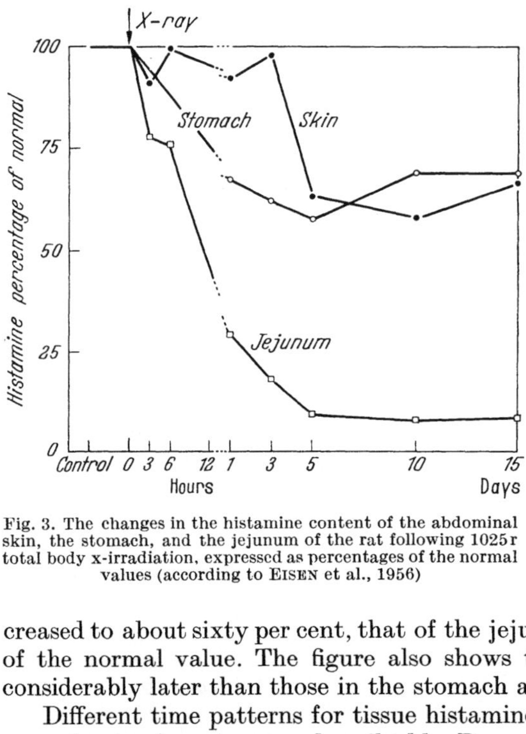

Fig. 3. The changes in the histamine content of the abdominal skin, the stomach, and the jejunum of the rat following 1025 r total body x-irradiation, expressed as percentages of the normal values (according to EISEN et al., 1956)

Different time patterns for tissue histamine changes following x-irradiation in several animal species were described by BEAUMARIAGE and LECOMTE (1957, 1958). Different organs in the same animal were also found to behave differently. Thus, three hours after irradiation there already appeared a significant fall in the histamine content of the lung and jejunum of the rabbit and chick, while in the rat the histamine content of the jejunum fell only forty eight hours after exposure, no changes in the lung histamine having been found. Skin histamine changes, which were simultaneous with those of the lung and jejunum in the rabbit, appeared twenty-four hours after exposure in the rat and were absent in the chick.

In man, skin histamine content seems also to be decreased by irradiation (FELDBERG and LOESER, 1954). In mice, however, no lessening in skin histamine content was found after irradiation (700 r). On the contrary, a small increase of histamine among female mice was actually found forty-eight hours after irradiation, males showing no alterations (BEAUMARIAGE, 1960a, b).

Ionizing radiations (β-rays from a Sr^{90} source) were reported to have no influence on the skin histamine content of rats (UNGAR and DAMGAARD, 1954), and air pockets made on the back of β-irradiated rats when washed one to one hundred and twenty hours after exposure also did not indicate any release of histamine (ROSENTHAL et al. 1960). These observations were not confirmed by EISEN and WILSON (1957) who have shown that the histamine content of the skin of β-irradiated rats began to decrease after twenty hours but such decrease did not become pronounced until the fifth day. On the tenth day the histamine content had fallen to forty-three per cent of the value of control samples of non-irradiated skin taken from the same animal.

Blood histamine alterations following x-irradiation have also been reported. Two hours after a 600 r irradiation the plasma histamine of exposed rats was found to be increased. In similarly irradiated rats there was found a fall in blood pressure correlating with the appearance of histamine in blood plasma which strongly suggested that the released histamine was responsible for the lowered blood pressure (WEBBER and STEGGERDA, 1949). Different results in blood histamine changes after x-irradiations were obtained by BAXTER et al. (1954), for in swine treated with total body x-irradiation of 400 r, the blood histamine fell steadily from the pre-radiation level until the thirteenth day post-irradiation. The histamine content then rose gradually. Only when a flash burn was added to the same amount of radiation did a rise in blood histamine content above pre-irradiation values occur in the second day. This was followed by a continuous decrease until the thirteenth day. There appeared to be a definite parallelism between the fall in blood histamine content and increasing severity of the symptoms of acute radiation illness. While the changes in blood histamine also were parallel to the decrease in the myeloid series of cells, this did not entirely account for the lowering of blood pressure.

In man, the variations in blood histamine were followed in patients submitted to x-ray therapy. SEGAL (1939) found that pretreatment plasma histamine of patients with tumours was normal, but increased during the treatment. LASSER and STENSTROM (1954) also reported elevated blood histamine levels in patients undergoing roentgen therapy. During the first four treatment days the blood histamine level was higher than in any other period of the therapy. Thereafter it fell and remained rather constant. A heightened blood histamine content after x-ray treatment was also found by CATTANEO and PELOCCHINO (1956). Divergent findings have been presented by FOCHEM et al. (1956), who determined the blood histamine content of thirty women on the sixth and tenth days following x-irradiation, but the great individual variation prevented them from reaching any conclusion on changes in blood histamine as caused by the treatment. They consider that the great individual variation appearing in SEGAL's (1939) data should also have prevented him from inferring an increase in plasma histamine of his x-ray treated patients.

Urinary excretion of histamine has been used to study the histamine releasing action of x-radiation, a two-fold increase in urinary excretion of histamine of rats submitted to x-rays having been detected (LEITCH and HALEY, 1955). It has been further shown that the amount of histamine excreted by rats is independent of the radiation dosage within the 600—1200 r range studied; significant levels of urinary excretion of histamine were detected only during the first twenty four hours post-irradiation. A latency in cell damage by irradiation was indicated by the doubling of urinary histamine content with each subsequent collection period, although during the first two collection periods (0—6 and 6—12 hours) the histamine excreted was already significantly raised (LEITCH et al., 1956).

The influence of x-rays on mast cells has been studied by several authors. SYLVEN (1940) found that very few if any mast cells were encountered in x-ray treated human carcinomas, while non-treated pieces presented a great number of these cells. Rat connective tissue mast cells were found to be altered one or two days after x-radiation, but their number remained unchanged. Mouse and hamster mast cell alterations appearing from three to five days after exposure were described by SMITH and LEWIS (1953). An increase in the number of atypical cells accompanied by a reduction in their total number following whole-body x-irradiation were reported by SMITH and LEWIS (1954) and MAYNARD et al. (1955). Rat mast cell changes were correlated with the whole-body radiation dose and the post-irradiation time (COMTE et al., 1956). After 75 r, during the first twenty-four hours a transient increase was followed by a slight decrease in the number of mast cells. After larger doses (150—600 r), mast cells decreased in number during the first two weeks following the exposure.

Histamine content alterations of x-irradiated rats were shown to be accompanied by mast cell changes (EISEN et al., 1956). On the fifth post-irradiation day in the subcutaneous connective tissue there was a lowered histamine content corresponding to a diminished number of mast cells; on the tenth day when the histamine content reached its lowest point mast cells were practically absent, and on the sixteenth day when the histamine content was already increasing, new mast cells were developing. In the stomach and jejunum, x-irradiation did reduce the histamine content, although the histamine they contain is not connected to mast cells and is not released by compound 48/80 (MOTA et al., 1956). β-irradiation influenced mast cell changes of the subcutaneous tissue of the rat in a similar way (EISEN and WILSON, 1957). Mast cell alterations in rat mesentery after large whole-body x-ray doses (3000 r) were described by VAN DEN BRENK (1958b) as early as one hour; they were maximal at twenty-four hours and remained so for the next four days. These x-ray induced changes were different from those caused by compound 48/80 since clear vacuolation and cell disruption were practically absent. With higher doses (4000 r) up to fifty per cent of the cells presented an abnormal appearance. Fourteen days and as late as four to eight weeks after irradiation, abnormal mast cells were still in excess but there also was a general reduction in the total number of mast cells.

An increase in the number of mast cells of tissues after irradiation has also been referred to. In their report on the pathologic changes caused by atomic bombs in Japan, LIEBOW et al. (1949) state that mast cells were found in relatively large numbers in the bone marrow and lymph nodes of irradiated casualties. In patients exposed to radiation coming from an accidental nuclear reaction one presented a large number of mast cells in almost all tissues, while another presented a smaller but nevertheless definite increase in number of these cells (HEMPELMANN et al., 1952). An increase in the number of mast cells in hematopoietic tissue of irradiated mice has been reported by ARVY et al. (1952) and in the thymus of irradiated hamsters (KELSALL and CRABB, 1952).

Some of the conflicting results reported on the alterations of the number of mast cells following irradiation may be explained by the difficulties met by PETTERSSON (1954) when evaluating his results on the reaction of mast cells of the guinea pig to irradiation. These difficulties came from the great individual variation met in the mast cell counts in non-irradiated control animals and from the highly significant difference in mast cell number between different zones of the same animal. Taking into account these differences and using each animal as its own control, PETTERSSON (1954) found a fifty per cent decrease of mast cells of the skin of guinea pigs from three to six weeks after a total-body irradiation of 660 r.

The production of local and systemic radiation effects has been attributed to histamine released by x-radiation (ELLINGER, 1951). The release of histamine by x-rays has been clearly demonstrated but some experimental evidences do not seem to support the histamine theory of the radiation syndrome. Thus, radiation lethality is considerably increased in rats chronically depleted of their tissue histamine by compound 48/80; acute depletion of tissue histamine has less influence on radiation lethality. Notwithstanding chronic depletion of tissue histamine, the rats developed radiation changes significantly earlier than controls, the skin erythema was more intense and final tissue damage was considerably increased (VAN DEN BRENK, 1957, 1958a). After β-irradiation, prior depletion of skin histamine also did not affect the severity of the subsequent ulceration (EISEN and WILSON, 1957). On the other hand, irradiated rats respond to intraperitoneal injection of compound 48/80 by severe shock symptoms and their mast cells also respond in a normal manner. Irradiated rat skin reacts normally to intradermal injection of histamine, coumpound 48/80, croton oil and a second dose of x-rays (VAN DEN BRENK, 1958b). β-irradiation also did not diminish the histamine liberating properties of compound 48/80 in the rat and the combination of compound 48/80 and irradiation did not decrease the skin histamine any more than compound 48/80 alone (EISEN and WILSON, 1957). No confirmation was thus provided to UNGAR and DAMGAARD'S (1954) report that the wheal formation induced by intradermal injections of 48/80 is prevented by previous β-irradiation.

Anti-histamine drugs have usually been of no avail in the treatment of radiation syndrome. Although LOFSTROM and NURNBERGER (1946) reported that in eighteen cases developing radiation sickness treated with Benadryl all were improved but one, other reports on a negative action of anti-histamines have been made. BROWN and HUNTER (1948) found Anthisan of no value in the treatment of radiation sickness. HALEY and HARRIS (1950) have even found a synergistic action of several anti-histamine drugs to radiation. X-ray lethality of guinea pigs was increased by daily subcutaneous administration of Benadryl, Thephorin, Neo-antergan, Neo-hetramine, Antistin, Phenergan after irradiation, while sensitization to roentgen erythema by anti-histamines was reported by PRATESI et al. (1952).

B. Mechanical stimulation (traumatic shock)

Low blood pressure is a common feature in shock states. A toxemic theory for certain types of shock has been developed and histamine held responsible for the lowering of the blood pressure under such conditions. Its release during shock would explain the blood pressure alterations then occurring. Some experimental evidences supporting the possibility of the participation of histamine in traumatic shock conditions was supplied by the demonstration that histamine is actually released by mechanical stimulation; pinching and pricking isolated pieces of skin of animals and human beings released histamine, the amount liberated being directly proportional to the degree of stimulation (ROSENTHAL and MINARD, 1939). By making human skin biopsies before and after mechanical stimulation, NILZEN (1947) has also shown that shortly after the stimulus was applied the histamine content of the skin was reduced. In dogs, MINARD (1937) found that blood returning from a traumatized leg contained a distinctly greater concentration of histamine than the venous blood coming from the normal extremity; the histamine content of arterial and normal venous blood before and after the animal was in profound shock was not changed. Such an increase in blood histamine by trauma was also reported by KOSLOWSKI et al. (1952) after pressing a hind leg of rats for two hours.

Notwithstanding these demonstrations of histamine release by mechanical stimulation and trauma, the histamine toxemic theory of shock has most frequently not been supported by the evidences obtained from traumatic shock conditions. Thus, after traumatic shock having been induced in dogs by striking their thigh with a hammer, HOLT and MACDONALD (1934) have been unable to demonstrate the presence of any blood pressure depressing substance in the blood coming from the traumatized area and the blood pressure was not reduced to a shock level without there being a loss of plasma and blood from the injured tissues sufficient in itself to account for the effects observed. In a comparison made between the histamine content of the blood coming from normal and traumatized limbs of rats, no significantly increased amounts of histamine were released from the damaged tissues (MACDONALD and WOOLFE, 1938). CHAMBON et al. (1943), when following the development of fatal traumatic shock inflicted in dogs, have not found any alterations in blood histamine content before and after trauma. During surgical shock, DRAGSTEDT and MEAD (1937) also failed to find a vasodepressor "toxin" in the blood and lymph of dogs, and in a series of patients in varying types of shock, ROSE and BROWNE (1940) have even found a marked diminution in the histamine content of the blood when shock state was established.

The lack of participation of histamine as a causal agent in the establishment of traumatic shock states was also evidenced by the verification that the depletion of tissue histamine with repeated injections of compound 48/80 did not change the survival time of adrenalectomized rats submitted to hind legs trauma. All animals died within twentyfour hours either pre-treated with 48/80 or not, although all of them had shown a marked increase in blood histamine after the trauma (SPUZIC and HALPERN, 1959). Pre-treatment with anti-histamine drugs did not influence the fatal outcome of traumatic shock inflicted in rats (JOURDAN and CHATONNET, 1943) and was also ineffective in delaying the onset of irreversible stages of hemorrhagic shock induced in dogs (INGRAHAM and WIGGERS, 1947).

C. Cold

PELLERAT and MURAT (1945) have shown that cold may release histamine since local freezing by ethyl chloride decreased significantly the histamine content of the skin, while the venous blood coming from the freezed area contained an increased histamine content. This histamine release could not be attributed to anesthesia since cutaneous anesthesia with procaine-adrenaline did not change the skin histamine content. ZIEMKE (1949) also found an increase in venous blood of rabbits submitted to local freezing.

II. Release of histamine by organic compounds

Several organic substances can liberate histamine from tissues and many unexpected reactions which follow their administration can be attributed to the release of histamine. STEINER (1934) has shown that repeated intramuscular injections of benzene (0.3 ml) into guinea pigs usually leads to a fatal reaction resembling acute anaphylactic shock. Death is due to to respiratory failure caused by bronchospasm, the lungs being emphysematous and presenting small hemorrhagic areas. Toluene, xylene and petroleum ether can also induce such a reaction, while ethyl ether and ethyl alcohol were found to be ineffective. Repeated injections (3 to 4) are necessary apparently to produce an area of inflammation from which the substance is absorbed in sufficient amounts to produce bronchospasm. Inhalation of these substances produced the same result, no preparatory injections being then necessary. Rats also are susceptible to this benzene reaction but require more injections than do guinea pigs.

While in the benzene reaction as described by STEINER (1934), histamine release can only be implied from the symptoms observed, BARTOSCH (1936) was able to demonstrate that a biologically active substance resembling histamine is released when 0.02 ml of hexane, heptane, octane, benzene, toluene, xylene, petroleum ether are injected into the trachea of a perfused guinea pig lung. Hexane, heptane and octane released more histamine than benzene, xylene and petroleum ether; mustard oil (allyl isothiocyanate) as well as the volatile anesthetics ether, chloroform and ethyl chloride did not cause the appearance of histamine into the perfusate. GARAN (1938), using the same method, confirmed the observations made by BARTOSCH (1936) and verified that from two to five minutes after the inhalation of several organic compounds a biologically active substance resembling histamine appeared in the perfusion fluid, maximum release occurring ten to fifteen minutes later. Xylene was found to be the most potent histamine releasing substance followed by toluene, benzene, hexane and heptane. Acrolein and chloroform have shown little histamine releasing activity while mustard oil and chloracetone were inactive.

Volatile anesthetics, as shown by KELLAWAY and TRETHEWIE (1939), do liberate histamine from the perfused dog lung but only when administered in high concentrations above those used for anesthesia. Thus, chloroform liberated histamine when the dog lung was ventilated with air containing chloroform in a concentration over four per cent. In the usual anesthetic concentrations – two to two and a half per cent—chloroform was inactive. Ether, also, realesed histamine only in concentrations from nineteen to forty-four per cent. With ethyl chloride, concentrations above twenty per cent were necessary for histamine to be detected in the perfusate, below this level it was inactive. Ethylene and nitrous oxide, even when administered in pure form, caused only trivial outputs of histamine. TRETHEWIE (1941) demonstrated that chloroform injected intraportally, in a dose sufficient to produce a concentration of the same order as that occurring in anesthesia, caused release of histamine from the perfused liver of the dog. When applied to dog skin samples, either "in situ" or removed from the body, chloroform, xylene or turpentine also released histamine (LAMBERT and ROSENTHAL, 1943).

An inhibitory action of ether and urethane on histamine release has been reported by KATZ (1940). Perfused lungs from sensitized guinea pigs released no detectable amounts of histamine upon injection of the antigen when the perfusion fluid contained ether or urethane in concentrations above 0.25 per cent. Inhaled ether led to the same results. When previously put in contact with ether or urethane, lung lobes, uterine horns or seminal vesicles, from sensitized guinea pigs incubated with the antigen, also did not release histamine, although the animals were well sensitized as shown by control experiments. The ether concentrations inhibiting histamine release are well below those found to liberate histamine by the specific action of ether.

Release of histamine by turpentine was shown by SPECTOR and WILLOUGHBY (1957, 1959a), when studing the inflammatory action of this substance. By assaying the exudate produced in the pleural cavity of the rat after injection of turpentine and by depleting the body stores of histamine or pre-treating the animals with the anti-histamine mepyramine, they came to the conclusion that histamine is released but only in the initial steps of the inflammation.

III. Release of histamine by metals

Mercuric chloride (2 to 10 mg per cent) injected into the perfusion fluid of the isolated gut of the cat and rabbit released a histamine-like substance which appeared in the perfusate in concentrations from 0.02 mg to 0.1 mg per cent (HEUBNER and Bachmann, 1937; Bachmann, 1938). Some relationship between the amount of mercuric chloride injected into a perfused liver of the dog and the histamine liberated was found by Feldberg and Kellaway (1938); 200 mg of mercuric chloride released 23 per cent of the histamine contained in the liver, 40 mg, 18 per cent and 15 mg, 3 per cent. Mercuric oxycyanide was also found to release histamine from the perfused gut of the cat (Bachmann, 1938), while mercuric cyanide liberated histamine from the isolated guinea pig gut and desensitized to antigen the gut from a sensitized animal (Parrot and Richet, 1944).

Other metals studied, gold chloride, zinc chloride and potassium cyanide, did not release histamine from the gut of the cat (Heubner and Bachmann, 1937). Arsenic also does not release histamine (Heubner and Bachmann, 1937; Bachmann, 1938) and the dermatitis appearing during the treatment with neo-arsphenamine, an arsenic compound, seems to be due to release of histamine by sensitization of the patients to the drug (Tarras-Wahlberg, 1937b). Simon and Staub (1937) have been able to sensitize guinea pigs by lymphatic ganglion injection of neo-arsphenamine. Ten days after the injection, a second injection of the drug induced an anaphylactic shock state in the animal with a heightened blood histamine content.

References

Abramson, H. A.: Whealing response of human skin to ultraviolet light and the histamine theory of allergic reactions. Proc. Soc. exp. Biol. (N. Y.) **43**, 410 (1940).

Antônio, A.: Inhibition of histamine release from the hind legs of the rat by "in vitro" heating at 45° C. IV. Meeting of the "Associação Latino-Americana de Ciências Fisiológicas". Ribeirão Prêto, July, 1961.

Arvy, L., J. A. Boiffard et M. Gabe: Déterminisme de la labrocytose provoquée par les rayons X dans les organes lymphöides de la souris. C. R. Soc. Biol. (Paris) **146**, 1537 (1952).

Bachmann, H.: Über die Freisetzung von Histamin bei Gewebeschädigungen durch Gifte. Naunyn-Schmiedeberg's Arch. exp. Path. Pharmak. **190**, 23 (1938).

Ballani, G. K., C. D. Jha, and R. K. Sanyal: Histamine and 5-hydroxytryptamine after cutaneous burn in mice and rats. J. Pharm. Pharmacol. **11**, 512 (1959a).

— Y.K. Sinha, and R.K. Sanyal: Effect of cutaneous burn on histamine and 5-hydroxytryptamine in mice. J. Pharm. Pharmacol. **11**, 192 (1959b).

Barsoum, G. S., and J. H. Gaddum: The pharmacological estimation of adenosine and histamine in blood. J. Physiol. (Lond.) **81**, 1 (1935).

— — The effect of cutaneous burns on the blood histamine. Clin. Sci. **2**, 357 (1936).

Bartosch, R.: Über die Freisetzung von Histamin durch chemisch bekannte Substanzen. Naunyn-Schmiedeberg's Arch. exp. Path. Pharmak. **181**, 176 (1936).

Baxter, H., J. A. Drummond, B. Rose, L. G. Stephens-Newsham, and R. G. Randall: Blood histamine levels in swine following total-body X-irradiation and a flash burn. Ann. Surg. **139**, 179 (1954).

Beaumariage, M. L.: Teneur en histamine de la peau chez la souris adulte exposée au rayonnement X. C. R. Soc. Biol. (Paris) **154**, 1533 (1960a).

— Teneur en histamine de la peau du souriceau et irradiation par rayons X. C. R. Soc. Biol. (Paris) **154**, 2135 (1960b).

—, et J. Lecomte: Teneur en histamine des tissus du lapin irradié par rayons X. C. R. Soc. Biol. (Paris) **151**, 1976 (1957).

— — Irradiation par rayons X et libération de l'histamine tissulaire. Arch. int. Pharmacodyn. **116**, 257 (1958).

Behrmann, V. G., V. Schelling, and F. W. Hartman: Blood histamine levels in experimental burns. Amer. J. Physiol. **145**, 483 (1946).

Bennet, D. W., and A. N. Drury: Further observations relating to the physiological activity of adenine compounds. J. Physiol. (Lond.) **72**, 288 (1931).

Birke, G., H. Dunér, S. O. Liljedahl, B. Pernow, L. O. Plantin, and L. Troell: Histamine, catechol amines and adrenocortical steroids in burns. Acta chir. scand. **114**, 87 (1958).

Brown, W. M., and R. B. Hunter: Antihistamine drugs and radiation sickness. Brit. med. J. **1948 II**, 984.

Cattaneo, R., and A. M. Pelocchino: Roentgentherapy and pyridoxine: blood histamine changes. Minerva med. **2**, 190 (1956).

Chambon, M., F. Jourdan et P. Martin: Sur la teneur du sang en histamine au cours du choc traumatique experimental chez le chien chloralosé. C. R. Soc. Biol. (Paris) **137**, 482 (1943).

Claesson, S., L. Juhlin, and G. Wettermark: The action of ultraviolet light on skin with and without horny layer. The effect of 48/80 and methotrimeprazine. Acta derm.-venereol. (Stockh.) **39**, 3 (1959a).
— G. Wettermark, and L. Juhlin: Action of ultraviolet light on skin: effect of the histamine liberator 48/80 and methotrimeprazine. Nature (Lond.) **183**, 1451 (1959b).
Code, C. F., and A. D. MacDonald: The histamine-like activity of blood. Lancet **1937 II**, 730.
Comte, F. P., G. S. Melville jr., and A. C. Upton: Effects of graded doses of whole-body X-irradiation on mast cells in the rat mesentery. Amer. J. Physiol. **187**, 160 (1956).
Dekanski, J.: The effect of cutaneous burns on histamine in mice. J. Physiol. (Lond.) **104**, 151 (1945).
— The effect of severe burns and some protein-precipitants on skin histamine in cats. J. Physiol. (Lond.) **106**, 33 (1947).
Dragstedt, C. A., and F. B. Mead: A pharmacologic study of the toxemia theory of surgical shock. J. Amer. med. Ass. **108**, 95 (1937).
Dunér, H., S. O. Liljedahl, and B. Pernow: Does the urinary excretion of imidazole acetic acid reflect the endogenous histamine metabolism in man? Acta physiol. scand. **51**, 41 (1961).
Eisen, V. D., R. E. Ellis, and C. W. M. Wilson: The effect of X-irradiation on tissue histamine in the rat. J. Physiol. (Lond.) **133**, 506 (1956).
—, and C. W. M. Wilson: The effect of β-irradiation on skin histamine and vascular responses in the rat. J. Physiol. (Lond.) **136**, 122 (1957).
Ellinger, F.: Über die Entstehung eines den Blutdruck senkenden und den Darm erregenden Stoffes aus Histidin durch Ultraviolettstrahlung. Naunyn-Schmiedeberg's Arch. exp. Path. Pharmak. **136**, 129 (1928).
— Weitere Untersuchungen über die Entstehung des Lichterythems. Naunyn-Schmiedeberg's Arch. exp. Path. Pharmak. **149**, 343 (1930).
— Die Entstehung von Histamin aus Histidin durch Bestrahlung. Naunyn-Schmiedeberg's Arch. exp. Path. Pharmak. **175**, 97 (1934).
— Die Histaminhypothese der biologischen Strahlenwirkungen. Schweiz. med. Wschr. **81**, 61 (1951).
Feldberg, W., and C. H. Kellaway: The liberation of histamine by staphylococcal toxin and mercuric chloride. Aust. J. exp. Biol. med. Sci. **16**, 249 (1938).
—, and A. A. Loeser: Histamine content of human skin in different clinical disorders. J. Physiol. (Lond.) **126**, 286 (1954).
Ferluga, J., u. P. Stern: Beziehungen zwischen Histamin und Verbrennung. Allergie u. Asthma **6**, 329 (1960).
Fochem, K., K. Formanek u. W. Smetana: Zum Verhalten des Histaminblutspiegels nach Röntgenbestrahlung unter besonderer Berücksichtigung des chemischen Nachweises des Histamins. Wien. med. Wschr. **106**, 543 (1956).
Garan, S. C.: Histamin-Freisetzung in der Lunge durch Reizstoffbeatmung. Naunyn-Schmiedeberg's Arch. exp. Path. Pharmak. **188**, 250 (1938).
Gunnar, R. M., and R. E. Weeks: Effect of tripelennamine hydrochloride on burn shock. Arch. Path. **47**, 594 (1949).
Haley, T. J., and D. H. Harris: The effect of several antihistamine drugs on mortality due to x-irradiation. Stanf. med. Bull. **8**, 1 (1950).
Hempelmann, L. H., H. Lisco, and J. G. Hoffman: The acute radiation syndrome: a study of nine cases and a review of the problem. Ann. intern. Med. **36**, 457 (1952).
Heubner, W., u. H. Bachmann: Über die Freisetzung von Histamin durch Quecksilber. Klin. Wschr. **16**, 279 (1937).
Hildebrandt, F.: Das Auftreten gefäßerweiternder Substanzen nach Kurzwellenbestrahlung. Naunyn-Schmiedeberg's Arch. exp. Path. Pharmak. **190**, 197 (1938).
— Über den Einfluß der Kurzwellen, der Diathermie und des Fango auf den Histamingehalt im Blut und Gewebe. Klin. Wschr. **19**, 270 (1940).
Holt, R. L., and A. D. MacDonald: Observations on experimental shock. Brit. med. J. **1934 I**, 1070.
Holtz, P.: Die Entstehung von Histamin aus Histidin durch Bestrahlung. Naunyn-Schmiedeberg's Arch. exp. Path. Pharmak. **175**, 97 (1934).
Ingraham, R. C., and H. C. Wiggers: Treatment of impending hemorrhagic shock with an antihistamine agent. Fed. Proc. **5**, 50 (1947).
Jourdan, F., et J. Chatonnet: La médication antihistaminique dans le choc traumatique expérimental. C. R. Soc. Biol. (Paris) **137**, 559 (1943).
Kalz, F., and C. Bower: The effect of iontophoresis of antihistaminics on ultraviolet and grenz ray erythema. Dermatologica (Basel) **101**, 29 (1950).
Katz, G.: The action of anesthesia on the histamine release in anaphylactic shock. Amer. J. Physiol. **129**, 735 (1940).
Kawaguchi, S.: Über den Einfluß der Lichtstrahlen auf den Gesamt-Cholesteringehalt der Haut. Biochem. Z. **221**, 232 (1930).

KELLAWAY, C. H., H. F. HOLDEN, and E. R. TRETHEWIE: Tissue injury by radiant energy and the liberation of histamine. Aust. J. exp. Biol. med. Sci. **16**, 331 (1938).
—, and W. A. RAWLINSON: Studies on tissue injury by heat; influence of anoxia. Aust. J. exp. Biol. med. Sci. **22**, 63 (1944).
—, and E. R. TRETHEWIE: Tissue injury by volatile and gaseous anaesthetics. Aust. J. exp. Biol. med. Sci. **17**, 225 (1939).
KELSALL, M. A., and E. D. CRABB: Increased mast cells in the thymus of X-irradiated hamsters. Science **115**, 123 (1952).
KISIMA, H.: Über die Bedeutung des Histamins für Verbrennungsgifte. Fukuoka Acta med. **31**, 49 (1938).
KLINE, P. R., and R. L. BAER: Nature of inhibition of ultraviolet erythema by pyribenzamine. J. invest. Derm. **10**, 397 (1948).
KOSLOWSKI, L., W. MARGGRAF u. W. SCHEELE: Histaminämie nach Muskeltraumen (crush-syndrom). Experimentelle Untersuchungen. Klin. Wschr. **30**, 365 (1952).
LAMBERT, E., and S. R. ROSENTHAL: Study of skin histamine (with some results of splanchnic nerve stimulation). Proc. Soc. exp. Biol. (N. Y.) **52**, 302 (1943).
LASSER, E. C., and K. W. STENSTROM: Elevation of circulating blood histamine in patients undergoing deep roentgen therapy. Amer. J. Roentgenol. **72**, 985 (1954).
LEITCH, J. L., V. G. DEBLEY, and T. J. HALEY: Endogenous histamine excretion in the rat as influenced by x-ray irradiation and compound 48/80. Amer. J. Physiol. **187**, 307 (1956).
—, and T. J. HALEY: Effect of 48/80 and x-irradiation on urinary histamine in the rat. Fed. Proc. **14**, 363 (1955).
LEWIS, T.: The blood vessels of the human skin and their responses. London: Shaw 1927.
LIEBOW, A. A., S. WARREN, and E. DECOURSEY: Pathology of atomic bomb casualities. Amer. J. Path. **25**, 853 (1949).
LOFSTROM, J. E., and C. E. NURNBERGER: Irradiation sickness: histamine effect treated with benadryl; a preliminary report. Amer. J. Roentgenol. **56**, 211 (1946).
LOOS, H. O.: Über die Beziehungen des Histamins zur Entzündung. II. Der Nachweis der Vermehrung eines histaminartigen Stoffes in der entzündeten Kaninchenhaut. Arch. Derm. Syph. (Berl.) **164**, 199 (1931).
MACDONALD, A. D., and G. WOOLFE: Blood histamine in traumatic shock. J. Physiol. (Lond.) **93**, 58 P (1938).
MACINTOSH, F. C., and W. D. M. PATON: The liberation of histamine by certain organic bases. J. Physiol. (Lond.) **109**, 190 (1949).
MAYNARD, F. L., G. B. WEST, R. KAGAN, and P. FULTON: Mast cells and histamine content in mesentery and cheek pouch of the hamster. Anat. Rec. **121**, 336 (1955).
MINARD, D.: Histamine-like substances in blood following trauma. Amer. J. Physiol. **119**, 375 (1937).
MONGAR, J. L., and H. O. SCHILD: Effect of temperature on the anaphylactic reaction. J. Physiol. (Lond.) **135**, 320 (1957).
MOTA, I., W. T. BERALDO, A. G. FERRI, and L. C. U. JUNQUEIRA: Action of 48/80 on the mast cell population and histamine content of the wall of the gastro-intestinal tract of the rat. Ciba Foundation Symposium on Histamine, page 47. London: Churchill 1956.
NILZEN, A.: Studies in histamine (H substance) with special reference to conditions obtaining in urticaria and related skin-changes. Acta derm.-venereol. (Stockh.) **27**, suppl. 17 (1947).
PARROT, J. L., et G. RICHET: Action du cyanure de mercure sur les organes isolés du cobaye. Un nouveau type de libération de l'histamine. C. R. Soc. Biol. (Paris) **138**, 364 (1944).
PARTINGTON, M. W.: The vascular response of the skin to ultraviolet light. Clin. Sci. **13**, 425 (1954).
PELLERAT, J., et M. MURAT: Variations de la teneur cutanée en histamine sous l'influence du froid et dans certaines dermatoses. C. R. Soc. Biol. (Paris) **139**, 1141 (1945).
— — et M. A. VÉDRINE: Action préventive de la crème au Phénergan sur les brûlures expérimentales. Bull. Soc. franç. derm. syphil. **57**, 446 (1950).
PETTERSSON, T.: The effect of x-ray total-body irradiation on the mast cell count in skin. An experimental investigation on guinea pigs. Acta path. microbiol. scand. Suppl. 102 (1954).
PRATESI, F., M. MATTEINI, and M. PAOLETTI: First observations on cutaneous reaction to x-rays after local intra-arterial injection of antihistamine drugs. Margin. derm. (Firenze) **4**, 117 (1952).
ROCHA E SILVA, M., and A. ANTÔNIO: Release of bradykinin and the mechanism of production of a "thermic edema" (45° C) in the rat's paw. Med. Exp. **3**, 371 (1960).
—, and S. R. ROSENTHAL: Release of pharmacologically active substances from the rat skin "in vivo" following thermal injury. J. Pharmacol. exp. Ther. **132**, 110 (1961).
ROSE, B., and J. S. L. BROWNE: Alterations in the blood histamine in shock. Proc. Soc. exp. Biol. (N. Y.) **44**, 182 (1940).
— — Studies on the blood histamine in cases of burns. Ann. Surg. **115**, 390 (1942).

ROSENTHAL, S. R., and D. MINARD: Experiments on histamine as the chemical mediator for cutaneous pain. J. exp. Med. **70**, 415 (1939).
— F. R. HUNTER, F. J. FINAMORE, and I. N. ROMAN: On an "in vivo" method of collection of difusates from skin. Arch. int. Pharmacodyn. **126**, 43 (1960).
— C. SAMET, R. J. WINZLER, and S. SHKOLNIK: Substances released from the skin following thermal injury. I. Histamine and proteins. J. clin. Invest. **36**, 38 (1957).
ROSS, A.: Activity of the anti-histamine drugs — A method of assessment in man. Lancet **1951 II**, 62.
SANYAL, R. K.: Histamine and 5-hydroxytryptamine metabolism after superficial skin burns Int. Arch. Allergy **21**, 326 (1962).
SEGAL, G.: Variations du taux d'histamine chez les malades soumis à un traitement par rayons x. C. R. Soc. Biol. (Paris) **131**, 1079 (1939).
SELYE, H.: An experimental model illustrating the pathogenesis of the diseases of adaptation. J. clin. Endocrinol. **14**, 997 (1954).
SEVITT, S.: The failure of anti-histamine drugs to influence the local vascular changes in experimental burns. Brit. J. exp. Path. **30**, 540 (1949).
— J. P. BULL, C. N. D. CRUICKSHANK, and JACKSON MACG: Failure of an anti-histamine drug to influence the course of experimental human burns. Brit. med. J. **1952 II**, 57.
SIMON, A., et A. M. STAUB: Libération de substances histaminiques au cours des réactions allergiques provoquées par l'arsénobenzol chez le cobaye. C. R. Soc. Biol. (Paris) **125**, 815 (1937).
SMITH, D. E., and Y. S. LEWIS: Effects of total-body x-irradiation on the tissue mast cell. Proc. Soc. exp. Biol. (N. Y.) **82**, 208 (1953).
— — Influence of total-body x-irradiation upon tissue mast cell number. Proc. Soc. exp. Biol. (N. Y.) **85**, 306 (1954).
SPECTOR, W. G., and D. A. WILLOUGHBY: Histamine and 5-hydroxytryptamine in acute experimental pleurisy. J. Path. Bact. **74**, 57 (1957).
— — Experimental suppression of increased capillary permeability in thermal burns in rats. Nature (Lond.) **182**, 949 (1958).
— — The demonstration of the role of mediators in turpentine pleurisy in rats by experimental suppression of the inflammatory changes. J. Path. Bact. **77**, 1 (1959a).
— — Experimental suppression of the acute inflammatory changes of thermal injury. J. Path. Bact. **78**, 121 (1959b).
SPUZIC, I. V., et B. N. HALPERN: Rôle de l'histamine dans de choc traumatique. C. R. Soc. Biol. (Paris) **153**, 1108 (1959).
STEINER, P. E.: Fatal pseudo-anaphylaxis by intramuscular injection of benzene and related substances. J. Immunol. **27**, 525 (1934).
SYLVÉN, B.: Studies on the liberation of sulphuric acids from the granules of the mast cells in the subcutaneous connective tissue after exposure to roentgen and gamma rays. Acta radiol. (Stockh.) **21**, 206 (1940).
TARRAS-WAHLBERG, B.: Über den Histamingehalt der Haut nach Ultraviolettbestrahlung. Klin. Wschr. **16**, 958 (1937a).
— Blood-histamine in salvarsan-dermatites. Acta derm.-venereol. (Stockh.) **18**, 284 (1937b).
TRETHEWIE, E. R.: Experiments on the problem of "free" and "bound" histamine and acetylcholine. Aust. J. exp. Biol. med. Sci. **16**, 225 (1938).
— The liberation of pharmacologically active substances from tissues by chloroform. Aust. J. exp. Biol. med. Sci. **19**, 175 (1941).
UNGAR, G., et M. BOLGERT: Libération d'une substance histaminique à la suite de l'inhalation de vapeurs irritantes. C. R. Soc. Biol. (Paris) **129**, 929 (1938).
—, and E. DAMGAARD: Inhibition of inflammatory response in beta-irradiated skin. Proc. Soc. exp. Biol. (N. Y.) **87**, 383 (1954).
VAN DEN BRENK, H. A. S.: Radiation lethality and local tissue damage in histamine depleted rats. Nature (Lond.) **180**, 1467 (1957).
— Radiation lethality in histamine depleted rats. Brit. J. exp. Path. **39**, 300 (1958a).
— Observations on mast cell changes, histamine release and local tissue damage in rats following x-irradiation. Brit. J. exp. Path. **39**, 356 (1958b).
VUGMAN, I.: Factors influencing histamine liberation from isolated rat diaphragm by compound 48/80. Thesis, Ribeirão Prêto 1961.
WEBBER, R. P., and F. R. STEGGERDA: Histamine in rat plasma; correlation with blood pressure changes following x-irradiation. Proc. Soc. exp. Biol. (N. Y.) **70**, 261 (1949).
WILHELM, D. L., and B. MASON: Rationale of antihistaminic therapy in thermal injury. An experimental evaluation in the guinea-pig. Brit. med. J. **1958 II**, 1141.
ZIEMKE, H.: Bluthistaminspiegel und örtliche Erfrierung. Naunyn-Schmiedeberg's Arch. exp. Path. Pharmak. **206**, 288 (1949).

Section C

Histamine Release by Basic Compounds

By

ADOLFO M. ROTHSCHILD

With 10 Figures

I. Introduction

The demonstration that histamine, a normal constituent of animal tissues could be released in its pharmacologically active form in animals submitted to peptone or anaphylactic shock, led to extensive studies of other conditions in which this release could occur. The first demonstration of a direct histamine releasing action of a drug possessing basic groups in its molecule, was given by ALAM et al. (1939), who showed that curarine could release considerable amounts of histamine from dog muscle *in vivo*. Subsequent work by different groups of investigators showed that a great number of basic organic compounds, some having quite simple chemical structures, could provoke the release of histamine from non-sensitized tissues (SCHILD and GREGORY, 1947; MACINTOSH and PATON, 1949; ROCHA E SILVA and SCHILD, 1949, etc.). An important early outcome of these studies was the differentiation of this action from drug allergy, a condition which is also characterized by the release of histamine following exposure to certain organic compounds; however, in contrast to the basic histamine releasers, these act only on sensitized tissues. As shown in Table 1, the list of basic histamine releasers includes now over one hundred compounds, some only active in the experimental animal but others possessing considerable activity in the human subject, where they can give rise to "histaminic" symptoms such as flushing, tachycardia, itching, edema, gastrointestinal distress and bronchospasm. Several drugs of clinical importance, including curarizing agents, opium alkaloids, atropine, quinine, antibiotics, chloroquine and trypanocidal amidines have been shown to be potentially able to elicit these reactions (LEWIS, 1927; KIRK and HENRY, 1944; WEST, 1938; GROB et al. 1947; SALTER and WHITE, 1949). Effective preventive or curative measures for the control of these side effects are available, and have been reviewed along with the discussion of proper skin tests to foretell histamine release in the human subject (COLLIER, 1956; COLLIER and MACAULEY, 1952; PATON, 1959).

Besides its clinical interest, the study of basic histamine releasing compounds is of importance to the pharmacologist because they often possess comparatively simple structures, that can be varied at will, enabling the determination of structure-activity relationships. Such studies have been made by several investigators: their results have led PATON (1957), to generalize "that histamine liberation appears when basic groups in a molecule are multiplied at sufficiently spaced distances, or when single groups are attached to substituted aromatic rings; too low or too high a basicity depresses activity, but bulk and complexity of a molecule favours it".

The demonstration that in some species like the rat and the cat, histamine release by basic compounds and by antigen-antibody reactions had several biochemical features in common, (CHAKRAVARTY et al. 1959, MOTA and ISHII, 1960), drew the interest of investigators toward studies about the mechanism of action of such compounds. Since basicity is an invariable feature of such releasers, many authors have considered their action as a direct effect on acidic cellular histamine receptors from which the amine would be dislodged by an ion-exchange type of reaction (PATON, 1956; MACINTOSH, 1956; KÜTTNER et al. 1961; AMANN and WERLE, 1956). A different view has been favoured by UVNÄS (1961), who believes that highly effective basic histamine releasing agents like compound 48/80, activate lytic phospholipases, located in the membrane of the mast cell, thereby provoking alterations of permeability leading to the release of intracellular ingredients. The activation of tissue proteases by compound 48/80 and other basic histamine releasing agents has been demonstrated (UNGAR and DAMGAARD, 1955), and considered as evidence in favour of the proteolytic theory of histamine release first suggested by ROCHA E SILVA in 1941. This theory, in its more recent aspect (UNGAR et al. 1961), admits that "chemical" histamine releasers as well as certain factors generated during the anaphylactic reaction activate proteinases in tissue or plasma capable of destroying protein "anchoring" sites for histamine, thus loosening its intracellular ties and allowing its escape into the surrounding medium.

A dependence on cellular metabolism has been shown to condition the histamine-releasing action of 48/80 and related compounds in the rat and the cat *in vitro* (ROTHSCHILD et al., 1961, DIAMANT and UVNÄS, 1961, WESTERHOLM, 1960). This type of relationship however, does not seem to control the action of all basic histamine releasers and in special not of those which are only active at comparatively high concentrations. Future work will show whether unspecific cytotoxic effects are the responsible factors for histamine release in such instances. Unlike the more subtle effects evoked by compound 48/80 and its analogues, these effects may have relatively little bearing on the mechanism responsible for histamine release in anaphylaxis.

II. Methods for the determination of histamine release

A brief discussion of the methods which have been employed for the study of the histamine releasing activity of basic organic compounds on animal tissues *in vivo* and *in vitro*, is presented below. Since species and organ variability are factors which influence histamine releasing activity, it is useful to test this activity in different species and on different structures whenever possible. Among others, such detailed studies have recently been made with adrenochrome (LECOMTE and FISCHER, 1957), and morpholin-ethylmorphine (CAHEN and AUBRON, 1960). The importance of the direct evaluation of histamine releasing ability in the human species by means of skin tests must also be emphasized: this test is specially useful in the screening of compounds of possible clinical application (COLLIER, 1956).

1. Increase in body fluid histamine

The most inequivocal evidence for the histamine releasing capacity of a compound is the demonstration of its ability to increase the histamine in the circulating blood (MACINTOSH and PATON, 1949; PATON, 1957). Dilution in the blood and other body fluid compartments, as well as the enzymatic destruction of released histamine are however, factors which limit the applicability of this method to the more active releasers. Useful measures to increase the sensitivity of the method consist in restricting the venous outflow from the region of the injection (ALAM et al. 1939; SCHACHTER, 1952; MONGAR and WHELAN, 1953), or pretreating the experimental animal with inhibitors of histaminase like iproniazid

(WASER and ITZBICKI, 1959), or aminoguanidine (SCHAYER et al., 1954; HALPERN 1960). It is interesting to note that CODE et al. (1961), have shown that in the sensitized rat, the injection of antigen increases the histaminolytic activity of plasma; such an effect could possibly also result from treatment with chemical liberators: experimental evidence for this is however lacking. The effects of basic releasers on histamine levels in urine have been observed by WILSON (1954), in normal rats, and by SCHAYER et al. (1954a, b, 1955), in rats having C^{14}-labelled tissue histamine stores. Increased levels of amine have also been observed in the peritoneal fluid of rats treated with compound 48/80 or other basic releasers (FAWCETT, 1954; SMITH, 1958a).

2. Decrease in tissue-bound histamine

FELDBERG and TALESNIK (1953), showed that repeated injections of the powerful releaser compound 48/80 into rats, resulted in successive decreases of the histamine content of skin and muscle, so that after six or eight days up to 90% of the amine had disappeared from these sites. As shown in Table 1, such effects can also be evoked by other basic releasers which are active in the rat. Decreased levels of bound histamine have also been observed in the skin of cats following treatment with licheniformin (MACINTOSH and PATON, 1949), in the liver of dogs receiving d-tubocurarine (REID, 1950), or atropine (BURSTEIN and PARROT, 1949), and in the blood platelets of rabbits treated with reserpine or 5-hydroxytryptamine (BURKHALTER et al. 1960). Histamine "depleted" rats have been used by FELDBERG and TALESNIK (1953), to study the role of histamine in photosensitization reactions, and by ROCHA E SILVA and ROTHSCHILD (1955) and BROCKLEHURST et al. (1955) to investigate the role of the amine in sensitivity to passive cutaneous anaphylaxis. MOULTON et al. (1957), have used this approach to determine whether the cutaneous response evoked by certain purine derivatives in the human subject was due to histamine release. They injected doses of compound 48/80 into a localized site of the skin of the forearm until the injection failed to produce the wheal and flare response of histamine. The purine compound under study was then injected into the depleted area and its effects compared with those produced at an untreated region. 48/80 treated, histamine depleted rats have been used to investigate the role of histamine in wound healing (BOYD and SMITH, 1959), and in the autograft and homograft reaction (BOYD and SMITH, 1960).

3. Histamine release from perfused organs and tissue fragments

The perfusion of isolated organs with histamine liberators with the ensuing demonstration of histamine in the collected perfusates, is a technique which combines a reasonably "physiological" working condition with some of the characteristics of straight *in vitro* techniques. Experimental details of the perfusion of cat skin, muscle or lung have been described by FELDBERG and PATON (1951); the perfusion of the isolated cat's paw was reported by HÖGBERG et al. (1956). The effect of d-tubocurarine on the histamine stores of dog's liver has been studied both *in vivo* and on the isolated perfused organ by REID (1950), who has made the interesting observation that curare, while highly effective in the intact animal, was entirely inactive on the isolated preparation. Technical details for the study of the effects of basic histamine releasers on the perfused dog skin have been presented by FELDBERG and SCHACHTER (1952), and similar data has been described for the perfused guinea pig lung and hindquarters (FELDBERG and MONGAR, 1954), as well as for the hindquarters of the rat (ROCHA E SILVA and SCHILD, 1949). Perfusion techniques are sensitive means for the detection of histamine releasing ability of basic compounds; their major drawback becomes evident when comparisons between the activity of two or more compounds are to be made: in such cases, the progressive exhaustion of the releasable histamine changes the condition of the preparation after each contact with the releasing agent, at least as far as histamine stores are concerned; it is therefore usually necessary to employ several identical preparations and alternate the order of the additions when potency ratios between two or more compounds are sought. An experimental design, based on a four point assay using the Latin square has been devised for the assay of the histamine releasing action of anaphylatoxin (ROCHA E SILVA and ROTHSCHILD, 1956). This design accounts for the tachyphylactic effect induced by repeated contact with the releasing agent; with suitable modifications it could easily be adapted to the determination of histamine releasing potency of basic compounds using perfusion techniques.

The use of tissue fragments, minces or homogenates offers useful means for the screening of suspected histamine releasers. Such methods are of special importance when comparisons of potencies are desired, since in these tests each compound can be assayed on the same material and under exactly the same conditions. These characteristics also make these methods the technique of choice when information about the effects of physical and chemical factors on the histamine releasing process is desired. The first detailed description of a technique using tissue fragments for the study of the histamine releasing activity of a basic compound was presented in 1949, by ROCHA E SILVA and SCHILD. Figure 1 taken from their data shows that histamine release from rat diaphragm by d-tubocurarine *in vitro*, is a measurable process in which relatively large quantities of histamine, amounting to 2/3 of the total amine content of the muscle, are released and rapidly diffuse from the tissue into the incubation medium. As shown by Figures 2 and 3, if the concentration of the releaser is reduced below 0.5 mg/ml, the rate of release of histamine is greatly retarded, but if the concentration is increased above 1.0 mg/ml, the rate of release is not increased any further. At the maximum rate, the liberation of histamine from rat's diaphragm can be treated as a simple diffusion process and a "diffusion coefficient" of histamine through muscle can be calculated. A value of 3.0×10^{-5} cm^2/min. at 37°C, which is of the same order of magnitude as that of urea has been obtained (ROCHA E SILVA and SCHILD, 1949). A detailed study of the distribution of histamine among the symmetrical halves of the rat diaphragm has been made by VUGMAN (1961), who showed that there was an equivalent content of the amine in each hemidiaphragm, but that the distribution among different parts of each hemidiaphragm was rather irregular. On the basis of histological studies, these differences were explained by the peculiar distribution of mast cells along muscle fibers, with a preferential disposition at the insertion of the ligaments, the phrenic nerve and the vicinity of blood vessels.

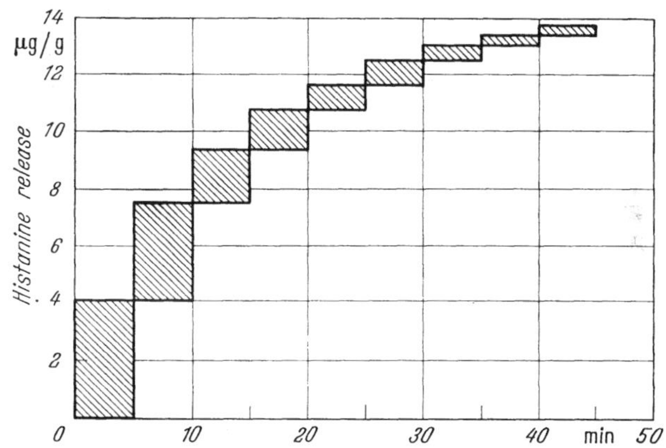

Fig. 1. Total histamine released from a diaphragm which was left during successive periods of 5 min in solutions of D-tubocurarine (1:1000) in Tyrode solution. (According to ROCHA E SILVA and SCHILD, 1949)

Histamine release by compound 48/80 was found to be proportional to the amine content of the tissue, so that results could be conveniently expressed as percentage of total histamine liberated after treatment with the releaser. This type of presentation resulted in less spreading among the results of identical experiments and a reduction of the experimental error (VUGMAN, 1961).

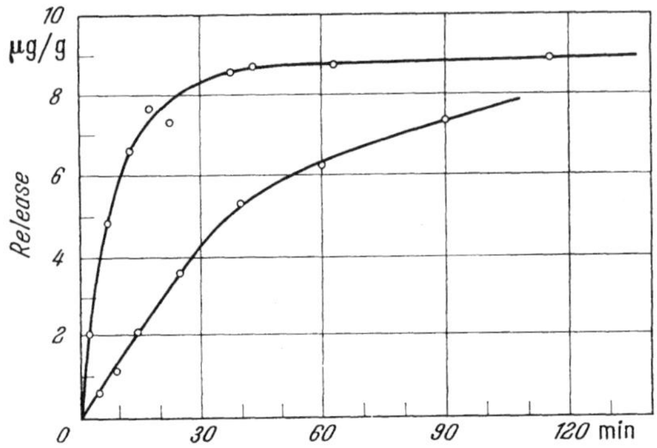

Fig. 2. Rates of release of histamine with concentrations of 1:1000 (upper curve) and 1:4000 D-tubocurarine (lower curve). (According to ROCHA E SILVA and SCHILD, 1949)

The use of free mast cells obtained from washings of the peritoneal cavity of rats offers efficient means for screening new histamine releasing agents and for studying their mechanism of action. This technique has been employed using either the whole peritoneal fluid cell population (LAGUNOFF and BENDITT, 1960; UVNÄS et al. 1961; VAN ARSDEL and BRAY, 1961; ROTHSCHILD, 1962a), or a purified mast cell fraction obtained by submitting the peritoneal washings to differential centrifugation in media possessing a density gradient (ARCHER, 1958; UVNÄS and THON, 1959; MOTA and DIAS DA SILVA, 1960). Isolated mast cells are also convenient

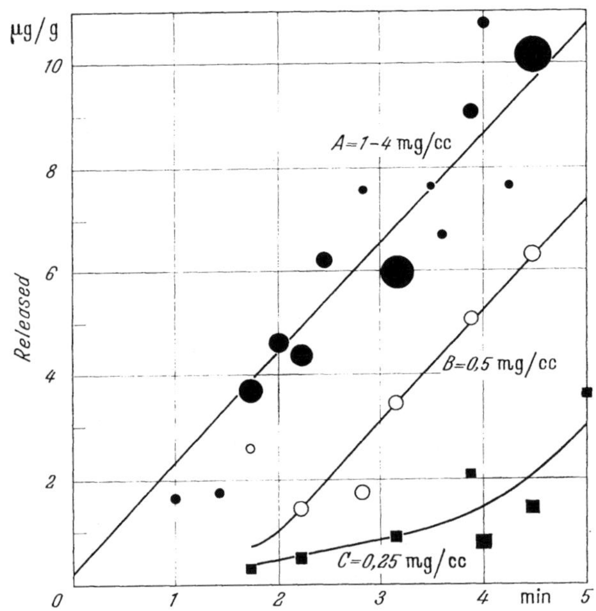

Fig. 3. Summary of 106 individual measurements of histamine release by curarine. Large circles represent mean values, the area of each circle being proportional to the number of observations. Black circles: histamine release with concentrations of curarine of 1 mg/ml or more; white circles: 0.5 mg/ml; squares: 0.25 mg/ml. The slope of line A has been used for the calculation of the diffusion constant of histamine. (According to ROCHA E SILVA and SCHILD, 1949)

substrates in studies using histamine releasing agents which interfere with the biological assay of the amine (ROTHSCHILD, 1961a). Thus, it became possible to study the histamine releasing action of catechol amines and their ring chloro-analogs at concentrations which antagonize the action of histamine on the guinea pig ileum, without having to resort to chromatographic separations. For this purpose, residual, rather than released histamine was estimated, and compared with the amine content of controls incubated in the absence of the releasing agent. Blanks showed that a negligible loss of bound histamine occurs during the removal from the peritoneal cavity and during washing or incubation in the absence of the releasing agent. A double washing by centrifugation with buffer after incubation, was sufficient to remove all interfering materials (adrenaline and other amines), which in these experiments were utilized in concentrations as high as 10 mg/ml. This technique has also been used to investigate the inhibitory action of histamine on its own release by compound 48/80: it was found that the amine at concentrations of 3 mM inhibited by 50% the releasing action of compound 48/80 (ROTHSCHILD, 1962).

The use of rat tissues whose rich skin and muscle stores of histamine are specially sensitive to the action of most basic releasers, has led to significant knowledge about the mechanism of action of these agents (MOTA and ISHII, 1960; CHAKRAVARTY, 1960; ROTHSCHILD et al. 1961; DIAMANT and UVNÄS, 1961). Noteworthy results have however also been obtained *in vitro* employing tissues from other species. Thus, MONGAR and SCHILD (1952, 1953, 1956, 1957a), and MONGAR (1957), have published the results of studies about the action of chemical liberators on guinea-pig lung slices, minces, homogenates and subcellular fractions, and brought insights into structural and environmental requirements for the activity of these compounds. Similar studies in other species have employed chopped cat skin (WESTERHOLM, 1960a, b), dog liver homogenates (HAGEN, 1954; GROSSBERG and GARCIA-AROCHA, 1954; MCILREATH, 1959), rabbit's whole blood (MCINTIRE et al. 1951) and rabbit's platelets (HUMPHREY and JAQUES, 1955; WAALKES et al. 1959; BURKHALTER et al. 1960; ROTHSCHILD and GARCIA LIMA, 1962).

4. Pharmacodynamic effects of endogenous released histamine

An important group of indirect methods for the determination of histamine releasing activity is based on the observation of the pharmacodynamic effects of liberators evoked by the histamine which they set free. Thus, effects of endogenous histamine on the circulation (MACINTOSH and PATON, 1949; FELDBERG and MILES, 1953), on smooth muscle and gastric secretion (FELDBERG and HOLMES, 1941), have served as indexes of histamine releasing activity. Since these effects are reproduced by the administration of histamine itself, they are discussed in chapter II, of this book. However, certain differences between the symptoms produced by exogenous histamine and those due to the action of the endogenous amine following its release from tissues exposed to a basic liberator, deserve further comment. Thus, it has been observed that repeated treatment with a histamine releaser will result in successively decreasing "histaminic" responses. This tachyphylactic effect which, as a rule, is not observed when histamine itself is administered, is due to the progressive exhaustion of the tissue stores of the amine available for release by the liberator. This is often observed, even in cases where subsequent assay for residual tissue histamine reveals that the total stores of the amine have only been decreased to a small extent (PATON, 1957).

Characteristic differences are exhibited by the hypotensive responses elicited in the cat and the dog by basic histamine liberators and by the amine itself. MACINTOSH and PATON (1949), have shown that a latency period of 20–25 seconds preceedes the onset of the hypotension induced by the liberator, the "delayed depressor response"; in contrast, the response to histamine becomes apparent a few seconds after intravenous administration. An interesting observation discussed by PATON (1957), is that the generalized itching observed after the administration of a diamidine to a human subject cannot be reproduced even by the highest tolerable intravenous doses of histamine. In the experimental animal as well, it is a common observation that certain localized effects of a releaser cannot be reproduced by exogenous histamine even when administered in doses higher than those expected to exist in the tissue under examination. Such results have led to the concept of "intrinsic histamine", (DALE, 1948), e.g. histamine which, by being released within the receptor cells provokes an intense pharmacological activity which cannot be reproduced by exogenous histamine because it would be impossible to built up high enough local levels of the amine. Observations showing that certain effects of histamine liberators cannot be effectively antagonized by antihistaminics have also been explained in this way. More recent observations have shown however, that highly active histamine releasing compounds like 48/80, do not owe their inflammatory or anaphylactoid effects to histamine release alone, but rather to the concomitant liberation or formation of other vasoactive and smooth muscle active agents, such as 5-hydroxytryptamine and/or slowly reacting substances (HALPERN et al. 1959; WEST, 1961; JORI et al. 1961; CHAKRAVARTY, 1960). Also, although up to now experimental evidence for this is lacking, formation of bradykinin shown to occur in anaphylaxis (BERALDO, 1950; LAHIRI and BROCKLEHURST, 1961) might result from the action of highly active chemical releasers of the 48/80 type. These observations should be taken into consideration in the evaluation of histamine release by indirect tests and emphasize the usefulness of the highly specific pharmacological antagonists (anti-histamines, antiserotonins, etc.), in studies concerning the relationship between auto-pharmacological agents and basic histamine releasing compounds (JORI et al. 1961).

III. Survey of basic compounds possessing histamine releasing activity in animal and man

Table 1 presents a survey of basic compounds of natural and synthetic origin which have been tested for histamine releasing activity. Structural, rather than pharmacological similarities were the predominant criteria for placing a compound into a given group. The species, the biological structure and the response obtained in each test are given; in order to present a picture of the potencies of the compounds listed, threshold dosages or concentrations are indicated in most instances. Data permitting exact comparisons between activities require the testing of drugs in the same species and under identical experimental conditions; such observations are available for several groups of compounds (MACINTOSH and PATON, 1949; MCINTIRE et al. 1951; SCHACHTER, 1952; MONGAR and SCHILD, 1953; COLLIER, 1956; PARRATT and WEST, 1957; PATON, 1957; ROTHSCHILD, 1962 a).

IV. Characteristics of the histamine releasing action of basic compounds

1. Specificity

The action of basic compounds does not have the absolute species specificity exhibited by certain high molecular weight histamine releasers like polyvinylpyrrolidone which is only active in the dog, dextran or ovomucoid which act only in rats, or horse serum whose activity is confined to the cat. Although a relative dependence on the species is shown by some basic releasers, it can be stated that in general, a basic compound active as a histamine releaser in one

Table 1. *Survey of basic compounds tested for histamine releasing activity in the animal and in man*

Abbreviations: Aeros. = aerosol; cont. = content; Decr. = decreased; Del. hypotens. = Delayed hypotensive response (MacIntosh and Paton, 1949); H = histamine; Incr. = increased; perf. = perfusion; permeab. = permeability; secr. = secretion; subcell. = subcellular; Trip. resp. = triple response (Lewis, 1927).

Compound	Dose or concentration	Species	Biological structure	Experimental evidence	Reference
Ammonia	—	G. pig	Lung, *in vivo* (aeros.)	Decr. H. cont.	64
Ammonia	0.15 M	Rat	Diaphragm, *in vitro*	H. release	193
Ammonia	1 M	Rat	Mesentery mast cells, *in vivo*	H. release + Degranul.	174
Aliphatic amines					
Methyl to dodecylamines	0.1—10 mM	G. pig	Lung (chopped)	H. release	130, 134, 135
Octylamine	50—1000 μg	Cat	Skin, muscle, lung (perf.)	H. release	60
Octylamine	2 mg	G. pig	Hindquarters (perf.)	H. release	60
Octylamine	100 μg/ml	G. pig	Lung (subcell. partic.)	H. release	132
Octylamine	50—200 μg/ml	G. pig	Mesentery mast cells, *in vitro*	Morphol. alterations	143
Octylamine	—	Dog	Liver (subcell. partic.)	H. release	74
Octylamine	1 mg/ml	Man	Skin	Trip. resp.	130
Octylamine	20 μg/ml	Man	Skin (particles)	H. release	133
Octylamine	1—5 mg	Rat	Hindquarters, lung (perf.)	H. release	60
Octylamine	20—100 μg/kg	Rat	Urine, *in vivo*	Incr. H. cont.	242
C_{12} to C_{18}	0.1—0.2 mM	Rabbit	Whole blood, *in vitro*	H. release	124
Decylamine	500 μg/kg	Rat	Urine, *in vivo*	Incr. H. cont.	242
Decylamine	20 μg/ml	Rat	Mesentery mast cells, *in vitro*	Degranul.	87
Cyst (e) inamide	—	Man	Skin	Trip. resp.	104
Cyst (e) inamide	5—10 mg	Rat	Hindquarters (perf.)	H. release	108
Neoarsphenamine	25 mg	Cat	Skin (perf.)	H. release	187
Neoarsphenamine	100 mg/kg	Cat	Whole animal	No Del. hypotens.	118
Thiamine	40 mg/lg	Cat	Whole animal	No Del. hypotens.	118
Thiamine	—	G. pig	Bronchioli	Constriction	208
Procaine	12 mg/kg	Cat	Whole animal	No Del. hypotens.	118
6-methoxy-4-quinolylethyl amine	4 mg/kg	Cat	Whole animal	No Del. hypotens.	118
Diamines (C_6 to C_{12})	1 mg/kg	Cat	Whole animal	Del. hypotens.	118
Cadaverine	—	Man	Skin	Trip. resp.	104
Diaminooctane	13 mg/kg	Cat	Plasma, *in vivo*	Incr. H. cont.	118
Diaminooctane	8 mg/kg	Cat	Vascular system	Incr. hematocr.	118
Diaminooctane	15 mg/kg	Dog	Plasma, *in vivo*	Incr. H. cont.	118

Table 1 (Continuation)

Compound	Dose or concentration	Species	Biological structure	Experimental evidence	Reference
Diaminooctane	1—10 mg/ml	Man	Skin	Trip. resp.	118
Diaminodecane	—	Cat	Whole animal	Del. hypotens.	49
Diaminodecane	10—200 μg/ml	Dog	Liver (subcell. partic.)	H. release	73
Diaminodecane	—	Rat	Mesentery mast cells, *in vivo* and *in vitro*	Degranul.	19, 119, 171
Diaminodecane	75 mg/kg	Rat	Bone marrow mast cells	Decrease	21
Arylalkyl amines					
Phenethylamine	10 mg	Cat	Skin (perf.)	H. release	163
Phenethylamine	—	Man	Skin	Trip. resp.	163
Tyramine	10 mg	Cat	Skin (perf.)	H. release	163
Tyramine	—	Man	Skin	Trip. resp.	163
Amphetamine	10 mg	Cat	Skin (perf.)	H. release	163
Amphetamine	—	Man	Skin	Trip. resp.	163
Amphetamine	5 mg/kg	Rat	Plasma, *in vivo*	Incr. H. cont.	232
Ephedrine	—	Cat	Skin (perf.)	No effect	163
Adrenaline	—	Cat	Plasma, *in vivo*	Incr. H. cont.	47
Adrenaline	20 μg/kg/min	Dog	Plasma, *in vivo*	Incr. H. cont.	233
Adrenaline	—	Man	Plasma, *in vivo*	Incr. H. cont.	216
Adrenaline	200 μg	Man	Plasma, *in vivo*	Incr. H. cont.	213, 215
Adrenaline	2.5—10 μg	Man	Arm (*in vivo* perf.)	No effect	131
Adrenaline	5 μg/ml	Rat	Lung (perf.)	H. release	96
Adrenaline	100 μg/ml	Rat	Diaphragm, *in vitro*	No effect	131
Adrenaline	5—2000 μg/ml	Rat	Periton. fluid mast cells, *in vitro*	No effect	184
Adrenaline	100 μg/kg	Rat	Urine, *in vivo*	Incr. H. cont.	242
Levoarterenol	10 μg/kg/min	Dog	Plasma, *in vivo*	Incr. H. cont.	40
Levoarterenol	2 mg/ml	Rat	Periton. fluid mast cells	No effect	184
Isoproterenol	2 mg/ml	Rat	Periton. fluid mast cells	No effect	184
Synephrine	—	Man	Plasma, *in vivo*	Incr. H. cont.	214
Priscoline	2 mg	Cat	Skin (perf.)	H. release	187
Adrenochrome	25—50 mg/kg	Cat	Whole animal	No Del. hypotens.	113
Adrenochrome	5—15 mg/kg	Dog	Whole animal	No Del. hypotens.	113
Adrenochrome	50—250 μg	Man	Skin, *in vivo*	No effect	113
Adrenochrome	0.5—1 mg	Rabbit	Skin, *in vivo*	No effect	113
Adrenochrome	1—4 mg	Rat	Hindquarters (perf.)	No effect	113
Dichloroepinephrine	750 μg/ml	Rat	Periton. fluid mast cells	H. release	184
Dichlorolevo-arterenol	750 μg/ml	Rat	Periton. fluid mast cells	H. release	184

Table 1 (Continuation)

Compound	Dose or concentration	Species	Biological structure	Experimental evidence	Reference
Dichloroisoproterenol (DCI)	750 μg/ml	Rat	Periton. fluid mast cells	H. release	184
L-1935[1]	0.5—2.5 μg	Cat	Skin (perf.)	H. release	62
L-1935	1 mg/kg	Cat	Whole animal	Del. hypotens	34
L-1935	250 μg/kg	Dog	Whole animal	Del. hypotens	77
L-1935	1 mg/kg	Dog	Plasma, *in vivo*	Incr. H. cont.	77
L-1935	2—100 μg	Man	Skin	Trip. resp.	34, 111
L-1935	100—500 μg/kg	Man		Anaphylactoid symptoms	109
L-1935	—	Man	Plasma, *in vivo*	Incr. H. cont.	109
L-1935	—	Man	Skin, *in vivo*	Decr. H. cont.	126
L-1935	—	Man	Asthmatic subject	Asthm., crisis	114
L-1935	20 mg/kg/day	Mouse	Skin, *in vivo*	Decr. H. cont.	238
L-1935	20 mg/kg/day	Hamster	Skin, *in vivo*	Decr. H. cont.	238
L-1935	10—200 μg	Rat	Hindquarters (perf.)	H. release	62
L-1935	7 mg/kg	Rat	Mast cells, *in vivo*	Degranul.	6
L-1935	10 mg/kg	Rat	Plasma, *in vivo*	Incr. H. cont.	6, 78
L-1935	10 mg/kg	Rat	Urine, *in vivo*	Incr. H. cont.	6
L-1935	10 mg/kg	Rat	Skin, *in vivo*	Decr. H. cont.	238
Cp. 48/80[2]	10 μg/kg	Cat	Whole animal	Del. hypotens.	44, 160
Cp. 48/80	500 μg/kg	Cat	Plasma, *in vivo*	Incr. H. cont.	160
Cp. 48/80	2 μg	Cat	Skin and muscle (perf. *in vivo*)	H. release	55, 56
Cp. 48/80	50 μg/ml	Cat	Skin, *in vivo*	Decr. H. cont.	202
Cp. 48/80	100 μg	Cat	Hindquarters (perf.)	H. release	13
Cp. 48/80	1 μg/ml	Cat	Skin (chopped)	H. release	240, 241
Cp. 48/80	2—4 μg	Cat	Paw (perf.)	H. release	32, 85
Cp. 48/80	10—20 μg	Cat	Sciatic nerve (perf.)	H. release	63
Cp. 48/80	5—20 μg	Cat	Stomach, *in vivo*	Incr. acid. secr.	201
Cp. 48/80	40 μg	Cock	Skin capillaries, *in vivo*	Incr. permeab.	112
Cp. 48/80	100 μg/kg	Dog	Whole animal	Hypotens.	7, 44, 170
Cp. 48/80	0.5 mg/kg	Dog	Whole animal	Anaphylactoid symptoms	161
Cp. 48/80	200 μg	Dog	Skin (perf. *in vivo*)	H. release	56
Cp. 48/80	500 μg	Dog	Skin, *in vivo*	Decr. H. cont.	59

[1] 3-(4-hydroxyphenyl)-3(4-hydroxy-3 methyl phenyl)-1-methyl propylamine.
[2] Condensation product of p-methoxy-phenethyl methyl amine and formaldehyde.

Table 1 (Continuation)

Compound	Dose or concentration	Species	Biological structure	Experimental evidence	Reference
Cp. 48/80	—	Dog	Str. muscle, liver, *in vivo*	H. release	150
Cp. 48/80	10—200 μg/ml	Dog	Liver (subcell. particles)	H. release	73, 123, 140
Cp. 48/80	—	Dog	Portal circulat., *in vivo*	Hypertens.	170
Cp. 48/80	10—20 μg	Dog	Sciatic nerve (perf.)	H. release	63
Cp. 48/80	0.5 mg/kg	Dog	Stomach, *in vivo*	Incr. acid secr.	161
Cp. 48/80	25 μg/kg	Dog	Cephalic venous circul.	Hypertens.	227
Cp. 48/80	1 mg/ml	G. pig	Lung, diaphragm, skin, smooth muscle, *in vitro*	H. release	129, 145
Cp. 48/80	1 mg/ml	G. pig	Lung (chopped)	H. release	130, 135, 136
Cp. 48/80	500 μg	G. pig	Lung (perf.)	H. release	60
Cp. 48/80	0.1 mg/ml	G. pig	Lung (subcell. particles)	H. release	132
Cp. 48/80	2.5—5 mg/kg	G. pig	Skin capillaries, *in vivo*	Incr. permeab.	57, 127
Cp. 48/80	20—50 mg/kg	G. pig	Skin, *in vivo*	Decr. H. cont.	204
Cp. 48/80	2.5 mg/kg	G. pig	Plasma, *in vivo*	No effects	143
Cp. 48/80	10 mg/kg	G. pig	Plasma, *in vivo*	Incr. H. cont.	204
Cp. 48/80	130 μg/ml	G. pig	Ileum, *in vitro*	Motor effects	58
Cp. 48/80	7.5 mg/kg	G. pig	Mesentery mast cells, *in vivo*	No effects	143
Cp. 48/80	4 mg/kg	G. pig	Stomach, *in vivo*	Ulceration	204
Cp. 48/80	3—5%	G. pig	Bronchioli, *in vivo*, aeros.	Spasm	53, 156, 197
Cp. 48/80	1—8 mg/kg/d	Hamster	Whole animal	Anaphylactoid symptoms	157
Cp. 48/80	1—24 mg/kg/d	Hamster	Skin, *in vivo*	Decr. H. cont.	238
Cp. 48/80	1—5 μg/ml	Hamster	Mesentery mast cells, *in vitro*	Degranul.	19
Cp. 48/80	0.01 μg	Man	Skin	Triple resp.	11, 52, 104, 160, 200
Cp. 48/80	300 μg i. a.	Man	Plasma, *in vivo*	Incr. H. cont.	198
Cp. 48/80	100 μg i. a.	Man	Cephalic venous circul.	Hypertension	199, 200
				Subject. sympt.	196
Cp. 48/80	2.5—10 mg/kg	Mouse	Whole animal	Anaphylactoid symptoms	173
Cp. 48/80	20 mg/kg/d	Mouse	Skin, *in vivo*	Decr. H. cont.	238
Cp. 48/80	—	Mouse	Mast cell granules	H. release	237
Cp. 48/80	0.5—2 mg	Rabbit	Skin (perf.)	H. release	188
Cp. 48/80	1—5 mg	Rabbit	Liver, intestine (perf.)	No effect	188
Cp. 48/80	1 mg/kg	Rabbit	Skin capillaries, *in vivo*	No effect	188
Cp. 48/80	2 mg/kg	Rabbit	Plasma, *in vivo*	No effect	188
Cp. 48/80	200 μg	Rabbit	Skin, *in vivo*	Decr. H. cont.	110

Table I (Continuation)

Compound	Dose or concentration	Species	Biological structure	Experimental evidence	Reference
Cp. 48/80	200 μg/ml	Rabbit	Isolated platelets	No effect	88
Cp. 48/80	—	Rabbit	Blood basophils, *in vitro*	Decr. number	20
Cp. 48/80	1 mg/kg	Rat	Whole animal	Anaphylactoid symptoms	59
Cp. 48/80	1 mg/kg	Rat	Skin, *in vivo*	Decr. H. cont.	22, 59, 142, 179
Cp. 48/80	200 μg/kg	Rat	Plasma (normal and diabetic, *in vivo*)	Incr. H. cont.	70
Cp. 48/80	150 μg/kg	Rat	Plasma (hypothermia)	Incr. H. cont.	80
Cp. 48/80	20—100 μg/kg	Rat	Urine, *in vivo*	Incr. H. cont.	191,115,189,242
Cp. 48/80	5 μg	Rat	Hindquarters, gut (perf.)	H. release	12, 13, 238
Cp. 48/80	1—5 mg/kg	Rat	Liver, duodenum, stomach, *in vivo*	No effect	59, 141
Cp. 48/80	2 mg/kg/d	Rat	Spleen, *in vivo*	No effect	158
Cp. 48/80	—	Rat	Tongue, *in vivo*	Decr. H. cont.	6, 18, 142, 158
Cp. 48/80	—	Rat	Scrotum, lips, ear, *in vivo*	Decr. H. cont.	6
Cp. 48/80	10—30 μg/ml	Rat	Skin, muscle, lung, *in vitro*	H. release	33, 45, 145, 181
Cp. 48/80	1—5 mg/kg	Rat	Periton. fluid, *in vivo*	Incr. H. cont.	51, 205
Cp. 48/80	0.5—20 μg/ml	Rat	Periton. fluid mast cells, *in vitro*	H. release	3, 184, 223, 224
Cp. 48/80	—	Rat	Subcut. tissue particles	H. release	140
Cp. 48/80	—	Rat	Liver (subcell. particles)	No effect	140
Cp. 48/80	—	Rat	Liver (subcell. particles)	No effect	74
Cp. 48/80	1 mg/kg	Rat	Stomach, *in vivo*	Incr. acid secr. ulcers	59, 204
Cp. 48/80	3 mg/kg	Rat	Stomach, *in vivo*	Incr. pepsinog. secr.	98
Cp. 48/80	5 mg/kg	Rat	Connect. tissue mast cells, *in vivo*	Degranul.	12,13,51,139,158
Cp. 48/80	20—100 μg/ml	Rat	Mesentery mast cells, *in vitro*	Degranul.	139, 172
Cp. 48/80	100—500 μg/d	Rat	Skin, tongue, oesophagus, cardia mast cells, *in vivo*	Decrease	142
Cp. 46/108[1]	1 mg/kg	Dog	Whole animal	Hypotension	7
Cp. 46/108	25 μg/ml	Rat	Perit. fluid mast cells, *in vitro*	H. release	183
α-aminobenzylmethyl-sulfone	30 mg/kg	Cat	Whole animal	No Del. hypotens	118
α-aminobenzyl-p-sulfon-amide (Marfanil)	30 mg/kg	Cat	Whole animal	No Del. hypotens	118
Indolamines					
Tryptamine, 5-hydroxy-tryptamine	2.5 mg	Cat	Skin, muscle (perf.)	H. release	61

[1] Condensation product (Dimer), of p-methoxiphenethylmethylamine and formaldehyde.

Table 1 (Continuation)

Compound	Dose or concentration	Species	Biological structure	Experimental evidence	Reference
Tryptamine, 5-hydroxy-tryptamine	2 mg	Dog	Skin (perf.)	H. release	61
Tryptamine, 5-hydroxy-tryptamine	—	Rat	Body tissues, *in vivo*	Decr. H. cont.	16, 61
5-hydroxytryptamine	—	Rabbit	Blood platelets, *in vivo*	H. release	24
5-hydroxytryptamine	40 μg/ml	Rabbit	Blood platelets, *in vitro*	No effect	24
Anti-histamines (see also phenothiazine derivatives)					
Antazoline	—	G. pig	Lung, *in vitro*	H. release	4
Antazoline	50 μg/ml	G. pig	Mesentery mast cells, *in vitro*	Degranul.	146
Antazoline	—	Man	Lung, *in vitro*	H. release	4
Diphenhydramine	—	G. pig	Lung, *in vitro*	H. release	4
Diphenhydramine	1 mM	G. pig	Diaphragm, mesentery, skin, *in vitro*	H. release	146
Diphenhydramine	100 μg/ml	G. pig	Mesentery mast cells, *in vitro*	Degranul.	146
Diphenhydramine	—	Dog	Skin (chopped)	H. release	217
Diphenhydramine	—	Rat	Skin, *in vivo*	Decr. H. cont.	146
Diphenhydramine	3 mM	Rat	Diaphragm, mesentery, skin, *in vitro*	H. release	146
Mepyramine	1 mM	G. pig	Skin, muscle, mesentery, *in vivo*	H. release	146
Mepyramine	3 mM	Rat	Skin, muscle, mesentery, *in vivo*	H. release	146
Chloropheniramine, Bromodipheniramine, Isothipendyl, Metapyrilene, Tripelenamine, Phenindamine	50—200 μg/ml	G. pig	Mesentery mast cells, *in vivo*	Degranul.	146
2359 R.P.[1]	—	Man	Plasma, *in vivo*	Incr. H. cont.	166
2786 R.P.[2]	—	Man	Plasma, *in vivo*	Incr. H. cont.	166
Phenothiazine derivatives					
Promethazine	12.5 μg/ml	G. pig	Mesentery mast cells, *in vitro*	Degranul.	146
Promethazine	—	Rat	Mesentery mast cells, *in vitro*	Degranul.	86, 207
Promethazine	—	Rat	Skin, *in vivo*	Decr. H. cont.	89
Promazine, Chlorpromazine	45 μg/ml	Rat	Mesentery mast cells, *in vitro*	Degranul.	86

[1] N-dimethylamino ethyl-N-benzylaniline.
[2] N-p-methoxybenzyl-N-dimethylamino ethylaminopyrine.

Table 1 (Continuation)

Compound	Dose or concentration	Species	Biological structure	Experimental evidence	Reference
Chlorpromazine	10 mg/kg	Rat	Mesentery mast cells, *in vivo*	Degranul.	103
Chlorpromazine	10 mg/kg	Rat	Plasma, *in vivo*	Incr. H. cont.	232
Pyrathiazine	—	Rat	Body tissues, *in vivo*	Decr. H. cont.	195
Amides					
Arfonad (Trimetaphan)	10 μg	Cat	Skin (perf.)	H. release	163
Arfonad (Trimetaphan)	—	Dog	Whole animal	Hypotension	168
Arfonad (Trimetaphan)	—	Dog	Skin, *in vivo*	Inflamm. resp.	128
Arfonad (Trimetaphan)	—	Dog	Plasma, *in vivo*	Incr. H. cont.	122
Arfonad (Trimetaphan)	—	G. pig	Skin, *in vivo*	Inflamm. resp.	128
Arfonad (Trimetaphan)	—	Man	Skin	Trip. resp.	128
Arfonad (Trimetaphan)	—	Man	Stomach, *in vivo*	Incr. acid secr.	165
1665 T.S.[1]	1 mg/kg	Dog	Plasma, *in vivo*	Incr. H. cont.	14
1665 T.S.[1]	0.1 mg/kg	Dog	Whole animal	Del. hypotens.	14
Meprobamate	—	Man	Skin	Allergic resp.	8, 95
Disulfiram (Antabuse)	—	Man	—	—	218
Sulphanilamide	4 mg/ml	Cat	Skin (perf.)	No effect	187
Nicotinamide	4 mg/kg	Cat	Whole animal	No Del. hypotens.	118
Amidines (Monoamidines)					
1-sulfonamide-6-amidino-hexane	6 mg/kg	Cat	Whole animal	Del. hypotens.	118
p-benzamidinomethyl-sulfone	5 mg/kg	Cat	Whole animal	Del. hypotens.	118
p-benzamidinoethylsulfone	6 mg/kg	Cat	Whole animal	Del. hypotens.	118
p-benzamidinopropylsulfone	4 mg/kg	Cat	Whole animal	Del. hypotens.	118
m-benzamidinomethyl-sulfone	5 mg/kg	Cat	Whole animal	Del. hypotens.	118
m-benzamidinoethylsulfone	5 mg/kg	Cat	Whole animal	Del. hypotens.	118
p-benzamidinophenyl-sulfone	1 mg/kg	Cat	Whole animal	Del. hypotens.	118
p-benzamidinobenzyl-sulfone	3 mg/kg	Cat	Whole animal	No Del. hypotens.	118
p-benzamidinosulfonamide	9 mg/kg	Cat	Whole animal	Del. hypotens.	118

[1] Sebacic diamide of 4-phenyl-4-aminoethyl-N-methylpiperidine.

Table 1 (Continuation)

Compound	Dose or concentration	Species	Biological structure	Experimental evidence	Reference
p-benzamidinoethyl ether	6 mg/kg	Cat	Whole animal	Del. hypotens.	118
p-benzamidino-β-amido-pyridyl sulfone	8 mg/kg	Cat	Whole animal	Del. hypotens.	118
p-amidinoaniline	6 mg/kg	Cat	Whole animal	Del. hypotens.	118
Benzamidine	18 mg/kg	Cat	Whole animal	No Del. hypotens.	118
Diamidines					
1-5-diamidino-pentane	—	Rat	Mesentery mast cells, *in vivo*	Degranul.	171
1-10-diamidinodecane	15 mg/kg	Dog	Plasma, *in vivo*	Incr. H. cont.	118
1-8-diamidino-octane	1.2 mg/kg	Cat	Whole animal	Del. hypotens.	118
1-16-diamidino-hexadecane	1.5 mg/kg	Cat	Whole animal	Del. hypotens.	118
β,β′-diamidinonaphtalene	3 mg/kg	Cat	Whole animal	Del. hypotens.	118
p,p′-dibenzamidinosulfone	0.3 mg/kg	Cat	Whole animal	Del. hypotens.	118
Stilbamidine[1]	300 μg/kg	Cat	Whole animal	Del. hypotens.	118
Stilbamidine[1]	7.5 mg/kg	Dog	Plasma, *in vivo*	Incr. H. cont.	177
Stilbamidine[1]	—	Man	Skin	Triple resp.	104
Stilbamidine[1]	50 μg/ml	Rat	Mesentery mast cells, *in vitro* and *in vivo*	Degranul.	139, 171
Stilbamidine[1]	125 mg/kg	Rat	Peritoneal fluid, *in vivo*	Incr. H. cont.	205
Stilbamidine[1]	1 mg/ml	Rat	Diaphragm, *in vitro*	H. release	177
Propamidine[2]	300 μg/kg	Cat	Whole animal	Del. hypotens.	118
Propamidine[2]	5 mg	Cat	Skin, muscle (perf.)	H. release	55
Propamidine[2]	10—200 μg/ml	Dog	Liver (subcell. particles)	H. release	73
Propamidine[2]	20 mg/kg	Rat	Skin, *in vivo*	Decr. H. cont.	59
Propamidine[2]	5 mg	Rat	Hindquarters (perf.)	H. release	12
Propamidine[2]	125 μg/kg	Rat	Mesent. mast cells, *in vivo*	Degranul.	12, 171
Propamidine[2]	150 μg/kg	Rat	Urine, *in vivo*	Incr. H. cont.	242
Propamidine[2]	1 mg/ml	G. pig	Ileum, *in vitro*	H. release	58
Guanidines					
Guanidine	18 mg/kg	Cat	Whole animal	No Del. hypotens.	118
Creatinine	7 mg/kg	Cat	Whole animal	No Del. hypotens.	118
N-guanidyl-N′-Phenyl-guanidine	3.5 mg/kg	Cat	Whole animal	No Del. hypotens.	118

[1] p,p′-diamidino-stilbene.
[2] Propyl-1,3-bis-p-amidino phenyl ether.

Table 1 (Continuation)

Compound	Dose or concentration	Species	Biological structure	Experimental evidence	Reference
1-amino-4-guanidinobutane	30 mg/kg	Cat	Whole animal	No Del. hypotens.	118
1,5-diguanidinopentane	2.5 mg/kg	Cat	Whole animal	Del. hypotens.	118
1,10-diguanidinodecane (Synthalin)	1 mg/kg	Cat	Whole animal	Del. hypotens.	118
1,18-diguanidinooctadecane	7 mg/kg	Cat	Whole animal	Del. hypotens.	118
Diisothioureas					
1,6-hexyl-diiso-thiourea	2 mg/kg	Cat	Whole animal	Del. hypotens.	118
1,16-hexadecyldiisothiourea	2 mg/kg	Cat	Whole animal	Del. hypotens.	118
Basic aminoacids, peptides and proteins (see also antibiotics)					
Arginine, lysine, carnosine, ornithine	100 mg/kg	Cat	Skin (perf.)	H. release	48
5-hydroxy-tryptophane	100 μg/kg	Rabbit	Platelets, *in vivo*	Decr., *in vivo*	24
5-hydroxy-tryptophane	2 μg/ml	Rabbit	Platelets, *in vitro*	No effect	24
Polylysine	—	Cat	Plasma, *in vivo*	Incr. H. cont.	65
Polylysine	—	Dog	Plasma, *in vivo*	Incr. H. cont.	65
Polylysine	—	Dog	Liver (homogenate)	H. release	65
Protamine	—	Cat	Plasma, *in vivo*	Incr. H. cont.	65
Protamine	—	Dog	Plasma, *in vivo*	Incr. H. cont.	65
Protamine	—	Dog	Liver (homogenate)	H. release	65
Protamine	1—4 mg/kg	Rat	Periton. fluid, *in vivo*	Incr. H. cont.	205
Protamine	10 μg/kg	Rat	Periton. fluid cells, *in vitro*	H. release	3
Spermine	50 μg	G. pig	Ileum, *in vitro*	Motor effects	2
Spermine	—	Man	Skin	Triple resp.	104
Quaternary ammonium compounds					
d-Tubocurarine	600 μg/kg	Cat	Whole animal	Del. hypotens.	118
d-Tubocurarine	5—15 mg	Cat	Skin, muscle (perf.)	H. release	55
d-Tubocurarine	20 mg	Cat	Stomach (spinal animal)	Incr. ac. secr.	55
d-Tubocurarine	—	Dog	Muscle (perf.)	H. release	1, 192
d-Tubocurarine	—	Dog	Whole animal	Hypotension	169
d-Tubocurarine	0.5—2 mg/kg	Dog	Bronchioli, *in vivo*	Spasm	102
d-Tubocurarine	—	Dog	Liver, *in vivo*	Decr. H. cont.	169

Table 1 (Continuation)

Compound	Dose or concentration	Species	Biological structure	Experimental evidence	Reference
d-Tubocurarine	—	Dog	Liver, lung (perf.)	No effect	169
d-Tubocurarine	—	Dog	Whole animal	Dessensiti. vs. anaphyl. shock	151
d-Tubocurarine	1 mg/ml	Dog	Intestine, *in vitro*	H. release	58
d-Tubocurarine	—	G. pig	Bronchioli, *in vivo*	Spasm	120, 235
d-Tubocurarine	6 mg/ml	G. pig	Diaphragm, aorta, uterus, heart, g-intest., tract, lung, spleen, *in vitro*	H. release	129
d-Tubocurarine	1 mg/ml	G. pig	Ileum, *in vitro*	H. release	58
d-Tubocurarine	—	Man	Bronchioli, *in vivo*	Spasm	234, 235
d-Tubocurarine	35 mg	Man	Plasma (perfused arm), *in vivo*	Incr. H. cont.	131
d-Tubocurarine	100 μg	Man	Skin	Triple resp.	37, 38, 72, 209
d-Tubocurarine	—	Man	Skin (isolated particles)	H. release	133
d-Tubocurarine	50 units	Man	Stomach, *in vivo*	Incr. ac. secr.	72
d-Tubocurarine	1 mg/ml	Rat	Diaphragm, *in vitro*	H. release	176
d-Tubocurarine	25 mg/kg	Rat	Peritoneal fluid, *in vivo*	H. release	205
d-Tubocurarine	1 mg/ml	Rat	Periton. fluid mast cells, *in vitro*	H. release	3, 30
d-Tubocurarine	—	Rat	Mesentery mast cells, *in vivo*	Degranul.	171
o-methyl-d-tubocurarine	600 μg/kg	Cat	Whole animal	Del. hypotens.	118
o-methyl-d-tubocurarine	250 μg	Rabbit	Skin capillaries, *in vivo*	Incr. permeab.	35
o-ethyl-d-tubocurarine	1 mg/ml	Rat	Periton. fluid mast cells, *in vitro*	H. release	30
Comps. 15[1] and 20[2]	1 mg	Cat	Whole animal	Del. hypotens.	37
Comps. 15[1] and 20[2]	15 mg	G. pig	Bronchioli, *in vivo*	Spasm	37
Dihydroerythriodine	2 mg/kg	Dog	Bronchioli, *in vivo*	No effect	102
Dihydroerythriodine	2 mg/kg	Dog	Whole animal	Hypotension	102
Dihydroerythriodine	13—200 μg	Man	Skin	Triple resp.	163
Dihydroerythriodine	—	Rat	Diaphragm, *in vitro*	H. release	163
Bebeerine	1 mg/ml	Rat	Periton. fluid cells, *in vitro*	H. release	30
Methylbebeerine	—	Dog	Muscle (perf.)	H. release	192
o-methylbebeerine	200 μg/ml	Rat	Periton. fluid cells, *in vitro*	H. release	30
Hexamethonium	70 mg/kg	Cat	Whole animal	Del. hypotens.	162
Hexamethonium	—	Rat	Diaphragm, *in vitro*	H. release	177
Decamethonium	4 mg/kg	Cat[3]	Whole animal	No hypotens.	118

[1] Decamethylene bis (1:2:3:4-dimethoxy-1(3:4′-dimethoxybenzyl)-2-methylisoquinolinium dimethosulfate (Laudexium, laudolissin).
[2] Decamethylene bis (1:2:3:4-tetrahydro 6:7:8: trimethoxy-2-methylisoquinolinium diiodide).
[3] After induced paralysis of autonomic ganglia.

Table 1 (Continuation)

Compound	Dose or concentration	Species	Biological structure	Experimental evidence	Reference
Dodecamethonium . . .	5 mg/kg	Cat[3]	Whole animal	Del. hypotens.	118
Succinylcholine	—	Cat	Skin (perf.)	H. release	163
Succinylcholine	—	Man	Skin	Triple resp.	163
Gallamine (Flaxedil) . . .	—	Man		No histaminic effects	69
Trimethyloctylammonium (curaryl)	10 mg	Rabbit	Skin capillaries	Incr. permeab.	35
Cetyltrimethylammoni. Br.	4 mg/kg	Cat	Whole animal	No hypoten.	118
Polybrene (Hexatrimetrine)	2 mg/kg	Cat	Plasma, *in vivo*	Incr. H. cont.	9
Polybrene (Hexatrimetrine)	2 mg/kg	Dog	Plasma, *in vivo*	Incr. H. cont.	9
Polybrene (Hexatrimetrine)	—	Dog	Whole animal	Hypotension	93
Polybrene (Hexatrimetrine)	—	Rat	Mesentery mast cells	Degranul.	93
Alkaloids and synthetic analogues					
Morphine, apomorphine, codeine, thebaine . . .	3 mg/kg	Cat	Whole animal	Del. hypotens.	50, 55
Morphine, apomorphine, codeine, thebaine . . .	2—10 mg	Cat	Skin, muscle (perf.)	H. release	55
Morphine, apomorphine, codeine, thebaine . . .	20 mg/kg	Cat	Plasma, *in vivo*	Incr. H. cont.	50, 55
Morphine	—	Dog	Whole animal	Anaphylactoid symptoms	67
Morphine	1.5 mg/kg	Cat	Whole animal plasma		47a
Morphine	—	Man	Skin	Triple resp.	116,149,186,210
Morphine	—	Man	Skin (subcell. particles)	H. release	133
Morphine	0.1 mM	Rabbit	Whole blood, *in vitro*	H. release	124
Morphine	—	Rat	Diaphragm, *in vitro*	H. release	149
Morphine	1 mg	Rat	Hindquarters (perf.)	H. release	12
Morphine	20 mg/kg/d	Rat	Feet pads, ears, *in vivo*	H. release	158
Morphine	20 mg/kg/d	Rat	Mesentery mast cells, *in vivo*	Degranul.	12, 158
Morphine	20 mg/kg/d	Rat	Skin H, *in vivo*	No effect	158
Morpholinethylmorphine .	4 mg/kg	Dog	Whole animal	Anaphylactoid symptoms	28
Morpholinethylmorphine .	4 mg/kg	Dog	Plasma, *in vivo*	Incr. H. cont.	28
Morpholinethylmorphine .	2 mg/kg	Rat	Whole animal	Anaphylactoid symptoms	28

[3] After induced paralysis of autonomic ganglia.

Table 1 (Continuation)

Compound	Dose or concentration	Species	Biological structure	Experimental evidence	Reference
Meperidine (Demerol) . .	15 mg/kg	Cat	Plasma, *in vivo*	Incr. H. cont.	187
Meperidine (Demerol) . .	50 μg	Cat	Skin (perf.)	H. release	187
Meperidine (Demerol) . .	500 μg	Dog	Skin (perf.)	H. release	187
Meperidine (Demerol) . .	5 mg/kg	Dog	Plasma, *in vivo*	Incr. H. cont.	243
Meperidine (Demerol) . .	5 mg/kg	Man	Skin	Triple resp.	27
Nalorphine	—	Cat	Skin (perf.)	H. release	163
Nalorphine	—	Man	Skin	Triple resp.	163
Papaverine	5 mg	Cat	Muscle (perf.)	H. release	55
Strychnine	—	Dog	Hindquarters, tongue (perf.)	H. release	192
Atropine	1 mg	Cat	Skin (perf.)	H. release	187
Atropine	15 mg/kg	Cat	Plasma, *in vivo*	Incr. H. cont.	187
Atropine	—	Dog	Plasma, *in vivo*	Incr. H. cont.	25
Atropine	—	Dog	Liver, *in vivo*	Decr. H. cont.	25
Atropine	2 mg	Dog	Skin (perf.)	H. release	187
Atropine	—	Man	Skin	Triple resp. urticar.	116, 211
Sinomenine	1.5 mg/kg	Dog	Plasma, *in vivo*	Incr. H. cont.	15, 121
Sinomenine	—	Dog	Skin, liver, muscle, *in vivo*	Decr. H. cont.	150
Sinomenine	—	Man	Skin	Trip. resp.	121
Sinomenine	—	Rat	Skin, *in vivo*	Decr. H. cont.	89
Reserpine	5 mg/kg	G. pig	Lung, *in vivo*	Decr. H. cont.	231
Reserpine	5 mg/kg	G. pig	Brain, gut H, *in vivo*	No effect	231
Reserpine	5 mg/kg	Mouse	Skin, *in vivo*	No effect	231
Reserpine	5 mg/kg	Mouse	Subcut. mastocytoma, *in vivo*	H. release	231
Reserpine	5 mg/kg	Rabbit	Plasma, *in vivo*	Incr. H. cont.	231
Reserpine	1—3 μg/ml	Rabbit	Blood platelets, *in vitro*	No effect	24
Reserpine	0.3 μg/ml	Rabbit	Blood platelets, *in vitro*	H. release	231
Reserpine	5 mg/kg	Rabbit	Brain, H, *in vivo*	No effect	24
Reserpine	5 mg/kg	Rabbit	Lung, liver, heart, kidney, H, *in vivo*	No effect	24
Reserpine	5 mg/kg	Rabbit	Whole blood, *in vivo*	Decr. H. cont.	24
Reserpine	0.5—2 mg	Rat	Hindquarters (perf.)	No effect	13
Reserpine	—	Rat	Skin, tongue, lung, liver, H, *in vivo*	No effect	158
Reserpine	—	Rat	Spleen, *in vivo*	H. release	158
Reserpine	1 mg/kg	Rat	Plasma, *in vivo*	Incr. H. cont.	232
Oxypanamine	0.25 mg/kg	Dog	Plasma, *in vivo*	No effect	138
Quinine	1 mg	Cat	Skin (perf.)	H. release	187
Quinine	50 mg/kg	Cat	Plasma, *in vivo*	Incr. H. cont.	187

Table 1 (Continuation)

Compound	Dose or concentration	Species	Biological structure	Experimental evidence	Reference
Quinine	10 mg/kg	Dog	Whole animal	Hypotension	102
Quinine	10 mg/kg	Dog	Bronchioli, *in vivo*	Spasm	102
Quinine	—	Man	Skin	Triple resp.	211
Purine bases, nucleosides, nucleotides					
Guanosine, inosine, inosinic acid	250 μg	Rat	Hindquarters (perf.)	H. release	147
Inosine	25 μg	G. pig	Skin capillaries	Incr. permeab.	147
Inosine	25 μg	Mouse	Skin capillaries	Incr. permeab.	147
Inosine	25 μg	Rabbit	Skin capillaries	Incr. permeab.	147
Xanthine, xanthosine	5 μg	Man	Skin	Triple resp.	147
Caffeine	25 mg	Cat	Skin (perf.)	No effect	187
Piperidine derivatives					
γ, γ' dipiperidyl	2.5 mg/kg	Cat	Whole animal	Del. hypotens.	118
α, γ' dipiperidyl	4 mg/kg	Cat	Whole animal	No Del. hypotens.	118
Pyridinium compounds					
N-hexadecylcarbomethoxy-pyridine	2 mg	Cat	Whole animal	Del. hypotens.	125
N-hexadecylcarbomethoxy-pyridine	0.1 mM	Rabbit	Whole blood, *in vitro*	H. release	124
N-hexadecylcarbomino-pyridine	2 mg	Cat	Whole animal	Del. hypotens.	125
N-hexadecylcarbomino-pyridine	0.1 mM	Rabbit	Whole blood, *in vitro*	H. release	124
Dyes					
Trypaflavine	—	Dog	Whole animal, *in vivo*	Hypertension	105
Trypaflavine	—	Man	Skin	Triple resp.	104
Trypaflavine	2.5 mg	Rat	Hindquarters, (perf.)	H. release	105
Trypan blue	—	Dog	Plasma, *in vivo*	Incr. H. cont.	40a
Trypan blue	—	Dog	Liver, *in vivo*	Decr. H. cont.	40a
Toluidine blue	10 μg/ml	Dog	Liver (homogenate)	H. release	123
Toluidine blue	4 mg/kg	Rat	Peritoneal fluid, *in vivo*	H. release	174, 205

Table 1 (Continuation)

Compound	Dose or concentration	Species	Biological structure	Experimental evidence	Referenes
Anti-malarials (see also alkaloids)					
Atebrine	5 mg	Rat	Hindquarters (perf.)	H. release	105
Chloroquine	0.5 mg/kg	Dog	Whole animal	Hypotension	105
Chloroquine	0.2 mg	Man	Skin	Triple resp.	105
Chloroquine	0.25 mg	Rabbit	Skin capillaries	Incr. permeab.	105
Chloroquine	2 mg	Rat	Hindquarters (perf.)	H. release	105
Paludrine	4 mg/kg	Cat	Whole animal	Del. hypotens.	118
Antibiotic bases					
Antrycide	—	Cat	Skin (perf.)	H. release	55
Aureomycin	75 μg/ml	Rat	Mesentery mast cells	Degranul.	153
Bacitracin, penicilin, achromycin	500 μg/ml	Rat	Mesentery mast cells	No effect	153
Polymyxin B	5—45 mg/kg	Hamster	Skin, *in vivo*	Decr. H. cont.	238
Polymyxin B	5—45 mg/kg	Mouse	Skin, *in vivo*	Decr. H. cont.	238
Polymyxin B	—	Rat	Whole animal	Anaphylactoid symptoms	26
Polymyxin B	0.4 μg/ml	Rat	Mesentery mast cells	Degranul.	153, 158
Polymyxin B	5—15 mg/kg/d	Rat	Skin, feet, spleen, lung, liver, *in vivo*	Decr. H. cont	158
Polymyxin B	2—10 mg/kg	Dog	Whole animal	Hypotension	163
Polymyxin B	2 mg/kg	Cat	Whole animal	Del. hypotens.	163
Licheniformin	0.3 mg/kg	Cat	Whole animal	Del. hypotens.	118
Licheniformin	30 mg/kg	Cat	Plasma, *in vivo*	Incr. H. cont.	118
Licheniformin	—	Cat	Skin, *in vivo*	Decr. H. cont.	118
Licheniformin	—	Cat	Stomach, *in vivo*	Incr. ac. secr.	118
Licheniformin	100 μg/ml	Man	Skin	Triple resp.	118

References for Table 1

1. ALAM et al. (1939)
2. AMANN and WERLE (1956)
3. ARCHER (1958)
4. ARUNLAKSHANA (1953)
5. ARVY (1956)
6. ARVY et al. (1956)
7. BALTZLY et al. (1949)
8. BARNES (1957)
9. BEAUJEAN and LECOMTE (1960)
10. BERALDO (1950)
11. BERNSTEIN and FEINBERG (1956)
12. BHATTACHARYA and LEWIS (1956a)
13. BHATTACHARYA and LEWIS (1956b)
14. BIGNAMI (1962)
15. BINET and QUIVY (1957)
16. BINET and QUIVY (1958)
17. BODMAN (1952)
18. BONIN and JASMIN (1959)
19. BOREUS (1960)
20. BOSEILA and ASBOE-HANSEN (1959)
21. BRAUNSTEINER et al. (1957)
22. BROCKLEHURST et al. (1955)
23. BRODIE et al. (1955)
24. BURKHALTER et al. (1960)
25. BURSTEIN and PARROT (1949)
26. BUSHBY and GREEN (1955)
27. BUTLER (1951)
28. CAHEN and AUBRON (1960)
29. CARMO and DIAS DA SILVA (1962)
30. CARVALHO et al. (1962)
31. CASS and MARSHALL (1962)
32. CHAKRAVARTY et al. (1959)
33. CHAKRAVARTY (1960)
34. CHARLIER et al. (1954)
35. CHEYMOL et al. (1951)
36. CODE et al. (1961)
37. COLLIER and MACAULEY (1952)
38. COLLIER (1956)
39. COMROE and DRIPPS (1946)
40. COPPOLA and DIPALMA (1962)
40a. CZARNECKI et al. (1950)
41. DALE (1948)
42. DANON and MOUSSATCHÉ (1961)
43. DARLOW (1955)
44. DEWS et al. (1953)
45. DIAMANT and UVNÄS (1961)
46. DIAS DA SILVA et al. (1962)
47. EICHLER and BARFUSS (1940)
47a. EICHLER and SPEDA (1940)
48. ELDRIDGE and PATON (1954)
49. ELLIS et al. (1954)
50. EVANS et al. (1952)
51. FAWCETT (1954)
52. FEINBERG et al. (1954)
53. FEINBERG and STERNBERGER (1956)
54. FELDBERG and HOLMES (1941)
55. FELDBERG and PATON (1951)
56. FELDBERG and SCHACHTER (1952)
57. FELDBERG and MILES (1953)
58. FELDBERG and SMITH (1953)
59. FELDBERG and TALESNIK (1953)
60. FELDBERG and MONGAR (1954)
61. FELDBERG and SMITH (1954)
62. FELDBERG and LECOMTE (1955)
63. FELDBERG and GREENGAARD (1956)
64. GARAN (1938)
65. GARCIA-AROCHA et al. (1953)
66. GERENDAS et al. (1958)
67. GERSHON and SHAW (1958)
68. GERTNER (1955)
69. GOODMAN and GILMAN (1955)
70. GOTH et al. (1957)
71. GRAHAM et al. (1955)
72. GROB et al. (1947)
73. GROSSBERG and GARCIA-AROCHA (1954)
74. HAGEN (1954)
75. HAGEN et al. (1959)
76. HALPERN (1956)
77. HALPERN et al. (1956)
78. HALPERN et al. (1957)
79. HALPERN et al. (1959a)
80. HALPERN et al. (1959b)
81. HALPERN (1960)
82. HARRIS et al. (1961)
83. HIGGINBOTHAM and DOUGHERTY (1956)
84. HIGGINBOTHAM (1958)
85. HÖGBERG et al. (1956)
86. HÖGBERG and UVNÄS (1957)
87. HÖGBERG and UVNÄS (1960)
88. HUMPHREY and JAQUES (1955)
89. IRINO (1958)
90. JAQUES and KÜTTNER (1961)
91. JORI et al. (1961)
92. JUNQUEIRA and BEIGUELMAN (1953)
93. KIMURA et al. (1959)
94. KIRK and HENRY (1944)
95. KLOTZ and BERNSTEIN (1957)
96. KOCH and SZERB (1950)
97. KÖKSAL (1953)
98. KOWALEWSKI (1960)
99. KÜTTNER et al. (1961)
100. LAGUNOFF and BENDITT (1960)
101. LAHIRI and BROCKLEHURST (1961)
102. LANDMESSER (1947)
103. LE BLANC (1958)
104. LECOMTE and BORENSZTAJN (1953)
105. LECOMTE (1955a)
106. LECOMTE (1955b)
107. LECOMTE (1955c)
108. LECOMTE (1955d)
109. LECOMTE (1956a)
110. LECOMTE (1956b)
111. LECOMTE (1957)
112. LECOMTE and BEAUMARIAGE (1957)
113. LECOMTE and FISCHER (1957)
114. LECOMTE and PETIT (1960)
115. LEITCH and HALEY (1955)
116. LEWIS (1927)
117. MACALUSO et al. (1961)
118. MAC INTOSH and PATON (1949)
119. MAC INTOSH (1956)
120. MAHFOUZ (1949)
121. MAYEDA (1953)
122. MCCUBBIN and PAGE (1952)
123. MCILREATH (1959)
124. MCINTIRE et al. (1951)
125. MCINTIRE (1962)
126. MELON and LECOMTE (1958)

127. Miles and Miles (1952)
128. Mitchell et al. (1951)
129. Mongar and Schild (1952)
130. Mongar and Schild (1953)
131. Mongar and Whelan (1953)
132. Mongar and Schild (1956)
133. Mongar (1956)
134. Mongar (1957)
135. Mongar and Schild (1957a)
136. Mongar and Schild (1957b)
137. Mongar and Schild (1958)
138. Moran et al. (1959)
139. Mota et al. (1953)
140. Mota et al. (1954)
141. Mota et al. (1956a)
142. Mota et al. (1956b)
143. Mota and Vugman (1956)
144. Mota (1959)
145. Mota and Ishii (1960)
146. Mota and Dias da Silva (1960)
147. Moulton et al. (1957)
148. Moussatché and Danon (1958)
149. Nasmyth and Stewart (1950)
150. Nishiyama et al. (1957)
151. Nitescu et al. (1959)
152. Norton (1954)
153. Norton and deBeer (1955)
154. Osler et al. (1959)
155. Papacostas and Loew (1959)
156. Papacostas et al. (1959)
157. Parratt and West (1957a)
158. Parratt and West (1957b)
159. Parrot and Laborde (1951)
160. Paton (1951)
161. Paton and Schachter (1951)
162. Paton (1956)
163. Paton (1957)
164. Paton (1959)
165. Payne (1955)
166. Pellerat and Murat (1946)
167. Quastel and Wheatley (1933)
168. Randall et al. (1949)
169. Reid (1950)
170. Reuse (1953)
171. Riley (1953)
172. Riley and West (1955a)
173. Riley and West (1955b)
174. Riley (1959)
175. Rocha e Silva (1941)
176. Rocha e Silva and Schild (1949)
177. Rocha e Silva (1952)
179. Rocha e Silva and Rothschild (1955)
179. Rocha e Silva and Rothschild (1956)
180. Rocha e Silva (1959)
181. Rothschild et al. (1961)
182. Rothschild (1961)
183. Rothschild (1962)
184. Rothschild (1962a)
185. Rothschild and Garcia Lima (1962)
186. Salter and White (1949)
187. Schachter (1952)
188. Schachter (1953)
189. Schayer and Smiley (1954)
190. Schayer et al. (1954)
191. Schayer et al. (1955)
192. Schild and Gregory (1947)
193. Schild (1949)
194. Selye (1949)
195. Shelesnyak and Kraicer (1959)
196. Sicuteri and Monfardini (1958)
197. Sicuteri et al. (1958)
198. Sicuteri et al. (1959)
199. Sicuteri et al. (1960)
200. Sicuteri (1961)
201. Smith (1953a)
202. Smith (1953b)
203. Smith and Lewis (1957)
204. Smith (1958)
205. Smith (1958a)
206. Smith (1958b)
207. Smith (1958c)
208. Smith et al. (1955)
209. Sniper (1952)
210. Sollmann and Pilcher (1917)
211. Sollmann (1948)
212. Sömjen and Uyldert (1955)
213. Staub (1946)
214. Staub and Bauer (1948)
215. Surkes (1948)
216. Szilagyi et al. (1960)
217. Tasaka (1957)
218. Troquet and Lecomte (1960)
219. Ungar and Damgaard (1955)
220. Ungar et al. (1961)
221. Uvnäs and Thon (1959)
222. Uvnäs (1961)
223. Uvnäs and Thon (1961)
224. Van Arsdel and Bray (1961)
225. Vane (1949)
226. Viana and Brandão (1962)
227. Virno et al. (1956)
228. Vogt (1957)
229. Vugman (1961)
230. Vugman and Rothschild (1961)
231. Waalkes et al. (1959)
232. Waser and Itzbicki (1959)
233. Went and Varga (1952)
234. West (1935)
235. West (1938)
236. West (1949)
237. West (1955)
238. West (1958)
239. West (1961)
240. Westerholm (1960a)
241. Westerholm (1960b)
242. Wilson (1954)
243. Zeppa et al. (1961)

species will also show effects in another, although often only at considerably different dosages or concentrations. Thus, compound 48/80 which is active in the tissues of the cat (Paton, 1951) and of the rat (Feldberg and Talesnik,

1953), at the microgram level, will only act on the tissues of the guinea-pig *in vitro* at concentrations of 100 μg to 1 mg/ml and *in vivo* in doses of 10 mg/kg (SMITH, 1958). Amounts of compound 48/80, 200 to 400 times greater than those required to release 80 to 90 percent of the histamine contained in isolated rat

Table 2. *Approximate threshold doses (mg), for release of histamine by octylamine, morphine, d-tubocurarine and 48/80 from perfused tissues.* (According to MONGAR, 1956)

	Octylamine	Morphine	d-Tubocurarine	48/80
Guinea pig lung	0.7	>20	3.5	0.5
Guinea pig limbs	1.0	3	0.2	0.05
Rat lung	0.3	3	1.1	0.2
Rat limbs	1.1	3	0.1	0.001
Cat lung	1.0	—	0.7	0.1

Table 3. *Threshold concentrations (μg/ml) for release of histamine by octylamine and 48/80 from isolated skin particles.* (According to MONGAR, 1956)

	Man	Rat	Dog	Cat	Mouse	Guinea pig	Rabbit
Octylamine . .	20	20	45	50	65	80	90
48/80.	40	80	30	1	100	80	10

mast cells (UVNÄS and THON, 1959), are wholly ineffective when tested on rabbit platelet suspensions (HUMPHREY and JAQUES, 1955), even though the abundant

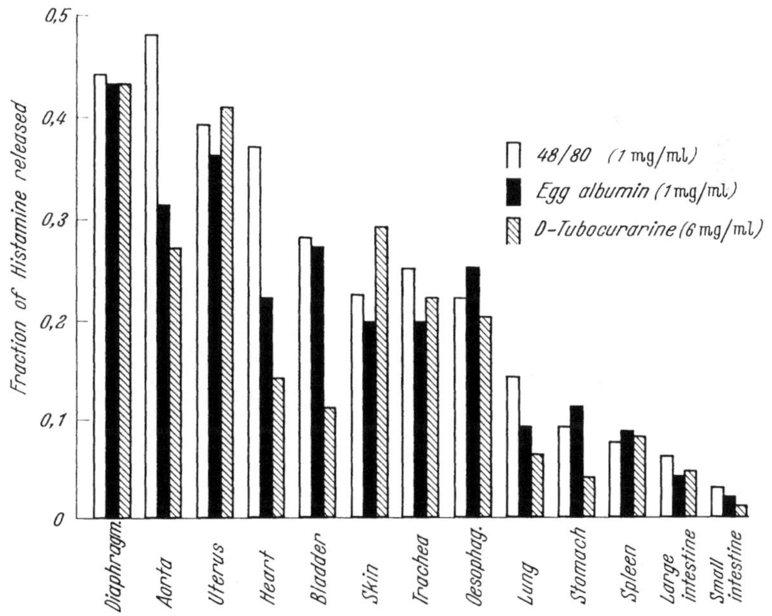

Fig. 4. Parallelism of histamine release by antigen and chemical releasers from thirteen guinea-pig tissues. (According to MONGAR and SCHILD, 1952)

histamine stores of these particles are easily mobilized by other basic releasers like morphine and octadecylamine (MCINTIRE et al. 1951). Compound 48/80 does however have a histamine-releasing effect when tested on the perfused rabbit's ear (SCHACHTER, 1953).

Organ and tissue specificity are another feature of the action of basic histamine releasers. Thus, MOTA et al. (1956), have shown that the organs of the lower gastro-intestinal tract of the rat, although containing histamine did not respond to 48/80 treatment in contrast to the skin or muscle of this species, whose histamine stores are readily exhausted by the compound. This difference is paralleled by observations showing that the histamine stores of the lower gastrointestinal tract are not bound to mast cells, and possibly are not succeptible to the action of basic histamine releasers (CASS and MARSHALL, 1962). Examples of surveys of the effects of species or tissue variations on the action of basic histamine releasers, are presented in Tables 2 and 3 and in Figure 4.

2. Temperature dependence

The effect of temperature on the *in vitro* release of histamine from subcellular dog liver fractions has been investigated by GROSSBERG and GARCIA-AROCHA (1954), who used diamino-decane, propamidine and compound 48/80 as releasing agents and showed that the action of these compounds was decreased when the temperature was lowered; this effect had a Q_{10} of approximately 2 and was interpreted as an indication that an enzymatic step was involved in the release of histamine from its intragranular confinement. Low temperatures have been shown to inhibit the release of histamine from guinea pig lung slices and rat skin fragments submitted to the action of compound 48/80 (Fig. 5), as well as the releasing effect of d-tubocurarine acting on the isolated rat diaphragm (Fig. 6).

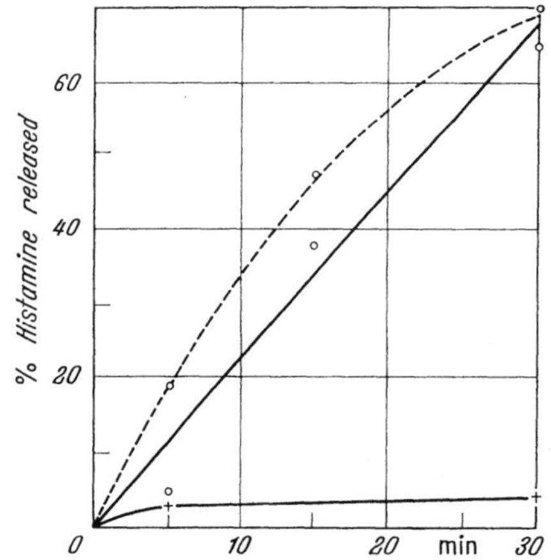

Fig. 5

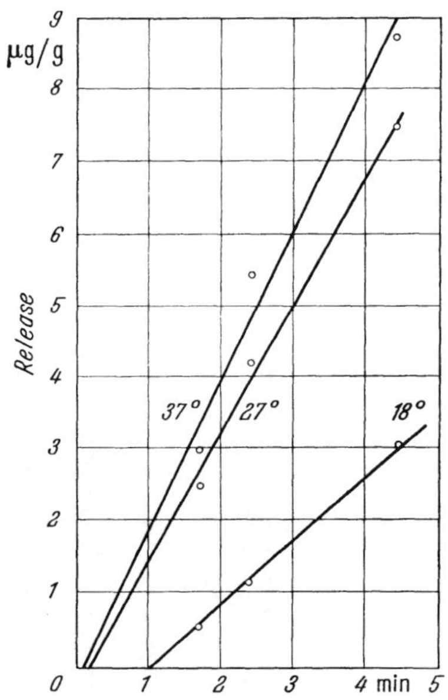

Fig. 6

Fig. 5. Effect of temperature on the release of histamine from guinea-pig lung slices and rat skin fragments by compound 48/80 (10^{-3} by wt.), in Tyrode medium (ROTHSCHILD, 1962). ○- - - - -○ guinea-pig lung, 37° C; +———+ guinea pig lung, 0—2° C; ○———○ rat skin, 37° C; +———+ rat skin, 0—2° C

Fig. 6. Effect of temperature on the rate of release of histamine by d-tubocurarine (1:1000) from rat diaphragm *in vitro*. (According to ROCHA E SILVA and SCHILD, 1949)

The effect of low temperature on mast cell degranulation by compound 48/80, a process shown to be associated with histamine release (MOTA et al. 1953), has been studied by JUNQUEIRA and BEIGUELMAN (1955). They showed that in the isolated rat mesentery, degranulation was inhibited by temperatures below 15° C, a result which agrees with other features of this process characterizing it as an enzyme-dependent reaction (MOTA and ISHII, 1960, ROTHSCHILD et al. 1961; DIAMANT and UVNÄS, 1961). A similar temperature dependence has been shown to condition the histamine releasing action of compound 48/80 on chopped cat skin (WESTERHOLM, 1960 a). The inhibitory effect of low temperatures on histamine release by basic compounds is apparently not exhibited *in vivo*. HALPERN and co-workers (1960), have shown that in rats whose rectal temperature had been lowered to 14°C, histamine release by compounds 48/80 and L-1935 was enhanced, while the release induced by dextran was greatly reduced. The reason for these differences remains unexplained. The irreversible blockade of histamine release and mast cell degranulation in tissues pre-heated to 45° C for 20—30 minutes, is an interesting feature of the *in vitro* action of certain basic histamine releasers in the rat (MOTA and ISHII, 1960; VUGMAN, 1961), but not in the guinea pig (MONGAR and SCHILD, 1957 b; MOTA, 1959); the cause of this effect is not clear.

3. pH dependence

Histamine release as well as mast cell alterations by basic compounds are pH dependent processes. An optimum at pH 7.5 has been observed for the action of compound 48/80 on the tissues of the cat (WESTERHOLM, 1960 a), the dog (GROSSBERG and GARCIA-AROCHA, 1954) and the rat (JUNQUEIRA and BEIGUELMAN, 1955; HÖGBERG and UVNÄS, 1960; VUGMAN, 1961). Since the action of compound 48/80 in these species is linked to cell metabolism, it is probable that metabolic requirements condition the optimal activity observed at pH 7.5, pH may however also influence histamine release by basic compounds by affecting the ionization of the releaser. Results of SCHILD (1949), showing that the *in vitro* release of histamine from the isolated rat diaphragm by ammonia only becomes apparent above pH 8.2, as well as data of MONGAR (1957), showing that the histamine releasing activity of mono- and diamines on guinea pig lung slices, is greatly increased when the pH of the medium is shifted from 7.0 to 8.5 (Fig. 7), bring experimental support for this hypothesis.

Since it is improbable that metabolic activity is enhanced at these high pH levels, it is reasonable to admit that an increase of histamine release can also occur as a consequence of a raise in the level of the unionized form of the basic agent. As suggested by MONGAR (1957), this form has greater liposolubility and therefore greater penetrating power into the lipoid boundaries of mast cells.

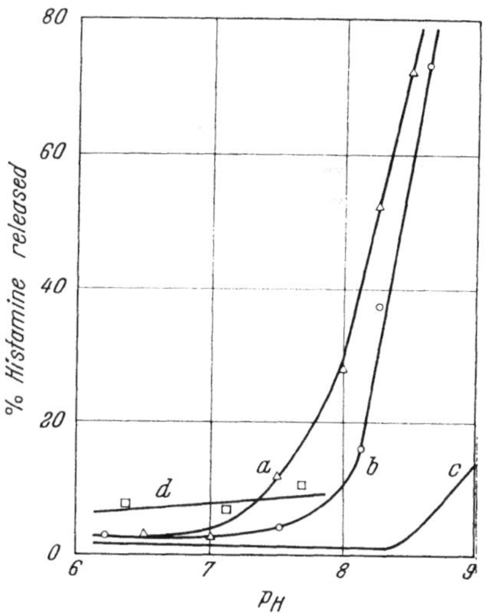

Fig. 7. Effect of pH on histamine release by a), octylamine (0.2 mg/ml); b) decamethylene diamine (0.2 mg/ml); c) Tyrode solution; d) dodecyl trimethyl ammonium chloride (0.2 mg/ml). (According to MONGAR, 1957)

4. Effects of metal ions

A requirement for calcium ions, both for the release of histamine and the degranulation of mast cells by compound 48/80 in the rat, has been demonstrated by HÖGBERG and UVNÄS (1960), CHAKRAVARTY (1960), MOTA and ISHII (1960) and VUGMAN (1961). These results have been confirmed by ROTHSCHILD (1962) in fluoride-treated tissue and, as shown in Fig. 8, an additional requirement for magnesium ions has been demonstrated.

A different picture is seen when the effect of calcium lack on the histamine releasing action of 48/80 on guinea pig tissues is examined. MONGAR and SCHILD (1958), as well as MOTA (1959), have shown that in lung slices depleted of calcium by versene treatment, amine release proceeded as well as in untreated controls. Although the reasons for these variations remain unexplained, they indicate that different mechanisms may be operative in histamine release by 48/80 in rat and guinea pig tissues respectively. It seems possible that in the rat, lack of Ca and Mg prevents histamine release by interfering with normal cell metabolism, since both cations are important co-factors of a series of metabolic enzymes. In addition, Ca is essential for the activation of humoral enzyme systems involved in complement fixation, a phenomenon which, under certain circumstances, has been shown to be associated with histamine release (OSLER et al., (1959).

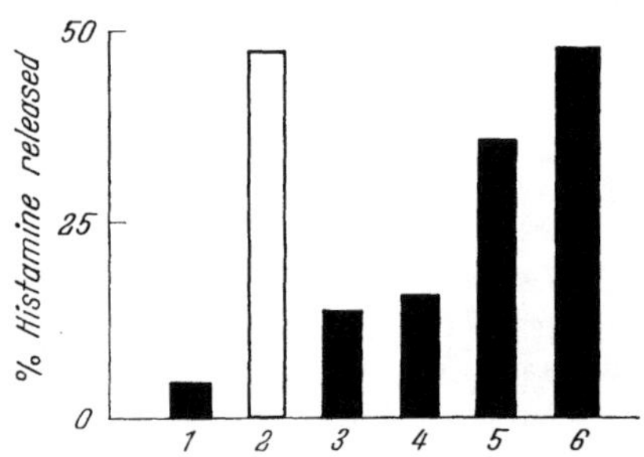

Fig. 8. Inhibition of the histamine releasing action of compound 48/80 (2×10^{-5} by wt.) in fluoride-treated rat diaphragm, *in vitro*. Reactivation by calcium and magnesium. (ROTHSCHILD, 1962). All samples except those of column 2 were preincubated for 20 min at 37° C in Krebs-Ringer phosphate buffer, pH 7.3, containing 40 mM NaF, rinsed, and reincubated for 20 min in fresh buffer containing respectively: 1. no 48/80; 2. 48/80; 3. 48/80; 4. 48/80 + $MgCl_2$ (1.5 mM); 5. 48/80 + $CaCl_2$ (4.7 mM); 6. 48/80 + $MgCl_2$ (1.5 mM) + $CaCl_2$ (4.7 mM)

5. Effects of ionic strength

NORTON (1954), has shown that the action of compound 48/80 on rat mesentery mast cells, is considerably reduced in a medium of low ionic strength, obtained by dilution of Tyrode fluid with distilled water. The results of her work, although allowing the interesting conclusion that a limited decrease in the osmolarity of the medium does not lead to spontaneous histamine release, do not clarify whether a decrease in total ionic strength or deficiency in a component of the diluted Tyrode medium were the cause for the inhibition of the action of 48/80. McILREATH (1959), has studied the effect of hypertonicity on the release of histamine from dog liver particles and the isolated perfused cat's paw. He showed that when basic releasers like 48/80, stilbamidine, toluidine blue or diaminodecane were employed, significantly less histamine was discharged from preparations tested in hypertonic (1.2 M sucrose), rather than isotonic media. In contrast, this difference was not apparent when surface active compounds (saponin or taurocholate) were used as histamine releasers.

6. Effects of metabolic inhibitors

MOTA and ISHII (1960), showed that sodium cyanide as well as sulfhydryl group reagents like monoiodoacetate, ethylmaleinimide and others, inhibited histamine release from rat skin exposed to compound 48/80, *in vitro*. Inhibitors of oxidative phosphorylation like dinitrophenol, thionembutal, sodium salicylate and sodium oleate are also effective inhibitors of this release as well as of the degranulation of mast cells in rat tissues exposed to compound 48/80 (ROTHSCHILD et al. 1961; DIAMANT and UVNÄS, 1961). Similar inhibitory effects of anoxia and dinitrophenol have been demonstrated for histamine release from cat skin (WESTERHOLM, 1960 a); they indicate that metabolic factors, most probably adenosinetriphosphate (ATP) or a closely related metabolic intermediate, are essential elements for the unfolding of the histamine releasing process. This conclusion, which had been postulated for the release of histamine in *in vitro* anaphylaxis (Moussatché and Danon, 1958), received support from observations by Westerholm (1960 b), Rothschild et al. (1961) and Diamant and Uvnäs (1961), showing that the inhibition produced by inhibitors of oxidative phosphorylation could be overcome by the presence of glucose, but not of Krebs cycle intermediates, in the incubation medium (Table 4). Since these inhibitory substances would not be expected to affect the utilization of glucose for the glycolytic synthesis of ATP, it is probable that the breakdown of this sugar by

Table 4. *Release of histamine from isolated rat diaphragm by compound 48/80 (20 μg/ml). Influence of glucose and other metabolites on the inhibition induced by 2:4-dinitrophenol (DNP). Figures within parentheses refer to the number of experiments performed.* (According to Rothschild et al., 1961)

Addition to medium	Per cent histamine released ± s.e.	
	total	total—blank
—	43.6 ± 2.7 (6)	38.3
Glucose, 4.5 mM	51.3 ± 2.8 (6)	45.2
DNP, 0.03 mM	35.5 ± 3.8 (6)	31.0
DNP, 0.03 mM + glucose, 4.5 mM	43.5 ± 3.2 (6)	39.0
DNP, 0.3 mM	8.5 ± 2.9 (4)	4.8
DNP, 0.3 mM + glucose, 4.5 mM	48.2 ± 5.6 (4)	43.7
DNP, 0.3 mM + succinate, 5 mM	8.3 ± 1.1 (3)	3.8
DNP, 0.3 mM + fumarate, 5 mM	4.1 ± 2.2 (3)	2.1
DNP, 0.3 mM + acetate, 5 mM	4.6 ± 1.6 (2)	2.3
DNP, 0.3 mM + pyruvate, 5 mM	3.5 ± 2.8 (3)	1.5
DNP, 0.3 mM + D-xylose, 4.5 mM	8.7 ± 1.8 (3)	3.4

the Embden-Meyerhof cycle is sufficient to supply the mast cell with the metabolites required for the histamine releasing process. This view is substantiated by observations (Rothschild et al. 1961), showing that in the presence of glucose and dinitrophenol, respiratory activity of rat diaphragm as measured in the Warburg apparatus is strongly depressed, while histamine release by 48/80 is preactically of the same level as that observed in normally respiring controls.

Similar considerations have been shown to apply to other conditions of histamine release, for instance that which follows the action of antigen on sensitized lung tissue (Rothschild, 1961; Danon and Moussatché, 1961) or that induced by anaphylatoxin in guinea pig lung tissue (Rothschild, 1961), and in isolated blood platelets (Rothschild and Garcia Lima, 1962). Smith (1958a), had suggested that the release of histamine from mast cells is a secretory function. Such functions are endergonic processes which require cellular metabolic activity (ATP), for their normal course; this consideration brings into focus a new aspect of the relationship between mast cell function and histamine release. It is however pertinent to note that the link between energy metabolism and histamine release may not control all cases in which this release occurs. Thus, it has been shown that the action of decylamine (Högberg and Uvnäs, 1960) and of dichlorocatecholamine derivatives (Rothschild, 1962), on rat mast cells can take place, in dinitrophenol treated tissues, in the absence of glucose, that is, under conditions in which ATP levels are presumably strongly depressed. Similar results have been reported by Mongar and Schild (1957 a) and by Mota (1959) for the effects of octylamine and compound 48/80 on guinea pig lung histamine. An additional difference observed by Mongar and Schild (1957), is that in the presence of monoiodoacetate, histamine release from guinea pig lung by 48/80 *in vitro,* is actually enhanced. The biochemical basis of this effect remains unknown; its explanation would be of value for the understanding of the mechanism of action of the basic histamine releasing agents on rat and guinea pig mast cells, respectively.

7. Effects of anti-histaminic agents

An inhibitory effect of diphenhydramine, mepyramine, as well as other anti-histaminics, on histamine-release and mast cell degranulation by compound 48/80, has been demonstrated by MOTA and DIAS DA SILVA (1960). The mechanism of this inhibition is not clear but it is interesting to note that in addition to their inhibitory power, anti-histamines have been shown to be effective histamine releasers from rat and guinea pig tissues when employed at higher concentrations (MOTA and DIAS DA SILVA, 1960). A similar double effect has been recently observed with DCI, the ring chlorinated analogue of isoproterenol, acting on isolated rat peritoneal fluid mast cells (ROTHSCHILD, 1962 a).

8. Hormonal influences

Adrenalectomized rats show an increased sensitivity to histamine releasers paralleled by an increased susceptibility to histamine (SELYE, 1949; HALPERN, 1956). These conclusions are confirmed by the demonstration that cortisone counteracts the effects of the adrenalectomy, both in relation to the increased sensitivity to histamine and to the releasing activity of the substances studied (SELYE, 1949).

3—10 mM adrenaline, nor-adrenaline, isoproterenol and tyramine have been shown to block the histamine releasing action of compound 48/80 on isolated rat peritoneal fluid mast cells (ROTHSCHILD, 1962). These effects, like those of dinitrophenol, were only observed in glucose-free media, an indication that they may have a common origin, i.e. the blockade of oxidative phosphorylation. Effects of tyramine on oxygen consumption of brain slices have been described by QUASTEL and WHEATLEY (1933).

The histamine releasing actions of adrenaline and laevoarterenol have been investigated by different workers, with contradictory results (Table 1). According to WENT and VARGA (1952), it is possible that the increased histaminaemia which undoubtedly occurs on dogs infused with adrenaline, has an indirect, reflex origin. Indirect confirmatory results to strengthen these conclusions have been afforded by *in vitro* observations showing that adrenaline had no direct histamine releasing effect on rat (MONGAR and WHELAN, 1953; ROTHSCHILD, 1962) or human and guinea pig tissues (MONGAR and WHELAN, 1953). These results stand in contradiction with those of KOCH and SZERB (1950), who obtained an abundant release of histamine from rat lungs perfused with adrenaline.

Insulin has been shown not to affect the histamine releasing activity of compound 48/80 in the rat (GOTH et al., 1957; DIAS DA SILVA and BERALDO, 1962), even when given after alloxan treatment leading to a pronounced diabetic state. Earlier results (VUGMAN and ROTHSCHILD, 1961), had indicated that insulin, both alone and in the presence of glucose, could enhance histamine release by 48/80 acting on the isolated diaphragm from alloxan diabetic rats. These results however, could not be confirmed when other groups of animals were employed (VUGMAN, 1962). Thus, although glucose metabolism will, under certain circumstances (ROTHSCHILD et al., 1961), enhance histamine release by 48/80, the dependence on insulin of this process remains unproven.

Thyroxin has been shown to inhibit the degranulation of rat mesentery mast cells by compound 48/80 *in vitro*. This effect may in part, be related to the uncoupling activity of this hormone, since glucose was able to reduce the blocking effect by 50% (DIAMANT and UVNÄS, 1961).

9. Interaction with acidic cell components

Several authors have demonstrated the formation of salts or complexes between basic histamine liberators and biologically occurring acidic compounds like heparin (MOTA et al., 1953; GERENDÁS et al., 1948; PARROT and LABORDE, 1951; AMANN and WERLE, 1956; JAQUES and KÜTTNER, 1961), organic phosphates (DARLOW, 1955), strandin (HARRIS et al., 1961), and nucleic acids (PATON, 1956). Histamine itself is also able to combine with heparin, and the "histamine-heparinates" thus formed can be decomposed by compounds like 48/80, basic proteins (protamine, clupein, salmine) and other basic histamine liberators (AMANN and WERLE, 1956). This reaction, in which histamine is set free by ion-exchange, has been proposed as a model for the action of histamine releasers on tissues (PATON, 1956; SMITH, 1958 b; KÜTTNER et al. 1961). Results showing that heparin as well as histamine are found in the same subcellular granular fraction isolated, either from subcutaneous rat tissue (KÖKSAL, 1953) or from murine mastocytomas (HAGEN et al. 1959), have been cited as additional evidence in favour of this view. The most serious objection to this simple but attractive mechanism has been raised by MACINTOSH (1956), who has pointed out that observations of PATON (1951) and FELDBERG and PATON (1951), showed that one molecule or rather, one basic unit of compound 48/80, could release up to 100 molecules of histamine from the perfused cat skin. Another objection to the ion-exchange theory of histamine release is the dependence of the action of 48/80, in the rat and cat, on cell metabolism whose functioning would presumably not be a requisite for a simple displacement reaction between two bases.

Another aspect of the interaction of basic releasers with acidic cell components has been investigated by HIGGINBOTHAM (1958); he has shown that some of these compounds react with heparin or heparinlike tissular components to form insoluble complexes (see chapter III, section G.), which are apparently taken up by fibroblasts, where, after a period of storage, they are gradually digested by micellophagosis. This process may play a role in the local detoxification of endogenous or exogenous basic compounds (HIGGINBOTHAM and DOUGHERTY, 1956), and could also explain the refractoriness towards the effects of basic histamine liberators *in vivo*, which sets in much before the histamine stores of the tissues are exhausted (PATON, 1957).

10. Effects on subcellular particles

Much, but by no means all, of the histamine of the animal body is located in the mast cells of connective tissue (GRAHAM et al. 1955; MOTA et al., 1956; CASS and MARSHALL, 1962), where it is bound to the metachromatic granules found in the cytoplasm of this cell (MOTA et al. 1954; SMITH and LEWIS, 1957; HAGEN et al. 1959). The question as to whether histamine release is the consequence of processes taking place within the histamine-enclosing granule or in the cellular cytoplasm, has been studied by comparing the response to histamine releasers, of the intact mast cell with that of its isolated, subcellular granules. GROSSBERG and GARCIA-AROCHA (1954) isolated such granules from whole dog liver homogenates as well as from sheep liver capsular tissue, and showed that histamine release by several basic compounds had the same features, e.g. temperature, pH and concentration dependence, which characterize this process in the intact cell. MONGAR and SCHILD (1956), isolated the mitochondrial fraction of guinea pig lung homogenates and showed that it contained the largest portion of the histamine of the tissue. Both octylamine and compound 48/80 were able to release histamine from such particles at approximately the same levels of concentration at which these agents act on whole tissue; however, the time course of the release was found to be more rapid in the mitochondrial fraction. It was also observed that octylamine and compound 48/80 were at least 10 times more active on particles suspended in a Tyrode, rather than in a sucrose medium; this may have been due to the low pH of the sucrose medium, and is an indication that some of the requisites for the action of chemical releasers on whole tissue have to be fulfilled for their full activity at the subcellular level. As discussed previously, the action of compound 48/80 on guinea pig lung tissue does not seem to require metabolic activity by the tissue (MONGAR and SCHILD, 1957 a) and, although the temperature dependence of this process has been demonstrated, (Figure 5), its enzymatic nature has not been proven. This contrasts with the action of 48/80 and of antigen on rat and cat tissues in which histamine release is definitely linked to cellular metabolic processes. More detailed studies about the effects of compound 48/80 on subcellular fractions from rat or cat tissues may therefore reveal whether the enzymatic character of its action is concerned with active membrane transport of the releaser into the mast cell, or the functioning of specific enzymatic mechanisms of the metachromatic granules. The results of histochemical studies concerning the enzymatic activity of this material have been summarized by RILEY (1959), who has stated that "the mast cell granule is more than a mere chemical polymerization of heparin, or even of heparin and histamine: it is a metabolically active organelle which responds to changes in its environment as an intracellular osmometer, and acting in this way, is capable of liberating its content."

11. Structure-activity relationships

The vast majority of histamine releasing substances whose action occurs independently of immunological mechanisms are basic compounds. As shown in Table 1, the basic groupings responsible for this activity are found in aliphatic

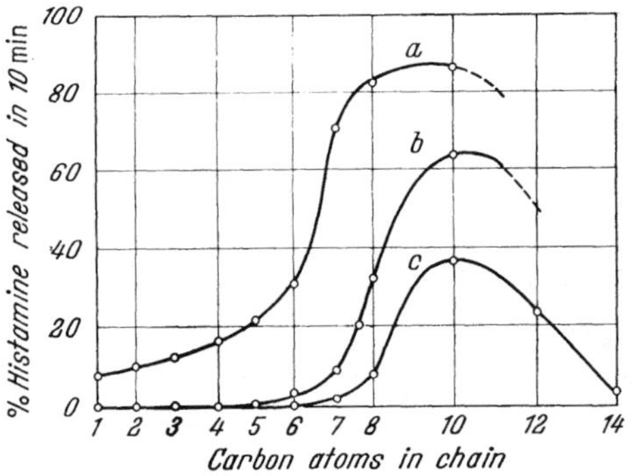

Fig. 9. Effect of chain length on histamine release from minced guinea-pig lung by equimolar solution of mono amines $C_nH_{2n+1}NH_2 \cdot HCl$: a) 10^{-2} M; b) 10^{-3}M; c) 5×10^{-4}M. (According to MONGAR and SCHILD, 1953)

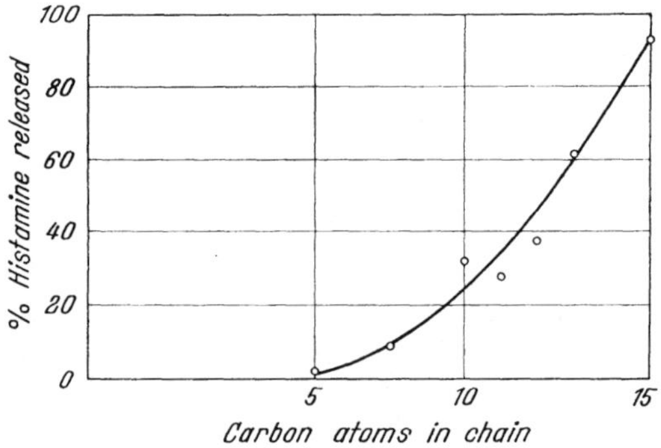

Fig. 10. Histamine release from minced guinea-pig lung by 1 mM solutions of straight-chain aliphatic diamines of various chain lengths. The amount released in 15 min is expressed as % of the total tissue histamine. (According to MONGAR, 1957)

amines, amides, amidines, guanidines, thio-ureas, as well as in a large number of heterocyclic compounds containing nitrogen. Basicity *per se* however, is not a sufficient property for histamine releasing activity: other structural characteristics are needed. To illustrate this, results showing that discrete structural alterations can lead to considerable changes in histamine releasing activity, are shown below.

MONGAR and SCHILD (1953) and MONGAR (1957) have studied the effect of chain length in monoamines and diamines acting on minced guinea pig lung. Their results (Figure 9 and 10), indicate that while in the diamine series, histamine release increases steadily with increasing chain length, monoamines have optimal activity at C_{10} but become less active with increasing numbers of carbon atoms.

MCINTIRE et al. (1951), have used straight chain aliphatic amines as histamine releasing agents from rabbit whole blood *in vitro*. They found a similar relationship as that shown in Figures 9 and 10, although maximal activity was only reached at considerably higher chain lengths, e.g. with octadecylamine.

The effect of increasing substitution of the hydrogen atoms of the amino groups of amines by alkyl radicals has been investigated by MCINTIRE et al. (1951), using N-methyl substituted derivatives of octadecylamine. They found that the primary amine was a highly active histamine releasing agent, the secondary amine had considerably less activity, while the tertiary and quaternary amines were entirely inactive. The relatively greater releasing activity of secondary over tertiary amines also becomes apparent when compound 48/80 (a secondary amine), and its N-methylated analogue, compound M-96 (BALTZLY et al. 1949), are compared. As shown in Table 5, at the 5.0 μg/ml level, the tertiary amine was one half as active, while at a lower level (0.5 μg/ml), this difference was even greater.

MCINTIRE et al. (1951), have compared the activities of the three β-substituted pyridinium compounds depicted below; they found that the carbo-methoxy

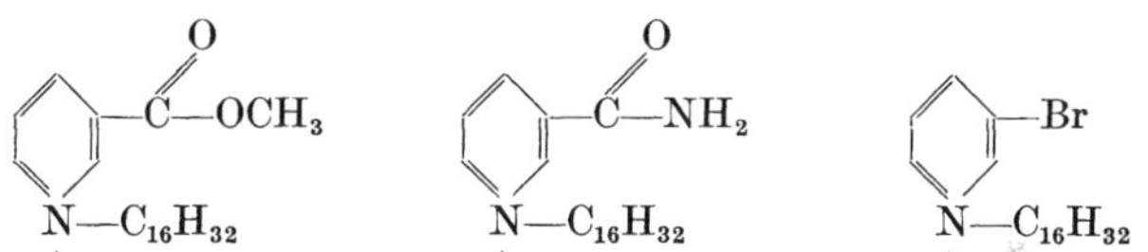

(I) (II) (III)

derivative (I) had by far the greatest activity, the carboamine (II) and halogen (III) substituted compounds being almost inactive.

The comparison of the histamine releasing properties of two closely related opium alkaloids, morphine (IV) and codeine (V) (MCINTIRE et al. 1951), has shown that the methylation of the phenolic group of morphine results in a decrease in histamine releasing activity.

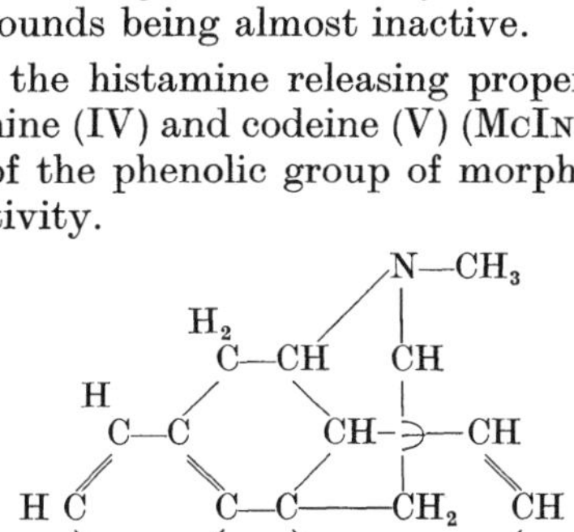

IV R = H: morphine

V R = CH_3: codeine

The substitution of the phenolic hydroxyl groups of catecholamines by chlorine atoms has been shown (ROTHSCHILD, 1962 a) to result in a marked increase in histamine releasing activity. This effect has been studied in the mast cells of the peritoneal fluid of rats, and is shown in Table 6, where it can also be seen that changes in the substituents of the nitrogen atom do not lead to histamine releasing

Table 5. *Activities of 48/80 and related compounds on the release of histamine from the peritoneal fluid mast cells of the rat*

Compound	Formula	Dose μg/ml	Per cent histamine retained[1]
48/80[2]	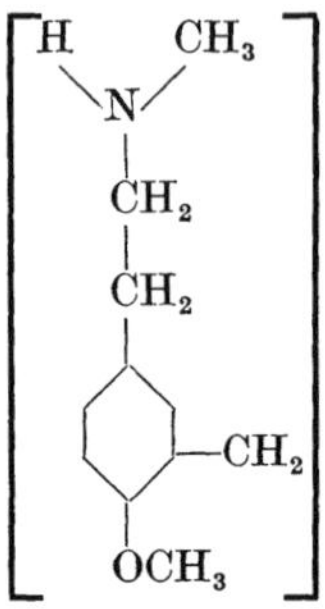 3 or 4	0.5	21
		5.0	15
46/108[2]	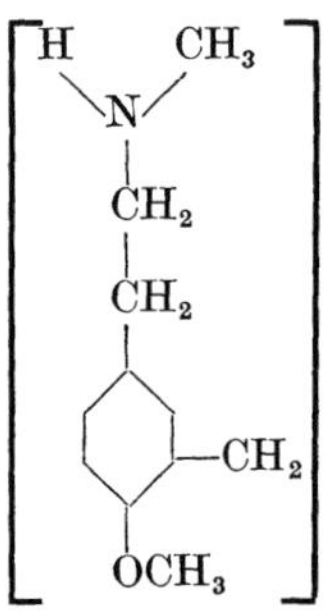 2	5.0	64
		25.0	54
		100.0	51
M-96[2]	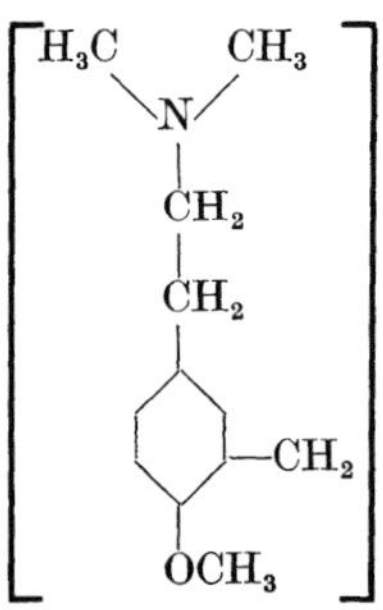 3 or 4	0.5	79
		5.0	57
		25.0	14
		100.0	15
M-92[2]	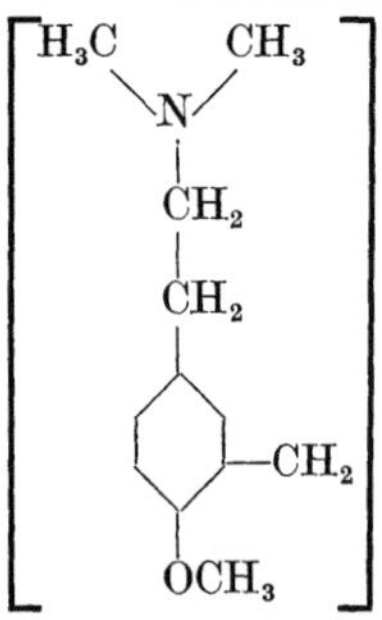 2	5.0	82
		25.0	49
		100.0	30

[1] Following 15 minute incubation at 37° C in Krebs-Ringer phosphate buffer (0.1% glucose). Each result is the average of three determinations.

[2] Gently supplied by Dr. R. Baltzly, The Wellcome Research Laboratories, Tuckahoe 7, New York.

activity; in contrast, the replacement of the phenolic hydroxyl groups by chlorine atoms produced compounds of comparatively strong histamine releasing capacity.

The effect of the degree of polymerization on the histamine releasing activity of polymers of p-methoxyphenethyl methylamine and formol (compounds 48/80 and 46/108, BALTZLY et al. 1949), has been examined by ROTHSCHILD (1962). Table 5 shows that compound 46/108 (a dimer), was considerably less active a releaser than compound 48/80 (a mixture of higher polymerization products). A similar relationship prevails for the relative activities of compounds M-92 and M-96 (BALTZLY et al. 1949), respectively a dimeric and a higher polymeric condensation product of formaldehyde and p-methoxyphenethyl dimethyl amine. These results confirm observations on the relative potency of these compounds in producing the delayed depressor response in dogs (BALTZLY et al. 1949 and BALTZLY, 1962, personal communication).

Table 6. *Effect of catecholamines and their ring chloro-analogs on the in-vitro release of histamine from cells of rat peritoneal fluid. Figures within parentheses refer to the number of experiments performed* (According to ROTHSCHILD, 1962a)

Amine	Histamine retained (%) Mean ± s.e.
Epinephrine, 10 mM	100 ± 0 (3)
Epinephrine, 3 mM	109 ± 11 (4)
Dichloroepinephrine, 3 mM	8 ± 2 (4)
Dichloroepinephrine, 1 mM	107 ± 12 (3)
Arterenol, 10 mM	90 ± 27 (3)
Arterenol, 3 mM	89 ± 8 (5)
Dichloroarterenol, 3 mM	10 ± 5 (4)
Dichloroarterenol, 1 mM	77 ± 15 (3)
Isoproterenol, 10 mM	93 ± 13 (2)
Isoproterenol, 3 mM	94 ± 16 (3)
Dichloroisoproterenol, 3 mM	3 ± 2 (4)
Dichloroisoproterenol, 1 mM	101 ± 12 (3)

V. Effects of basic histamine releasers other than the release of histamine

An examination of the pharmacological properties of the compounds listed in Table 1, will reveal that histamine releasing capacity is found among compounds having the most diverse major pharmacological activities. The discussion of such effects would overstep the scope of this sub-chapter; however, certain features of the pharmacodynamic activity of basic compounds, apparently related to histamine release, will be considered.

1. Morphological alterations of mast cells

The loss of cytoplasmic metachromatic granules of the mast cells exposed to basic histamine releasers, has been demonstrated both *in vivo* and *in vitro*. Such effects, which in the rat are indistinguishable from the morphological alterations induced by antigen on the mast cells of sensitized tissue, are described in Chapter 3, Section F of this book. According to UVNÄS (1961), histamine release by basic compounds is invariably accompanied by such morphological alterations; this view however, is not shared by SMITH (1958 a), who has presented evidence that the intraperitoneal administration of toluidine blue or protamine sulfate to rats leads to a copious release of histamine into the peritoneal cavity, but to no concomitant alterations of mesentery mast cell morphology. This result seems to be restricted to a few compounds only, since the histamine releasing action of compound 48/80, d-tubocurarine or stilbamidine was invariably accompanied by widespread mast cell degranulation (SMITH, 1958 a). MACALUSO et al. (1961) have presented observations which they interpret as an indication that treatment with histamine liberators does not lead to degranulation, but rather to the partial loss of the metachromatic staining capacity of the mast cells of the rat. According to these authors, pre-treatment with compound 48/80, protamine or lysozyme, inhibits the metachromatic staining of mesentery mast cell granules when low concentrations (0.01 %) of dye (toluidine blue), are used. In contrast to the sensitivity of untreated cells, which are fully stained at 0.01 % dye, the stain only appears in the treated specimens when 1 % toluidine blue is employed. Such conclusions are in direct contradiction to the results of MOTA et al. (1953), RILEY (1959), and others, which clearly show the typical picture of metachromatically stained granules, scattered around 48/80 or stilbamidine-treated rat mesentery mast cells. Mast cell degranulation and histamine release are therefore generally regarded as associated processes (UVNÄS, 1961). Yet, it should be noted, that according to SMITH (1958 b), "extensive disruption of mast cells leading to death does satisfy the requirements for the concept that these cells play a major and continuous role in meeting the organism's requirements for histamine, heparin and 5-hydroxytryptamine." It may well be that the extensive degranulation observed following 48/80 action on rat mast cells, represents an exaggeration of a process which, while not microscopically apparent under physiological conditions, follows a qualitatively similar mechanism. Support for this assumption is brought forth by observations showing that in the rat, mast cell degranulation as well as histamine release are processes with similar requirements for metabolic activity (UVNÄS, 1961; ROTHSCHILD et al. 1961).

Relativelly few observations about the effects of basic histamine releasers on mast cells of species other than the rat have been reported. MOTA (1959), has shown that in the guinea pig mesentery, histamine release by octylamine is not accompanied by the extrusion of mast cell granules; rather, a loss of the contours of the intracellular metachromatic granular material occurs ("fusion"). It seems to us that this could be indicative of an osmotic swelling of the granule, similar to that described in rat mesentery mast cells exposed to toluidine blue (SMITH, 1958 b). WEST (1958), and PARRATT and WEST (1957 a, b), have compared the *in vivo* effects of compounds L-1935, 48/80 and polymyxin B on mast cell alterations and histamine release in rat, hamster and mouse. Their results indicate that while all three compounds were relatively active histamine releasers in the mouse and the hamster, they induced only discrete and patchy morphological alterations of the subcutaneous tissue mast cell of these species. This contrasted with the widespread degranulation and marked histamine release induced by much smaller doses of compounds 48/80 and L-1935 in the mast cells of the rat (see Table 1).

2. Release of heparin

An increased coagulation time, probably due to the release of heparin, has been reported in the blood of dogs (PATON, 1951), but not of rats (MOTA et al. 1953), injected with basic histamine liberators. In commenting about these differences, MOTA et al. (1953) point out the difficulty met with in the histologic fixation of the dog mast cell as compared with that of the rat mast cell; this may indicate a looser binding of heparin to its intracellular anchoring sites in the former species. The absence of free heparin in the blood of 48/80 treated rats could however, also be due to its release in a bound, inactive form, e.g. as a component of insoluble particle debris which, by being disposed off locally by macrophages and fibroblasts, would prevent the access of heparin to the circulation (RILEY, 1959; HIGGINBOTHAM and DOUGHERTY, 1956).

3. Release of 5-hydroxytryptamine (serotonin)

The concomitant release of histamine and 5-hydroxytryptamine is a characteristic feature of the action of compound 48/80 (PARRATT and WEST, 1957 b), and of compound L-1935 (HALPERN et al. 1957, 1959) in the rat. In contrast, polymyxin B, although a powerful releaser of histamine in this species, will not liberate 5-hydroxytryptamine (PARRATT and WEST, 1957 b). An opposite effect has been demonstrated for reserpine; this alkaloid, while being a powerful "depleter" of tissue serotonin (BRODIE et al. 1955; BHATTACHARYA and LEWIS, 1956), has only a very slight direct histamine releasing action in the rat (PARRATT and WEST, 1957 b).

A histamine releasing effect of reserpine in the rabbit has been described *in vivo*, but not *in vitro* (BURKHALTER et al. 1960); it is probable that this action is mediated by serotonin, since reserpine is an effective releaser of this amine from platelets, and serotonin in turn, has been shown by FELDBERG and SMITH (1953), to liberate histamine from animal tissues.

4. Release of slow reacting substances

PATON (1951), demonstrated the release of a substance, active on smooth muscle, which could be clearly differentiated from histamine, in the plasma of cats and dogs injected with compound 48/80. Recent studies (CHAKRAVARTY et al. 1959; CHAKRAVARTY, 1960), have brought additional information about the mechanism of release and the probable chemical nature of this principle, termed SRS = slow reacting substance. Thus, the perfusion of the isolated cat's paw with 1—10 micrograms of compound 48/80 led to the release of SRS, evidenced by its action on the atropine and mepyramine-treated guinea-pig ileum, on which it produced a slowly-developing and long-lasting contraction not unlike that evoked by bradykinin. Chemical tests have, however permitted the clearcut differentiation of SRS from both bradykinin and substance P. It seems to be a lipoidical substance, possibly a fatty acid derivative, similar but not identical to the "Darmstoff" described by VOGT (1957). Unlike histamine, SRS is not present in the untreated mast cell but rather, arises as a consequence of an enzymatic process which can be initiated either by 48/80 or by antigen acting on sensitized tissue (CHAKRAVARTY, 1960).

5. The pharmacology of compound 48/80

A brief survey of certain pharmacological properties of this compound is included in this discussion, not because they are a consequence of histamine release, but rather for the opposite reason, for pharmacological effects of 48/80 unconnected with histamine release are often encountered in experimental work with this compound. The first proof of such an effect was provided by DEWS et al. (1953), with the demonstration that the strong antagonistic action exerted by 48/80 on the contractile response of frog skeletal muscle to acetylcholine, could not be reproduced by high doses of histamine, and could therefore not be due to endogenous, released histamine. A direct ganglion-blocking action of compound 48/80 has been demonstrated by GERTNER (1955), using the perfused superior cervical ganglion of the cat. Analysis of this block showed that, while the release of acetylcholine from the pre-ganglionic endings was not interfered with, sensitivity of the ganglion cells to this mediator was significantly reduced. According to CHARLIER et al. (1954), compound L-1935, a potent histamine releasing butylamine derivative, has a similar ganglionic blocking activity, which apparently is due to direct competition with acetylcholine. SÖMJEN and

Uyldert (1955), have shown that 48/80 causes marked paralysis in rabbits and, under certain conditions, in rats as well. A direct action on the muscle was ruled out and a neuromuscular blocking action was postulated. The nature of this blockade remains unclear: in contrast to that of d-tubocurarine, it was not antagonized by choline esterase inhibitors so that it probably did not arise as a consequence of a competition with end-plate acetylcholine; a direct depolarizing action was also ruled out since no stimulating effect upon denervated rat muscle could be observed.

Mota and Vugman (1956), studied the effects of compound 48/80 in the guinea pig *in vivo*. They showed that the toxic action observed could not be attributed to histamine release or mast cell alterations, which were entirely absent at the dosage levels employed. Treated animals displayed spasmodic contractions of the extremities and respiratory failure and died within 2 to 3 minutes; in contrast to the picture shown after death by histamine, collapsed lungs were found at necropsy. In the rabbit, an animal whose histamine depots are also rather resistant to release by compound 48/80, the intravenous injection of 2.25 mg/kg elicited a severe respiratory depression followed by a marked fall of blood pressure (Papacostas and Loew, 1959). The later could be shown to be due, not to a direct effect of 48/80, but rather to a reflex reaction to the respiratory failure. Here again, lethal doses of histamine produced effects which could be clearly differentiated from those induced by compound 48/80.

A condition of motor excitement, termed "delirium ambulatorium," in mice receiving an intraventricular injection of 48/80 has been described (Rocha e Silva, 1959). Intracerebral injections of histamine or 5-hydroxytryptamine failed to reproduce these effects; they were not reduced but rather potentiated by anti-histaminics possessing the phenothiazine nucleus. Pentobarbital readily abolished this action of 48/80, but atropine enhanced it to a marked extent. The effect of atropine has been further studied by Carmo and Dias da Silva (1962), who showed that the alkaloid was able to induce a condition of motor excitement similar to that caused by 48/80. The effects of both substances were of a tachyphylactic nature and crossed desensitization was obtained. According to Rocha e Silva (1959), 48/80 may exert its central effects by provoking the release of catecholamines from brain depots. This release could possibly be due to an indirect effect of 48/80, involving a primary release of histamine which could, in turn, liberate the catecholamines.

Toxicity studies by Papacostas et al. (1959), have shown that in contrast to wide variations in the susceptibility of different species to histamine and anaphylaxis, the differences in the intravenous LD_{50} of 48/80 in the mouse, rat, guinea pig and rabbit respectively, are quite small. The outstanding feature of the toxicity observed in all species tested was a severe depression of the respiration with ensuing gasping, convulsions, prostration and death. Thus, the primary toxic action of compound 48/80 even in the rat, in which it has such outstanding histamine releasing effects, is apparently unrelated to the liberation of the amine. This is an almost paradoxical situation for no other single compound has been more intensively studied in the past by those interested in the investigation of the mechanism of histamine release. These efforts have certainly resulted in a better understanding of the process of histamine release by basic compounds. Whether they have also been an important aid towards the elucidation of the mechanism of histamine release in anaphylaxis and allergy, will only become clear when all the facets of these processes are known. It is unquestionable however, that compound 48/80 is the most typical and most powerful of the "chemical" basic histamine releasers, and as such deserves its position of importance as a pharmacological prototype.

References

ALAM, M., G. V. ANREP, G. S. BARSOUM, M. TALAAT, and E. WIENINGER: Liberation of histamine from skeletal muscle by curare. J. Physiol. (Lond.) **95**, 148 (1939).

AMANN, R., u. E. WERLE: Über Komplexe von Heparin mit Histamin und anderen Di- und Polyaminen. Klin. Wschr. **34**, 207 (1956).

ARCHER, G. T.: Release of histamine from mast cells by tissue extracts. Nature (Lond.) **182**, 727 (1958).

ARUNLAKSHANA, O.: Histamine release by antihistaminics. J. Physiol. (Lond.) **119**, 47 P (1953).

ARVY, L.: Action de doses répétés d'un dérivé de la méthylamine sur la richesse du tissu conjonctif et des ganglions lymphatiques en labrocytes chez le rat. C. R. Soc. Biol. (Paris) **150**, 2071 (1956).

— B. N. HALPERN et T. NEVEU: Modifications morphologiques de labrocytes et corrélations avec la mise en liberté de l'histamine endogène après injection d'une butylamine substitutive (1935 L) donnée de propriétés histamino-libératrices chez le rat. C. R. Soc. Biol. (Paris) **150**, 2074 (1956).

BALTZLY, R., J. S. BUCK, E. J. DE BEER, and F. A. WEBB: A family of long-acting depressors. J. Amer. chem. Soc. **71**, 1301 (1949).

BARNES, J.: Toxic reactions to meprobamate. J. Irish med. Ass. **41**, 119 (1957).

BEAUJEAN, M., et J. LECOMTE: Sur l'activité histamino-libératrice du polybrène. C. R. Soc. Biol. (Paris) **154**, 437 (1960).

BERALDO, W. T.: Formation of bradykinin in anaphylactic and peptone shock. Amer. J. Physiol. **163**, 283 (1950).

BERNSTEIN, I. L., and S. M. FEINBERG: Liberation of histamine from human skin. Effect of an anti-histamine and hydrocortisone on the activity of the histamine liberator, compound 48/80. J. Allergy **27**, 231 (1956).

BHATTACHARYA, B. K., and G. P. LEWIS: The release of 5-hydroxytryptamine by histamine liberators. Brit. J. Pharmacol. **11**, 202 (1956a).

— — The effects of reserpine and compound 48/80 on the release of amines from the mast cells of rats. Brit. J. Pharmacol. **11**, 411 (1956b).

BIGNAMI, G.: Pharmacological studies about a new derivative possessing histamine-releasing action, the sebacic diamide of 4-phenyl-4-amino ethyl-N-methylpiperidine (1665 I.S.). Farmaco **17**, 24 (1962).

BINET, L., et D. QUIVY: Libération d'héparine dans le chien traité par l'alkaloïde sinoménine. C. R. Acad. Sci. (Paris) **244**, 1579 (1957).

— — Sur la libération d'histamine déterminée chez le rat par l'injection locale de 5-hydroxytryptamine dans diverses conditions expérimentales. C. R. Acad. Sci. (Paris) **247**, 75 (1958).

BODMAN, R. I.: Evaluation of two synthetic curarizing agents in conscious volunteers. Brit. J. Pharmacol. **7**, 409 (1952).

BONIN, A., et G. JASMIN: Dosage de l'histamine chez le rat traité au 48/80. Rev. canad. Biol. **18**, 53 (1959).

BOREUS, L. O.: A comparison of mast cell reactions in rat, hamster and guinea pig. Acta physiol, scand. **49**, 251 (1960).

BOSEILA, A. W., and G. ASBOE-HANSEN: Influence of compound 48/80, protamine and other substances on rabbit basophils in vitro. Proc. Soc. exp. Biol. (N. Y.) **101**, 198 (1959).

BOYD, J. F., and A. N. SMITH: The effect of histamine and a histamine-releasing agent (compound 48/80) on wound healing. J. Path. Bact. **78**, 379 (1959).

— — The effect of compound 48/80 on the autograft and homograft reaction. Brit. J. exp. Path. **41**, 259 (1960).

BRAUNSTEINER, H. VON, E. MITSOTAKIS u. N. THUMB: Über die Wirkung von Diamino-decan auf Mastzellen und basophile Leucozyten. Blut **3**, 255 (1957).

BROCKLEHURST, W. E., J. H. HUMPHREY, and W. L. M. PERRY: The role of histamine in cutaneus antigen-antibody reaction in the rat. J. Physiol. (Lond.) **129**, 205 (1955).

BRODIE, B. B., A. PLETSCHER, and P. A. SHORE: Evidence that serotonin has a role in brain function. Science **122**, 968 (1955).

BURKHALTER, A., V. H. COHN JR., and P. A. SHORE: Effect of reserpine, serotonin and 5-hydroxyptamine on rabbit platelet histamine in vivo and in vitro. Biochem. Pharmacol. **3**, 328 (1960).

BURSTEIN, M., et J. L. PARROT: Elévation de l'histaminémie chez le chien à la suite de l'injection d'une forte dose d'atropine. C. R. Soc. Biol. (Paris) **143**, 251 (1949).

BUSHBY, S. R. M., and A. F. GREEN: The release of histamine by polymyxin B and polymyxyn E. Brit. J. Pharmacol. **10**, 215 (1955).

BUTLER, E. B.: Case of hypersensitivity to pethidine in woman in labour. Brit. med. J. **1951 II**, 715.

CAHEN, R., et S. AUBRON: Effet histaminogène de la morpholinéthyl morphine. C. R. Acad. Sci. (Paris) **251**, 3111 (1960).

CARMO, R. J., and W. DIAS DA SILVA: Effect of the intracerebral injection of compound 48/80 in the rat. Study of its mechanism of action. Ciência e Cultura **14**, 241 (1962).

CARVALHO, P., A. P. CORRADO, A. M. ROTHSCHILD, and O. VITAL BRAZIL: Unpublished results (1962).

CASS, R., and P. B. MARSHALL: Effect of adrenocortical hormones on tissue histamine and 5-hydroxytryptamine. Arch. int. Pharmacodyn. **136**, 311 (1962).

CHAKRAVARTY, N.: The mechanism of histamine release in anaphylactic reaction in guinea pig and rat. Acta physiol. scand. **48**, 146 (1960).

CHAKRAVARTY, N. R., B. HÖGBERG, and B. UVNÄS: Mechanism of the release by compound 48/80 of histamine and of a lipid soluble smooth muscle stimulating principle ("SRS"). Acta physiol. scand. **45**, 255 (1959).

CHARLIER, R., M. J. DALLEMAGNE et E. PHILIPPOT: Propriétés hypotensives d'une butyl amine substituée. Arch. int. Pharmacodyn. **100**, 127 (1954).

CHEYMOL, J., J. THUILLIER, and P. MOUILLÉ: So-called histaminogenic effects of natural and synthetic curares. Ann. pharm. franç. **9**, 705 (1951).

CODE, C. F., D. T. CODY, M. HURN, J. C. KENNEDY, and M. J. STRICKLAND: The simultaneous release of histamine and a histamine-destroying factor during anaphylaxis in rats. J. Physiol. (Lond.) **156**, 207 (1961).

COLLIER, H. O. J.: Release of histamine-clinical considerations. Ciba Found. Symp. on Histamine, p. 155. London: Churchill 1956.

—, and B. MACAULEY: The pharmacological properties of "Laudolissin", a long acting curarizing agent. Brit. J. Pharmacol. **7**, 398 (1952).

COMROE, J. H., and R. D. DRIPPS: The histamine like actions of curare and tubocurarine injected intracutaneously and intraarterially in man. Anesthesiology **7**, 260 (1946).

COPPOLA, J. A., and J. R. DIPALMA: Histamine as a factor in tolerance to levarterenol. Amer. J. Physiol. **202**, 114 (1962).

CZARNECKI, E., J. KIERSZ et E. MIETKIEWSKI: Changements survenues dans le sang à la suite du choc consécutif aux injections de colorants. Int. Arch. Allergy **1**, 285, 292 (1950).

DALE, H. H.: Antihistamine substances. Brit. med. J. **1948 II**, 281.

DANON, A. P., and H. MOUSSATCHÉ: Influence of anabolic glycolysis on release of histamine in the guinea pig and rat anaphylactic reaction in vitro. Nature (Lond.) **192**, 361 (1961).

DARLOW, G.: Reaction between histamine liberators and phosphates. J. Physiol. (Lond.) **131**, 13 P (1955).

DEWS, P. B., A. L. WNUCK, R. V. FANELLI, A. E. LIGHT, J. A. TALLABEN, S. NORTON, C. H. ELLIS, and E. J. DE BEER: The pharmacology of n° 48/80, a long-acting vaso depressor drug. J. Pharmacol. exp. Ther. **107**, 1 (1953).

DIAMANT, B., and B. UVNÄS: Evidence for energy requiring processes in histamine release and mast cell degranulation in rat tissues induced by compound 48/80. Acta physiol. scand. **53**, 315 (1961).

DIAS DA SILVA, W., A. D. L. FERNANDES, and W. T. BERALDO: Release of histamine by dextran and its inhibition by carbohydrates and inhibitors of anaphylaxis. Ciência e Cultura **14**, 239 (1962).

EICHLER, O., u. F. BARFUSS: Histamingehalt im Blut bei Infusion von Adrenalin und Histamin. Naunyn-Schmiedeberg's Arch. exp. Path. Pharmak. **195**, 245 (1940).

—, u. G. SPEDA: Histamin im Plasma und Atmung. Naunyn-Schmiedeberg's Arch. exp. Path. Pharmak. **195**, 153 (1940).

ELDRIDGE, E., and W. D. M. PATON: The release of histamine from cat's isolated perfused skin by amino-acids. J. Physiol. (Lond.) **124**, 27 P (1954).

ELLIS, C. H., A. VAN HARREVELD, and F. J. WOLFGRAM: A study of the hemodynamic actions of histamine and 1,10-diaminodecane in cats. Arch. int. Pharmacodyn. **97**, 287 (1954).

EVANS, A. G. J., P. A. NASMYTH, and H. C. STEWART: The fall of blood pressure caused by intravenous morphine in rat and cat. Brit. J. Pharmacol. **7**, 542 (1952).

FAWCETT, D. W.: Cytological and pharmacological observations on the release of histamine by mast cells. J. exp. Med. **100**, 217 (1954).

FEINBERG, S. M., A. R. FEINBERG, J. REBHUN, and S. MALKIEL: Liberation and depletion of histamine from human skin. Comparison of effects of specific antigens and a new histamine liberator, compound 48/80. Quart. Bull. Northw. Univ. med. Sch. **28**, 246 (1954).

—, and L. A. STERNBERGER: Action of histamine liberator compound 48/80 in the guinea pig. J. Allergy **26**, 170 (1955).

FELDBERG, W., and P. GREENGAARD: Release of histamine from the perfused sciatic nerve by 48/80. J. Physiol. (Lond.) **133**, 63 P (1956).
—, and B. HOLMES: The effect of muscular contraction and of curarine on acid gastric secretion in cats. J. Physiol. (Lond.) **99**, 3 P (1941).
—, and J. LECOMTE: Release of histamine by a substituted butylamine (L. 1935): Comparison with compound 48/80. Brit. J. Pharmacol. **10**, 254 (1955).
—, and A. A. MILES: Regional variations of increased permeability of skin capillaries by a histamine liberator and their relation to the histamine content of the skin. J. Physiol. (Lond.) **120**,205 (1953).
—, and J. L. MONGAR: Comparison of histamine release by compound 48/80 and acetylcholine on perfused tissues. Brit. J. Pharmacol. **9**, 197 (1954).
—, and W. D. M. PATON: Release of histamine from skin and muscle in the cat by opium alkaloids and other histamine liberators. J. Physiol. (Lond.) **114**, 490 (1951).
—, and M. SCHACHTER: Histamine release by horse serum from skin of the sensitized dog and the nonsensitized cat. J. Physiol. (Lond.) **118**, 124 (1952).
—, and A. N. SMITH: Release of histamine by tryptamine and 5-hydroxytryptamine. Brit. J. Pharmacol. **8**, 406 (1953).
—, — The role of histamine release for the motor effects of histamine liberators on the guinea pig ileum preparation. J. Physiol. (Lond.) **124**, 219 (1954).
—, and J. TALESNIK: Reduction of tissue histamine by compound 48/80. J. Physiol. (Lond.) **120**, 550 (1953).
GARAN, R. S.: Histamin-Freisetzung in der Lunge durch Reizstoffbeatmung. Naunyn-Schmiedeberg's Arch. exp. Path. Pharmak. **188**, 250 (1938).
GARCIA-AROCHA, H., J. G. ASHWIN, and A. L. GROSSBERG: Release of histamine by protamine and polylysine. Abstr. Comm. XI. Int. Physiol. Congr. Montreal, p. 378 (1953).
GERENDÁS, M., I. CSEFKO, and M. D. F. UDVARDY: Histamine-Heparin-thrombin chain mechanism. Nature (Lond.) **162**, 257 (1948).
GERSHON, S., and F. H. SHAW: Morphine and histamine release. J. Pharm. Pharmacol. **10**, 22 (1958).
GERTNER, S. B.: The effect of compound 48/80 on ganglionic transmission. Brit. J. Pharmacol. **10**, 103 (1955).
GOODMAN, L. S., and A. GILMAN: The pharmacological basis of therapeutics. P. 616. New York: Macmillan 1955.
GOTH, A., W. L. NASH, M. NAGLER, and J. HOLMAN: Inhibitors of histamine release in experimental diabetes. Amer. J. Physiol. **191**, 25 (1957).
GRAHAM, H. T., O. H. LOWRY, N. WAHL, and M. K. PRIEBAT: Mast cells as sources of tissue histamine. J. exp. Med. **102**, 307 (1955).
GROB, D., J. L. LILIENTHAL JR., and A. M. HARVEY: On certain vascular effects of curare in man. The "histamine" reactions. Johns Hopk. Hosp. Bull. **80**, 299 (1947).
GROSSBERG, A. L., and H. GARCIA-AROCHA: Histamine liberation in vitro and mode of binding of histamine in tissues. Science **120**, 762 (1954).
HAGEN, P.: The intracellular distribution of histamine in dog's liver. Brit. J. Pharmacol. **9**, 100 (1954).
— R. J. BARRNETT, and F. L. LEE: Biochemical and electron microscopic study of particles isolated from mastocytoma cells. J. Pharmacol. exp. Ther. **126**, 91 (1959).
HALPERN, B. N.: Histamine release by long chain molecules. Ciba Found. Symposium on Histamine, p. 92. London: Churchill 1956.
— Substances histamino-libératrices et processus de libération de l'histamine endogène. Actualités pharmacol. **13**, 109 (1960).
— M. BRIOT, P. LIACOPOULOS, T. NEVEU et H. BRANELLEC: Propriétés histamino-libératrices d'une butylamine substituée (1935 L) chez le chien. C. R. Soc. Biol. (Paris) **150**, 1302 (1956).
— M. LIACOPOULOS-BRIOT, T. NEVEU et P. LIACOPOULOS: Propriétés histamino-libératrices d'une butylamine substituée, le 1935 L chez le rat. C. R. Soc. Biol. (Paris) **151**, 853 (1957).
— P. LIACOPOULOS et M. LIACOPOULOS-BRIOT: Recherches sur les substances exogènes et endogènes agissant sur la perméabilité capillaire et leurs antagonistes. Arch. int. pharmacodyn. **119**, 56 (1959a).
— T. NEVEU et A. BRANELLEC: Modalités de la libération d'histamine par diverses substances histamino-libératrices en hypothermie profonde. C. R. Soc. Biol. (Paris) **153**, 14 (1959b).
HARRIS, A. F., A. SAIFTER, and S. R. WEINTRAUB: Interaction of compound 48/80 and stilbamidine with Strandin. Proc. Soc. exp. Med. **107**, 35 (1961).
HIGGINBOTHAM, R. D.: Studies on the functional interrelationship of fibroblasts and ground substance imunopolysaccharides. Ann. N. Y. Acad. Sci. **73**, 186 (1958).
—, and T. F. DOUGHERTY: Fate of shed mast cell granules. Proc. Soc. exp. Biol. **92**, 256 (1956).
HÖGBERG, B., G. THUFVESSON, and B. UVNÄS: Histamine liberation produced in the perfused paw of the cat by 48/80 and extracts from jellyfish (Cynea capillata) and Eelworm (Ascaris Lumbricoides) from swine. Acta physiol. scand. **38**, 135 (1956).

Högberg, B., and B. Uvnäs: Fragmentation of mast cells by some phenothiazine derivates. Acta chem. scand. **11**, 1092 (1957).
— — Further observations on the disruption of rat mesentery mast cells caused by compound 48/80, antigen-antibody reaction, lecithinase A and decylamine. Acta physiol. scand. **48**, 133 (1960).
Humphrey, J. H., and R. Jaques: The release of histamine and 5-hydroxytryptamine (serotonin) from platelets by antigen-antibody reactions in vitro. J. Physiol. (Lond.) **128**, 9 (1955).
Irino, S.: Effect of histamine releasers and of anti-inflammatory drugs on the egg-white edema of rat's hind paws in relation to skin histamine. Acta Med. Okayama **12**, 93 (1958).
Jaques, R., u. K. Küttner: Selektive Farbstofferdrängung an biogenen Polyelektrolyten als Modell für die Liberation biogener Amine. Helv. physiol. pharmacol. Acta **19**, 335 (1961).
Jori, A., A. P. Bentivoglio, and S. Garattini: The mechanism of the local inflammatory reaction induced by compound 48/80 and dextran in rats. J. Pharm. Pharmacol. **13**, 617 (1961).
Junqueira, L. C. U., and B. Beiguelman: Studies on the in vitro action of compound 48/80, a formaldehyde condensation product on rat mast cells. Tex. Rep. Biol. Med. **13**, 69 (1953).
Kimura, E. T., P. R. Young, and D. M. Ebert: Further studies on hexadimethrine bromide (polybrene) — an antiheparin agent. Toxicol. appl. Pharmacol. **1**, 560 (1959).
Kirk, R., and A. J. Henry: Observations on the toxicity of stilbamidine. Ann. trop. Med. Parasit. **38**, 99 (1944).
Klotz, S. D., and C. Bernstein: Allergy to meprobamate with some observations regarding the tranquilizing drugs. Sth. med. J. (Bgham, Ala.) **50**, 1478 (1957).
Koch, J., and J. Szerb: Liberation of histamine by adrenaline from isolated lung. Arch. int. Pharmacodyn. **81**, 91 (1950).
Köksal, M.: Extraction of a heparin-like substance from mast cell granules in mouse connective tissues. Nature (Lond.) **172**, 733 (1953).
Kowalewski, K.: Effect of a histamine liberator and of serotonin on plasma pepsinogen in rats. Arch. int. Pharmacodyn. **129**, 71 (1960).
Küttner, K., H. Majer, G. Huber u. R. Jaques: Untersuchungen an Ionenaustauschmodellen zum Verständnis der Physiologie biogener Amine. Austauschversuche an einem Schwefelsäuregruppen tragenden Harz zum Verständnis von sogenannten Histamin-Liberationsvorgängen. Experientia (Basel) **17**, 371 (1961).
Lagunoff, D., and E. P. Benditt: Mast cell degranulation and histamine release observed in a new in vitro system. J. exp. Med. **112**, 571 (1960).
Lahiri, S. C., and W. E. Brocklehurst: Bradykinin and anaphylactic shock. Brit. J. Pharmacol. **17**, 5 (1961).
Landmesser, C. M.: Study of bronchoconstrictor and hypotensive actions of curarizing drugs. Anesthesiology **8**, 506 (1947).
Le Blanc, J.: Effect of chlorpromazine on number of mast cells and of certain formed elements of blood. Proc. Soc. exp. Biol. (N. Y.) **97**, 238 (1958).
Lecomte, J.: Libération d'histamine par certains dérivés d'acridine. C. R. Soc. Biol. (Paris) **149**, 1060 (1955a).
— Pouvoir histamino-libérateur de la chlorpromazine. C. R. Soc. Biol. (Paris) **149**, 1693 (1955b).
— Libération de l'histamine endogène chez l'homme. Arch. int. Pharmacodyn. **101**, 375 (1955c).
— Propriétés anti-histaminiques des dérivés décarboxylés de la cystéine (cystéamine et cystamine). Arch. int. Physiol. **63**, 291 (1955d).
— Endogenous histamine liberation in man. Ciba Foundation Symposium on Histamine, p. 173. London: Churchill 1956a.
— Déplétion en histamine et phénomène d'Arthus chez de lapin. Int. Arch. Allergy **8**, 343 (1956b).
— Liberation of endogenous histamine in man. J. Allergy **28**, 102 (1957).
—, et M. L. Beaumariage: Réactions anaphylactiques cutanées locales du Coq. C. R. Soc. Biol. (Paris) **151**, 1452 (1957).
—, et L. Borensztajn: Libération d'histamine et intradermoréaction tuberculinique chez l'homme. Acta allerg. (Kbh.) **6**, 89 (1953).
—, et P. Fischer: Sur la libération de l'histamine tissulaire provoquée par l'adrénochrome et ses dérivés. Arch. int. Physiol. Biochim. **65**, 396 (1957).
—, et J. M. Petit: Effets de l'histamine et des processus d'histamino-libération sur la fonction pulmonaire. Int. Arch. Allergy **17**, 10 (1960).
Leitch, J. L., and T. J. Haley: Effect of 48/80 and X-irradiation on urinary histamine in the rat. Fed. Proc. **14**, 363 (1955).
Lewis, T.: The blood vessels of the human skin and their responses. London: Shaw & Son, 1927.
Macaluso, M. P., A. Salerno, and A. Friscia: Researches on the so-called degranulation of mast cells produced by histamine liberators. Boll. Soc. ital. Biol. sper. **37**, 21 (1961).

MacIntosh, F. C.: Histamine and intracellular particles. Ciba Found. Symposium on Histamine p. 20. London: Churchill 1956.
—, and W. D. H. Paton: The liberation of histamine by certain organic bases. J. Physiol. (Lond.) **109**, 190 (1949).
Mahfouz, M.: Fate of tubo-curarine in the body. Brit. J. Pharmacol. **4**, 295 (1949).
Mayeda, H.: Release of histamine by sinomenine. Jap. J. med. Sci. IV. Pharmacol. **3**, 62 (1953).
McCubbin, J. W., and I. H. Page: Nature of the hypotensive action of a thiophanium derivative (Ro 2-2222) in dogs. J. Pharmacol. exp. Ther. **105**, 437 (1952).
McIlreath, F. J. jr.: Some evidence concerning the mode of binding of histamine. Canad. J. Biochem. **37**, 151 (1959).
McIntire, F. C.: Personal communication 1962.
— L. W. Roth, and M. Sproull: Histamine release in rabbit blood by simple molecules, inhibition and reaction rate studies. Amer. J. Physiol. **167**, 233 (1951).
Mélon, J., et J. Lecomte: Influence de la libération pharmacodynamique de l'histamine cutanée sur les réactions anaphylactiques locales de type immédiat. Acta allerg. (Kbh.) **12**, 245 (1958).
Miles, A. A., and E. M. Miles: Vascular reactions to histamine, histamine liberators and leukotaxine in the skin of guinea pigs. J. Physiol. (Lond.) **118**, 228 (1952).
Mitchell, R., P. J. Newman, D. MacGillivray, and B. B. Clark: Evaluation of histamine liberator activity illustrated by a thiophanium compound, Ro 2-2222. Fed. Proc. **10**, 325 (1951).
Mongar, J. L.: Measurement of histamine-releasing activity. Ciba Found. Symposium on Histamine, p. 74. London: Churchill 1956.
— Effect of chain length of aliphatic amines on histamine potentiation and release. Brit. J. Pharmacol. **12**, 140 (1957).
—, and H. O. Schild: A comparison of the effects of anaphylactic shock and of chemical histamine releasers. J. Physiol. (Lond.) **118**, 461 (1952).
— — Quantitative measurement of the histamine releasing activity of a series of monoalkyl amines using minced guinea pig lung. Brit. J. Pharmacol. **8**, 103 (1953).
— — Effect of antigen and organic bases on intra-cellular histamine in guinea pig lung. J. Physiol. (Lond.) **131**, 207 (1956).
— — Inhibition of the anaphylactic reaction. J. Physiol. (Lond.) **135**, 301 (1957a).
— — Effect of temperature on the anaphylactic reaction. J. Physiol. (Lond.) **135**, 320 (1957b).
— — The effect of calcium and pH on the anaphylactic reaction. J. Physiol. (Lond.) **140**, 272 (1958).
—, and R. F. Whelan: Histamine release by adrenaline and D-tubocurarine in the human. J. Physiol. (Lond.) **120**, 146 (1953).
Moran, N. C., G. P. Quinn, and W. M. Butler jr.: An analysis of the histamine-like actions of oxypanamine. J. Pharmacol. exp. Ther. **125**, 85 (1959).
Mota, I.: Effect of antigen and octylamine on mast cells and histamine content of sensitized guinea pig tissues. J. Physiol. (Lond.) **147**, 425 (1959).
— W. T. Beraldo, and L. C. U. Junqueira: Protamine-like property of compound 48/80 and stilbamidine and their action on mast cells. Proc. Soc. exp. Biol. (N. Y.) **83**, 455 (1953).
— — A. G. Ferri, and L. C. U. Junqueira: Intracellular distribution of histamine. Nature (Lond.) **174**, 698 (1954).
— — — — Action of 48/80 on the mast cell population and histamine content of the wall of the gastrointestinal tract of the rat. Ciba Found. Symposium on Histamine, p. 47. London: Churchill 1956b).
—, and W. Dias da Silva: The anti-anaphylactic and histamine releasing properties of the anti-histamines. Their effects on the mast cells. Brit. J. Pharmacol. **15**, 396 (1960).
— A. G. Ferri, and S. Yoneda: The distribution of mast cells in the digestive tract of laboratory animals; its bearing on the problem of the localization of histamine in tissues. Quart. J. micr. Sci. **97**, 251 (1956a).
—, and T. Ishii: Inhibition of mast cell disruption and histamine release in rat anaphylaxis in vitro. Comparison with compound 48/80. Brit. J. Pharmacol. **15**, 82 (1960).
—, and I. Vugman: Action of compound 48/80 on the mast cells and histamine content of guinea pig tissues. Brit. J. Pharmacol. **11**, 304 (1956).
Moulton, R., W. G. Spector, and D. A. Willoughby: Histamine release and pain production by xanthosine and related compounds. Brit. J. Pharmacol. **12**, 365 (1957).
Moussatché, H., and A. P. Danon: Influence of oxidative phosphorylation inhibitors on the histamine release in the anaphylactic reaction in vitro. Experientia (Basel) **14**, 414 (1958).
Nasmyth, P. A., and H. C. Stewart: The release of histamine by opium alkaloids. J. Physiol. (Lond.) **111**, 19 P (1950).
Nishiyama, R., K. Tasaka, and S. Irino: The sites of action of some histamine releasing substances in the dog. Acta Med. Okayama **11**, 133 (1957).

NITESCU, I. I., M. GRINSPAN, and M. CIRSTEA: Interaction of curare and anaphylactic shock in the dog. Stu. Genet. Fisiol. (Bucarest) **4**, 127 (1959).

NORTON, S.: Quantitative determination of mast cell fragmentation by compound 48/80. Brit. J. Pharmacol. **9**, 494 (1954).

—, and E. J. DEBEER: Effect of some antibiotics on rat mast cells in vitro. Arch. int. Pharmacodyn. **102**, 352 (1955).

OSLER, A. G., H. G. RANDALL, B. M. HILL, and Z. OVARY: The participation of complement in the formation of anaphylatoxin. J. exp. Med. **110**, 311 (1959).

PAPACOSTAS, C. A., and E. R. LOEW: Cardiovascular and respiratory effects of lethal doses of histamine and compound 48/80 in rabbits. Proc. Soc. exp. Biol. (N. Y.) **100**, 604 (1959).

— —, and G. B. WEST: Studies on the toxicology of a histamine liberator, compound 48/80. Arch. int. Pharmacodyn. **120**, 353 (1959).

PARRATT, J. R., and G. B. WEST: Histamine liberation in the hamster. Arch. int. Pharmacodyn. **113**, 209 (1957a).

— — Release of 5-hydroxytryptamine and histamine from tissues of the rat. J. Physiol. (Lond.) **137**, 179 (1957b).

PARROT, J. L., et C. LABORDE: Captation de l'histamine par l'héparine. C. R. Soc. Biol. (Paris) **145**, 1047 (1951).

PATON, W. D. M.: Compound 48/80, a potent histamine liberator. Brit. J. Pharmacol. **6**, 499 (1951).

— The mechanism of histamine release. Ciba Found. Symposium on Histamine, p. 59. London: Churchill 1956.

— Histamine release by compounds of simple chemical structure. Pharmacol. Rev. **9**, 269 (1957).

— The effects of muscle relaxants other than muscular relaxation. Anesthesiology **20**, 453 (1959).

—, and M. SCHACHTER: The influence of an anti-histamine drug on the release of histamine in the unanesthetized dog. Brit. J. Pharmacol. **6**, 509 (1951).

PAYNE, J. P.: Histamine release during controlled hypotension with arfonad. Proc. World Congr. Anesthesiology, p. 180 (1955).

PELLERAT, J., et M. MURAT: Action des anti-histaminiques de synthèse sur l'histaminémie. C. R. Soc. Biol. (Paris) **140**, 297 (1946).

QUASTEL, J. H., and A. H. WHEATLEY: The effects of amines on oxidations of the brain. Biochem. J. **27**, 1609 (1933).

RANDALL, L. O., W. G. PETERSON, and G. LEHMANN: The ganglionic blocking action of thiophanium derivatives. J. Pharmacol. exp. Ther. **97**, 48 (1949).

REID, G.: Liberation of histamine and heparin by tubocurarine and its circulatory effects in the dog. Aust. J. exp. Biol. med. Sci. **28**, 465 (1950).

REUSE, J. J.: Modifications circulatoires au cours du choc anaphylactique et après administration d'un libérateur d'histamine (composé 48/80). Arch. int. Pharmacodyn. **93**, 122 (1953).

RILEY, J. F.: The effects of histamine-liberators on the mast cells of the rat. J. Path. Bact. **65**, 471 (1953).

— The mast cells. Edinburgh and London: Livingstone 1959.

—, and G. B. WEST: Tissue mast cells. Studies with a histamine liberator of low toxicity (compound 48/80). J. Path. Bact. **69**, 269 (1955a).

— — Histamine liberation in the rat and mouse. Arch. int. Pharmacodyn. **102**, 304 (1955b).

ROCHA E SILVA, M.: Concerning the mechanism of anaphylactic and tryptic shock. J. Immunol. **40**, 399 (1941).

— Unexpected reactions in pharmacology. Thesis, São Paulo (1952).

— Central effects produced by injection of 48/80 into the cerebral ventricles of mice. Brit. J. Pharmacol. **14**, 243 (1959).

—, and A. M. ROTHSCHILD: Anaphylatoxin, histamine depletion and skin reactions in the rat. Nature (Lond.) **175**, 987 (1955).

— — Experimental design for bioassay of a material inducing strong tachyphylactic effect (anaphylatoxin). Brit. J. Pharmacol. **11**, 252 (1956).

—, and H. O. SCHILD: Release of histamine by D-tubocurarine from the isolated diaphragm of the rat. J. Physiol. (Lond.) **109**, 448 (1949).

ROTHSCHILD, A. M.: Effect of metabolic inhibitors on the release of histamine by anaphylatoxin and by antigen in vitro. Experientia (Basel) **17**, 555 (1961).

— Unpublished results (1962).

— Effect of catecholamines and their chloroanalogues on the in vitro release of histamine from rat peritoneal fluid cells. Biochem. Pharmacol. **11**, 979 (1962a).

—, and E. GARCIA LIMA: Effect of dinitrophenol and glucose on the release of histamine and of serotonin from rabbit platelets by anaphylatoxin in vitro: To be published (1962).

— I. VUGMAN, and M. ROCHA E SILVA: Metabolic studies on the release of histamine by compound 48/80 in the rat diaphragm. Biochem. Pharmacol. **7**, 248 (1961).

SALTER, W. T., and M. L. WHITE: Morphine sensitivity. Anesthesiology **10**, 553 (1949).
SCHACHTER, M.: The release of histamine by pethidine, atropine, quinine and other drugs. Brit. J. Pharmacol. **7**, 646 (1952).
— Anaphylaxis and histamine release in the rabbit. Brit. J. Pharmacol. **8**, 412 (1953).
SCHAYER, R. W., and R. L. SMILEY: Binding and release of radioactive histamine in intact rats. Amer. J. Physiol. **177**, 401 (1954).
— K. J. DAVIS, and R. L. SMILEY: Evaluation of histamine release in rats by analysis of urine. Amer. J. Physiol. **181**, 484 (1955).
— K. Y. WU, and R. L. SMILEY: Sources of urinary histamine in the rat. Amer. J. Physiol. **179**, 481 (1954).
SCHILD, H. O.: Release of histamine by ammonia. Nature (Lond.) **164**, 24 (1949).
—, and R. A. GREGORY: Liberation of histamine from striated muscle by curarine, strychnine and related substances. Abstr. Comm. XVII. Intern. Congr. Physiol. Oxford, p. 208 (1947).
SELYE, H.: Effect of ACTH and cortisone upon an anaphylactoid reaction. Canad. med. Ass. J. **61**, 553 (1949).
SHELESNYAK, M. C., et P. F. KRAICER: La pyrathiazine est un anti-histaminique capable de provoquer le déciduone utérin par libération d'histamine dans l'organisme. C. R. Acad. Sci. (Paris) **248**, 2126 (1959).
SICUTERI, F., and R. MONFARDINI: Protected histamine release in man, first therapeutical experiments with 48/80. Comm. III. Intern. Congr. Allergol. Paris (1958).
— M. RICCI et G. FRANCHI: Asthme provoquée dans le cobaye par des aérosols de l'histamino-libérateur, 48/80. Particularités symptomatologiques et histologiques. Comm. III. Intern. Congr. Allergol. Paris (1958).
— Biologia e chimica della liberazione di istamina. Edizioni La Settimana Medica, Firenze (1961).
— —, and E. ROMAGNOLI: Behaviour of pressure and pulse of cerebral fluid in man during release of histamine by compound 48/80. Acta allerg. (Kbh.) **15**, 222 (1960).
— L. SALVINI, G. FRANCHI, and S. VIOLA: Variations in the heparinemia and histaminemia during the action of the histamine releaser 48/80 in man. G. Clin. med. **60**, 1378 (1959).
SMITH, A. N.: The effect of compound 48/80 on gastric secretion in the cat. J. Physiol. (Lond.) **119**, 233 (1953a).
— Release of histamine by the histamine liberator compound 48/80 in cats. J. Physiol. (Lond.) **121**, 517 (1953b).
— The experimental production of gastric ulcers by histamine releasing substances. Brit. J. Surg. **46**, 157 (1958).
SMITH, D. E.: Nature of the secretory activity of the mast cell. Amer. J. Physiol. **193**, 573 (1958a).
— Dynamics of release of histamine from tissue mast cells. Science **128**, 207 (1958b).
— Influence of anti-histamine on mast cells disruption following X-irradiation. Proc. Soc. exp. Biol. (N. Y.) **97**, 872 (1958c).
—, and Y. S. LEWIS: Electron microscopy of the tissue mast cells. J. biophys. biochem. Cytol. **3**, 9 (1957).
SMITH, J. A., A. H. LIND, and R. I. RYZOFF: Production of bronchoconstriction by thiamine in guinea-pigs. Fed. Proc. **14**, 141 (1955).
SNIPER, W.: The estimation and comparison of histamine release by muscle relaxants in man. Brit. J. Anaesth. **24**, 232 (1952).
SOLLMANN, T.: A Manual of Pharmacology. London and Philadelphia: Saunders 1948.
—, and J. D. PILCHER: Endermic reactions. J. Pharmacol. exp. Therap. **9**, 309 (1917).
SÖMJÉN, G., and I. E. UYLDERT: The effect of compound 48/80 on mammalian skeletal muscle. Brit. J. Pharmacol. **10**, 413 (1955).
STAUB, H.: Die Adrenalin-Histaminregulation, gleichzeitig Beitrag zum Antistinmechanismus. Helv. physiol. pharmacol. Acta **4**, 539 (1946).
—, u. H. BAUER: Sympatolhistaminämie bei Psychopathie und vegetativer Störung. Schweiz. med. Wschr. **78**, 1249 (1948).
SURKES, A.: Bluthistaminbestimmungen nach intravenöser Adrenalininjektion bei allergischen und neurovegetativen Störungen. Schweiz. med. Wschr. **78**, 662 (1948).
SZILÁGYI, T., A. KOVER, and B. CSABA: Effect of hypothermia on histamine release induced by epinephrine infusion. Amer. J. Physiol. **199**, 272 (1960).
TASAKA, K.: Histamine release and its inhibition by anti-histamines. Folia pharmacol. jap. **53**, 1029 (1957).
TROQUET, J., and J. LECOMTE: On the histamine nature of complications caused by disulfiran. Rev. belge Path. **27**, 180 (1960).
UNGAR, G., and E. DAMGAARD: Tissue reaction to anaphylactic and anaphylactoid stimuli; proteolysis and release of histamine and heparin. J. exp. Med. **101**, 1 (1955).
— T. YAMURA, J. B. ISOLA, and S. KOBRIN: Further studies on the role of proteases in the allergic reaction. J. exp. Med. **113**, 359 (1961).

UVNÄS, B.: Mechanism of histamine release from mast cells. Chemotherapia (Basel) **3**, 137 (1961).
—, and I. L. THON: Isolation of "biologically intact" mast cells. Exp. Cell Res. **18**, 512 (1959).
— — Evidence for enzymatic histamine release from isolated rat mast cells. Exp. Cell. Res. **23**, 45 (1961).
VAN ARSDEL, P., and R. E. BRAY: On the release of histamine from rat peritoneal mast cells by compound 48/80. Effect of metabolic inhibitors. J. Pharmacol. exp. Ther. **133**, 319 (1961).
VANE, J. R.: Some pharmacological actions of paludrine. Brit. J. Pharmacol. **4**, 14 (1949).
VIANA, H. M., and D. BRANDÃO: Effects of phenothiazines and nonphenothiazine antihistaminics on tissue slices. Ciência e Cultura **14**, 235 (1962).
VIRNO, M., S. B. GERTNER, and D. BOVET: Action of histamine on the jugular pressure and cerebral circulation of the dog; effects of anti-histaminic drugs and a histamine liberatory agent. J. Pharmacol. exp. Therap. **118**, 63 (1956).
VOGT, W.: The chemical nature of Darmstoff. J. Physiol. (Lond.) **137**, 154 (1957).
VUGMAN, I.: Factors which influence the release of histamine from the isolated diaphragm of the rat by compound 48/80. Thesis, Faculdade de Medicina de Ribeirão Prêto, Brazil (1961).
— Influence of insulin and of glucose on the liberation of histamine from the isolated diaphragm of the rat by compound 48/80. Ciência e Cultura **14**, 239 (1962).
—, and A. M. ROTHSCHILD: Effect of glucose and insulin on the histamine release by compound 48/80 from alloxan diabetic rats. Acta physiol. lat.-amer. **11**, 108 (1961).
WAALKES, T. P., H. COBURN, and L. L. TERRY: The effect of reserpine on histamine and serotonin. J. Allergy **30**, 408 (1959).
WASER, P. G., and J. ITZBICKI: Effects of psychotropic drugs on blood histamine in rat. Experientia (Basel) **15**, 197 (1959).
WENT, I., u. E. VARGA: Experimentelle Untersuchungen über die chemische Gegenregulation des Blutdruckes. Acad. Sci. Hung. **3**, 377 (1952).
WEST, G. B.: Histamine in mast cell granules. J. Pharm. Pharmacol. **7**, 80 (1955).
— Comparison of the release of histamine and 5-hydroxytryptamine from tissues of the rat, mouse and hamster. Int. Arch. Allergy **13**, 336 (1958).
— Chemical nature and possible role of mediators in allergic reactions. Int. Arch. Allergy **18**, 56 (1961).
WEST, R.: The pharmacology and therapeutics of curare and its constituents. Proc. roy. Soc. Med. **28**, 565 (1935).
— The actions of curarine on the respiratory mechanism. J. Physiol. (Lond.) **91**, 437 (1938).
— Bronchospasm and antihistamine drugs. Proc. roy. Soc. Med. **42**, 625 (1949).
WESTERHOLM, B.: In vitro release of histamine from cat skin by compound 48/80. Acta physiol. scand. **50**, 41 (1960a).
— The influence of anoxia on 48/80 induced histamine release from cat skin. Acta physiol. scand. **50**, 300 (1960b).
WILSON, C. W. M.: Factors influencing the urinary excretion of histamine in the rat. J. Physiol. (Lond.) **126**, 141 (1954).
ZEPPA, R., D. GROSSKREUZ, and K. SUGIOKA: Histamine release into the circulation by meperidine (Demerol). Proc. Soc. exp. Biol. (N. Y.) **106**, 794 (1961).

Section D

Release of Histamine in Anaphylaxis

By

M. Rocha e Silva

With 12 Figures

I. Historical survey

A. Origin of the histamine theory

As the main characteristics of anaphylaxis in most species of animals and of human allergy involve reactions of smooth muscle, increased capillary permeability (edema formation) and hemodynamic changes with a predominance of fall in arterial blood pressure, it was natural to look for a principle present in the body having such pharmacodynamic actions. Among the endogenous principles known to physiologists in the earliest days of anaphylaxis, only histamine would fit the prerequisites as a mediator of the anaphylactic reactions. However as the complex picture of anaphylaxis emerged from the many-sided studies on its mechanism, it became more and more clear that histamine could not explain all symptoms which are typical of anaphylaxis. In 1941, Dragstedt defined anaphylaxis as a phenomenon of "auto-intoxication by physiologically active substances." Therefore, besides histamine, many other endogenous principles might participate in the phenomenon, and at least one more principle, heparin, was shown to be released in dog's anaphylaxis, explaining the decreased coagulability of the blood which is a typical occurrence in this species of animals. Today, though histamine still is the most important mediator of the anaphylactic reaction in some species, as the guinea pig and the dog, we have to look for newly identified principles such as 5-HT and bradykinin (or a slowly reacting principle) in the genesis of anaphylaxis. Other endogenous principles, as acetylcholine, catechol amines or adenylic compounds, could play a rather subsidiary or questionable role in the anaphylactic reaction in all species of animals or in human allergy.

That histamine might play a role in anaphylaxis was already suggested as early as 1910-11, by the fundamental experiments by Dale and Laidlaw on the physiological action of β-imidazolylethylamine. "*It may be noted that the symptoms and post-mortem examination in the guinea pig correspond in a suggestive manner with those described by several workers as the effect of poisoning in the animal by Witte's peptone, or by serum or other protein in the sensitized guinea pig (anaphylactic shock).*" The analysis of the mechanism of death of a guinea pig, submitted to anaphylactic shock, as done by Auer and Lewis (1910); Auer (1910); Biedl and Kraus (1909,10); Anderson and Schultz (1909-1910); Schultz and Jordan (1911), indicated that the main cause was an acute constriction of the bronchiolar tree immobilizing the lung in deep inspiration and this could be reproduced by injection of a suitable dose of histamine in normal guinea pigs (Dale and Laidlaw, 1910). Furthermore, it was shown by Dale (1913) that the phenomenon is mainly peripheral occurring in the isolated perfused lungs taken from a sensitized guinea pig. Again, in this isolated preparation, histamine would produce an immobilization of the lung comparable in all details with the effect of the antigen (DALE, 1920). The other symptoms of *in vitro* anaphylaxis, as first described by SCHULTZ (1910) in the isolated guinea pig intestine or by DALE (1912-13) in the isolated guinea pig uterus, could also be reproduced by the addition of histamine to the bath containing the isolated normal organ (DALE, 1912-13). These preliminary evidences led DALE to the conviction that the effect of the antigen was mainly directed to the effector structures, independent of any participation of the blood constituents, since washing out of traces of blood from the *in vitro* reacting structures would not impair but in some cases improve the reaction elicited by adding the antigen to the sensitized isolated organ. The occurrence of the phenomenon of desensitization (or "anti-anaphylaxis") following repeated additions of the antigen would indicate that a mediator is set free when the antigen meets the antibody anchored to the reacting structure. Given all the evidences on the similarity between the effects of histamine upon normal animals and of the antigen upon a sensitized guinea pig, it became an attractive possibility to consider histamine as a mediator to explain anaphylaxis. This possibility, however, was presented in a very cautious way by DALE (1920) and only as late as 1929, could DALE himself digress on the possibility of histamine playing a role in some physiological or pathological reactions. Between these two dates, LEWIS (1924-27) had adduced evidences for the release of an H-substance from the skin submitted to injury or to the allergen in sensitized individuals; on the other hand, BEST, DALE, DUDLEY and THORPE (1927) succeeded in obtaining histamine, as such, from alcoholic extracts of fresh liver and lung, and DALE and DUDLEY (1929) isolated histamine in the form of a picrate from the spleen of the horse and the ox. These findings allowed a definite statement by DALE (1929): "*In the guinea pig in which death is produced by contraction of the bronchioles, isolated samples of plain muscle give a direct response to application of the antigen in high dilutions; the histamine, we must suppose, is liberated from, or in the immediate neighbourhood of the reacting cells. Isolated plain muscle from the anaphylactic dog, on the other hand, gives no significant response to the antigen . . . Yet, when the antigen is injected into the circulation of the whole anaphylactic dog, there is a general vascular and plain muscle reaction strongly similar to that produced by histamine.*"

These analogies were so meaningful that they constituted for many years the sole basis of the so-called "histamine theory of anaphylaxis", according to which most of the symptoms of anaphylaxis in the different species and also of skin allergy in humans, could be explained by a release of histamine from previous stores in the sensitized cells submitted to the aggression by the antigen. Since these cells might be freed from plasma or blood and still give the anaphylactic reaction, the "histamine theory" or "cellular theory" appeared to exclude any participation of other blood-borne principles as *protein digests* (RICHET, 1909; VAUGHAN, 1913; DOERR and MOLDOVAN, 1912; DOERR, 1913; BRONFENBRENNER, 1915; JOBLING et al. 1914,15; and many others), *apotoxin* (RICHET, 1909-1912), or *anaphylatoxin* (FRIEDBERGER, 1909-11; FRIEDEMANN, 1909; BORDET, 1913; BESREDKA et al. 1913 and others), which could not possibly be formed in isolated organs in the absence of even traces of blood. However, the first demonstrations that histamine is actually released from cells in conditions of anaphylactic shock only appeared in the literature in the earliest thirties following the work by DRAGSTEDT and GEBAUER-FUELNEGG (1932) and BARTOSCH, FELDBERG and NAGEL (1932,33).

We have divided (ROCHA E SILVA, 1957) the history of participation of histamine in anaphylaxis in three distinct periods:

a) From its discovery in 1907, till the first demonstration, in 1932, of its release from sensitized cells by contact with the antigen; this period might be called the "phase of analogies";
b) From 1932 to the appearance of the first potent synthetic anti-histaminics, in 1937-39 (BOVET and STAUB, 1937; STAUB, 1939), which brought forward the possibility of testing on sound pharmacological basis the nature of the mediator (s) released in anaphylaxis and allergy; during this period the evidences in favor of a release of histamine accumulated (SPINELLI, 1932; DRAGSTEDT et al. 1932,36,40; BARTOSCH et al. 1932,33; DALY et al. 1935; BARTOSCH, 1935; UNGAR and PARROT, 1936; CODE, 1939,44; SCHILD, 1939; KATZ, 1940, and others);
c) The modern phase, in which the limitations of the histamine theory became apparent and new mediators, such as 5-HT, "slowly reacting substances" and/or bradykinin became potentially important to explain many facets of the symptoms which could not be explained by histamine alone. It is no fortuitous coincidence that the mode of action of anaphylatoxin by a release of histamine only became clear in the third period, since the availability of highly specific histamine antagonists, such as mepyramine (neo-antergan) was of decisive importance to prove the histaminic nature of the shock elicited by anaphylatoxin in the guinea pig (HAHN and OBERDORF, 1950; ROCHA E SILVA et al. 1951; HAHN and LANGE, 1956).

A subdivision of this modern phase, might be proposed in order to stress the importance of the discovery of the localization of histamine in the mast cell granules (RILEY and WEST, 1952,53; MOTA, 1953) leading to a new trend in the studies of its liberation by damage to mast cells, covering the period from 1952 to the present days. This period will be dealt with by other contributors to this book.

B. Limitations of the histamine theory

Before going into the detailed study of the participation of histamine in the different species of animals, a general survey of the difficulties usually encountered in the applicability of the histamine concept should be briefly discussed.

The histamine theory involves the following basic statements:

a) histamine reproduces, in certain animal species, the complex of symptoms characteristic of the anaphylactic crisis;
b) histamine is encountered in the so-called shock organs in quantities to explain the most marked effects produced locally, in the event of its liberation;
c) there is much experimental evidence that histamine is liberated from the tissues after the injection of the antigen;
d) there is a general parallelism between the sensitivity of the different animal species to histamine and to anaphylactic shock (SCHMIDT and STAEHELIN, 1929).

These are, so to speak, the postulates of the histamine theory of anaphylactic shock. They are fulfilled in certain animal species but not in others, but even in those species which are most frequently given as examples of the applicability of the histamine conception, there are exceptions or discrepancies which can be formulated as follows:

1) differences in degree between the most characteristic symptoms developed after the injection of the antigen and that of histamine;
2) histamine sometimes produces an effect just the opposite of the one produced by the antigen;

3) discrepancies regarding the experimental conditions under which the reaction to histamine and to the antigen are brought forward, especially in relation to specific inhibitors, such as anti-histaminics.

In the course of the foregoing discussion we will give examples illustrating each one of these discrepancies. Some are still unsolved, some could be overcome by the introduction of the concept of multiple mediators, others are of minor importance and not strong enough to disregard histamine as an important mediator of the anaphylactic reaction.

II. Anaphylaxis in the guinea pig

A. Humoral versus cellular theory

In spite of the strong analogies between the effects of histamine when injected intravenously in the guinea pig and those typical of anaphylaxis in this animal species, as first indicated in two publications by Dale and Laidlaw (1910-11), at the beginning of the second decade of this century, two apparently opposing conceptions were conflicting in the endeavor to explain anaphylaxis in the guinea pig. According to Friedemann (1909) and Friedberger (1909) the incubation of the specific precipitate with the serum of a normal guinea pig could generate a toxin, which has been named "anaphylatoxin" or "serotoxin". This "humoral theory" was strongly sponsored by the Belgian immunologist, Jules Bordet, who contributed a great deal to the development of this concept of the mechanism of anaphylaxis. According to Bordet (1913), it was not necessary to use the specific precipitate to generate anaphylatoxin, the incubation of the normal serum of a guinea pig with agar or starch being sufficient to activate a principle which would provoke a symptomatology, in the guinea pig itself, very similar to that of anaphylaxis. Since this subject will be dealt with in another section of this book, I limit my comments to the main historical concerns of this conception.

The other view was sponsored by Dale (1913-1920) on the basis of experiments made on the isolated organs of the guinea pig. According to these, the stimulating action of the antigen upon sensitized smooth muscle structures of the guinea pig, such as the bronchiolar tree (Auer and Lewis, 1910) or the isolated intestine (Schultz, 1910), or uterus (Dale, 1913) would result in the release of histamine by damage of the cells in direct contact with the antigen. Since the effects of anaphylatoxin on the isolated smooth muscle were not very constant and differed by many details from the effects produced by the antigen, Dale and Kellaway (1922) adduced considerable evidence against participation of anaphylatoxin or of any blood-borne principle in the anaphylactic reaction of the guinea pig.

B. Release of histamine in in vitro anaphylaxis

In the subsequent years, the balance shifted in favor of the cellular theory of anaphylaxis as evidences accumulated to show that histamine is present in normal organs (Best et al. 1927; Dale and Dudley, 1929), as well as by the convincing evidence of a histamine release presented by Bartosch, Feldberg and Nagel, (1932,33); Bartosch (1935); Feldberg (1937); Daly, Peat and Schild (1935) in experiments of lung perfusion and by Ungar and Parrot (1936) and Schild (1939) by using a more simplified procedure of suspending pieces of organs of a sensitized guinea pig in a "shock fluid" containing small concentrations of the antigen.

In the experiments by Bartosch et al. (1932), the substance released by perfusing the guinea pig lung with the antigen was identified with histamine by its action upon the guinea pig gut, the blood pressure of the cat and by its capacity of releasing adrenaline from the adrenal gland of the cat. Estimated as histamine, amounts of the order of 0.05 to 4.0 μg were found in the perfusates. In confirmation of those findings, DALY, PEAT and SCHILD (1935) have shown that the yield of histamine in the perfusates of 38 guinea pigs varied from 0.17 to 12.8 μg with an average of 4.49 μg total, using egg white as antigen. With horse serum the yields were consistently lower, from 0 to 1.13 μg (averaging 0.246 μg). The analysis presented by SCHILD (1936 a) indicated that the bronchiolar constriction was not the cause but the consequence of the release of histamine: if the spasm is prevented by adrenaline, the release of histamine takes place as well; on the other hand, a broncho-constriction produced by barium chloride, agar, kaolin, K^+ and Ca^{++} resulted in no release of histamine.

The amounts released under these conditions were consistently low, with an average of 5 to 10 μg of histamine, about one hundredth of the quantity of histamine necessary to produce the bronchomotor effects of anaphylactic shock in the intact guinea pig. As SCHILD (1936 a) commented: "*The available evidence does not permit us to state definitely that histamine is the only or even the main cause of the anaphylactic reaction in the guinea-pig's lung.*"

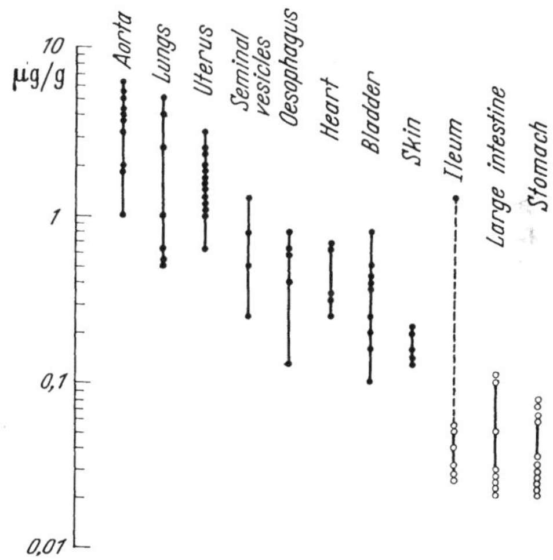

Fig. 1. Release of histamine (μg/g of tissue) from various organs in anaphylactic shock (according to SCHILD, 1939)

The system was simplified by UNGAR and PARROT (1936), who have shown the release of a substance indistinguishable from histamine by simply suspending a piece of lung *in vitro* in a fluid containing the antigen (PARROT, 1938). Later on, SCHILD (1939) utilized a similar technique to demonstrate the release of histamine from isolated pieces of several organs: aorta, skin, lung, uterus, seminal vesicle, intestine, stomach, heart, bladder, etc., taken from sensitized animals and submitted *in vitro* to the contact of the antigen (Fig. 1). Using slices of skin suspended *in vitro* in contact with the antigen, EMMELIN, KAHLSON and LINDSTRÖM (1941) have likewise demonstrated the release of histamine when the pieces were taken from a sensitized animal.

Concerning the origin of the released histamine, it became obvious that it could only spring from previous stores of the amine in the treated organs or tissues. By perfusing only one lung, BARTOSCH (1935) could show that the "released plus the residual" histamine would sum up the "total histamine" which could be extracted from the other, unperfused lung. On the other hand, the possibility of the amine being formed from the histidine contained in the antigen, was disproved by SCHILD (1936 a) on the basis of a simple calculation of the maximum of histidine existing in the amounts of antigen utilized.

In more recent studies on the release of histamine in *in vitro* anaphylaxis or by the action of chemical releasers, a perfect balance sheet could be drawn equating the sum of histamine "released + residual" with the "total" histamine previously contained in the assayed material (MONGAR and SCHILD, 1956,57,58; MOTA, 1958 a; ROTHSCHILD et al., 1961; VUGMAN, 1961).

Table 1 gives an example of the balance existing between released, residual and total histamine from chopped, sensitized lungs submitted to *in vitro* anaphylaxis and from rat diaphragm in contact with compound 48/80.

Table 1. *Balance sheet of released, residual and total histamine* (μg/g)

A. Release by compound 48/80, under different experimental conditions, from hemidiaphragms of the same rat (according to VUGMAN, 1961)

Experiment N°	Hemidiaphragm 1				Hemidiaphragm 2			
	Spont. release A	Release by 48/80 B	Residue C	Total A+B+C	Spont. release A	Release by 48/80 B	Residue C	Total A+B+C
I	0.4	1.1	14.4	15.9	0.5	6.3	9.4	15.2
II	0.5	6.1	18.0	24.6	0.4	1.7	21.0	23.1
III	0.8	5.9	21.3	28.0	1.7	6.6	19.2	27.5
IV	1.8	1.3	14.6	17.7	1.9	2.5	12.5	16.9
V	2.0	1.3	17.9	21.2	1.9	3.6	18.8	24.3
VI	1.7	2.6	17.8	22.1	1.2	1.0	21.6	23.8
VII	2.1	1.2	22.5	25.8	1.0	1.6	24.0	26.6
VIII	0.7	8.9	12.0	21.6	0.4	11.5	10.6	22.5
IX	1.0	11.6	10.6	23.2	1.9	4.3	18.0	24.2
Average	1.22	4.44	16.57	22.23	1.21	4.34	17.23	22.79

B. Release by antigen (egg albumin) from chopped guinea pig lung (according to MONGAR and SCHILD, 1957 a)

	Spont. release A	Release by antigen B	Residue C	Total A + B + C
	0.05	1.17	1.57	2.79
	0.04	1.10	1.60	2.74
	0.04	1.11	1.68	2.83
	0.04	1.32	1.43	2.79
	0.05	1.15	1.40	2.60
	0.04	1.25	1.60	2.89
Average	0.043	1.183	1.547	2.773

C. Quantitative aspects of the histamine release

The great limitation of the significance of these findings has always been the minute amounts which could be released from an entire lung in the mentioned experiments. Those amounts could not explain *per se* the death of a guinea pig if the conditions prevailing *in vitro* were verified *in vivo*. We have thought that this discrepancy might be explained by the participation of some constituents of the blood, such as anaphylatoxin, which might play a role in the genesis of the symptoms through its ability of releasing histamine (ROCHA E SILVA, 1952,54,56). Anaphylatoxin, obtained by activation of the guinea pig serum with agar, is able to release much larger amounts of histamine than the antigen itself under comparable conditions. In experiments of lung perfusion with agar-anaphylatoxin amounts varying from 14.3 μg to 103 μg per lung could be obtained (ROCHA E SILVA, ARONSON and BIER, 1951; ROCHA E SILVA and ARONSON, 1952) (Fig.2).

Since bronchospasm in the guinea pig produced by anaphylaxis is stronger than that produced by anaphylatoxin, as shown by DALE and KELLAWAY (1922), and at the same time the amounts of histamine released by the antigen are much smaller, DALE (1953) suggested that this would be a clear cut demonstration that anaphylatoxin could not participate in the genesis of the anaphylactic symptoms and indicated that the histamine liberated from the lung by anaphylatoxin would come from different sites and in particular from the endothelial cells; on the contrary, the histamine released in anaphylaxis ("intrinsic histamine") would derive from the sensitized muscle cells and therefore, though in relatively smaller quantities, would be more efficient than that released by anaphylatoxin. This argument of "intrinsic histamine" (Dale, 1948, 50) lost much of its strength by the discovery that histamine is mainly confined to mast cells (see Riley and West, Chapter 1, Section E) and that the histamine released in anaphylaxis and by anaphylatoxin comes mainly from its stores in the lung mast cells (Mota 1958a, 59; Mota and Vugman, 1956). However, it appears evident now that the effects of anaphylaxis or that of anaphylatoxin upon the isolated guinea pig lung are quantitatively as well as qualitatively different, not only in relation to the amounts of histamine actually released but also to the action of anti-histaminics. It appears that the bronchospasm induced by anaphylatoxin can be totally prevented by small doses of anti-histaminics, being therefore a pure histamine effect, though the spasm induced by the antigen is more resistant to the inhibitory action of anti-histaminics (Giertz and Schmutzler, 1960; Giertz et al., 1961; Hahn et al., 1961, and Chapter 3, Section E). Since in both cases histamine derives from the same source (mast cells) it is in both cases "extrinsic" to the plain muscles of the bronchiolar tree and the discrepancy mentioned shows that other substance(s) are probably involved in the anaphylactic reaction. This point will be further discussed below (D).

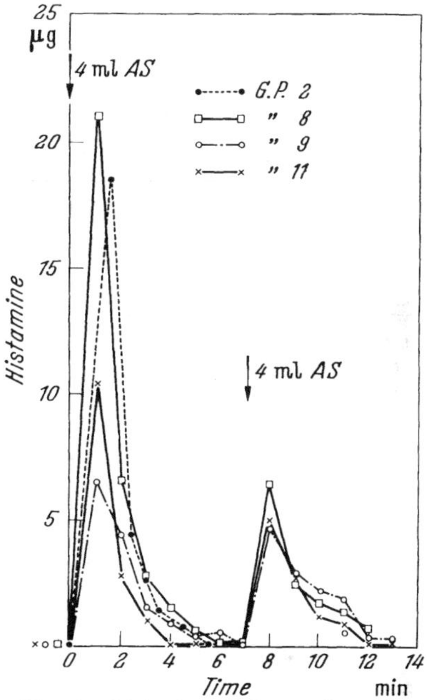

Fig. 2. Histamine discharges from four guinea-pig lungs perfused with Tyrode's solution. At the arrows, 4 ml of agar activated guinea-pig serum injected. The first injections released about twice as much histamine as the second ones (according to Rocha e Silva, 1952)

In other manifestations of anaphylaxis in the guinea pig, histamine may also play a role. It has been shown that the isolated guinea pig heart responds to histamine or to the antigen in a similar manner (Wilcox and Andrus, 1938; Andrus and Wilcox, 1939) with sharp inotropic and chronotropic positive reactions. The constricting effect upon the coronary bed could be obtained with both agents. By taking records of electrical changes in the atria of the guinea pig heart, as well as comparing the effects of histamine with those of anaphylaxis, it was shown recently (Feigen et al. 1960; Vaughan Williams, 1961) that there is a striking analogy between both effects. There could also be demonstrated a release of histamine from the isolated heart of the guinea pig in perfusion experiments with the antigen (Feigen et al., 1960). With the isolated auricle from sensitized guinea pigs, Greeff et al. (1959) demonstrated positive inotropic and chronotropic reactions by addition of the antigen, strikingly similar to the effects produced by histamine. Also anaphylatoxin elicited similar reactions which were blocked by anti-histaminics but unaltered by BOL, dihydroergotamine, hexamethonium or reserpine.

D. Release of other agents

The limitations of the histamine theory as applied to the guinea pig were evidenced by the experiments described by Schild (1936b, 49, 56) upon the isolated uterus of the sensitized guinea pig. Following the addition of 4 mg of histamine the isolated sensitized uterus contracts maximally and returns slowly to the normal tone, becoming refractory to new additions of histamine; the further addition of the antigen, however, still produced a strong contraction as shown in Fig. 3.

From sensitized guinea pig lungs, perfused with the antigen, CAMPBELL and NICOLL (1940) obtained a material which stimulated the normal rat uterus and consequently differed from histamine.

The denervated iris of several species of animals, including the guinea pig, the rabbit and the dog, contracts during anaphylactic shock and the mediator appears to differ from histamine (BENDER, 1943).

Another argument to limit the importance of histamine in *in vitro* anaphylaxis was derived from the use of highly specific anti-histaminics, such as mepyramine

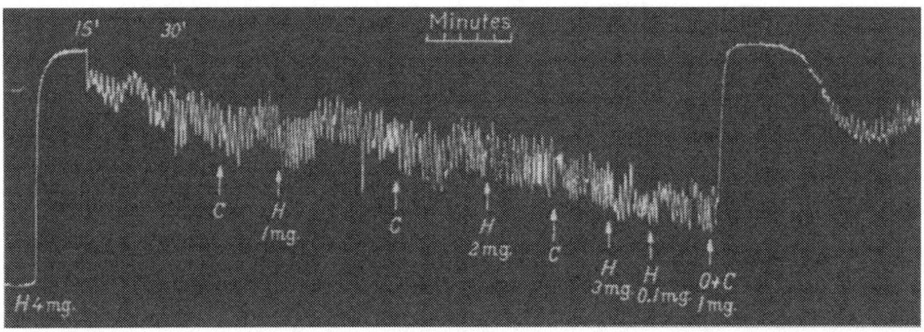

Fig. 3. Contractions of the isolated uterus of a guinea-pig which had been previously sensitized to egg albumin. Uterus suspended in 20 ml bath in Ringer's solution. Addition of histamine to the bath at first produces contraction, but gradually the muscle relaxes in spite of the continued presence of histamine and shows no more response to further addition of histamine acid phosphate (H) or sodium acid phosphate (C). When, however, the specific antigen, egg albumin (O) is added, it contracts maximally. This experiment shows that it is possible to abolish the response to extrinsic histamine and yet preserve the anaphylactic response of plain muscle (according to SCHILD, 1949)

(neo-antergan). In the isolated ileum or in preparations of trachea rings from strongly sensitized guinea pigs, HAWKINS and ROSA (1956) verified that the response to the antigen (egg white) was not very much affected by concentrations of the anti-histaminic (mepyramine) which would block the effects elicited by large doses of histamine. Again, the explanation of "intrinsic histamine" could not be upheld because the histamine is released from mast cells present in the connective tissues surrounding the reacting structures and would be therefore "extrinsic" to the muscle fibers.

DALE (personal communication, 1957) agreed to this view, in the case it had been demonstrated *"that all the histamine involved in the reaction comes thus from mast cells, rather than from the reacting plain muscle cells themselves. If so, my suggested contrast between intrinsic histamine could seem to be eliminated, all the histamine, if it really came from the mast cells, would be extrinsic."* Participation of other factors which might be released in association with histamine might explain the discrepancies, as indicated below.

In experiments done *in vivo* with aerosols of the antigen or by simple intravenous injection of the antigen, there is a generally accepted evidence that even the least active anti-histaminics fully prevent the acute shock, by relieving the pulmonary emphysema (STAUB and BOVET, 1937; ROSENTHAL and BROWN, 1940; HALPERN, 1942, 47; BOVET and WALTHERT, 1944; MAYER et al., 1945; FEINBERG et al., 1950 and many others). Nevertheless, the anti-histaminics are less effective in preventing the so-called protracted shock (by intraperitoneal injection of the antigen) and a certain percentage of the animals which survive the acute shock by treatment with anti-histaminics will die later on with a more chronic symptomatology of peritoneal hemorrhages, hypotension, without signs of respiratory distress (HAHN et al., 1961). Furthermore, in guinea pigs which have been partially depleted of their histamine and serotonin by a combined treatment with reserpine plus 48/80, prior to the challenge with the antigen, the shock observed was of undiminished strength (LIBRO and MARIANI, 1961). It appears quite obvious that if the immediate death produced by a release of histamine is prevented, other endogenous toxic principles will act to kill a certain percentage of animals. On the nature of such principles playing a subsidiary role in the genesis of the anaphylactic symptoms in the guinea pigs, only a few speculative statements can be presented.

"SRS" or *"SRS-A."* KELLAWAY and TRETHEWIE (1940) reported the release of a slowly reacting substance (SRS) from the perfused lung of the sensitized guinea pig. By using a highly specific anti-histaminic (mepyramine) BROCKLEHURST (1953,56,60) demonstrated the presence of a principle resistant to that inhibitor, in perfusates from the guinea pig lung after the injection of the antigen. This material "SRS-A" produced a slow contraction of the guinea pig ileum and could sharply be distinguished from 5-HT, bradykinin or substance-P, as indicated in Table 2.

Its polypeptide nature was questioned since proteolytic enzymes did not destroy its activity. Though being a stimulator of the human bronchiolar muscles, it was found to be inactive upon the isolated bronchiolar muscles of the cat, dog, rabbit and guinea pig (BROCKLEHURST, 1956, 1960). A similar principle was described by CHAKRAVARTY, HÖGBERG and UVNÄS (1959), CHAKRAVARTY (1960) and CHAKRAVARTY and UVNÄS (1960) with the name of "SRS," as being released in conditions in which mast cells are damaged and histamine released. Apparently, this principle is a lipid-soluble material sharply distinguishable from bradykinin or substance-P, because it is inactive upon the rat's uterus. Attempts to purify SRS from normal swine lungs have been also described (LINN et al., 1961). Taking

Table 2. *Pharmacological differentiation between SRS-A and other substances* (according to MONGAR and SCHILD, 1962)

Preparation	SRS-A		Prosta-Glandin	Irin	Darm-stoff	Brady-Kinin	Sub-stance P	5-Hydroxy-tryptamine	Oxy-tocin
	B	C	C	C	C	B	B	B	B
Guinea-pig ileum .	+	+	+	+	+	+	+	+	0
Rabbit intestine .	+	+	+	+	+	+			
Rat colon . . .	0	+	+	+					
Guinea-pig uterus	0	0	+		+				+
Rat uterus . . .	0	0	+	0	+	+		+	+
Human bronchioles	+					0	0		
Cat trachea . . .	0							+	
Rabbit B.P.. . .	0		+		0	+	+	+	
Cat B.P.	0	0	+						

+: Contraction of plain muscle or fall of B.P.; 0: no effect observed; B: Data from BROCKLEHURST; C: data from CHAKRAVARTY.

advantage of the fatty acid-like properties of SRS, an active material was extracted by chloroform from acidified aqueous solutions, separating it from histamine and possibly from other contaminant active materials; evaporation of the solvent yielded about 50 mg of a lipid concentrate from 1 kg of wet tissue. This material contracted the guinea pig ileum at a level of 0.025–0.125 μg/ml of bathing fluid. Since SRS does not act upon the bronchiolar muscles of the guinea pig, it could not explain the discrepancies presented above about the relative inefficiency of anti-histaminics upon the anaphylactic bronchospasm in this species of animals. A final clarification of the chemical nature of this material still awaits further experimentation.

Serotonin. In conditions of acute anaphylactic shock in guinea pigs, ENGELHARDT and SCHWABE (1960) found a decrease in the 5-HT content of the spleen and intestine, but not in the lungs or the brains of guinea pigs. In protracted shock only the spleen showed any significant decrease. In experiments of lung perfusion only small or negligible amounts of 5-HT could be found in the perfusates after the injection of the antigen (GIERTZ and SCHMUTZLER, 1960).

Bradykinin. Regarding formation of bradykinin in conditions of *in vitro* or *in vivo* anaphylaxis, it has been shown by HAWKINS and ROSA (1959) and more recently by LAHIRI and BROCKLEHURST (1961) that there occurs an increase of activity in conditions of lung perfusion or in the plasma of guinea pigs submitted to anaphylaxis. As much as 40 ng/ml of bradykinin were found in the blood of guinea pigs submitted to anaphylaxis (LAHIRI and BROCKLEHURST, 1961). This result agrees with the finding of LIBRO and MARIANI (1961) showing an increase from a normal value of 0.4 μg/g to 3.5 μg/g of bradykinin extractable from the lungs of guinea pigs submitted to anaphylactic shock.

The bradykininogen content of guinea pig's plasma is sharply reduced after onset of anaphylactic shock (BROCKLEHURST, 1962, personal communication). According to FELDBERG (1961) the properties of bradykinin, its high activity, ready activation from plasma proteins and rapid inactivation would make it a very suitable candidate for an anaphylactic transmitter. "*It is to be hoped that specific antagonists of bradykinin will become available by means of which its role in anaphylaxis can be tested*" (MONGAR and SCHILD, 1962).

The participation of bradykinin in aggravating the bronchiolar constriction in the guinea pig became a strong possibility since it has been shown by COLLIER et al. (1960) that this polypeptide is extremely potent in inducing bronchiolar constriction *in vivo* in the guinea pig. Though COLLIER and SHORLEY (1960) were unable to prevent the bronchiolar constriction induced by anaphylaxis, with anti-pyretic agents, such as acetylsalicylic acid, antipyrine, which strongly and specifically prevent the bronchiolar spasm produced by bradykinin, the participation of this polypeptide in anaphylaxis is an interesting possibility in view of the results quoted in the literature about the favorable effect of salicylate in such conditions (CAMPBELL, 1948; SMITH and HUMPHREY, 1949; LEPPER et al. 1950). Nevertheless it is more likely that salicylate might interfere with the mechanism of histamine liberation (TRETHEWIE, 1951; HAINING, 1956b; MONGAR and SCHILD, 1957a and others) or with the antigen-antibody reaction (LEPPER et al. 1950; COBURN and KAPP, 1943).

E. Enzymatic mechanism of histamine release

There are many indications that the release of histamine from the sensitized guinea pig lung by the contact of the antigen involves a sequence of enzymatic reactions. The phenomenon is temperature dependent, shows an optimum of pH at 7.8 and is blocked by inhibitors presumably acting by antagonizing enzymatic mechanisms. When the temperature is lowered to 2° C at the moment of the addition of the antigen, histamine is not released from pieces of the guinea pig lung. Also removal of Ca^{++} ions reduces considerably or abolishes the release of histamine from guinea pig lungs by the antigen (MONGAR and SCHILD, 1957a). MONGAR and SCHILD (1957b) investigated the effect of a previous heating of the sensitized tissues on the subsequent histamine release by contact with the antigen. If the tissue (guinea pig lung, ileum or uterus) is kept for 25 minutes at 42°—43°C the capacity of releasing histamine on further contact with the antigen is completely and irreversibly lost. To explain this phenomenon, it has been suggested that an enzymatic system highly sensitive to temperature would be damaged or otherwise inactivated by such mild heat treatment. If this were true, this enzymatic system would have a higher activation energy (45.000 calories) than that usually found in isolated enzyme systems. Complement in plasma, and also the precursor of anaphylatoxin would require a much higher temperature (56° C) to be inactivated. However, as suggested by OSLER et al. (1959a), this sole criterion would not be sufficient to exclude complement for intracellular anaphylatoxin formation, since in the conditions of the cells, the thermic requirements to inactivate a biological system might be quite distinct from conditions prevailing in plasma.

Opinions diverge on the nature of the enzymes or the enzymatic system involved. It was for a long time known that anoxia can prevent the release of histamine from sensitized lung (PARROT, 1942) and that mercury cyanide interferes with the *in vitro* anaphylactic reaction of the isolated guinea pig gut (PARROT and RICHET, 1944). These preliminary experiments called attention to the possibility of participation of respiratory enzymes in the mechanism of release. From the observation that iodoacetate in concentrations up to 1 mM inhibits the release of histamine, MONGAR and SCHILD (1955) concluded that some oxidation-reduction enzymes requiring free SH-groups might play an important role. Other substances, such as cyanide, antipyretics, phenol, cinnamate, urethane, etc., which in different molar concentrations can prevent the release of histamine without affecting desensitization due to the combination of the antigen with the antibody, were also tried by MONGAR and SCHILD (1957a) and discussed by SCHILD (1959). From these experiments the scheme of Fig. 4 was drawn:

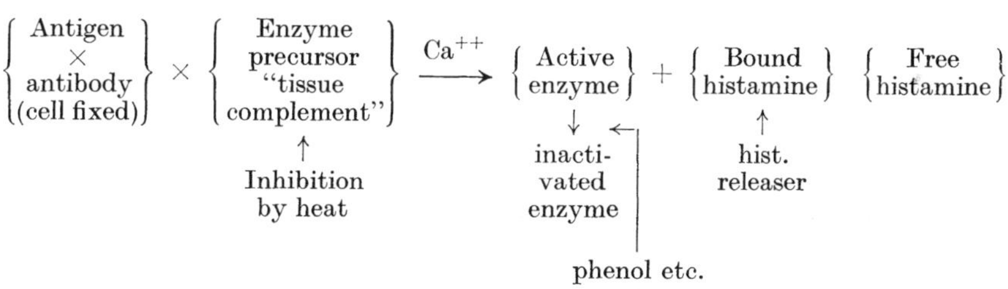

Fig. 4. Mechanism of histamine release in guinea-pigs in anaphylactic shock (according to MONGAR and SCHILD, 1957b, and SCHILD, 1959)

A questionable increase in respiration during *in vitro* anaphylactic shock in slices of the guinea pig lung was demonstrated by MOUSSATCHÉ and DANON (1957) and also a potentiating effect by succinate and an inhibition by malonate. From such results MOUSSATCHÉ and DANON (1958) concluded that activation of a respiratory enzyme from the cytochrome chain, depending upon the Krebs cycle would be operative in the chain of events leading to the release of histamine in anaphylaxis. Similar results and conclusions were presented by YAMASAKI et al. (1960). It can, however, be argued whether the SH-enzymes which participate in the mechanism of histamine release actually belong to the respiratory system, or if they are proteolytic in nature, since some of the cathepsins depend upon free SH-groups to be operative.

Along this line it is interesting to note that HAYASHI et al. (1960) described release of a protease in tissue culture of monocytes from sensitized rabbits, following *in vitro* addition of the homologous antigen. The protease had an optimum pH of 7.5 and was inhibited by SH-reagents and reactivated by cysteine. Protease activation occurs simultaneously with morphological changes in the cytoplasm of the cultured cells (HAYASHI et al., 1955; HAYASHI, 1956). For a review of this subject see UNGAR and HAYASHI (1958). In a series of papers HERBERTS (1949,55) has demonstrated an increased proteolysis in extracts from guinea pig's lungs, after addition of the antigen. This proteolytic activity was increased by cysteine in low concentration (0.02%) and inhibited by higher concentrations (0.2%). A number of thiol compounds blocked the proteolytic activity (HERBERTS and DRESSLER, 1955). These results and those reported by HAYASHI et al. (1960) would point to an enzyme similar to cathepsin C which needs cysteine to be active. However, a closer analysis utilizing synthetic substrates would be desirable. In contrast, AUSTEN and BROCKLEHURST (1961a) attributed a chymotrypsin-like character to the enzyme or enzymes which are presumably activated in the guinea pig lung by contact with the antigen, because the release of histamine in such conditions is significantly blocked by synthetic substrates specific for chymotrypsin. Recently BENDITT and ARASE (1959) have found a chymotrypsin-like enzyme in the peritoneal mast cells of rats. An enhancement of the histamine release as seen with succinate, could be observed with other dibasic organic acids, having no relationship to the tricarboxylic cycle of Krebs, such as glutaric, adipic, pimelic or maleic acid. The structural configuration required for a dibasic acid to enhance anaphylactic reaction in the guinea pig, according to AUSTEN and BROCKLEHURST (1961b) is quite specific: the carboxyl groups should be separated by a two carbon chain, and must be free or fixed in the *cis* position. Monobasic acids from valeric to dodecanoic acids inhibit the release of histamine and the inhibitory activity increases with the carbon chain length; the introduction of a polar group into the hydrocarbon residue diminishes or abolishes the inhibitory capacity (AUSTEN and BROCKLEHURST, 1961b). The inhibition of the histamine release by another polycarboxylic acid, derived from salicylic acid by polymerization with formaldehyde (polymethylene salicylic acid) was described by FERNÖ et al. (1960). Nonetheless, an anti-rat γ-globulin which releases histamine from isolated mast cells is potentiated by chymotrypsin substrates and its histamine releasing activity is not affected by succinate (AUSTEN and HUMPHREY, 1961).

That the phenomenon of histamine release might require the production of high energy phosphate bonds (ATP) was suggested by the experiments by MOUSSATCHÉ and DANON (1958) showing that 2,4-dinitrophenol and other phenol derivatives, which can uncouple the respiration from the production of ATP, are strong inhibitors of the release of histamine by basic compounds such as 48/80 (HÖGBERG and UVNÄS, 1957; UVNÄS, 1958; ROTHSCHILD, VUGMAN and ROCHA E SILVA, 1961) and sinomenine (YAMASAKI, 1961), acting upon histamine rich structures such as the diaphragm, the mesentery or the skin of the rat. As the problem will be extensively studied in Chapter 3, Section H, only a mention is needed in connection with the release of histamine in anaphylaxis of the guinea pig.

On the basis of the inhibition of the anaphylactic release of histamine from the guinea pig lung by carbon monoxide (CO) and antimycin, as well as the reversal of the inhibition by CO, when the slices were exposed to light, MOUSSATCHÉ and DANON (1958) suggested a participation of the cytochrome system in the mechanism of release. AUSTEN and BROCKLEHURST (1961c), however, were unable to find any inhibitory effect by CO and even the effects of cyanide and anoxia were questioned on the basis that cyanide is active only if added immediately before the antigen, and that malonic acid, a competitive inhibitor of succinic dehydrogenase, did not affect the release at all in contrast with what has been demonstrated by MOUSSATCHÉ and DANON (1958). These discrepancies might be explained by the fact that AUSTEN and BROCKLEHURST (1961c) did not take into consideration the fact that the glucose present in Tyrode can revert almost totally the inhibitory effect of cyanide, anoxia and 2,4-dinitrophenol as shown by several workers (Westerholm, 1960; Diamant, 1960; Rothschild, Vugman and Rocha e Silva, 1961; Prouvost-Danon and Moussatché, 1961). This controversy indicates: a) that the cytochrome chain would be required as an indispensable step of the phenomenon, in aerobiose *but in the absence of glucose*, a rather artificial situation; and b) that glucose constitutes an important substrate either for the production of high energy phosphate bonds or in some still undisclosed step in the chain of events leading to histamine release.

The scheme of Fig. 5 is an attempt to visualize such a complex mechanism as the release of histamine and breakdown of mast cells. It appears likely that enzymes of the carbohydrate metabolism cycle are required for the production of

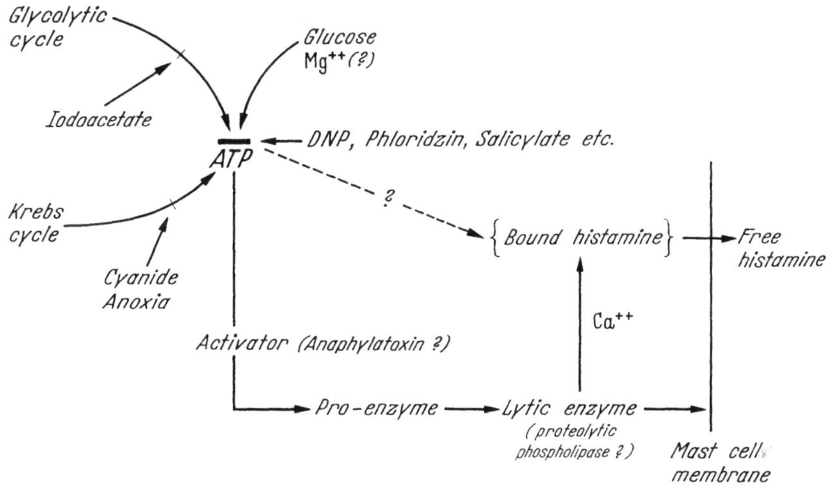

Fig. 5. Possible chain of events in the mechanism of histamine release, showing enzymes of the carbohydrate metabolism and activation of a lytic enzyme which might be responsible for the breakdown of the mast cell membrane

high energy bonds (ATP ?) and that this constitutes an indispensable step for the activation of a lytic enzyme, the nature of which is still controversial (proteolytic ?, phospholipase ?).

To end this subject it should be mentioned that the release of histamine from the guinea pig lung depends upon the integrity of its cellular structure, since it has been shown by Mongar and Schild (1957a) that the release by the antigen will not take place if the lung tissues are desintegrated and the granules collected by centrifugation. Those granules, however, release histamine if treated with basic compounds, such as 48/80. Another difference between the action of 48/80 and anaphylaxis in the lung of the guinea pig is the fact that iodoacetate does not block but rather potentiates the release by the former and blocks totally the release by anaphylaxis. As far as anaphylatoxin is concerned its mechanism of action upon the guinea pig lung is similar to that produced by anaphylaxis (Rothschild, 1961) and especially the mast cells are altered in a very similar way by either agent (Frenger and Gemählich, 1958; Gemählich et al. 1958; Mota, 1959). It has also been shown by Moussatché and Danon (1956) that p-chloromercuribenzoate antagonizes not only the *in vitro* anaphylactic reaction (Schultz-Dale), but also the effect of anaphylatoxin upon the isolated normal guinea pig ileum; and also by Haining (1956b) that salicylate and HPCA (3-hydroxy-2-phenylcinchoninic acid) prevents the constriction of the guinea pig ileum put in contact with the antigen or with anaphylatoxin *in vitro*.

Heating the guinea pig ileum at 45° C for 15 minutes, however, abolishes the anaphylactic reaction, but does not prevent the effect of formed anaphylatoxin (MOTA, 1959; BERALDO et al. 1961).

In spite of the many coincidences which might induce one to consider anaphylatoxin as a possible mediator in the chain of events leading to the release of histamine in anaphylaxis, it has been repeatedly argued that it could not be so because a tissue completely desensitized to anaphylatoxin still gives a maximal contraction with the antigen (GREISMAN, 1958; MOTA, 1959; GREEFF et al., 1959). *In vivo*, when anaphylatoxin is repeatedly given to a sensitized guinea pig it can reduce or abolish the subsequent shock produced by an injection of the antigen (HALPERN et al. 1956a; FRENGER et al., 1958), in spite of earlier negative reports in the literature (BESREDKA, 1920; DALE and KELLAWAY, 1922). The arguments derived from immunologic studies are going to be discussed in other Sections of this Chapter (E, F).

III. Anaphylaxis in the rabbit

A. Applicability of the histamine theory to the rabbit's anaphylaxis

The histamine theory of anaphylaxis met with difficulties when applied to the rabbit (ROCHA E SILVA, 1942). It is known that the injection of histamine in the anesthetized rabbit normally produces a rise in blood pressure (DALE and LAIDLAW, 1910, 11; ACKERMANN and KUTSCHER, 1910; FELDBERG, 1937), although the administration of the antigen to the sensitized animal is almost invariably followed by a steep fall in arterial blood pressure. This fact was known since the earliest days of anaphylaxis and studied in a systematic way by ARTHUS (1909, 21), AIRILA (1914), COCA (1919), LARSON and BELL (1919) and DRINKER and BRONFENBRENNER (1924), who have explained this phenomenon as due to stagnation of blood in the venous circulation by spasm of the pulmonary vessels. A contribution of the vagus nerve to this effect was demonstrated by ROCHA E SILVA (1940 b) in experiments in which section of the vagi during the hypotension provoked by anaphylaxis promptly restored the initial level of blood pressure.

It is difficult, however, to reproduce by an injection of histamine the typical and peculiar pattern of symptoms occurring in the rabbit's anaphylaxis (BALLY, 1929; GROVE, 1932). When injected intravenously, histamine produces a generalized spasm of the arterial and venous system with a consequent rise in arterial blood pressure. It is to be noted that the antigen in a sensitized rabbit can also produce a spasm in the circulatory apparatus, though the main symptom is a fall in blood pressure (VALLERY-RADOT, 1937). Under certain circumstances the effect of the antigen could be even reverted into a hypertensive one similar to that elicited by histamine, when the animal had been previously submitted to a persistent vaso-dilation by repeated constrictions and releases of the trunk of the pulmonary artery (ROCHA E SILVA, 1940 b). It seems evident that the antigen produces also a dual effect with the predominance of a fall in arterial blood pressure due to its peculiar effect upon the pulmonary artery bed. If this mechanism is rendered inoperative as by the procedure described above a predominance of the hypertensive effect can be observed.

An increased tone of the arteriolar system in the sensitized rabbit was shown in experiments by FRIEDBERGER and SEIDENBERG (1927) by perfusing the isolated rabbit's ear with Ringer-Locke solution. A similar result was obtained in a more systematic way, by ABELL and SCHENK (1938) using a transparent moat chamber (Clark's) adapted to the rabbit's ears after repeated injections of the antigen into sensitized animals. Besides arteriolar contraction with obliteration of the lumen, increased adherence of leukocytes to the endothelium of the blood vessels and leukocyte migration occurred. Particularly interesting was the fact that the leukocytes became sticky, adhering to form clumps or emboli and in certain cases stoppage of the circulation could be observed. Endothelial destruction with blood extravasation was seen in most severe reactions. These observations gave the experimental basis to start a rational analysis of the mechanism of anaphylaxis in the rabbit and of the so-called ARTHUS reaction (local anaphylaxis).

B. Changes in blood histamine

The rabbits present a peculiarity which played a decisive role in the studies of the mechanism of anaphylaxis in this species. Among the experimental animals it shows the highest content of histamine in the blood (TARRAS-WAHLBERG, 1936; CODE, 1937; CODE and ING, 1937; ROSE and WEIL, 1939; ROSE, 1941; ROSE and BROWNE, 1941; MINARD, 1941, and CODE, 1952). As much as 2 to 7.3 μg per ml have been estimated in the rabbit's blood. This histamine was thought to be confined to leukocytes (CODE and ING, 1937) but it was finally demonstrated to be held mainly by platelets (MINARD, 1941; ZON, CEDER and CRIGLER, 1939). Under certain circumstances, as by contact with the antigen, this histamine diffuses to plasma and disappears from circulating blood (ROSE and WEIL, 1939; ROSE, 1941). DRAGSTEDT et al. (1940 a) calculated from *in vitro* experiments that the amount of histamine which could be liberated *in vivo* from rabbit's blood cells would be about 0.1 to 0.3 mg per kg of body weight. This amount would be insufficient to explain the severity of anaphylactic shock in a certain percentage of rabbits, in so far as the effects of histamine upon the blood pressure are in the opposite direction, as discussed above. However, it might be argued: a) that other sources of histamine are available *in vivo* and SCHACHTER (1953) has shown that histamine is released from the rabbit's ear in considerable amounts when the isolated organ is perfused with the antigen; b) that histamine released *in loco* in the lung of the rabbit by the clumped white blood elements and platelets would be much more effective in producing spasm of the pulmonary bed than the histamine injected intravenously; c) other factors as the mechanical obstruction of the pulmonary bed with the formation of microthrombi of leukocytes and platelets might play a role to aggravate the stagnation in the right heart and the venous system; furthermore, the mechanical obstruction of the pulmonary vessels can be aggravated by a plugging of the capillaries with the abundant specific precipitate formed. The presence of the specific precipitate in microemboli occluding the pulmonary small vessels was demonstrated by measurement of radioactivity, using I^{131} labelled antigen (DIXON, 1953) or by challenging the sensitized animal with the antigen made visibly detectable by conjugation with fluorescein (MCKINNON et al. 1957; MCKINNON, 1959); d) as far as the fall in blood pressure is concerned it has been shown recently by LECOMTE (1959,60), LECOMTE and TROQUET (1960) that bradykinin might be a mediator since butazolydine (phenylbutazone) would block both effects of bradykinin and the fall in blood pressure characteristic of the anaphylactic shock in the rabbit. Bradykininogen was found to fall in rabbits, submitted to anaphylaxis (LECOMTE, 1961; DINIZ and CARVALHO, 1963; LAMBERT et al., 1964). Furthermore, when locally applied to the mesentery of rabbits, bradykinin can start vascular changes which resemble those of anaphylaxis (HUGHES and LECOMTE, 1960); e) some minor discrepancies might also be explained by the release of 5-HT, since its presence in rabbit's platelets has been demonstrated by RAND and REID (1952) and its release by the antigen-antibody reaction shown by HUMPHREY and JAQUES (1953,55) *in vitro*, and by WAALKES et al. (1957) in the intact animal. In the rabbit, serotonin appears to come exclusively from platelets (UDENFRIEND and WAALKES, 1959). Following accumulation of the platelets in the lung capillaries after the injection of the antigen, the total histamine and serotonin extractable from the lung tissue are greatly increased (WEISSBACH et al., 1957; WAALKES and COBURN, 1960), their values returning to normal as the platelets return to circulation.

It is difficult to assess the relative importance of these factors in the genesis of the anaphylactic shock in the rabbit and the following discussion will be mainly aimed to give a balance of the present evidence concerning the possible mediators involved in such circumstances.

C. Release in vitro

The diffusion of histamine from blood cells to plasma under the condition of anaphylaxis, led KATZ (1940) to develop an interesting and useful technique to study quantitatively the release of histamine in rabbit's anaphylaxis. Rabbits sensitized to egg white were bled by cardiac puncture and the heparinized blood was submitted *in vitro* to contact with the antigen. The plasma separated by centrifugation showed marked increase in the amount of histamine which had diffused from its stores in the cells. These findings have been confirmed and extended by several workers (DRAGSTEDT et al. 1940 a; ROSE and BROWNE, 1941; EICHBAUM and ROCHA E SILVA, 1943). Due to its extreme simplicity, this technique has been applied to study the factors which enhance or interfere with the histamine release owing to the facility of having duplicate samples submitted to varying experimental conditions. The release of histamine by peptone (GOTZL and DRAGSTEDT, 1942), by trypsin (DRAGSTEDT and ROCHA E SILVA, 1941), by papain (ROCHA E SILVA and ANDRADE, 1943), by toxic materials derived from hydatic fluid, Ascaris extracts and so forth (GRAÑA and ROCHA E SILVA, 1945; ROCHA E SILVA, GRAÑA and PORTO, 1945; ROCHA E SILVA, 1950) snake venoms (ROCHA E SILVA and ESSEX, 1942) and the antagonistic action of heparin (DRAGSTEDT, WELLS and ROCHA E SILVA, 1942), of salicylate and HPCA (HAINING, 1956 b), as well as the effect of polysaccharides such as dextran and inulin (HAINING, 1955, 1956a; ROTHSCHILD, unpublished results) on the histamine release in rabbit's blood, were studied with that simple technique devised by KATZ. Still with this *in vitro* technique, MCINTIRE et al. (1949,50,52) showed the importance of calcium ions and also the inefficiency of basic compounds to release histamine from rabbit's blood cells. With this technique, MCINTIRE et al. (1951,57) found a certain relationship between the ability of aliphatic amines in releasing histamine and the length of their carbon chains. By methylation of the amino group, the compounds acquire the property of blocking the release of histamine by octadecylamine and by the antigen-antibody reaction.

With a 2×10^{-4} molar concentration of octadecylamine the release of histamine from rabbit's blood cells is rapid and reaches completion in 1 to 2 minutes. The release by the antigen shows a lag period lasting for 1.5 to 2.5 minutes after which the curve is very similar to that obtained with octadecylamine. (Fig. 6). Compounds containing a pyridinium ion and a long carbon chain such as β-carbomethoxy-N-(n-hexadecyl) pyridinium ion will block both the release by octadecylamine and by the antigen. The soya bean trypsin inhibitor (SBI) while blocking the release of histamine by trypsin did not substantially affect the release by the antigen (MCINTIRE et al. 1950; MCINTIRE, 1956). Nor did fibrinolysin (plasmin) or streptokinase, even in large concentrations, produce any substantial shift of histamine from rabbit's blood cells to plasma. This, according to MCINTIRE et al. (1952) and McIntire (1956), would invalidate the conception that histamine is released in anaphylaxis by activation of plasma fibrinolysin (Ungar, 1956). It is to be noted that the experiments by Ungar et al. (1949-58) were mainly done on guinea pigs, showing a high correlation between activation of proteolytic enzymes, or proteases (Ungar et al. 1961) and release of histamine. However, even in this species it has been contended by Burdon et al. (1961) that there is no such parallelism between plasmin activation and production of anaphylactic symptoms. In the rabbit, this lack of parallelism, between *in vivo* fibrinolysis and the severity of the symptoms was also shown by Gans and Krivit (1961) using the specific inhibitor ε-amino caproic acid to prevent activation of plasminogen to plasmin, *in vivo*. It is to be noted, however, that because fibrinolysin does not release histamine this will not invalidate the fact that other proteolytic enzymes do release it as trypsin or papain, from rabbit's platelets (Dragstedt and Rocha e Silva, 1941; Dragstedt et al., 1942; Rocha e Silva and Andrade, 1943; Humphrey and Jaques, 1953,55) or trypsin, from the guinea pig lung (Rocha e Silva, 1939, 40 a; Trethewie, 1942, and others) or chymotrypsin which has been attributed to be the agent to release histamine in anaphylaxis (Austen and Brocklehurst, 1960) or to damage mast cells in rat's mesentery (Keller, 1961,62).

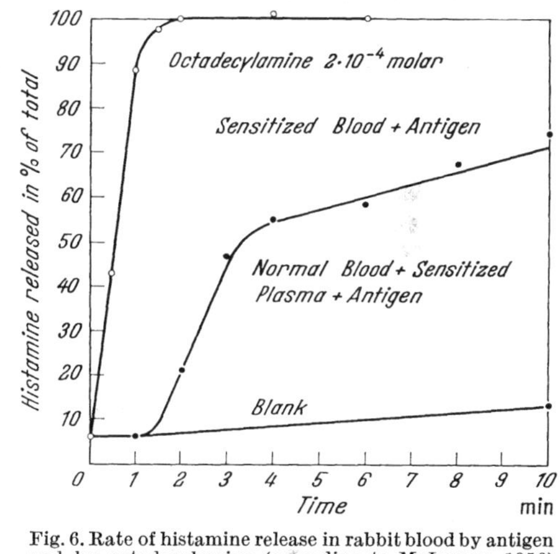

Fig. 6. Rate of histamine release in rabbit blood by antigen and by octadecylamine (according to McIntire, 1956)

However, the clear cut experiments by McIntire (1956) have indeed shown that fibrinolysin is a poor releaser of histamine and therefore a conception based on its activation to explain histamine release has been thoroughly invalidated. The assumption of a simple displacement mechanism of histamine from its ionic bindings with acid polysaccharides such as heparin, appears to be as well invalidated by the fact that such a strong releaser of histamine, as 48/80, is completely inert when tested upon rabbit's blood or isolated platelets (Humphrey and Jaques, 1955). Activation of anaphylatoxin under these conditions might be more significant since, as shown above, dextran, agar and inulin can activate the releasing system in rabbit's plasma (Haining, 1955,56 a; Rothschild, unpublished results).

A certain correlation between the shift of histamine from cells to plasma with lysis of sheep red cells was demonstrated by Carryer and Code (1950) in samples of blood taken from rabbits immunized to sheep red cells. The significance of this correlation, however, is difficult to assess, since the two phenomena (hemolysis and histamine release) have entirely different sites and duration, as the released histamine comes from platelets and takes only a few minutes to be complete, while hemolysis was read after incubation for 1 hour. One might be inclined to infer that complement participates in the process of release, but this again is a controversial matter, as shown below.

A more elaborate technique to study the shift of histamine from platelets to plasma, in contact with the antigen, was described by Humphrey and Jaques (1955). The platelets were separated from the blood and resuspended, after washing with Tyrode solution, in heparinized plasma, which had been submitted to several experimental procedures, such as heating at 56° C for 30 minutes, or treatment with several reagents such as oxalate, versene, or citrate to remove calcium ions. If the antigen-antibody mixture was added directly to the suspension of platelets in Tyrode solution, no release was observed. The mixture had to be added to the recomposed system "platelets + plasma". Calcium ions were found to be necessary for the release; addition of the proper amount of calcium chloride was sufficient to reverse the inhibition of the release by the previous treatment with oxalate or versene (EDTA), but not if the plasma was previously treated with citrate. Trypsin, but not 48/80, rapidly and completely released histamine from platelets suspended in Tyrode's solution. The basic releaser 48/80, even in amounts of the order of 200 μg/ml did not release histamine, in conditions in which the antigen-antibody complex did work. Treatment of plasma with agar in conditions suggestive of activation of anaphylatoxin was followed by a histamine release when the system "platelets + activated plasma" was recomposed. From these experiments, the following sequence of events was outlined by HUMPHREY and JAQUES, (1955):

$$\left\{\begin{matrix}\text{Antigen}\\ \times\\ \text{Antibody}\end{matrix}\right\} \xrightarrow{Ca^{++}} \left\{\begin{matrix}\text{Fixation of}\\ \text{some component}\\ \text{of complement}\end{matrix}\right\} \longrightarrow \left\{\begin{matrix}\text{Activation}\\ \text{of}\\ \text{protease}\end{matrix}\right\} \longrightarrow \left\{\begin{matrix}\text{Histamine}\\ \text{and serotonin}\\ \text{release}\end{matrix}\right\}$$

At variance with the results described above, are the findings of BARBARO (1961) on the isolated rabbit's platelets treated with the specific precipitate + diluted plasma. The shift of histamine was observed to parallel the amount of antibody in the specific precipitate bearing no relationship to complement activity as measured by hemolysis of sensitized sheep red cells. Since in these experiments the release was relatively independent of heating the plasma to 56° C and of the treatment with zymosan (which even reduced the release), it can be suspected that some anaphylatoxin already formed by diluting the plasma was operating in the conditions of BARBARO's experiments. In a more recent report, BARBARO (1962) demonstrated that the plasma factor is multi-component. After incubation of immune precipitates with plasma, neither the supernatant plasma nor the washed precipitates when added separately to the suspension of platelets will give a full release of histamine. If the washed precipitates are added back to the supernatant plasma there occurs as much release as in the control. These findings indicate the presence of at least two components in plasma that are involved in histamine release. Besides calcium ions, a requirement for Mg^{++} was also demonstrated.

D. Release in vivo

When the antigen is given intravenously into the intact anesthetized rabbit, profound changes in the content of blood histamine take place, not confined to a simple shift of histamine from blood cells to plasma. Sometimes these changes faithfully reflect the alterations in the count of white blood cells and platelets in the circulation and their confinement to the capillary network of certain organs as the lung, the liver or the skin. The final result is invariably a sharp drop of the total content of histamine in the circulating blood as first demonstrated by ROSE and WEIL (1939). Concomitantly with the fall in blood histamine, a slight and sometimes significant rise in plasma histamine occurred. A correlation between the decrease in blood histamine and the severity of anaphylactic shock was described by ROSE (1941).

Since histamine in rabbit's blood is mainly confined to the WBC and especially to platelets, it was an obvious and expected consequence that any agent producing a removal of such elements from circulation would produce a decrease in the histamine extractable from rabbit's blood. ROSE (1941) has shown a close correlation between the leukopenia which occurs in anaphylaxis and the fall in blood histamine. The removal of WBC occurring in anaphylaxis might be the consequence of the clumping of leukocytes observed *in vivo* in the experiments of ABELL and SCHENCK (1938) with a transparent chamber adapted to the rabbit's ears. Concomitant with the removal of leukocytes there invariably occurs a sharp drop in platelet counts in the circulating blood. The immunologic mechanism underlying agglutination of platelets in rabbits and guinea pigs was restudied recently by SIQUEIRA and NELSON (1961), who concluded that the complex, antigen-antibody-complement, has a specific "receptor site" on the surface of platelets. Platelets were not agglutinated after heating at 56°C for 15 minutes, nor after treatment with trypsin or with chymotrypsin. Versene (EDTA) inhibited the agglutination of platelets, but citrate or heparin did not affect it (SIQUEIRA and NELSON, 1961).

The earlier experiments described above, combined with the fact that the lung of the rabbit plays a major role in the production of the symptoms, led DRAGSTEDT et al. (1940 b) to perform experiments of lung perfusion with rabbit blood to which the antigen and the antibody were added in optimal proportions. A sharp decrease of the WBC counts correlated with the decrease of total histamine could be observed after a first passage through the lung. With the demonstration that histamine is mainly bound to platelets (MINARD, 1941; ZON, CEDER and CRIGLER, 1939), it would be expected that the clumping of leukocytes and their segregation in the lung's capillaries parallel the removal of platelets in the DRAGSTEDT et al. (1940b) experiments. Along that line, KOPELOFF and KOPELOFF (1941) and KINSELL et al. (1941) found a correlation between the thrombocytopenia and the severity of anaphylactic shock in the *Rhesus* monkey and the rabbit, suggesting that a breakdown of platelets might be correlated with the shift of histamine from cells to plasma.

As changes in total blood histamine reflect the removal of WBC and platelets from circulation, such alterations would be expected in many circumstances in which there occur leukopenia and thrombocytopenia (QUICK et al., 1946). In fact, it has been shown that peptone (GOTZL and DRAGSTEDT, 1942), polysaccharides such as liver glycogen (ROCHA E SILVA, GRAÑA and PORTO, 1945), products from hydatid fluid (GRAÑA and ROCHA E SILVA, 1945) or Ascaris extracts (ROCHA E SILVA, GRAÑA and PORTO, 1945) induce changes in the total blood histamine similar to those occurring in anaphylactic shock. These changes are more likely to be correlated with variations of platelet counts than with leukocytes (ROCHA E SILVA, 1950). This was taken as additional evidence that histamine is mainly bound to platelets, confirming the views of MINARD (1941) and ZON, CEDER and CRIGLER (1939). However, there was a substantial difference between the phenomenon as observed by the injection of glycogen or polysaccharides extracted from Ascaris and hydatic fluid, on one side, and the changes induced by anaphylaxis on the other side. The polysaccharides studied, especially liver glycogen, did not produce shock-like symptoms in the rabbit and no shift of blood histamine when added *in vitro* to the blood samples was observed. The injection of glycogen into the intact rabbit produced the segregation of platelets in the lung as could be judged by the increase of the histamine content of this organ, after intravenous injection of glycogen (ROCHA E SILVA, 1950), (Fig. 7).

Therefore, the conclusion was drawn that a simple decrease in blood histamine and segregation of platelets into the lung capillaries would not *per se* explain the symptoms of anaphylaxis, but that the release of histamine (and, now we know, of serotonin as well) might be critical in the production of the symptoms (pulmonary artery constriction, dilatation of the right heart and fall in blood pressure).

Furthermore, it was shown that glycogen, when given previously to a sensitized rabbit, was able to abolish the symptomatology of anaphylaxis (ROCHA E SILVA et al, 1945). Now that we know that the aggregates in the lung of rabbits submitted to anaphylaxis are full of the specific precipitate (McKINNON, 1959), we can think that a concomitant formation of the precipitate embedded into the disintegrating clumps of leukocytes and platelets might constitute an important factor for the genesis of the symptoms. In that case, the inhibition of the shock by a previous injection of glycogen receives a simple explanation since in these circumstances the precipitate will not be forming in such an intimate contact with the blood cells as to permit their disintegration from previously formed clumps in the lung's capillaries.

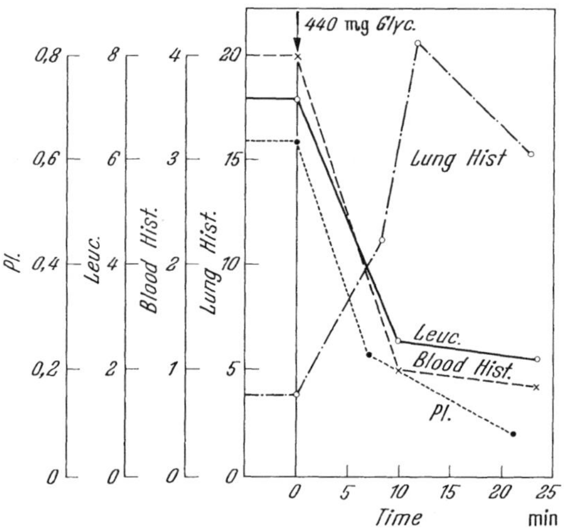

Fig. 7. Variations of leucocytes, platelets, blood histamine, and lung histamine, after the injection of 440 mg of liver glycogen per kg of body weight, in a "thoracic rabbit" (inferior vena cava and thoracic aorta clamped just above the diaphragm) (according to ROCHA E SILVA, 1950)

A reconsideration of this mechanism including a possible participation of serotonin was presented recently by WAALKES and COBURN (1959,60) and WAALKES et al. (1959), and an experiment showing the increase of serotonin and histamine in rabbit lungs during anaphylaxis was also described by UDENFRIEND and WAALKES (1959). Formation of micro-emboli of platelets and leukocytes in the production of myocarditis in rabbits submitted to hypersensitivity experiments was observed by HUGHES and TONKS (1959).

It is very unlikely that the main constituents of such emboli, as seen in the rabbit should be constituted of aggregates of the precipitated antigen-antibody, as postulated by McKINNON et al. (1957) and McKINNON (1959). The hyaline emboli seen by WALTER et al. (1961) and WALTER and FRANK (1961) were mainly constituted of a fibrinoid material. The formation of such micro-emboli is not confined to the lungs, as BURRAGE and IRWIN (1953) described plugging of the liver capillaries with micro-emboli, in guinea pigs and rabbits submitted to anaphylaxis (for a revision, see IRWIN, WEILLE and BURRAGE, 1955). Even the injection of histamine produced the appearance of white emboli, red blood cell aggregates and thrombose in the rabbit's lung capillaries (BURRAGE et al. 1954) and in the spiral ligament of the cochlea in guinea pigs (IRWIN et al. 1955).

To sum up, one might suggest that in the rabbit and possibly in other species, 1) the release of histamine is connected with some kind of breakdown of the white blood elements; 2) the clumping of the white blood elements is a constant event during anaphylactic and peptone shock; 3) histamine might constitute a localizing factor for the capture of leukocytes and platelets which have already begun to clump in the peripheral circulating blood; 4) obstruction of the small vessels and capillaries depends upon two main factors, one chemical, probably histamine, and the other mechanical, the agglutinated white blood elements.

On the basis of newly acquired evidences one might add serotonin (UDENFRIEND and WAALKES, 1959) and bradykinin (LECOMTE, 1961; BROCKLEHURST and LAHIRI, 1962) as possible mediators.

In as much as the two main theories (cellular and humoral) are concerned, the experiments with the rabbit's blood provide a system in which participation of plasma in the mechanism of release from cells (platelets) has been demonstrated beyond doubt. Again, no essential conflicting evidence can be adduced in favor of either one theory, since the mechanism of release could involve a plasma (or humoral) component and a cell element (platelets) and the activation of a "plasma releaser(s)", acting as an intermediary, might contribute to reconcile the apparently conflicting views of the humoral and cellular theories.

IV. Arthus phenomenon and PCA

Before going further in the study of the participation of histamine in anaphylaxis in other animal species, a brief consideration of the possible role played by histamine in some local phenomena elicited by the interaction of the antigen with the antibody might be of interest. Four different local phenomena should be considered:

a) the Arthus phenomenon (AP)
b) the passive cutaneous anaphylaxis (PCA)
c) the reverse Arthus phenomenon (RAP) and also
d) anaphylactoid reactions by soluble antigen-antibody complexes.

Methods of observation: The evidences in favor or against participation of histamine in these local phenomena are mainly indirect by the use of anti-histaminics and the observation of the intensity of the reaction. Considerable use has been made, in this connection, of the production of a blue spot in the site of the challenging injection, after the intravenous injection of a blue dye, such as trypan, pontamine sky, Evans or Geigy blue. As this reaction is highly non-specific, being produced by many agents which might release histamine, serotonin or bradykinin, considerable caution is necessary in the interpretation of a positive reaction, (see Circulatory effects of histamine). It is generally accepted that a blockade of the reaction by anti-histaminics should be considered a good evidence of a participation of histamine. However, in certain cases the reaction produced by a typical histamine releaser, such as 48/80, can be more resistant to the action of anti-histaminics than that elicited by histamine itself (Miles and Miles, 1952). Now, we know that 5-HT (Rowley and Benditt, 1956; Sparrow and Wilhelm, 1957, and others) in the rat, and bradykinin (Bhoola et al. 1960) in the guinea pig, and possibly in all animal species, increase capillary permeability giving a positive blue test. Though there are indications of an earlier use of the blue test to show increased capillary permeability, the first reference of the use of trypan blue to demonstrate a skin reaction in sensitized guinea pigs and rabbits receiving the antigen by intracutaneous injection, is due to Ramsdell (1928). The local injection of histamine also produces a blue spot after the intravenous injection of trypan blue. These experiments have been confirmed by Bier and Rocha e Silva (1939 a,b); Rocha e Silva and Bier (1939) and Rocha e Silva and Dragstedt (1941). In these experiments, histamine must be injected in small concentrations (1 to 8 μg) to induce a homogenous blue spot, since higher concentrations (up to the mg) as those utilized by Menkin (1939) produce a white area surrounded by a pale blue. However, since the endogenous histamine, acting locally at the place of its release (mast cells) in direct contact with the small vessels and capillaries, can induce a different pattern of reactions, it is altogether difficult or impossible to decide whether a blue spot is due to a release of histamine or of other capillary-active principles, judging only by the appearance of the blue spot.

Using the criterion of localization of the blue spot in areas of the skin with highest histamine contents (Feldberg and Miles, 1953), as well as the effect of a previous depletion of the skin by intraperitoneal injection of 48/80 (Feldberg and Talesnik, 1953), additional evidences of the participation of a release of histamine in some local skin reactions could be obtained as, for instance, a diminution or abolition of the skin reactions produced by egg white or hematoporphyrin and light (Feldberg and Talesnik, 1953). However, since it has been shown that depletion of histamine from skin depends upon destruction of mast cells and since it was demonstrated that the content of 5-HT can also drop by a previous treatment with 48/80 (See other Chapters of this book), the question persists whether histamine might be the only, or one of the multiple mediators released in such circumstances. It is possible, by the combined use of different kinds of depleters (48/80, reserpine, dextran, polymyxin, and so forth) to attempt to eliminate one or more of the known and possible mediators, but the results even under the best possible conditions can be dubious since the number of possibilities has not yet been exhausted, as polypeptides (bradykinin, angiotensin, substance-P, etc.) might be involved in such local inflammatory reactions and for them we have no specific inhibitors or reagents yet. Again the evidence given by the action of antihistaminics appears to be the only one acceptable to prove or disprove a participation of histamine in these local reactions. For a critical analysis of the method, see Halpern et al. (1956 b, 58).

A. Arthus phenomenon

The first demonstration of anaphylaxis in the rabbit was the production of a local aseptic inflammation by repeated injections of horse serum in the skin (Arthus and Breton, 1903; Arthus, 1903). After a few weeks of repeated subcutaneous injections the aseptic inflammation evolves through a phase of strong edema and leukocytic migration, into necrosis and scar formation. This "Arthus phenomenon" can also be elicited in guinea pigs (Cannon and Marshall, 1941) though the accidents of bronchiolar constriction are a serious obstacle to the reproduction of a local chronic reaction in the guinea pig. The intensity of the local inflammation appears to depend upon the presence of circulating antibodies and as early as 1924, Opie showed a parallelism between the precipitin titer and the intensity of the skin reaction. This has been restudied and confirmed by Fischel and Kabat (1947) and Benacerraf and Kabat (1950).

By an ingenious experiment, Auer (1920) had demonstrated that the phenomenon results from the combination of the circulating antigen with the antibody locally formed. In rabbits sensitized to horse serum, the skin was treated with xylene after the injection of a massive dose of the antigen intravenously. In the areas of the skin tested with xylene, a severe inflammatory reaction with all characteristics of an Arthus phenomenon developed, while in the control animals the xylene only produced a mild irritating reaction. This fact would indicate the passage of the antigen through the capillaries of the skin rendered more permeable by the action of xylene. The possibility of a direct cytotoxic action of the complex antigen-antibody upon the skin structure was ruled out by the experiments of Aronson (1933) and Meyer and Loewenthal (1937) showing the inocuity of this complex in tissue culture even when the cells of a sensitized animal were cultivated in a nutrient medium containing plasma of the same animal to which the antigen was added (Rich, Lewis and Gay, 1940). The production of a typical Arthus phenomenon appeared to depend upon the organization of the tissue starting with rupture of small vessels, hemorrhage and edemae. Rich and Follis (1940) have demonstrated in the cornea of rabbits previously sensitized with horse serum or egg white, that the phenomenon can only be seen by the local application of the antigen when the cornea of one side had been previously submitted to a contact with irritating agents and developed an intensive artificial vascularization. The avascularized tissues of the other cornea will not develop a typical ARTHUS phenomenon. More recently, it has been shown that morphological changes can be reproduced in the normal avascular cornea following a local injection of antigen + antibody (GERMUTH et al. 1959) but the alterations described could hardly be called a typical Arthus reaction. On the basis of experiments of ABELL and SCHENCK (1938) mentioned above, with the chamber adjusted to the rabbit's ear and the accumulation of blood elements in organs perfused with the total blood to which optimal amounts of antigen and antibody were added (DRAGSTEDT et al., 1940 b), one might assume that the first step in the production of an ARTHUS phenomenon is an accumulation of leukocytes and platelets, with production of microthrombi, stagnation of the blood and hemorrhage in the skin area when the antigen is applied locally (ROCHA E SILVA, 1950; STETSON and GOOD, 1951).

A similar mechanism might hold for the SHWARTZMAN phenomenon, since it has been shown that clumping of leukocytes and platelets occurs in the skin at the site of preparation with the meningococcus toxin after the intravenous challenging injection with the same toxin, polysaccharides or anti-platelet serum (ROCHA E SILVA and MARTINS DA SILVA, 1946; ROCHA E SILVA, 1952). Agglutination of platelets occurred with fresh serum from normal rabbits and guinea pigs, mixed with agents which are known to prepare and provoke a SHWARTZMAN reaction, such as dextrans and soluble antigens of *S. typhosa* (SIQUEIRA and NELSON, 1961). The profound analogy between the development of an ARTHUS phenomenon and a SHWARTZMAN reaction has been stressed by STETSON (1951).

However, the real importance of a release of histamine to account for the phenomena leading to the hemorrhagic ARTHUS or SHWARTZMAN phenomena is difficult to evaluate. It might be reasonable to postulate that an initial release of histamine from clumped platelets, which lyse in the intimacy of the small vessels and capillaries, might trigger the whole reaction by increasing vascular permeability and facilitating a filtration of circulating antibodies into the skin area treated with the antigen. In this connection it is interesting to note that anti-histaminics have a partial inhibitory effect upon the acute symptoms of the ARTHUS reaction in guinea pigs (OVARY and BIER, 1953) and rabbits (BENACERRAF and FISCHEL, 1949). One has to assume that release of proteolytic enzymes or other agents, such as vaso-active polypeptides, might also play a role in the genesis of the phenomenon (STETSON, 1951; ZWEIFACH et al., 1961; ANTOPOL and CHRYSSANTHOU, 1963).

B. Passive cutaneous anaphylaxis

Another interesting feature of the local anaphylactic phenomenon is the so-called "passive cutaneous anaphylaxis" (PCA) first described by BIOZZI, MENÉ and OVARY (1948) by injecting the antibody locally and a few hours later giving a mixture of the antigen + Geigy blue intravenously (see also OVARY, 1958). A seepage of blue into the cutaneous area would be an indication of the increased capillary permeability elicited by the reaction of minute amounts of antigen entering into contact with the areas treated with the antibody. As shown by OVARY and BRIOT (1951), the intracutaneous injection into guinea pigs of such minute amounts of rabbit anti-egg albumin corresponding to 0.003 μg of antibody-N can already induce a local seepage of dye after the intravenous injection of a mixture of antigen plus Geigy Blue. However, the evidences that histamine participates in this reaction are indirect or circumstantial. The increased capillary permeability as seen by diffusion of dye into the skin is by no means specific for histamine, and the antihistaminics are effective in blocking the PCA only in guinea pigs. The "passive cutaneous anaphylaxis" induced in rats is unimpaired when anti-histaminics are previously injected (BROCKLEHURST et al. 1955,60) or when the skin is depleted from its histamine content by a treatment with 48/80 (ROCHA E SILVA and ROTHSCHILD, 1955). Polysaccharides, such as agar or dextran, when previously injected intravenously, would partially deplete the blood from its pro-anaphylatoxin content and abolish the production of the PCA in rats (ROCHA E SILVA and ROTHSCHILD, 1955). Experiments of depletion of complement by injection of specific precipitates, antigen followed by antibody, polysaccharides, such as zymosan, have been described by BIER et al. (1955) and OSLER et al. (1957).

A relationship between production of PCA and anaphylatoxin formation was recently postulated by OSLER et al. (1959). A further discussion on the immunologic mechanism of production of PCA and the ARTHUS reaction would transcend the limits of this Chapter. The relationship with anaphylatoxin activation will be discussed in another section of this Book, (Chapter 3, E.).

The similarity of the skin changes in local anaphylaxis and by injection of proteolytic enzymes (trypsin) and also the parallel changes of skin histamine in such conditions, has been studied by CRAPS and INDERBITZIN (1957), INDERBITZIN (1959) and INDERBITZIN and DOBRIČ (1959).

C. Reverse Arthus phenomenon

The possibility of obtaining a vascular phenomenon similar to the ARTHUS reaction, by inverting the order of injections was described by OVARY and BIER (1952,53) in guinea pigs and rabbits, by preparing the skin with the specific antibody and injecting the antigen + Geigy Blue intravenously. This phenomenon which has been called a "Reverse ARTHUS phenomenon" (RAP) could be differentiated from a typical "passive cutaneous anaphylaxis" (PCA) not only by its morphological characteristics (absence of vascular reactions in PCA contrasting with the hemorrhages and necrosis in RAP), but also by the absence of latency for the first and requirement of a long latent period for PCA. Though the RAP depends upon circulating antibodies diffusing from the site of injection and starts immediately after the intravenous injection of the antigen, the so-called PCA requires 30 minutes to a few hours after the intracutaneous injection of the antibody, and is a much more superficial skin reaction mimicking the evanescent response characteristic of a histamine liberation. On the other hand, both reactions PCA and RAP differ by important quantitative data as far as the amount of the antibody is concerned; while the former can be elicited with such minute amounts of antibody (rabbit anti-egg albumin) corresponding to 0.003 μg of antibody-N, the latter needs much higher concentrations of antibody injected locally, corresponding to 5-10 μg of antibody-N. On the other hand, if the antibody is prepared with horse serum it will elicit a strong RAP and it is entirely ineffective in promoting PCA in the guinea pig skin (OVARY and BRIOT, 1951; OVARY and BIER, 1953). Though the independence of both reactions has been repeatedly postulated, SIQUEIRA and BIER (1961) have shown that the concomitant production of PCA enhances RAP elicited by intravenous injection of an immune complex, unrelated to the immune system utilized for PCA. These conditions are reminiscent of AUER'S (1920) experiments mentioned above.

The evidence in favor or against participation of histamine in a RAP are almost the same as those obtained for PCA. In the guinea pig, the anti-histaminics will reduce the intensity of the reaction (OVARY and BIER, 1953) although in the rat, they are completely ineffective to mitigate either reaction. For a detailed review of these local phenomena, see OVARY (1958).

D. Soluble antigen-antibody complexes

When the specific precipitate, washed a number of times with 0.15 M NaCl is redissolved by the addition of an excess antigen, the soluble complex formed will produce symptoms similar to those of anaphylaxis when injected into normal guinea pigs and rabbits (GERMUTH, JR. and MCKINNON, 1957; WEIGLE et al., 1960), smooth muscle contraction (TRAPANI et al. 1958) and cutaneous lesions, ranging in intensity from a simple increase in capillary permeability to edema and hemorrhages (COCHRANE and WEIGLE, 1958; ISHIZAKA and CAMPBELL, 1958; ISHIZAKA et al. 1959). Some of the symptomatology of serum sickness can also be reproduced by the injection of soluble antigen-antibody complexes (MCCLUSKEY and BENACERRAF, 1959). A strong similarity between the passive ARTHUS phenomenon and the skin lesions produced by the soluble complexes has been stressed by COCHRANE and WEIGLE (1958). It does not appear that the toxic material present in such complexes could be identified with anaphylatoxin, since washing the precipitate would entirely remove this soluble protein fraction of plasma, but it seems likely that the toxic effects on guinea pigs might be due to a release of histamine since anti-histaminics have been found to prevent shock in guinea pigs (WEIGLE et al., 1960).

A release of histamine from perfused guinea pig lungs by such complexes has been reported (GARCIA-AROCHA and MCILREATH, 1959) though damage to mast cells could not be detected (MOTA, 1961). Participation of complement in the biological actions of soluble complexes has been postulated on the basis that they are able to almost completely remove complement from circulation when injected in guinea pigs (WEIGLE et al., 1960). However, the mechanism of action and the release of mediators are still highly controversial. Anyway, the possibility of producing anaphylactoid reactions by injecting an antigen-antibody mixture without any latent period, opens up a new possibility for the study of the intimate mechanism of anaphylaxis itself.

V. Anaphylaxis in the dog

A. The Richet phenomenon

Among the many intriguing questions about the phenomenon of anaphylaxis, one of no small interest is that attached to the meaning of the name itself. To a physiologist, the word *Anaphylaxis* (absence of protection) sounds like the wrong connotation for a misunderstood reaction of the cell to a variety of unrelated materials. To the immunologist the term is still misleading, but the phenomenon can be understood as a more rational reaction or accident in the course of immunization. Hematologists, pharmacologists, clinical men and surgeons, may each have a different view of the phenomenon, but for all of them the meaning of the term has been lost in the course of time, and it would not be superfluous here to trace its origin to the heroic times when PORTIER and RICHET performed the crucial experiments which gave origin to the word, *Anaphylaxis*. In 1902, RICHET and his collaborator PORTIER, were studying the venoms of the tentacles of the sea-actinias (*Physalia*) on dogs, in a Mediterranean cruiser at the expense of Prince Albert of Monaco (PORTIER and RICHET, 1902). These coelenterates contain a poison to which RICHET gave the name of "actino-congestine", because the symptoms to a first injection of a sufficiently large dose of the extracts consisted in generalized congestion of the abdominal vessels, with hyperemia, hemorrhages in the intestinal tract, and profuse bloody diarrhea, and eventual collapse and death. If the dog survived a first treatment, the subsequent injection of the same or smaller dose might produce much severer, though similar symptoms: "*An exceptionally vigorous dog received in a first injection* 0.1 *cc of a glycerinated extract without any symptom. Twenty days later, as it was in excellent condition, the same dose of* 0.1 *cc was reinjected. A few seconds afterwards, the animal presented considerable discomfort, with a difficult respiration; in continuation it walked with difficulty, lay down upon its flanks and presented diarrhea and vomited; the animal became unconscious and died after* 25 *minutes*". It appeared to RICHET, that instead of becoming protected or immunized by the first injection, the dog had developed a reverse condition to which the name of Anaphylaxis was applied: "*When the phenomenon had been solidly established from the experimental standpoint, M.* RICHET *decided to baptize it. I tried to persuade him of the inutility of creating a neologism, since there was already so many in the scientific literature, and especially as we had forgotten our Greek.-'You may be right', answered Richet, 'if the phenomenon we have discovered is only a rarity, but if it presents a certain general interest we have to have a name for it'. - At this moment he approached a small blackboard hidden under the stairs and asked me if I knew the Greek word for 'immunity', 'protection'. - No, I answered, I might have known it but I have forgotten.' - 'It is φυλαξις (phylaxis) and now let us affix a privative α (a)' - The resulting word 'aphylaxis' not being very euphonious we decided to adopt the word 'anaphylaxie' (anaphylaxis). At that moment we could not dream of the great value attached to this expression*". (PORTIER, 1952). When one considers the extraordinary amplitude given to this expression to indicate all kinds of accidents occurring during the process of immunization to such a great variety of antigenic materials, one has to accept the evidence that a considerable deviation from the initial meaning occurred in the course of time. According to RICHET, the word of anaphylaxis was proposed to indicate "*that many venoms display the remarkable capacity of increasing, instead of decreasing, the sensitivity of an organism to its action*". Therefore, in the mind of the discoverers of the phenomenon of anaphylaxis this concept was inseparable from the idea of a primary toxicity of the causative agent.

The demonstration that the phenomenon might be reproduced in the dog by the re-injection of non-toxic materials, such as serum proteins or egg-albumin, was done by ARTHUS (1909-10). By that time, it was already possible to describe the phenomenon in terms of an antigen x antibody interaction, since similar phenomena were regularly obtained in rabbits and guinea pigs with antigenic materials (ARTHUS, 1903; ARTHUS and BRETON, 1903; THEOBALD SMITH, 1906; OTTO, 1906,07; ROSENAU and ANDERSON, 1906 and many others). Also in human beings, the so-called serum sickness was explained on a basis of an interaction of horse serum with preformed circulating antibodies (PIRQUET and SCHICK, 1905). This situation had an enormous and decisive impact upon the earliest theories and nomenclature proposed to explain and connote the newly discovered phenomena. The simple interpretation identifying the "anaphylactic antibody" with precipitins (DOERR and RUSS, 1909) rendered unnecessary and cumbersome the terminology proposed by RICHET (1909-12) of formation of an "apotoxine" as a consequence of the interaction of the venom (actino-congestine) upon a hypothetical "toxogenine" formed by the previous injection of the toxic material. Other variants on the name of anaphylactic antibody such as "anaphylactin", "sensibilizine" or "allergin" became likewise obsolete (DALE, 1913).

B. Symptoms in dog's anaphylaxis

In 1910, BIEDL and KRAUS showed that the main symptom of anaphylaxis in the dog was a steep fall in the systemic blood pressure. The heart continued to beat, with an accelerated rhythm, while the blood accumulated in the peripheral vessels with a sharp decrease in the cardiac output. In 1910, PEARCE and EISENBREY pointed to stagnation of the blood in the liver and portal region, with reduction of volume of the kidneys and spleen. Electrocardiographic records made by EISENBREY and PEARCE (1912) and by ROBINSON and AUER (1913) indicated that there was no damage to the heart.

As early as 1910, MANWARING defined the liver of the dog as the main "shock organ" in anaphylaxis, since its exclusion from circulation by ligatures upon the thoracic aorta and caval vein just above the diaphragm prevented the precipitous fall of blood pressure, while ligatures upon the spleen, adrenals, stomach and intestinal segments had no appreciable effect on the outcome of anaphylactic shock. It was also demonstrated by VOEGTLIN and BERNHEIM (1911) and DENECKE (1914) that removal of the liver by an ECK fistula would prevent anaphylactic shock in the dog. Though, in more recent times, a typical anaphylactic shock was shown to be eventually elicited in the liverless dog (WATERS, MARKOWITZ and JAQUES, 1938), the importance of the liver as the main site of the anaphylactic reaction in this animal species could not be overshadowed. And here again, the similarity of the symptomatology of anaphylaxis with that obtained by an intravenous injection of histamine in the dog was pointed out by DALE (1920-29) as explaining anaphylaxis on the basis of a release of endogenous histamine from sensitized liver cells by contact with the antigen. Nonetheless, the final demonstration of a participation of histamine in dog anaphylaxis came much later as will be discussed below.

The predominant role played by the liver as the shock organ in the dog, was confirmed and extensively studied by WEIL (1912-17) who concluded that stagnation of blood in the portal region is quantitatively sufficient to explain the fall in blood pressure. No less than 61.5% of the total blood of a dog submitted to anaphylactic shock could be confined in the liver. From many necropsies, WEIL (1917) concluded: "*The condition of the liver dominates the pathological impression and presents a picture which is rarely, if ever seen under any other circumstances. The organ is tremendously swollen. Its color is intensively cyanotic. Upon section the cut surface bleeds freely*". The gastro-intestinal symptoms appeared to WEIL to be secondary to blood stagnation in the portal region. All attempts to demonstrate the release or formation of a mediator to explain the symptomatology of anaphylaxis in the dog, were unsuccessful. Even when massive quantities of blood were transferred from a dying animal to a normal one, it failed to reproduce in the latter the typical symptoms of anaphylaxis (WEIL, 1917).

The condition in which the liver is found in anaphylactic shock has always been taken as an example of the predominant participation of the smooth muscle sphincters of the suprahepatic veins, which would contract under the action of a mediator released *in loco*. In fact, the enormous increase in size of the liver of the dog, with stagnation of blood in the portal region, constitutes an excellent illustration of the truth contained in the theory of "strategic points" in the circulatory apparatus to explain species differences in several kinds of shock, such as anaphylactic, peptone, histamine and by bacterial toxins. The presence of sphincters of smooth muscle in the liver sinusoids and in the opening of the hepatic veins into the caval veins has been discussed in another Section (see Circulatory effects of histamine). The direct demonstration of the importance of the liver of the dog submitted to anaphylactic and peptone shock was given by the technique of injecting a plastic material (vinyl-acetate) into the hepatic vessels at the peak of the symptoms (THOMAS and ESSEX, 1949). A generalized constriction of the medium and larger veins could be visualized in confirmation of the idea that, among the common laboratory animals, the dog shows this peculiarity in the liver circulation.

On the other hand, the occurrence of such a predominant symptom of venous constriction in the liver of the dog would in itself indicate the participation of a smooth muscle stimulating substance released locally in spite of the failure of many early attempts to detect such a mediator in the circulating blood of dogs dying of anaphylaxis.

A first demonstration of the release of a mediator in anaphylaxis among dogs was presented by MANWARING et al. (1924, 1925) by transplanting the liver of a sensitized dog to the circulation of a normal one. When the antigen was injected, an increase in intracystic pressure and a fall in blood pressure in the normal (non sensitized) animal were observed.

I have always been puzzled by the lack of data in the literature trying to reproduce the above experiments by simply perfusing the isolated sensitized dog's liver with the antigen to detect free histamine and heparin in the perfusates. Actually, in a relatively recent publication, DALE (1953) revealed that he had tried it himself and failed to show any release of histamine *in vitro*, by perfusing the liver with the antigen. We had similar difficulties in perfusing the liver of the dog with Tyrode solution to which the antigen was added. With peptone also only traces of histamine can be released in perfusion experiments of the dog's liver, using Tyrode as vehicle. These negative results make the old experiments by MAUTNER and PICK (1915, 1922) showing a *Lebersperre* in experiments of liver perfusion with saline or Tyrode solution, difficult to understand. It is possible that in the experiments of the Viennese workers, the initial washing of the liver was not extensive enough to remove portions of blood which can be essential for the release of a smooth muscle stimulating substance. On the contrary, the success of MANWARINGS experiments depended upon having the liver abundantly perfused with the normal blood of the donor animal. The significance of these facts will be discussed later on. Nonetheless, we have to render homage to the correct biological intuition of MAUTNER and PICK attributing such a great importance to the circulatory spasm in the dog's liver to explain many kinds of shock, a concept which has been largerly confirmed by morphological and physiological observations (AREY and SIMONDS, 1920; JAFFÉ, 1924; DEAN and WEBB, 1924; AREY, 1941; THOMAS and ESSEX, 1949, and many others).

We had, however, to wait until the early thirties to have a convincing demonstration of the appearance of a histamine-like material in free form in the peripheral circulation of dogs submitted to anaphylactic shock.

Histamine: In 1932, DRAGSTEDT and GEBAUER-FUELNEGG identified histamine in the lymph of the thoracic duct in a dog submitted to anaphylactic shock. Later on, DRAGSTEDT (1940) described the genesis of these experiments: "*When the late* GEBAUER-FUELNEGG *and I began our work in* 1932, *we were aware that we would be called upon to traverse a cemetery of departed hopes. The circumstantial evidence indicating that the anaphylactic reaction was mediated by some toxin resembling histamine, was, however, so convincing that we were persuaded to look for incriminating evidence in spite of the many negative results in the literature*".

The reasons to look upon the lymph to demonstrate a release of histamine were the following: a) the obvious participation of the liver in the phenomenon; b) the increased flow of lymph in the thoracic ducts as shown previously by PETERSEN and LEVINSON (1923) and c) the demonstration by SIMONDS and BRANDES (1927) that removal of the liver stops the increased flow of lymph in the thoracic duct, indicating that the extra lymph appearing as a consequence of anaphylactic shock comes from the liver.

The material appearing in the lymph in these experiments was identified with histamine because it was dialysable, resisted boiling in acid medium, could be inactivated by coupling with sulfanilic acid and displayed the pharmacological activities typical of histamine (GEBAUER-FUELNEGG and DRAGSTEDT, 1932).

Later on, DRAGSTEDT and MEAD (1936,37) showed that a similar material appeared in the circulating blood immediately after the fall in blood pressure elicited by the antigen in sensitized dogs and also by the injection of peptone. Besides producing the typical pharmacological effects of histamine, the active material was destroyed by histaminase (DRAGSTEDT and MEAD, 1936,37).

By utilizing a specific method for histamine extraction from total blood or plasma, CODE (1939) confirmed the preliminary results by DRAGSTEDT and GEBAUER-FUELNEGG (1932), DRAGSTEDT and MEAD (1936) showing that during anaphylactic shock in guinea pigs and dogs, histamine appears in the circulating blood (see also OJERS et al., 1939). In the dog, the concentrations of histamine appearing in the blood at the maximum of the fall in arterial blood pressure, somehow paralleled the severity of the symptoms. In moderate shocks, with a rapidly recovering arterial blood pressure, the peaks of histamine did not go above the 0.2 μg per ml level; in the severest shocks, peaks of 0.5 to 1.0 μg per ml of histamine could be found. An example is given in Fig. 8.

Though in CODE's experiments, histamine, as such, could be identified in the circulating blood of dogs submitted to anaphylaxis, suggesting a correlation between its concentration and the intensity of the primary fall in arterial blood pressure, two important questions were left behind: a) the origin of this histamine, and b) the cause of death in those animals in which histamine had already disappeared long before the fatal outcome. The first question was soon answered by OJERS, HOLMES and DRAGSTEDT (1941) showing the considerable decrease of liver histamine when fragments taken before and after shock were compared for their histamine contents. In one experiment, the histamine content before the injection of the antigen was as high as 60 μg per gm. After the onset of the shock another fragment of the same liver showed a value as low as 6 μg/g. This reduction, calculated for the whole liver amounted to 2.3 mg of histamine. In other experiments in which the shock was particularly severe, the drops were of the order of 4.8 mg of histamine for the whole organ. These amounts were enough to explain the main symptoms, considering that, when released *in loco* in the proximity of the sphincters of the suprahepatic veins, the concentration of the released histamine would be maximal. Similar experiments with peptone indicated that in that kind of shock there also occurs a considerable drop of the histamine content in the liver of dogs (HOLMES, OJERS and DRAGSTEDT, 1941).

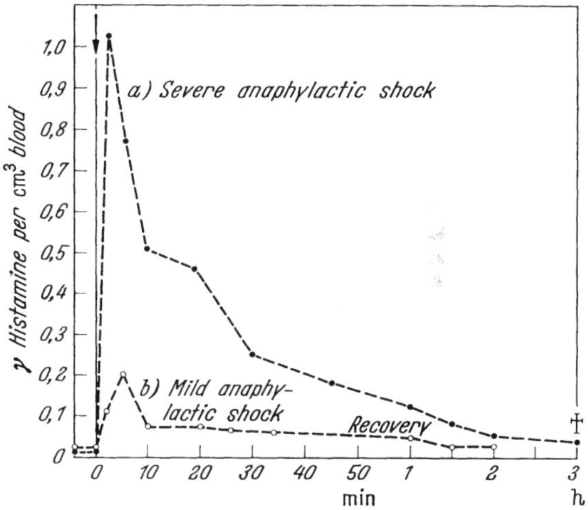

Fig. 8. Blood histamine changes during anaphylactic shock in unanesthetized dogs. At the arrow the antigen was given intravenously. *a* Severe reaction; by twenty minutes the animal was deep in shock; intravenous fluids and adrenaline were given but despite these death occurred just after the three hour mark. *b* Mild reaction; the animal recovered completely within two hours (according to CODE, 1939)

Though the major release of histamine in dog's anaphylaxis occurs from the liver, other stores of histamine, presumably in mast cells of the skin, the spleen and the ears are also strongly depleted (of more than 40 % of their previous content) in dogs sensitized to egg white and horse serum, following the challenge with the antigen (AKCASU and WEST, 1960). Serotonin (5-HT) was not released to any appreciable extent, in spite of the fact that this amine was present in the organs which reacted to the antigen with a large release of histamine (AKCASU and WEST, 1960).

The other question, in reference to why a certain percentage of animals die well after the blood histamine has returned to normal, remains unanswered even now. One might speculate that the enormous quantities of histamine flooding the liver and portal region might produce an irreversible damage upon the lining of the capillary vessels with continuous extravation of plasma fluid, micro-hemorrhages through the intestinal walls with a generalized involvement of the capillary bed throughout the body. Other factors, as mechanical obstruction of the liver capillaries with microthrombi of leukocytes and platelets might create in the liver of the dog a situation similar to that of the lung of the rabbit in anaphylaxis (ROCHA E SILVA, 1950). As a matter of fact, in a small percentage of animals dying of anaphylactic shock or by extracts of Ascaris, only discrete or small concentrations of histamine could be detected in the circulating blood (CODE, 1939; ROCHA E SILVA and GRAÑA, 1946 a; ROCHA E SILVA et al. 1946 c). It is understandable that histamine is by no means the only factor involved and it can, at most, constitute the trigger factor to localize in the liver, and therefore in the whole splanchnic area, stagnation of blood and vascular (venules) and capillary permeation further aggravated by other factors such as the mechanical plugging and local disintegration of the blood elements. This mechanical plugging of capillaries, first seen in the rabbit's anaphylaxis, might constitute a basic phenomenon in anaphylaxis in all species, including human allergy. The fact that, even after histamine, micro-emboli could be found in the circulation of other organs in the rabbit and the guinea pig and directly observed in the spiral ligament of the guinea pig's cochlea (BURRAGE and IRWIN, 1953; BURRAGE et al., 1954; IRWIN, WEILLE and BURRAGE, 1955) precludes the idea that formation of an antigen-antibody precipitate is a condition *sine qua non* of the plugging of capillaries by micro-emboli in these kinds of shock.

In 1946, we had the opportunity of studying, with the late DR. GRAÑA, the mechanism by which ASCARIS extracts *(Ascaris suum)* produce an extremely severe kind of shock in the normal dog. Since dogs are invariably infested with related worms and since it has been observed the occurrence of crossed sensitization to helminths (BRUNNER et al,. 1944) and given the extraordinary similarity between the shock produced by ASCARIS extracts and that by the antigen in a sensitized dog, we thought that the underlying mechanism in this kind of shock should be the same as in true anaphylaxis (ROCHA E SILVA et al., 1946 c). Therefore, we did not call it anaphylactoid, but "anaphylaxis-like" to indicate this conceptual difference with other kinds of shock, as those produced by peptone or bacterial toxins.

The advantage of working with *Ascaris suum* extracts was the facility of finding the worms, and the extreme severity of the reactions produced in a large percentage of normal dogs, abbreviating therefore the experiment by excluding the phase of preparation of the animal. Furthermore, with the ASCARIS extracts, many of the contingencies of the anaphylactic shock would be excluded, and the experiments could be done in a more reproducible way.

In some animals, the injection of extracts corresponding to a small fraction of a single worm, produced dramatic events, such as vomiting, bloody diarrhea, collapse and eventually death of the animal. A more detailed analysis indicated that the liver and the portal region were remarkably filled with dark blood and at a direct inspection of the opened abdomen the liver increased in size while the blood stagnated in the whole portal region. When pieces of liver were taken before and at 10 to 20 minutes after the injection of the ASCARIS extracts, reductions of the order of 20 μg of histamine per gram of liver were observed. Calculated for the whole organ, these variations would indicate a discharge of histamine from the liver of the order of milligrams, that is, amounts comparable to those obtained by HOLMES, OJERS and DRAGSTEDT, (1941) in true anaphylaxis. Furthermore, by taking samples of blood stagnated in the portal system and comparing their histamine contents with those in the femoral vein blood, enormous differences were found. (Fig. 9). When the peripheral histamine had already returned to normal levels, the portal vein histamine was still high (ROCHA E SILVA and GRAÑA, 1946 a).

Another feature of this kind of shock is the extreme incoagulability of the blood because of the release of large amounts of heparin from the liver, a situation identical to what occurs in anaphylaxis, as we are going to discuss below. The participation of the liver in the shock by ASCARIS extracts was confirmed by GRAÑA et al., 1947 and THOMAS and ESSEX, 1949.

Recently, BERALDO et al. (1961) adduced evidence to show that the release of histamine by ASCARIS extracts in the guinea pig could be ascribed to a sensitization phenomenon. The subject will be discussed in full in another Section

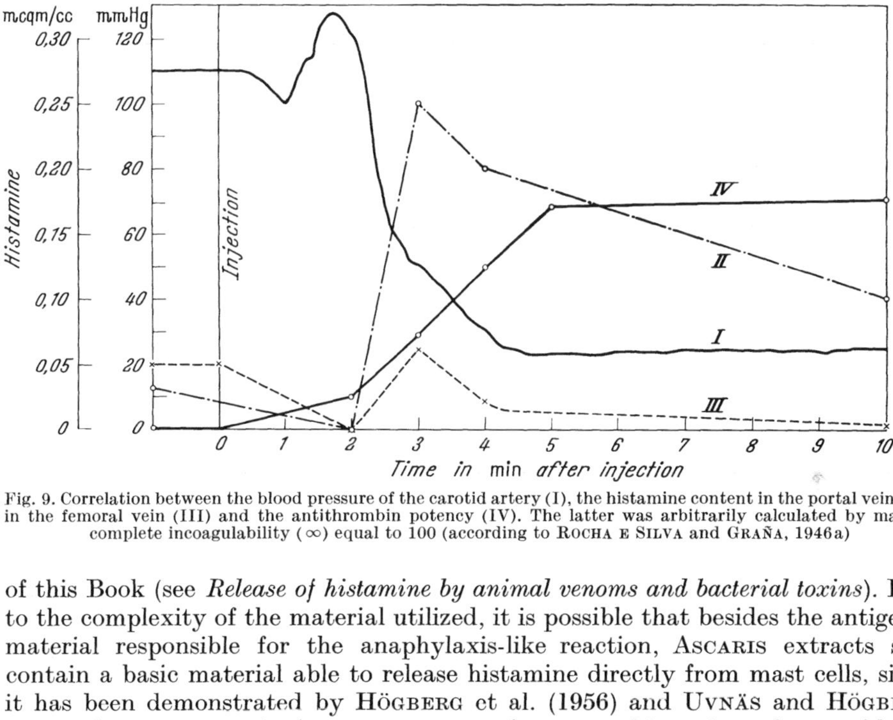

Fig. 9. Correlation between the blood pressure of the carotid artery (I), the histamine content in the portal vein (II), in the femoral vein (III) and the antithrombin potency (IV). The latter was arbitrarily calculated by making complete incoagulability (∞) equal to 100 (according to ROCHA E SILVA and GRAÑA, 1946a)

of this Book (see *Release of histamine by animal venoms and bacterial toxins*). Due to the complexity of the material utilized, it is possible that besides the antigenic material responsible for the anaphylaxis-like reaction, ASCARIS extracts still contain a basic material able to release histamine directly from mast cells, since it has been demonstrated by HÖGBERG et al. (1956) and UVNÄS and HÖGBERG (1958) the occurrence in ASCARIS extracts of a potent histamine releaser of basic character.

Whatever be the ultimate mechanism by which ASCARIS extracts release histamine from dog's liver, they were utilized in our laboratory as tools to study some of the conditions of this release. For comparison, we have utilized animals sensitized to horse serum. We have also compared it with the shock produced by peptone. Because enormous amounts of histamine appeared to be released *in vivo* from a single organ, we decided to do experiments of liver perfusion, under varying experimental conditions, starting with Tyrode solution. Injecting the ASCARIS extracts after a prolonged perfusion with Tyrode caused no obvious release of histamine or heparin. By using defibrinated blood (kept unclotted by citrate), small but detectable amounts of histamine could be obtained, but the amounts were surprisingly and dispairingly small. When citrated blood was utilized a sharp reduction of the WBC and platelet counts were observed (ROCHA E SILVA et al., 1946 c) and the volume of the liver somehow increased in size.

The blood elements were found forming clumps inside of the vessels of the organs, and microthrombi of platelets with few leukocytes were easily detected by staining, with Giemsa, smears of pieces of liver taken immediately after the injection of the extracts. The situation was impressively similar to that seen in the lungs of the rabbit following the injection of the antigen. Those clumps, in the experiments where no histamine or heparin appeared, were stable and could be easily detected by a Giemsa staining of smears obtained by impressions of pieces of liver.

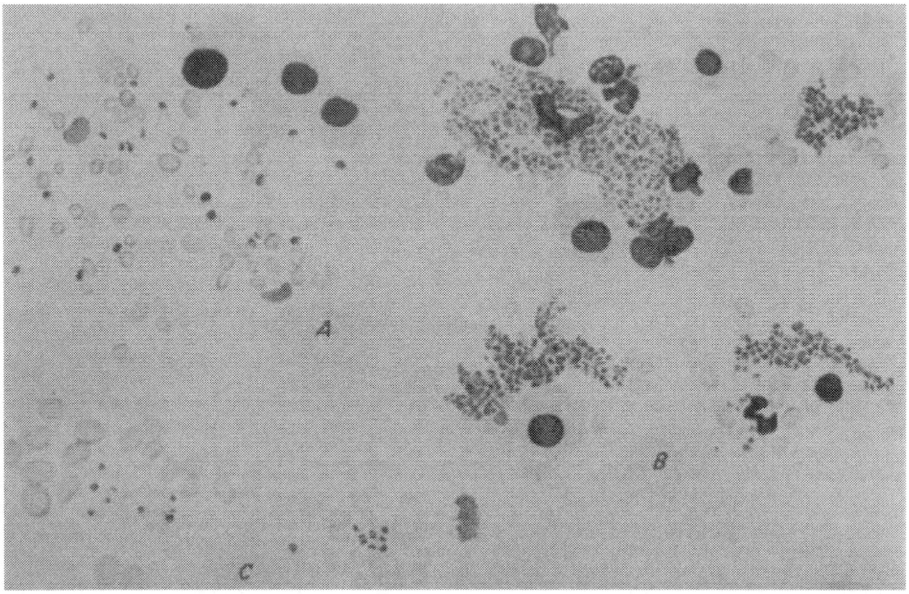

Fig. 10. *A* Smear of a piece of normal dog liver, taken directly into a 3.8% solution of sodium citrate. Stained by May-Grünwald. Note the homogeneous distribution of platelets among red cells. (450 × enlargement). *B* Impression over slide of a piece of liver of a dog submitted to shock by injection of the antigen from Ascaris lumbricoides. Enormous clumps of platelets are seen in the slides, made with a fragment of liver taken before two minutes after the injection of the shocking agent (450 × enlargement). *C* Impression over slide of a piece of the liver of the same animal, ten minutes after the injection of the Ascaris antigen. The clumps previously seen, are entirely desintegrated and in their place only remains of platelets or ghosts of clumps can be seen (450 × enlargement) (according to Rocha e Silva, 1950)

The same technique of making smears of liver fragments taken before and after the onset of shock was applied to the intact dog in *in vivo* experiments. Impressions on slices stained with Giemsa showed considerable clumping of leukocytes and platelets immediately after the injection of the extracts. To a certain extent in correlation with the discharge of histamine and heparin, these clumps or microthrombi would disintegrate in a sort of explosive way, a few minutes after the onset of the shock, coinciding with the appearance of a peak of histamine and heparin in the circulating blood or in the samples taken from the portal vein (Rocha e Silva et al., 1946 c; Rocha e Silva, 1950).

Fig. 10 shows the microthrombi in three stages of the phenomenon, immediately after the injection of the agent (antigen or Ascaris extracts), at the moment when they start to disintegrate, and some time after, when the blood pressure started to return to normal.

These experiments combined with the failure of obtaining but traces of histamine from the isolated dog liver when perfused with Tyrode solution or citrated blood, appeared to indicate that something was still lacking in our perfusion experiments to be comparable to the *in vivo* conditions. In Toronto, in 1946, we had the opportunity of utilizing the newly developed technique of keeping the blood for perfusion in the most natural conditions possible, using recipients covered with silicone to collect the blood without any anti-coagulant. By injecting peptone together with this silicone protected blood, enormous amounts of histamine and heparin could be released in one stroke (Fig. 11) (ROCHA E SILVA, SCROGGIE, FIDLAR and JAQUES, 1947). Later on, SCROGGIE and JAQUES (1949) succeeded in releasing histamine and heparin from the liver of a sensitized

Table 3. *Attempted comparison of quantities of histamine and heparin released by antigen in vivo and the isolated liver* (according to SCROGGIE and JAQUES, 1949)

Experiment	Number of dog	Estimated blood volume	% Histamine release	% Heparin release*
Perfusion of liver *in situ* with antigen	70	1860	390	73
	66	1090	54	27
Perfusion of *isolated* liver				
Antigen in blood	84	1200	32	1.4
	79	1250	25	3.8
	88	580	26	—
	78	530	27	2.5
	83	1450	5.0	2.2
	87	1290	4.1	0
Antigen in Tyrode's	89	840	84	17
	101	780	42	23.5

$$* \text{ Histamine (heparin) release} = \frac{\text{measured release}}{\text{estimated release}} \times 100.$$

Measured release = actual assay value for histamine or heparin.

Estimated release = value obtained by multiplying the average maximal level of histamine (0.29 μg/ml) or heparin (0.024 mg/ml in the blood during severe anaphylactic shock in the intact dog by the blood volume of the dog from which the liver was removed.

animal by the injection of the antigen, keeping the liver in the best possible condition, *in situ* as seen in Table 3.

The conditions of SCROGGIE and JAQUES' experiments were different from ours, since we did perfuse part of the liver after thorough washing with Tyrode solution. It is possible that in the experiments by SCROGGIE and JAQUES, some collections of intact blood might have remained in the *in situ* preparation. On the other hand, in their experiments, oxygenation of the perfusing fluid was intentionally maintained at high levels. This problem, however, is still open to further experimentation.

Heparin: The mechanism by which histamine is liberated from the liver of the dog can only be understood by analysing other features of the shock in this species of animals. One of the most characteristic events of anaphylaxis in the dog is the increase in clotting time of the blood. ARTHUS (1909) and BIEDL and KRAUS (1910) were the first to indicate this incoagulability of the blood during anaphylactic shock in the dog. HOWELL (1925) assumed that this incoagulability of the blood was due to an increase of the anti-thrombin titer. This idea was further substantiated by experiments of QUICK (1936) on the shock produced by peptone. A deficiency in fibrinogen, platelets and prothrombin as a cause of the incoagulability was suggested by EAGLE, JOHNSTON and RAVDIN (1937). The final demonstration that heparin released from the liver is the factor responsible for the blood incoagulability in anaphylactic and peptone shock was given almost simultaneously by WATERS, MARKOWITZ and JAQUES (1938) using the protamine test for estimating heparin in the blood, and by the histochemical evidence presented by WILANDER (1938) identifying the granules of EHRLICH's mast cells, in the liver of the dog, as depots of heparin. After peptone (WILANDER, 1938) and anaphylactic shock (JAQUES and WATERS, 1941) these granules in the liver become rarer and paler.

Liberation of histamine in anaphylactic shock in the dog appears to be correlated with the release of heparin. Although there is no strict parallelism, it seems likely that the release of both substances depends upon an analogous mechanism. When no heparin appears in the blood, it is extremely difficult to find any increase in blood histamine. There is, however, a difference in the time of disappearance of both agents. Heparin being less diffusible is retained longer in the circulation and therefore long after histamine has disappeared from the peripheral blood, it still remains incoagulable. On the other hand, the peak of heparin in the blood appears a little later than that of histamine (JAQUES and WATERS, 1941). When the experiment is done *in vitro*, with the isolated liver perfused with silicone protected blood plus peptone, both peaks coincide, as shown in Fig. 11. This striking coincidence is now understandable on the basis that not only heparin but also histamine comes from depots in the liver mast cells (See RILEY and WEST, Chapter 1, Section E).

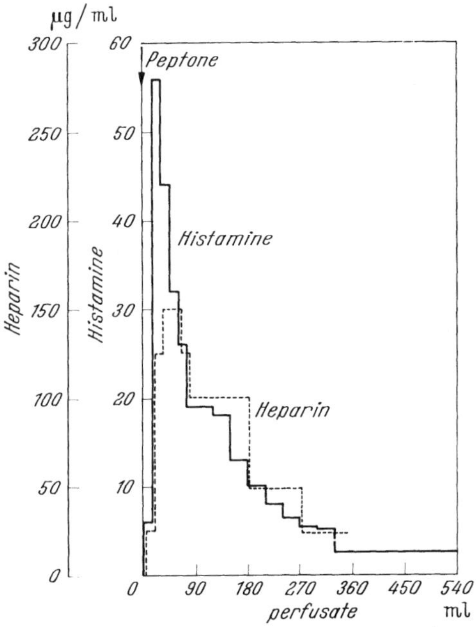

Fig. 11. Liver perfusion (dog) with silicone blood + peptone. Discharge of histamine and heparin after passage of the blood through the liver. Note the sharp peak (56 gµ histamine per ml of perfusate) occurring before the first 50 ml of blood passed through (according to ROCHA E SILVA et al., 1947)

Mast cells: A direct approach to the problem of histamine and heparin release from dog liver mast cells, was presented by GROSSBERG and GARCIA-AROCHA (1954), and related *in extenso* by MACINTOSH (1956). Though a release of histamine was easily obtained by basic compounds such as 48/80, diaminodecane (DA_{10}), propamidine, di-isothionate, toluidine blue and some basic proteins like clupein sulphate, protamine or the basic polypeptide polylysine (n=15), no histamine or heparin releasing activity could be obtained from liver particles obtained from sensitized animals by *in vitro* addition of the antigen or after passive sensitization of the particles themselves. With anaphylatoxin no success was obtained either (GROSSBERG and GARCIA-AROCHA, 1954). Since the problem of the release by basic compounds is treated in another section of this book, only a brief mention is needed here of the interesting experiments by GARCIA-AROCHA and collaborators in Montreal.

The participation of mast cells in the intact dog submitted to anaphylaxis and/or the injection of basic releasers (compound 48/80 and d-tubocurarine) was studied by AKCASU and WEST (1960). Widespread damage to mast cells in the liver, the spleen and the skin, could be observed in these conditions. If a dose of 48/80 (1 mg/kg intravenously) was given under the protection of mepyramine maleate (5 mg/kg) considerable depletion of the histamine stores apparently had a protective effect against the challenge with horse serum, up to 12 to 13 days after the injection of the chemical releaser. In order to obtain a typical shock with release of histamine after a first injection of 48/80, an interval of 17 to 19 days was needed, though a second injection of 48/80, after 15 to 16 days will produce a maximum release of histamine. These results indicated the need of a larger time interval for the production of anaphylactic shock, after depletion of the histamine stores by the first injection of 48/80, and were interpreted as indicating a necessity of replenishment of the newly formed mast cells, not only of its histamine stores, but also of a supply of antibody which could take longer to migrate inside the newly formed mast cells. On the other hand, the mast cells of the liver appeared more vulnerable to the action of the antigen than those present in the skin and spleen, thus confirming the predominant role of the liver in dog's anaphylaxis. In no case was there any substantial or detectable release of serotonin (AKCASU and WEST, 1960).

Other mediators: In no other species has the demonstration of a release of proteolytic (or fibrinolytic) activity been evidenced so conclusively as in the dog submitted to anaphylaxis and related shocks (peptone, ASCARIS extracts, bacterial toxins, etc.). As early as 1904, NOLF (1938,46) performed a clear cut experiment to show fibrinolysis in peptone shock. If, immediately after the injection of peptone and before the blood becomes incoagulable, the liver is temporarily removed from the circulation by simply compressing the hepatic vessels, the blood will coagulate; but shortly afterwards, the clot will redissolve. In order to observe this fibrinolytic effect we have devised the technique of adding increasing concentrations of protamine to blood samples taken immediately and at certain intervals after shock (ROCHA E SILVA, ANDRADE and TEIXEIRA, 1946 b). As the protamine neutralizes the heparin, which is released during anaphylactic and peptone shock, the clot is formed, but if the mixture is incubated for a few hours, it will redissolve, indicating the release or activation of the fibrinolytic system of the blood. The phenomenon of activation of this system could be correlated with the intensity of shock and shows the phenomenon of decreased intensity (desensitization) when the injection of the antigen or peptone is repeated several times. Table 4 shows a typical result obtained with the "protamine fibrinolytic test."

A conspicuous fibrinolytic effect can be observed, without addition of protamine, if the circulation of the animal submitted to the peptone injection is confined to the upper part of the body (thoracic animal) by simply clamping aorta and inferior vena cava just above the diaphragm (NOLF, 1946; ROCHA E SILVA et al., 1946 a). This would indicate that the activator of the fibrinolytic system derives probably from the lung. As fibrinolysis observed in such conditions (thoracic animal) is extremely rapid to occur, it has been suggested that the presence of heparin, even when blocked by an optimal amount of protamine, might constitute a disturbing factor in the redissolution of the coagulum.

It is difficult to assess the importance of the fibrinolytic enzyme for the severity of anaphylactic and peptone shock. Fibrinolysin (or plasmin) can produce by itself a kind of shock which has been attributed to the formation of an intermediary named *vascularin* by GUEST et al. (1947). However, the participation of vasoactive polypeptides released under those circumstances cannot be ruled out (BACK et al., 1963). In 1950 BERALDO demonstrated that a bradykinin-like material is formed *in vivo* and *in vitro*, by anaphylaxis and peptone. Likewise, the treatment of dog's plasma *in vitro* with streptokinase, a material known to activate plasmin, releases bradykinin. However, the maximum of bradykinin recovered *in vivo*, from the blood of dogs submitted to anaphylactic shock, was obtained at a later stage when the blood pressure started to return to normal. Experiments of estimation of bradykininogen in our laboratory are in progress.

Table 4. *Estimation of heparin and fibrinolysis in the blood samples of a dog subjected to peptone shock* (according to ROCHA E SILVA, ANDRADE and TEIXEIRA, 1946b)

Amounts of protamine added γ/0.5 ml)	Blood samples after several intervals following the injection of 300 mgm of peptone per kilo of body-weight:							
	Before	Ist injection				2nd injection		3rd injection
	I	II	III	IV	VI	VII	VIII	IX
100 clot. time (min)	10	12	13	10	8	20	15	10
100 fibrinolysis	0	++++	++++	++++	0	++++	0	0
50 clot. time min)	8	11	12	8	7	14	9	10
50 fibrinolysis	0	+++	++++	+++	0	++	0	0
25 clot. time (min)	5	8	10	7	9	13	7	8
25 fibrinolysis	0	+	+++	+++	0	0	0	0
10 clot. time (min)	5	6	11	9	10	12	5	5
10 fibrinolysis	0	++	+++	0	0	0	0	0
0 clot. time (min)	4	∞	∞	∞	∞	∞	∞	∞
0 fibrinolysis	0	—	—	—	—	—	—	—

++++, Total fibrinolysis in less than 1 hr.; +++, total fibrinolysis in less than 2 hr.; ++, total fibrinolysis in less than 3 hr; +, partial fibrinolysis; 0, no fibrinolysis for at least 24 hours. The minimum clotting time indicates the optimum amount of protamine and therefore the amount of heparin present in the blood samples.

VI. Other species

Rats. Some aspects of the relationship between histamine and anaphylaxis in the rat, such as the effect of adrenalectomy and sensitization with *Pertussis* vaccine, have been already studied in another Chapter (Action upon the Circulatory Apparatus, Chapter 2, Section E) and will be further discussed by MOTA (Chapter 3, Section F).

By using adjuvants, such as alum-precipitated horse serum or *Bordetella* (*haemophilus*) *pertussis* vaccine, MOTA (1957,58 b) has demonstrated an increase in plasma histamine following anaphylactic shock. Likewise, MARUNO (1958) obtained small increases in the whole blood of rats submitted to anaphylactic shock with horse serum. These findings were confirmed by CODE et al. (1961) by estimating histamine in whole blood and plasma during anaphylaxis in rats sensitized to crystalline ovoalbumin + suspension of *Pertussis* vaccine or with horse serum given on four successive days after adrenalectomy (without *Pertussis*). Blood was withdrawn by cardiac puncture, or under pentobarbital sodium anesthesia, through a polyethylene tubing inserted into the superior vena cava. In all cases the concentration of histamine rose significantly during anaphylactic shock from normal levels of 0.078 μg/ml (vena cava blood) or 0.136 μg/ml (cardiac puncture) to mean values of 0.733 μg/ml to 1.950 μg/ml when challenged with ovoalbumin or to 0.680 μg/ml in the adrenalectomized animals challenged with horse serum. Fig. 12 gives a time course of the changes of total blood histamine in control and sensitized rats submitted to anaphylactic shock.

The increases in plasma histamine of sensitized rats challenged with egg albumin were even more conspicuous, from a mean value of 0.046 μg/ml to 2.360 μg/ml (CODE et al. 1961).

The exact source of the histamine liberated during anaphylactic shock in rats is not known. BROCKLEHURST (1960) did not detect hitamin e in the perfusates of lung, liver or hind quarters of sensitized rats after addition of the antigen to the perfusion system. Since damage to mast cells can be detected in the omentum of sensitized rats submitted to anaphylaxis (MOTA, 1957,58 b; HÖGBERG and UVNÄS, 1960) the abdominal organs appear to be the most likely alternative. The small bowel shows striking vascular changes during anaphylaxis (CODE et al., 1961).

The mast cells normally present in the serous tissue of the peritoneal cavity of rats are destroyed by an intraperitoneal injection of distilled water. A similar destruction of mast cells can be obtained by giving normal rats intraperitoneally, rabbit anti-egg albumin serum and 3 hours later an intravenous injection of the antigen. If Evans blue is administered simultaneously with the antigen, a blue coloration of the peritoneum can be observed indicating increased vascular

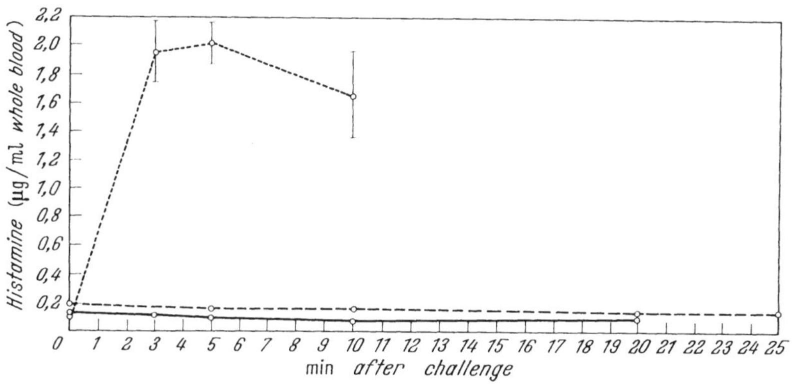

Fig. 12. The concentration of histamine in the blood of sensitized and unsensitized rats after challenge by intravenous injection of a solution of antigen or of 0.9% NaCl solution; blood withdrawn by venous catheter. —— Sensitized, saline-challenged; — — — unsensitized, antigen-challenged; ------ sensitized, antigen-challenged. Vertical bars show 2 × S.E. of mean (according to Code et al., 1961)

(capillary) permeability. This coloration was diminished or absent in the peritoneum of rats which were similarly sensitized and challenged but were preactivated with distilled water. Similar results were obtained when the rat skin was used as the site of antigen-antibody reaction after destruction of the mast cell population by an intradermal injection of distilled water (DRAPER and SMITH, 1961). From those experiments one might infer that rupture of mast cells can be of primary importance to initiate the vascular changes which follow the antigen-antibody reaction.

Opinions diverge on the real significance of the release of histamine to explain the symptoms of anaphylaxis in this species of animals. In rats, with their skin stores of histamine depleted by a previous treatment with 48/80, the anaphylactic reaction was strongly reduced, according to MOTA, though when Polymyxin B and X-ray irradiation were employed to deplete the histamine stores, the anaphylactic reaction was unchanged (SANYAL and WEST, 1958 a). Furthermore, the so-called "passive cutaneous anaphylaxis" (PCA) was not even diminished by depletion of the skin histamine by a previous treatment with 48/80 (ROCHA E SILVA and ROTHSCHILD, 1955) nor by an intensive treatment with anti-histaminics (BROCKLEHURST et al., 1955,60), though a partial depletion of the anaphylatoxin percursor (pro-anaphylatoxin) in the circulating blood by injection of agar and starch or dextran will prevent the onset of PCA (ROCHA E SILVA and ROTHSCHILD, 1955). The same is true as regards complement in the circulating blood (BIER et al., 1955). Apparently, other mediators are preponderant in producing tissue changes leading to PCA in rats. This question was mentioned previously and will be discussed more extensively by GIERTZ and HAHN (Chapter 3, Section E).

Recently RAPP (1961) has described the release of a slow reacting substance (SRS) during anaphylaxis in the peritoneal cavity of rats, and BROCKLEHURST and LAHIRI (1962) found an increase of free bradykinin in the blood of rats submitted to anaphylactic shock.

Mice. Anaphylaxis in mice is not influenced by antihistaminics. As mice are so insensitive to histamine, it is doubtful whether a simple release of histamine might explain the lethal effect after anaphylaxis. It is true that a previous treatment of the animals with the *Pertussis* vaccine increases both their susceptibility to anaphylaxis and to histamine. However, the toxicity of serotonin (5-HT) is also enhanced by this treatment. Adrenalectomized mice, like *Pertussis* treated animals become more sensitive to histamine and anaphylaxis. Cortisone and other adrenal steroids protect *H. Pertussis*-treated animals from fatal anaphylaxis, from histamine and from serotonin. It might be thought that *Pertussis* vaccine induces, in mice and rats, changes mimicking removal of the adrenals. However, increased susceptibility of mice to histamine can be observed in animals with normal adrenal glands or unimpaired adrenal function. These points have been already discussed in Chapter 2, Section E (Circulatory Effects of Histamine).

Participation of serotonin (5-HT) to explain the SCHULTZ-DALE reaction in the isolated uterus of the mouse, which is insensitive to histamine, was postulated by FINK (1956). There is a general acceptance that some of the manifestations of anaphylaxis in rodents might be due to a release of serotonin (5-HT) though the proofs are only circumstantial. Some evidences are against it, as for instance the participation of serotonin in the uterus contraction *in vitro*. In spite of the fact that the anaphylactic reaction is entirely blocked by minute doses of antiserotonin agents such as LSD, the alleged mediator (5-HT) was not found in the uterus of the mice (UDENFRIEND and WAALKES, 1959).

Other species. References on the participation of histamine in anaphylaxis in the monkey (BROCKLEHURST, 1960), the horse and the calf (CODE and HESTER, 1939) and the fowl (LECOMTE and BEAUMARIAGE, 1956,58) are given in the Bibliography. See also SANYAL and WEST, 1958 b.

References

ABELL, R. G., and H. P. SCHENCK: Microscopic observations on the behavior of living blood vessels of the rabbit during the reaction of anaphylaxis. J. Immunol. **34**, 195 (1938).

ACKERMANN, D., u. F. KUTSCHER: Die physiologische Wirkung einer Secalebase und des Imidazolyläthylamins. Z. Biol. **54**, 387 (1910).

AIRILA, Y.: Über die Ursache der tödlichen Blutdrucksenkung im akuten anaphylaktischen Schock beim Kaninchen. Skand. Arch. Physiol. **31**, 388 (1914).

AKCASU, A., and G. B. WEST: Anaphylaxis in the dog. Int. Arch. Allergy **16**, 326 (1960).

ANDERSON, J. F., and W. H. SCHULTZ: The cause of serum anaphylactic shock and some methods of alleviating it. Proc. Soc. exp. Biol. (N. Y.) **7**, 32 (1909—1910).

ANDRUS, E. C., and H. B. WILCOX: Effects of anaphylaxis upon coronary arteries in the isolated heart. J. exp. Med. **69**, 545 (1939).

ANTOPOL, W., and C. P. CHRYSSANTHOU: Possible significance of bradykinin in Shwartzman and related phenomena. Ann. N. Y. Acad. Sci. **104**, 346 (1963).

AREY, L. B.: Throttling veins in livers of certain mammals. Anat. Rec. **81**, 21 (1941).

—, and J. P. SIMONDS: The relation of smooth muscle in the hepatic veins to shock phenomena. Anat. Rec. **18**, 219 (1920).

ARONSON, J. D.: Tissue culture studies on the relation of the tubercullin reactions to anaphylaxis and the Arthus phenomenon. J. Immunol. **25**, 1 (1933).

ARTHUS, M.: Injections répétées de sérum de cheval chez le lapin. C. R. Soc. Biol. (Paris) **40**, 817 (1903).

— La séro-anaphylaxie du lapin. Arch. int. Physiol. **7**, 471 (1909).

ARTHUS, M.: La séro-anaphylaxie du chien. Arch. int. Physiol. **9**, 179(1910).
— De l'Anaphylaxie à l'Immunité. Paris: Masson et Cie. 1921.
—, et M. BRETON: Lésions cutanées produites par les injections de sérum de cheval chez le lapin anaphylactisé. C. R. Soc. Biol. (Paris) **55**, 1478 (1903).
AUER, J.: The effect of vagus section upon anaphylaxis in guinea pigs. J. exp. Med. **12**, 638 (1910).
— Local autoinoculation of the sensitized organism with foreign proteins as a cause of abnormal reactions. J. exp. Med. **32**, 427 (1920).
—, and P. A. LEWIS: The physiology of the immediate reaction of anaphylaxis in the guinea pig. J. exp. Med. **12**, 151 (1910).
AUSTEN, K. F., and W. E. BROCKLEHURST: Inhibition of the anaphylactic release of histamine from chopped guinea pig lung by chymotrypsin substrates and inhibitors. Nature (Lond.) **186**, 866 (1960).
— — Anaphylaxis in chopped guinea pig lung. I. Effect of peptidase substrates and inhibitors. J. exp. Med. **113**, 521 (1961a).
— — II. Enhancement of the anaphylactic release of histamine and slow reacting substance by certain dibasic acids and inhibition by dibasic fatty acids. J. exp. Med. **113**, 541 (1961b).
— — Anaphylaxis in chopped guinea pig lung. III. Effect of carbon monoxide, cyanide salicylaldoxime, and ionic strength. J. exp. Med. **114**, 29 (1961c).
—, and J. H. HUMPHREY: Release of histamine from rat peritoneal mast cells by antibody against rat-γ-globulin. J. Physiol. (Lond.) **158**, 37 P (1961).
BACK, N., P. S. GUTH, and A. E. MUNSON: On the relationship between plasmin and kinin. N. Y. Acad. Sci. **104**, 53 (1963).
BALLY, L. H.: Anaphylaxis. IX. Physiological studies of the hypersensitive rabbit. J. Immunol. **17**, 223 (1929).
BARBARO, J. F.: The release of histamine from rabbit platelets by means of antigen-antibody precipitates. I. The participation of the immune complex in histamine release. J. Immunol. **86**, 369 (1961).
— The release of histamine from rabbit platelets by means of antigen-antibody precipitates. II. The role of plasma in the release of histamine. J. Immunol. **86**, 377 (1961).
— The release of histamine from rabbit platelets by means of antigen-antibody precipitates. Fed. Proc. **21**, 273 (1962).
BARTOSCH, R.: Über die Herkunft des Histamins bei der Anaphylaxie des Meerschweinchens. Klin. Wschr. **1**, 307 (1935).
— W. FELDBERG u. E. NAGEL: Das Freiwerden eines histaminähnlichen Stoffes bei der Anaphylaxie des Meerschweinchens. Pflügers Arch. ges. Physiol. **230**, 129 (1932).
— — — Versuche über das Freiwerden eines histaminähnlichen Stoffes aus der durchströmten Lunge sensibilisierter Meerschweinchen. Pflügers Arch. ges. Physiol. **231**, 616 (1933).
BENACERRAF, B., and E. E. FISCHEL: Effect of phenergan (N-dimethyl-amino-2-propyl-1. Thiodiphenylamine, 3277 RP) on the Arthus reaction in rabbits. Proc. Soc. exp. Biol. (N.Y.) **71**, 349 (1949).
—, and E. A. KABAT: A quantitative study of the Arthus phenomenon induced passively in the guinea pig. J. Immunol. **64**, 1 (1950).
BENDER, M. B.: The reaction of the smooth muscle of the denervated iris in anaphylaxis. A comparative study in the guinea pig, rabbit, dog, cat and monkey. J. Immunol. **47**, 483 (1943).
BENDITT, E. P., and M. ARASE: An enzyme in mast cells with properties like chymotrypsin. J. exp. Med. **110**, 451 (1959).
BERALDO, W. T.: Formation of bradykinin in anaphylactic and peptone shock. Amer. J. Physiol. **163**, 283 (1950).
— W. DIAS DA SILVA, and J. PUDLES: Antigenic properties of purified fractions from Ascaris Lumbricoides var. summ on naturally sensitized guinea pig. Brit. J. Pharmacol. **17**, 236 (1961).
BESREDKA, A.: Anaphylatoxine et anaphylaxie. Ann. Inst. Pasteur **34**, 334 (1920).
— H. STRÖBEL et F. JUPILLE: Anaphylatoxine, peptoxine et peptone dans leurs rapports avec l'anaphylaxie. Ann. Inst. Pasteur **27**, 185 (1913).
BEST, C. H., H. H. DALE, H. W. DUDLEY, and W. V. THORPE: The nature of the vasodilator constituents of certain tissue extracts. J. Physiol. (Lond.) **62**, 397 (1927).
BHOOLA, K. D., J. D. CALLE, and M. SCHACHTER: The effect of bradykinin, serum kallikrein and other endogenous substances on capillary permeability in the guinea pig. J. Physiol. (Lond.) **152**, 75 (1960).
BIEDL, A., u. R. KRAUS: Experimentelle Studien über Anaphylaxie. Wien. Klin. Wschr. **22**, 363 (1909).
— — Experimentelle Studien über Anaphylaxie. Wien. Klin. Wschr. **23**, 385 (1910).

BIER, O., and M. ROCHA E SILVA: Histamine as the primary cause of the increased capillary permeability in inflammation. Proc. III. Intern. Congr. Microbiol., New York, p. 767 (1939a).
— — Untersuchungen über Entzündung. I. Mechanismus der Erhöhung der Capillarpermeabilität bei der Entzündung, mit besonderer Berücksichtigung der Rolle des Histamins. Virchows Arch. path. Anat. **303**, 325 (1939b).
— M. SIQUEIRA, and A. G. OSLER: Studies on mechanism of hypersensitivity phenomena; effect of *in vivo* antigen-antibody reactions on passive cutaneous anaphylaxis in rat. Int. Arch. Allergy **7**, 1 (1955).
BIOZZI, G., G. MENÉ et Z. OVARY: L'histamine et la granulopexie de l'endothélium vasculaire. Rev. Immunol. (Paris) **12**, 320 (1948).
BORDET, J.: Le méchanisme d'anaphylaxie. C. R. Soc. Biol. (Paris) **74**, 225 (1913).
— Gélose et anaphylatoxine. C. R. Soc. Biol. (Paris) **74**, 877 (1913).
BOVET, D., et A. M. STAUB: Action protectrice des éthers phénoliques au cours de l'intoxication histaminique. C. R. Soc. Biol. (Paris) **124**, 547 (1937).
—, et F. WALTHERT: Structure chimique et activité pharmacodynamique des anti-histaminiques de synthèse. Ann. pharm. franç. II. suppl. au n. 4 (1944).
BROCKLEHURST, W. E.: Occurrence of an unidentified substance during anaphylactic shock in cavy lung. J. Physiol. (Lond.) **120**, 16 P (1953).
— A slow reacting substance in anaphylaxis-(SRS-A) In: Ciba Foundation Symposium on Histamine. London: J. and A. Churchill 1956.
— The release of histamine and formation of slow reacting substance(SRS-A) during anaphylactic shock. J. Physiol. (Lond.) **151**, 416 (1960).
— J. H. HUMPHREY, and W. L. M. PERRY: The role of histamine in cutaneous antigen-antibody reactions in the rat. J. Physiol. (Lond.) **129**, 205 (1955).
— — — Cutaneous antigen-antibody reactions in the rat. J. Physiol. (Lond.) **150**, 489 (1960).
—, and S. C. LAHIRI: The production of bradykinin in anaphylaxis. J. Physiol. (Lond.) **160**, 15 P (1962).
BRONFENBRENNER, J.: Specific parenteral digestion and its relation to phenomena of immunity and anaphylaxis. J. Lab. clin. Med. **16**, 573 (1915).
— The nature of anaphylatoxin. J. exp. Med. **21**, 480 (1915).
— On the mechanism of anaphylaxis and anti-anaphylaxis. Proc. Soc. exp. Biol. (N. Y.) **13**, 19 (1915).
BRUNNER, M., I. ALTMAN, and K. BOWMAN: Canine sensitivity to Ascaris antigen. J. Allergy **15**, 2 (1944).
BURDON, K. Z., J. P. MCGOVERN, G. D. BARKIN, and W. M. MYERS: Fibrinolysis and anaphylaxis. I. Activation of blood fibrinolysin during anaphylactic shock in guinea pigs. J. Allergy **32**, 55 (1961).
BURRAGE, W. S., and J. W. IRWIN: Microscopic observations of the pulmonary arterioles, capillaries and venules of living mammals before and during anaphylaxis. J. Allergy **24**, 289 (1953).
— — J. I. GALLEMORE, and D. M. K. WANG: Effects of histamine and epinephrine on the small pulmonary blood vessels of living rabbits. J. Allergy **25**, 293 (1954).
CAMPBELL, B.: Inhibition of anaphylactic shock by acetylsalicylic acid. Science **108**, 478 (1948).
—, and P. A. NICOLL: Studies on in vitro anaphylaxis and release of an active non-histamine material from sensitized guinea pig lung. J. Immunol. **39**, 103 (1940).
CANNON, P. R., and C. E. MARSHALL: Studies on the mechanism of the Arthus phenomenon. J. Immunol. **40**, 127 (1941).
CARRYER, H. M., and C. F. CODE: Release of histamine during hemolytic reactions in the blood of rabbits. Proc. Soc. exp. Biol. (N. Y.) **73**, 452 (1950).
CHAKRAVARTY, N.: The occurrence of a lipid-soluble smooth-muscle stimulating principle ("SRS") in anaphylactic reaction. Acta physiol. scand. **48**, 167 (1960).
—, and B. UVNÄS: Histamine and a lipid-soluble smooth muscle stimulating principle ("SRS") in anaphylactic reaction. Acta physiol. scand. **48**, 302 (1960).
— B. HÖGBERG, and B. UVNÄS: Mechanism of the release by compound 48/80 of histamine and of a lipid-soluble smooth muscle stimulating principle ("SRS"). Acta physiol. scand. **45**, 255 (1959).
COBURN, A. F., and E. M. KAPP: The effect of salicylates on the precipitation of antigen with antibody. J. exp. Med. **77**, 173 (1943).
COCA, A. F.: The perfusion experiment in the study of anaphylaxis. J. Immunol. **4**, 219 (1919).
COCHRANE, C. G., and W. O. WEIGLE: The cutaneous reaction to soluble antigen-antibody complexes. A comparison with the Arthus phenomenon. J. exp. Med. **108**, 591 (1958).
CODE, C. F.: The source in blood of the histamine-like constituent. J. Physiol. (Lond.) **90**, 349 (1937).
— The histamine-like activity of white blood cells. J. Physiol. **90**, 485 (1937).
— The histamine content of the blood of guinea pigs and dogs during anaphylactic shock. Amer. J. Physiol. **127**, 78 (1939).

CODE, C. F.: The mechanism of anaphylaxis and allergic reactions. An evaluation of the role of histamine in their production Ann. Allergy **2**, 427 (1944).
— The mechanism of anaphylactic and allergic reactions: an evaluation of role of histamine in their production. Collect. Papers Mayo Clinic and Mayo Foundation. **36**, 766 (1944).
— Histamine in blood. Physiol. Rev. **32**, 47 (1952).
— D. T. CODY, M. HURN, J. C. KENNEDY, and M. J. STRICKLAND: The simultaneous release of histamine and a histamine destroying factor during anaphylaxis in rats. J. Physiol. **156**, 210 (1961).
—, and H. R. HESTER: The blood histamine during anaphylactic shock in the horse and calf. Amer. J. Physiol. **127**, 71 (1939).
—, and H. R. ING: The isolation of histamine from the white cell layer of centrifuged rabbit blood. J. Physiol. **90**, 501 (1937).
COLLIER, H. O. J., and P. G. SHORLEY: Analgesic antipyretic drugs as antagonists of bradykinin. Brit. J. Pharmacol. **15**, 601 (1960).
— J. A. HOLGATE, M. SCHACHTER, and P. G. SHORLEY: The broncho-constrictor action of bradykinin. Brit. J. Pharmacol. **15**, 290 (1960).
CRAPS, L., and T. INDERBITZIN: Anaphylaxie cutanée et protéolyse. Dermatologica (Basel) **114**, 218 (1957).
— — Histamine cutanée et réactions inflammatoires. Arch. belges Derm. **1**, 1 (1957).
— — L'histamine dans la peau humaine, normale et pathologique. Int. Arch. Allergy Applied Immunol. **7**, 140 (1957).
DALE, H. H.: The anaphylactic reaction of plain muscle in the guinea pig. J. Pharmacol. exp. Ther. **4**, 167 (1912—1913).
— The effect of varying tonicity on the anaphylactic and other reactions of plain muscles. J. Pharmacol. exp. Ther. **4**, 517 (1913).
— The biological significance of anaphylaxis. Proc. roy. Soc. B. **91**, 126 (1920).
— On some chemical factors in the control of circulation. Croonian Lectures. II. and III. Lancet **216**, 1232, 1285 (1929).
— Antihistamine substances. Brit. med. J. **1948II**, 281.
— The pharmacology of histamine with a brief survey of evidence for its occurrence, liberation and participation in natural reactions. Ann. N. Y. Acad. Sci. **50**, 1017 (1950).
— Action and uses of antihistamine drugs as applied to dermatology. Brit. J. Dermatol. **62**, 151 (1950).
— Adventures in Physiology, p. 387. London: Pergamon Press 1953.
—, and H. W. DUDLEY: The presence of histamine and acetylcholine in the spleen of the ox and the horse. J. Physiol. (Lond.) **68**, 97 (1929).
—, and C. H. KELLAWAY: Anaphylaxis and anaphylatoxins. Phil. Trans. B **211**, 273 (1922).
—, and P. P. LAIDLAW: The physiological action of β-iminazolylethylamine. J. Physiol. (Lond.) **41**, 318 (1910).
— — Further observations on the action of β-iminazolylethylamine. J. Physiol. (Lond.) **43**, 182 (1911).
DALY, I. B., S. PEAT, and H. O. SCHILD: The release of a histamine-like substance from the lungs of guinea pig during anaphylactic shock. Quart. J. exp. Physiol. **25**, 33 (1935).
DEAN, H. R., and R. A. WEBB: The morbid anatomy and histology of anaphylaxis in the dog. J. Path. Bact. **27**, 51 (1924).
DENECKE, G.: Über die Bedeutung der Leber für die anaphylaktische Reaktion. Z. Immun.-Forsch. **20**, 501 (1914).
DIAMANT, B.: The influence of anoxia and glucose on histamine liberation caused by a principle in Ascaris suis. Acta physiol. scand. **50**, suppl. **175**, 34 (1960).
DINIZ, C. R., and I. F. CARVALHO: A micromethod for determination of bradykinogen under several conditions. Ann. N. Y. Acad. Sci. **104**, 77 (1963).
DIXON, F. J.: The use of I^{131} in immunologic investigation. J. Allergy **24**, 547 (1953).
DOERR, R.: Allergie und Anaphylaxie. Handb. pathog. Mikroorganismen, (Jena) **2**, 947 (1913).
—, u. J. MOLDOVAN: Die Wirkungen eiweißfällender Kolloidlösungen auf warmblütige Tiere und ihre Beziehungen zu anaphylaktischen Prozessen. Biochem. Z. **41**, 27 (1912).
—, u. V. K. RUSS: Der anaphylaktische Immunkörper und seine Beziehung zum Eiweißantigen. Z. Immun.-Forsch. **3**, 181 (1909).
DRAGSTEDT, C. A.: The physiological significance of histamine. Quart. Bull. Northw. Univ. med. Sch. **14**, 1 (1940).
— Anaphylaxis. Physiol. Rev. **21**, 563 (1941).
— M. R. ARELLANO, and A. H. LAWTON: The relationship of histamine to anaphylaxis in the rabbit. Science **91**, 617 (1940a).
— — — and G. P. YOUMANS: Passive sensitization of rabbit's blood. J. Immunol. **39**, 537 (1940b).
—, and E. GEBAUER-FUELNEGG: Studies in Anaphylaxis. I. The appearance of a physiologically active substance during anaphylactic shock. Amer. J. Physiol. **102**, 512 (1932).

DRAGSTEDT, C. A., and F. B. MEAD: Role of histamine in canine anaphylaxis. J. Pharmacol. exp. Ther. **57**, 419 (1936).
— — Peptone shock. J. Pharmacol. exp. Ther. **59**, 429 (1937).
—, and M. ROCHA E SILVA: Effect of trypsin upon blood histamine of rabbits. Proc. Soc. exp. Biol. (N. Y.) **47**, 420 (1941).
— J. A. WELLS, and M. ROCHA E SILVA: Inhibitory effect of heparin upon histamine release by trypsin, antigen and proteose. Proc. Soc. exp. Biol. (N. Y.) **51**, 191 (1942).
DRAPER, L. R., and D. E. SMITH: A function for tissue mast cells. Science **134**, 842 (1961).
DRINKER, C. K., and J. BRONFENBRENNER: The pulmonary circulation in anaphylactic shock. J. Immunol. **9**, 387 (1924).
EAGLE, H., C. G. JOHNSTON, and I. S. RAVDIN: On the prolonged coagulation time subsequent to anaphylactic shock. Bull. Johns Hopk. Hosp. **60**, 428 (1937).
EICHBAUM, F., and M. ROCHA E SILVA: Failure of ascorbic acid to influence the variations of the histamine content of rabbit's blood during anaphylactic shock. Rev. bras. Biol. **3**, 39 (1943).
EISENBREY, A. B., and R. M. PEARCE: A study of the action of the heart in anaphylactic shock in the dog. J. Pharmacol. exp. Ther. **4**, 21 (1912).
EMMELIN, N., G. S. KAHLSON, and K. LINDSTRÖM: Liberation of histamine from skin during anaphylactic reaction in guinea pig. Acta physiol. scand. **2**, 78 (1941).
ENGELHARDT, G., u. U. SCHWABE: Über eine 5-Hydroxytryptamin-Freisetzung unter der anaphylaktischen Reaktion des Meerschweinchens. Naunyn-Schmiedeberg's Arch. exp. Path. Pharmak. **239**, 170 (1960).
— — Bei der anaphylaktischen und allergischen Reaktion freigesetzte Wirkstoffe. Klin. Wschr. **38**, 145 (1960).
FEIGEN, G. A., E. M. VAUGHAN WILLIAMS, J. K. PETERSON, and C. B. NIELSEN: Histamine release and intracellular potentials during anaphylaxis in the isolated heart. Circulat. Res. **8**, 713 (1960).
FEINBERG, S. M., S. MALKIEL, T. B. BERNSTEIN, and B. J. HARGIS: Histamine antagonists. Comparative experimental studies of certain antihistaminic compounds. J. Pharmacol. exp. Ther. **99**, 195 (1950).
— —, and A. R. FEINBERG: The antihistamines. Chicago: The Year Book Publishers 1950.
FELDBERG, W.: Ergebnisse tierexperimenteller Untersuchungen über die Physiologie des Histamins. Volume Jubilaire, Prof. J. Demoor (Liège) 1937.
— Histamine and anaphylaxis. Ann. Rev. Physiol. **3**, 671 (1941).
— On some physiological aspects of histamine. J. Pharm. Pharmacol. **6**, 281 (1954).
— Allergische Reaktionsmechanismen. Arch. klin. exp. Derm. **213**, 343 (1961).
—, and A. A. MILES: Regional variations of increased permeability of skin capillaries induced by a histamine liberator and their relation to the histamine content of the skin. J. Physiol. (Lond.) **120**, 205 (1953).
—, u. E. SCHILF: Histamin. Seine Pharmakologie und Bedeutung für die Humoralphysiologie. Berlin: Verlag Julius Springer 1930.
—, and J. TALESNIK: Reduction of tissue histamine by compound 48/80. J. Physiol. (Lond.) **120**, 550 (1953).
FERNÖ, O., B. HÖGBERG, and B. UVNÄS: The inhibitory action of a polycarboxylic acid on the disruption of mast cells and liberation of histamine produced by compound 48/80, Ascaris extract, antigen-antibody reaction on phospholipase A. Acta pharmacol. (Kbh.) **17**, 18 (1960).
FINK, M. A.: Anaphylaxis in the mouse: possible relation of the Schultz-Dale reaction to serotonin release. Proc. Soc. exp. Biol. (N. Y.) **92**, 673 (1956).
FISCHEL, E. E., and E. A. KABAT: Quantitative study of the Arthus phenomenon induced passively in the rabbit. J. Immunol. **55**, 337 (1947).
FRENGER, W., u. M. GEMÄHLICH: Studien zur Morphologie der Gewebsmastzellen beim Meerschweinchen nach einem Anaphylatoxin-Schock unter wechselnden Bedingungen. III. Congr. Intern. Allergol., Paris 1958.
— F. SCHEIFFARTH u. M. GEMÄHLICH: Untersuchungen zum Wirkungsmechanismus des Anaphylatoxin. II. Mitteilung. Ablauf der passiven Anaphylaxis beim Meerschweinchen. Z. Immun.-Forsch. **115**, 367 (1958).
FRIEDBERGER, E.: Kritik der Theorien über die Anaphylaxie. Z. Immun.-Forsch. **2**, 208 (1909).
— Weitere Untersuchungen über Eiweißanaphylaxie. Z. Immun.-Forsch. **3**, 692; **4**, 636 (1910).
— Die Anaphylaxie. Fortschr. dtsch. Klin. **2**, 620 (1911).
— Anaphylaxie mit besonderer Berücksichtigung ihrer Bedeutung für Infektion und Immunität. Dtsch. med. Wschr. **37**, 481 (1911).
—, u. S. SEIDENBERG: Versuche mit Serum an isolierten Gefäßpräparaten normaler anaphylaktischer Tiere. Z. Immun.-Forsch. **51**, 276 (1927).

FRIEDEMANN, U.: Weitere Untersuchungen über den Mechanismus der Anaphylaxie. Z. Immun.-Forsch. **2**, 591 (1909).
GANS, H., and W. KRIVIT: Study of fibrinogen and plasminogen concentrations in rabbits during anaphylactic shock. J. Lab. clin. Med. **58**, 259 (1961).
GARCIA-AROCHA, H.: Cit. in MACINTOSH (1956).
—, and F. J. MCILREATH: Production of anaphylaxis in vivo and in vitro by soluble antigen-antibody complexes. Abstr. Comm. XXI. Intern. Congr. Physiol. Sci. 103 (1959). Buenos Aires.
GEBAUER-FUELNEGG, E., and C. A. DRAGSTEDT: Studies in anaphylaxis. II. The nature of a physiologically active substance appearing during anaphylactic shock. Amer. J. Physiol. **102**, 520 (1932).
GEMÄHLICH, M., W. FRENGER u. L. SCHEIFFARTH: Untersuchungen zur Morphologie der Mastzellen im Anaphylatoxinschock beim Meerschweinchen. Int. Arch. Allergy **13**, 370 (1958).
GERMUTH, F. G. JR., and G. E. MCKINNON: Studies of the biological properties of antigen-antibody complexes in unsensitized normal guinea pigs. Bull. Johns Hopk. Hosp. **101**, 13 (1957).
— A. E. MAUMENEE, J. A. PRATT-JOHNSON, L. B. SENTERFIT, C. E. VAN ARMAN, and A. D. POLLACK: Observations on the site and mechanisms of antigen-antibody interaction in anaphylactic hypersensitivity. In: Mechanisms of Hypersensitivity. Henry Ford Hospital, International Symposium. Boston, Toronto: Little, Brown & Co. 1959.
GIERTZ, H., F. HAHN, I. JURNA u. W. SCHMUTZLER: Vergleichende Untersuchungen über den anaphylaktischen Schock und den Anaphylatoxinschock am intakten Meerschweinchen. Naunyn-Schmiedeberg's Arch. exp. Path. Pharmak. **242**, 65 (1961).
—, u. W. SCHMUTZLER: Über Freisetzung von Wirkstoffen aus der isolierten Meerschweinchenlunge im anaphylaktischen und Anaphylatoxin-Schock. Naunyn-Schmiedeberg's Arch. exp. Path. Pharmak. **238**, 103 (1960).
GOTZL, F. R., and C. A. DRAGSTEDT: Peptone shock in rabbits. J. Pharmacol. exp. Ther. **74**, 33 (1942).
GRAÑA, A., F. C. MANN, and H. E. ESSEX: Influence of the liver on the shock produced by extracts of certain parasites. Amer. J. Physiol. **148**, 243 (1947).
—, and M. ROCHA E SILVA: Effect of hydatid fluid on histamine content of rabbit blood. Amer. J. Physiol. **143**, 314 (1945).
GREEFF, K., B. G. BENFEY u. A. BOKELMAN: Anaphylaktische Reaktionen am isolierten Herzvorhofpräparat des Meerschweinchens und ihre Beeinflussung durch Antihistaminica, BOL, Dihydroergotamin und Reserpin. Naunyn-Schmiedeberg's Arch. exp. Path. Pharmak. **236**, 421 (1959).
GREISMAN, S. E.: The role of anaphylatoxin during in vitro anaphylaxis. J. Immunol. **81**, 214 (1958).
GROSSBERG, A. L., and H. GARCIA-AROCHA: Histamine liberation in vitro and mode of binding histamine in tissues. Science **120**, 762 (1954).
GROVE, E.: On the role of unstriped muscle in acute anaphylaxis in the rabbit. J. Immunol. **23**, 125, 147, 150 (1932).
GUEST, M. M., R. C. MURPHY, S. R. BODNAR, A. G. WARE, and W. H. SEEGERS: Physiological effects of a plasma protein: blood pressure leucocyte concentration, smooth and cardiac muscle activity. Amer. J. Physiol. **150**, 471 (1947).
HAHN, F., H. GIERTZ u. W. SCHMUTZLER: Studien über die anaphylaktische und anaphylaktoide Histaminfreisetzung in der Meerschweinchenlunge. Int. Arch. Allergy **18**, 62 (1961).
—, u. A. LANGE: Das Anaphylatoxin. Eine alte Theorie der Anaphylaxie in neuer Sicht. Dtsch med. Wschr. **81**, 1269 (1956).
— A. OBERDORF: Antihistaminica und anaphylaktoide Reaktionen. Z. Immun.-Forsch. **107**, 528 (1950).
HAINING, C. G.: Histamine release in rabbit blood by dextran and dextran sulphate. Brit. J. Pharmacol. **10**, 87 (1955).
— Activation of rabbit serum protease by dextran sulphate. Brit. J. Pharmacol. **11**, 107 (1956a).
— Inhibition of histamine release by sodium salicylate and other compounds. Brit. J. Pharmacol. **11**, 357 (1956b).
HALPERN, B. N.: Les antihistaminiques de synthèse. Essais de chimiothérapie des états allergiques. Arch. int. Pharmacodyn. **68**, 339 (1942).
— Experimental research on new series of chemical substances with powerful antihistaminic activity; thiodiphenylamine derivatives. J. Allergy **18**, 263 (1947).
— Recherches sur une nouvelle série chimique de corps doués de propriétés antihistaminiques et anti-anaphylactiques: les dérivés de la thiodiphénylamine. Arch. int. Pharmacodyn. **74**, 314 (1947).

HALPERN, B. N., P. LIACOPOULOS et M. BRIOT: Méchanisme de protection du cobaye contre le choc anaphylactique mortel par l'anaphylatoxine. Acta allerg. (Kbh.) **10**, 9 (1956a).
— — — Aspects qualitatifs et quantitatifs de l'antagonisme des anti-histaminiques de synthèse à l'égard de l'histamine, des substances histamino-libératrices et de la réaction anaphylactique. C. R. Soc. Biol. (Paris) **150**, 313 (1956b).
— — et M. LIACOPOULOS-BRIOT: Recherches sur les substances exogènes agissant sur la perméabilité capillaire et leurs antagonistes. Arch. int. Pharmacodyn. **119**, 56 (1959).
— M. LIACOPOULOS-BRIOT et P. LIACOPOULOS: Recherches sur les modalités de la protection croisée exercée par les diverses substances histamino-libératrices chez le rat albino. C. R. Soc. Biol. (Paris) **152**, 285 (1958).
HAWKINS, D. F., and L. M. ROSA: Some discrepancies in the histamine theory of anaphylaxis in smooth muscle. In: Ciba Foundation Symposium on Histamine. London: J. & A. Churchill Ltd. 1956.
— — Some observations on the release of a substance active on the rat's uterus from guinea pig lung during anaphylactic shock. Int. Arch. Allergy **14**, 312 (1959).
HAYASHI, H.: Review concerning trigger mechanism of allergic inflammation. Mie med. J. **6**, 195 (1956).
—, et al.: Experimental studies on rheumatic inflammation. Mie med. J. **4**, suppl. 2 (1955).
— A. TOKUDA, and K. UDAKA: Biochemical study of cellular antigen-antibody reaction in tissue culture. I. Activation and release of a protease. J. exp. Med. **112**, 237 (1960).
HERBERTS, G.: A study of the mechanism of allergy. II. In vitro experiments of the proteolytic effect in tissue extracts. Acta Soc. Med. upsalien. **54**, 387 (1949).
— Proteolytic activity in organ extracts after anaphylactic shock. With special regard to the action of thiols. Acta Soc. Med. upsalien. **60**, 246 (1955).
—, u. O. DRESSLER: Hemmung des anaphylaktischen Prozesses mit organischen Schwefelverbindungen. Acta Soc. Med. upsalien. **60**, 187 (1955).
HÖGBERG, B., G. THUFVESSON, and B. UVNÄS: Histamine liberation produced in the perfused paw of the cat by 48/80 and extracts from jelly fish (Cyanea capillata) and eelworm (Ascaris lumbricoides) from swine. Acta physiol. scand. **38**, 135 (1956).
—, and B. UVNÄS: The mechanism of disruption of mast cells produced by compound 48/80. Acta physiol. scand. **41**, 345 (1957).
— — Further observations on the disruption of rat mesentery mast cells caused by compound 48/80, antigen-antibody reaction, lecithinase A and decylamin. Acta physiol. scand. **48**, 133 (1960).
HOLMES, C. A., G. OJERS, and C. A. DRAGSTEDT: Liver histamine during peptone shock in dogs. Proc. Soc. exp. Biol. (N. Y.) **46**, 576 (1941).
HOWELL, W. H.: The purification of heparin and its presence in the blood. Amer. J. Physiol. **71**, 553 (1925).
HUGHES, A., and R. S. TONKS: The role of micro-emboli in the production of cardiaditis in hypersensitivity experiments. J. Path. Bact. **77**, 207 (1959).
HUGHES, J., et J. LECOMTE: Action de la bradykinine déposée au contact des vaisseaux mésentériques du lapin. C. R. Soc. Biol. (Paris) **154**, 1523 (1960).
HUMPHREY, J. H., and R. JAQUES: Liberation of histamine and serotonin from platelets by antigen-antibody reactions in vitro. J. Physiol. (Lond.) **119**, 43 P (1953).
— — The release of histamine and 5-HT (serotonin) from platelets by antigen-antibody reactions (in vitro). J. Physiol. (Lond.) **128**, 9 (1955).
INDERBITZIN, T.: The effect of acute and delayed cutaneous allergic reactions on the amount of histamine in the skin. Int. Arch. Allergy **7**, 140 (1957).
— Histamine in allergic responses of the skin. In: Mechanisms of Hypersensitivity. Henry Ford Hospital, International Symposium, p. 493. Boston, Toronto: Little, Brown & Co. 1959.
—, and V. DOBRIČ: Histamine in skin anaphylaxis. Int. Arch. Allergy **14**, 325 (1959).
IRWIN, J. W., F. L. WEILLE, and W. S. BURRAGE: Small blood vessels during allergic reactions. Ann. Otol. (St. Louis) **64**, 1164 (1955).
ISHIZAKA, K., and D. H. CAMPBELL: Biological activity of soluble antigen-antibody complexes. I. Skin reactive properties. Proc. Soc. exp. Biol. **97**, 635 (1958).
— T. ISHIZAKA, and D. H. CAMPBELL: The biological activity of soluble antigen-antibody complexes II. Physical properties of soluble complexes having skin-irritating activity. J. exp. Med. **109**, 127 (1959).
JAFFÉ, W. G. (1924): Cit. In: FELDBERG and SCHILF (1930).
JAQUES, L. B., and E. T. WATERS: The identity and origin of the anticoagulant of anaphylactic shock in the dog. J. Physiol. (Lond.) **99**, 454 (1941).
JOBLING, J. W., and W. PETERSEN: The mechanism of anaphylatoxin formation. Studies on ferment action. XV. J. exp. Med. **20**, 37 (1914).
— —, and A. A. EGGSTEIN: Studies on ferment action. XXIII. The mechanism of anaphylactic shock. J. exp. Med. **22**, 401 (1915).

KATZ, G.: Histamine release from blood cells in anaphylaxis in vitro. Science **91**, 221 (1940).
—, and S. COHEN: Experimental evidence for histamine release in allergy. J. Amer. med. Ass. **117**, 1782 (1941).
KELLAWAY, C. H., and E. R. TRETHEWIE: The liberation of a slow reacting smooth muscle stimulating substance in anaphylaxis. Quart. J. exp. Physiol. **30**, 121 (1940).
KELLER, R.: Ergebnisse immunologischer Untersuchungen an isolierten Mastzellen. Int. Arch. Allergy **19**, 387 (1961).
— Mast cells and anaphylaxis. Experientia (Basel) **18**, 286 (1962).
KINSELL, L. W., L. M. KOPELOFF, R. L. ZWEMER, and N. KOPELOFF: Blood constituents during anaphylactic shock in the monkey. J. Immunol. **42**, 35 (1941).
KOPELOFF, N., and L. M. KOPELOFF: Blood platelets in anaphylaxis. J. Immunol. **40**, 471 (1941).
LAHIRI, S. C., and W. E. BROCKLEHURST: Bradykinin and anaphylactic shock. Brit. J. Pharmacol. **17**, 5 (1961).
LAMBERT, P. H., OTTO-SERVAIS, Mme., J. SALMON et J. LECOMTE: Sur le rôle du complement dans le choc anaphylactique du lapin. Intern. Arch. Allergy **24**, 27 (1964).
LARSON, W. P., and E. T. BELL: The perfusion experiments in the study of cellular anaphylaxis. J. infect. Dis. **24**, 185 (1919).
LECOMTE, J.: Bradykinine et choc anaphylactique du lapin. Acta allerg. (Kbh.) **14**, 408 (1959).
— Bradykinine et réactions anaphylactiques du Lapin. C. R. Soc. Biol. (Paris) **154**, 1118 (1960).
— Consommation des kininogènes plasmatiques an cours du choc anaphylactique du lapin. Compt. rend. soc. biol. **155**, 1411 (1961).
—, et M. L. BEAUMARIAGE: Rôle de l'histamine dans le choc anaphylactique du coq. Arch. int. Pharmacodyn. **107**, 117 (1956).
— — Le choc anaphylactique du coq. Rôle de l'histamine dans son déterminisme. Int. Arch. Allergy **13**, 145 (1958).
—, et J. TROQUET: Antagonisme entre bradykinine et phenylbutazone chez le lapin. C. R. Soc. Biol. (Paris) **154**, 1115 (1960).
LEPPER, M. H., E. R. CALDWELL JR., P. K. SMITH, and B. F. MILLER: Effects on anaphylactic shock of salicylates, aminopyrine and other compounds. Proc. Soc. exp. Biol. (N. Y.) **74**, 254 (1950).
LEWIS, T.: Vascular reactions of the skin to injury. I. Reaction to stroking. Heart **11**, 119 (1924).
— Vascular reactions of the skin to injury. IV. An irresponsive condition of the vessels. Heart **13**, 153 (1926).
— Blood vessels of the human skin and their responses. London: Shaw and Sons Ltd. 1927.
LIBRO, V., e L. MARIANI: Un trattamento con reserpina e con 48/80 non modifica lo shock anafilattico della cavia. Atti Accad. med. lombarda **16**, 244 (1961).
LINN, B. O., C. H. SHUNK, K. FOLKERS, O. GAULEY, and H. J. ROBINSON: SRS-S concentrates from normal swine lung without anaphylaxis. Biochem. Pharmacol. **8**, 338 (1961).
MCCLUSKEY, R. T., and B. BENACERRAF: Localization of colloidal substances in vascular endothelium. A mechanism of tissue damage. II. Experimental serum sickness with acute glomerulonephritis induced passively in mice by antigen-antibody complexes in antigen excess. Amer. J. Pathol. **35**, 275 (1959).
MCINTIRE, F. C.: The mechanism of histamine release. In: Ciba Foundation Symposium on Histamine, p. 416. London: J. & A. Churchill 1956.
— R. K. RICHARDS, and L. W. ROTH: Histamine release inhibition in vitro and antianaphylactic effects in vivo of some chemical compounds. Brit. J. Pharmacol. **12**, 39 (1957).
— L. W. ROTH, and R. K. RICHARDS: The in vitro release of histamine from the blood cells of sensitized rabbits: relationship to blood coagulation mechanism. Amer. J. Physiol. **159**, 332 (1949).
— —, and M. SPROULL: In vitro histamine release from sensitized rabbit blood cells. Evidence against participation of fibrinolysin. Proc. Soc. exp. Biol. (N. Y.) **73**, 605 (1950).
— — — Histamine release in rabbit blood by simple molecules; inhibition and reaction rate studies. Amer. J. Physiol. **167**, 233 (1951).
— — — Mechanism of anaphylaxis in the rabbit. Further evidence against plasma protease mechanism. Proc. Soc. exp. Biol. (N. Y.) **81**, 691 (1952).
MACINTOSH, F. C.: Histamine and intracellular particles. In: Ciba Foundation Symposium on Histamine. London: J. & A. Churchill, Ltd. 1956.
MCKINNON, G. E.: Role of in vivo antigen-antibody precipitation in hypersensitivity reactions. In: Mechanisms of Hypersensitivity, Henry Ford Hospital, International Symposium. Boston, Toronto: Little, Brown & Co. 1959.
— E. C. ANDREWS, R. H. HEPTINSTALL, and F. G. GERMUTH JR.: An immunhistologic study on the occurrence of intravascular antigen-antibody precipitation and its role in anaphylaxis in the rabbit. Bull. Johns Hopk. Hosp. **101**, 258 (1957).
MANWARING, W. H.: Der physiologische Mechanismus des anaphylaktischen Schocks. Z. Immun.-Forsch. **8**, 1 (1910).

Manwaring, W. H., V. M. Hosepian, J. R. Enright, and D. R. Porter: Hepatic reactions in anaphylaxis. XI. Effects of deheparization in canine anaphylaxis. J. Immunol. **10**, 567 (1925).

— — F. I. O'Neil, and H. B. Moy: The hepatic anaphylatoxin studied by hepatic transplantation and blood transfusion. J. Amer. med. Ass. **83**, 2092 (1924).

— — — — Hepatic reactions in anaphylaxis. X. The hepatic anaphylatoxin. J. Immunol. **10**, 575 (1925).

Maruno, Y.: Studies on histamine metabolism and adrenal cortical activity in allergic reactions. I. Histamine metabolism in rats following sensitization. Ann. paediat. jap. **4**, 109 (1958).

— Studies on histamine metabolism and adrenal cortical activity in allergic reactions. II. Histamine metabolism in rats following anaphylactic and other form of shock. Ann. paediat. jap. **4**, 124 (1958).

Mautner, H., u. E. P. Pick: Über die durch „Schockgifte" erzeugten Zirkulationsstörungen. Münch. med. Wschr. **62**, 1141 (1915).

— — Über die durch „Schockgifte" erzeugten Zirkulationsstörungen. II. Das Verhalten der überlebenden Leber. Biochem. Z. **127**, 72 (1922).

Mayer, R. L., C. P. Huttrer, and C. R. Scholz: Antihistaminic and antianaphylactic activity of some α-pyridinoethylenediamines. Science **102**, 93 (1945).

Menkin, V.: A note on the differences between histamine and leukotaxine. Proc. Soc. exp. Biol. (N. Y.) **40**, 103 (1939).

Meyer, K., u. H. Loewenthal: Untersuchungen über Anaphylaxie an Gewebskulturen. Z. Immun.-Forsch. **54**, 420 (1937).

Miles, A. A., and E. M. Miles: Vascular reaction to histamine, histamine-liberator and leukotaxine in the skin of guinea pigs. J. Physiol. (Lond.) **118**, 228 (1952).

Minard, D.: The presence and distribution of histamine in blood. Amer. J. Physiol. **132**, 327 (1941).

Mongar, J. L., and H. O. Schild: Inhibition of anaphylaxis. J. Physiol. (Lond.) **130**, 40 P (1955).

— — Effects of antigen and organic bases on intracellular histamine in guinea pig lung. J. Physiol. (Lond.) **131**, 207 (1956).

— — Inhibition of the anaphylactic reaction. J. Physiol. (Lond.) **135**, 301 (1957a).

— — Effect of temperature on the anaphylactic reaction. J. Physiol. (Lond.) **135**, 320 (1957b).

— — The effect of calcium and pH on the anaphylactic reaction. J. Physiol. (Lond.) **140**, 272 (1958).

— — Cellular mechanisms in anaphylaxis. Physiol. Rev. **42**, 226 (1962).

Mota, I.: Mast cell damage by anaphylaxis, peptone shock and compound 48/80. Thesis, University of S. Paulo, Brazil (1953).

— Action of anaphylactic shock and anaphylatoxin on mast cells and histamine in rats. Brit. J. Pharmacol. **12**, 453 (1957).

— Mast cells and anaphylaxis. J. Physiol. (Lond.) **140**, 6 P (1958a).

— Mast cells and histamine in rat anaphylaxis. The effect of Haemophilus pertussis. Nature (Lond.) **182**, 1021 (1958b).

— Effect of the antigen-antibody reaction on mast cells and histamine content of sensitized guinea pig tissues. J. Physiol. (Lond.) **147**, 425 (1959).

— The mechanism of action of anaphylatoxin. Its effect on guinea pig mast cells. Immunology **2**, 403 (1959).

— Mechanism of action of antigen-antibody complexes: their effect on mast cells. Nature (Lond.) **191**, 572 (1961).

—, and I. Vugman: Effects of anaphylactic shock and compound 48/80 on the mast cells of guinea pig lung. Nature (Lond.) **177**, 427 (1956).

Moussatché, H., and A. P. Danon: Inhibition by sulfhydril blocking agents of the guinea pig gut reaction to anaphylaxis and to anaphylatoxin. Naturwissenschaften **10**, 227 (1956).

— — On the action of succinate and malonate upon the histamine released during the anaphylactic reaction in vitro. Naturwissenschaften **44**, 330 (1957).

—, and A. Prouvost-Danon: Influence of oxidative phosphorylation inhibitors on the histamine release in the anaphylactic reaction in vitro. Experientia (Basel) **14**, 414 (1958).

Nolf, P.: The coagulation of the blood. Medicine (Baltimore) **17**, 381 (1938).

— Recherches anciennes et récentes sur la coagulation du sang. Arch. méd. belges **5**, 1 (1946).

Ojers, F., C. A. Holmes, and C. A. Dragstedt: The histamine content of the blood of guinea pigs and dogs during anaphylactic shock. Amer. J. Physiol. **127**, 78 (1939).

— — — The relation of the liver histamine to anaphylactic shock in dogs. J. Pharmacol. exp. Ther. **73**, 33 (1941).

Opie, E. L.: The relation of antigen to antibody in the Arthus phenomenon. J. Immunol. **9**, 255 (1924).

OSLER, A. G., M. M. HAWRISIAK, Z. OVARY, M. SIQUEIRA, and O. G. BIER: Studies on the mechanism of hypersensitivity phenomena: II. The participation of complement in passive cutaneous anaphylaxis of the albino rat. J. exp. Med. **106**, 811 (1957).
— H. G. RANDALL, B. M. HILL, and Z. OVARY: Studies on the mechanism of hypersensitivity phenomena. III. The participation of complement in the formation of anaphylatoxin. J. exp. Med. **110**, 311 (1959a).
— — — — Some relationships between complement, passive cutaneous anaphylaxis and anaphylatoxin. In: Mechanism of Hypersensitivity. Henry Ford Hospital, International Symposium. Boston, Toronto: Little, Brown & Co. 1959b.
OTTO, R.: Das Theobald-Smith-Phänomenon der Serumüberempfindlichkeit. Gedenk. Rud. Leuthold. Berlin 1906.
— Zur Frage der Serumüberempfindlichkeit. Münch. med. Wschr. **54**, 1665 (1907).
OVARY, Z.: Immediate reaction in the skin of experimental animals provoked by antigen-antibody interaction. Progr. Allergy **5**, 459 (1958).
—, and O. G. BIER: Quantitative study of Arthus reaction and of cutaneous anaphylaxis induced passively in the rat. Proc. Soc. exp. Biol. (N. Y.) **81**, 584 (1952).
— — Quantitative studies on passive cutaneous anaphylaxis in the guinea pig and its relationship to the Arthus phenomenon. J. Immunol. **71**, 6 (1953).
—, et M. BRIOT: Nouvelle méthode de dosage de l'anticorps anaphylactique et son rapport avec l'azote de l'anticorps. Ann. Inst. Pasteur **81**, 670 (1951).
PARROT, J. L.: Les manifestations de l'anaphylaxie et les substances histaminiques. Paris: Baillière edit. 1938.
— Sur la réaction cellulaire de l'anaphylaxie. Son caractère aérobie. C. R. Soc. Biol. (Paris) **136**, 361 (1942).
—, et G. RICHET: Action du cyanure de mercure sur les organes isolés du cobaye. Un nouveau type de libération d'histamine. C. R. Soc. Biol. (Paris) **138**, 364 (1944).
PEARCE, R. M., and A. B. EISENBREY: The physiology of anaphylactic shock in the dog. J. infect. Dis. **7**, 565 (1910).
PETERSEN, W. F., and S. A. LEVINSON: Endothelial permeability; role of endothelium in canine anaphylactic shock. J. Immunol. **8**, 349 (1923).
PIRQUET, C. v., u. B. SCHICK: Serumkrankheit. Leipzig und Wien 1905.
PORTIER, P.: Naissance de l'anaphylaxie. Presse méd. **60**, 679 (1952).
—, et C. RICHET: De l'action anaphylactique de certains venins. C. R. Soc. Biol. (Paris) **54**, 170 (1902).
— — Nouveaux faits d'anaphylaxie ou sensibilization aux venins par doses réitérées. C. R. Soc. Biol. (Paris) **54**, 548 (1902).
PROUVOST-DANON, A., and H. MOUSSATCHÉ: Influence of anaerobic glycolysis on release of histamine in the guinea pig and rat anaphylactic reaction in vitro. Nature (Lond.) **192**, 361 (1961).
QUICK, A. J.: On the coagulation defect in peptone shock. A consideration of antithrombines. Amer. J. Physiol. **116**, 535 (1936).
— R. K. OTA, and T. D. BARONOSKY: On the thrombocytopenia of anaphylactic and peptone shock. Amer. J. Physiol. **145**, 273 (1946).
RAMSDELL, S. G.: The use of trypan blue to demonstrate the immediate skin reaction in rabbits and guinea pigs. J. Immunol. **15**, 305 (1928).
RAND, M., and G. REID: On presence in rabbit serum of thrombotonin, thrombocytin or serotonin. Aust. J. exp. Biol. med. Sci. **30**, 153 (1952).
RAPP, H. J.: Release of a slow reacting substance (SRS) in the peritoneal cavity of rats by antigen-antibody interaction. J. Physiol. (Lond.) **158**, 35 P (1961).
RICH, A. R., and R. H. FOLLIS: Studies on the site of sensitivity in the Arthus phenomenon. Bull. Johns Hopk. Hosp. **66**, 106 (1940).
— W. H. LEWIS, and L. N. GAY: Cit. in RICH and FOLLIS (1940).
RICHET, C.: De la réaction anaphylactique in vitro. C. R. Soc. Biol. (Paris) **61**, 1005 (1909).
— (1909—1912). See RICHET (1930).
— L'Anaphylaxie. Paris: Félix Alcan 1930.
RILEY, J. F., and G. B. WEST: Histamine in tissue mast cells. J. Physiol. (Lond.) **117**, 72 P (1952).
— — The presence of histamine in tissue mast cells. J. Physiol. (Lond.) **120**, 528 (1953).
ROBINSON, G. C., and J. AUER: Disturbances of the heart beat in the dog caused by serum anaphylaxis. J. exp. Med. **18**, 410 (1913).
ROCHA E SILVA, M.: Libération de l'histamine par la perfusion du poumon du cobaye au moyen de la trypsine. C. R. Soc. Biol. (Paris) **130**, 186 (1939).
— Beiträge zur Pharmakologie des Trypsins. I., II. Naunyn-Schmiedebergs Arch. exp. Path. Pharmak. **194**, 335 (1940a).
— Anaphylaxis in the rabbit. J. Immunol. **38**, 333 (1940b).

ROCHA E SILVA, M.: The histamine theory of anaphylactic shock with special reference to anaphylaxis in the rabbit. Arch. Path. **33**, 387 (1942).
— The role played by leukocytes and platelets in anaphylactic and peptone shock. Ann. N. Y. Acad. Sci. **50**, 1045 (1950).
— Concerning the mechanism of anaphylaxis and allergy. Brit. med. J. **1952I**, 779.
— Anaphylatoxin and histamine release. Quart. Rev. Allergy 8, 220 (1954).
— Histamine release by naturally occurring substances. In: Ciba Foundation Symposium on Histamine. London: J. & A. Churchill Ltd. 1956.
— Histamine. Triangle (En.) **3**, 1 (1957).
—, and S. O. ANDRADE: Histamine and proteolytic enzymes. Liberation of histamine by papain. J. biol. Chem. **149**, 9 (1943).
— — and R. M. TEIXEIRA: Coagulation defect in the shocks produced by trypsin, peptone and Ascaris extracts. Exp. Med. Surg. **4**, 260 (1946a).
— — — Fibrinolysis in peptone and anaphylactic shock in the dog. Nature (Lond.) **157**, 801 (1946b).
—, and M. ARONSON: Histamine release from the perfused lung of the guinea pig by serotoxin (anaphylatoxin). Brit. J. exp. Path. **33**, 577 (1952).
— — and O. G. BIER: Histamine release by anaphylatoxin. Nature (Lond.) **168**, 465 (1951).
—, u. O. BIER: Untersuchungen über Entzündung. II. Zusätzliche Versuche über die Beziehungen von Menkinschem Leukotaxin zum Histamin. Virchows Arch. path. Anat. **303**, 337 (1939).
—, and C. A. DRAGSTEDT: Observations on the trypan blue capillary permeability test in rabbits. J. Pharmacol. exp. Ther. **73**, 405 (1941).
—, and H. E. ESSEX: The effect of animal poisons (rattle-snake venom and trypsin) on the blood histamine of guinea pig and rabbits. Amer. J. Physiol. **135**, 372 (1942).
—, and A. GRAÑA: Anaphylaxis-like shock produced by Ascaris extracts. I. The changes in the histamine content and the coagulability of the blood in guinea pigs and in dogs. Arch. Surg. **52**, 523 (1946a).
— — Anaphylaxis-like shock produced by Ascaris extracts. II. The mechanism of shock induced in dogs. Arch. Surg. **52**, 713 (1946b).
— — and A. PORTO: Inhibitory effect of glycogen upon anaphylactic shock in the rabbit. Proc. Soc. exp. Biol. (N. Y.) **59**, 57 (1945).
—, and E. MARTINS DA SILVA: (1946). Cit. In: ROCHA E SILVA, M. (1952).
— A. PORTO, and S. O. ANDRADE: Anaphylaxis-like reaction produced by Ascaris extracts. III. The role played by leucocytes and platelets in the genesis of shock. Arch. Surg. **53**, 199 (1946c).
— and A. M. ROTHSCHILD: Anaphylatoxin, histamine depletion and skin reactions in the rat. Nature (Lond.) **175**, 987 (1955).
— A. E. SCROGGIE, E. FIDLAR, and L. B. JAQUES: Liberaction of histamine and heparin by peptone from the isolated dogs liver. Proc. Soc. exp. Biol. (N. Y.) **64**, 141 (1947).
ROSE, B.: Studies on the histamine content of the blood and tissues of rabbit during anaphylactic shock. J. Immunol. **42**, 161 (1941).
—, and J. S. L. BROWNE: Studies on the release of histamine from the blood of the rabbit by addition of horse serum or egg albumin. J. Immunol. **41**, 403 (1941).
—, and P. WEIL: Blood histamine in the rabbit during anaphylactic shock. Proc. Soc. exp. Biol. (N. Y.) **42**, 494 (1939).
ROSENAU, M. J., and J. F. ANDERSON: A study of the cause of sudden death following the injection of horse serum. U. S. Hyg. Lab. Bull. **29**, 95 (1906).
ROSENTHAL, S. R., and N. BROWN: Thymoxyethyldiethylamine as an antagonist of histamine and of anaphylactic reactions. J. Immunol. **38**, 259 (1940).
ROTHSCHILD, A. M.: Effect of metabolic inhibitors on the release of histamine by anaphylatoxin and by antigen. Experientia, (Basel) **17**, 555 (1961).
— I. VUGMAN, and M. ROCHA E SILVA: Metabolic studies on the release of histamine by compound 48/80 in the rat diaphragm. Biochem. Pharmacol. **7**, 248 (1961).
ROWLEY, D. A., and E. P. BENDITT: 5-Hydroxytryptamine and histamine as mediators of the vascular injury produced by agents which damage mast cells in rats. J. exp. Med. **103**, 399 (1956).
SANYAL, R. K., and G. B. WEST: Anaphylactic shock in the albino rat. J. Physiol. (Lond.) **142**, 571 (1958a).
— — The relationship of histamine and 5-hydroxytryptamine to anaphylactic shock in different species. J. Physiol. (Lond.) **144**, 525 (1958b).
SCHACHTER, M.: Anaphylaxis and histamine release in the rabbit. Brit. J. Pharmacol. 8, 412 (1953).
SCHILD, H. O.: Histamine release and anaphylactic shock in isolated lungs of guinea pigs. Quart. J. exp. Physiol. **26**, 165 (1936a).

SCHILD, H. O.: The reaction of the guinea pig's uterus immersed in a histamine solution to histamine and anaphylaxis. J. Physiol. (Lond.) **86**, 51 P (1936b).
— Histamine release in anaphylactic shock from various tissues of the guinea pig. J. Physiol. (Lond.) **95**, 393 (1939).
— The experimental evidence for the use of antihistaminic drugs in allergic conditions. Proc. roy. Soc. Med. **42**, 623 (1949).
— Histamine release and anaphylaxis. In: Ciba Foundation Symposium on Histamine. London: J. & A. Churchill Ltd. 1956.
— Mechanism of the anaphylactic reaction as studied by means of inhibitors. In: Mechanisms of Hypersensitivity. Henry Ford Foundation, International Symposium, p. 243. Boston, Toronto: Little, Brown & Co. 1959.
SCHMIDT, G. W., u. A. STAEHELIN: Histaminempfindlichkeit und anaphylaktische Reaktionen. Z. Immun.-Forsch. **60**, 222 (1929).
SCHULTZ, W. H.: Physiological studies in anaphylaxis. I. The reaction of smooth muscle of the guinea pig sensitized with horse serum. J. Pharmacol. exp. Therap. **1**, 549; II. Reaction of smooth muscle from guinea pigs rendered tolerant to large doses of serum. J. Pharmacol. exp. Ther. **2**, 221 (1910).
—, and H. E. JORDAN: Physiological studies in anaphylaxis. III. A microscopie study of the anaphylactic lung of the guinea-pig and mouse. J. Pharmacol. exp. Ther. **2**, 375 (1911).
SCROGGIE, A. E., and L. B. JAQUES: The release of histamine and heparin by antigen from the isolated perfused liver of the sensitized dog. J. Immunol. **62**, 103 (1949).
SIMONDS, J. P., and W. W. BRANDES: Anaphylactic shock and mechanical obstruction of the hepatic veins in the dog. J. Immunol. **13**, 11 (1927).
SIQUEIRA, M., and O. G. BIER: Hemorrhagic reactions at sites of passive cutaneous anaphylaxis. Anaphylaxis in guinea pig after intravenous inoculation of unrelated immune complex. Proc. Soc. exp. Biol. (N. Y.) **107**, 779 (1961).
—, and R. A. NELSON JR.: Platelet agglutination by immune complexes and its possible role in hypersensitivity. J. Immunol. **86**, 516 (1961).
SMITH, THEOBALD: Discussion on Hypersusceptibility. J. Amer. med. Ass. **47**, 1010 (1906).
SMITH, W., and J. H. HUMPHREY: The effect of sodium salicylate upon hypersensitivity reaction. Brit. J. exp. Path. **30**, 560 (1949).
SPARROW, E. M., and D. L. WILHELM: Species differences in susceptibility to capillary permeability factors: histamine 5-HT and compound 48/80. J. Physiol. (Lond.) **135**, 51 (1957).
SPINELLI, A.: Démonstration de la mise en liberté de substances type histamine du poumon isolé du cobaye en choc anaphylactique. Boll. sez. ital. soc. int. microbiol. **4**, 257 (1932).
STAUB, A. M.: Recherches sur quelques bases synthétiques antagonistes de l'histamine. I. Ann. Inst. Pasteur **63**, 400 (1939).
—, et D. BOVET: Action de la thymoxyéthyldiéthylamine (929 F) et des éthers phénoliques sur le choc anaphylactique du cobaye. C. R. Soc. Biol. (Paris) **125**, 818 (1937).
STETSON, C. A.: Studies on the mechanism of the Shwartzman phenomenon: certain factors involved in the production of the local hemorrhagic necrosis. J. exp. Med. **93**, 489 (1951).
—, and R. A. GOOD: Studies on the mechanism of the Shwartzman phenomenon; evidence for the participation of polymorphonuclear leucocytes in the phenomenon. J. exp. Med. **93**, 49 (1951).
STETSON, C. A. JR.: Similarities in the mechanism determining the Arthus and Shwartzman phenomena. J. exp. Med. **94**, 347 (1951).
TARRAS-WAHLBERG, B.: On the presence and appearance of histamine in blood and lungs. Skand. Arch. Physiol. **93**, suppl. 1 (1936).
THOMAS, W. D., and H. E. ESSEX: Observations on the hepatic venous circulation with special reference to the sphyncteric mechanism. Amer. J. Physiol. **158**, 303 (1949).
TRAPANI, I. L., J. S. GARVEY, and D. H. CAMPBELL: Stimulating action of soluble antigen-antibody complexes on normal guinea pig smooth muscle. Science **127**, 700 (1958).
TRETHEWIE, E. R.: Injury by trypsin. Aust. J. exp. Biol. med. Sci. **20**, 49 (1942).
— The influence of sodium salicylate and acetylsalicylic acid on the release of histamine in anaphylaxis. Aust. J. exp. Biol. med. Sci. **29**, 443 (1951).
UDENFRIEND, S., and T. P. WAALKES: On the role of serotonin in anaphylaxis. In: Mechanisms of Hypersensitivity. Henry Ford Hospital, International Symposium, p. 219. Brown, Toronto: Little 1959.
UNGAR, G.: Mechanism of histamine release. In: Ciba Foundation Symposium on Histamine. London: J. & A. Churchill, Ltd. 1956.
—, and E. DAMGAARD: Protein breakdown in thermal injury. Proc. Soc. exp. Biol. (N. Y.) **87**, 378 (1954).
— — Inhibition of inflammatory response in beta-irradiated skin. Proc. Soc. exp. Biol. (N. Y.) **87**, 383 (1954).

UNGAR, G., and E. DAMGAARD: Tissue reactions to anaphylactic and anaphylactoid stimuli, proteolysis and release of histamine and heparin. J. exp. Med. **101**, 1 (1955).
— — and F. P. HUMMEL: Activation of profibrinolysin by antigen-antibody reaction and by anaphylactoid agents; its relation to complement. J. exp. Med. **98**, 291 (1953).
—, and H. HAYASHI: Enzymatic mechanisms in allergy. Ann. Allergy **16**, 542 (1958).
—, and S. H. MIST: Release of serum fibrinolysin by specific antigen, peptone and certain polysaccharides. J. exp. Med. **90**, 38 (1949).
—, et J. L. PARROT: Recherches sur le choc anaphylactique in vitro. Mise en liberté d'une substance active par le poumon isolé du cobaye sensibilisé. C. R. Soc. Biol. (Paris) **129**, 753 (1936).
— T. YAMURA, J. B. ISOLA, and S. KOBRIN: Further studies on the role of proteases in the allergic reactions. J. exp. Med. **113**, 359 (1961).
UVNÄS, B.: The mechanism of histamine liberation. J. Pharm. Pharmacol. **10**, 1 (1958).
—, and B. HÖGBERG: Inhibiting action of Allicin on degranulation of mast cells produced by 48/80, a histamine liberator from Ascaris, lecithinase A and antigen. Acta physiol. scand. **44**, 157 (1958).
VALLERY-RADOT, P.: L'anaphylaxie humaine et expérimentale. Paris: Masson et Cie. 1937.
VAUGHAN, W. T.: Protein split products in relation to immunity and disease. Philadelphia: Lea & Febiger 1913.
VAUGHAN WILLIAMS, E. M.: The action of quinidine, acetyl choline and anaphylaxis interpreted from simultaneous records of contraction and intracellular potentials in the heart. In: The Scientific Bases of Medicine, p. 302. Ann. Rev. University of London. The Athlone Press 1961.
VOEGTLIN, C., and B. M. BERNHEIM: The liver in its relation to anaphylactic shock. J. Pharmacol. exp. Ther. **2**, 507 (1911).
VUGMAN, I.: Fatores que influem na libertação da histamina do diafragma isolado do rato pelo composto 48/80. Tese, Ribeirão Prêto (Faculty of Medicine) (1961).
WAALKES, T. P., and H. COBURN: The role of platelets and the release of serotonin and histamine during anaphylaxis in the rabbit. J. Allergy **30**, 394 (1959).
— — Studies on the relationship of the release of serotonin and histamine by chemical means to anaphylaxis in the rabbit. J. Allergy **31**, 395 (1960).
— — and L. L. TERRY: The effect of reserpine on histamine and serotonin. J. Allergy **30**, 408 (1959).
— H. WEISSBACH, J. BOZICEVICH, and S. UDENFRIED: Serotonin and histamine release during anaphylaxis in the rabbit. J. clin. Invest. **36**, 1115 (1957).
— — — — Further studies on release of serotonin and histamine during anaphylaxis in the rabbit. Proc. Soc. exp. Biol. (N. Y.) **95**, 479 (1957).
WALTER, J. B., and J. A. FRANK: The relationship of hyaline emboli to other manifestations of anaphylaxis. Brit. J. exp. Path. **42**, 609 (1961).
— —, and J. W. IRWIN: Hyaline emboli in the microcirculation of rabbits during anaphylaxis. Brit. J. exp. Path. **42**, 603 (1961).
WATERS, E. T., J. MARKOWITZ, and L. B. JAQUES: Anaphylaxis in the liverless dog and observations on the anticoagulant of anaphylactic shock. Science **87**, 582 (1938).
WEIGLE, W. O., C. G. COCHRANE, and F. J. DIXON: Anaphylactogenic properties of soluble antigen-antibody complexes in the guinea pig and rabbit. J. Immunol. **85**, 469 (1960).
WEIL, R.: The nature of anaphylaxis and the relations between anaphylaxis and immunity. J. med. Res. **27**, 497 (1912).
— Studies in anaphylaxis. J. med. Res. **30**, 87 (1914).
— Anaphylaxis in dogs. J. Immunol. **2**, 525 (1917).
WEISSBACH, H., T. P. WAALKES, and S. UDENFRIEND: Presence of serotonin in lung and its implication in the anaphylactic reaction. Science **125**, 235 (1957).
WESTERHOLM, B.: The influence of anoxia on 48/80 induced histamine release from cat skin. Acta physiol. scand. **50**, 300 (1960).
WILANDER, O.: Chemistry and physiology of heparin. Skand. Arch. Physiol. **15**, 89 (1938).
WILCOX, H. B., and E. C. ANDRUS: Anaphylaxis in the isolated heart. J. exp. Med. **67**, 169 (1938).
YAMASAKI, H.: Mechanism of histamine release by antigen and chemical substances as studied by means of inhibitors. Folia pharmacol. jap. **59**, 171 (1961).
— S. MURAOKA, and K. ENDO: Energy metabolic aspect of histamine release in anaphylaxis. Jap. J. Pharmacol. **10**, 21 (1960).
ZON, L., E. CEDER, and C. W. CRIGLER: The presence of histamine in the platelets in the rabbit. U. S. Publ. Hlth. Rept. **54**, 1978 (1939).
ZWEIFACH, B. W., A. L. NAGLER, and W. TROLL: Some effects of proteolytic inhibitors on tissue injury and systemic anaphylaxis. J. exp. Med. **113**, 437 (1961).

Section E

Makromolekulare Histaminliberatoren

(Eiklar, Dextran, Polyvinylpyrrolidon, Tween 20, Anaphylatoxin)

Von

H. GIERTZ und F. HAHN

Die makromolekularen Histaminliberatoren sind Stoffe, die nur bei bestimmten Tierspecies, meist einer einzigen, Histamin (teilweise in Kombination mit Serotonin) freisetzen und dadurch für diese Tierart hochgiftig werden, während sie sonst keine besonderen pharmakologischen Wirkungen besitzen. Sie werden daher von allen übrigen Tierarten auch in hohen Dosen vertragen. Einige von ihnen finden sogar als Blutersatzstoffe Verwendung.

Man darf annehmen, daß sich der Mechanismus der Histaminfreisetzung bei diesen Stoffen von der Wirkung der sonstigen Histaminliberatoren unterscheidet, bei denen die Wirkung nicht artspezifisch begrenzt und für gewöhnlich noch mit anderen pharmakologischen Wirkungen verknüpft ist. Die makromolekularen Stoffe haben weder, wie viele niedermolekulare Histaminliberatoren, einen basischen Charakter, noch gleichen sie in ihrer Wirkung den histaminliberierenden Fermenten oder tierischen Giften, bei denen die Histaminfreisetzung nur eine Teilerscheinung sehr weitgehender Zellzerstörung ist.

Man hat wiederholt die Wirkung der makromolekularen Stoffe mit der Wirkung von Antigen-Antikörperkomplexen verglichen oder auch, wie im Falle des Anaphylatoxins, in noch engere Beziehungen zur Anaphylaxie gesetzt. Die durch die makromolekularen Stoffe ausgelösten Reaktionen werden daher meist auch als „anaphylaktoide Reaktionen" bezeichnet (JASMIN, 1956; LÉGER, MASSON und PRADO, 1947c). Jedoch spielen weder natürliche noch erworbene Antikörper hierbei eine Rolle. Überhaupt ist der Ausdruck „anaphylaktoid" fragwürdig, solange man nicht weiß, worauf die spezifische Empfindlichkeit einiger Tierarten gegenüber bestimmten makromolekularen Stoffen beruht und ob der durch sie ausgelöste Mechanismus der Aminfreisetzung in ähnlichen Bahnen verläuft wie der anaphylaktische. Trotzdem halten wir mangels eines besseren Wortes an diesem Ausdruck für die im folgenden zu besprechenden Erscheinungen fest, möchten ihn aber zugleich hierauf begrenzt wissen. Denn in seiner ursprünglichen, sehr viel umfassenderen Bedeutung (HANZLIK und KARSNER, 1920, 1924a, b, c; HANZLIK, KARSNER und FETTERMAN, 1920) erscheint uns der Begriff „anaphylaktoid" weniger umrissen. Umfaßt er doch eine Reihe von Reaktionen, die man durch hauptsächlich intravenöse Injektion heterogenster Substanzen auslösen kann. Das nach unserer Meinung Charakteristische der anaphylaktoiden Reaktionen, nämlich die speciesabhängige spezifische Stoffempfindlichkeit und die vermittelnde Rolle aminartiger Überträgerstoffe, dürfte hier in den allermeisten Fällen fehlen. Dies ergibt sich auch aus neueren Untersuchungen von HILDEBRAND (1958a, b), der zwei auch in der Symptomatik verschiedene Gruppen von anaphylaktoiden Reaktionen unterscheidet, von denen nur die eine auf Wirkstoff-(Histamin-)freisetzung beruht.

Die Anaphylaxieähnlichkeit der anaphylaktoiden Reaktionen wird dadurch eingeschränkt, daß die Symptome von den anaphylaktischen Symptomen abweichen können, besonders bei der Ratte (West, 1961a). Dies könnte darauf beruhen, daß bei den anaphylaktoiden Reaktionen nur ein Teil der für die Anaphylaxie charakteristischen Reaktionen, nämlich die Aminfreisetzung, die bei der Rattenanaphylaxie anscheinend sogar nur eine untergeordnete Rolle spielt, in Gang gesetzt wird. Die vorliegenden Probleme werden von der Tatsache nicht berührt, daß einige der makromolekularen Stoffe (Dextran, Ovomucoid und anscheinend auch PVP) auch als Antigene fungieren (Lit.: Hahn, 1961) und damit bei bestimmten Tierarten (auch anderen als der Ratte) echte Anaphylaxie hervorbringen können.

Die makromolekularen Stoffe erzeugen durch wiederholte Verabreichung eine Toleranz. Man spricht auch von Desensibilisierung, Tachyphylaxie oder Refraktärzustand, obwohl diese Ausdrücke bereits für andere Vorgänge vergeben sind. Anders als bei der Anaphylaxie wird die Toleranz gegen makromolekulare Stoffe hauptsächlich als Erschöpfung des Gewebes an disponiblen Wirkstoffen aufgefaßt. Damit läßt sich auch erklären, daß sie nicht spezifisch begrenzt ist, sondern als Kreuztoleranz auf andere Stoffe übergreifen kann, die bei der gleichen Tierart aminliberierend wirken. Auch niedermolekulare Aminliberatoren können gegen die makromolekularen Stoffe eine Toleranz hervorbringen. Schwieriger ist die Toleranzerzeugung durch makromolekulare Stoffe gegen niedermolekulare Aminliberatoren. Ob allerdings die Toleranzsteigerung ausschließlich durch Wirkstoffverarmung des Gewebes zu erklären ist, erscheint bei dem augenblicklichen Stand unseres Wissens noch nicht sicher. Einige Beobachtungen, auf die wir im folgenden zurückkommen werden, lassen sich mit dieser Auffassung nicht vereinbaren.

A. Die anaphylaktoide Reaktion der weißen Ratte

Die Kardinalsymptome der anaphylaktoiden Reaktion bei der Ratte sind die typisch lokalisierten Ödeme (an Pfoten, Nase, Ohren, Zunge und Genitalorganen). Die Ödembildung wird eingeleitet durch Hyperämie an den Prädilektionsstellen und durch generalisierten Pruritus. Dieses Bild tritt am reinsten nach i. p. Injektion der auslösenden Stoffe auf, während i.v. Cyanose und Kollaps im Vordergrund stehen und die Ödembildung maskieren können. Subcutan läßt sich, von extrem hohen Dosen abgesehen, die Ödembildung nur durch Injektion in die Prädilektionsstellen hervorrufen, wobei das Ödem auf den injizierten Bezirk beschränkt bleibt, in seltenen Fällen und unter besonderen Bedingungen aber auch auf andere Prädilektionsstellen überspringen kann.

Die beiden typischen bei der Ratte anaphylaktoid wirkenden Stoffe sind Hühnereiklar und Dextran. Lokalisierte Ödeme lassen sich bei der Ratte durch lokale oder intraperitoneale Injektion auch zahlreicher anderer Stoffe makro- und niedermolekularer Natur, wie z. B. Globin, Glykogen, Testisextrakt, Hyaluronidase, Proteasen, Ricin, Formalin, Kaolin, niedermolekulare Aminliberatoren u. a. (Jasmin, 1956a, b), Carrageenin (Winter u. Mitarb., 1962), Dextrine (Veilleux, 1963) sowie auch durch physikalische Eingriffe (Erhitzung der Pfote) hervorbringen. Als Modelle für Entzündungsvorgänge spielen sie in der experimentellen Pathologie und Pharmakologie eine große Rolle, obwohl es sich sicher nicht bei allen diesen Vorgängen um echte Entzündungen handelt (zur Kritik vgl. Varga u. Mitarb., 1963). Die meisten dieser Ödemreaktionen sind nicht als anaphylaktoid aufzufassen, da ihnen entweder die eine oder die andere der charakteristischen Eigenschaften, die Wirkstofffreisetzung oder die artspezifische Gebundenheit oder das Freisein von sonstigen toxischen Effekten, fehlt. Eine Ausnahme bilden vielleicht das Glykogen, die Dextrine und das Globin, die jedoch noch nicht ausreichend untersucht sind.

Bei der folgenden Darstellung haben wir uns für eine getrennte Behandlung des Eiklar- und Dextranödems entschieden, obwohl sie sich pathogenetisch und symptomatisch sehr ähneln. Weil sich aber viele Arbeiten nur mit dem Eiklarödem, das zuerst entdeckt wurde, andere nur mit dem Dextranödem beschäftigen, so hätte nach unserer Meinung die gemeinsame Behandlung die Übersichtlichkeit beeinträchtigt. Außerdem entsprechen sich beide Ödemformen nicht vollständig, so daß bis zu einem gewissen Grade auch sachliche Gründe die Trennung rechtfertigen. Alle Arbeiten, in denen beide Ödemformen gleichwertig behandelt sind, sind im Eiklarkapitel ausführlich besprochen und werden im Dextrankapitel kurz erwähnt.

I. Das Eiklarödem

Eiklar war die Substanz, an der die anaphylaktoide Reaktion der Ratte entdeckt wurde, und zwar von SELYE (1937). Schon in den vorausgehenden Jahrzehnten wurden von verschiedenen Autoren Ratten mit Eiereiweißpräparaten behandelt mit dem Ziel, eine Anaphylaxie zu erzeugen. Offenbar wurde aber das typische Ödem nicht beobachtet (ALMON und PARSONS, 1937; NOVY und DE KRUIF, 1917e; PARKER und PARKER, 1924; PRATT, 1935).

Noch 1939 hat MOLOMUT ausdrücklich eine primäre Toxicität der von ihm benutzten Eiklarpräparate in Abrede gestellt. Nur PARKER und PARKER haben schon 1924 eine Giftwirkung von Eiklar bei nicht mit Eiklar vorbehandelten Ratten beschrieben. Aber das typische Ödem tritt in der Schilderung der Symptome nicht auf. Die mitgeteilten Symptome entsprechen nach unseren heutigen Kenntnissen (SANYAL u. WEST, 1958) mehr den anaphylaktischen Symptomen bei dieser Tierart. PRATT (1935) erwähnt Fußödeme als Zeichen anaphylaktischer Reaktion bei der Ratte, ohne dabei einen ausdrücklichen Unterschied zwischen den beiden von ihm benutzten Antigenen, nämlich Eiklar und Pferdeserum, zu machen.

1. Allgemeine Symptomatologie

10 Jahre nach der Entdeckung durch SELYE wurde das Eiklarödem von LÉGER, MASSON und PRADO (1947b, c) weiter bearbeitet. Danach tritt das typische Ödem nach 0,15 ml Eiklar pro Ratte i. p. bei 50 % der Tiere auf. Mit steigenden Dosen erhöht sich mehr der Prozentsatz der befallenen Tiere als die Intensität der Reaktion. Die Intensität zeigt starke, von der Dosis unabhängige Schwankungen (ARRIGONI-MARTELLI und KRAMER, 1958; EICHENBERGER, SCHMIDHAUSER und RUFENER, 1952; KRAMER, 1956b). Mit einiger Regelmäßigkeit erhält man das Ödem innerhalb 60—90 min nach Gaben von 1—3 ml Eiklar pro Tier. I.v. tritt das Ödem schon nach 10—30 min ein, sofern die schon erwähnten allgemeinen Reaktionen dabei nicht im Vordergrund stehen. Das Ödem schwindet im Verlauf von 4—6 Std wieder. Ein tödlicher Ausgang ist selten. Die genauere Untersuchung deckt als Begleitsymptome ein Absinken der Körpertemperatur und, besonders bei i. v. Injektion, einen Abfall des Blutdruckes auf (HALPERN, 1956; MASSON, CORCORAN und FRANCO-BROWDER, 1958). Die Ödembildung ist von einem Plasmaverlust in der Blutbahn begleitet, der sich durch Bluteindickung zu erkennen gibt (HALPERN, 1949b, 1956; HALPERN und BRIOT, 1949). Gefäßerweiterung und Erhöhung der Capillarpermeabilität sind somit die kardinalen pathogenetischen Faktoren der Eiklarreaktion bei der Ratte. Weitere Kennzeichen der Permeabilitätssteigerung der Gefäße sind der hohe Eiweißgehalt der Ödemflüssigkeit (nach HALPERN, 1956, 30—35 g/l) und die Anfärbung der ödematösen Bezirke durch vorher i.v. injizierte Farbstoffe (Evansblau und Trypanblau), die an die Albumine gebunden werden und mit diesen aus der Gefäßbahn austreten (MENKIN, 1938). Die Blaufärbung der Haut tritt etwas früher ein als das Ödem und hält länger an (HALPERN, 1956). Im großen und ganzen geht sie aber mit der Ödembildung und der Hämokonzentration parallel (BENDITT, BADER und LAM, 1955; HALPERN und BRIOT, 1950; PARRATT und WEST, 1958). Die Zunahme der Farbkonzentration in Haut und Pfoten ist nach quantitativen Farbstoffbestimmungen im Gewebe mit einer Abnahme der Farbstoffkonzentration in Herz, Lunge und Gehirn verbunden (BEACH und STEINETZ, 1961).

Auch der Jancsó-Test (JANCSÓ, 1947, 1961), die Anlagerung kolloidaler Teilchen (Tusche) an die Gefäßwand und deren nachträgliche Speicherung in den Endothelien und schließlich in den perivasculären Phagocyten („Endothelaktivierung", „Phagocytosestimulierung") fällt positiv aus. Namentlich GÖZSY und KÁTÓ haben diesem Phänomen eine Reihe von Untersuchungen gewidmet (1957a, b). Einige Beobachtungen, auf die noch zurückzukommen sein wird, könnten dafür sprechen, daß die Ödembildung und die Vorgänge der Tusche- resp. Farbstoffspeicherung nicht immer miteinander streng gekoppelt sind und daß vielleicht verschiedene Mechanismen im Spiele sind.

Der Eiweißgehalt der Ödemflüssigkeit ist etwas niedriger als im Serum, aber von gleicher Zusammensetzung mit Ausnahme eines etwas geringeren Gehaltes an γ-Globulinen und einer leichten Vermehrung der α-Globuline (FORMANEK, HÖLLER u. STOKLASKA, 1961). Serotonin-, Histamin- und Hyaluronidaseödem verhalten sich ähnlich. Die Eiweißzusammensetzung spricht ebenso wie die Zellfreiheit der Ödemflüssigkeit dafür, daß beim Eiweißödem keine echte Entzündung, sondern nur eine Transsudation infolge einer Permeabilitätssteigerung vorliegt (vgl. auch KRAMER, 1956a). Nur in der Postödemphase kommt es zu einer Leukocytenemigration (KLEIN, 1951; RIECHERT u. KLEIN, 1951). Das Formalinödem verhält sich jedoch wie ein entzündliches Ödem, ausgezeichnet durch hohen γ-Globulin- und niedrigen Albumingehalt.

Für zahlreiche Untersuchungen ist auch das zuerst von GROSS (1950a) und WILHELMI und DOMENJOZ (1951b) angegebene Verfahren benützt worden, das Eiklar subcutan in die Dorsalseite der Pfote zu injizieren. Andere ziehen die Plantarseite vor (KÜCHLE und WEGENER, 1952). Man injiziert 0,06—0,1 ml Eiklar in verdünnter oder unverdünnter Form. Man erhält auf diese Weise eine lokalisierte, von Dosis und Konzentration abhängige Ödembildung, die sich gut messen läßt. Hierfür sind verschiedene Verfahren angegeben worden: Grobe Schätzung, Wägung der abgeschnittenen Pfote (HALPERN und BRIOT, 1950; KRANTZ, CARR u. a., 1949), Plethysmographie (BUTTLE u. Mitarb., 1957; HALPERN und BRIOT, 1949; HARRIS u. SPENCER, 1962; HILLEBRECHT, 1954), Bestimmung des Wassergehaltes in der Pfote (ROWLEY und BENDITT, 1956) oder ein radiometrisches Verfahren durch Injektion von J^{131}-markiertem Albumin in die Blutbahn, welches in das Ödem übertritt (FRIES, 1958). Durch Injektion von Eiklar in die Pfote läßt sich der Austritt von i. v. injiziertem Evansblau auf den injizierten Bezirk lokalisieren.

Es gibt auch ein Verfahren (GÖZSY u. KÁTÓ, 1957a; HALPERN, 1956; HALPERN, LIACOPOULOS-BRIOT u. LIACOPOULOS, 1958), bei dem die für die Ödembildung wenig empfindliche Bauchhaut zur intradermalen Injektion von Eiklar benutzt wird. Als Test dient die Blaufärbung an der Innenseite der Haut nach gleichzeitiger i.v. Evansblau-Injektion. Es läßt sich also durch die intradermale Eiklarinjektion auch an anderen als den Prädilektionsstellen eine spezifische Permeabilitätssteigerung durch Eiklar erzielen. Das Verfahren eignet sich besonders gut zur Bestimmung von Eiklarschwellendosen und ihrer Beeinflussung durch verschiedene Maßnahmen.

Die Empfindlichkeit der Ratten gegen Eiklar hängt offenbar nicht vom Alter, aber möglicherweise vom Geschlecht ab (LÉGER, MASSON u. PRADO, 1947b, c). In einem kleinen Prozentsatz findet sich eine angeborene Resistenz (VAN CAUWENBERGE, LAPIÈRE u. a., 1958), in gesetzmäßiger Weise bei Wistarratten (HARRIS u. WEST, 1961).

Über die Toleranz nach wiederholten Gaben von Eiklar gehen die Angaben auseinander. Mit täglichen i.p. Eiklargaben erzielte SELYE (1937) schon nach 4 Tagen eine Toleranz, LÉGER, MASSON und PRADO (1947c) nach 9 Tagen noch keine deutliche Gewöhnung. KRAMER (1956b) sah erst am 16. Tage eine vollständige Toleranz, EICHENBERGER, SCHMIDHAUSER und RUFENER (1952) erst am 35. Tag ein Minimum an Ödemneigung. Auch durch lokale Injektion von Eiklar (Dextran, Pepton, Hyaluronidase) in die Pfote oder durch Vorerhitzung der Pfote tritt Ödemschutz gegenüber nachträglicher i.p. Injektion von Eiklar oder Dextran ein (HOENE, 1954; HOENE, LABBÉ und SELYE, 1952). Ovomucoid erzeugt i. v. bei der 2. Gabe, 3 Wochen nach der ersten, wieder ein Ödem, während Testisextrakt von Stieren bei der ersten Injektion ein Ödem, bei der zweiten aber eine schwere Allgemeinreaktion auslöst (BENDITT, BADER u. ARASE, 1953). Eine Resistenz gegen

Eiklar (oder Ovomucoid) läßt sich ferner durch länger dauernde Vorbehandlung mit Dextran erzeugen, gleichzeitig mit einer Toleranz gegen Dextran (HALPERN, LIACOPOULOS-BRIOT und LIACOPOULOS, 1958; KRAMER, 1956b; PARRATT und WEST, 1957e; WEST, 1957a).

Über den umgekehrten Vorgang liegt nur eine Mitteilung von GÖZSY u. KÁTÓ (1957a) vor. Sie konnten allerdings nach 13tägiger Vorbehandlung mit Eiklar noch immer intradermal mit Dextran eine Tusche- und Trypanblauspeicherung in der Bauchhaut erzielen. Da die intradermale Dextranreaktion auch nach Vorbehandlung mit Dextran erhalten blieb, stehen ihre Versuche im Widerspruch zu ähnlich angelegten Versuchen anderer Autoren (HALPERN, LIACOPOULOS-BRIOT u. LIACOPOULOS, 1958). Eine mögliche Erklärung liegt darin, daß nicht genügend lange vorbehandelt worden ist, weshalb auch alle aus solchen negativen Toleranzversuchen gezogenen Schlußfolgerungen (insbesondere über die Rolle von Überträgerstoffen) mit Vorsicht aufgenommen werden müssen. Dagegen stimmt die Beobachtung von GÖZSY und KÁTÓ, daß nach Vorbehandlung mit 48/80 durch Eiklar kein Ödem mehr ausgelöst werden kann, Eiklar aber keine Toleranz gegen 48/80 erzeugt, mit den Beobachtungen anderer Autoren (HALPERN, LIACOPOULOS-BRIOT u. LIACOPOULOS, 1958; JASMIN, 1956a, b; PARRATT u. WEST, 1957e) überein. Aber auch mit 48/80 tritt die Resistenz gegen Eiklar oft erst nach langer Vorbehandlung ein (FELDBERG u. TALESNIK, 1953; KRAMER, 1956b).

2. Ursächlicher Faktor des Eiklars

Wir verdanken LÉGER, MASSON und PRADO (1947b) den Nachweis, daß unter den verschiedenen Fraktionen des Eiklars (HEKTOEN u. COLE, 1928) nur das Ovomucoid die ödemerzeugende Wirksamkeit bei der Ratte besitzt. Mit Rücksicht auf das Dextran ist es von Interesse, daß es sich um ein Glucoproteid handelt mit einem Molekulargewicht von etwa 29000 (HALPERN und BRIOT, 1952b). Werden Zucker- und Eiweißkomponente voneinander getrennt, so erweisen sich beide für sich allein als unwirksam. Ovomucoid ist wirksam in Dosen von 50 mg/kg i.p. (ARRIGONI-MARTELLI und KRAMER, 1958). Subcutan bekommt man eine Lokalreaktion mit Konzentrationen von 50 μg/ml (ROWLEY und BENDITT, 1956). Intradermal genügt, auf Stickstoff berechnet, 1 μg für die Evansblaureaktion (HALPERN, 1956).

Pferde- oder Rinderserum vermag bei der Ratte die toxischen Eiklarphänomene nicht hervorzurufen (BENDITT, BADER u. LAM, 1955; LÉGER, MASSON u. PRADO, 1947c). Die noch zu besprechende histaminliberierende Wirkung des Eiklars bei der Ratte fehlt beim Hund. Eiklar setzt jedoch auch bei der Katze Histamin frei. Die Wirkung bei der Katze ist aber an einen anderen, nämlich koktolabilen Faktor gebunden als bei der Ratte, wo er koktostabil ist (SCHACHTER u. TALESNIK, 1952).

3. Histamin- und Eiklarödem

Die schon von LÉGER und MASSON (1947) erörterte Möglichkeit einer Histaminfreisetzung durch Eiklar wurde von SCHACHTER und TALESNIK (1952) durch den Nachweis einer Histaminvermehrung im Plasma, die über 60 min anhielt, bestätigt. Ovomucoid setzt an der isolierten Rattenhaut ähnlich wie 48/80 Histamin frei (BENDITT, BADER u. a., 1954). Außerdem gelang dieser Nachweis auch im Durchströmungsversuch mit Eiklar an der hinteren Körperhälfte der Ratte (PARRATT und WEST, 1957e). Vorher hatte allerdings LECOMTE (1957) in der gleichen Versuchsanordnung negative Ergebnisse mit Eiklar wie mit Dextran, positive nur mit der Substanz 1935 L. Die Histaminfreisetzung durch Eiklar (und Dextran) geht langsamer vor sich als durch 48/80 oder Polymyxin B (PARRATT und WEST, 1957e). Damit hängt wohl zusammen, daß sich nach Kramer (1956b) die Eiklar- und Dextranödeme langsamer entwickeln, aber auch länger anhalten als die Ödeme durch 48/80. Die Vermehrung des Histamins im Plasma geht nach FELDBERG und TALESNIK (1953) mit einer Abnahme des Histamingehaltes in der Haut des Bauches und Schenkels um 45 resp. 38 % nach i.p. Injektion von 2 ml Eiklar einher. PARRATT und WEST (1957e) fanden dagegen nur in der Pfotenhaut und an den

Ohren, nicht aber in der Bauchhaut eine deutliche Abnahme. In vitro ließ sich an der Cutis und Subcutis der Pfote eine maximale Histaminabnahme um $^{1}/_{3}$ des Ausgangswertes erzielen. Dieser Effekt konnte selbst durch 10fache Steigerung der wirksamen Eiklardosen nicht mehr erhöht werden (BENDITT, BADER und LAM,1955).

Das Histamin stammt aus den Mastzellen, die unter der Wirkung des Eiklars resp. Ovomucoids und des Dextrans besonders in den vom Ödem betroffenen Gebieten ihre Granula ausstoßen und an Größe abnehmen und die besonders zahlreich an den Prädilektionsstellen sind (BENDITT, BADER u. a., 1954; BENDITT, BADER und LAM, 1955; FELDBERG und TALESNIK, 1953; ROWLEY und BENDITT, 1956). Histamin und Serotonin üben diese Wirkung nicht aus. Es handelt sich also nicht um Sekundäreffekte freigesetzter Amine oder des Ödems. PARRATT und WEST (1957e) denken allerdings auch an sekundäre Veränderungen, weil sie nicht nur die perivasculären, sondern auch von den Blutgefäßen entfernte Zellgruppen betroffen fanden. Die Mastzellen in der Subcutis des Bauches sind nach PARRATT und WEST (1957e) bei i. p. Injektion nicht betroffen, wohl aber die mesenterialen Zellen (schon 1931 von WEBB beschrieben). BENDITT, BADER und LAM (1955) fanden auch eine zeitliche Beziehung zwischen Mastzellveränderungen, Histaminverarmung und Ödembildung in der dorsalen Haut der Pfote. An isolierten Rattenmastzellen fanden LAGUNOFF und BENDITT (1960) im Gegensatz zu der Wirkung von 48/80 oder Polymyxin B keine Degranulation mit Histaminfreisetzung durch Ovomucoid und Dextran. Auch KELLER und BEEGER (1961) sahen eine Schwellung, Granulafreisetzung und Vacuolisierung durch Zugabe von Hühnereiweiß nur an isolierten Mastzellen sensibilisierter Ratten.

Aus den Beobachtungen über die Histaminabnahme in der Haut und aus den Befunden über die Histaminfreisetzung aus isolierten Hautstücken, in Durchströmungspräparaten und aus isolierten Mastzellen geht hervor, daß Ovomucoid (und Dextran) schwächere Histaminliberatoren sind als die basischen Liberatoren (48/80, 1935 L, Polymyxin B).

Eine Histamintheorie des Eiklarödems setzt voraus, daß man mit Histamin die gleichen Erscheinungen wie mit Eiklar hervorrufen kann. Dies trifft jedoch nur in beschränktem Maße zu (LÉGER, MASSON und PRADO, 1947b), am wenigsten für die i. v. Injektion, bei der sich die Ratte bekanntlich als sehr wenig histaminempfindlich erweist. Nur subcutan bekommt man mit Histamin ein lokalisiertes Ödem, z. B. in der Pfote, aber in auffallend hohen Dosen (100 μg) (PARRATT und WEST, 1957e). Die niedermolekularen Histaminliberatoren dagegen, sowohl 48/80 (DEWS, WNUCK u. a., 1953) als auch Polymyxin B (BUSHBY und GREEN, 1955), rufen Ödembildung an den typischen Stellen auch schon bei i. p. Injektion in Dosen von 5 mg/kg hervor. Bei lokaler Applikation in die Pfote wirkt schon 1 μg von beiden Stoffen (PARRATT und WEST, 1957b, e). Man könnte zugunsten einer Histamintheorie des Rattenödems annehmen, daß die Histaminliberatoren unabhängig von der Zuführungsart lokal eine so hohe Histaminkonzentration durch Entbindung des Gewebshistamins hervorrufen, wie sie durch exogenes Histamin nur bei lokaler Applikation erzeugt werden kann. Der Histamingehalt der Haut sinkt unter 48/80 oder Polymyxin B nach einmaliger Gabe um 80 % oder mehr (BUSHBY und GREEN, 1955; KRAMER, 1956b). Ob die schwächer histaminfreisetzende Wirkung von Eiklar oder Dextran aber dazu ausreicht, ist eine andere Frage.

Auf die zahlreichen Versuche, mit Antihistaminica das Eiklarödem zu hemmen (ACKERMANN, EICHENBERGER u. a., 1962; CHEN und WICKEL, 1952; CLARK und MACKAY, 1949b; FISCHER und FREY, 1951; GROSS, 1950a, b; HALPERN, 1949a, b; HALPERN und BRIOT, 1949; KÜCHLE und WEGENER, 1952; LÉGER und MASSON,

1947; Léger, Masson und Prado, 1947b; Rothlin und Cerletti, 1955; Wilhelmi und Domenjoz, 1950/51), soll hier nicht im einzelnen eingegangen werden. Die wichtigsten Befunde für die Frage nach der ursächlichen Bedeutung des Histamins für das Ödem sind folgende: Antihistaminica wirken nur in hohen und oft schon toxischen Dosen (Léger und Masson, 1947; Léger, Masson und Prado, 1947a). Es bestehen starke Unterschiede in der Wirkung. Eine besonders starke Wirkung sollen das Promethazin (Halpern, 1949a, b; Halpern und Briot, 1949) und das 7-Chlor-10-β-dimethylaminoäthyl-10,11-dihydro-11-oxo-5-dibenzo-[b,e] [1,4]-diazepin HCl (Ackermann, Eichenberger u. a., 1962) haben. Die Wirkung der Antihistaminica richtet sich gegen alle Symptome der Eiklarvergiftung mit Ausnahme der Hypothermie. Promethazin hat auch eine Schutzwirkung gegen die noch zu besprechende letale Wirkung von Eiklar bei nebennierenlosen Ratten. Halpern und Briot (1950) vertraten die Auffassung, daß die Schutzwirkung dieses Stoffes mit seiner starken Antihistaminwirkung zusammenhänge. Aus anderen Beobachtungen geht aber hervor, daß ein gesetzmäßiger Zusammenhang zwischen der Antieiklar- und der Antihistaminwirkung bei der Prüfung mehrerer Antihistaminica nicht besteht. Allerdings sind solche Versuche nicht beweisend, die sich auf einen Vergleich der Antieiklarwirkung bei der Ratte mit der antiletalen Wirkung auf die Histaminvergiftung des Meerschweinchens stützen und die besonders starke Differenzen ergeben haben, z. B. bei der Prüfung von Mepyramin und Diphenhydramin (Friedlaender, Feinberg und Feinberg, 1947; Léger und Masson, 1947; Léger, Masson und Prado, 1947b). Denn es ist möglich, daß hierbei auch die Verschiedenartigkeit der Testobjekte eine Rolle spielt.

Ein brauchbares Vorgehen besteht darin, die Antihistaminwirkung bei der Ratte sowohl am Eiklarödem als auch am Histaminödem zu prüfen. Dabei kann zwar zugunsten der Histamintheorie die Feststellung angeführt werden, daß die gleiche Dosis eines Antihistaminicums (Mepyramin) zur Hemmung des Eiklar- und des Histaminödems ausreicht (Léger und Masson, 1947; Parratt und West, 1958). Ferner zeigen manche Antihistaminica, z. B. Promethazin, Phenindamin und Mepyramin in ihren relativen Wirkungsunterschieden ein ähnliches Verhalten gegenüber Eiklar wie gegenüber Histamin. Aber solche Übereinstimmungen verlieren an Beweiskraft, wenn andere Befunde ein abweichendes Verhalten von Antihistaminica gegenüber dem Eiklar- und dem Histaminödem ergeben. Beispiele dieser Art lassen sich ebenfalls aus dem Material von Parratt und West (1958) entnehmen. Sie können dafür sprechen, daß ohne die Annahme einer weiteren Wirkungskomponente der Antihistaminica ihre Wirkung beim Eiklarödem nicht voll zu erklären ist.

Da derartige Abweichungen durch die weiter unten besprochene Serotoninfreisetzung eine Erklärung finden, soll hier nur kurz auf Auffassungen hingewiesen werden, nach denen die Wirkung der Antihistaminica mit „unspezifischen“ Wirkungen auf die Gefäßwand, z. B. nach Gözsy und Kátó (1957a, b, 1959b) auf die sog. Endothelaktivierung (Klebrigkeit der Endothelien) zusammenhängen könne. Ein gewisses Argument für diese Möglichkeit liefern Versuche dieser Autoren. Danach ist es möglich, trotz Vorbehandlung mit Eiklar, Dextran oder 48/80 durch intradermale Injektion von Dextran oder 48/80 noch eine Tusche- und Trypanblauspeicherung zu erzielen, die durch Antihistaminica blockierbar ist. Da aber die Erschöpfung der Amindepots durch Aminliberatoren nie vollständig ist, so fehlt derartigen Versuchen die letzte Beweiskraft gegen die Möglichkeit, daß unter gewissen Bedingungen doch noch eine Wirkstofffreisetzung zustandekommt.

Es ist andererseits nicht von der Hand zu weisen, daß die bekannten Nebenwirkungen der Antihistaminica auch eine unterstützende Rolle spielen könnten. Läßt sich doch das Eiklarödem auch durch zahlreiche andere Medikamente beeinflussen, so z. B. durch Sympathicomimetica, Corticoide, Calcium, Lokalanaesthetica, Pyrazole, Morphin, Cinchophen, Azulene, Eisensalze, Hyaluronidasehemmstoffe, Mutterkornalkaloide, Propylenglycol, 2-Dimethylaminoäthanol, Proteasen u. a. m. (Adamkiewicz, Rice u. McColl, 1955; Beiler, Brendel u.

Martin, 1955; Bickhardt u. Heite, 1954; Bludau u. Heite, 1954; Chen u. Wickel, 1952; Cronheim u. Toekes, 1959; Domenjoz, 1952, 1953, 1960; Domenjoz, Mörsdorf u. a., 1955, 1957; Fabinyi-Szebehely, Hahn u. Szebehely, 1953; Fischer u. Frey, 1951; Flandre u. Mitarb., 1963; Frey u. Fischer, 1956; Fries, 1958; Gaddum u. Hameed, 1954; Gibertini, Vecchati u. Giberti, 1951; Gross, 1950a, b; Haas, Hohagen u. Kollmannsperger, 1953; Halpern, 1949b; Halpern u. Briot, 1950; Heilmeyer, Frey u. Fischer, 1951, 1952; Heite u. Höland, 1956; Hillebrecht, 1954; Kramer, 1953, 1956a; Küchle u. Wegener, 1952; Martin, 1957; Martin, Brendel u. Beiler, 1953, 1954; Meier, Gross u. Desaulles, 1951; Riechert u. Barghorn, 1954; Riechert u. Klein, 1951; Scheiffarth u. Berg, 1952; Stern u. Milin, 1956; Van Cauwenberge, Lapière u. a., 1958; Wilhelmi, 1949, 1952; Wilhelmi u. Domenjoz, 1951a, b; Winder, Wax u. Been, 1957). Für die Pyrazole wurde ein antihistaminärer Wirkungsmechanismus diskutiert (Jaques u. Domenjoz, 1950/51; Wilhelmi u. Pulver, 1955).

Noch verwickelter stellen sich die Verhältnisse in den Versuchen von Irino (1958) dar, welcher findet, daß eine Hemmung des Eiweißödems verursacht sein kann 1. durch Histaminliberatoren, 2. durch Stoffe, welche die Freisetzung von Histamin hemmen und 3. durch Stoffe die beides bewirken. Salicylat, Aminopyrin, Butazolidin, Cortison und Guajazulen sind Hemmstoffe des Eiweißödems, welche (wie auch Phenergan in kleinen Dosen) die Eigenschaft besitzen, die Hemmung des Eiklarödems durch Vorbehandlung mit einer Dextrangabe zu potenzieren und andererseits die Freisetzung von Histamin durch Dextran zu hemmen, ohne selbst den Histamingehalt der Haut zu ändern. Irgapyrin und große Phenergandosen, welche sowohl histaminliberierende Wirkungen als auch hemmende Wirkungen auf die Histaminfreisetzung und schließlich auch Antihistaminwirkungen besitzen, ferner das Hauthistamin leicht vermindern, sind relativ starke Ödemhemmer. Nach Adrenalektomie und Hypophysektomie nimmt die ödemhemmende Wirkung von Salicylat und Aminopyrin ab, von Cortison zu. Guajazulen bleibt in seiner Wirkung unverändert.

Büch u. Wagner-Jauregg (1962) haben gezeigt, daß Substanzen mit ödemerzeugender Wirkung (bei subplantarer Injektion) in der Lage sind, bei intraperitonealer Injektion die Ödembildung durch eine Reihe subplantar injizierter Stoffe zu hemmen, und zwar durch eine „Reizwirkung". Gegenüber dem durch PVP an der Rattenpfote ausgelösten Ödem sind in abnehmender Reihenfolge u. a. folgende Stoffe wirksam: Flavine, Äscin, NaOH, Ovalbumin, Dextran, Formalin, PVP. Ödemerzeugende und ödemhemmende Wirksamkeit gehen parallel.

Stärkere Bedenken gegen die ausschließliche Rolle des Histamins beim Eiklarödem entstanden aus der Beobachtung, daß bei wiederholter Vorbehandlung mit Eiklar die Abnahme der Ödembereitschaft nicht mit der Abnahme der Histaminvorräte parallel geht. Die Histaminvorräte in der Haut sinken unter der Wirkung von Histaminliberatoren schon nach wenigen Injektionen auf einen Endwert ab, der sich trotz fortgesetzter Behandlung mit den Liberatoren nicht mehr ändert. Dieser Endwert liegt beim Eiklar mit 60 % der Norm noch sehr hoch, während er bei den basischen Liberatoren (48/80) unter 10 % der Norm beträgt. Alle Autoren stimmen darin überein, daß weder mit der Eiklarvorbehandlung noch mit dem stärker auf die Histamindepots wirkenden 48/80 die Eiklarresistenz zu dem Zeitpunkt der maximalen Histaminausschöpfung der Gewebe auftritt, sondern erst mehrere Tage nach fortgesetzter Vorbehandlung mit den Liberatoren (Adamkiewicz und Adamkiewicz, 1959b; Feldberg und Talesnik, 1953; Kramer, 1956b; Lecomte und Van Cauwenberge, 1955). Auffallend ist auch, daß bei täglicher Eiklargabe der Histamingehalt der Haut weniger, die Ödembereitschaft aber schneller abnimmt als bei täglicher Dextrangabe (Kramer, 1956b). Angesichts dieser Umstände verliert selbst die Tatsache an Beweiskraft für eine ausschließliche Rolle des Histamins, daß die stärkeren Histaminliberatoren 48/80 und 1935 L leichter eine Toleranz gegen Eiklar und Dextran erzeugen, als umgekehrt die makromolekularen Stoffe gegen 48/80 oder 1935 L (Halpern, Liacopoulos-Briot und Liacopoulos, 1958).

Van Cauwenberge, Lecomte und Vliers (1957) sehen ein weiteres Argument gegen die alleinige Rolle des Histamins darin, daß während des anaphylaktoiden Ödems nicht wie nach Histamininjektion eine Stimulierung des Hypophysen-Nebennieren-Systems auftritt.

4. Serotonin und Eiklarödem

Die Schwierigkeiten, die sich einer ausschließlichen Histamintheorie des Eiklarödems in den Weg stellen, scheinen wenigstens bis zu einem gewissen Grade durch den Nachweis überwunden, daß gleichzeitig mit Histamin auch Serotonin frei wird. Als erste haben BENDITT, BADER und LAM (1955) sowie PARRATT und WEST (1957b) an das Serotonin gedacht, nachdem vorher schon BENOS (1954) für das Dextranödem eine sogenannte „vasodepressive Substanz" in Betracht zog. Auch BOIS u. SELYE (1956) beschreiben die Ähnlichkeit der Serotonin- und Eiklar- resp. Dextranwirkung bei i.v., i.p. und subcutaner Anwendung an Ratten. Serotonin ist in der Rattenhaut in großer Menge enthalten (PARRATT und WEST, 1957c). Daß Serotonin durch Eiklar freigesetzt wird, läßt sich aus der Abnahme des Serotoningehaltes in der Haut, aus Perfusionsversuchen an der isolierten hinteren Rattenhälfte (PARRATT und WEST, 1957c), sowie aus Versuchen an isolierten, inkubierten Hautstücken (MEDAKOVIĆ, 1959) entnehmen. Die Freisetzung des Serotonins erfolgt im Durchströmungsversuch ähnlich wie die des Histamins mit einer deutlichen Verzögerung gegenüber der Wirkung von 48/80. Serotonin ist auch in der Ödemflüssigkeit nachweisbar, nicht dagegen Histamin, obwohl auch dieses frei wird (PARRATT und WEST, 1957c).

Das Serotonin scheint bei der Ratte als regulativer Faktor der Gefäßpermeabilität eine besondere Rolle zu spielen. Gegenüber der permeabilitätssteigernden Wirkung von Serotonin ist die Ratte viel empfindlicher als z. B. das Meerschweinchen, während das Umgekehrte gegenüber Histamin der Fall ist (SPARROW u. WILHELM, 1957). Serotonin erzeugt subcutan in einer Konzentration von 1 μg/ml in die Pfote injiziert ein Ödem und einen positiven Farbstofftest (BENDITT u. ROWLEY, 1956; PARRATT u. WEST, 1957c, e; VAN CAUWENBERGE, LECOMTE u. VLIERS, 1957; WEST, 1957a, b, 1961a). Diese Konzentration ist mit 200 μg/ml Histamin äquieffektiv. JORI, BENTIVOGLIO u. GARATTINI (1961) bezeichnen Serotonin in einer Konzentration von 2,5 μg/ml als etwa äquieffektiv im Farbstofftest mit einer Histaminkonzentration von 1 mg/ml. Andere Autoren geben allerdings ein anderes Verhältnis der permeabilitätssteigernden Wirkung der beiden Amine an, was mit unterschiedlichen Testmethoden zusammenhängen kann. Nach SPARROW und WILHELM (1957) ist Serotonin 11mal wirksamer als Histamin, nach HALPERN, LIACOPOULOS-BRIOT und LIACOPOULOS (1958) 30mal wirksamer.

Die Serotoninwirkung tritt auch auf an Tieren, deren Haut vorher histaminarm durch Vorbehandlung mit Polymyxin B gemacht worden ist. Nach Erschöpfung des Gewebsserotonins durch Reserpin setzen Histaminliberatoren noch Histamin frei. Es wurde daraus von PARRATT und WEST (1957e) der Schluß gezogen, daß die Wirkung des Serotonins nicht auf dem Umwege über eine Histaminfreisetzung zustande kommt. SPARROW und WILHELM (1957) vertreten jedoch die Auffassung, daß mindestens ein Teil der Gefäßwirkung von Serotonin durch Freisetzung von Histamin bedingt ist. Im gleichen Sinne sprechen die Versuche von BINET und QUIVY (1956, 1957, 1958b), wonach Serotonin nach Injektion in die Rattenpfote zu einer schwachen Histaminliberierung führt. Diese Frage bedarf noch weiterer Prüfung.

THEOBALD und DOMENJOZ (1958) sind der Meinung, daß dem Serotonin nur eine accessorische Rolle für die Ödementstehung zukomme, weil sie durch i.p.-Injektion mit Serotonin keine Ödeme an den Acren erhalten konnten. Auch die i.v.-Injektion von Serotonin-Histamingemischen (im Verhältnis der beim Ödem freigesetzten Mengen) führt nach MASSON, CORCORAN u. FRANCO-BROWDER (1958) nicht zum Ödem (nur zur Hyperämie und Blutdrucksenkung). Man muß jedoch, wie auch beim Histamin schon erwähnt, daran denken, daß die Ödembildung an so hohe Aminkonzentrationen im Gewebe gebunden ist, wie sie vielleicht nur durch Freisetzung an Ort und Stelle (also gewissermaßen "intrinsic") entstehen können.

Nur die Mäusehaut enthält von allen untersuchten Tierarten noch viel Serotonin, wenn auch wesentlich weniger als die Rattenhaut. Es ist darum interessant, daß außer Ratten nur noch Mäuse eine Reaktion nach Injektion von Dextran oder Eiklar zeigen. Es kommt zwar nicht zum Ödem, aber zur Blaufärbung an den Extremitäten, wenn vorher Evansblau i.v. injiziert wurde (WEST, 1957a).

Bei der Ratte macht nach PARRATT und WEST (1957c) die Serotoninmenge in der Haut mehr als die Hälfte der gesamten Serotoninmenge im Körper aus. Histamin- und Serotoninverteilung gehen nicht parallel. Die Haut aller Körperteile enthält Serotonin. Die Prädilektionsstellen der Ödembildung scheinen nicht besonders ausgezeichnet zu sein. Nach WEST (1957a) sollen sich aber die bedeutenderen Veränderungen im Gehalt an Serotonin und Histamin nach i.p. Injektion von Eiklar oder Dextran in der Haut des Fußrückens der Pfote und des Ohres finden. Die Abnahme an beiden Aminen kann mehr als 50 % der vorhandenen Amine in den empfindlichen Hautstellen betragen.

Serotonin und Histamin sind in der Rattenhaut im Verhältnis 1 : 16–1 : 26 enthalten (BENDITT, WONG u. a., 1955; ROWLEY und BENDITT, 1956). In diesem Verhältnis werden sie offenbar auch freigesetzt. Trotzdem wird man annehmen müssen, daß das Serotonin mit seiner 200fach stärkeren ödemerzeugenden Wirkung eine größere Bedeutung als das Histamin in diesem Mischungsverhältnis hat.

Das Serotonin ist nach PARRATT u. WEST (1957c, d) (anders als das Histamin) im Gegensatz zur Auffassung von BENDITT, WONG u. a. (1955) in der Rattenhaut nur teilweise in den Mastzellen lokalisiert. Besonders bemerkenswert ist es, daß die innere Schicht der Bauchhaut und Fußrückenhaut viel Mastzellen und Histamin enthält, während das Serotonin hauptsächlich in der mastzellfreien äußeren Bauchhaut und den Pfotenballen konzentriert ist (PARRATT u. WEST, 1957c). Daher stammt auch, ebenfalls im Gegensatz zum Histamin, das durch Eiklar oder Dextran freigesetzte Serotonin überwiegend (vielleicht zu 80%) nicht aus den Mastzellen. Die Mastzellveränderungen nach Eiklar und Dextran werden im Gegensatz zu der Wirkung von 48/80 und Polymyxin B von WEST (1957a) als relativ gering bezeichnet, da es sich mehr um eine bloße Degranulation als um einen kompletten Zerfall (disruption) handelt. Das könnte für die vorwiegende Bedeutung des Serotonins sprechen, wenn nicht sicher stünde, daß auch Histamin in relativ großen Mengen freigesetzt wird, und zwar auch lokal in der Haut. Noch schwieriger wird das Problem durch die neuerlichen Feststellungen von KÁTÓ u. GÖZSY (1962) sowie GÖZSY u. KÁTÓ (1963). Danach verursacht Dextran in Dosen bis zu 300 mg/kg (i.v. oder i.p.) keine oder eine nur sehr geringe Mastzellschädigung, in einer Dosis von 600 mg/kg i.v. einen Mastzellzerfall in der Extremitäten- und Bauchhaut von etwa 40%. Die gleichen Autoren beobachteten nach 48/80 einen erheblich stärkeren Mastzellzerfall. Bereits nach etwa 8 mg/kg Dextran i.v. entstanden maximale Ödeme, während nach 48/80 (100 μg/kg) zwar ein Mastzellzerfall, aber keine Ödeme auftraten. Der Mastzellzerfall ging der Ödembildung voraus. Nach hohen Dextrandosen entwickelt sich das Ödem deutlich langsamer als bei kleinen Dosen (GÖZSY u. KÁTÓ, 1960a, 1963; KÁTÓ u. GÖZSY, 1962). Gemeinsam mit LAAFF ermittelten wir in noch unveröffentlichten Versuchen etwa die gleiche Schwellendosis wie GÖZSY u. KÁTÓ (zwischen 6 und 15 mg/kg i.v.) für die Ödembildung; nach 15 mg/kg setzte diese sehr rasch ein und erreichte das Maximum deutlich früher als bei Verwendung höherer Dosen (120 oder 300 mg/kg i.v.), obwohl hier das Maximum eher niedriger lag. Die Verzögerung der Ödembildung nach hohen Dextrandosen könnte man auf die allgemeinen Kreislaufsymptome (siehe oben) zurückführen. Die Histaminausschüttung ins Plasma nimmt nach unseren Versuchen mit der Dextrandosis zu und ist bereits bei Verwendung der Schwellendosen nachweisbar. BERALDO u. Mitarb. (1962) stellen für das Dextranödem die Mastzellruptur in den Vordergrund. Sie finden nach Injektion von Dextran in die Lippenhaut ähnliche Veränderungen wie nach 48/80 und zeigen, daß nach vorheriger Mastzellentfernung aus dem Gewebe die Dextranreaktion ausbleibt. Mesenterial- oder Hautfragmente zeigen auch in vitro nach Kontakt mit Dextran eine starke Ruptur der Mastzellen (48% der Zellen).

Welche Auskunft geben nun die Toleranzversuche über die Bedeutung des Serotonins? Ähnlich wie Histamin ist auch das Serotonin keineswegs im Gewebe völlig erschöpft, wenn durch geeignete Vorbehandlung (z. B. mit Dextran) gegen Eiklar eine Resistenz erzielt worden ist (PARRATT und WEST, 1957e; WEST, 1957a). Die Tatsache, daß 48/80 zu diesem Zeitpunkt noch ein Ödem hervorbringt, könnte damit erklärt werden, daß es als stärkerer Aminliberator wirkt. Es setzt bekanntlich nicht nur Histamin, sondern auch Serotonin frei (BHATTACHARYA und LEWIS, 1956). Von größerer Bedeutung sind die Versuche mit Polymyxin B und Reserpin. Polymyxin B, das den Histamingehalt der Haut maximal, den Serotoningehalt nur etwa um 20 % herabsetzt (BUSHBY und GREEN, 1955), hemmt nur die Ödembildung durch Polymyxin B, nicht durch Eiklar, Dextran und 48/80. Reserpin, das den Serotoningehalt weitgehend erschöpft, den Histamingehalt nur wenig beeinflußt (PARRATT und WEST, 1957d; WEST, 1957b), hemmt die Ödembildung durch Eiklar, Dextran und 48/80 (PARRATT und WEST, 1957e). Reserpin selbst macht kein Ödem (CRAPS und INDERBITZIN, 1961) oder höchstens ein schwaches Ödem (MÖRSDORF, 1959a, 1961a). Eigentümlicherweise wurde auch die Ödembildung durch Polymyxin B nach der Reserpinvorbehandlung vermindert gefunden (CRAPS und INDERBITZIN, 1961; PARRATT und WEST, 1957e). Vielleicht wirkt also auch das Polymyxin B nicht nur über Histamin, sondern auch über die geringe Serotoninmenge, die es (vielleicht aus den Mastzellen) freisetzt. Die ödemhemmende Wirkung von Reserpin ist mehrfach beschrieben worden (ARRIGONI-MARTELLI und KRAMER, 1958; MEDAKOVIĆ, 1959; RIECHERT und ESCHBACH, 1955). Die Vorbehandlung mit 48/80 schließlich setzt die Wirkung von Eiklar, Dextran, 48/80 und Polymyxin B herab. Bei keiner der drei Vorbehandlungsmethoden ist, wie zu erwarten, die ödembildende Wirkung von Histamin und Serotonin aufgehoben (PARRATT und WEST, 1957e).

Durch die Serotonintheorie erscheint auch die Wirkung der Antihistaminica in einem neuen Licht. Bei der Prüfung einer Reihe von solchen Substanzen kamen PARRATT und WEST (1958) zu dem Ergebnis, daß die Wirkung auf das Eiklar- und Dextranödem mehr mit der Wirkung auf das Serotonin- als auf das Histaminödem parallel geht. Die Antihistaminica wirken also mehr durch ihre Antiserotoninkomponente. Daß dies jedoch nicht durchgängig der Fall ist, zeigt das Verhalten von Trimeprazin, das in den Versuchen von PARRATT und WEST starke Hemmwirkung auf Eiklar- und Dextranödem mit starker Antihistamin- und schwacher Antiserotoninwirkung im Ödemtest vereinigt. Ein besonders starker Hemmstoff des Eiklarödems ist nach diesen Autoren Methotrimeprazin, das sowohl starke Antihistamin- als auch starke Antiserotonineigenschaften hat. Sehr schwach wirkt Mepyramin, das sich durch ein relatives Überwiegen der Antihistamin- über die Antiserotoninwirkung auszeichnet.

Häufig sind wegen ihrer starken ödemhemmenden Wirkung Promethazin und Chlorpromazin untersucht worden (COURVOISIER, FOURNEL u. a., 1953; MASSON, CORCORAN und FRANCO-BROWDER, 1958; PARRATT und WEST, 1958; STONE, WENGER u. a., 1961; VIAUD, 1954). Auch sie haben beide sowohl eine Antiserotonin- als auch eine Antihistaminwirkung (BENDITT und ROWLEY, 1956; DOEPFNER und CERLETTI, 1957; GYERMEK, LÁZÁR und CSÁK, 1956; LÉCOMTE, 1955; PARRATT und WEST, 1958; STONE, WENGER u. a., 1961). Beide Substanzen wirken nach PARRATT und WEST (1958) auf das Histaminödem genau so stark wie auf das Serotoninödem. Von Promethazin sind dabei doppelt so große Dosen notwendig wie von Chlorpromazin (8 statt 4 mg/kg).

EICHENBERGER, SCHMIDHAUSER und RUFENER (1952) beobachteten, daß unter fortgesetzter Eiklarbehandlung die ödematösen Reaktionen zwar nicht verschwanden, aber allmählich gegen Promethazin resistent wurden. Dieser Befund verdient eine Nachprüfung, denn er könnte darauf hinweisen, daß an dem Eiklarödem noch ein anderer pathogenetischer Mechanismus beteiligt ist als die Freisetzung von Aminen und daß sich der Körper gegen diesen Mechanismus besonders langsam resistent machen läßt.

Anders verhalten sich die beiden Stoffe gegenüber der toxischen Wirkung von Histamin und Serotonin am Meerschweinchen. Hierbei erweist sich Promethazin als ein relativ stärkerer Histaminantagonist als Chlorpromazin (SCHMID, ZICHA u. a., 1959; VIAUD, 1954). Das ist nach HALPERN, LIACOPOULOS und LIACOPOULOS-BRIOT (1959) nicht nur am Meerschweinchen, sondern auch an der Ratte der Fall, wenn man nicht die allgemeine Histamintoxicität, sondern die Wirkung des Histamins auf die Gefäßpermeabilität an der Bauchhaut im Farbstoffversuch zugrunde legt. Die permeabilitätssteigernde Wirkung von Histamin auf die Capillaren der Ratte und des Meerschweinchens wird durch Antihistaminica (in Mol ausgedrückt) in der Reihenfolge Promethazin > Mepyramin > Chlorpromazin gehemmt. Im gleich angelegten Test mit Serotonin aber, der allerdings nur an der Rattenhaut durchführbar ist, lautet die Reihenfolge: Chlorpromazin > Promethazin > Mepyramin. Eine Differenz gegenüber den oben zitierten Versuchen von PARRATT und WEST besteht auch in dem Verhalten von Mepyramin. Nach PARRATT und WEST ist nämlich Mepyramin nicht nur gegenüber dem Serotoninödem, sondern auch gegenüber dem Histaminödem selbst in einer höheren Dosis (10 mg/kg) schwächer wirksam als Chlorpromazin und Promethazin. Die Versuche von HALPERN sind auf Dosis-Wirkungskurven, die von PARRATT und WEST auf jeweils einer einzelnen Dosis aufgebaut. Ferner läßt sich aus den Versuchen von PARRATT und WEST nicht entnehmen, ob Promethazin oder Chlorpromazin stärker auf das Eiklar- (resp. Dextran-)ödem wirkt, da beide Stoffe in den verwendeten Dosen eine komplette Hemmung ergaben, also überschwellig gewesen sein können.

Wichtig ist die Feststellung, daß die Lysergsäurederivate (LSD und BOL 148) zu den stärksten Hemmstoffen des Eiklarödems gehören (DOEPFNER und CERLETTI, 1957; HALPERN, LIACOPOULOS und LIACOPOULOS-BRIOT, 1959; PARRATT und WEST, 1957a, e; STONE, WENGER u. a., 1961; WEST, 1957a). BOL 148 hemmt auch das Ödem durch Dextran, 48/80, Serotonin und auch durch Polymyxin B, nicht dagegen das Ödem durch Histamin (auch nicht das Ödem durch Hyaluronidase und Formaldehyd, die beide weder durch Histamin noch durch Serotonin bedingt zu sein scheinen). Gegenüber der permeabilitätssteigernden Wirkung von Serotonin und makromolekularen Stoffen ist LSD noch wirksamer als Chlorpromazin, gegenüber der Histaminwirkung noch schwächer als Chlorpromazin (HALPERN, LIACOPOULOS und LIACOPOULOS-BRIOT, 1959). Nach DOEPFNER und CERLETTI (1957, 1958) nimmt die Wirkung gegenüber Serotonin am Rattenuterus in folgender Reihenfolge ab: LSD, Phenothiazinderivate (Promethazin, Chlorpromazin), Piperidinderivate (Thenalidin). Danach scheint die Antiserotoninwirkung am Rattenuterus mit der Antieiklar- und Antidextranwirkung an der Ratte im Ödemtest parallel zu gehen (ROTHLIN und CERLETTI, 1955). Eine ähnliche Reihenfolge besteht auch in der Wirkung auf das Serotoninödem. LSD ist auch von voller Schutzwirkung gegenüber der Eiklarwirkung am adrenalektomierten Tier (MEDAKOVIĆ, 1959). Daß die Phenothiazine als Serotoninantagonisten unter den Antihistaminica besonders hervorragen, geht aus zahlreichen Untersuchungen hervor (BENDITT und ROWLEY, 1956; DOEPFNER und CERLETTI, 1957; GYERMEK, LÁZÁR und CSÁK, 1956; PARRATT und WEST, 1958; SCHMID, ZICHA u. a., 1959; STONE, WENGER u. a., 1961). Dazu gehört auch das Cyproheptadin, das nach STONE, WENGER u. a. (1961) dem LSD als Antagonist des Serotoninödems mindestens ebenbürtig ist.

Bemerkenswert ist nun aber, daß nach STONE, WENGER u. a. (1961) die starken Serotoninantagonisten (außer LSD und Cyproheptadin noch das Hydroxindasol) das Serotoninödem stärker hemmen als das Eiklarödem. Chlorpromazin, Promethazin, Trimeprazin und Thenalidin sind gegen Eiklarödem gleich oder stärker wirksam als gegenüber dem Serotoninödem, eine Tatsache, die sich auch aus den Versuchen von PARRATT und WEST (1958) ergibt. Nur BOL 148 hemmte in den Versuchen von PARRATT und WEST das Serotoninödem stärker als das Eiklarödem. Vielleicht darf man darin den Ausdruck der Beteiligung des Histamins am Eiklarödem erblicken. In ähnlichem Sinne spricht die Beobachtung von ROWLEY und BENDITT (1956), wonach weder Dibenamin, ein Serotoninantagonist (GADDUM und HAMEED, 1954), noch Pyrilamin, ein Histaminantagonist, sondern erst beide zusammen die Ovomucoidwirkung hemmen. Auch der Blutdruckabfall durch Ovomucoid läßt sich nach MASSON, CORCORAN und FRANCO-BROWDER (1958) mit reinen oder überwiegenden Serotoninantagonisten (z. B. Phenoxybenzamin oder BOL 148) ebensowenig vollständig hemmen wie mit überwiegend antihistaminartig wirkenden Stoffen, wohl aber z. B. durch BOL 148 + Promethazin. Eine gewisse Wirksamkeit zeigte dagegen Chlorpromazin mit seinen doppelten Wirkungskomponenten. Unaufgeklärt bleibt jedoch, warum gewisse Serotonin-Antimetaboliten ohne Wirkung auf das Eiklar- oder Dextranödem sind (PARRATT und WEST, 1958). Nach BEACH und STEINETZ (1961) schützt BOL 148 nur teilweise gegen die Eiklareffekte (Evansblaukonzentration im Gewebe), Chlorpromazin wesentlich, Pyrilamin wenig. Nach HILLEBRECHT (1959) sprechen auch die Wirkungen von Valmorin (Chlorphenoxazin) und dem Serotoninantagonisten UML 491 (einem Lysergsäurederivat) beim Eiweiß- und Serotoninödem für die Rolle des Serotonins beim Eiweißödem.

Iproniazid, das durch Hemmung des Serotoninabbaues das Eiklar- oder Ovomucoidödem verstärken müßte, hat eigentümlicherweise ähnlich wie Reserpin eine ödemhemmende Wirkung (ARRIGONI-MARTELLI u. KRAMER, 1958). Diese steht vielleicht im Zusammenhang mit der antiphlogistischen Iproniazidwirkung, auf die DOMENJOZ (1952) hingewiesen hat. Auch Pentamidin hemmt das Eiweißödem (COHEN u. BOISMARE, 1961).

Nach MASSON, CORCORAN und FRANCO-BROWDER (1958) verhalten sich die verschiedenen Antagonisten gegenüber der Blutdruckwirkung von Ovomucoid genauso wie gegenüber der Blutdruckwirkung von Serotonin-Histamingemischen im Verhältnis 1 : 5—1 : 15. Es wird daraus gefolgert, daß außer Histamin und Serotonin keine weiteren Stoffe an der Ovomucoidwirkung beteiligt sind.

Den möglichen Anteil von Histamin am Gesamteffekt haben ROWLEY und BENDITT (1956) zu berechnen versucht. Sie fanden, daß die Zunahme des Wassergehaltes in der Pfote nach Ovomucoid durch Dibenamin von 5,5% auf 1,2—2,5% herabgesetzt werden kann, und nehmen an, daß dieser Resteffekt auf Histamin beruht.

Der Mechanismus, der zur Histamin- bzw. Serotoninfreisetzung durch Eiklar führt, ist noch unbekannt. Die Frage, ob eine Proteaseaktivierung die vermittelnde Rolle spielen könne, wurde von KRAMER (1958) mit negativem Ergebnis untersucht. Proteolytische Enzyme hemmen sogar das Eiklarödem (ADAMKIEWICZ, RICE und MCCOLL, 1955; BEILER, BRENDEL und MARTIN, 1955; MARTIN, BRENDEL und BEILER, 1953, 1954). MÖRSDORF (1960) erzielte keine eindeutige Wirkung auf den Transaminasegehalt des Serums nach Applikation von Eiklar in die Rattenpfote. Diese Feststellungen sprechen gegen die Anschauungen von UNGAR (UNGAR und DAMGAARD, 1955; UNGAR, DAMGAARD und HUMMEL, 1952, 1953; UNGAR und MIST, 1949). Von besonderer Bedeutung ist der Befund, daß das Ödem und die Histaminfreisetzung unter Eiklar- oder Ovomucoideinwirkung durch Insulin verstärkt, durch Alloxan und 2-Deoxyglucose gehemmt wird (ADAMKIEWICZ und LANGLOIS, 1958; GOTH, 1959; GOTH, NASH u. a., 1957; KONDO, 1959; SANYAL, 1960b; SANYAL, SPENCER und WEST, 1959). Die Untersuchungen sind jedoch hauptsächlich mit Dextran durchgeführt worden und sollen daher eine eingehende Besprechung im Dextrankapitel erfahren.

Schon vor Jahren hat JANCSÓ (1947), neuerdings wieder ZEMPLÉNYI u. LOJDA (1960) auf die Bedeutung des Histamins für die sog. „Endothelaktivierung" hingewiesen. In diesem Zusammenhang ist von Interesse, daß GÖZSY und KÁTÓ (1957a, b) die Tusche- oder Trypanblauspeicherung durch gewisse „RES-Aktivatoren" oder durch Dextran, 48/80, Histamin und Serotonin mit Mepyramin und Promethazin unterdrücken konnten, während die mit Eiklar, 48/80, Dextran, Serotonin und Histamin hervorgerufenen Ödeme nur durch Promethazin hemmbar waren. Die zur Zeit noch schwer zu deutenden Versuchsergebnisse können vielleicht ein Hinweis darauf sein, daß an den Speicherphänomenen und der Ödembildung Histamin und Serotonin in einem unterschiedlichen Verhältnis beteiligt sind. Die Auffassung der Autoren, daß die mit der Speicherung verbundenen Vorgänge ohne die Vermittlung von Überträgerstoffen zustande kämen, müßte in Anbetracht der positiven Wirksamkeit von Histamin oder

Serotonin noch genauer geprüft werden. Übrigens wird von den gleichen Autoren später (GÖZSY u. KÁTÓ, 1960b) das Serotonin für die „Endothelaktivierung" und nicht für die Ödembildung verantwortlich gemacht.

Neuerdings halten es auch BONACCORSI u. WEST (1963) für möglich, daß die Steigerung der Capillarpermeabilität durch intradermale Injektion von Dextran oder Ovomucoid (nachgewiesen im Farbstofftest) nicht durch Vermittlung von Histamin oder Serotonin zustandekommt, sondern vielleicht durch eine direkte Wirkung auf die Capillaren, wie von GÖZSY u. KÁTÓ (1957a) bereits diskutiert wurde. Am ehesten scheint da für die Beobachtung zu sprechen, daß nach Erschöpfung der Histamindepots in der Haut durch Vorbehandlung mit 48/80 oder Polymyxin B die Reaktion auf Dextran und Ovomucoid früher zur Norm zurückkehrt als der Histamingehalt der Haut und die Reaktionsfähigkeit auf 48/80. Allerdings laufen die Veränderungen in der Dextran- resp. Ovomucoidempfindlichkeit nach der Vorbehandlung mit den Histaminliberatoren ziemlich parallel mit Veränderungen in der Histamin- und Serotoninempfindlichkeit. Die auffallende vorübergehende Abnahme der Histaminempfindlichkeit nach 48/80 wurde auch von HARVEY (1961) sowie von GUTH u. Mitarb. (1961) beschrieben.

Man könnte sich daher vielleicht auch fragen, ob die Veränderungen der Dextran- resp. Ovomucoidempfindlichkeit nicht direkt durch die Veränderungen in der Aminempfindlichkeit bedingt sind. Dann müßte man allerdings auch die Möglichkeit erörtern, daß Dextran resp. Ovomucoid auch nach 48/80 noch Histamin freisetzen kann, jedoch aus anderen Quellen als 48/80. Hinweise hierauf liefern die neueren Beobachtungen über die Bedeutung der nichtmastzellgebundenen Amine (CASS u. MARSHALL, 1962) und über das Ausbleiben des Mastzellzerfalls nach kleinen (7,9 mg/kg), aber zu starken Ödemen führenden Dextrandosen im Gegensatz zu 48/80 (KÁTÓ u. GÖZSY, 1962; GÖZSY u. KÁTÓ, 1963). Im gleichen Sinne läßt sich auch deuten, daß nach BONACCORSI u. WEST (1963) Reserpinvorbehandlung die Dextran- und Ovomucoidreaktion im Farbstofftest verhindert, nicht aber die Reaktion auf 48/80, Histamin und Serotonin; denn MORAN u. WESTERHOLM (1963) finden, daß Reserpin keine sichere Wirkung auf die Mastzellen hat und doch Serotonin aus der Haut freisetzt. Auch ist damit zu vereinbaren, daß nach BONACCORSI u. WEST (1963) die Vorbehandlung mit Dextran die Gefäßreaktion auf Dextran und Ovomucoid verhindert, wobei der Histamin- und Serotoningehalt der Haut nur leicht abnimmt und die Reaktion auf 48/80, Histamin und Serotonin nicht beeinflußt wird.

5. Eiklarödem und innere Sekretion

Durch Nebennierenexstirpation wird die Eiklar- und Ovomucoidreaktion erheblich verstärkt und in Richtung vorherrschender allgemeiner Schocksymptome verschoben (LÉGER und MASSON, 1948; SELYE, 1937). Meist ist der Ausgang letal (HALPERN, 1956; HALPERN und BRIOT, 1949; HOENE, LABBÉ und SELYE, 1952). Die LD_{50} beträgt 2 ml/kg des 1:12,5 verdünnten Eiklars, während normalerweise 20 ml/kg 1:1 verdünnt i.p. vertragen werden (CHEN und WICKEL, 1952). Hypotonie und Hypothermie sind verstärkt. Während nach manchen Autoren (RIECHERT und KLEIN, 1951; SCHEIFFARTH und BERG, 1952; SELYE, 1937) das Ödem verstärkt und verlängert ist, nehmen andere eine Reduktion der Ödemwirkung infolge des niedrigen Blutdruckes an (VAN CAUWENBERGE, LAPIÈRE u. a., 1958). Die auch von HALPERN vertretene Auffassung, daß die abnehmende Ödemneigung die Folge eines zu geringen Filtrationsdruckes sei, ist nicht vereinbar mit dem Vorhandensein einer sogar verstärkten Hämokonzentration.

Die Wirkung der Adrenalektomie auf das Ödem beruht nach SELYE (1949) auf dem Wegfall der Glucocorticoide. Viertägige Vorbehandlung mit Cortison hat bei adrenalektomierten Tieren eine hemmende und sogar antiletale Wirkung auf die Eiklarreaktion. DOCA soll den tödlichen Ausgang nur verzögern und die lokale Reaktion sogar verstärken. Auch das Serotoninödem soll durch Cortison gehemmt und durch DOCA gefördert werden (BOIS u. SELYE, 1956). In der Folgezeit ist die Wirkung von Cortison vielfach sowohl bei normalen als auch bei adrenalektomierten Tieren, aber mit uneinheitlichem Ergebnis nachgeprüft worden. Manche fanden nur eine mäßige (CHEN und WICKEL, 1952; GROSS, 1950a, b; WILHELMI und DOMENJOZ, 1951b) oder keine sichere Wirkung (HILLEBRECHT, 1954), während sich andere für eine Schutzwirkung bei normalen und adrenalektomierten Tieren aussprechen (FREY und FISCHER, 1956; GIBERTINI, VECCHATI und GIBERTI, 1951;

HEILMEYER, FREY und FISCHER, 1952; VAN CAUWENBERGE, LAPIÈRE u. a., 1958). Die fehlende Hemmwirkung von DOCA wird von allen Autoren bestätigt (GIBERTINI, VECCHATI und GIBERTI, 1951; GROSS, 1950a, b; HALPERN, 1949a; HALPERN und BRIOT, 1950; HEILMEYER, FREY und FISCHER, 1952), die ödemverstärkende Wirkung jedoch nur von MEIER, GROSS und DESAULLES (1951). Ebenso uneinheitlich sind die Berichte über die Wirkung von ACTH (HEILMEYER, FREY und FISCHER, 1952; HILLEBRECHT, 1954; WILHELMI und DOMENJOZ, 1951b). Die negativen Ergebnisse mit Cortison lassen sich wahrscheinlich darauf zurückführen, daß nicht immer genügend lange, d. h. 4 Tage, vorbehandelt worden ist. Allerdings liegen auch positive Befunde nach kurzfristiger Behandlung mit einer einmaligen hohen Gabe (50 mg/kg) vor (GROSS, 1950a, b). ACTH soll hingegen in einmaliger Dosis optimal wirksam sein. Adrenalektomie verstärkt den Plasmaverlust nach Eiklar i.p. und Cortison hemmt ihn (WILLIAMS, 1954).

Die einmalige Injektion von Eiklar ist nach 3 Std von einer Abnahme der Ascorbinsäure in der Nebenniere gefolgt. Sie steht jedoch in keinem Zusammenhang mit einer Freisetzung von 17-Hydroxycorticosteroiden, da das Nebennierencholesterin und die Bluteosinophilen keine Abnahme, die Blutcorticosteroide keine Zunahme erfahren (VAN CAUWENBERGE, LAPIÈRE u. a., 1958; VAN CAUWENBERGE, LECOMTE u. VLIERS, 1957). Dagegen steigen die Blutcorticoide an, wenn Eiklar alle 8 Tage wiederholt gegeben wird. Als Ursache dieses Anstiegs kommt eine erhöhte Hormonsekretion oder ein verminderter Hormonverbrauch in Betracht.

Für die Beziehungen zwischen Rattenödem und Nebenniere sind zahlreiche Untersuchungen von Interesse, die sich mit der Bedeutung der Nebenniere und ihren Hormonen für die Wirkung und den Stoffwechsel von Histamin und Serotonin befassen, auf die aber an dieser Stelle nur summarisch hingewiesen werden kann. Hierbei sollen auch nur Arbeiten erwähnt werden, die sich speziell mit den Verhältnissen bei der Ratte befassen. Lange bekannt ist die Steigerung der Histamintoxicität nach Adrenalektomie (VOEGTLIN u. DYER, 1925; SCOTT, 1927; CRIVELLARI, 1927a, b; MARMORSTON-GOTTESMAN u. GOTTESMAN, 1928) und der Antagonismus von Adrenalin und mehr noch von Rindenextrakt gegen diese Empfindlichkeitssteigerung (PERLA u. MARMORSTON-GOTTESMAN, 1931). Das Gewebshistamin nimmt nach Adrenalektomie zu (ROSE u. BROWNE, 1941; WILSON, 1941; MARSHALL, 1943; HICKS u. WEST, 1958 a, b (auch Serotoninvermehrung); BARTLET u. LOCKETT, 1959; TELFORD u. WEST, 1961b; TELFORD, 1963). Corticosteroide verändern in Abhängigkeit von ihrer glucocorticoiden Wirksamkeit den Histamin- und auch Serotoningehalt der Gewebe, indem sie insbesondere in der Haut eine Verminderung herbeiführen (HICKS u. WEST, 1958a, b; TELFORD u. WEST, 1960). Die Beeinflussung des Gewebsserotonins durch Adrenalektomie ist auch von GARATTINI u. Mitarb., 1961 untersucht und diskutiert worden, allerdings in anderen Geweben als der Haut. Dabei wurde keine Verminderung gefunden. Das Blutserotonin nimmt ab (MEDAKOVIĆ u. SPUŽIĆ, 1959). Über Steigerung der Serotonintoxicität durch Adrenalektomie, gemessen an der Temperatursenkung und Blutdrucksenkung, berichten GARATTINI u. Mitarb., (1961). Die Beziehungen zwischen Temperatursenkung durch Serotonin und der Nebenniere sind ferner von HOFFMAN (1959) untersucht worden.

Die Frage, ob die Glucocorticoidwirkung auf das Histamin in erster Linie auf Hemmung der Histidindecarboxylase, Aktivierung der Histaminase oder Verminderung der Histaminbindungsfähigkeit des Gewebes beruht, ist Gegenstand zahlreicher Untersuchungen (SCHAYER, 1955, 1956a, b, 1957; SCHAYER u. SMILEY, 1954; SCHAYER, SMILEY u. DAVIS, 1955, 1956; SCHAYER, DAVIS u. SMILEY, 1955; SCHAYER, ROTHSCHILD u. BIZONY, 1959; TELFORD u. WEST, 1960, 1961, 1963a, b; KARADY, ROSE u. BROWNE, 1940; TELFORD, 1963). Für die Wirkung auf das Serotonin scheint eine Hemmung der 5-Hydroxytryptophandecarboxylase nicht in Betracht zu kommen (PARROT u. LABORDE, 1961; TELFORD u. WEST, 1961a). Über eine Verminderung der Aufnahme von Serotonin in verschiedene Organe bei adrenalektomierten Ratten schreiben GARATTINI u. Mitarb. (1961). Adrenalektomie beeinflußt nicht die Aktivität der Monoaminoxydase und Caeruloplasminoxydase, die beide für den Serotoninmetabolismus von Wichtigkeit sind (GARATTINI u. Mitarb., 1961). Auf die widersprüchlichen Ergebnisse der Untersuchungen über die Corticoidwirkungen auf die Mastzellen hinsichtlich Zahl und Morphologie sei ebenfalls hingewiesen (ASBOE-HANSEN, 1952, 1954, 1958, 1959; SCHOCH u. GLICK, 1953; SMITH u. LEWIS, 1954). Besondere Beachtung dürfte in Zukunft die Arbeit von CASS u. MARSHALL (1962) verdienen, nach denen der Angriffspunkt des Cortisons am nicht-mastzellgebundenen Histamin und Serotonin liegt und die Aminentleerung der Mastzellen sekundär ist.

Cortison, Hydrocortison und ACTH hemmen nicht die permeabilitätssteigernde Wirkung von lokal injiziertem Serotonin (VAN CAUWENBERGE, LAPIÈRE u. a., 1958). Cortison beeinflußt auch nicht das Histaminödem (HALPERN, 1956).

Aber auch der Wegfall der sympathicomimetischen Amine nach der Adrenalektomie kommt als Ursache der erhöhten Eiklartoxicität in Betracht (VAN CAUWENBERGE, LAPIÈRE u. a., 1958). Die folgenden Beobachtungen zeigen, daß dabei in erster Linie an das Adrenalin zu denken ist. Eiklar und Dextran bewirken bei Ratten eine Abnahme des Adrenalins (nicht des Noradrenalins) in der Nebenniere (LECOMTE, DRESSE und VAN CAUWENBERGE, 1960). Adrenalin, viel weniger das Noradrenalin, hat an normalen und adrenalektomierten Tieren einen stark hemmenden Einfluß auf die Eiklarsymptome, d. h. auf Ödem, Schock und Tod (CLARK und MACKAY, 1949a, b; HALPERN, 1949a, b; HALPERN und BRIOT, 1950; MEIER, GROSS und DESAULLES, 1951; PARRATT und WEST, 1958). Die Wirkung ist optimal, wenn Adrenalin gleichzeitig mit Eiklar gegeben wird (CHEN und WICKEL, 1952). Noradrenalin hat nur $^1/_{25}$ der Wirkung von Adrenalin (CLARK und MACKAY, 1949a). Besser wirkt es bei lokaler Applikation in die Pfote (GROSS, 1950b). Ephedrin ist unwirksam (HALPERN und BRIOT, 1950). Sehr wichtig ist die Feststellung von HALPERN (1949a, b), wonach die Adrenalinwirkung nicht auf seiner Gefäßwirkung beruht, sondern auf einer noch unbekannten Stoffwechselwirkung. Für diese kommt ein oxydatives Zwischenprodukt, jedoch nicht Adrenochrom in Betracht. Die Befunde von HALPERN machen es verständlich, daß das Adrenalin sehr lange wirkt und daß das Noradrenalin trotz seiner stärkeren Gefäßwirkung so schwach wirksam ist (PARRATT und WEST, 1958). Wenn es also auf ein Abbauprodukt des Adrenalins ankommt, so besteht auch kein Widerspruch mehr zwischen der Adrenalinwirkung und der Tatsache, daß auch Adrenolytica eine ödemhemmende Wirkung besitzen (RIECHERT und BARGHORN, 1954; RIECHERT und ESCHBACH, 1955; ROWLEY und BENDITT, 1956). Diese beruht übrigens zum Teil auf der Antiserotoninwirkung.

Umgekehrt wie die Nebennierenentfernung wirkt sich die Schilddrüsenentfernung auf die Eiklarreaktion aus. Es wurde beobachtet (LÉGER und MASSON, 1948; LÉGER, MASSON und PRADO, 1947a, b), daß 12tägige Behandlung mit Thyroxin die Eiklarwirkung ähnlich wie die Adrenalektomie verstärkt und verändert. Thyreoidektomie hingegen schwächt sie ab. PARRATT und WEST (1960) haben die gleichen Beobachtungen außer auf Eiklar auch noch auf die Wirkung von Dextran, 48/80, Polymyxin B, Histamin und Serotonin ausdehnen können. Thyroxin steigert die Eiklarletalität von Null auf 60 %. Besonderes Interesse verdient der Hinweis darauf, daß sich unter Thyroxin Ödeme und Blutungen im Magen-Darmtrakt einstellen und daß dadurch eine Annäherung an die anaphylaktischen Symptome bei der Ratte (SANYAL und WEST, 1958) eintritt. Thyroxin wirkt offenbar so, daß es die Histaminaseaktivität im Darm hemmt und dadurch zu einer Histaminanhäufung im Körper führt. Der Histamingehalt im Gewebe nimmt zwar nur leicht zu, aber die Erhöhung des Blutspiegels hält länger an, und die Ausscheidung im Harn ist 5—10fach erhöht. Die Freisetzung von Histamin oder Serotonin durch Eiklar oder Dextran wird dagegen durch Thyroxin nicht gesteigert.

SPENCER u. WEST (1962) haben die Bedeutung der Schilddrüse für die anaphylaktoide Reaktion der Ratte auf Eiklar und Dextran noch weiter untersucht und außer Thyroxin auch Trijodthyronin und außer der Thyreoidektomie auch die Wirkung antithyreoidaler Substanzen in die Betrachtung einbezogen. Dabei machten sie die Beobachtung, daß die Auswirkungen des Hyper- und des Hypothyreoidismus vorübergehender Natur sind, d. h. daß trotz fortgesetzter Behandlung mit Thyroxin oder Trijodthyronin die anfängliche Steigerung der durch intraperitoneale Injektion von Eiklar oder Dextran ausgelösten Reaktion wieder zurückgeht, und umgekehrt trotz fortgesetzter Behandlung mit Methylthiouracil oder bei thyreoidektomierten Tieren die reduzierte anaphylaktoide Reaktion sich allmählich wieder mehr oder weniger normalisiert. Als Ursache dieser Kompensationsvorgänge konnte im ersten Fall eine Hypertrophie, im zweiten Fall eine Hypotrophie der Nebennierenrinde festgestellt werden. Die Bedeutung der Nebennierenrinde für die Schilddrüsenwirkung wird durch den Befund unterstrichen, daß gleichzeitige Gaben von Glucocorticoiden (Hydrocortison und Prednisolon) die Thyroxinwirkung aufheben. Die Autoren gehen noch einen Schritt weiter, indem sie überhaupt die ganze Schilddrüsenwirkung auf die anaphylaktoide Reaktion als einen indirekten, über die Nebennierenrinde ablaufenden Vorgang ansehen. Das Schilddrüsenhormon soll zunächst durch Förderung des Corticoidabbaus in der Leber und damit durch Senkung des Corticoidspiegels im Gewebe die von ihnen ebenfalls nachgewiesene vorübergehende Zunahme der Histamin- und Serotoninempfindlichkeit, des Gehaltes der Gewebe an Histamin und der Histaminausscheidung im Urin (s. a. SPENCER u. WEST, 1961, 1963) bewirken, bis durch erhöhte ACTH-Ausschüttung die kompensatorische Hypertrophie der Nebennierenrinde einsetzt und die Auswirkungen auf die Aminempfindlichkeit wieder rückgängig macht. Bei Hypothyreoidismus folgt einer anfänglichen Vermehrung des Corticoidspiegels (durch Hemmung der Steroidreduktase in der Leber) eine Wiederabnahme durch verminderte ACTH-Ausschüttung. Während Nebennierenentfernung die Thyroxinwirkung verstärkt, schwächt Hypothyreoidismus die verstärkte anaphylaktoide Reaktion adrenalektomierter Ratten nicht ab, wahrscheinlich infolge des Mangels an peripheren Corticosteroiden. Weibliche Ratten mit ihren größeren Nebennieren zeigen unter Thyroxin eine stärkere Hypertrophie der Nebennierenrinde und entwickeln infolgedessen einen geringeren Grad von Dextranempfindlichkeit.

Die mit der anfänglichen Zunahme und späteren Abnahme der Dextranempfindlichkeit unter Thyroxin einhergehende Vermehrung und Wiederabnahme (SPENCER u. WEST, 1961, 1962, 1963; vgl. auch GOTZL u. DRAGSTEDT, 1940) des Histamin- und Serotoningehaltes im Haut- und Darmgewebe wird als ausreichende Basis für eine vorübergehend vermehrte Freisetzung von Aminen angesehen. Die Histaminausscheidung im Urin steigt an, um — vor allem bei Weibchen — später wieder abzufallen. Thyroxin bewirkt zwar eine Hemmung der Histaminaseaktivität im Ileum um 45%, SPENCER u. WEST glauben jetzt jedoch, daß diese nicht ausreicht, um die erhöhte Aminempfindlichkeit und das langsamere Wiederabfallen des unter Dextran erhöhten Bluthistamins zu erklären. Die Verlangsamung der Blutzirkulation im schweren Schock soll eher als Ursache des verzögerten Histaminschwunds in Betracht kommen.

Die neben der verlangsamten Ausscheidung festzustellende Erhöhung des Histaminspiegels nach Dextran erreicht unter Thyroxin doppelt so hohe Werte wie ohne Thyroxin.

Oestrogene Hormone und Testosteron schwächen das Rattenödem ab; Progesteron, Parathormon, Entfernung der Hypophyse oder der Geschlechtsdrüsen sowie Schwangerschaft sind ohne Einfluß (LÉGER u. MASSON, 1948). Die Thymektomie, die Ratten auch unempfindlicher gegen Histamin und gegen verschiedene Formen des Stress macht (vgl. WELTMAN u. SACKLER, 1961), soll im Gegensatz zu früheren Befunden (LÉGER u. MASSON, 1948) Ödem und Cyanose abschwächen (COMSA, 1959). Eine besonders starke Reaktion auf Eiklar sollen Thymusextrakte bei thymektomierten Tieren auslösen.

Splenektomie schwächt die Eiklarreaktion ab (SANYAL, 1960a). Dieser Effekt verläuft mehr über eine Veränderung der Histamin- und Serotonintoxicität und hat auch keine Beziehungen zu gewissen Veränderungen des Histamin- und Serotoningehaltes in der Haut.

II. Das Dextranödem

Dextran ist ein bakterielles Polysaccharid, das als kolloidaler Bestandteil von Plasmaersatzmitteln (Macrodex, Expandex, Dextraven u. a.) dient. Es wird als hochmolekularer Schleim von Leuconostoc mesenteroides und dextranicum produziert und muß durch Hydrolyse zu Produkten mit niedrigerem Molekulargewicht für den klinischen Gebrauch abgebaut werden. Das Molekulargewicht der Handelspräparate weist stets eine erhebliche Streuung auf und lag im Mittel in den letzten Jahren gewöhnlich zwischen 70000 und 80000 (GRÖNWALL, 1957; SQUIRE, BULL u. a., 1955).

Die Eigenschaften des Dextrans hängen weitgehend davon ab, wie die Zuckereinheiten (Glucose) miteinander verknüpft sind. Die Zuckermoleküle sind α-glykosidisch hauptsächlich in Form von 1:6-Bindungen kettenförmig aneinander gelagert. Hinzu kommen 1:4-, 1:3- und vielleicht noch 1:2-Bindungen, durch die in wechselnder Proportion je nach Herkunft des Dextrans und den Züchtungsbedingungen des Bakterienstammes und dem Grad der Hydrolyse Verzweigungen entstehen. Über die Abhängigkeit der im folgenden zu besprechenden Phänomene von diesen chemisch-konstitutionellen Faktoren sind wir im allgemeinen noch wenig unterrichtet. Meist wurden die klinischen Dextranpräparate verwendet. Angaben über das Molekulargewicht und sonstige Eigenschaften fehlen oft. Auch die antigene Natur des Dextrans hängt von der chemischen Struktur ab, worauf jedoch hier nicht weiter eingegangen werden soll (vgl. COULSON u. STEVENS, 1961; KABAT, 1957, 1958, 1960; KABAT u. BEZER, 1958). Die neueste Tendenz geht dahin, Präparate mit eingeengtem Molekulargewichtsbereich, mit geringerem mittlerem Molekulargewicht (ungefähr 40000) und möglichst geringem Verzweigungsgrad zu schaffen (Näheres siehe: HAHN, 1961).

Dextran wirkt toxisch nur bei der Ratte und nicht bei anderen Tierarten (BLOOM u. WILLCOX, 1951; LECOMTE u. BEAUMARIAGE, 1956; WEST, 1957a). Einen noch zu besprechenden Sonderfall stellt die histaminliberierende Wirkung von Dextran und Dextransulfat im Kaninchenblut in vitro dar.

1. Allgemeine Symptomatologie

Daß das Dextran bei der Ratte praktisch genauso wirkt wie das Eiklar, wurde offenbar zuerst von PULASKI beobachtet und 1951 zum ersten Mal von VOORHEES, BAKER und PULASKI (1951) sowie von MORRISON, RICHARDSON und BLOOM (1951) und MORRISON, BLOOM und RICHARDSON (1951) beschrieben. Die Ähnlichkeit der Symptome ergibt sich auch aus den folgenden Untersuchungen, besonders aus denen von BRIOT und HALPERN (1952a) und HALPERN (1956, 1960a). Vasodilatation und erhöhte Capillarpermeabilität bilden auch hier die pathogenetische Grundlage (MARSHALL und HANNA, 1957). Die Ödemreaktion scheint allerdings stärker als nach Eiklar zu sein (HALPERN und BRIOT, 1952b). Der Eiweißgehalt der Ödemflüssigkeit ist höher, wohl als Folge einer stärkeren Permeabilitätssteigerung der Capillaren, aber qualitativ gleich (FORMANEK, HÖLLER und STOKLASKA, 1961).

Nach intravenöser Injektion von J^{131}-Ovalbumin tritt beim Dextranödem mehr markiertes Ovalbumin in die Ödemflüssigkeit aus als beim Hyaluronidaseödem. Die Ovalbuminkonzentration erreicht im ersten Fall in der Ödemflüssigkeit höhere Werte als im Serum. RÉDEI (1962) sieht in diesem Befund den Ausdruck einer Hemmung des Abtransports von Ovalbumin in der Lymphe durch Dextran.

Auffallend ist, daß die Hämokonzentration im Gegensatz zu verschiedenen Autoren (EDLUND, LÖFGREN u. VÄLI, 1952; KITCHIN, SMITH u. a., 1954; LEVY u. DE VAILLANCOURT, 1960) von MORRISON, RICHARDSON und BLOOM (1951) vermißt wurde. Sie fanden eine Blutverdünnung trotz Ödembildung. Gleichzeitig war Dextran chemisch im Blute nachzuweisen. Allerdings ist dies die normale Reaktion auf Dextran bei Tieren, die nicht dextranempfindlich sind. Vielleicht spielt auch bei der Ratte dieser Vorgang als konkurrierender Faktor mit hinein und kann unter besonderen Bedingungen sichtbar werden. In der Tat führt Dextran beim Alloxandiabetes (GOTH, NASH u. a., 1957), wo die Ödembildung verhindert ist, zu einer Blutverdünnung. Andere Beobachtungen könnten im gleichen Sinne sprechen, wie die Abnahme der Plasmaeiweißkonzentration (LEVY u. DE VAILLANCOURT, 1960) oder die Tatsache, daß auch bei der Ratte Dextran als Plasmaersatzmittel bei Blutverlust wirksam sein soll (MORRISON, LUNDY u. ESSEX, 1952). Leider fehlen Untersuchungen, die uns Auskunft geben über die Verweildauer des Dextrans und seiner Fraktionen im Blute der Ratte und seinen Übertritt durch die Capillarwand der einzelnen Gefäßgebiete einschließlich der ödematösen Bezirke.

Auch der Menkin-Test ist zu vielen Untersuchungen herangezogen worden (COURVOISIER u. DUCROT, 1955; EDLUND, LÖFGREN u. VÄLI, 1952; HALPERN, 1956; HALPERN, LIACOPOULOS u. BRIOT, 1956a; KÁTÓ u. GÖZSY, 1956; MARSHALL u. HANNA, 1957; MORRISON, RICHARDSON u. BLOOM, 1951). Ödembildung und Farbstoff- bzw. Tuschespeicherung laufen auch hier im allgemeinen parallel (GÖZSY u. KÁTÓ, 1957a; HALPERN, 1956; PARRATT u. WEST, 1957e). GÖZSY und KÁTÓ (1959a) haben jedoch neuerdings auf einen Unterschied im Auftreten des Dextranödems und der Tuschespeicherung hingewiesen. Sie fanden, daß die Tuschespeicherung an den Stellen stattfindet, wo sich später die Ödeme entwickeln. Aber während des Vorhandenseins von Ödemen findet eine Tuschespeicherung nicht mehr statt. Während der Ödeme ist auch das Verschwinden der Tuscheteilchen aus der Blutbahn verzögert. Eine Deutung dieser Befunde wird von den Autoren nicht gegeben.

Eine andere Frage ist, ob die speziell mit Dextran untersuchte Diuresehemmung mit der Ödembildung zusammenhängt. Das Ödem ist von KITCHIN, SMITH u. a. (1954) als Ursache der Diuresehemmung in Betracht gezogen worden. Von diesen Autoren wurde auch vermutet, daß die von ERSPAMER und OTTOLENGHI (1953) beschriebene antidiuretische Wirkung subcutaner Serotoningaben auf einem solchen Mechanismus beruhen könne. GREEFF und CONTZEN (1960) haben aber gezeigt, daß der Effekt des Dextrans auf die Niere wahrscheinlich auf einer direkten Wirkung des freigesetzten Histamins beruht. Die Diuresehemmung ist durch Antihistaminica und nicht durch Reserpin blockierbar und verhält sich somit anders als das Ödem, das stärker durch Reserpin hemmbar ist und bei dem auch nach diesen Versuchen das Serotonin die wichtigere Rolle spielt.

Auch die Dextranwirkung ist selten tödlich. Das Ödem klingt gewöhnlich nach 3–4 Std. ab. Die tödlichen Dosen betragen 2–3 g/kg i.v. oder i.p. (HALPERN, 1956; KITCHIN, SMITH u. a., 1954), während zur Ödemerzeugung gewöhnlich 150–600 mg/kg i. p. verabreicht werden (KÁTÓ und GÖZSY, 1960c; MORRISON, RICHARDSON und BLOOM, 1951; STUCKI und THOMPSON, 1958). Auch beim Dextran finden wir i.v. ein Zurücktreten der Ödembildung gegenüber den allgemein-toxischen Erscheinungen. Von Interesse ist, daß der Blutdruckabfall nach 600 mg/kg Dextran i.v. bei normalen oder mit Äther narkotisierten Ratten mäßig ist oder fehlt, während in der Barbituratnarkose ein starker Abfall auftritt. Die Tatsache, daß gleichzeitig mit einem starken Blutdruckabfall in Barbituratnarkose auch der Austritt von Evansblau aus der Blutbahn ins Gewebe gehemmt ist, könnte im Sinne der auch von HALPERN (1956) vertretenen Auffassung sprechen, wonach der Filtrationsdruck eine wichtige Rolle für die extravasalen Erscheinungen der anaphylaktoiden Reaktion spielt. Jedoch fehlen Angaben über das Verhalten der Hämokonzentration bei den verschiedenen narkotischen Zuständen.

Während Dextran (1,6 g/kg) innerhalb 5–15 min in Euthermie einen Blutdruckabfall bewirkt, der dann einer Blutdrucksteigerung mit einem Maximum nach 60 min weicht, verursacht 48/80 innerhalb von 5–10 min einen Blutdruckabfall von längerer Dauer. In Hypothermie bewirkt Dextran einen zunehmenden Blutdruckanstieg, während 48/80 einen raschen Anstieg erst nach einer initialen Senkung zeigt (VUKOBRATOVIĆ, 1961).

Durch subcutane Injektion in die empfindlichen Bezirke der Haut werden lokalisierte Ödeme schon mit so kleinen Dosen wie 0,05—0,1 (HALPERN, 1956; ROWLEY u. BENDITT, 1956), 0,01 (EDLUND, LÖFGREN u. VÄLI, 1952) oder sogar nur 0,006 mg (PARRATT u. WEST, 1957e) ausgelöst. SELYE (1954) beobachtete auch ein Überspringen der Reaktion von der Injektionsstelle auf andere empfindliche Stellen der Haut. Dieses Überspringen kann nach SANYAL, SPENCER und WEST (1959) durch Insulin ausgelöst werden. Besonders klein sind die Dextrandosen, die bei normalen (0,9—2 μg) und bei adrenalektomierten Tieren (0,3 μg) ausreichen, um intradermal in der Bauchhaut die Evansblaureaktion auszulösen (HALPERN, 1956). JASMIN (1956b) verpflanzte ein Ohr in die Rückenhaut der Ratte und zeigte an dem Auftreten der Tuschereaktion nach Dextrangabe, daß die Prädilektionsstelle (in diesem Falle das Ohr) unabhängig von der nervösen oder vasalen Versorgung ist.

Die wenigen Untersuchungen über die Abhängigkeit der Dextranwirkung von der Struktur und dem Molekulargewicht haben eine gewisse Unabhängigkeit vom Molekulargewicht innerhalb eines Bereiches von 25000–170000 (VOORHEES, BAKER und PULASKI, 1951) bzw. von 20000–400000 (HAHN, LANGE und GIERTZ, 1954) ergeben. Andererseits zeigte sich ein gewisses Optimum der Wirkung bei dem Molekulargewicht 100000. Die toxische Wirkung erlischt bei extremen Molekulargewichtswerten, nämlich 6000 einerseits und 2000000 (HALPERN, 1956) andererseits. Bei Dextran mit dem Molekulargewicht 10000 war nach EDLUND, LÖFGREN und VÄLI (1952) eine hundertfach höhere Dosis zur lokalen Farbreaktion nötig als bei dem klinischen Dextran. Nach den gleichen Autoren sind Dextrane mit starkem Verzweigungsgrad toxischer als weniger verzweigte. Schwefelsäureester des Dextrans sind ohne Wirkung bei der Ratte. Nur BINET und QUIVY (1956) fanden eine Histaminabnahme in der Rattenpfote nach Injektion von Dextransulfat. Ob bei derartigen Differenzen der Grad der Sulfatierung eine Rolle spielt, ist bisher nicht bekannt. Dextransulfat verursacht beim Meerschweinchen Krämpfe und Kreislaufkollaps ohne Beteiligung von Histamin (WALTON und RICKETTS, 1954).

Eigentümliche Befunde wurden mit 3 verschiedenen Dextranen gleichen mittleren Molekulargewichtes (72000) erhoben (GÖZSY u. KÁTÓ, 1960a; KÁTÓ u. GÖZSY, 1960b). Die Autoren ermittelten sehr niedrige Schwellenwerte für die Ödembildung (1—8 mg/kg) und beobachteten, daß die Wirkung mit steigender Dosis abnimmt und bei einer bestimmten, von der Art des Dextrans abhängigen, nach oben und unten scharf begrenzten Dosis bis auf Null sinkt, um bei weiterer Dosissteigerung wieder aufzutreten. Diese nicht wirksame Zwischendosis soll zusammen mit einem Antihistaminicum ein Ödem auslösen. Zur Erklärung dieser Erscheinungen werden (in jeder Charge in unterschiedlicher Proportion) 2 Dextranfraktionen angenommen, die eine mit einer ödemfördernden, die andere mit einer ödemhemmenden Wirkung. Inzwischen sind diese Befunde allerdings nicht bestätigt worden (JASMIN, BOIS u. SU, 1962; HARRIS u. WEST, 1963).

Die schon von anderen Autoren (KITCHIN, SMITH u. a., 1954; PARRATT und WEST, 1957e) kurz erwähnte Resistenz einzelner Wistarratten gegen Dextran (und Eiklar) ist neuerdings von HARRIS und WEST (1961), HARRIS, KALMUS und WEST (1963) und WEST (1961b) einer eingehenderen Studie unterzogen worden. Sie findet sich bei etwa 25% der Tiere als erbliche Eigenschaft. Bisher konnte bei der Untersuchung der verschiedensten als Ursache in Betracht kommenden Faktoren (Blutzucker, Gewicht der Nebennieren, Serotoningehalt der Haut, Histamintoxicität u. a.) der Mechanismus dieser Resistenz nicht aufgeklärt werden. Die Resistenz konnte auch nicht durchbrochen werden durch Maßnahmen, die die Dextranreaktion bei normalempfindlichen Tieren verstärken (Insulin, Chlorpropamid, Adrenalektomie, Stress).

Auch serologische Befunde (Eiweißgehalt des Serums, Anaphylatoxinbildung durch Serum mit Dextran, antigene Wirksamkeit des Serums im Anaphylaxieversuch an Meerschweinchen, Sensibilisierbarkeit der Ratten durch Pferdeserum) zeigten keinen Unterschied zwischen dextranempfindlichen und unempfindlichen Ratten (HARRIS, 1963; HARRIS u. WEST, 1963). Andere Rattenstämme (August, Hooded Lister, Sprague Dawley) lieferten keine resistenten Kolonien. Resistente Ratten lassen auch die Farbstoff-(Azovanblau-)Akkumulation in der Haut vermissen, wenn nach der intravenösen Farbstoffinjektion Dextran oder Ovomucoid intradermal in die Bauchhaut injiziert wird (BONACCORSI u. WEST, 1963). Intradermale Injektion von Histamin, Serotonin und 48/80 ist dagegen wie bei normalen Ratten wirksam.

In der Frage der Toleranz durch Vorbehandlung mit wiederholten Dextrangaben waren die ersten Angaben widersprechend (MORRISON, RICHARDSON und BLOOM, 1951; VOORHEES, BAKER und PULASKI, 1951). Aus den Versuchen von PARRATT und WEST (1957e), die in 5 Tagen insgesamt 6,45 g/kg Dextran in ansteigenden, meist 2mal täglich verabreichten i.p. Dosen gaben und damit eine Toleranz erzielten, geht hervor, daß eine lange bzw. intensive Vorbehandlung nötig ist. Die Toleranz hält etwa 3 Tage an und greift auch auf Eiklar über. Dextranresistente Ratten sind dagegen empfindlich für 48/80, 1935 L und Polymyxin B (HALPERN, LIACOPOULOS-BRIOT und LIACOPOULOS, 1958; PARRATT und WEST, 1957e), während umgekehrt 48/80 in wiederholten Gaben nicht nur gegen 48/80, sondern auch gegen Dextran, Eiklar und Polymyxin B schützt (JASMIN, 1956a, b; PARRATT und WEST, 1957e). Anders lautende Angaben, wonach Dextran bis zu einem gewissen Grade auch gegen 48/80 schützen soll (MARSHALL und HANNA, 1958), sind vielleicht auf die kurzfristige Versuchsanordnung (z. B. 2mal 600 mg/kg Dextran i. v. im Abstand von 53 min und 63 min später 200 μg/kg 48/80) zurückzuführen. Bei der üblichen Prüfung auf Resistenz wird die Prüfinjektion 24 Std nach der letzten Gabe des toleranzerzeugenden Stoffes durchgeführt. Aber auch die Resistenz gegen Dextran durch 48/80 erfordert eine längere Vorbehandlung, wie aus den Versuchen von KRAMER (1956b) hervorgeht, der erst nach 30tägiger Vorbehandlung mit 48/80 eine Dextranresistenz erzielte, wobei die Tiere aber noch unvermindert auf 48/80 reagierten. Die Dextranresistenz durch Dextran entwickelte sich in diesen Versuchen erst nach 14–18 Tagen mit 2mal täglich 300 mg/kg Dextran.

MARSHALL und HANNA (1957) fanden im Blutdruckversuch nach einer i.v. Gabe von 600 mg/kg Dextran, daß sich erst nach 10 min eine Resistenz entwickelte, die nur für 50 min verfolgt wurde. Es erscheint zweifelhaft, ob bei dieser Art des Vorgehens der gleiche Mechanismus erfaßt wird wie bei dem üblichen Vorgehen mit täglichen Gaben. Auf die Besonderheiten der Versuchsanordnung ist es wohl auch zurückzuführen, daß HOENE, LABBÉ und SELYE (1952) schon nach einer lokalen Injektion von Dextran (Eiklar, Pepton, Hyaluronidase) die injizierte Stelle gegen die Wirkung nachfolgender i.p. Injektionen von Dextran oder Eiklar für 5 Tage schützen konnten.

2. Histamin und Dextranödem

Zur Frage der Histaminfreisetzung durch Dextran haben verschiedene Autoren unabhängig voneinander Stellung genommen (HAHN, LANGE und GIERTZ, 1954; HAHN und WELLMANN, 1952; HALPERN, 1956, 1960a; HALPERN und BRIOT, 1952a, 1954b; HALPERN, BRIOT u. a., 1955). Nach i.v. Injektion von 5 ml/kg 6%iger Dextranlösung wurde eine Histaminvermehrung im Blut (vgl. auch: PARRATT und WEST, 1960) und im Plasma gefunden (HAHN, LANGE und GIERTZ, 1954; HAHN und WELLMANN, 1952). Die Vermehrung im Plasma hielt über 2 Std. an. Im Plasma wurden höhere Anstiege erzielt als im Blut, weil im Blut die als Histaminträger in Betracht kommenden weißen Blutelemente abgenommen hatten. In noch unveröffentlichten Versuchen erzielten wir gemeinsam mit WIRTH an einem größeren Tiermaterial 10–20 min nach 300 mg/kg Dextran i. v. im Mittel einen Anstieg auf etwa das 15fache (0,75 μg/ml) der Norm (0,05 μg/ml) im Plasma. Nach einer 6fach höheren Dextrandosis erzielten HALPERN und BRIOT (1954b) eine Vermehrung des Histamins um das 41fache der Norm. Nach mehrfachen Dextrangaben bleibt der Histaminanstieg aus. HALPERN errechnet, daß 10–20% des Histaminvorrats in der Haut genügen würden, um den von ihm gefundenen Histaminanstieg zu ergeben. Daß das Histamin aus der Haut stammt, wurde von HALPERN und BRIOT (1952a) durch den Nachweis einer „explosiven“ Histaminfreisetzung an isolierten Hautstücken in vitro nach Zusatz von Dextran (nicht PVP) wahrscheinlich gemacht. Die Freisetzung erfolgt nur bei 37°, nicht bei tiefen Temperaturen. Dextran führt außerdem zu einer Herabsetzung des Histamingehaltes in der Haut (BINET und QUIVY, 1957, 1958a; HALPERN, LIACOPOULOS und LIACOPOULOS-BRIOT, 1959; KRAMER, 1956b; LECOMTE, 1957; PARRATT und WEST, 1957e). Diese Abnahme kann an den empfindlichen Stellen des Körpers (Fußrücken, Pfoten, Ohren) nach einer einzigen Dextrangabe 44–58% betragen (PARRATT und WEST, 1957e). Die Abnahme in der Haut des Bauches geht anscheinend langsamer vor sich. Sie beträgt erst nach 3maligen Dextrangaben 36% (HALPERN und BRIOT, 1954a). Danach sinkt der Histamingehalt trotz weiterer Dextrangaben nicht mehr weiter ab. An den empfindlichen Stellen des Körpers ist der Histamingehalt nach 3maligen Dextrangaben noch weiter abgesunken, und zwar an den Pfotenballen um 75 %, an den Ohren um 88 % und an den Fußrücken allerdings nur um 65 %. An der durchströmten hinteren Körperhälfte der Ratte läßt sich mit Dextran im Gegensatz zu den negativen Befunden von LECOMTE (1957) wie mit 48/80, Polymyxin B und 1935 L eine Histaminfreisetzung nachweisen (HALPERN, LIACOPOULOS und LIACOPOULOS-BRIOT, 1957; PARRATT und WEST, 1957e).

Die Histaminfreisetzung ist von einer Hyperkaliämie begleitet, die durch Promethazin gehemmt wird, also wahrscheinlich eine Folge der Histaminwirkung ist (HALPERN, BRIOT u. a., 1955).

Dextran ist wie Ovomucoid ein schwächerer Histaminliberator als 48/80, Polymyxin B und 1935 L (HALPERN, LIACOPOULOS und LIACOPOULOS-BRIOT, 1957; PARRATT und WEST, 1957e). Dies prägt sich auch in der Höhe der durch diese Stoffe erzielten Histaminspiegel im Plasma aus (HALPERN, LIACOPOULOS-BRIOT und LIACOPOULOS, 1958). Vorbehandlung mit Dextran hebt nur die histaminliberierende Wirkung von Dextran auf, nicht die von 48/80 oder 1935 L. Umgekehrt wird die histaminliberierende Wirkung von Dextran durch alle 3 Substanzen aufgehoben (HALPERN, LIACOPOULOS-BRIOT und LIACOPOULOS, 1958). Ob Dextran stärker wirkt als Ovomucoid, wie es nach den Beobachtungen über das Verhalten des Hauthistamins und anderen Beobachtungen scheint (KRAMER, 1956a), ist nicht genauer untersucht. Auch gemessen an der Histaminausscheidung im Urin sind Dextran und Hühnereiweiß schwächere Histaminliberatoren als 48/80 oder Sinomenin (KONDO, 1959).

Die stärker histaminliberierende Wirkung der basischen Liberatoren kommt auch bei der Bestimmung des „labilen“ Histamins nach HALPERN, BIOZZI u. a. (1953) zum Ausdruck. Ein Maß für diese Wirkung ist die Schwellendosis der Liberatoren, die intradermal injiziert an der Bauchhaut die Evansblaureaktion auslöst. Vorbehandlung mit Dextran erhöht die Schwellendosen von Dextran und Ovomucoid, nicht die von 48/80 oder 1935 L. Wiederholte Gaben von 1935 L oder 48/80 erhöhten dagegen die Schwellendosen von Dextran ebenso wie von 1935 L und 48/80.

Bezüglich der Herkunft des Histamins und der Veränderungen an den Mastzellen gelten die Ausführungen im Eiklarkapitel. PARRATT und WEST (1957e) fanden mit Dextran, daß auch bei wiederholten Gaben die Mastzellveränderungen nicht stark waren. Mastzellveränderungen im Mesenterium ließen sich nicht nur nach i.p. Injektion (PARRATT und WEST, 1957e), sondern auch nach subcutaner Injektion nach KELLER (1957a, b) nachweisen. Auffallend ist die Beobachtung dieser Autoren, daß sich die hauptsächlichen Veränderungen nicht in der Nachbarschaft der Gefäße, sondern in ferner liegenden Gebieten befanden. Die Veränderungen waren ähnlich wie nach Injektion von Trypsin, Wasser, Pepton und im Tourniquet-Schock, obwohl die Symptome differieren. Nur nach Dextran- und Wasserinjektion sowie im Tourniquet-Schock war die Gesamtausscheidung von Histamin im Urin erhöht.

Nach CORBASCIO (1958) nehmen unter Dextran auch die Granula in den epitheloiden Nierenzellen ab, ohne daß sich dabei der Histamingehalt der Niere verändert.

Ähnlich wie beim Eiklarödem wurde ursprünglich auch in der Wirkung der Antihistaminica mehr oder weniger ein Beweis für die überwiegende Rolle des Histamins beim Dextranödem erblickt. Allerdings fiel auch hier schon von vornherein auf, daß nur einzelne Antihistaminica wirksam sind. Zum Beispiel wurde darauf hingewiesen, daß nur Phenindamin, nicht Tripelennamin und Diphenhydramin wirksam sind (MORRISON, BLOOM und RICHARDSON, 1951; MORRISON, RICHARDSON und BLOOM, 1951). Später wurde das Promethazin hervorgehoben (BRIOT und HALPERN, 1952b; HALPERN und BRIOT, 1952b), das sich ähnlich wie beim Eiklar gegen alle Symptome der Dextranvergiftung der Ratte einschließlich der letalen Wirkung bei adrenalektomierten Tieren (HALPERN, 1956) richtet. Ausgenommen ist nur die Hypothermie. Auch STUCKI und THOMPSON (1958), ferner LECOMTE, VAN CAUWENBERGE und VLIERS (1959) bestätigen die starke Wirkung von Promethazin. Aber das Promethazin wird übertroffen von Chlorpromazin (BOHNSTEDT und LANZ, 1956; COURVOISIER und DUCROT, 1955; COURVOISIER, FOURNEL u. a., 1953), obwohl seine Antihistamineigenschaften relativ schwächer ausgeprägt sind. Noch wirksamer ist Levopromazin (KÁTÓ und GÖZSY, 1960a,

1961a). Von GÖZSY und KÁTÓ (1960c) und von ODA u. Mitarb. (1961) wird die Wirkung weiterer Phenothiazinderivate auf das Dextranödem beschrieben. Hervorgehoben wird ferner die Wirkung von Theophenopiperidin (ROTHLIN und CERLETTI, 1955). Andererseits ist Mepyramin, das besonders starke Antihistamineigenschaften hat, von der geringsten Wirksamkeit (BRIOT und HALPERN, 1952b; COURVOISIER und DUCROT, 1955; HALPERN, LIACOPOULOS und LIACOPOULOS-BRIOT, 1959). Im großen und ganzen finden wir hier ähnliche Verhältnisse wie beim Eiklarödem vor. Auch das Piperazinderivat Cinnarazin ist beim Dextranödem nur schwach wirksam (HALPERN, STIFFEL u. Mitarb., 1963).

Eine eigentümliche Auffassung über die Wirkung der Antihistaminica auf das Dextranödem haben neuerdings KÁTÓ und GÖZSY (1961b) geäußert. Danach sollen die Antihistamine in der Weise wirken, daß sie das injizierte Dextran chemisch binden. Sie stützen sich hauptsächlich auf den Befund, daß bei gleichzeitiger Injektion von Dextran und Antihistaminica keine Hemmung der Capillarwirkung von Histamin oder Serotonin durch das Antihistaminicum stattfindet.

Ähnlich wie beim Eiklar mag es hier genügen, nur kurz auf die Versuche hinzuweisen, das Dextranödem mit antiphlogistisch wirksamen Stoffen zu beeinflussen. Zur Theorie des Dextranödems tragen sie nur verhältnismäßig wenig bei. Untersucht wurden: Lokalanaesthetica, Salicylsäure, Pyrazole, Isonicotinsäurehydrazid, Coffein, Narkotica und Alkohole, BAL, Ketobemidon, Polykieselsäuren, Chlorthenoxazin u. a. (ANTWEILER, 1955; BINET u. QUIVY, 1958a; COURVOISIER u. DUCROT, 1955; DOMENJOZ, 1952, 1953, 1955, 1960; DOMENJOZ, THEOBALD u. MÖRSDORF, 1955; EDLUND, LÖFGREN u. VÄLI, 1952; FRANK, 1955; HARRIS u. SPENCER, 1962; HERTTING u. STOKLASKA, 1957; KEMPER u. AMELIN, 1959; KITCHIN, SMITH u. a., 1954; KRAMER, 1955, 1956a; LECOMTE, 1958; LECOMTE, VAN CAUWENBERGE u. VLIERS, 1959; MEYER, 1963; MORRISON, RICHARDSON u. BLOOM, 1951; ROWLEY u. BENDITT, 1956; VAN CAUWENBERGE, LECOMTE u. LAPIÈRE, 1958). Zum Teil haben diese Untersuchungen auch dazu gedient, Unterschiede zwischen den Ödemarten festzustellen. So ließ sich z. B. das Dextranödem vom Eiklarödem (FREY u. FISCHER, 1956; HALPERN u. BRIOT, 1952b; KRAMER, 1955, 1956a; LECOMTE, VAN CAUWENBERGE u. VLIERS, 1959) oder vom Formalinödem (DOMENJOZ, 1952; DOMENJOZ, THEOBALD u. MÖRSDORF, 1955; HERTTING u. STOKLASKA, 1957, 1959; HILLEBRECHT, 1959; KADATZ, 1957; MÖRSDORF, 1959a, 1960; PARRATT u. WEST, 1957e; STENGER, 1958, 1959) differenzieren.

Ein besonderer entzündungshemmender Stoff, der das Dextran- und Eiklarödem sowie in geringerem Maße auch das Hyaluronidase-, Formalin- und Histaminödem hemmt, ist das Guajazulen, das von YAMASAKI u. Mitarb. (1958) sowie UDA (1960) untersucht worden ist. Es unterdrückt auch die passive cutane Anaphylaxie der Ratte. Hervorzuheben ist besonders seine hemmende Wirkung auf die Histaminfreisetzung, durch die es die Abnahme des Hauthistamins nach großen Dosen von Dextran verhindert und die Ausscheidung von Histamin im Urin nach zahlreichen Histaminliberatoren, darunter auch Dextran und Eiklar vermindert. Zur Deutung der ödemhemmenden Wirkung wird auch eine Hemmung der Serotoninfreisetzung, ferner auch eine Antihistaminwirkung, eine Antihyaluronidasewirkung und eine permeabilitätssenkende Wirkung auf die Capillaren angenommen. Guajazulen soll seine Wirkung eher einer direkten Wirkung auf die Zellen als einer indirekten Wirkung über die Nebennieren verdanken.

Die nicht direkt bewiesene Hemmung der Serotoninfreisetzung wird vermutet, weil Guajazulen mit der ödemhemmenden Wirkung von Reserpin, das die Serotonindepots der Haut entleert, interferiert. Ein Anteil an dem Dextranödem wird auch einer Hyaluronidaseaktivierung zugesprochen.

Große Ähnlichkeit mit der Guajazulenwirkung besitzen auch einige, dem Guajazulen chemisch verwandte Lumisantoninderivate (YAMASAKI, KONDO, UDA, YAMAMOTO u. ENDO, 1960, 1961). Unter diesen ragt das Methylpyrophosphosantoninat besonders hervor, dessen ödemhemmende und anaphylaxiehemmende Wirkung die des Guajazulens übertrifft und das sich durch besonders geringe allgemeine Toxicität auszeichnet.

Die Ödemhemmung durch Salicylat, Aminopyrin, Cortison und Phenergan soll wohl mit einer Hemmung der Histaminfreisetzung, nicht aber mit einer Hemmung der Serotoninfreisetzung verknüpft sein. YAMASAKI, KONDO u. UDA (1960) beschreiben auch 3 Acetanilidderivate und 2 Pyrazolonderivate mit ödemhemmenden Eigenschaften, u. a. auch gegenüber dem Dextranödem. Alle diese Stoffe, ferner die als Kontrollsubstanzen verwendeten Stoffe aus der gleichen chemischen Gruppe (Phenacetin, Acetanilid, Aminopyrin, Aminopropylon, Butazolidin) hemmen die Histaminausscheidung im Urin nach i.p. Injektion von Ovomucoid bei der Ratte.

Hinsichtlich des Wirkungsmechanismus, der der Histaminfreisetzung durch Dextran zugrunde liegt, ist zunächst die Feststellung von Interesse, daß sowohl an der isolierten Rattenhaut (Halpern und Briot, 1952a) als auch am intakten Tier die Histaminfreisetzung durch Hypothermie gehemmt wird, wie verschiedene Autoren gezeigt haben (Halpern, 1960a; Halpern, Neveu und Branellec, 1959; Vukobratović, 1958, 1961; Vukobratović und Bata, 1957). Dagegen wird die Histaminvermehrung im Plasma durch 48/80 durch die Hypothermie sogar erheblich verstärkt. Es scheint also ein fundamentaler Unterschied in der Wirkung dieser beiden Histaminliberatoren vorzuliegen. Im Falle des Dextrans wäre, ähnlich wie bei einer Antigen-Antikörperreaktion, an die Beteiligung eines enzymatischen Prozesses zu denken.

Eine Aktivierung von Proteasen scheint jedoch hierbei nicht in Betracht zu kommen. Dextran aktiviert im Rattenserum die proteolytischen Prozesse nicht (Kramer, 1955, 1958). Positive Ergebnisse am Meerschweinchenserum (Kramer, 1958; Olesen, 1959) können hier außer Betracht bleiben. Eine Veränderung der Plasminaktivität findet während des Ödems nicht statt (Levy u. De Vaillancourt, 1960). Eine Proteaseaktivierung in verschiedenen Serumarten vermißte Haining (1956a). Gegen die Proteasetheorie des Dextranödems kann auch angeführt werden, daß Streptokinase kein Ödem macht und Trypsin das Dextranödem hemmt (Beiler, Brendel u. Martin, 1955; Cohen, Graff u. Kleinberg, 1955). Der Mechanismus der hemmenden Trypsinwirkung ist nach Martin (1957) durch "spreading increase" gegeben. Von Fermentgiften wirken Monojodessigsäure und 2,4-DNP stärker auf das Formalinödem als auf das Dextranödem, NaF auf beide gleich (Stenger, 1959). Die Zunahme des Gesamtaminosäurengehaltes im entzündeten Pfotengewebe nach lokaler Dextran- oder Serotoninapplikation könnte zwar Folge einer gesteigerten Proteolyse sein, doch kann der Grund für die Anhäufung freier Aminosäuren im Entzündungsgebiet auch in einem vermehrten Antransport oder gedrosselten Abtransport liegen (Kalbhen, 1963a).

Nach eigenen, gemeinsam mit Wirth durchgeführten Versuchen zeigt die Histaminfreisetzung ins Plasma durch Dextran (300 mg/kg i.v.) und durch 48/80 (200 μg/kg i.v.) etwa den gleichen zeitlichen Verlauf: Nach 10—20 min ist das Maximum (das etwa 15fache des normalen Plasmahistaminspiegels) erreicht, schon 2 min nach der Injektion ist das Plasmahistamin auf etwa 50% des Maximums erhöht. Beiden histaminliberierenden Substanzen ist gemeinsam, daß sie im Gegensatz zur Rattenanaphylaxie (vgl. Code, Cody u. Mitarb., 1961a, b; Cody u. Mitarb., 1963) keine Histaminaseaktivierung im Plasma bewirken.

Weil Rattenserum ein guter Anaphylatoxinbildner ist, hat Rocha e Silva (1956) den Gedanken geäußert, daß das Anaphylatoxin eine vermittelnde Rolle bei der Histaminfreisetzung durch Dextran spielen könne. Der Nachweis, daß das Dextran mit Rattenserum Anaphylatoxin bildet, wurde von Hahn (1954b) geführt. Dieses Anaphylatoxin wirkt auf Meerschweinchen in typischer Weise. Es erzeugt auch ein Ödem bei Ratten, das aber auf Dextranreste zurückzuführen ist. Mit Inulin bereitetes Anaphylatoxin ist unwirksam. Außerdem erzeugt ein niedermolekulares Dextran (Molekulargewicht 20000) Ödeme bei der Ratte, aber kein Anaphylatoxin mit Rattenserum (Hahn, Lange und Giertz, 1954). Die Ödembildung bei der Ratte kann also nicht auf intermediärer Anaphylatoxinbildung beruhen. Zu dem gleichen Ergebnis gelangten auch Halpern, Briot und Neveu (1954a, b). Sie fanden, daß Polymere von Dextran, die bei der Ratte unwirksam sind, noch ein Anaphylatoxin bilden, das auf Meerschweinchen wirkt; ferner daß Agaranaphylatoxin kein Ödem erzeugt; und schließlich, daß Serum von Ratten, die gegen Dextran tolerant gemacht worden sind, doch noch Anaphylatoxin bildet. Hereditär dextranresistente Wistarratten haben ein Serum, das sich zur Anaphylatoxinbildung wie Serum dextranempfindlicher Ratten eignet (Harris u. West, 1963). Nach Parratt und West (1957e) ist Anaphylatoxin, mit Dextran und Rattenserum hergestellt, am Durchströmungspräparat hinsichtlich der Histamin- und Serotoninfreisetzung nicht wirksamer als Dextran allein. Damit soll die Möglichkeit nicht ausgeschlossen sein, daß der Histaminfreisetzung durch Dextran primär eine Reaktion zwischen Dextran und bestimmten Eiweißkörpern der Ratte zugrunde liegt, für die es mehrere Hinweise gibt (PILLEMER, BLUM u. a., 1954; PILLEMER, SCHOENBERG u. a., 1955; PONDER und PONDER, 1960; RICKETTS, 1952).

Das gleiche Thema berühren noch zwei Angaben der Literatur, die allerdings das Ovomucoid betreffen. LAGUNOFF und BENDITT (1960) untersuchten, ob Ovomucoid in Kombination mit Rattenserum statt mit einfacher Salzlösung auf isolierte Mastzellen wirken könne, fanden aber auch dabei keine Wirkung. LECOMTE (1957) erhielt eine histaminliberierende und ödembildende Wirkung von Ovomucoid im Durchströmungsversuch auch nicht durch Mischung des Ovomucoids mit Rattenheparinplasma. Beachtung verdienen ferner die Versuche von ARCHER (1959a, b). Der Verfasser beschreibt ein histaminliberierendes Prinzip, das er durch Behandlung von Rattenserum mit Dextran erhielt und das auf Ratten wirkte. Sera von adrenalektomierten Tieren waren wirksamer als normale. Dextrosezugabe verhinderte die Bildung dieses Prinzips. Auch in komplementinaktivem Serum bildet sich die Substanz. Sie läßt sich auch mit Hilfe der β- oder γ-Globulinfraktion gewinnen. Ähnliche Ergebnisse liefert auch Zymosan, das bei Ratten kein Ödem erzeugt. Die Darstellung dieses Prinzips unterliegt also anderen Bedingungen als die des Anaphylatoxins. ARCHER vermutet, daß es sich um ein Histon oder ein Abbauprodukt des Histons handelt.

Neuerdings glauben auch ADAMKIEWICZ u. SACRA (1963), die vermittelnde Rolle bei der Entstehung der anaphylaktoiden Dextranreaktion einem Serumfaktor zuschreiben zu können, der sich durch intravenöse Übertragung kleiner Serummengen (0,5 ml) dextranvorbehandelter Ratten auf normale Ratten nachweisen läßt. Um Dextranreste, wie es GÖZSY u. KÁTÓ (1960a) bei ähnlichen Versuchen angenommen haben, soll es sich dabei nicht handeln, zumal der Serumfaktor (als „TARIF" = transferable anaphylactoid reaction inducing factor bezeichnet) erst 60 min nach der intravenösen Dextraninjektion (120 mg/kg) seine volle Wirksamkeit erlangt. Präsensibilisierung mit Dextran soll diesen Faktor verstärken. Gemeinsam mit LAAFF gelang es uns nicht, die Ergebnisse von ADAMKIEWICZ u. SACRA zu reproduzieren, allerdings konnten wir weder das gleiche Dextran noch den gleichen Rattenstamm verwenden. In diesem Zusammenhang ist vielleicht ein Hinweis auf die Arbeit von FORMANEK u. HÖLLER (1959) angebracht, die durch Injektion von homologem Serum nicht vorbehandelter Ratten in die Rattenpfote ein Ödem erzeugen konnten.

Vielleicht bringen in Zukunft die wichtigen Befunde über den Zusammenhang des Dextran- und Ovomucoidödems mit Veränderungen im Kohlenhydratstoffwechsel tiefere Einblicke in den Mechanismus der Histaminfreisetzung. 1956 berichteten ADAMKIEWICZ und LANGLOIS über eine sensibilisierende Wirkung von Insulin gegen Dextran. So bewirken z. B. 20 E Insulin, daß unterschwellige Dosen von Dextran in der Plantarseite der Pfote zu schweren anaphylaktoiden Reaktionen führen (ADAMKIEWICZ und LANGLOIS, 1957). Insulin sensibilisiert die Pfoten auch gegen die sonst unwirksamen Injektionen von Dextran unter die Rückenhaut. Es durchbricht ferner die ödemhemmende Wirkung einer 4tägigen Cortisonbehandlung. Diese Insulinwirkung besteht auch an spinalisierten Ratten (ADAMKIEWICZ, LANGLOIS und POIRIER, 1958). Nach 25tägiger Vorbehandlung mit 48/80 ist auch nach Insulin kein Dextraneffekt mehr vorhanden (ADAMKIEWICZ und LANGLOIS, 1958). Nach SANYAL, SPENCER und WEST (1959) verläuft das Bild der Dextranvergiftung unter Insulin nicht nur heftiger als ohne Insulin, sondern ist häufig mit schweren Darmblutungen, die zum Tode führen, verknüpft. Es kommt zum Überspringen einer lokal (in der Pfote) ausgelösten Reaktion auf andere Pfoten, auf Ohren oder Schnauze. Außer der Wirkung von Dextran wird auch die Wirkung von Eiklar und Glycogen verstärkt (ADAMKIEWICZ und LANGLOIS, 1958; KONDO, 1959). Auch Tolbutamid, das den Blutzucker senkt, sensibilisiert gegen Dextran. Seine Wirkung ist an die Gegenwart von Insulin gebunden (ADAMKIEWICZ, FITKO und FORTIER, 1960). Glucagon hat keine Wirkung auf den sensibilisierenden Insulineffekt. Es soll überhaupt keine Wirkung auf das Dextranödem haben (ADAMKIEWICZ und ADAMKIEWICZ, 1959a). Aber Blutzuckerbestimmungen fehlen in diesen Untersuchungen.

Neuerdings fanden allerdings LEFEBVRE und VAN CAUWENBERGE (1962) einen Hemmeffekt des Glucagons auf das lokal ausgelöste Dextran-, Histamin- und Formalinödem. Diese Wirkung beruht wahrscheinlich auf einer Freisetzung von Nebennierenmarkhormonen durch Glucagon, denn sie wird durch Adrenalektomie und durch Adrenolytica verhindert.

Insulin führt zu einer verstärkten Mastzelldegranulation unter Dextran und Eiklar und bedingt dadurch auch eine stärkere Vermehrung des Plasmahistamins (GOTH, NASH u. a., 1957; RÉDEI, NAGY und KARÁDY, 1961). Wichtig für das Verständnis dieser Insulinwirkung ist die Tatsache, daß sich die sensibilisierende Insulinwirkung nicht auf andere Histaminliberatoren wie 48/80 und Polymyxin B erstreckt (GOTH, NASH u. a. 1957; SANYAL, SPENCER und WEST, 1959).

Das Gegenstück, die Hemmung des Dextranödems durch den experimentellen Alloxandiabetes, wurde zuerst von GOTH, NASH u. a. (1957) (vgl. auch BERALDO u. Mitarb., 1962) beschrieben, nachdem schon EDLUND, LÖFGREN und VÄLI (1952) eine angeblich an subdiabetische Dosen gebundene Hemmwirkung des Alloxans erwähnt haben. Insulin wirkt hier antagonistisch (ADAMKIEWICZ und ADAMKIEWICZ, 1959b; GOTH, NASH u. a. 1957). Auch die Alloxanwirkung erstreckt sich nicht auf das Ödem durch 48/80, wohl aber auf das Eiklarödem (vgl. auch KONDO, 1959). Alloxan verhindert auch die Histaminfreisetzung durch Dextran oder Eiklar, nicht aber die durch 48/80 (GOTH, NASH u. a., 1957). Ferner wird auch der Austritt von i.v. injiziertem Evansblau in die Rückenhaut an der Stelle intradermal injizierten Dextrans durch Alloxan gehemmt (BERALDO u. Mitarb., 1962). Allerdings ist am isolierten Zwerchfell von alloxandiabetischen Ratten auch eine Hemmung der Histaminliberation durch 48/80 beobachtet worden, die durch Glucose und Insulinzugabe normalisiert wurde (VUGMAN und ROTHSCHILD,1961). Das Hauthistamin wird durch den Diabetes nicht herabgesetzt (GOTH, NASH u. a., 1957). Wie die Histaminfreisetzung, so ist auch die Mastzelldegranulation durch Dextran bei den alloxandiabetischen Tieren gehemmt (RÉDEI, NAGY und KARÁDY, 1961).

Durch die Veränderungen im Zuckerstoffwechsel wird offenbar nicht die Wirkung der Überträgerstoffe Histamin und Serotonin betroffen. Die Wirkung von in die Pfote injiziertem Histamin und Serotonin sowie Polymyxin B und 48/80 bleibt durch Insulin unbeeinflußt (SANYAL, 1960b; SANYAL, SPENCER und WEST, 1959). Jedoch wird die i.p. Histamintoxicität erhöht (SANYAL, 1960b). Serotonin und Histamin vermögen auch nicht an 48/80 vorbehandelten Ratten die sensibilisierende Insulinwirkung gegenüber Dextran wiederherzustellen. Eine direkte Wirkung von Insulin auf die Gefäßpermeabilität oder eine Histaminfreisetzung durch Insulin ist auszuschließen (ADAMKIEWICZ und LANGLOIS, 1958; GOTH, NASH u. a., 1957). Insulin beeinflußt nicht den Dextranspiegel im Blute bei Katzen (RÈDEI, NAGY und KARÁDY, 1961). Bei Ratten liegen keine Befunde darüber vor. Aber nach Beobachtungen an Mastzellen von Ratten scheint es so zu sein, daß durch einen verminderten Blutzucker die Permeabilität der Zellmembranen für Polysaccharide bzw. Ovomucoid gefördert und durch Steigerung des Blutzuckers gehemmt wird. Man denkt an eine Kompetition zwischen Glucose und den polysaccharidartigen Makromolekülen (auch das Ovomucoid enthält ja einen Zuckerkomplex) um die an der Zuckeraufnahme beteiligten Transportmechanismen der Zellen (ADAMKIEWICZ und ADAMKIEWICZ, 1960). Dafür spricht, daß Glucose und andere Monosaccharide, ganz besonders 2-Deoxyglucose, das Dextran- bzw. Ovomucoidödem (nicht das Ödem nach 48/80) hemmen (GOTH, 1959, 1961). Auch neuere Versuche mit U-C^{14}-markierter Glucose und U-C^{14}-markiertem Dextran an insulinbehandelten Tieren sprechen dafür (ADAMKIEWICZ u. BATA, 1962). Auf die Ähnlichkeit mit der Wirkung von Oligosacchariden auf die Antigen-Antikörperreaktion zwischen Dextran und Dextran-Antikörpern (KABAT, 1956) wäre in diesem Zusammenhang auch hinzuweisen. Nach BERALDO u. Mitarb. (1962) läßt sich auch die intradermale Dextranwirkung im Evansblautest durch gleichzeitige Injektion von Glucose in Mischung mit Dextran hemmen. In vitro ließ sich zeigen, daß die Histaminfreisetzung durch Dextran aus Hautstücken durch Glucosezugabe zur Suspensionsflüssigkeit verhindert wird. Parallel hiermit geht ein Ausbleiben des Mastzellzerfalls in Haut- und Mesenterialstückchen. Die hemmende Wirkung anderer Zucker ist an strukturelle Verwandtschaft zur Glucose gebunden (Xylose, Mannose, Fructose, Maltose, Galaktose).

Aufgrund dieser Tatsachen läßt sich eine Theorie der Dextran- und Ovomucoidwirkung formulieren, welche besagt, daß beide Stoffe auf den normalen Wegen des Zuckerstoffwechsels in die Mastzellen und vielleicht auch in andere Zellen eindringen und dort als körperfremde Faktoren den normalen Zuckerstoffwechsel stören und damit zu einer Zellschädigung und Histaminfreisetzung führen (Goth, 1959).

Beraldo u. Mitarb. (1962) geben unseres Wissens erstmalig auch Hinweise darauf, daß gewisse intermediäre Stoffwechselprodukte, möglicherweise aus dem glykolytischen Stoffwechsel, unabhängig vom Krebscyclus, in die Dextranreaktion eingeschaltet sind. Zusatz von bekannten Stoffwechselinhibitoren (Jodacetat, N-Äthylmaleimid, Nicotinamid, Mepyramin, DNP, Ca-Mangel, Erwärmung auf 45° C), von denen bekannt ist, daß sie Histaminfreisetzung und Mastzellzerfall durch 48/80 oder durch Anaphylaxie bei der Ratte unterdrücken, hemmen beides auch im Falle der Dextranreaktion in vitro an der Haut oder dem Mesenterium. Glucose hebt die DNP-Wirkung auf in Konzentrationen, die die Histaminfreisetzung am nicht durch DNP gehemmten Gewebe ebenfalls erhöhen. Hierdurch wird gezeigt, daß der Mechanismus, der zur Histaminfreisetzung durch Dextran führt, ähnliche Stufen durchläuft wie bei der Wirkung von 48/80 oder der anaphylaktischen Reaktion der Ratten.

Bemerkenswert sind in diesem Zusammenhang die neuen Untersuchungen von Kalbhen (1963b), der im entzündeten Gewebe 2 Std nach der Dextrangabe einen starken Abfall der Uridindiphosphatglucose und vor allem der Glykolysephosphate und einen Anstieg des Diphosphopyridinnukleotids beobachtete. Er faßt diese Veränderungen vor allem als Ausdruck einer gesteigerten Glykolyse auf.

3. Serotonin und Dextranödem

Die Überlegungen und Tatsachen, die gegen eine ausschließliche oder auch nur überwiegende Rolle des Histamins für das Dextranödem sprechen, sind im Prinzip ähnlich wie die im Kapitel über das Eiklarödem dargelegten. Einige der dort referierten Befunde betreffen in gleicher Weise das Dextran- und das Eiklarödem. Erwähnt sei nur, daß man auch hier auf die Diskrepanz zwischen Histaminabnahme in der Haut nach wiederholten Dextrangaben und dem Auftreten der Gewöhnung an Dextran gestoßen ist (Kramer, 1956b). Hinzuzufügen sind noch die Beobachtungen von Halpern (1956), wonach Promethazin bei adrenalektomierten Tieren die Dextrangiftigkeit nicht komplett aufhebt, wohl aber die Giftigkeit von injiziertem Histamin, die bei adrenalektomierten Tieren bekanntlich auch erhöht ist (Crivellari, 1927). Durch Histaminverarmung läßt sich bei adrenalektomierten Tieren die Dextrantoxicität nur in dem gleichen Maße reduzieren wie durch Promethazin, aber nicht vollständig aufheben.

Auch die Gründe, die für eine überwiegende Rolle des Serotonins sprechen und die von Parratt und West (1957e) und West (1957a, b, 1961a) zusammengefaßt worden sind, gelten für das Dextranödem in gleicher Weise wie für das Eiklarödem: Das Vorkommen von Serotonin in der Rattenhaut, seine Freisetzung durch Dextran, das Vorhandensein in der Ödemflüssigkeit, die Hemmung der Ödembildung durch Vorbehandlung mit Reserpin oder 48/80 und nicht mit Polymyxin B und die wesentlich stärkere ödembildende Wirksamkeit von Serotonin im Vergleich zu Histamin.

Ein Hinweis auf die Freisetzung von Serotonin ist die Tatsache, daß der Serotoningehalt in der Haut durch Dextran herabgesetzt wird. PARRATT und WEST (1957e) haben gezeigt, daß nach i.p. Injektion von 300 mg/kg Dextran Serotonin und Histamin in der Haut des Fußrückens, der Pfoten und der Ohren etwa in dem gleichen Maße abnehmen wie nach 24 ml/kg Eiklar. Die Abnahme des Serotonins in der Pfote nach Dextran wird neuerdings von MÖRSDORF (1959a, 1961a,b) und von SUPEK, JOVIĆ und KECKES (1961) bestätigt. Sie ist auch mit Terpentinöl, nicht mit Formalin nachweisbar.

Im Gegensatz zu Reserpin bewirkt allerdings weder Dextran noch 48/80, noch Polymyxin B eine Mehrausscheidung von 5-Hydroxyindolessigsäure. JASMIN (1960) schließt aus diesem Befund, daß eine Serotoninbeteiligung an der anaphylaktoiden Reaktion fraglich sei.

Nach HALPERN, LIACOPOULOS und LIACOPOULOS-BRIOT (1957) sinkt der Serotoningehalt in der Bauchhaut nach 5 Dextraninjektionen um etwa 50%. Nach PARRATT und WEST ist nach einer Injektion eine Abnahme in der Bauchhaut noch nicht nachweisbar, während in den empfindlichen Bezirken der Haut das Serotonin um 50% oder mehr absinkt. Nach wiederholten Dextrangaben ändert sich in diesen Bezirken der Haut der Serotoningehalt nicht mehr wesentlich, während der Histamingehalt an einzelnen Stellen (Ohren und Pfoten) noch weiter abnimmt. Es ist also für die Frage nach den Ursachen der Dextrantoleranz nicht uninteressant, daß sich die Erschöpfung der mobilisierbaren Serotoninvorräte in den empfindlichen Stellen der Haut noch schneller vollzieht als die Abnahme der Histaminvorräte und daß im Zustande der Dextrantoleranz noch sehr viel Serotonin in der Haut enthalten ist. Die Gewöhnungsversuche scheinen danach auch für eine reine Serotonintheorie das gleiche Dilemma aufzudecken wie für eine reine Histamintheorie.

Der direkte Beweis für die Serotoninfreisetzung durch Dextran ließ sich ähnlich wie für Eiklar im Durchströmungsversuch erbringen. HALPERN, LIACOPOULOS und LIACOPOULOS-BRIOT (1957) fanden am Durchströmungspräparat eine Freisetzung von Serotonin und Histamin im Verhältnis 1:17 nach Dextran und 1:12 nach 1935 L.

Im Hinblick auf die Wirkung der sogenannten Antihistaminica auf das Dextranödem und die Abhängigkeit dieser Wirkung von ihren Antiserotonineigenschaften gelten die Ergebnisse von PARRATT und WEST (1958) sowie DOEPFNER und CERLETTI (1957), die bereits im Eiklarkapitel ausführlich erwähnt wurden. Einige Untersuchungen (COURVOISIER und DUCROT, 1955; HALPERN, LIACOPOULOS und LIACOPOULOS-BRIOT, 1959), die sich nur mit dem Dextranödem beschäftigen, lassen ebenfalls die schwache Wirkung von Mepyramin erkennen. Aus diesen und anderen Untersuchungen (BOHNSTEDT und LANZ, 1956; COURVOISIER, FOURNEL u. a., 1953; JASMIN, 1957; KRAMER, 1955; STUCKI und THOMPSON, 1958; VIAUD, 1954) geht auch die starke Schutzwirkung von Chlorpromazin und Promethazin hervor. COURVOISIER und DUCROT (1955) fanden auch, daß quarternäre Ammoniumbasen von beiden Stoffen noch volle Antihistamineigenschaften haben, aber nicht mehr antiödematös wirken. Im allgemeinen gilt allerdings das Dextranödem als schwerer hemmbar als das Eiklarödem. Keine Einmütigkeit herrscht aber darüber, ob das Chlorpromazin wirksamer ist als Promethazin gegenüber dem Dextranödem. Während COURVOISIER und Mitarbeiter das Chlorpromazin pro Gewichtseinheit 10fach wirksamer fanden, ist nach HALPERN, LIACOPOULOS und LIACOPOULOS-BRIOT (1959) in der Wirkung auf das Ödem und die Hämokonzentration kein Unterschied vorhanden, in dem an der Bauchhaut durchgeführten Farbstofftest das Promethazin sogar überlegen. Wenn man nach HALPERN und Mitarb. annimmt, daß das Promethazin auch an den Rattencapillaren relativ stärkere Antihistamineigenschaften hat als das Chlorpromazin, so ist der meist angenommene Parallelismus zwischen Antiödem- und Antiserotonineigenschaften in diesem Falle nicht festzustellen. Nur im Falle des Mepyramin mit seinen (nach

Halpern) stärksten Antihistamin- und schwächsten Antiserotonineigenschaften besteht dieser Zusammenhang. Vielleicht sind Abweichungen der genannten Art ein Hinweis darauf, daß neben dem Serotonin auch dem Histamin eine Bedeutung für das Dextranödem zukommt. Man könnte in diesem Sinne auch die Befunde von Kramer und Arrigoni-Martelli (1958) deuten, welche bei der Prüfung von 5 verschiedenen Phenothiazinderivaten keinen Parallelismus zwischen der Wirkung auf das Dextranödem und der Antiserotoninwirkung am Rattencolon fanden, wenn man nicht im Sinne einer späteren Deutung dieser Autoren (Arrigoni-Martelli und Kramer, 1958) die Verschiedenartigkeit der Testorgane für dieses abweichende Verhalten verantwortlich machen will.

Einer Deutung entzieht sich vorläufig die Mitteilung von Hertting und Stoklaska (1959), welche beobachteten, daß die Chlorpromazinwirkung auf das Dextranödem durch Denervierung der Pfote gehemmt wird.

Auf die starke Schutzwirkung der spezifischen Serotoninantagonisten (LSD und BOL 148), die auch für das Dextranödem gilt, wurde schon beim Eiklar hingewiesen (Halpern, Liacopoulos und Liacopoulos-Briot, 1959; Parratt und West, 1958). Auch nach Stenger (1958) soll LSD zu einer kompletten Hemmung des Dextranödems führen. Nach Gelfand und West (1961) wirken 2 Lysergsäurederivate, nämlich das Butanolamid und das Propanolamid der 1-Methyl-Lysergsäure, welche starke Antiserotonineigenschaften besitzen, auf das Dextranödem und das Ödem durch 48/80, nicht aber auf das Histaminödem hemmend.

Neuerdings haben aber Craps und Inderbitzin (1961) mit Hilfe eines Pontaminblautestes beobachtet, daß BOL 148 erst in Kombination mit Mepyramin die Dextranwirkung komplett hemmt. UML (1-Methyllysergsäure) hemmt das Serotoninödem stärker als Cyproheptadin. Es ist jedoch gegenüber dem Dextranödem schwächer wirksam als Cyproheptadin, das außer dem Serotonin- auch das Histaminödem hemmt (Jori, Bentivoglio und Garattini, 1961). Solche Beobachtungen sprechen ähnlich wie die schon beim Eiklar erwähnten Befunde von Rowley und Benditt (1956) für eine Mitwirkung des Histamins bei der Entstehung des Dextranödems.

Reserpinvorbehandlung hemmt auch das Dextranödem (Arrigoni-Martelli und Kramer, 1958; Parratt und West, 1957e). Mörsdorf und Fehres (1959) und Mörsdorf (1959b) betonen, daß eine längere Vorbehandlung notwendig ist. Nach Craps und Inderbitzin (1961) macht die Vorbehandlung mit Reserpin nicht nur gegen Dextran, 48/80 und 1935 L, sondern auch gegen Polymyxin B unempfindlich. Die Autoren betonen, daß hieraus keine definitiven Schlüsse gezogen werden können, weil die Tiere in diesem Zustande durch das Reserpin stark sedativ beeinflußt sind. Die Tatsache, daß das Reserpin keine Wirkung auf die Gefäßpermeabilität hat, veranlaßt die Autoren, eine Freisetzung des Serotonins in einer inaktiven Form unter der Wirkung von Reserpin anzunehmen. Nach 3maliger Reserpinbehandlung (je 3 mg/kg) nahm der Serotoningehalt in dem Pfotengewebe um 55 %, die Stärke des Dextranödems um 54 % ab. Nach einmaliger Reserpingabe zeigte der Serotoningehalt und die Ödembereitschaft noch keine Veränderung (Mörsdorf, 1959b, 1960/61). Vorbehandlung mit wiederholten Gaben von Reserpin schwächt auch die Wirkung von Dextran auf die Tuschespeicherung in den Gefäßen ab (Saito, 1958).

Die Untersuchungen über die Auswirkung, die eine Hemmung des Serotoninabbaus durch Iproniazid zur Folge hat, haben zu schwer deutbaren Ergebnissen geführt. Nach Arrigoni-Martelli und Kramer (1958) kommt es meist zu einer Ödemhemmung (Dextran und Ovomucoid). Nach Mörsdorf (1959b, 1960/61) wird das Dextranödem nicht beeinflußt, das Formalinödem gehemmt. Offenbar ist das eine Dosisfrage, da nach Setnikar u. Mitarb. (1959) hohe Dosen von Iproniazid das Dextranödem, wenn auch schwächer als das Formalinödem, hemmen. Nach Georges, Herold und Cahn (1958) hemmt Iproniazid das Dextran- und nicht das Serotoninödem. Nach den gleichen Autoren soll Reserpin das Serotoninödem hemmen und nicht das

Dextranödem. Schließlich wird noch darüber berichtet, daß Serotonin i.p. das Dextranödem antagonistisch beeinflußt (GEORGES u. HEROLD, 1957). Nach SETNIKAR u. Mitarb. (1959) ist der Iproniazideffekt wie auch der Serotonineffekt von der Nebenniere abhängig. Allerdings soll der Iproniazideffekt nicht durch Hemmung des Serotoninabbaus zustande kommen. Vielmehr soll Iproniazid vielleicht den Corticoidabbau in der Leber hemmen, während Serotonin die Sekretion der Nebennierenhormone beeinflußt. Von verschiedenen Amidinen hemmten vor allem das Propamidin und das Pentamidin, aber auch das Dibrompropamidin, Stilbamidin und Hexamidin das Dextranödem. Durch Pentamidin werden auch das Serotonin-, Eiweiß- und Kaolinödem, nicht aber das Histaminödem gehemmt (COHEN u. BOISMARE, 1961).

Man kommt zusammenfassend zu dem Ergebnis, daß auch für das Dextranödem die Serotonintheorie nicht alle Erscheinungen erklären kann und daß neben dem Serotonin auch dem Histamin wahrscheinlich eine nicht zu vernachlässigende Bedeutung zukommt (CRAPS und INDERBITZIN, 1961).

VOGEL und MAREK (1961) konnten mit LSD (i.v.) nur das Serotoninödem, nicht aber das Dextran- und Ovomucoidödem gut hemmen. Ergotamin dagegen wirkte nicht nur auf das Serotonin-, sondern auch auf das Dextran- und Ovomucoidödem, aber auch auf zahlreiche andere Ödemarten. Die gegensätzliche Wirkung von LSD auf das Serotonin- und Dextranödem wurde auch schon von MÖRSDORF und FEHRES (1959) beschrieben. Unseres Erachtens lassen aber diese Ergebnisse die daraus gezogene Schlußfolgerung von der untergeordneten Bedeutung des Serotonins beim Dextranödem nicht zwingend zu. Die einseitige Wirkung des LSD auf das Serotoninödem wird verständlich, wenn man für das Dextranödem auch noch dem Histamin eine wichtige Rolle zuspricht. Die gewissermaßen unspezifische Wirkung des Ergotamins könnte über eine gefäßkontrahierende Wirkung laufen.

4. Dextranödem und innere Sekretion

Durch Exstirpation der Nebennieren wird auch die Dextranwirkung verstärkt. Es kommt zu schweren Schocksymptomen mit meist tödlichem Ausgang (BRIOT und HALPERN, 1952a; HALPERN, 1956; HALPERN und BRIOT, 1952b). Die LD_{50} von Dextran wird von 2 g/kg i.v. auf 0,03 g/kg gesenkt. Lokal injiziert erzeugen extrem kleine Dosen (0,6 mg) Ödem. Die tödliche Kreislaufstörung ist mit Sequestration des Blutes und Stase in den Capillaren und unvollkommenem venösen Rückfluß verbunden (SWINGLE, FEDOR u. a., 1953).

PARRATT (1957) und PARRATT und WEST (1960) beschreiben ein ähnliches tödliches Vergiftungsbild durch Dextran bei Ratten nach Thyroxinbehandlung. Die Wirkung der Schilddrüsenhormone und der antithyreoidalen Substanzen sowie der Thyreoidektomie auf die Dextranreaktion hat eine eingehende Untersuchung durch SPENCER u. WEST (1962) erfahren. Hierüber wurde ausführlich im Eiklarkapitel referiert (siehe dasselbe).

Über die Wirkung von Cortison, das in wiederholten Gaben das Dextranödem bei normalen Tieren verhindern soll, haben als erste MORRISON, RICHARDSON und BLOOM (1951) und EDLUND, LÖFGREN und VÄLI (1952) berichtet. Weitere Untersuchungen führten zu ungleichen Resultaten. Nach DOMENJOZ wird das Dextranödem weniger als das Eiklarödem durch Cortison und ACTH beeinflußt (DOMENJOZ, 1955). Keine sicheren Ergebnisse erhielten LECOMTE, VAN CAUWENBERGE und VLIERS (1959) mit Cortison, Hydrocortison und ACTH, sowie HALPERN (1956) mit Cortison (ferner auch STUCKI und THOMPSON, 1958). Als wirksam erwiesen sich Δ1-Hydrocortison (LECOMTE, VAN CAUWENBERGE und VLIERS, 1959) und Triamcinolon (SELYE, 1955). Nach VUKOBRATOVIČ (1958) hemmt Cortison die Histaminfreisetzung durch Dextran. Eine andere Cortisonwirkung besteht darin, daß es die Wiederbeladung des Gewebes mit mobilisierbarem Histamin verhindert, wenn dieses durch Dextran erschöpft worden ist (HALPERN, 1956, 1960a; HALPERN, BIOZZI, BRIOT und BENACERRAF, 1953). Der Effekt entspricht dem schon vorher an Hunden mit Tween 20 festgestellten (GOTH, ALLMAN u. a., 1951; GOTH, HOLMAN und COPENHAVER, 1952).

Auch die Ergebnisse mit Cortison bei adrenalektomierten Tieren sind nicht eindeutig ausgefallen. Es stehen sich negative Ergebnisse mit einmaligen Cortisongaben (COURVOISIER und DUCROT, 1955) und positive mit wiederholten Gaben (SWINGLE, FEDOR u. a., 1953) gegenüber. Die Auffassung von SELYE, BAJUSZ und NADASDI (1958), wonach negative Befunde von ungenügend langer Cortisonbehandlung herrühren, scheint durch diese Befunde gestützt. Doch ließ sich die Behandlungsdauer durch Verwendung einer wäßrig-alkoholischen Lösung erheblich abkürzen (SWINGLE, FEDOR u. a., 1953). DOMENJOZ (1952) beobachtete auch, daß es eine optimale Dosierung von Cortison gibt, die bei 2mal 10 mg/kg liegt.

Im Gegensatz zum Ovomucoid ruft Dextran in einmaliger Dosis (Macrodex Poviet 0,5 bis 1 ml/100 g) eine beträchtliche Vermehrung der totalen 17-Hydroxycorticosteroide und der totalen Corticosteroide im Plasma hervor. Das Fehlen einer Abnahme der Nebennieren an Ascorbinsäure und Cholesterin spricht gegen die Möglichkeit einer verstärkten sekretorischen Tätigkeit der Nebennierenrinde, d. h. mehr für Verminderung des Verbrauchs an Hormonen in der Peripherie (LECOMTE, VAN CAUWENBERGE u. VLIERS, 1959).

Über die Wirkung des Adrenalins beim Dextranödem wird berichtet, daß es in Dosen von 2mal 100 μg/kg wirksam sei, jedoch weniger als Promethazin. Bei adrenalektomierten Tieren richtet sich die Wirkung gegen die allgemeinen Schocksymptome. Der Tod wird aber nur verzögert (BROCKLEHURST, 1960; COURVOISIER und DUCROT, 1955). Im Gegensatz zu adrenalektomierten Tieren wird die Wirkung auf das Ödem nach i.p. Gaben von Dextran bei normalen Tieren als sehr stark bezeichnet (STUCKI und THOMPSON, 1958). Die negative Wirkung von Noradrenalin (COURVOISIER und DUCROT, 1955) spricht gegen die Annahme einer ursächlichen Bedeutung der Vasoconstriction für die ödemhemmende Adrenalinwirkung. Untersuchungen über die Bedeutung von Abbauprodukten des Adrenalins liegen für das Dextranödem nicht vor, außer einer Mitteilung von LECOMTE (1958), wonach Adrenochrom das Dextranödem durch einen toxischen Effekt hemmen soll. Der Nachprüfung wert erscheint die Angabe von VUKOBRATOVIĆ (1958), daß das Adrenalin die Histaminfreisetzung durch Dextran hemmen soll. Es wäre denkbar, daß dieser Effekt durch die blutzuckersteigernde Wirkung von Adrenalin zustande kommt. Nach J. SCHMIDT (1963) hemmt Adrenalin subcutan das (subplantar erzeugte) Dextranödem, schwächer auch das Serotoninödem, Noradrenalin in der gleichen Dosis (1 mg/kg) subcutan nur das Dextranödem, und zwar in geringerem Grade. Subplantar (100 μg) wirkt Noradrenalin auch auf das Serotoninödem, und zwar sogar stärker als auf das Dextranödem und in beiden Fällen stärker als Adrenalin. Die Rolle des Blutzuckereffektes der subcutanen Adrenalininjektion wäre auch bei der Diskussion dieser Versuche zu berücksichtigen.

SANYAL, SPENCER und WEST (1959) haben den Blutzucker ebenfalls zur Deutung gewisser hormonaler Effekte herangezogen. Sie weisen darauf hin, daß ödemverstärkende Faktoren, wie Thyroxinbehandlung, Adrenalektomie und Hypophysektomie, als gemeinsames eine blutzuckersenkende Wirkung haben. Von Interesse ist in diesem Zusammenhang auch, daß Fasten bei adrenalektomierten Tieren den Dextraneffekt erhöht (JASMIN u. BOIS, 1959). Die Tatsache jedoch, daß Thyroxin auch die Wirkung von Histamin und Serotonin verstärkt (PARRATT u. WEST, 1960), was bei der Insulinwirkung nicht der Fall ist, läßt zum mindesten für das Thyroxin einen anderen Mechanismus als einen, der durch Blutzuckersenkung zustande kommt, wahrscheinlicher erscheinen.

MOELLER (1955) beobachtete, daß Nierenexstirpation die Ratten vor dem Dextranödem schützt. Nach SELYE (1955) ist dieser Schutz durch den Operations-Stress bedingt und tritt daher nicht auf, wenn die Nebennieren mit entfernt werden. Werden die Ratten nephrektomiert und adrenalektomiert und mit Cortison + DOCA substituiert, so tritt die gleiche Ödemreaktion nach Dextran auf wie bei normalen Tieren (JASMIN u. BOIS, 1958). Sie wird durch Vorbehandlung mit 48/80 auch bei den nebennieren- und nierenlosen Tieren verhindert. Die Niere ist also selbst nicht an den Vorgängen der Ödembildung beteiligt.

B. Die anaphylaktoide Reaktion des Hundes

I. Polyvinylpyrrolidon

Polyvinylpyrrolidon (Kollidon; PVP) wurde 1943 von Hecht und Weese als Plasmaersatzmittel in die Therapie eingeführt (siehe auch Reppe, 1954). Es ist, meist als 3,5%ige Lösung, unter verschiedenen Namen im Handel: Periston, Subtosan, Plasdone, Polyvidone u. a. Schon die genannten Autoren haben in ihrer Einführungsarbeit festgestellt, daß das PVP von den gebräuchlichen Laboratoriumstieren, so vor allen von Kaninchen, Katzen, Affen (auch vom Hahn, Lecomte und Beaumariage, 1956) vertragen wird mit Ausnahme des Hundes. Ob auch andere Arten der Canidenfamilie gegenüber PVP empfindlich sind, scheint nicht untersucht zu sein. Die Symptome der Vergiftung sind die eines akuten Gefäßschocks, sehr ähnlich dem anaphylaktischen Schock und dem Peptonschock (Halpern und Briot, 1953a).

Das Vergiftungsbild wurde erstmalig genauer beschrieben von Loubatières (1948). Er beobachtete 3 min nach 0,175 g/kg PVP i.v. einen Schock mit Koma, Durchfällen und Lähmung der hinteren Extremitäten. Der Zustand hielt bis zu 2 Std. an und führte zu vollständiger Erholung nach 3 Std. Im Mittelpunkt stand ein Blutdruckabfall, der bis auf 40 % des Ausgangswertes ging und sich plateauartig für 1 Std auf dieser Höhe hielt, wenn in Narkose (Morphin-Numal oder Morphin-Chloralose) 0,75 g/kg injiziert wurden. Hecht und Weese sahen nach 15 ml/kg der 3,5%igen Lösung (mittleres Molekulargewicht 25000) nur einen mäßigen Blutdruckabfall. Nach Perlmutt, Parkins und Vars (1953) kommt es nach 3 ml/kg der 3,5%igen Lösung (mittleres Molekulargewicht 81000) regelmäßig zu einem Abfall des Blutdruckes um 33%. Gegenüber kleineren Dosen (0,03–0,5 ml/kg) wurden große individuelle Empfindlichkeitsunterschiede beobachtet. Als schockauslösende Dosen werden ferner angegeben: 0,2 ml/kg der 25%igen Lösung (Halpern und Briot, 1953a); 5 ml/kg (Binet und Burstein, 1949), 3,8 ml/kg (Besse und Patay, 1953), 1 ml/kg (Marshall und Hanna, 1957) jeweils der 3,5%igen Lösung. Der Blutdruckabfall ist begleitet von einer Milzkontraktion und Abnahme des Nierenvolumens (Besse und Patay, 1953). Der Druck in der Portalvene steigt unter Schwellung der Leber an (Halpern, 1956).

Wenig bekannt ist bisher über die Abhängigkeit der Wirkung vom Molekulargewicht. Das klinische PVP hat ein mittleres Molekulargewicht von 25000–30000 mit außerordentlich starker Streuung. Die verschiedenen Kollidonfraktionen werden durch K-Werte (Viscositätskoeffizient nach Fikentscher) charakterisiert. Hieraus läßt sich das mittlere Molekulargewicht errechnen (vgl. z. B.: Ravin, Seligman und Fine, 1952). Perlmutt, Parkins und Vars (1953) fanden, daß Kollidon K 21 (Molekulargewicht 20500) so wirksam ist wie K 33,5 (Molekulargewicht 81000). K 62 (Molekulargewicht 560000) hatte dagegen nur unbedeutende Effekte. Das monomere Vinylpyrrolidon war wirkungslos.

Bei den eben angegebenen Zahlen für die Molekulargewichte handelt es sich um das sog. Gewichtsmittel, von dem das Zahlenmittel zu unterscheiden ist. Das Gewichtsmittel liegt zwischen dem Zahlenmittel und dem 3fachen des Zahlenmittels. Je geringer der Unterschied, desto kleiner die Streuung des Molekulargewichts (Squire, Bull u. a., 1955). Leider werden in den meisten Arbeiten keine Angaben darüber gemacht, ob das Zahlen- oder Gewichtsmittel gemeint ist.

Zu dem Blutdruckabfall kommen als weitere Symptome: Pruritus, Rötung der Haut und Steigerung der Hauttemperatur (Halpern und Stiffel, 1955), nach 30–60 min Ödeme an Schnauze, Ohren und Pfotenballen hinzu. Bei schwerem Schock treten Prostration, Hypothermie und blutige Diarrhoe auf (Halpern und Briot, 1953a). Wir haben also neben der Gefäßerweiterung auch eine erhöhte Capillarpermeabilität vor uns, die sich auch durch Hämokonzentration, Eiweißaustritt und Durchtritt von Farbstoffen, die an die Eiweißkörper adsorbiert sind, zu erkennen gibt. Die Magensekretion ist gesteigert. Der Eiweißgehalt der Ödemflüssigkeit entspricht praktisch dem Plasma (HALPERN, 1956).

Die intradermale Injektion führt zu papulo-erythematöser Reaktion. Die befallenen Stellen färben sich mit i.v. injiziertem Evansblau an (HALPERN u. BRIOT, 1953a). Andere Autoren finden nach i.v. Injektion von PVP eine intensive und diffuse Blaufärbung der Haut (HANNA u. MARSHALL, 1957; MARSHALL u. HANNA, 1957, 1958).

Umstritten ist das Verhalten der Blutgerinnungszeit, die nach LOUBATIÈRES (1948) verlängert wird, nach BESSE und PATAY (1953) aber nicht. Nach QUIVY (1956) verändert sich auch die Plasmagerinnungszeit nach blutdrucksenkenden Dosen von PVP nicht.

Eigentümlich ist die Angabe von MORRISON, LUNDY und ESSEX (1952), wonach PVP bei Hunden als Plasmaersatzmittel brauchbar sein soll. Nach LOUBATIÈRES (1948) verstärkt jedoch PVP den hämorrhagischen Schock des Hundes. PERLMUTT, PARKINS und VARS (1953) beobachteten bei entbluteten Hunden durch PVP einen verzögerten Blutdruckanstieg im Vergleich zu einfacher Salzlösung, eine stärkere Blutverdünnung und bei rascher Infusion Todesfälle. Bei sehr langsamer Injektion scheint allerdings PVP vom Hunde vertragen zu werden (CUNY u. QUIVY, 1948; HECHT u. WEESE, 1943). Von Einfluß ist auch die Narkose. Äther, im Gegensatz zur Barbituratnarkose, hemmt den Blutdruckabfall durch PVP (HANNA u. MARSHALL, 1957).

Bei wiederholter Gabe kommt es anscheinend ziemlich schnell zu einer Toleranz gegen PVP. Tiere, die eine hohe, schockauslösende Dosis überstanden haben, reagieren auf eine 2. Dosis, wenn diese unmittelbar danach folgt, nicht mehr (HALPERN, 1956; HECHT und WEESE, 1943; LOUBATIÈRES, 1948; PERLMUTT PARKINS und VARS, 1953). 24 Std. nach der ersten Injektion ist die Reaktionsfähigkeit wieder vorhanden. Das ist insofern bemerkenswert, als nach dieser Zeit die Mastzellen nicht regeneriert sein können, so daß die Toleranzsteigerung wie z. B. auch beim Tween und Anaphylatoxin (siehe dort) nicht nur auf einer Mastzellzerstörung beruhen kann. MARSHALL und HANNA (1957) beobachteten eine Toleranz bei der zweiten Gabe, wenn sehr hohe Dosen (350 mg/kg i.v.) im Abstand von $1-1^1/_2$ Std. hintereinander gegeben wurden. Wenn aber 35 mg/kg und $1-1^1/_2$ Std. später 350 mg/kg verabreicht wurden, kam es beidesmal zu schweren Reaktionen. Eine gewisse Toleranz gegen 350 mg/kg entwickelte sich nach vorausgehender wiederholter Behandlung mit ansteigenden Dosen innerhalb 30 Std.

Interessant sind die Beobachtungen (MARSHALL u. HANNA, 1957) mit dialysiertem PVP. Hierbei werden die Fraktionen mit einem Molekulargewicht bis zu 10000—15000 entfernt. Unvorbehandelte Tiere reagieren hierauf mit Blutdruckabfall wie auf undialysiertes PVP. Vorbehandelte Tiere zeigen keinen Blutdruckabfall auf dialysiertes PVP, wohl aber allgemeine Erscheinungen wie Erythem und Ödem. Auf nichtdialysiertes PVP reagieren sie auch mit Blutdruckabfall. Es wird angenommen, daß die Blutdruckreaktion im Gegensatz zu den allgemeinen Erscheinungen eine um so größere Zahl kleinerer Moleküle erfordert, je größer die Toleranz ist. Die Toleranz erscheint als ein Prozeß, der sich am „vasodepressorischen System" abspielt und der besonders die kleineren, dialysierbaren Moleküle betrifft.

Nicht ganz durchsichtig sind die Ergebnisse von WALTON, RICHARDSON und THOMPSON (1959). Sie beobachteten eine Toleranz, wenn sehr hohe Dosen (600—700 mg/kg), die zu schweren hypotensiven Reaktionen führen, überstanden worden waren. Aber sie gaben beim zweiten Mal kleinere Dosen (100—150 mg/kg). Dosen dieser Größenordnung (50—350 mg/kg) sollen nach ihren Angaben bei unvorbehandelten Hunden bisweilen schon tödliche Reaktionen auslösen können.

Daß die PVP-Vergiftung des Hundes auf einer Histaminfreisetzung beruht, erscheint durch eine Reihe von Tatsachen gestützt. Hier ist in erster Linie zu erwähnen, daß es nach HAHN und WELLMANN (1952) durch Injektion von PVP bei Hunden zu einer Histaminvermehrung im Blut und im Plasma kommt. Die Vermehrung im Plasma erreichte nach 350 mg/kg PVP nach 5—10 min maximal das 6fache, im Durchschnitt das 3,2fache des Ausgangswertes. Die Histaminvermehrung durch Kollidon fehlte bei Ratten, während umgekehrt Dextran bei Hunden wirkungslos war. Eine Injektion der halben Dosis bedingt, daß 2 Std. später die volle Dosis keine Histaminvermehrung mehr erzeugt.

Im Blut stieg das Histamin im Mittel um das 3fache, maximal um das 5fache an. Für die Frage, inwieweit das Ergebnis im Blut durch Verschiebungen cellulärer Elemente, die als Histaminträger in Frage kommen, beeinflußt wurde, sind folgende Befunde wichtig: Im Gegensatz zu LOUBATIÈRES fand sich, gemessen an der Erythrocytenzahl, keine Bluteindickung. Auch die Thrombocyten blieben konstant. Dagegen sanken die Leukocyten und Lymphocyten ab. Auch BESSE und PATAY (1953) fanden keine Hämokonzentration, aber eine Abnahme der Leukocyten, besonders der Neutrophilen.

Schon vorher haben BINET und BURSTEIN (1949) Versuche mitgeteilt, die die Rolle einer vasodepressorischen Substanz beim PVP-Schock des Hundes wahrscheinlich machten. Sie fanden, daß die Vasodilatation in der Pfote, die den Blutdruckabfall nach PVP begleitet, nach intraarterieller Injektion in die Pfote ausbleibt, während sie andererseits nach i.v. Injektion von PVP auch an der denervierten Pfote auftritt.

Die Histaminvermehrung im Plasma findet ihre prinzipielle Bestätigung durch die Versuche von HALPERN und BRIOT (1953a, b). Die Autoren beobachteten allerdings schon nach kleineren Dosen (0,2 ml/kg der 25%igen Lösung) beträchtlich höhere Histaminanstiege im Plasma, nämlich auf 350 μg/l bei Normalwerten von weniger als 20 μg/l. Das Maximum wird nach 5 min erreicht. Danach fällt der Histaminspiegel innerhalb etwa 2 Std. wieder zur Norm ab. Eine zweite Injektion 1 Std. nach der ersten ist wirkungslos und selbst nach 6 Tagen noch vermindert wirksam.

Die Frage nach der Abhängigkeit der histaminfreisetzenden Wirkung von der Molekülgröße haben in noch unveröffentlichten Versuchen GIERTZ, HAHN und SCHMUTZLER untersucht. Gemessen an der Steigerung des Plasmahistaminspiegels ließ sich über einen weiten Dosenbereich (25–350 mg/kg i.v.) kein signifikanter Unterschied zwischen den Kollidonchargen K 17, K 25 und K 30 (Zahlenmittel Mn der Molekulargewichte 6670, 14400 und 22000) feststellen.

Die Histaminvermehrung im Plasma erreichte in diesen Versuchen ihr Maximum nach 2–5 min, nach 80 min waren die Werte wieder normal. Die Vermehrung des Histamins betrug im Mittel maximal das 16fache der Normalwerte.

In Versuchen an der Hundehaut in vitro fanden SCHMUTZLER und GIERTZ (1962), daß bei PVP-Konzentrationen von 0,5–4 % durch alle Kollidonchargen einschließlich K 90 (Mn = 197000) unabhängig von ihrem Molekulargewicht gleich viel Histamin freigesetzt wurde. Erst bei niedrigeren Konzentrationen als 0,5 % fanden sich Unterschiede. Diese bestanden jedoch dann nicht, wenn die PVP-Lösungen der verschiedenen Kollidonchargen auf etwa gleiche *molare* Konzentrationen eingestellt waren. Dann waren sogar die Schwellendosen gleich.

Aus der Mitochondrienfraktion der Hundeleber ließ sich nur mit kleinmolekularem PVP (K 17), nicht dagegen mit höhermolekularen PVP-Fraktionen eine Histaminfreisetzung erzielen.

WALTON, RICHARDSON und THOMPSON (1959) finden sehr große Histaminmengen, mit einer chemischen Methode bestimmt, im Plasma des Hundes nach PVP: z. B. nach 100 mg/kg PVP, 2,1 μg/ml statt des normalen Wertes von $<$0,022—0,063 μg/ml. Mehr oder weniger starke Erhöhungen des Histaminspiegels beobachteten die Autoren auch nach Gummi arabicum, von dem bekannt ist (BUSQUET u. VISCHNIAC, 1929), daß es bei Hunden schockartige Reaktionen auslöst; ferner aber auch nach Stärke und Dextran sowie, wie zu erwarten, auch nach 48/80. Nur nach PVP war der Schock häufig tödlich. Bei Dextran und Stärke fehlten schockartige Reaktionen fast ganz. Es fehlte also eine Beziehung zwischen dem Histaminspiegel und dem Grad der hypotensiven Reaktionen. Dieses Mißverhältnis fand seinen Ausdruck auch noch in der weiteren interessanten Beobachtung, daß die Blutdrucksenkung bei allen Stoffen geringer war als nach den Plasmahistaminwerten zu erwarten gewesen wäre. Dies ergab sich aus Kontrollversuchen mit Histamininjektionen. Auch die Befunde von BEHRMANN u. HARTMANN (1955), die einen niedrigeren Capillarwiderstand sowohl nach PVP als auch nach Dextran beobachteten, haben wahrscheinlich nichts mit der spezifischen histaminliberierenden PVP-Wirkung zu tun.

Daß wiederholte Injektionen von PVP schließlich nicht mehr mit einer Erhöhung des Bluthistamins beantwortet werden, fanden auch DURIČIĆ, SAVIĆ u. a. (1959). Wichtig ist aber ihre Feststellung, daß dann immer noch ein anaphylaktischer Schock mit Histaminanstieg auslösbar ist. Das PVP verhält sich in dieser Hinsicht nach VUKOBRATOVIĆ (1959a, b) wie 1935 L. Beide Stoffe verhindern den anaphylaktischen Schock nicht, führen nur dazu, daß die Kreislaufreaktionen besser überstanden werden. CÎRSTEA und SUHACIU (1961b) bestätigen, daß der durch Pferdeserum ausgelöste anaphylaktische Schock durch PVP-Vorbehandlung nicht abgeschwächt wird, sie beobachteten jedoch eine Abschwächung des durch Hühnereiweiß ausgelösten anaphylaktischen Schocks. Das hängt wahrscheinlich damit zusammen, daß im anaphylaktischen Schock durch Hühnereiweiß genau wie nach PVP vor allem die Histamindepots der Haut betroffen sind (AKCASU, persönliche Mitteilung). Auch HALPERN (1960b) berichtet über eine Abschwächung des anaphylaktischen Schocks nach Vorbehandlung mit PVP und Tween 20. Nach Ablauf des anaphylaktischen Schocks reagieren die Hunde noch auf die Histaminliberatoren mit Blutdruckabfall. Auch zwischen 48/80 und PVP entwickelt sich nach MARSHALL und HANNA (1958) sowie auch nach HALPERN (1956) keine Kreuztoleranz. Nach HALPERN (1960b) kommt es wohl zur Kreuztoleranz zwischen PVP und Tween 20, nicht aber zwischen PVP und Tween 20 einerseits und 48/80 und 1935 L andererseits. Offenbar kommt es bei einer Schockform zu keiner vollständigen Erschöpfung der Histamindepots. Man muß außerdem annehmen, daß die einzelnen Histaminliberatoren auf die verschiedenen Histamindepots ungleich wirken oder auch daß das Histamin in den Depots nicht in einheitlicher Form vorliegt (HALPERN, 1956).

Interessant sind in dieser Hinsicht die Beobachtungen von NISHIYAMA, TASAKA und IRINO (1957). Nach diesen Autoren setzt PVP besonders viel Histamin aus der Haut frei. Es folgen die Leber und dann die Muskeln. Ähnlich ist die Wirkung von Sinomenin und Tween 20. Bei 48/80 hingegen ist die Wirkung auf Leber und Muskulatur am größten. Den in vivo gewonnenen Ergebnissen stehen allerdings in vitro Versuche mit Haut und Leber gegenüber, in denen sich keine wesentlichen Organunterschiede bei den einzelnen Stoffen ergaben. SCHMUTZLER und GIERTZ (1962) fanden dagegen auch in vitro eine deutliche Histaminfreisetzung aus der Haut, aber nicht aus Lebergewebe. ADANT (1954) konnte schon früher zeigen, daß der durch Antihistaminica hemmbare PVP-Schock am normalen und leberlosen Hund in gleicher Weise abläuft. Daß das Histamin durch Mastzellzerfall frei wird, geht aus den Untersuchungen von KAWAMOTO (1958) hervor. Auch hierbei steht die Wirkung auf die Haut bei PVP im Vordergrund. Auf die Lebermastzellen wirkt PVP (im Gegensatz zu Pepton) nur leicht. In der Lippenhaut waren die Veränderungen an der oberflächlichen Region stärker als in der Tiefe. In der geringen Wirkung des PVP auf die heparinreichen Mastzellen der Hundeleber ist wahrscheinlich auch die Ursache für das Ausbleiben einer starken Gerinnungshemmung im PVP-Schock zu suchen (QUIVY, 1956).

Über die Wirkung der Antihistaminica hat zuerst LOUBATIÈRES (1948) berichtet, der allerdings mit Phenbenzamin keine Wirkung erhielt. Positive Ergebnisse mit Mepyramin und Promethazin erzielten jedoch HALPERN (1956) und HALPERN und BRIOT (1953a). Promethazin ist voll wirksam gegen das Erythem, die Urticaria und den Pruritus. Es reduziert die Hämokonzentration und vermindert die Wasser- und Eiweißfiltration durch die Capillaren. Ebenso wird der Blutdruckabfall verhindert (vgl. auch CÎRSTEA und SUHACIU, 1961a) und die Schwellendosis für die Auslösung einer intracutanen Injektion von 1,2 μg PVP je nach Promethazindosis auf 500 und mehr als 6000 μg erhöht. Auf die gesteigerte Magensäuresekretion hat Promethazin keinen Einfluß. Promethazin hemmt auch die Temperatursteigerung der Haut, ohne sie ganz aufzuheben (HALPERN und STIFFEL, 1955). Die Wirkung des Promethazin wird von BESSE und PATAY (1953) bestätigt. Nach ihren Angaben sind Thiazinamium und Chlorpromazin ohne Wirkung.

Eine gewisse Abschwächung der PVP-Wirkung kann durch Vorbehandlung mit Cortison erzielt werden (PERLMUTT, PARKINS u. VARS, 1953). Adrenalin hat eine flüchtige Wirkung, wenn es während der Hypotension gegeben wird. Vorher gegeben ist es wirkungslos (BESSE u. PATAY, 1953).

LINDNER (1953) beschrieb ein Symptombild bei Hunden, das er durch verschiedene Injektionsarten und auch durch Inhalation mit einem Mischpolymerisat aus Vinylpyrrolidon und Vinylcaprolactam erhielt. Es sind die gleichen Symptome wie nach PVP. Die Giftigkeit beschränkt sich auf den Hund. Seine Angabe, daß im Serum nur eine sehr kleine Histaminvermehrung vorhanden war, kann vielleicht auf methodische Gründe und auf die mangelhafte Eignung des Serums für solche Untersuchungen zurückgeführt werden. Auch in diesen Versuchen waren Antihistaminica wirksam, wie besonders an der Hämokonzentration gezeigt werden konnte. Gewisse Beobachtungen, nämlich die geringere Ausprägung von Juckreiz und Ödemen nach hohen Dosen des Mischpolymerisats, bedürfen noch der Erklärung.

Polyvinylalkohol hat beim Hund keine schockauslösende Wirkung (LOUBATIÈRES, 1948).

Wenn auch PVP bei anderen Tierarten als dem Hund nach den bisherigen Feststellungen keine histaminfreisetzende Wirkung hat, so ist es in diesem Zusammenhang vielleicht doch von Interesse, kurz auf Beobachtungen einzugehen, wonach PVP auf den anaphylaktischen Schock des Meerschweinchens verstärkend zu wirken scheint. Eine solche Wirkung haben PAUTRIZEL und PAUTRIZEL-BEZIAN (1950) in vitro, nicht in vivo bei passiv sensibilisierten Meerschweinchen beobachtet. Nach HAHN, LANGE und GIERTZ (1954) läßt sich durch PVP, nicht durch Dextran, der Forssman-Schock bei Meerschweinchen verstärken. Nach unveröffentlichten Versuchen von GIERTZ, HAHN und SCHMUTZLER ist diese Wirkung besonders stark bei den niedermolekularen PVP-Fraktionen K 17 und K 26. Aber nur K 17 allein (nicht K 26) verstärkt auch nach diesen Untersuchungen den anaphylaktischen Schock aktiv sensibilisierter Meerschweinchen. Der Mechanismus dieser Wirkung ist noch nicht bekannt. Eine Verstärkung der Histaminwirkung oder eine Förderung der Histaminausschüttung scheint nicht vorzuliegen. Im Hinblick auf gewisse Zwischenfälle in der Klinik, die gerade das niedermolekulare Periston N (K 17) betreffen (Lit.: HAHN, 1954c), sind diese Beobachtungen vielleicht nicht ohne Interesse. Auch an die verstärkende Wirkung von Kollidon auf gewisse Antigen-Antikörperreaktionen (HAHN, 1954c; NEUZIL, PAUTRIZEL u. MARQUEVIELLE, 1949) wäre in diesem Zusammenhang zu denken. Andererseits hemmt PVP gewisse sog. „anaphylaktoide" schockartige Reaktionen (traumatischer Schock, Schock durch mikrobielle Gifte und durch Kongorotinjektion, BOVET, COURVOISIER u. DUCROT, 1947; MEIDINGER, 1947).

II. Tween 20

Zu den speziell bei Hunden durch Histaminfreisetzung blutdrucksenkenden Stoffen gehören auch Tween 20, 40, 60, 80. Die Tweene sind Polyalkylenderivate unvollständiger Fettsäureester von Hexitolanhydriden. KRANTZ, CARR u. a. (1948) führten den Histaminnachweis in Sera von Hunden, die 5 ml 5 % Tween 20 i.v. erhalten hatten. Diese Sera riefen im Gegensatz zum Verhalten vor der Tween-20-Injektion eine Kontraktion des Meerschweinchenjejunums hervor, die durch Tripelennamin hemmbar war. Ratten, Kaninchen, Affen, Huhn und Mensch reagieren nicht in dieser Weise auf Tween 20. Tween 20, das am eingehendsten untersucht wurde, ist das Polyoxyäthylenderivat des Sorbitanmonolaurats. Es erzeugt beim Hund i.v. außer Blutdrucksenkung Urticaria und Magensekretionssteigerung (GROSSMAN und ROBERTSON, 1948; JANCSÓ, 1947). Diphenhydramin soll eigentümlicherweise nicht nur die Urticaria, sondern auch die Sekretionssteigerung des Magens hemmen, so daß möglicherweise noch ein anderer Faktor als Histamin im Spiele ist (GROSSMAN und ROBERTSON, 1948). Intravenös läßt sich die Blutdrucksenkung mit Hautrötung und Pruritus schon durch 0,1 ml/kg der 5%igen Lösung hervorrufen (KRANTZ, CARR u. a., 1949). Intradermal erzeugen 0,01 ml einer 0,05–0,5%igen Lösung eine Quaddel. Außer beim Hund wirkt Tween 20 in diesem Sinne noch bei anderen Caniden, am stärksten beim Graufuchs (C. virginianus). Schwächer als der Hund reagiert der Wolf (C. lupus). Auch C. latrans und C. lupaster zeigen eine Reaktion. Resistent ist der Waschbär (Procyon lotor), ein entfernter Verwandter der Caniden.

Unwirksam sind Sorbitol, Sorbitan, Äthyllaurat und die hydrolysierte Polyoxyäthylenkette. Das Mannitanaloge von Tween 20 verhält sich wie Tween 20.

GOTH und Mitarb. fanden 5 min nach 0,1 mg/kg Tween 20 papierchromatographisch über 50 μg/100 ml Plasmahistamin (GOTH, ALLMAN u. a., 1951; GOTH, HOLMAN und COPENHAVER, 1952). Eine Vorbehandlung mit Cortison verhindert nicht die hypotensive Wirkung von Tween 20. Aber sie hemmt oder vermindert die Wirkung einer zweiten Injektion 24–48 Std. später. Damit haben die Autoren zum ersten Mal gezeigt, daß Cortison die Wiederbeladung des Gewebes mit Histamin verhindert.

Die gleichen Autoren (SLOMKA und GOTH, 1956a, b) untersuchten, ob sich eine gegenseitige Resistenz von 48/80 und Tween 20 erzielen läßt. Nach Vorbehandlung mit steigenden Dosen von 48/80 bis zur vollkommenen Toleranz gegen 48/80 reagieren die Hunde noch auf Tween 20 mit einem ausgesprochenen Blutdruckabfall. Da 48/80 bei dieser Art der Vorbehandlung (im Gegensatz zur Wirkung einmaliger hoher Gaben) keinen Histaminanstieg im Blute erzeugte, wird angenommen, daß die Resistenz gegen 48/80 durch 48/80 nicht auf der Erschöpfung der Histamindepots, sondern auf einem anderen Mechanismus beruht. Eine andere Deutung ermöglichen vielleicht die Untersuchungen von NISHIYAMA, TASAKA und IRINO (1957), nach denen Tween 20 die stärkste Histaminfreisetzung in der Haut, 48/80 aber in Leber und Muskel bewirkt. Andererseits setzt Tween 20 ebenso wie 48/80 Histamin aus Lebermitochondrien frei (SLOMKA und GOTH, 1956b). HALPERN (1960b) berichtet über eine Kreuztoleranz zwischen PVP und Tween 20. Nach CÎRSTEA und SUHACIU (1964) beruht die Toleranzsteigerung durch wiederholte Tweengaben nicht auf einer Entleerung der Histamindepots. Trotzdem läßt sich aber mit der Toleranzsteigerung gegen Tween auch eine Abschwächung des anaphylaktischen Schocks erzielen.

Im Zusammenhang mit der Histaminfreisetzung durch anaphylaktoide Substanzen beim Hund sei hier auch noch die toxische Wirkung von arteigenem, aber nicht „autologem", d. h. individuumgleichem Plasma beim Hund erwähnt, die auch auf Histaminfreisetzung beruht (BLISS, JOHNS und BURGEN, 1959; BLISS und STEWART, 1957; BLISS, STEWART und FULLER, 1958; BLISS und WALKER, 1959; LEVINSON, NEUWELT und NECHELES, 1960).

Als Beispiel einer Histaminfreisetzung durch artfremdes Serum kann die Histaminfreisetzung durch Pferdeserum bei der Katze dienen (FELDBERG u. SCHACHTER, 1952). Die toxische Wirkung des Rinderserums auf Meerschweinchen beruht offenbar nicht auf Histaminfreisetzung (HAHN u. OBERDORF, 1950; HANZLIK u. KARSNER, 1924c).

C. Das Anaphylatoxin

1. Geschichte und Einführung

FRIEDBERGER, der Entdecker des Anaphylatoxins (AT), war ein Verfechter der humoralen Theorie der Anaphylaxie. Auf der Basis dieser Theorie gelang es ihm im Jahre 1910, aus Meerschweinchenserum in vitro ein toxisches Prinzip von anaphylaxieartiger Wirkung darzustellen. Er nahm an, durch die Entstehung dieses Giftes in vivo werde der anaphylaktische Schock ausgelöst. Er nannte es daher „Anaphylatoxin".

FRIEDBERGER hat damit das Verdienst, erstmalig in einem Modellversuch die Möglichkeit einer humoralen anaphylaktischen Giftentstehung gezeigt zu haben, ohne daß freilich bis zum heutigen Tage die Existenz dieses Giftes bei der Anaphylaxie erwiesen werden konnte.

Wegen der ungeklärten Bedeutung des AT für die Anaphylaxie ersetzten einige Autoren den Begriff „Anaphylatoxin" durch „Serotoxin" (vgl. DOERR, 1929). Da jedoch auch in der neueren Literatur vorwiegend der Ausdruck „Anaphylatoxin" gebraucht wird, da eine Beteiligung dieses Stoffes an der Anaphylaxie auch heute noch diskutiert wird, und auch aus historischen Gründen verwenden wir im folgenden den Ausdruck Anaphylatoxin.

Abgesehen von der speziellen Problematik einer AT-Bildung in vivo hängt die Frage der AT-Beteiligung am anaphylaktischen Schock von der Gültigkeit der humoralen Theorie der Anaphylaxie ab. Da diese aber schon frühzeitig durch die celluläre Theorie (SCHULTZ, 1910; DALE, 1913) abgelöst wurde, ist es verständlich, daß die AT-Theorie schließlich in den Hintergrund trat.

Trotzdem hat die Beschäftigung mit dem AT noch einige Jahre das Aufkommen der zellulären Theorie überdauert. Die Kritik an der AT-Theorie der Anaphylaxie setzte nämlich nicht an der humoralphysiologischen Grundlage der Theorie an, sondern an den speziellen Vorstellungen FRIEDBERGERs über den Modus der AT-Bildung.

FRIEDBERGER (1910a) stellte das AT folgendermaßen her: Er inkubierte normales, komplementhaltiges Meerschweinchenserum mit Immunpräcipitaten und beobachtete, daß das Serum nach der Inkubation und nach dem Abzentrifugieren der Präcipitate bei intravenöser Injektion am Meerschweinchen anaphylaxieähnliche Symptome auslöste. Er nahm an, daß zur Giftbildung ein Antigen-Antikörper-Komplex und aktives Komplement erforderlich seien. In der Spaltung des Antigens mit Hilfe des Antikörpers und des Komplements sah er die Ursache der Giftentstehung.

Da FRIEDBERGER das AT für das Abbauprodukt eines eiweißartigen Antigens hielt, hatte seine Theorie der Anaphylaxie Beziehungen zu den älteren Anschauungen von VAUGHAN u. Mitarb. (1907, 1911) und von PFEIFFER u. MITA (1910). Die AT-Theorie der Anaphylaxie wurde in ihrer ursprünglichen Form zweifelhaft, als BORDET (1913a, b) durch Inkubation von Meerschweinchenserum mit dem Polysaccharid Agar AT erhielt. Der Einwand FRIEDBERGERs (FRIEDBERGER u. JOACHIMOGLU, 1917; FRIEDBERGER, LURÀ u. a., 1913), nur durch eiweißhaltige Verunreinigungen seien Polysaccharide in der Lage, AT zu bilden, wurde widerlegt (BORDET u. ZUNZ, 1915a; KOPACZEWSKI u. MUTERMILCH, 1914; LOEWIT u. BAYER, 1913; NATHAN, 1913a, b; SCHMIDT, 1917).

Ferner zeigte sich bald nach der Entdeckung des AT, daß nicht nur ein eiweißartiges Antigen, sondern auch der Antikörper für die AT-Bildung entbehrlich war. Meerschweinchenserum wurde nämlich durch die Inkubation mit Mikroorganismen und mit einer Reihe anderer eiweißhaltiger Stoffe auch dann giftig, wenn die serumspendenden Tiere nicht gegen diese Stoffe sensibilisiert waren (FRIEDBERGER, GOLDSCHMID u. a., 1911; FRIEDBERGER u. ITO, 1911; FRIEDBERGER u. KAPSENBERG, 1913; FRIEDBERGER, MITA u. KUMAGAI, 1913; FRIEDBERGER u. NATHAN, 1911). Grobe, die Antigennatur verändernde Eingriffe an den Kontaktstoffen beeinflußten nicht ihre Fähigkeit, mit Serum AT zu bilden (DOLD u. AOKI, 1912; FRIEDBERGER, GOLDSCHMID u. a., 1911). Die Teilnahme von spezifischen Antikörpern schien auch aus anderen Gründen unwahrscheinlich (MORESCHI u. VALLARDI, 1911; VON GONZENBACH u. HIRSCHFELD, 1912).

Gegen die von FRIEDBERGER aus verschiedenen Gründen (FRIEDBERGER, 1910; FRIEDBERGER u. ITO, 1911; FRIEDBERGER, LURÀ u. a., 1913; RITZ u. SACHS, 1917) postulierte Teilnahme des Komplements an der AT-Bildung ließen sich ebenfalls Einwände vorbringen. Alle damals bekannten Methoden zur Komplementinaktivierung stellen grobe Eingriffe in das kolloidale Milieu der Serumeiweiße dar (vgl. DOLD, 1920a, b; HIRSCHFELD u. KLINGER, 1914; LUMIÈRE u. MEYER, 1935c). Das Ausbleiben der AT-Bildung in derartig behandelten Sera braucht daher nicht auf der Komplementausschaltung zu beruhen, sondern könnte auch durch weitergehende Veränderungen der Serumeiweißkörper bedingt sein. Zudem berichteten einige Autoren (BIER, 1931; BRUGNATELLI, 1913; DOERR u. RUSS, 1912; DOLD, 1926a, b; RITZ und SACHS, 1917; SEITZ, 1911; ZUNZ, 1917/18) über Versuche, in denen die Komplementausschaltung und die Zerstörung des AT-Bildungsvermögens im Serum nicht parallel gingen. Auch die häufig beobachtete Komplementabnahme im Serum während der AT-Bildung beweist nicht die ursächliche Verknüpfung beider Vorgänge, zumal eine AT-Bildung ohne Komplementschwund beschrieben wurde (KOPACZEWSKI u. MUTERMILCH, 1914; VON GONZENBACH u. HIRSCHFELD, 1912).

Auf Grund dieser Einwände wurde die Friedbergersche Theorie durch die physikalische Theorie der AT-Bildung von SACHS (RITZ und SACHS, 1911; SACHS, 1920) abgelöst. Diese sucht allerdings nur die einleitenden Vorgänge bei der AT-Entstehung zu deuten und läßt für den weiteren Ablauf der AT-Bildung mehrere Möglichkeiten, darunter auch chemische oder enzymatische Reaktionen, offen. Dabei unterscheidet sie sich von den Friedbergerschen Vorstellungen dadurch, daß sie das Substrat der Giftbildung ins Serum verlegt. Als Rahmentheorie, die sich vor allem mit der Funktion der Kontaktstoffe befaßt, kann die Sachssche

Auffassung auch heute noch volle Gültigkeit beanspruchen. Im einzelnen ergeben sich folgende Möglichkeiten:

Die Kontaktstoffe könnten durch Adsorption eines antagonistischen Prinzips eine im Serum präformierte Giftwirkung freilegen oder aber eine chemische bzw. enzymatische Giftbildung ermöglichen. Auch dem Komplement, das nach unsern heutigen Kenntnissen eine Fermentfunktion besitzt und dessen Inaktivierung ebenso wie die AT-Bildung vom physikalischen Zustand der Kontaktstoffe abhängt, könnte im Rahmen dieser Auffassung ein Platz angewiesen werden, wenn auch nicht im Sinne der Friedbergerschen Vorstellung von der antigenauflösenden Wirkung des Komplements. Auf rein kolloidchemische Weise sollte aber im Rahmen der Sachsschen Theorie eine Giftbildung auch dadurch möglich sein, daß eine Zustandsänderung an den Serumeiweißkörpern (Globulinen), z. B. im Sinne einer Denaturierung oder Aggregatbildung, zustande käme.

Auf der Basis der physikalischen Theorie hielt die Mehrzahl der Autoren auch weiterhin daran fest, daß AT die anaphylaktische Noxe sein könne. Allerdings mußte man nun annehmen, daß in vivo das Antigen oder der Antigen-Antikörper-Komplex analog den Kontaktstoffen in vitro den Anstoß zur Giftbildung gäbe. Erst DALE und KELLAWAY (1922) haben diesen Glauben erschüttert und damit die AT-Forschung für fast 3 Jahrzehnte zum Erliegen gebracht. Sie waren die ersten, die mit größerem Nachdruck nicht nur die Bildung, sondern auch die Wirkung des AT untersuchten und mit den anaphylaktischen Vorgängen verglichen und dabei Unterschiede fanden, die ihnen mit der Annahme einer Beteiligung des AT an der Anaphylaxie unvereinbar schienen. Begünstigt wurde das Erlöschen des allgemeinen Interesses am AT dadurch, daß die celluläre Theorie der Anaphylaxie in der Zwischenzeit weiter gefestigt und als Histamintheorie (DALE, 1929) eine neue Gestalt bekam.

Es zeigte sich jedoch, daß eine Ablehnung der AT-Theorie vom Standpunkt der Histamintheorie nur insofern gerechtfertigt war, als das AT sicherlich nicht mit Histamin identisch ist (siehe unten). Auch eine Histaminvermehrung im Serum findet bei der AT-Bildung nicht statt (HAHN, LANGE und GIERTZ, 1954). Aber der Gedanke, daß das AT den Anstoß zu einer Histaminfreisetzung geben könne, taucht erst 1950 auf.

Als HAHN und OBERDORF (1950) diese Möglichkeit durch den Nachweis, daß der AT-Schock durch Antihistaminica gehemmt werden kann, in den Bereich der Wirklichkeit rückten, war der Boden für eine neue Epoche der AT-Forschung gegeben. Weitere Untersuchungen haben dann durch den gelungenen Nachweis einer Histaminfreisetzung durch AT aus isoliertem Gewebe (ROCHA E SILVA, BIER und ARONSON, 1951) und eines Anstiegs des Plasmahistamins nach AT-Injektion (HAHN, 1954) dieser Vorstellung Recht gegeben. Es zeigte sich dabei auch, daß einige der Befunde von DALE und KELLAWAY (1922), die einen qualitativen Unterschied in der Wirkung des echten Anaphylaxiegiftes — als welches Histamin anzusehen ist — und des AT zu ergeben schienen, nicht richtig interpretiert wurden.

Nach dem heutigen Stande der Forschung läßt sich das AT folgendermaßen definieren: AT ist der einzige bekannte spezifisch am Meerschweinchen wirkende Histaminliberator. Es hat gegenüber allen andern Histaminliberatoren die Eigenschaft, ein aus Blutserum bzw. -plasma entstehendes Prinzip zu sein. Dadurch kommt ihm ein besonderes biologisches Interesse zu.

Seine Darstellung erfolgt heute vor allem aus Rattenserum. Als Kontaktstoffe dienen neben den Immunpräcipitaten besonders Polysaccharide wie Agar, Inulin und Dextran. Die Kontaktstoffe werden in Konzentrationen von 0,1—1 mg/ml im Serum suspendiert, nicht gelöst, und nach einer Inkubationsdauer von etwa 1 Std. bei 37° C abzentrifugiert. Nach der Inkubation enthält das Serum AT.

Zur Bestimmung des AT-Gehaltes in einem Serum dient meist die intravenöse Injektion am Meerschweinchen oder die Testung der kontrahierenden Wirkung am Meerschweinchenileum. Letztere eignet sich jedoch nur zur Testung starker ATe aus Rattenserum, ferner ist fraglich, ob diese Wirkung tatsächlich ausschließlich auf einer Histaminliberation beruht (siehe unten). Am intakten Tier tritt nach intravenöser Injektion ein schwerer, meist tödlicher Schock auf, und zwar nach Dosen von 10–20 ml/kg AT-haltigen Meerschweinchenserums oder 2,5–10 ml/kg AT-haltigen Rattenserums.

2. Die Bildung des AT

Es ist nicht möglich, in dieser Übersicht den Inhalt der älteren Arbeiten im einzelnen zu referieren. Allein FRIEDBERGER und Mitarbeiter veröffentlichten annähernd 100 Mitteilungen über das AT. Die wichtigsten Ergebnisse der älteren Autoren sind in Zusammenfassungen zitiert (BORDET, 1919, 1921, 1924; DOERR, 1929, 1950/51; HAHN, 1960; HAHN und GIERTZ, 1960; HAHN und LANGE, 1956; ROCHA E SILVA, 1954, 1955).

a) Die Kontaktstoffe

Die Mannigfaltigkeit der Kontaktstoffe, mit denen sich AT bilden läßt, schließt die Möglichkeit aus, daß AT aus diesen Kontaktstoffen gebildet wird. Wie zuerst RITZ und SACHS (1911) vermuteten, muß es aus den Plasma- bzw. Serumbestandteilen entstehen.

Als Kontaktstoffe wurden benutzt: 1. Immunpräcipitate (z. B. FRIEDBERGER, 1910; OSLER, RANDALL u. a., 1959a, b; ROTHSCHILD und ROCHA E SILVA, 1954); dabei ist bemerkenswert, daß sich Immunpräcipitate aus Antisera vom Meerschweinchen schlechter als solche aus Antisera vom Kaninchen zur AT-Bildung im Meerschweinchenserum eignen (SUKIENNIKOWA, 1913;) 2. Mikroorganismen (z. B. DOLD und AOKI, 1912; FRIEDBERGER, GOLDSCHMID u. a., 1911; FRIEDBERGER und ITO, 1911; FRIEDBERGER und KAPSENBERG, 1913; NOVY, DE KRUIF und NOVY, 1917; RITZ und SACHS, 1911; SEITZ, 1911); 3. Eiweiße (Pferdeserum, Toxine usw.: DOERR und RUSS, 1912; FRIEDBERGER, MITA und KUMAGAI, 1913; FRIEDBERGER und NATHAN, 1911); 4. Polysaccharide (Agar: z. B. BORDET, 1913a, b; BORDET und ZUNZ, 1915; JOBLING und PETERSEN, 1914b; LOEWIT und BAYER, 1913; NATHAN, 1913a; NOVY und DE KRUIF, 1917a, b, c; ROTHSCHILD und ROCHA E SILVA, 1954); (Stärke: z. B. JOBLING und PETERSEN, 1914b; NATHAN, 1913b; ROTHSCHILD und ROCHA E SILVA, 1954; SCHMIDT, 1917); (Inulin: z. B. HAHN und OBERDORF, 1950; NATHAN, 1915); (Dextran oder Sephadex: z. B. HAHN, LANGE und GIERTZ, 1954; HALPERN, BRIOT und NEVEU, 1954a, b; FRIEDBERG, ENGELHARDT und MEINEKE, 1963, 1964); (Glykogen: z. B. GIERTZ, 1959; GIERTZ und HAHN, 1961; ROTHSCHILD und ROCHA E SILVA, 1954); (Zymosan: z. B. GIERTZ, 1959; GIERTZ und HAHN, 1961; GREISMAN, 1958; OSLER, RANDALL u. a., 1959b); (Bakterienpolysaccharide oder -lipopolysaccharide verschiedener Herkunft: z. B. ANTWEILER, 1961; GREISMAN, 1960; NETZER und VOGT, 1964; ROTHSCHILD und ROCHA E SILVA, 1954).

Andere Substanzen, die gelegentlich als Kontaktstoffe mit Erfolg zur AT-Bildung benutzt wurden, sind: Ein eiweißfreies Pektinpräparat (KOPACZEWSKI u. MUTERMILCH, 1914), Hefe (DA COSTA CRUZ, 1938), Na-Alginat und Polyvinylpyrrolidon (ROTHSCHILD u. ROCHA E SILVA, 1954), Liquoid (GIERTZ, 1959; OSLER, RANDALL u. a., 1959b) und Baumwollstaub (ANTWEILER, 1961).

Eine AT-Bildung durch Kaolin wurde ebenfalls beobachtet (BAUER, 1912; FRIEDBERG u. LENDLE, 1955; WASSERMANN u. KEYSSER, 1911), von andern Autoren aber bestritten (Lit. siehe DOERR, 1929; ROTHSCHILD u. ROCHA E SILVA, 1954). Die negativen Ergebnisse beruhen möglicherweise darauf, daß Kaolin wie auch bestimmte andere Kontaktstoffe (vgl. RITZ u. SACHS, 1911) fertiges AT unter Umständen entgiften kann.

Ebenfalls widersprüchlich sind die Angaben über eine AT-Bildung durch Pepton (Novy, De Kruif u. F. O. Novy, 1917; Rothschild u. Rocha e Silva, 1954). Besredka u. Mitarb. behaupteten, nur auf peptonhaltigem Agar gezüchtete Mikroorganismen seien zur AT-Bildung befähigt und nur mit peptonhaltigem Agar lasse sich AT bilden (Besredka u. Ströbel, 1911a, b; Besredka, Ströbel u. Jupille, 1911, 1913a, b). Es sind jedoch sowohl peptonfreier Agar (s. oben) als auch in peptonfreiem Milieu gezüchtete Mikroorganismen (Boehncke, 1912; Boehncke u. Bierbaum, 1912; Friedberger u. Girgolaff, 1911; Friedberger u. Kapsenberg, 1913; Joachimoglu, 1912; Szymanowski, 1913) zur AT-Bildung geeignet. Der Gedanke, Pepton sei an der AT-Bildung und damit an der Anaphylaxie beteiligt, geht auf Beobachtungen von Biedl u. Kraus (1910a, b) zurück. Diese Autoren hatten auf die Ähnlichkeit der Peptonwirkung mit dem anaphylaktischen Schock hingewiesen.

Über eine AT-Bildung aus anderen anorganischen Substanzen als Kaolin (Quarz, Talkum, Silikatgel, Kieselgur, Tricalciumphosphat, Bariumsulfat, Eisenarseniat oder -hydroxyd, Aluminiumhydroxyd u. a.) liegen nur ungenügende und teilweise widersprechende Angaben vor (Lit. s. Doerr, 1929; Friedberg u. Lendle, 1955; Mutermilch, 1912).

Ungeeignet zur AT-Bildung waren Heparin, Ovomucoid und sulfatierte Derivate von Agar, Stärke und Dextran sowie Alginsäure, Chondroitinschwefelsäure und Pektin (Conard und Mutsaars, 1949; Rothschild und Rocha e Silva, 1954). Das sulfatierte Polysaccharid Heparin hemmt sogar die AT-Bildung, allerdings erst in Konzentrationen, welche höher als die zur Gerinnungshemmung erforderlichen Konzentrationen sind (Giertz, Hahn, Jurna und Lange, 1958; Hahn, 1960; Rothschild und Rocha e Silva, 1954).

Haining (1956c) verwandte allerdings auch Dextransulfat mit Erfolg zur AT-Bildung. Ob ein sulfatiertes Polysaccharid zur AT-Bildung geeignet ist oder nicht, hängt vermutlich vom Grad der Sulfatierung ab. Auch der besonders gut zur AT-Bildung verwendbare Agar enthält Sulfatgruppen.

Welche Eigenschaften muß ein Stoff haben, damit er sich als Kontaktstoff zur AT-Bildung verwenden läßt? Eines ist sicher: Der physikalische Zustand der Kontaktstoffe ist für die AT-Bildung von großer Bedeutung. Zuerst zeigte Nathan (1913b, 1915), daß sich durch Stärkekleister besser als durch eine Aufschwemmung und durch eine Inulinaufschwemmung besser als durch eine Lösung AT herstellen läßt. Novy und De Kruif (1917a, b, c) erhielten bei Verwendung eines Sol-Gel-Gemisches von Agar leichter ein AT als durch Agar-Sol oder Agar-Gel. Gelöstes Pepton bildet schlechter als nicht gelöstes AT (Novy, De Kruif und F. O. Novy, 1917). Dold (1920a) faßte alle damals bekannten Befunde zusammen, aus denen die Bedeutung des physikalischen Zustandes der Kontaktstoffe für die AT-Bildung hervorgeht.

In neuerer Zeit berichteten Hahn, Lange und Giertz (1954), daß zwei Dextrane vom Molekulargewicht 20000 bzw. 400000 in pulverisierter Form zur AT-Bildung geeignet waren, daß aber in Lösung nur das höhermolekulare ein AT bilden konnte. Ferner beobachteten sie, daß sie durch ein Dextran vom Molekulargewicht 260000 in pulverisierter Form ein stärkeres AT erhielten als durch das gleiche Dextran in gelöster Form. Halpern, Briot und Neveu (1954a, b) fanden, daß von vier Dextranen mit den Molekulargewichten 6000, 35000, 230000 und 2000000 die am schlechtesten löslichen, — das waren die mit den mittleren Molekulargewichten, — am besten zur AT-Bildung geeignet waren. Osler, Randall u. a. (1959a) verwandten Dextranpräparate mit den Molekulargewichten 33300, 56400, 91700, 123900, 194000, 255000 und 412000. Nur die Dextrane mit den Molekulargewichten 33300, 194000 und 412000 waren als Kontaktstoffe verwendbar, und nur diese Präparate lösten sich im Gegensatz zu den übrigen nicht klar.

Lumière und Meyer (1935a, b) verwendeten verschiedene Stärkesorten zur AT-Bildung. Dabei erwies sich eine Körnchengröße von etwa 1 μ Durchmesser als besonders gut geeignet, größere Partikel waren schlechter wirksam. Rothschild u. Rocha e Silva (1954) stellten eine Abhängigkeit der AT-Bildung vom Polymerisationsgrad der verwendeten Stärke fest: Mit abnehmendem Polymerisationsgrad nahm auch die AT-Bildung ab. Nach Haining (1956c) sind Dextran und Dextransulfat vom Molekulargewicht von etwa 400000 zur AT-Bildung brauchbar, nicht dagegen Präparate von Molekulargewichten unter 10000. Alle letztgenannten Autoren geben die Löslichkeit ihrer Präparate nicht an.

b) Die Bedingungen für die AT-Bildung

Eine AT-Bildung erfolgt, wenn Serum oder Plasma mit einem der genannten Kontaktstoffe inkubiert wird. Es eignen sich jedoch nicht alle Serumarten zur AT-Bildung. Besonders geeignet ist Rattenserum (vgl. HAHN, LANGE und GIERTZ, 1954; HALPERN, BRIOT und NEVEU, 1954a, b; NOVY und DE KRUIF, 1917c; ROTHSCHILD und ROCHA E SILVA, 1954). Ein schwächeres AT läßt sich aus Meerschweinchenserum gewinnen (FRIEDBERGER, 1910; GIERTZ, 1959; GIERTZ, HAHN, OPFERKUCH und SCHMUTZLER, 1961; NOVY und DE KRUIF, 1917a; ROTHSCHILD und ROCHA E SILVA, 1954). Außerdem eignen sich noch Kaninchenserum und Pferdeserum zur AT-Bildung mit Hilfe von Kontaktstoffen, beide allerdings schlecht (ADANT, 1950; DOERR und RUSS, 1912; NOVY und DE KRUIF, 1917b; ZUNZ, 1917, 1918).

AT kann auch ohne die Vermittlung von Kontaktstoffen gebildet werden, und zwar vor allem durch Verdünnung von Rattenserum mit Wasser oder durch Dialyse von Rattenserum gegen Wasser (NOVY und DE KRUIF, 1917e; ROTHSCHILD und ROCHA E SILVA, 1954).

AT soll sich auch durch Ansäuern von Meerschweinchenserum und Abfiltrieren des Niederschlags, durch Ausschütteln mit Fettlösungsmitteln, durch Behandlung mit Jod (JOBLING u. PETERSEN, 1914a), durch Einleiten von Kohlendioxyd (BORDET u. MCKINLEY, 1925), durch Schütteln und durch Lagerung (DOLD, 1926a, b) bilden.

AT läßt sich im Plasma ebenso gut wie im Serum bilden. Zur Gerinnungshemmung wurden Hirudin, Heparin und Oxalat (letztere hemmen beide in hohen Dosen die AT-Bildung) verwandt (BORDET, 1921; FRIEDBERGER und KAPSENBERG, 1913; GIERTZ, 1959; GIERTZ und HAHN, 1958; GIERTZ, HAHN, JURNA und LANGE, 1958; HAHN, 1960; HIRSCHFELD und KLINGER, 1913; ROTHSCHILD und ROCHA E SILVA, 1954).

Sowohl Meerschweinchenserum (FRIEDBERGER und ITO, 1911) als auch Rattenserum (GIERTZ, 1959; GIERTZ, HAHN und LANGE, 1956a, b; HAHN, 1960; JONES, 1960) läßt sich in zwei Fraktionen zerlegen, von denen jede zur AT-Bildung unbrauchbar ist, die jedoch zusammen wie frisches Serum zur AT-Bildung geeignet sind.

Die Fraktionierung der Sera erfolgte auf verschiedene Weise. FRIEDBERGER u. ITO (1911) trennten Meerschweinchenserum in Mittelstück und Endstück auf. GIERTZ, HAHN u. Mitarb. verwandten die (modifizierte) Cohnsche Methode 10 zur Serumfraktionierung. Die beiden Fraktionen I-III-1,2,3 und III-0 aus Rattenserum erwiesen sich als zur AT-Bildung notwendig. JONES (1960) fällte die Euglobuline aus Rattenserum bei niedrigem pH und geringer Ionenstärke. Nur die ausgefällte Euglobulinfraktion und der Überstand zusammen waren durch Agar aktivierbar.

Die Fähigkeit von Serum oder Serumfraktionen zur AT-Bildung wird durch Erhitzen auf 56° C zerstört. Im Rattenserum beruht diese Zerstörung auf der Thermolabilität des mit der Fraktion III-0 fällbaren, zur AT-Bildung notwendigen Serumfaktors.

Die Möglichkeit, durch Erhitzung das AT-Bildungsvermögen von Serum aufzuheben, wurde zuerst von FRIEDBERGER (1910) für die Inkubation mit Immunpräcipitaten, von BORDET (1913a) und von NATHAN (1913a, b) für die Inkubation mit Polysacchariden und von NOVY u. DE KRUIF (1917e) für die Verdünnung mit Wasser beschrieben.

Bemerkenswert ist, daß bei Anwendung verschiedener Verfahren zur AT-Bildung die Angaben über die Hitzeempfindlichkeit des Serums etwas schwanken (vgl. NOVY u. DE KRUIF, 1917c, e; NOVY, DE KRUIF u. R. L. NOVY, 1917).

Die Geschwindigkeit der AT-Bildung ist stark temperaturabhängig. Sie hat einen Temperaturkoeffizienten über 2 (GIERTZ, 1959; GIERTZ und HAHN, 1957b, 1961; HAHN, 1960; ROCHA E SILVA, 1954; ROTHSCHILD und ROCHA E SILVA, 1954).

Die AT-Bildung durch Agar hat einen etwas anderen Zeitverlauf und eine andere Temperaturabhängigkeit als die AT-Bildung durch Verdünnung mit Wasser (ROTHSCHILD u. ROCHA E SILVA, 1954).

Die AT-Bildung in den nach GIERTZ, HAHN und LANGE (1956a, b) gewonnenen Rattenserumfraktionen ist bei einem pH von 5,3 oder weniger und 9,0 oder mehr stark gehemmt oder aufgehoben (GIERTZ und HAHN, 1957b, 1961). Nach NOVY und DE KRUIF (1917b) scheint auch die AT-Bildung im Kaninchenserum säureempfindlich zu sein.

In den Rattenserumfraktionen läuft die AT-Bildung auch dann ungestört ab, wenn sie in Ca-, Mg- und K-freier Pufferlösung oder in physiologischer Kochsalzlösung gelöst sind (GIERTZ, 1959; GIERTZ und HAHN, 1957b, 1961; HAHN, 1957). Die Bedeutung des Calciums für die AT-Bildung ist noch umstritten. Das durch Citrat gestörte AT-Bildungsvermögen des Serums läßt sich durch Ca-Zusatz nicht vollständig restituieren; durch einen Ionenaustauscher decalcifiziertes Serum hat ein normales AT-Bildungsvermögen (ROCHA E SILVA, 1952, 1954; ROTHSCHILD und ROCHA E SILVA, 1954). Oxalat in gerinnungshemmenden Dosen hemmt die AT-Bildung nicht (siehe oben). Andrerseits hemmt Na_3HEDTA die AT-Bildung (OSLER, RANDALL u. a., 1959a, b; VOGT, 1963), und diese Hemmung läßt sich durch Zugabe von Ca- und Mg-Ionen wieder aufheben.

Die AT-Bildung wird nicht nur durch Cl-Ionen (erhöhte Kochsalzkonzentration, vgl. FRIEDBERGER, LURÀ u. a., 1913) sondern auch durch alle andern untersuchten Anionen in bestimmter Ionenstärke gehemmt (ROTHSCHILD und ROCHA E SILVA, 1954).

Die eben hemmenden Konzentrationen betragen: Sulfat oder Chlorid 0,12 N; Jodid und Nitrat 0,06 N; Thiocyanid und Salicylat unter 0,06 N; Oxalat 0,04 N; Zitrat 0,03 N.

Von den Kationen zeigen Na, K und Li (als Chloride) keinen Unterschied in der Wirkung auf die AT-Bildung. Ca und Sr wirken stärker hemmend als Mg. Harnstoff hemmt in einer Konzentration von 0,25M, Glucose ist dagegen in der doppelten Konzentration unwirksam (ROTHSCHILD und ROCHA E SILVA, 1954).

Zn-Ionen hemmen die AT-Bildung wahrscheinlich deshalb, weil der mit der Fraktion III-0 isolierbare Serumfaktor zinkempfindlich ist (GIERTZ, 1959; GIERTZ und HAHN, 1957b, 1961; HAHN, 1957, 1960). Dementsprechend ist die Serumfraktion III-0, wenn sie nach HAHN und LANGE (1955) mit Zink gefällt wird, nicht zur AT-Bildung geeignet.

Die Zn-Wirkung beruht wahrscheinlich nicht auf einer SH-Gruppen-Blockierung, denn Jodacetat hemmt die AT-Bildung nicht und durch Cystein läßt sich die Zn-Wirkung nicht abschwächen (GIERTZ u. HAHN, 1961).

Außer durch die erwähnten Stoffe oder Maßnahmen wird die AT-Bildung durch Hydrocortison gehemmt (HERSHBERGER und HANSEN, 1958). Vorbehandlung von Ratten mit Hydrocortison oder Prednisolon beeinflußt dagegen das AT-Bildungsvermögen im Rattenserum nicht (JAQUES, 1961). Andrerseits hemmt Vorbehandlung der Ratten mit bestimmten Proteuspolysacchariden die AT-Bildung im Serum, obwohl diese Stoffe unwirksam sind, wenn sie in vitro Rattenserum zugesetzt werden (JAQUES, 1961). Auch Toluidinblau und Janusgrün sollen die AT-Bildung hemmen (CONARD und MUTSAARS, 1949).

Die Fraktion III-0 aus AT-haltigem Serum ist im Mittel um 0,09 g-% eiweißreicher als die gleiche Fraktion aus normalem Serum; umgekehrt ist die Fraktion I-III-1,2,3 aus AT-haltigem Serum um genau den gleichen Betrag eiweißärmer als I-III-1,2,3 aus normalem Serum (GIERTZ, 1959; GIERTZ u. HAHN, 1957a, 1961; HAHN, 1957, 1960; HAHN u. LANGE, 1955). Man könnte daher an eine durch die AT-Bildung bedingte Verschiebung von Eiweiß aus der Fraktion I-III-1,2,3 in die Fraktion III-0 denken.

c) Die Rolle proteolytischer oder anderer Fermente und des Komplements bei der AT-Bildung

JOBLING und PETERSEN (1914a, b) untersuchten als erste die Frage, ob bei Anwendung verschiedener Verfahren stets eine Proteolyse an der AT-Bildung beteiligt ist. Sie stellten fest, daß durch Inkubation von Serum mit Kontaktstoffen, die sich zur AT-Bildung eignen, der Antitrypsintiter des Serums absinkt (JOBLING und PETERSEN, 1914b). Sie führten diesen Befund auf eine Adsorption der Antitrypsine an die Kontaktstoffe zurück. Sie hielten die Antitrypsine für ungesättigte Fettsäuren; denn sie konnten auch durch Entfernung dieser Fettsäuren aus dem Serum (durch Ansäuern und Abfiltrieren oder durch Ausschütteln mit Fettlösungsmitteln) oder durch ihre chemische Veränderung (durch Jodierung) eine AT-Bildung erzielen (JOBLING und PETERSEN, 1914a). Ihre Auffassung wurde noch dadurch gestützt, daß sich so gewonnenes AT durch den Zusatz der entzogenen Fette wieder entgiften läßt.

Die Beobachtung von DOLD (1920a) und von DOLD und AOKI (1912), daß mit Ölen, Gallen oder Cholesterin vorbehandelte Bakterien zur AT-Bildung nicht mehr geeignet sind, könnte man so erklären, daß die Mikroorganismen nicht mehr Fettsäuren adsorbieren können.

JOBLING und PETERSEN gelang es jedoch nicht nachzuweisen, daß eine AT-Bildung stets mit einer Proteolyseaktivierung einhergeht. Gegen die von diesen Autoren trotzdem angenommene (vgl. auch BRONFENBRENNER, 1915) Verknüpfung von Proteolyseaktivierung und AT-Bildung sprechen auch andere Untersuchungen älterer Autoren, in denen keine Beziehung zwischen AT-Bildung und Eiweißabbau gefunden wurde (DALE und KELLAWAY, 1922; DE KRUIF und GERMAN, 1917; MISCH, 1919). BORDET und ZUNZ (1915b) betonen, daß selbst ein Parallelismus zwischen Proteaseaktivierung und AT-Entstehung kein Beweis für eine ursächliche Verknüpfung ist, sondern daß auch beide Prozesse nebeneinander herlaufen könnten.

In neuerer Zeit diskutiert vor allem ROCHA E SILVA mehrfach eine Proteolysebeteiligung an der AT-Bildung. Es gelang ihm jedoch nicht, eine solche Beteiligung nachzuweisen (ROCHA E SILVA, 1954, 1956; ROCHA E SILVA und ARONSON, 1952; ROTHSCHILD und ROCHA E SILVA, 1954).

Wie schon früher DE KRUIF und GERMAN (1917), so fanden auch ROCHA E SILVA u. Mitarb. sowie JONES (1960) eine stärkere Proteolyseaktivierung in agarbehandeltem Meerschweinchenserum als im Rattenserum, obwohl sich im Rattenserum besser AT bildet. In neueren Versuchen kamen auch UNGAR u. Mitarb. (UNGAR, YAMURA u. a., 1961), die früher stets eine Verknüpfung zwischen Proteolyse und AT-Aktivierung angenommen hatten (UNGAR, 1953, 1956; UNGAR u. DAMGAARD, 1955; UNGAR, DAMGAARD u. HUMMEL, 1953; UNGAR u. HAYASHI, 1958; UNGAR u. MIST, 1949), zu einem ähnlichen Ergebnis. Bemerkenswert ist auch, daß die Proteolyseaktivierung unter Bedingungen, die auch zur AT-Bildung führen, meist nur sehr gering ist (GEIGER, 1952; UNGAR, DAMGAARD u. HUMMEL, 1953; UNGAR u. MIST, 1949; UNGAR, YAMURA u. a., 1961).

Einige Hemmstoffe der Proteolyse beeinflussen die AT-Bildung nicht. Na-Salicylat und 3-Hydroxy-2-phenylcinchoninsäure, welche die Plasminaktivität hemmen (UNGAR und DAMGAARD, 1955; UNGAR, DAMGAARD und HUMMEL, 1952), stören in etwa den gleichen Konzentrationen die AT-Bildung nicht (HAINING 1956b). Auch Sojabohnentrypsininhibitor (SBTI) hemmt die AT-Bildung nicht (ROTHSCHILD und ROCHA E SILVA, 1954).

NETZER u. VOGT (1962) beobachteten eine AT-Bildung in Rattenplasma durch Streptokinase und durch Rinderplasmin. Die Autoren (VOGT, 1963a; NETZER u. VOGT, 1964) nehmen jedoch nicht an, daß durch die Plasminaktivität AT entsteht, da Antiplasmin die AT-Bildung durch Plasmin nicht hemmt. Sie glaubten vielmehr, daß eine Verunreinigung ihrer Präparate mit Bakterienlipopolysacchariden für die AT-Bildung verantwortlich ist.

Ein an der AT-Bildung beteiligtes Ferment könnte natürlich auch einen ähnlichen Charakter wie die Gerinnungsfermente haben, die nicht zum Auftreten niedermolekularer Stoffe führen und daher auch nicht durch Methoden nachweisbar sind, die auf der Bestimmung niedermolekularer Eiweißspaltprodukte beruhen.

Die Aktivierung der kininbildenden Fermente (Lit. s. LEWIS, 1960) und des von MILES u. Mitarb. beschriebenen Permeabilitätsfaktors PF/dil (MILES u. WILHELM, 1955; WILHELM, MILES u. MACKAY, 1955; WILHELM, MILL u. MILES, 1957) unterscheidet sich von der AT-Bildung vor allem dadurch, daß sie auch bei Verdünnung von Serum mit physiologischer Kochsalzlösung erfolgt, und zwar auch in Sera, die zur AT-Bildung ungeeignet sind. Im Gegensatz zu den Kininen wird AT durch Behandlung mit heißem Alkohol zerstört (ROCHA E SILVA, 1954). Der neuerdings von DAVIES und LOWE (1960, 1961, 1962a, b) beschriebene Permeabilitätsfaktor PF/P wird zwar durch einen ähnlichen Mechanismus wie das AT gebildet, er ist jedoch im Gegensatz zum AT kein Histaminliberator am Meerschweinchen.

Das Ausmaß der AT-Bildung geht parallel mit der Konzentration der beiden, zur AT-Bildung notwendigen, durch die Cohnsche Fraktionierung isolierbaren Serumfaktoren; ferner werden diese Faktoren durch die AT-Bildung aufgebraucht (GIERTZ, 1959; GIERTZ und HAHN, 1957b, 1958, 1961; HAHN, 1957, 1960). Es ist bisher nicht gelungen, die AT-Bildung in mehrere Etappen aufzuspalten (GIERTZ, 1959; GIERTZ und HAHN, 1961).

Man könnte aus diesen Ergebnissen vielleicht schließen, daß die AT-Bildung ein nichtenzymatischer Prozeß ist; doch die Möglichkeit, daß in den genannten Versuchen ein enzymatischer Faktor teilnimmt, der bei der Cohnschen Fraktionierung nicht von den beiden zur AT-Bildung notwendigen Serumfraktionen getrennt wird, ist nicht auszuschließen.

Nach neuesten Untersuchungen nimmt an der AT-Bildung ein Ferment teil, das neben dem für die AT-Bildung notwendigen Substrat (Anaphylatoxinogen) im Rattenplasma enthalten ist (STEGEMANN, VOGT und FRIEDBERG, 1964; VOGT, 1963a, b, 1964; VOGT und SCHMIDT, 1964). Über den Mechanismus der Aktivierung des Fermentes durch die Kontaktstoffe ist bisher nichts bekannt. Ein dem Ferment des Rattenplasmas ähnliches Enzym läßt sich aus Cobragift isolieren. Es führt zur AT-Bildung im Rattenplasma und auch im Schweineplasma und in einer durch Gelfiltration gewonnenen Rattenplasmafraktion, welche beide mit den üblichen Kontaktstoffen kein AT bilden und nur Anaphylatoxinogen enthalten. Dieses AT-bildende Enzym ist wahrscheinlich ein Metallferment und läßt sich von der Phospholipase A und den proteolytischen Enzymen des Cobragiftes trennen. Das Ferment wird durch Carbonylreagentien gehemmt. Ferner stören hohe Pyridoxalphosphatkonzentrationen (10^{-3}) die AT-Bildung.

Das in Abschnitt C 1 erwähnte Problem der Komplementbeteiligung an der AT-Bildung wurde neuerdings vor allem von OSLER und Mitarbeitern wieder aufgegriffen, die besonders eine Beteiligung der Komplementkomponente C′3 diskutieren.

Schon 1938 wurde von DA COSTA CRUZ ein Parallelismus zwischen C′3-Schwund und AT-Bildung im agarbehandelten Meerschweinchenserum beobachtet. OSLER, RANDALL u. a. (1959a, b) zeigten, daß auch die AT-Bildung im Rattenserum durch steigende Dosen von Immunpräzipitaten mit der C′3-Inaktivierung parallel ging. Erfolgte dagegen eine fast vollständige Komplementinaktivierung durch Immunpräcipitate in der Kälte, ohne daß auch die Komponente C′3 inaktiviert wurde, so wurde auch kein AT gebildet.

Nach OSLER u. Mitarb. sollen auch die Komplementkomponenten C′1, C′2 und C′4, wenn auch nur in Spuren, für die AT-Bildung notwendig sein; denn die Hemmwirkung des Na_3HEDTA auf die AT-Bildung und die C′3-Inaktivierung deuten die Autoren als Hemmung der Funktion der andern Komplementkomponenten durch Ca- und Mg-Entzug. Nach VOGT (1963a, b) ist jedoch Rattenplasma, das mit EDTA-Zusatz ultrafiltriert und dann durch Ultrafiltration mit Kochsalzlösung von EDTA befreit wurde, wieder zur AT-Bildung fähig, ohne daß divalente Kationen neu zugesetzt werden müssen. Dieses Verhalten spricht gegen die Auffassung, daß das EDTA durch Einwirkung auf das Komplement die AT-Bildung hemme.

OSLER u. Mitarb. sehen auch darin einen Hinweis auf die C'3-Beteiligung an der AT-Bildung, daß sich nach der Zerstörung von C'3 durch Formaldehyd und bei Gegenwart von Phlorizin, das die C'3-Inaktivierung hemmt, kein AT im Ratten- oder im Meerschweinchenserum bilden läßt. Weitere Hinweise auf eine Beteiligung der Komplementkomponente C'3 an der AT-Bildung finden sich in der Arbeit von RANDALL u. Mitarb. (1961).

Die Untersuchungen von OSLER u. Mitarb. gehen aus von Untersuchungen über die passive cutane Anaphylaxie der Ratte (BIER, SIQUEIRA u. OSLER, 1955), die ähnliche Beziehungen wie die AT-Bildung zur C'3-Funktion haben soll. Bei Ratten, deren Komplementtiter im Blut durch Injektion von Antigen-Antikörper-Komplexen gesenkt worden war, verlief nicht nur die passive cutane Anaphylaxie abgeschwächt, sondern es nahm auch das AT-Bildungsvermögen im Serum dieser Ratten ab. Eine Abnahme des AT-Bildungsvermögens im Serum von Meerschweinchen nach Injektion von Agar oder amboceptorbeladenen Erythrocyten (BORDET, 1919, 1921) und im Serum von Ratten nach Dextraninjektion (ROCHA E SILVA u. ROTHSCHILD, 1955) wurde schon früher beobachtet. GIERTZ, HAHN, JURNA u. LANGE (1958) fanden im Serum von Meerschweinchen im Forssman-Schock ein herabgesetztes AT-Bildungsvermögen. Alle diese Versuche könnten zwar im Oslerschen Sinne gedeutet werden, doch nehmen die genannten Autoren eine Abnahme der AT-Vorstufen durch eine in vivo erfolgte AT-Bildung an.

UNGAR (1953) hielt das fertige AT für identisch mit einer aktivierten Serofibrinokinase. Die Aktivierung soll komplementabhängig sein. Das Fehlen einer Plasminaktivierung bei der AT-Entstehung (s. oben) spricht gegen UNGARs Auffassung. Außerdem können auch solche Stoffe (48/80, Tween 20 u. a.) nach UNGAR die Serofibrinokinase aktivieren, die keine AT-Bildner sind.

Gegen die Annahme einer Komplementbeteiligung bei der AT-Bildung lassen sich einige Einwände erheben. Die Komplementkomponente C'1, die den Charakter einer Esterase hat (vgl. LEPOW, 1959), läßt sich durch den Esterasehemmstoff DFP (0,01 M) hemmen, nicht aber die AT-Bildung (BECKER, 1959). Nur mit o-p-Nitrophenyl-o-äthyl-phenylphosphonat (0,001 M) läßt sich die AT-Bildung hemmen, während fertiges AT durch diesen Stoff nicht zerstört wird (BECKER, 1962). In ammoniakbehandeltem Serum läßt sich trotz völligen C'4-Schwundes in vereinzelten Fällen ein AT bilden (GIERTZ, 1959). Die von GIERTZ, HAHN und LANGE (1956a) isolierten, zur AT-Bildung verwendbaren Serumfraktionen enthalten nur etwa $^1/_3$ des ursprünglichen Serumeiweißgehaltes (GIERTZ, 1959; GIERTZ und HAHN, 1957, 1958, 1961; HAHN, 1957, 1960; HAHN und GIERTZ, 1960) und nur noch wenig Komplement (GIERTZ, 1959; HAHN, 1960; HAHN und GIERTZ, 1960). Trotzdem sind sie ebenso gut wie das ursprüngliche Serum zur AT-Bildung geeignet. Allerdings sind in diesen Fraktionen vor allem die Komplementkomponenten C'1, C'2 und C'4 vermindert, in einzelnen Versuchen ließen sie sich überhaupt nicht mehr nachweisen. Der C'3-Titer ist dagegen im Mittel nur um eine Titerstufe abgesunken, so daß durch die Versuche eine Beteiligung von C'3 nicht ausgeschlossen ist.

Andererseits ist das Ausmaß der AT-Bildung in Serumfraktionen und im nativen Serum gleich, obwohl in den Fraktionen der C'3-Titer niedriger als im Serum ist. Trotz des niedrigeren Titers ist jedoch der C'3-Schwund durch die AT-Bildung in den Fraktionen geringer als im nativen Serum. Diese Befunde sprechen gegen eine C'3-Beteiligung an der AT-Bildung (GIERTZ, 1959; HAHN und GIERTZ, 1960).

Die Inkubation von Serum mit Dextran oder anderen Polysacchariden führt nicht nur zu einer AT-Bildung, sondern auch zu einer C'3-Inaktivierung durch den Properdinmechanismus (vgl. PILLEMER u. a., 1954, 1955). Es ist daher schwer zu entscheiden, ob die Veränderungen am C'3-Titer wirklich durch die AT-Bildung bedingt sind.

Zusammenfassend kann man über die Beteiligung der Proteolyse und des Komplements heute nur sagen, daß es sowohl Hinweise auf eine solche Beteiligung als auch eine Reihe von Gegenargumenten gibt. Sicher darf man nicht so weit gehen, im AT den Ausdruck einer Komplementzerstörung schlechthin zu sehen (CITRON, 1911; LEPOW, 1957).

d) Die kolloidchemischen Begleiterscheinungen der AT-Bildung

BORDET (1913a) lenkte als erster das Interesse der AT-Forschung auf die Möglichkeit, das AT sei das Ergebnis eines sich an den Globulinen abspielenden

Vergröberungsprozesses. Er beobachtete, daß Meerschweinchenserum sich während der AT-Bildung trüben kann und daß bei bestimmten Maßnahmen AT-haltiges Serum leichter als normales zur Trübung neigt (BORDET, 1913a, 1924). Er hielt das trübende Agens jedoch nicht für AT, denn auch nach Entfernung der Trübung blieb das Serum giftig; ferner ließ sich auch AT gewinnen, ohne daß es zur Trübung kam (BORDET, 1924). DOLD (1920a, b) fand, daß sich der Charakter der Trübung je nach Art des verwendeten Kontaktstoffes ändert und daß Trübungen durch Kontaktstoffe auch in solchen Sera auftreten, die nicht zur AT-Bildung geeignet sind. Demnach könnten die Trübungsphänomene (wie auch andere serologische Prozesse, vgl. SACHS und STILLING, 1917) zwar mit der AT-Bildung parallel laufen, brauchten aber nicht ursächlich damit verknüpft zu sein.

Es besteht aber auch die andere Möglichkeit, daß die sichtbaren Trübungsphänomene nur die nicht obligate Begleiterscheinung eines subvisiblen Vergröberungsprozesses an den Serumeiweißen sind. Der Giftungsprozeß könnte eine fortschreitende Teilchenvergrößerung sein, die über eine „optimale Labilisierung der Globuline" (HIRSCHFELD und KLINGER, 1913) hinaus bis zu einer „klärenden Ausflockung" mit Wirkungsverlust (vgl. DOLD, 1920a, b) gehen kann.

Als Ursache der Vergröberung kommt nach Ansicht der älteren Autoren entweder eine Adsorption labiler Globuline an die (nach DALE und KELLAWAY, (1922) durch Zentrifugieren aus dem Serum nicht völlig entfernbaren) Kontaktstoffe in Betracht (SCHMIDT, 1917) oder eine Zusammenballung der Globuline durch Veränderung des elektrischen Milieus infolge der stark negativen Ladung der Kontaktstoffe (KOPACZEWSKI, 1919; KOPACZEWSKI und GRUZEWSKA, 1920).

Aus Versuchen über die Filtrierbarkeit und Zentrifugierbarkeit des AT lassen sich keine eindeutigen Schlüsse auf die Größe des einzelnen AT-Teilchens ziehen. Stärke-AT aus Meerschweinchenserum soll Kieselgurfilter nicht passieren (DALE und KELLAWAY, 1922; SCHMIDT, 1917). Über die Filtrierbarkeit von Bakterien-AT sind die Ansichten geteilt (BRUGNATELLI, 1913; FRIEDBERGER und KONITZER, 1921). Agar-AT läuft angeblich durch normale, aber nicht durch besonders feinporige Kieselgurfilter hindurch (BORDET, 1925; DALE und KELLAWAY, 1922). Die Zentrifugierbarkeit von Stärke-AT (FRIEDBERGER und JOACHIMOGLU, 1917; SCHMIDT, 1917) und von Agar-AT (BORDET, 1925; LUMIÈRE und COUTURIER, 1925, 1926) ist umstritten. RITZ und SACHS (1918) erörterten auf Grund der damals vorliegenden Ergebnisse die Möglichkeit, die Zentrifugierbarkeit und Filtrierbarkeit könne von den zur AT-Bildung benutzten Kontaktstoffen abhängen.

Neuerdings versuchten GIERTZ, HAHN und SCHMUTZLER (noch unveröffentlicht), Dextran-AT aus Rattenserum mit Hilfe der Ultrazentrifuge auszuschleudern. Bei einer Dauer von 10 Std. und einer Beschleunigung von etwa 200000 g ergab sich kein Hinweis, daß AT-Teilchen gröber als die übrigen Serumeiweiße sind. Neuere Befunde (s. Abschnitt 3) machen wahrscheinlich, daß das AT-Molekül kleiner als die Moleküle der Serumproteine ist.

Allerdings haben ältere Autoren durch Zentrifugieren oder Filtrieren in manchen Fällen anscheinend eine Entgiftung AT-haltigen Serums erzielt. Bei der Durchsicht der älteren Literatur fällt auf, daß gerade das Stärke-AT am schlechtesten filtrierbar und am besten zentrifugierbar ist. Nach DALE und KELLAWAY (1922) verursacht aber gerade dieses AT viel häufiger Ödeme und Hämorrhagien als Bakterien- oder gar Agar-AT. Man muß an die Möglichkeit denken, daß diese für die AT-Wirkung uncharakteristischen Symptome (s. unten) möglicherweise durch vergröberte Teilchen zustande kommen, die nicht mit AT identisch sind. Es ist daher erklärlich, daß SCHMIDT (1917) die Trübung für die Giftigkeit seines Stärke-AT verantwortlich machte, indem er eine mechanische Schädigung oder Verstopfung der Lungencapillaren annahm (vgl. auch LUMIÈRE, 1924; LUMIÈRE u. COUTURIER, 1925). Andere Autoren führten allerdings die Neigung schwacher ATe zur Ödembildung auf die Notwendigkeit zurück, zur Schockauslösung große Serummengen zu injizieren (s. unten).

Wie Trübungen des Serums so können auch Veränderungen der Viscosität und der Oberflächenspannung mit der AT-Bildung einhergehen. Aber auch diese Vorgänge scheinen mit der AT-Bildung nicht ursächlich verknüpft zu sein (DALE und KELLAWAY, 1922; FRIEDBERGER und PUTTER, 1923; LUMIÈRE und MEYER, 1935a, b, c).

Auch wenn man nicht annimmt, das AT sei ein vergröbertes Eiweißaggregat, so könnte man sich doch vorstellen, daß denaturierende Prozesse an den Eiweißkörpern in irgendeiner Weise zur AT-Bildung notwendig sind. Es fällt nämlich auf, daß alle Vorgänge, die zur AT-Bildung führen sollen, mit Denaturierungsvorgängen an den Serumeiweißen einhergehen: Die Verdünnung mit Wasser, die Dialyse gegen Wasser, die Ansäuerung, die Behandlung mit Fettlösungsmitteln, die Einleitung von CO_2, das Schütteln und das Lagern. Immunpräcipitate stellen denaturierte Eiweißkörper dar. Die Polysaccharide können Eiweißkörper adsorbieren (z. B. das Properdin und die Komplementkomponente C'3, vgl. PILLEMER und Mitarbeiter, 1954, 1955) und führen dabei möglicherweise auch zu Denaturierungsvorgängen. SEELICH (1948) nahm an, daß an derartigen Kontaktstoffen „die primäre monomolekulare Adsorptionsschicht den Charakter eines denaturierten Proteins annimmt“. Er hält das Vorhandensein von denaturierten Eiweißkörpern für entscheidend wichtig für die AT-Bildung. ROCHA E SILVA (1954) sieht in der Herabsetzung der Ionenstärke und einer Negativierung des elektrischen Milieus durch die Kontaktstoffe den Anstoß zur AT-Bildung. Auch hierbei könnte es zu einer Eiweißdenaturierung kommen, wenn auch ROCHA E SILVA selbst den Effekt der Veränderungen im Ionenmilieu anders deutet (siehe unten).

Ein sehr interessantes Phänomen ist die Auslösung anaphylaxieähnlicher und anaphylatoxinähnlicher Effekte am Meerschweinchen durch die Injektion von aggregierten Gammaglobulinen (ISHIZAKA und Mitarbeiter, 1959, 1960, 1961). Die Frage, ob diese Untersuchungen eine Beziehung zur AT-Bildung und AT-Wirkung haben, wird zwar von ISHIZAKA (1963) diskutiert, ihre endgültige Aufklärung steht aber noch aus.

3. Die Natur des AT

In der älteren Literatur steht die Ansicht FRIEDBERGERs, das AT sei ein niedermolekulares Eiweißspaltprodukt, der Vorstellung gegenüber, das AT sei das Produkt eines sich an den Serumeiweißen abspielenden Vergröberungsprozesses. Wir haben bereits ausgeführt (siehe oben), daß AT kein aggregiertes oder vergröbertes Eiweißteilchen und auch kein gröberer Komplex aus den Kontaktstoffen und Eiweiß sein kann.

Die große Ähnlichkeit der AT-Wirkung mit dem Histaminschock und dem anaphylaktischen Schock (vgl. DALE und LAIDLAW, 1910) führte bald nach der Entdeckung des AT zu dem Versuch, eine Identität zwischen AT und Histamin nachzuweisen (FRIEDBERGER und JERUSALEM, 1910; FRIEDBERGER und MORESCHI, 1912). Dabei ergab sich vor allem, daß AT im Gegensatz zum Histamin nicht dialysabel ist. Aus späteren Versuchen kann man entnehmen, daß AT auch nicht den Charakter von Kininen oder Peptonen hat; denn es wandert nicht durch peptondurchlässige Membranen (HIRSCHFELD und KLINGER, 1913) und wird durch heißen Alkohol zerstört (ROCHA E SILVA, 1954). Der Entstehungsmodus des AT ist ebenfalls anders als bei diesen Stoffen (siehe oben). Ferner unterscheidet auch die auf eine einzige Tierart, nämlich das Meerschweinchen beschränkte Wirkung das AT von Kininen und Peptonen.

Neuerdings gelang es, Anaphylatoxin mit Hilfe der Gelfiltration von höhermolekularen Plasmaproteinen, zu denen auch seine Vorstufe, das Anaphylatoxinogen, gehört, zu trennen und es dadurch sehr erheblich anzureichern. Seinem Verhalten an basischen und sauren Ionenaustauschern nach ist es ein basisches, relativ hochmolekulares Polypeptid, das durch Proteinasen und Carboxypeptidase zerstört wird. Allerdings scheint die Frage, ob AT nicht doch ein Protein ist, noch nicht endgültig geklärt, denn es gelang nicht, es durch Ultrafilter zu filtrieren (FRIEDBERG, STEGEMANN und VOGT, 1963; STEGEMANN, VOGT und FRIEDBERG, 1964).

AT zeigt eine bemerkenswerte Stabilität gegenüber Einflüssen, die den labileren der beiden zur AT-Bildung notwendigen Serumfaktoren zerstören oder den Prozeß der AT-Bildung hemmen. AT ist weniger hitzeempfindlich als die mit der Fraktion III-0 isolierbare Vorstufe und wird erst bei Temperaturen von 65° C und mehr zerstört (FRIEDBERGER, 1910a; GIERTZ, HAHN und LANGE, 1956a, b; GIERTZ und HAHN, 1961; ROCHA E SILVA, 1954; ROTHSCHILD und ROCHA E SILVA, 1954). AT ist relativ unempfindlich gegen Säuerung und erheblich weniger säureempfindlich als seine Vorstufen (FRIEDBERGER und JERUSALEM, 1910; FRIEDBERGER und MORESCHI, 1912; GIERTZ, 1959; GIERTZ und HAHN, 1957b, 1958, 1961; HAHN, 1957; NOVY und DE KRUIF, 1917b; SCHMIDT und SCHÜRMANN, 1918). Nach STEGEMANN, VOGT und FRIEDBERG (1964) ist AT bei einem pH von 2 und einer Temperatur von 80° C für eine Stunde stabil.

In getrocknetem Zustand läßt sich AT angeblich auf 100°C erhitzen (FRIEDBERGER u. JERUSALEM, 1910). Gegen mehrfaches Einfrieren und Auftauen ist es wie seine Vorstufen unempfindlich (BOEHNCKE u. BIERBAUM, 1912). In gefriergetrocknetem Zustand ist es mindestens ein halbes Jahr haltbar. Ausschütteln von AT-haltigem Serum mit dem zehnfachen Äthervolumen oder Fällung mit dem zehnfachen Alkoholvolumen soll AT nicht zerstören (FRIEDBERGER u. JERUSALEM, 1910).

Das fertige AT besitzt nicht die Empfindlichkeit gegenüber Zinkionen, die eine seiner Vorstufen auszeichnet, denn es läßt sich mit Hilfe von Zinkionen ausfällen (HAHN und LANGE, 1955). Allerdings findet man nur etwa 30–50% der ursprünglichen AT-Aktivität des Serums in der Fraktion III-0 wieder, wobei es gleichgültig ist, ob diese Fraktion mit Zink oder bei niedriger Ionenstärke mit Alkohol gefällt wurde (GIERTZ, 1959; GIERTZ, HAHN und LANGE, 1956a, b). Ein geringer Anteil der AT-Aktivität fand sich auch in der Fraktion I-III-1,2,3. Es ist fraglich, ob der Rest sich durch die COHNsche Methode überhaupt nicht ausfällen läßt oder ob er auf andere Fraktionen verteilt ist.

Auch andere Versuche, das AT auszufällen, zeigen, daß es sich um einen relativ stabilen Eiweißkörper handelt. Bei 24stündiger Dialyse gegen Wasser fällt es nicht mit den Globulinen aus (FRIEDBERGER und JERUSALEM, 1910). Aus Rattenserum läßt es sich bei pH 5.2 und niedriger Ionenstärke nicht mit den Euglobulinen ausfällen (JONES, 1960). Es beginnt erst bei einer Na-Sulfat-Konzentration über 22% auszufallen, und erst bei einer Ammonsulfatsättigung von 65–70% fand sich das gesamte AT im Präcipitat (JONES, 1960; ROCHA E SILVA, 1954, 1956).

Sucht man Anhaltspunkte über die Natur des AT aus seinem Bildungsmechanismus zu gewinnen, kommt man zu dem Schluß, daß AT zwar möglicherweise durch einen fermentativen Mechanismus gebildet wird, daß aber die Beteiligung proteolytischer Fermente nicht erwiesen ist und daß AT selbst auch nicht den Charakter einer Protease hat. Diese Feststellung ist im Hinblick auf die bereits erwähnte Tatsache wichtig, daß manche proteolytischen Fermente Histamin freisetzen können (vgl. ROCHA E SILVA, 1940a, b). Da die AT-Bildung mit Hilfe von Kontaktstoffen sich nicht in Etappen zerlegen läßt, scheinen gewisse Möglichkeiten der AT-Entstehung unwahrscheinlich, wie z. B. die primäre Entfernung eines Hemmstoffes. Die Möglichkeit, daß AT das Produkt einer chemischen, nichtenzymatischen Reaktion zwischen zwei Eiweißkörpern ist, scheint uns nicht ausgeschlossen im Hinblick auf den Aufbrauch der an der AT-Bildung beteiligten beiden Serumfaktoren.

Das Kernproblem der AT-Entstehung ist die Frage, welche Bedeutung die Kontaktstoffe dabei haben. Eine umfassende Theorie müßte erklären, daß die AT-Bildung von einem optimalen physikalischen Zustand der Kontaktstoffe abhängt, daß sowohl Polysaccharide als auch eiweißartige Stoffe als Kontaktstoffe wirken können und daß sogar ohne Gegenwart von Kontaktstoffen durch rein physikalische Maßnahmen eine AT-Bildung möglich ist. Es ist unwahrscheinlich, daß der Kontaktstoff selbst ein Bestandteil des fertigen AT ist, weil eine AT-Bildung auch ohne die Anwesenheit von Kontaktstoffen möglich ist. Allerdings könnte man in diesem Fall daran denken, daß primär gefällte Globuline die Rolle der Kontaktstoffe übernehmen. Man müßte dann aber doch dem AT eine Teilchengröße zusprechen, die es nach den bereits erörterten Fakten (siehe oben) nicht hat. Es bleibt daher nur die Annahme, daß die Kontaktstoffe in gleicher Weise wie andere zur AT-Bildung führende Maßnahmen ein physikochemisches Milieu schaffen, in dem der zur AT-Bildung führende chemische Prozeß ablaufen kann.

Eine interessante Theorie hat Rocha e Silva (1954) aufgestellt. Er macht (wie schon früher Kopaczewski, 1919; Kopaczewski und Gruzewska, 1920) die Elektronegativität der Kontaktstoffe, insbesondere der Polysaccharide, für die Einleitung der AT-Bildung verantwortlich. Er nimmt an, daß durch die elektronegativen Polysaccharide die Ionenstärke verringert wird und dadurch eine Reaktion zwischen einem thermolabilen Serumfaktor („activator“) und einem zweiten Faktor („precursor“) zustande kommt. Rocha e Silva erörtert mehrere Möglichkeiten, wie sich die Elektronegativität der Kontaktstoffe auswirken könnte. Die Vorstellung, daß die AT-Bildung durch eine Herabsetzung der Ionenstärke zustande kommt, ist gut vereinbar mit dem Befund, daß sich AT durch Verdünnung mit Wasser, aber nicht durch Verdünnung mit physiologischen Salzlösungen aus Serum bilden läßt. Die Theorie von Rocha e Silva steht auch mit den Befunden von Giertz, Hahn und Lange (1956a, b) in Einklang: Der labile, in Fraktion III-0 enthaltene Serumfaktor könnte durch die Herabsetzung der Ionenstärke noch weiter labilisiert werden, so daß er eine Bindung mit einem zweiten, in der Fraktion I-III-1,2,3 enthaltenen Serumeiweiß eingeht.

1958 legte Rocha e Silva ein erweitertes Schema vor, das nicht nur die AT-Bildung erfaßte, sondern auch die Wirkung der basischen Histaminliberatoren einschloß. Im Serum soll der Prozeß der AT-Bildung etwa in der oben geschilderten Weise durch Herabsetzung der Ionenstärke ablaufen. Durch stark elektronegative Substanzen wie die sulfatierten Polysaccharide soll ein elektropositiver AT-Vorläufer blockiert und gegen die Aktivierung unempfindlich gemacht werden. So ließe sich die Hemmwirkung des Heparins auf die AT-Bildung erklären. In den Mastzellen soll der AT-Vorläufer in einer derartig durch Heparin blockierten Form vorliegen. Die basischen Histaminliberatoren sollen das Heparin von diesem Vorläufer verdrängen, dadurch AT aktivieren und so zur Histaminfreisetzung führen. Diese Auffassung entbehrt noch einer ausreichenden experimentellen Grundlage.

Da sich die Theorie Rocha e Silvas auf die Elektronegativität der polysaccharidartigen Kontaktstoffe stützt, kann sie die AT-Bildung durch Immunpräcipitate oder andere eiweißartige Kontaktstoffe nicht befriedigend erklären. Die andere Möglichkeit, ob nicht die AT-Bildung durch das Auftreten denaturierter Eiweiße eingeleitet wird, haben wir bereits erörtert. Mit dieser Vorstellung könnte man zwar alle Möglichkeiten der AT-Bildung auf einen Nenner bringen, es fehlt uns jedoch noch eine brauchbare Erklärung, wie die denaturierten Eiweiße die chemische Reaktion zwischen den zur AT-Bildung notwendigen Serumfaktoren in Gang setzen könnten. Es gibt Hinweise darauf (siehe oben), daß sich auch die eiweißartigen Stoffe in einem optimalen physikalischen Zustand befinden müssen, um eine AT-Bildung einzuleiten. Allen Theorien der AT-Bildung ist daher gemeinsam, daß physikochemisch aktive Oberflächen für die Einleitung der AT-Bildung von Bedeutung sind.

Die Frage, ob die AT-Bildung zur Entstehung eines einheitlichen Stoffes führt oder ob es verschiedene ATe gibt ist noch ungeklärt. Für die Existenz mehrerer ATe könnte die Beobachtung sprechen, daß die Vorstufen des AT je nach dem zur AT-Bildung angewandten Verfahren unterschiedlich hitzeempfindlich sein können (NOVY, DE KRUIF, 1917c, e; NOVY, DE KRUIF und NOVY, 1917) und daß bei einer AT-Bildung durch verschiedene Maßnahmen auch der Zeitverlauf und die Temperaturabhängigkeit verschieden sein können (ROTHSCHILD und ROCHA E SILVA, 1954). Aus der Tatsache, daß die Giftigkeit des gleichen Serums nach Inkubation mit verschiedenen Kontaktstoffen auch verschieden sein kann, darf man nicht ohne weiteres auf die unterschiedliche Identität der entstandenen ATe schließen (GIERTZ, 1959; GIERTZ und HAHN, 1961; ROTHSCHILD und ROCHA E SILVA, 1954); denn solche Unterschiede treten auch dann auf, wenn der gleiche Kontaktstoff im gleichen Serum in verschiedenem physikalischen Zustand angewandt wird.

4. Die Wirkung des AT

a) Die Wirkung des AT am intakten Tier und am isolierten Organ

Nur am Meerschweinchen läßt sich durch AT ein tödlicher Schock erzeugen. FRIEDBERGER sah die Lungenblähung, wie sie von AUER und LEWIS (1910) für den anaphylaktischen Schock beschrieben war, als typisches Symptom des AT-Schocks an. Diese Lungenblähung ist durch einen Bronchospasmus bedingt. Auch GRAETZ (1911) betonte, daß der anaphylaktische Schock und der Anaphylatoxinschock weder durch die Beatembarkeit noch pathologisch-anatomisch unterscheidbar seien.

Andere Autoren beobachteten dagegen auch Lungenödeme und Hämorrhagien nach AT und behaupteten, das Sistieren der Atmung ließe sich im anaphylaktischen Schock viel schwerer als im AT-Schock überwinden (BIEDL und KRAUS, 1910a, b; DALE und KELLAWAY, 1922; KRAUS und KIRSCHBAUM, 1913; LOEWIT, 1913; LOEWIT und BAYER, 1913; VON WORZIKOWSKI-KUNDRATITZ, 1913). Selbst FRIEDBERGER beobachtete gelegentlich Ödeme (FRIEDBERGER und VALLARDI, 1910). Er ließ daher durch seinen Mitarbeiter KUMAGAI speziell dieses Problem noch einmal an einem großen Tiermaterial bearbeiten.

KUMAGAI (1913) bestätigte, daß im AT-Schock häufiger als im anaphylaktischen Schock Ödeme und Hämorrhagien auftreten. Er führte das darauf zurück, daß zur Auslösung eines Schocks das Antigen in kleinen, das AT-haltige Meerschweinchenserum dagegen in großen Injektionsvolumina injiziert wurde. Er zeigte, daß der anaphylaktische Schock dem AT-Schock ähnlicher wurde, wenn das Antigen in einem größeren Flüssigkeitsvolumen gegeben wurde. Die beiden Schockformen glichen sich sogar völlig, wenn das Antigen in einer Serummenge injiziert wurde, die der zur Schockauslösung notwendigen Menge AT-haltigen Serums entsprach.

Aus den Versuchen von KUMAGAI (1913) könnte man schließen, daß der AT-Schock und der anaphylaktische Schock sich nicht grundsätzlich voneinander unterscheiden, daß also das vorherrschende Symptom die Lungenblähung infolge eines Bronchospasmus ist. Es scheint allerdings so, als ob ATe, die durch verschiedene Kontaktstoffe hergestellt wurden, sich auch dann in ihren Symptomen unterscheiden können, wenn die Injektionsvolumina etwa gleich sind.

Während Agar-AT stets eine Lungenblähung verursachte, führte Stärke-AT aus Meerschweinchenserum in manchen Fällen zu Ödemen und Hämorrhagien (DALE u. KELLAWAY, 1922; FRIEDBERGER u. JOACHIMOGLU, 1917; SCHMIDT, 1917). DALE und KELLAWAY erzielten sogar mit einer bestimmten Charge von Stärke-AT regelmäßig ein starkes Ödem mit Austritt blutiger Ödemflüssigkeit aus den Nasenlöchern. Dem Bacillen-AT räumten sie einen Platz zwischen Agar- und Stärke-AT ein. FRIEDBERGER und VALLARDI (1910) beobachteten häufiger ein hämorrhagisches Lungenödem nach AT, das mit Hilfe von amboceptorbeladenen Hammelerythrocyten oder Erythrocytenschatten hergestellt war.

Nach diesen Befunden scheint es, als ob sich ATe verschiedener Herkunft nicht stets in ihrer Wirkung glichen. In der neueren Literatur fehlt es an derartigen Angaben. Das liegt wohl daran, daß hier meist mit starken ATen aus Rattenserum oder mit solchen ATen aus Meerschweinchenserum gearbeitet wurde, die wie Agar- oder Dextran-AT stets eine Lungenblähung hervorrufen.

Nach den Ergebnissen am intakten Tier hätte es schon früher nahe gelegen, die AT-Wirkung an der isolierten Meerschweinchenlunge zu untersuchen. Obwohl die anaphylaktische Reaktion wie auch die Wirkung anaphylaxieähnlich wirkender Substanzen (z. B. Pepton, Histamin) wenige Jahre nach der Entdeckung des AT an der isolierten, mit Salzlösung durchströmten Meerschweinchenlunge untersucht wurden (BAEHR u. PICK, 1913), bezog man das AT in diese Versuche nicht ein. Die Versuche von DALE und KELLAWAY (1922) wurden zwar nicht am intakten Tier ausgeführt, die Bedingungen glichen jedoch insofern denen am intakten Tier, als die Lunge mit Blut durchströmt war.

Erst in jüngerer Zeit wurde die AT-Wirkung auf die isolierte Lunge, und zwar entweder nur die Histaminliberation oder außerdem auch die bronchospastische Wirkung und die Wirkung auf die Lungengefäße untersucht (siehe unten).

FRIEDBERGER und KUMAGAI (1914) suchten als erste eine AT-Wirkung am isolierten Darm nachzuweisen, hatten jedoch am Meerschweinchendarm keine eindeutigen Ergebnisse.

Im Hinblick auf die Versuche von SCHULTZ (1910) und von DALE (1913) ist es unverständlich, daß sie eine lähmende und nicht eine kontrahierende Wirkung des AT auf den Darm erwarteten. Sie benutzten daher auch wegen der zahlreichen Spontankontraktionen meist den Kaninchendarm.

DOLD u. BÜRGER (1914) beobachteten zwar am Meerschweinchendarm eine kontrahierende Wirkung des Bacillen-AT, dieses wirkte jedoch nicht stärker als normales Serum. Ferner waren die tonussteigernden Stoffe im Gegensatz zum AT koktostabil und dialysabel.

In neuerer Zeit untersuchte zuerst ADANT (1950) die AT-Wirkung am Meerschweinchendarm, jedoch infolge Verwendung ungeeigneter Sera ohne Erfolg. Alle andern Autoren, die am isolierten Meerschweinchenileum arbeiteten, benutzten hochwirksames AT aus Rattenserum, das stets eine Kontraktion bewirkt (FRIEDBERG, ENGELHARDT und MEINEKE, 1963, 1964; GREISMAN, 1958; MOTA, 1959; MOUSSATCHÉ und DANON, 1956; OSLER, RANDALL u. a., 1959a, b; ROCHA E SILVA, 1952, 1954; ROCHA E SILVA und ARONSON, 1952; ROCHA E SILVA und ROTHSCHILD, 1956; ROTHSCHILD und ROCHA E SILVA, 1954).

Die Latenzperiode bei der isometrischen Kontraktion des Meerschweinchendarms beträgt nach AT 5–15 sec und ist anscheinend umgekehrt proportional der AT-Dosis. In der gleichen Versuchsanordnung beträgt die Latenzperiode nach Histamin weniger als 3 sec, nach Antigenzugabe am sensibilisierten Darm 30 sec und mehr. An diesem Präparat verläuft die Dosis-Wirkungskurve für AT steiler als für Histamin (RANDALL u. Mitarb., 1961).

Am isolierten Uterushorn sahen DALE und KELLAWAY (1922) nach Stärke-AT keine, nach Bacillen-AT eine schwache und nach Agar-AT eine stärkere Kontraktion.

Während in ihren Versuchen am intakten Meerschweinchen das Serum völlig ungiftig, das AT-haltige gleiche Serum dagegen tödlich giftig war, ist der Wirkungsunterschied zwischen normalem und AT-haltigem Serum am Meerschweinchenuterus nicht so erheblich. Ferner wirkt am intakten Meerschweinchen durch Berkefeldfilter mittlerer Porengröße filtriertes Agar-AT kaum schwächer als unfiltriertes, während die Wirkung auf den Uterus durch eine solche Filtration erheblich abnimmt. Die Autoren sahen in ihren Befunden ein Argument für die Annahme, daß AT am intakten Tier nicht durch eine Kontraktion glatter Muskeln wirkt. Mit diesen und andern Befunden (s. unten) begründeten sie ihre ablehnende Haltung zur AT-Theorie der Anaphylaxie.

In jüngerer Zeit fanden auch CONARD und MUTSAARS (1949) eine kontrahierende Wirkung von Agar-AT aus Meerschweinchenserum auf den isolierten Meerschweinchenuterus. Auch Agar- oder Sephadex-AT aus Rattenserum ist stark wirksam (FRIEDBERG, ENGELHARDT und MEINEKE, 1963, 1964).

HASHIMOTO (1928) und neuerdings FRIEDBERG und LENDLE (1955) sowie FRIEDBERG, ENGELHARDT und MEINEKE (1963, 1964) beschrieben eine constrictorische AT-Wirkung auf die Gefäße des durchströmten Meerschweinchenhinterleibes und -hinterschenkels. SCHEIFFARTH, GEMÄHLICH u. a. (1958) beobachteten eine verengernde AT-Wirkung auf die Mesenterialgefäße des Meerschweinchens. FRIEDBERG, ENGELHARDT und MEINEKE (1963, 1964) sahen eine starke Wirkung von AT aus Rattenserum auf den isolierten Streifen der Art. pulmonalis des Meerschweinchens. Eine Durchströmungsminderung nach AT an der isolierten Meerschweinchenlunge wurde ebenfalls beobachtet (GIERTZ, HAHN, OPFERKUCH und SCHMUTZLER, 1961; GIERTZ und SCHMUTZLER, 1960; HAHN, GIERTZ und SCHMUTZLER, 1961). GREEFF und BOKELMANN (1959) fanden eine coronarverengernde Wirkung von Dextran-AT aus Rattenserum am LANGENDORFF-Präparat des Meerschweinchenherzens. Hier wie auch am Meerschweinchenvorhof verursachte das AT außerdem eine Zunahme der Schlagfrequenz und der Hubhöhe (GREEFF, BENFEY und BOKELMANN, 1959; GREEFF und BOKELMANN, 1959).

Einige Autoren beschrieben eine permeabilitätserhöhende Wirkung von AT auf die Capillaren der Meerschweinchenhaut (HALPERN, LIACOPOULOS und LIACOPOULOS-BRIOT, 1959; LIACOPOULOS, HALPERN und LIACOPOULOS-BRIOT, 1957; OSLER, RANDALL u. a., 1959a). Dieser Test ist besonders geeignet, um Vergleiche zwischen AT-Wirkung und cutaner Anaphylaxie anzustellen. Andererseits ist gerade in diesem Test die Eigenwirkung des normalen Serums besonders ausgeprägt (OSLER, RANDALL u. a., 1959a) und daher bei der AT-Testung sehr störend.

Aber auch an den meisten isolierten, glattmuskeligen Organen macht sich die Tatsache störend bemerkbar, daß auch normales, nicht AT-haltiges Serum bereits eine Kontraktion glatter Muskeln verursachen kann. Nur bei Verwendung starker ATe läßt sich die AT-Wirkung gut von der Serumeigenwirkung differenzieren. Für einen Vergleich schwächerer ATe mit stärkeren eignet sich daher praktisch nur der Versuch am intakten Tier.

b) Die Wirkung des AT auf das Blutbild

Von DALE und KELLAWAY (1922) wurde erstmals die Wirkung von AT (Stärke-, Bakterien- und Agar-AT aus Meerschweinchenserum) auf das Blut untersucht. Sie beschreiben einen Abfall der Leukocytenzahl im Schock, der vor allem durch einen Schwund der polymorphkernigen Leukocyten bedingt ist.

Da die Autoren einen solchen Leukocytenschwund auch im anaphylaktischen Schock und im Histaminschock beobachteten, sahen sie darin keine spezifische AT-Wirkung. Dementsprechend sahen sie auch keine Unterschiede in der Wirkung von Stärke-, Bacillen- und Agar-AT, wie sie hinsichtlich der anderen AT-Wirkungen sowohl am intakten Tier als auch am isolierten Organ zu beobachten waren.

In jüngerer Zeit bestätigten HAHN und LANGE (1956) diesen Sachverhalt mit Inulin-AT aus Meerschweinchenserum. Sie fanden jedoch auch, daß bereits normales Meerschweinchenserum einen Leukocytenschwund verursacht, allerdings nicht ganz so deutlich wie AT-haltiges Serum. Sie stellten keinen Zusammenhang zwischen dem Leukocytenschwund und der Schwere des Schocks fest. GIERTZ, HAHN, JURNA und SCHMUTZLER (1961) sowie GIERTZ, HAHN, SCHMUTZLER und KOLLMEIER (1964) sahen auch nach Dextran-AT aus Rattenserum einen Granulocytenschwund; normales Rattenserum bewirkte einen geringeren Schwund. Aus den Versuchen aller genannten Autoren ergibt sich also, daß AT-haltige Sera zwar einen Leukocytenschwund bewirken, daß dieser aber keine Beziehung zu den typischen AT-Wirkungen hat.

DALE und KELLAWAY (1922) fanden im AT-Schock im Gegensatz zum anaphylaktischen Schock und zum Histaminschock einen besonders ausgeprägten Thrombocytensturz. Auch nach HAHN und LANGE (1956) sinkt die Thrombocytenzahl durch Inulin-AT aus Meerschweinchenserum viel stärker als durch normales Serum ab. Giertz, Hahn, Jurna und Schmutzler (1961) sowie Giertz, Hahn, Schmutzler und Kollmeier (1964) beobachteten nur nach Dextran-AT aus Rattenserum, nicht aber im anaphylaktischen Schock und im Histaminschock einen statistisch gesicherten Thrombocytenschwund. Hahn und Lange (1956) sahen keinen Zusammenhang zwischen der Schwere des Schocks und dem Thrombocytensturz durch AT.

Man könnte bei solchen Versuchen daran denken, daß es nicht das AT, sondern die im Serum gelösten Kontaktstoffe sind, welche die Veränderungen im weißen Blutbild bewirken. Hahn, Lange u. Giertz (1954) sahen nämlich an der Ratte einen Abfall der Leukocyten- und Thrombocytenzahlen durch Dextran. Befunde an der Ratte mit Dextran sind jedoch nur unter starken Vorbehalten auf das Meerschweinchen zu übertragen, weil Dextran an der Ratte im Gegensatz zum Meerschweinchen eine starke Giftwirkung hat (s. Dextrankapitel).

Giertz, Hahn, Jurna und Schmutzler (1961) berichten auch über ein Ansteigen der Erythrocytenzahlen im AT-Schock. Diese AT-Wirkung weist wohl auf eine Bluteindickung im Schock hin, wie sie sich auch im anaphylaktischen Schock und im Histaminschock findet. Nach Injektion von normalem, nicht AT-haltigen Rattenserum sinkt die Erythrocytenzahl entsprechend der Blutverdünnung ab.

Da die weißen Blutzellen Histamin enthalten, sinkt durch den starken Abfall der Thrombocyten und Leukocyten der Gehalt des Blutes an cellulär gebundenem Histamin im AT-Schock erheblich ab. Daher entspricht bei dieser Schockform die Zunahme des Histaminspiegels im Gesamtblut nicht der Histaminausschüttung aus dem Gewebe ins Plasma (siehe folgenden Abschnitt) und ist trotz gleicher Plasmahistaminkonzentration geringer als bei anderen Schockformen (z. B. beim anaphylaktischen Schock durch Ovalbumin), die nicht mit einer solchen Abnahme der weißen Blutzellen einhergehen (Giertz, Hahn, Schmutzler und Kollmeier, 1964).

c) *Die Histaminfreisetzung durch AT*

Auf die Ähnlichkeit des AT-Schocks mit dem Histaminschock wurde bald nach der Entdeckung des AT hingewiesen (Kumagai, 1913). Es wurde auch experimentell geprüft, ob nicht AT und Histamin identisch seien (Friedberger und Moreschi, 1912; Friedberger, Szymanowski u. a., 1912). An eine Beteiligung des Histamins an der AT-Wirkung dachte jedoch niemand.

Die Erkenntnis, daß die typischen AT-Effekte durch eine Histaminfreisetzung vermittelt werden, wurde zuerst durch Versuche mit Antihistaminica gewonnen.

Im Jahre 1950 konnten Hahn und Oberdorf durch subcutane Vorbehandlung von Meerschweinchen mit Antazolin (1 mg/kg) oder Chlorpyramin (5,4 mg/kg) den Schock durch Inulin-AT aus Meerschweinchenserum verhindern. Eine intravenöse Vorbehandlung mit 10 μg/kg von Mepyraminmaleat reicht aus, den Schock des Meerschweinchens durch Dextran-AT aus Rattenserum zu verhindern. Die gleiche Antihistamindosis reicht auch aus, einen gleich schweren Schock (gemessen an der Todesrate) durch intravenöse Histamininjektion zu verhindern (Giertz, Hahn, Jurna und Schmutzler, 1961; Hahn, Giertz und Schmutzler, 1961).

Trotz der Aufhebung der letalen AT-Wirkung am intakten Tier durch Antihistaminica fanden wir neuerdings gemeinsam mit Bernauer und Schmutzler einen Wirkungsrest, wenn wir den Beatmungswiderstand registrierten. Solche antihistaminresistente Wirkung beobachteten wir auch nach Injektion von normalem Rattenserum, jedoch in erheblich geringerem Maße als nach AT. Hier liegt also ein Hinweis auf eine Komponente der AT-Wirkung vor, die nicht durch Histamin bedingt ist.

Auch am Herz-Lungen-Präparat des Meerschweinchens, welches mit Heparinblut oder Erythrocytensuspension in Tyrodelösung durchströmt wird, läßt sich die AT-Wirkung durch Antihistaminica nicht ganz aufheben, wobei auch in diesem

Fall der übrigbleibende Effekt über die Wirkung normalen Rattenserums hinausgeht.

Merkwürdigerweise ließ sich aber der AT-Effekt an der isolierten, mit Salzlösung durchströmten Lunge durch Antihistaminica vollständig aufheben bis auf einen Wirkungsrest, der sich aber mit der Wirkung normalen Rattenserums deckte (GIERTZ, HAHN, OPFERKUCH u. SCHMUTZLER, 1961; HAHN, GIERTZ u. SCHMUTZLER, 1961). Die Antihistamindosen, die an der isolierten Lunge zur Aufhebung der AT-Wirkung erforderlich sind, betragen aber etwa das 10fache der Dosen (Mepyraminmaleat 10 μg/ml statt 1 μg/ml), die zur Aufhebung einer gleich starken Histaminwirkung nötig sind. Dies steht im Gegensatz zu den oben erwähnten Versuchen am intakten Tier, wo man gleiche Antihistamindosen zur Hemmung des AT- und des Histaminschocks (gemessen an der Todesrate) benötigt. Diesen Unterschied zwischen intaktem Tier und isolierter Lunge kann man durch die Tatsache erklären, daß an der isolierten Lunge nach AT-Zufuhr nur endopulmonal freigesetztes Histamin wirksam wird (vgl. DALE, 1948).

Am isolierten Meerschweinchendarm wurden zwar sehr verschiedene Antihistaminkonzentrationen zur AT-Hemmung angewandt (von 0,001–1,0 μg/ml Mepyraminmaleat), doch ist die Wirkung des AT hier sicher leichter zu hemmen als an der isolierten Lunge (HAINING, 1956b; MOTA, 1959; ROTHSCHILD und ROCHA E SILVA, 1954). Allerdings scheint am isolierten Meerschweinchendarm und -uterus ein histaminunabhängiger Mechanismus beteiligt zu sein; denn am Uterus läßt sich die AT-Kontraktion weder durch Antihistaminica noch durch Desensibilisierung gegen Histamin hemmen; am Darm läßt sich zwar durch Antihistaminica die AT-Wirkung hemmen, doch nach einer unter bestimmten Bedingungen durchgeführten Desensibilisierung gegen Histamin erfolgt noch eine, allerdings abgeschwächte, Kontraktion durch Ratten-AT (VOGT und ZEMANN, 1964). Die Ergebnisse von VOGT und ZEMANN am Meerschweinchenuterus stimmen mit älteren Versuchen von CONARD und MUTSAARS (1949) überein.

Am isolierten Meerschweinchenvorhof wird die Amplitudenvergrößerung durch AT durch Mepyraminmaleat, Tripelennamin und Isothipendyl gehemmt. Die zur Hemmung notwendigen Antihistaminkonzentrationen sind hier (anders als an der isolierten Lunge) nicht höher als die zur Histaminhemmung nötigen Konzentrationen. Die AT-Tachykardie kann an diesem Präparat genauso wenig wie die Histamintachykardie durch Antihistaminica unterdrückt werden. Die Zunahme der Hubhöhe am LANGENDORFF-Herzen durch AT läßt sich wie am Vorhofpräparat hemmen (GREEFF, BENFEY und BOKELMANN, 1959; GREEFF und BOKELMANN, 1959). Das gleiche gilt für die Coronarverengerung durch AT, nach FRIEDBERG, ENGELHARDT und MEINEKE (1963, 1964) auch für die AT-Kontraktion des isolierten Pulmonalisstreifens.

Die Permeabilitätsänderung in den Capillaren der Meerschweinchenhaut durch AT ist ebenfalls durch Antihistaminica hemmbar (HALPERN, LIACOPOULOS und LIACOPOULOS-BRIOT, 1959; LIACOPOULOS, HALPERN und LIACOPOULOS-BRIOT, 1957). Dabei erwies sich Promethazin am wirksamsten, weniger wirksam Mepyramin und kaum wirksam Chlorpromazin. Die gleiche Reihenfolge der Wirkungsstärke zeigte sich gegenüber der Permeabilitätserhöhung durch Histamin, doch reichten hier geringere Dosen als zur Hemmung des AT-Effektes aus.

Eine Histaminfreisetzung durch AT wurde zuerst von ROCHA E SILVA und Mitarbeitern beschrieben. Sie beobachten nach 4 ml eines Agar-AT aus Meerschweinchenserum eine erhebliche Histaminfreisetzung aus der isolierten, mit Salzlösung durchströmten Meerschweinchenlunge, die in einem Fall nicht weniger als 103 μg innerhalb 10 min betrug (ROCHA E SILVA und ARONSON, 1952; ROCHA E SILVA, BIER und ARONSON, 1951). Eine geringere Histaminfreisetzung durch

Dextran-AT aus Ratten- oder Meerschweinchenserum beschrieben GIERTZ, HAHN, OPFERKUCH und SCHMUTZLER (1961). In diesen Versuchen wurde außer der Histaminfreisetzung und der Durchflußrate auch der Bronchospasmus gemessen. Die Stärke des Bronchospasmus ging der insgesamt freigesetzten Histaminmenge parallel (vgl. auch HAHN, GIERTZ und SCHMUTZLER, 1961). In kürzlich von FRICK, HALPERN und LIACOPOULOS (1961, 1962) beschriebenen Versuchen war die Histaminfreisetzung durch AT aus der isolierten Meerschweinchenlunge ebenfalls geringer als in ROCHA E SILVAs Untersuchungen.

Der Unterschied in dem von ROCHA E SILVA und den anderen Autoren beobachteten Ausmaß der Histaminfreisetzung mag daran liegen, daß verschiedene ATe und verschieden große Versuchstiere verwandt wurden. Ferner arbeiteten GIERTZ u. Mitarb. sowie FRICK u. Mitarb. ihre Perfusate vor der Histaminbestimmung auf, um störende, einen zu hohen Histamingehalt vortäuschende Faktoren auszuschalten.

Der zweite Weg, eine Histaminfreisetzung durch AT zu zeigen, wurde zuerst von HAHN (1954a) beschritten, der eine Erhöhung des Plasmahistaminspiegels im Schock durch Inulin-AT aus Meerschweinchenserum beobachtete. Diese Erhöhung fand sich vor allem bei solchen Tieren, die nach AT schwer oder tödlich schockten. Auch GIERTZ, HAHN, JURNA und SCHMUTZLER (1961) fanden eine Erhöhung des Plasmahistaminspiegels nach Dextran-AT aus Rattenserum. Diese war deutlich abhängig von der AT-Dosis und ging parallel mit der Todesrate.

Neuerdings wurde im AT-Schock eine stark erhöhte Histaminaseaktivität im Blut nachgewiesen, die zwar nicht so stark ist wie im anaphylaktischen Schock, aber normalerweise und auch nach Histamininjektion nicht zu beobachten ist (GIERTZ, HAHN, HAHN und SCHMUTZLER 1962; SCHMUTZLER, GIERTZ und HAHN, 1963; GIERTZ, HAHN und SCHMUTZLER, 1964). Schon während der Plasmagewinnung wird ein Teil des Plasmahistamins zerstört, so daß die früher angegebenen Werte allesamt zu niedrig sind. Der Plasmahistaminspiegel im AT-Schock läßt sich daher nur in Gegenwart eines Histaminasehemmstoffes (Aminoguanidinsulfat) bestimmen. Er betrug im Mittel von 30 Versuchen nach 5 ml/kg Dextran-AT aus Rattenserum etwa 1 μg/ml bei einer Letalität von etwa 90%. Die Histaminaseaktivität im Plasma von Tieren im AT-Schock war etwa 10mal höher als im normalen Meerschweinchenplasma und etwa 10mal niedriger als im Plasma von Tieren im anaphylaktischen Schock (GIERTZ, HAHN und SCHMUTZLER, 1964). Die Aktivierung der Histaminase erfolgt wahrscheinlich in der Leber durch die Vermittlung von Heparin (BERNAUER u. Mitarb., 1964).

Die hohen Histaminkonzentrationen im Plasma der AT-behandelten Tiere sind bemerkenswert, weil man solche Konzentrationen nur durch intravenöse Injektion von Histamindosen erreichen kann, die selbst eine Schockwirkung haben. Die Injektion von Histamindosen, wie sie aus der isolierten Lunge maximal freigesetzt werden, beeinflußt den Histaminspiegel dagegen nicht (H. HAHN, 1964).

Die gute Hemmbarkeit des AT-Schocks durch Antihistaminica und der stark erhöhte Histaminspiegel deuten darauf hin, daß am AT-Schock des intakten Tieres auch Histamin beteiligt ist, das aus andern Organen der Lunge zufließt, wofür sich in neueren, gemeinsam mit BERNAUER und SCHMUTZLER am Herz-Lungen-Präparat durchgeführten Versuchen auch weitere Anhaltspunkte ergaben.

Es gäbe noch eine weitere Möglichkeit, eine Histaminbeteiligung am AT-Schock nachzuweisen: die Untersuchung der AT-Wirkung an Tieren, deren Histamindepots mit Hilfe anderer Histaminliberatoren erschöpft sind. An andern Tierarten sind ähnliche Versuche durchgeführt worden (vgl. Dextran- und PVP-Kapitel). Dabei hat sich jedoch gezeigt, daß das bei verschiedenen Schockformen freigesetzte Histamin aus verschiedenen Organen stammen kann, so daß ein negativer Ausfall eines solchen Versuchs nichts besagt. Ferner besteht die Möglichkeit, daß die zur Vorbehandlung benutzten Histaminliberatoren eine Toleranzsteigerung bewirken, die nicht auf einer Entleerung der Histamindepots beruht. Daher spricht die Beobachtung von SCHEIFFARTH, FRENGER u. GEMÄHLICH (1958), daß eine Stilbamidinvorbehandlung den AT-Schock nicht beeinflußt, nicht gegen eine Histaminbeteiligung am AT-Schock, zumal die Autoren unseres Wissens nicht untersucht haben, ob Stilbamidin beim

Meerschweinchen überhaupt Histamin liberiert. Bei der Unempfindlichkeit für andere Histaminliberatoren ist das nämlich nicht wahrscheinlich.

Wie die chemische Histaminliberation an andern Tierarten so beruht auch die Histaminfreisetzung durch AT beim Meerschweinchen auf einer Schädigung der Mastzellen.

Im Jahre 1953 beschrieb RILEY als erster eine Mastzellschädigung durch AT, allerdings an Mastzellen der Ratte. Da es nur wenige Anhaltspunkte für eine AT-Wirkung an der Ratte gibt (s. unten) und die meisten Versuche eine Unwirksamkeit an dieser Tierart ergaben und da ferner diese Beobachtung von MOTA (1957) nicht bestätigt wurde, müßte die Wirkung von AT auf Rattenmastzellen noch einmal experimentell überprüft werden.

Ein Zerfall von Meerschweinchenmastzellen durch AT, und zwar von Mastzellen des Mesenteriums, wurde im Jahre 1957 von MOTA beschrieben. GEMÄHLICH, FRENGER und SCHEIFFARTH (1958) berichteten über eine Zerstörung der Mastzellen im AT-Schock, vor allem der Lungen-Mastzellen.

Die AT-Wirkung auf die Mastzellen des Meerschweinchenmesenteriums wird durch Jodacetat (0,001 Mol/l), p-Chlormercuribenzoat (0,001 Mol/l) oder Phenol (0,01 Mol/l) gehemmt (MOTA, 1959). In calciumfreier Tyrodelösung, die noch zusätzlich das calciumbindende Versen (Na-Salz der EDTA) enthielt, verlief die AT-Wirkung ungestört. Wurde das Mesenterium vor der AT-Gabe auf 45° C erhitzt, so verlief anschließend die Mastzellschädigung durch AT ebenfalls ungestört (MOTA, 1959); p-Chlormercuribenzoat (MOTA, 1959; MOUSSATCHÉ und DANON, 1956) und Phenol (MOTA, 1959) hemmen auch die AT-Kontraktion des isolierten Meerschweinchendarmes, während Erhitzung des Darmes auf 45° C eine nachfolgende AT-Kontraktion unbeeinflußt läßt (MOTA, 1959). Diese Parallelen zwischen der Mastzellschädigung und der Darmkontraktion durch AT deuten auf einen ursächlichen Zusammenhang hin. Nach ROTHSCHILD und BARRETO (1961) läßt sich die Histaminfreisetzungdurch AT aus Lungenschnitten vom Meerschweinchen durch NaCN, DNP und Sauerstoffmangel hemmen. Diese Hemmung bleibt jedoch bei Gegenwart von Glucose aus. An der Mitochondrienfraktion der Meerschweinchenlunge setzt Rattenanaphylatoxin kein Histamin frei (GIERTZ, REUTTER und SCHMUTZLER, 1964b).

Möglicherweise wirken auch das Na-Salicylat (4 mg/ml) und die 5-Hydroxyphenylcinchoninsäure (0,5 mg/ml) dadurch hemmend auf die Darmkontraktion durch AT (HAINING, 1956b), daß sie die Mastzellschädigung und damit die Histaminfreisetzung verhindern.

Nach SCHEIFFARTH u. Mitarb. hemmt Prednisonvorbehandlung die Mastzellschädigung durch AT; dadurch läßt sich möglicherweise die Hemmung des AT-Schocks durch Prednison oder Prednisolon erklären (FRENGER, SCHEIFFARTH u. GEMÄHLICH, 1958; SCHEIFFARTH, FRENGER u. a., 1958). Die gleichen Autoren diskutieren jedoch auch die Möglichkeit, daß die Wirkung der Prednisonvorbehandlung auf eine Hemmung der Histaminsynthese in den Mastzellen zurückzuführen ist. Andererseits fanden sie (GEMÄHLICH, FRENGER u. SCHEIFFARTH, 1958), daß nach Stilbamidinvorbehandlung der AT-Schock ungestört abläuft, obwohl auch diese Vorbehandlung die Mastzellschädigung durch AT hemmen soll. Auf welche Weise die Vorbehandlung mit einem Proteuspolysaccharid den AT-Schock abschwächt (JAQUES, 1961), ist bisher nicht bekannt.

Es liegt nahe anzunehmen, daß die schon in der älteren Literatur bekannte Wirkungsabnahme des AT bei wiederholter Gabe auf einer sukzessiven Entleerung der Histamindepots beruht. Diese Ansicht äußerten vor allem ROCHA E SILVA und ROTHSCHILD (1956), die das Phänomen gründlich am Meerschweinchenileum untersuchten. Weitere Versuche über die Wirkungsabnahme wiederholter AT-Gaben führten GREISMAN (1958) ebenfalls am isolierten Darm und GREEFF und Mitarbeiter (GREEFF, BENFEY und BOKELMANN, 1959; GREEFF und BOKELMANN, 1959) am isolierten Meerschweinchenvorhof durch. An allen isolierten Organen nimmt die AT-Wirkung bei wiederholter Gabe zunehmend bis zur völligen Unwirksamkeit nach etwa 3—6 Dosen ab. Mit der Ansicht, dieses Phänomen beruhe auf einer Entleerung der Histamindepots, lassen sich die Befunde von ROCHA E SILVA und ARONSON (1952) und ROCHA E SILVA, BIER und ARONSON (1951) gut vereinbaren, daß die Histaminfreisetzung aus der isolierten Lunge nach der ersten Gabe stets stärker als nach einer wiederholten Gabe ist. GIERTZ, HAHN u. a. (1961) zeigten, daß an der isolierten Lunge nicht nur die Histaminfreisetzung, sondern auch der Bronchospasmus nach der ersten AT-Gabe stets am stärksten war. FRICK und Mitarbeiter (FRICK, HALPERN und LIACOPOULOS, 1962; FRICK, LIACOPOULOS und HALPERN, 1961) behandelten Meerschweinchen 6 Tage lang mit steigenden Dosen Dextran-AT aus Rattenserum und fanden dann eine Abnahme des Histamingehaltes der Lunge auf durchschnittlich 25 % (9,8 μg/g) des normalen Wertes (38,6 μg/g). Im Dünndarm und in der Bauchhaut nahm dagegen der Histamingehalt nicht ab. Aus isolierten Lungen der AT-vorbehandelten Tiere ließ sich durch AT wesentlich weniger Histamin freisetzen als aus den Lungen normaler Tiere, und zwar auch dann, wenn die Versuche erst 14 Tage nach der letzten AT-Injektion durchgeführt wurden.

Es gibt jedoch Hinweise in der Literatur, daß die Wirkungsabnahme wiederholter AT-Gaben nicht nur auf einer fortschreitenden Zerstörung der Mastzellen, d. h. auf einer Entleerung der Histamindepots beruhen kann. Besonders bemerkenswert ist, daß die Toleranzsteigerung gegen AT nach einer AT-Gabe nur so kurze Zeit anhält, daß sich die Histamindepots in dieser Zeit unmöglich wieder auffüllen können. So dauert am isolierten Darm die Empfindlichkeitsminderung gegen AT nur etwa 30–40 min (ROCHA E SILVA, 1960).

Lediglich FRIEDBERGER (1910a) behauptete in seiner ersten Mitteilung über das AT, er habe mehrere Tage nach einer AT-Gabe eine Toleranzsteigerung gegen eine zweite Dosis beobachtet. Doch zwei Jahre später schrieb er (FRIEDBERGER, SZYMANOWSKI u. a., 1912), daß keine Empfindlichkeitsminderung gegen eine Zweitinjektion von AT zu beobachten sei, wenn diese 24 Std nach der Erstinjektion erfolge. Die Autoren weisen ausdrücklich darauf hin, daß SACHS und RITZ (zit. nach FRIEDBERGER, SZYMANOWSKI u. a., 1912) deshalb eine Empfindlichkeitsabnahme sahen, weil bei ihnen die Zeitintervalle zwischen beiden Injektionen kürzer (20—45 min) waren.

FRIEDBERG, ENGELHARDT und MEINEKE (1963, 1964) kamen ebenfalls zu dem Ergebnis, daß sowohl am intakten Tier als auch am isolierten Meerschweinchenileum und -uterus die Empfindlichkeitsminderung nur kurze Zeit anhält; schon eine halbe Stunde nach den ersten, zur Unempfindlichkeit des Testobjekts führenden Injektionen, läßt sich am isolierten Organ wieder ein AT-Effekt nachweisen. Am intakten Tier dauert die Unempfindlichkeit allerdings etwa 12 Std an. Dieser Unterschied zwischen dem isolierten Organ und dem intakten Organismus könnte vielleicht dadurch bedingt sein, daß beim intakten Tier das injizierte AT längere Zeit im Blute kreist, wogegen es am isolierten Organ gleich nach Ablauf der Kontraktion ausgewaschen wird.

Diese Befunde machen es wahrscheinlich, daß es auch eine Toleranzsteigerung gibt, die nicht durch eine Depotentleerung bedingt ist. Dementsprechend läßt sie sich auch nachweisen, ohne daß eine Zerstörung von Mastzellen erfolgt. MOTA (1959) bewahrte ein Stück Meerschweinchenmesenterium bei 15° C in AT-haltigem Serum auf. Bei dieser niedrigen Temperatur trat keine Mastzellschädigung auf, trotzdem aber wurde das Präparat unempfindlich gegen eine zweite AT-Einwirkung bei 37° C. Ferner ließ der gleiche Autor auf ein Stück Meerschweinchenmesenterium AT in Gegenwart von Phenol (0,001 Mol/l) einwirken. Die Mastzellen blieben dabei intakt, doch nach dem Auswaschen des AT und des Phenols war das Präparat gegen eine zweite AT-Gabe unempfindlich. Der gleiche Versuch ließ sich auch am Meerschweinchenileum durchführen, an dem die AT-Kontraktion durch Phenol gehemmt wird und an dem nach einer zweiten AT-Gabe in phenolfreiem Milieu die Kontraktion ausblieb, obwohl der Darm gegen Histamin normal empfindlich war.

Es soll hier noch einmal betont werden, daß diese Art der AT-Tachyphylaxie nicht eine Toleranzsteigerung durch Mastzellzerstörung ausschließt. Die bereits erwähnten Versuche von FRICK u. Mitarb. (1961, 1962) zeigen klar, daß eine länger dauernde Vorbehandlung mit AT eine Toleranzsteigerung durch Zerstörung der Mastzellen und Entleerung der Histamindepots verursacht. Allein aus der Tatsache, daß die AT-Tachyphylaxie nur kurz andauert und daß sich die AT-Kontraktion mehrmals wiederholen läßt, kann man keine schlüssigen Argumente gegen eine Histaminbeteiligung an der AT-Wirkung ableiten; denn durch eine einzige AT-Kontraktion werden wahrscheinlich nicht mehr als 2–5 % der Mastzellen des Darmes zerstört (ROCHA E SILVA, 1960).

d) *Wirkt AT auch an anderen Tierarten als am Meerschweinchen?*

Alle Autoren, die eine AT-Wirkung an anderen Tierarten als am Meerschweinchen nachzuweisen suchten, kamen bei Verwendung intakter Versuchstiere nicht zu eindeutig positiven Ergebnissen. Insbesondere ist nie ein tödlicher, durch Histaminfreisetzung bedingter Schock durch AT an einer anderen Tierart beobachtet worden, auch nicht an der Ratte, deren Serum ein sehr starkes, und am Kaninchen, dessen Serum ein schwaches AT bildet.

Nach KRAUS und KIRSCHBAUM (1913) war Agar-AT aus Meerschweinchenserum am Hund (40 ml i. v.) unwirksam, ebenso wenig wirkte die gleiche Dosis agarbehandelten Hundeserums. Die Autoren sahen auch keinen Effekt von Agar-AT aus Meerschweinchen- oder Kaninchenserum (20 ml/kg) am Kaninchen. NOVY und DE KRUIF (1917d) betonen, daß für Meerschweinchen hochtoxisches Rattenserum-AT an Kaninchen in Dosen von etwa 10–20 ml/kg völlig unwirksam war und daß Ratten mehr als das Hundertfache der für Meerschweinchen giftigen Dosis symptomlos vertrugen.

FRIEDEMANN (1909) beobachtete leicht anaphylaxieähnliche Symptome (Unruhe, Atemstörungen) an Kaninchen, die mit amboceptorbeladenen Rindererythrocyten inkubiertes Kaninchenserum erhielten. Manche Autoren (Lit. siehe DOERR, 1929) bezeichnen ihn deshalb als eigentlichen Entdecker des AT. ZUNZ und GELAT (1915) sowie ZUNZ und MOHILEVITCH (1916) fanden einen leichten Effekt von Agar- und Pararabin-AT aus Pferdeserum an Kaninchen. Sie betonen, daß das AT am Kaninchen nur in optimaler Dosierung wirksam sei, zu viel oder zu wenig sei unwirksam. Am Meerschweinchen wurden derartige Beobachtungen nicht gemacht, stets ging die Schwere des Schocks mit der Höhe der Dosis parallel.

Am isolierten Kaninchenherzen wurde von RYLANT (1923) eine Wirkung von Kaninchenserum-AT beobachtet, die der AT-Wirkung am Meerschweinchenherzen zwar ähnelt, aber nicht gleicht. Angeblich soll AT auch am Froschherzen Wirkungen entfalten (FRIEDBERGER u. MITA, 1911), die der Anaphylaxie des Froschherzens (KÖNIGSFELD, 1925) gleichen. Am Kaninchendarm sahen FRIEDBERGER u. Mitarb. eine uncharakteristische, nämlich lähmende Wirkung.

Die spärlichen Beobachtungen schwacher AT-Effekte am Kaninchen stehen negativen Befunden gegenüber und reichen daher nicht als Beweis für eine AT-Wirkung am Kaninchen aus. Sie verdienen jedoch im Lichte neuerer Untersuchungen Beachtung. Kaninchenplasma läßt sich nämlich durch eine Reihe von Maßnahmen, wie sie auch zur AT-Bildung geeignet sind, so aktivieren, daß es aus Kaninchenthrombocyten Histamin (und Serotonin) freisetzt. HAINING (1956b) weist zwar auf die Ähnlichkeiten im Bildungsmodus zwischen dem an Kaninchenthrombocyten wirksamen Histaminliberator und AT hin, hält beide jedoch nicht für identisch. Wir referieren daher über diesen AT-ähnlichen Stoff an anderer Stelle (s. u.).

Über eine eventuelle AT-Wirkung an der Ratte stehen in der neueren Literatur einigen negativen Befunden positive Ergebnisse gegenüber. RILEY (1953), der im Gegensatz zu MOTA (1957) eine Zerstörung der Mastzellen des Rattenmesenteriums durch AT beobachtete, betont, daß AT im Gegensatz zu anderen Histaminliberatoren nicht die Mastzellen der Subcutis schädige, so daß das Ausbleiben des Ödems (vgl. Eiklar- und Dextrankapitel) nicht gegen die Mastzellschädigung spricht. Gegen einen massiven Mastzellzerfall lassen sich die Befunde von HAHN, LANGE und GIERTZ (1954) bzw. von HALPERN, BRIOT und NEVEU (1954a, b) anführen, die keine Wirkung von Inulin- bzw. Agar-AT an der Ratte sahen. HAHN, LANGE und GIERTZ (1954) sowie MOTA (1957) fanden auch keine Erhöhung des Plasmahistaminspiegels bei der Ratte. Eine Vorbehandlung von Ratten mit Hämophilus-Pertussis-Vaccine machte Ratten nicht empfindlich gegen AT (GIERTZ, HAHN und SCHMUTZLER, unveröffentlicht), obwohl es sie gegen Histamin und Serotonin empfindlicher macht (Lit. siehe HAHN und GIERTZ, 1960) und eventuell auch die Freisetzung dieser Amine begünstigt (MOTA, 1958). SCHEIFFARTH, GEMÄHLICH u. a. (1958) sahen weder eine Wirkung von AT an der intakten Ratte noch an den Mesenterialgefäßen dieser Tierart bei lokaler Anwendung.

Hinweise auf eine AT-Wirkung an der Ratte sind allerdings die Befunde von FERLUGA (1960), FRIEDBERG, ENGELHARDT und MEINEKE (1963, 1964) sowie VOGT und ZEMANN (1964). Diese Autoren beobachteten an isolierten glattmuskeligen Rattenorganen (Duodenum, Ileum, Colon, Uterus, Streifen der Art. pulmonalis) Kontraktionen durch anaphylatoxinhaltiges Serum. Diese Kontraktionen sind nicht durch Antihistaminica, BOL 148, Reserpin oder Atropinsulfat zu hemmen. Die Bildung des an Rattenorganen wirksamen Stoffes läßt sich wie die AT-Bildung durch Vorerwärmung des Rattenserums auf 56°C, durch Heparin, durch Na-Citrat und durch Na_3HEDTA hemmen. Die Aktivität wurde durch einstündige Erwärmung des aktivierten Serums auf 69° C abgeschwächt und durch Chymotrypsinbehandlung aufgehoben. Trotz der Parallelen, die in der Wirkung und im Bildungsmechanismus zwischen der an Rattenorganen wirksamen Substanz und AT bestehen, betont FERLUGA (1960), daß er nichts Sicheres über die Identität der beiden Stoffe sagen kann. In einer späteren Veröffentlichung (FERLUGA, 1961) allerdings führt er die an Ratten nach Dextran-, Levan- und Inulininjektion von ihm beobachteten Hämorrhagien, Ödeme und Exsudationen im Gastrointestinalgebiet auf eine Vermittlung von in vivo entstehendem AT zurück. Bemerkenswert ist noch, daß an den glattmuskeligen Rattenorganen (Ileum, Uterus, A. pulmonalis) AT keine deutliche Tachyphylaxie zeigte (FRIEDBERG, ENGELHARDT und MEINEKE, 1963, 1964).

Während nach FERLUGA (1960) die von ihm untersuchten Polysaccharide in Abwesenheit humoraler Faktoren an isolierten Rattenorganen unwirksam sind, beschrieben neuerdings LENDLE und WEISSER (1962) eine Konstriktion der Gefäße des durchströmten Rattenhinterschenkels und eine Kontraktion des Rattenileums durch Dextran. Die spontane Automatie des Rattenuterus wurde dagegen durch Dextran gehemmt. Darin, daß auch Hühnereiweiß am Rattenhinterschenkel und am Rattenileum ähnlich, wenn auch keineswegs gleich wie Dextran wirkt, sehen die Autoren eine Beziehung zur anaphylaktoiden Reaktion der Ratte. Andererseits wirkten Dextran und Eiweiß am Rattenuterus völlig verschieden, und keine der untersuchten Reaktionen scheint nach den Untersuchungen der Autoren von einer Serotonin- oder Histaminfreisetzung abzuhängen.

AT aus Rattenserum bewirkt auch eine Erregung des Hühneramnions (FRIEDBERG, ENGELHARDT und MEINEKE, 1963, 1964).

5. Die biologische Bedeutung des AT

a) *Das AT und die Anaphylaxie des Meerschweinchens*

Die Friedbergersche Theorie, die im AT das Anaphylaxiegift sah und sogar eine Beteiligung des AT bei Infektionskrankheiten unterstellte (FRIEDBERGER, 1910b), ist ihrem Wesen nach eine humorale Theorie der Anaphylaxie. Aus dem Grundversuch der zellulären Anaphylaxietheorie, der Auslösung anaphylaktischer Reaktionen am isolierten, blutfreien Organ (DALE, 1913; SCHULTZ, 1910), ergibt sich jedoch, daß die Anaphylaxie nicht an die Anwesenheit eines aus dem Blute stammenden Anaphylaxiegiftes wie AT gebunden ist.

Bei dieser Sachlage könnte man sich höchstens fragen, ob auch bei dem cellulären Geschehen ein AT-ähnlicher Faktor, also eine Art Gewebs-AT, beteiligt wäre. Es sei hier auf Versuche von AUSTEN und BROCKLEHURST (1960) verwiesen, aus denen hervorgeht, daß an der anaphylaktischen Histaminfreisetzung aus isoliertem Gewebe ein C'3-artiger Faktor beteiligt ist. Selbst wenn man nicht annimmt, daß C'3 an der AT-Bildung beteiligt ist, ergibt sich hieraus zumindest, daß Plasmafaktoren möglicherweise auch im Gewebe vorkommen und dort bei der Anaphylaxie eine Rolle spielen. Aber direkte Anhaltspunkte für die Existenz eines Gewebs-AT gibt es nicht.

Eine weitere Möglichkeit einer AT-Beteiligung an der Anaphylaxie könnte darin bestehen, daß AT am intakten Tier als humoraler Faktor noch eine zusätzliche Rolle spielt, z. B. in der Form, daß die schon am isolierten Organ nachweisbare Histaminfreisetzung weiterhin verstärkt wird. Es gibt einige Hinweise auf eine verstärkende Wirkung humoraler Faktoren auf die anaphylaktische Reaktion isolierter Organe. MANWARING und KUSAMA (1917) beobachteten, daß unter bestimmten Umständen an der isolierten Meerschweinchenlunge der anaphylaktische Bronchospasmus bei Durchströmung mit Blut stärker als bei Durchströmung mit physiologischer Salzlösung war. UNGAR und DAMGAARD (1955) konnten, allerdings im Gegensatz zu BROCKLEHURST (1960), durch Serumzusatz zur Durchströmungsflüssigkeit die anaphylaktische Histaminfreisetzung aus der isolierten Meerschweinchenlunge erheblich verstärken.

Am Herz-Lungen-Präparat des Meerschweinchens wird in der Anaphylaxie etwa die gleiche Histaminmenge frei wie bei der Durchströmung mit Blut, wenn man das Präparat mit einer plasmafreien Erythrocytensuspension durchströmt. In diesen, gemeinsam mit BERNAUER u. SCHMUTZLER, von uns durchgeführten Versuchen betrug die anaphylaktische Histaminfreisetzung aus dem Herz-Lungen-Präparat nicht mehr als an der isolierten mit Salzlösung perfundierten Lunge. Diese Ergebnisse widersprechen der Auffassung, daß ein humoraler Faktor die anaphylaktische Histaminfreisetzung unterstützt.

Aus der mit Blut durchströmten anaphylaktischen Hundeleber wird mehr Histamin freigesetzt als aus einem mit physiologischer Salzlösung durchströmten Präparat. Es ist aber fraglich, ob man auch diesen Befund in Beziehung zum AT setzen kann. Wir kennen nämlich weder eine AT-Wirkung am Hund, noch eine AT-Bildung im Hundeplasma oder -serum. SCROGGIE und JAQUES (1949) deuten diesen Befund auch nicht wie ROCHA E SILVA (1954) als Ausdruck einer Beteiligung humoraler Faktoren an der anaphylaktischen Histaminfreisetzung; sie nehmen vielmehr an, daß bei der Durchströmung mit Blut die für die Histaminfreisetzung notwendige Integrität der Zellstruktur besser erhalten bleibt.

Als Argument gegen die Beteiligung von AT am anaphylaktischen Schock muß heute die Auffassung von DALE und KELLAWAY (1922) ausscheiden, wonach der AT-Schock nicht auf einem echten Bronchospasmus beruhe. Trotzdem verdient die Beobachtung dieser und anderer Autoren (BIEDL u. KRAUS, 1910a, b; KRAUS u. KIRSCHBAUM, 1913; LOEWIT u. BAYER, 1913), daß der Bronchialwiderstand im AT-Schock durch künstliche Beatmung leichter zu überwinden ist als im anaphylaktischen Schock, eine Diskussion an dieser Stelle; denn die Beteiligung des AT am anaphylaktischen Schock setzt auch eine genügende Wirkungsstärke des AT voraus. ROCHA E SILVA u. Mitarb. haben daher erneut die Wirkungsstärke des AT an der isolierten Lunge gemessen und mit den anaphylaktischen Vorgängen verglichen (ROCHA E SILVA u.

Aronson, 1952; Rocha e Silva, Bier u. Aronson, 1951). Als Maß der Schockintensität diente bei ihnen aber die Histaminfreisetzung. Sie fanden im AT-Schock eine stärkere Histaminliberation, als andere Autoren (Lit. s.: Hahn u. Giertz, 1960) im anaphylaktischen Schock der isolierten Lunge gefunden haben. Später allerdings fand Brocklehurst (1960) eine anaphylaktische Histaminfreisetzung aus der isolierten Meerschweinchenlunge, die so stark wie die von Rocha e Silva mit AT erzielte Histaminliberation war. Doch weder der eine noch der andere Befund erlaubt direkte Rückschlüsse auf die Intensität des Bronchospasmus, deren Messung den Versuchen von Dale und Kellaway zugrunde lag, da histaminunabhängige Mechanismen bei beiden Schockformen in Betracht zu ziehen sind. Giertz u. Mitarb. haben daher nicht nur die Histaminfreisetzung, sondern auch den Bronchospasmus gemessen und gezeigt, daß man auch mit AT einen ebenso starken Bronchospasmus bekommen kann, wenn man eine geeignete Dosis wählt, wie im anaphylaktischen Schock an der isolierten Lunge (Giertz, Hahn, Opferkuch u. Schmutzler, 1961; Giertz u. Schmutzler, 1960; Hahn, Giertz u. Schmutzler, 1961). Die Auffassung von Rocha e Silva, daß Dale und Kellaway ein zu schwaches AT verwendeten, war dadurch bestätigt. Irgendwelche Schlüsse über eine Beteiligung von AT am anaphylaktischen Schock lassen sich jedoch aus diesen Befunden, die durch Gegenüberstellung von anaphylaktischem und AT-Schock gewonnen wurden, nicht ziehen.

Eine wichtige, schon von Friedberger hervorgehobene Übereinstimmung zwischen AT-Bildung und anaphylaktischen Erscheinungen sind auffällige Parallelen in der Beziehung beider Vorgänge zum Komplement. So konnte schon Friedberger durch hypertonische Kochsalzlösung die AT-Bildung in vitro, die Komplementbindung und den anaphylaktischen Schock des Meerschweinchens hemmen.

Aber nicht nur der anaphylaktische, sondern auch der AT-Schock wird durch Kochsalzinjektion gehemmt, so daß man hier auch von einer Parallele zwischen AT-Wirkung und Anaphylaxie sprechen könnte. Allerdings wird auch der Peptonschock durch Kochsalzinjektion gehemmt (Ritz, 1912).

Sowohl die AT-Bildung als auch der anaphylaktische Schock können mit einem Komplementschwund einhergehen. Die Bedeutung solcher Parallelen ist jedoch deshalb gering, weil die Beteiligung des Komplements sowohl an der AT-Bildung (siehe oben) als auch an der Anaphylaxie (Ecker, Kovacs und Pillemer, 1939; Lepow, 1959; Rice, 1955) noch fraglich ist.

Das gilt auch für die Komplementkomponente C'3, der von Osler und Mitarbeitern ja eine besondere Bedeutung für dieAT-Bildung beigemessen wurde. Die Oslerschen Versuche gehen von der Beobachtung aus, daß bei einer immunologisch hervorgerufenen C'3-Armut des Blutes die passive cutane Anaphylaxie schlecht auslösbar und gleichzeitig das AT-Bildungsvermögen im Plasma der Versuchstiere vermindert ist (Bier, Siqueira und Osler, 1955; Osler, Hawrisiak und Ovary, 1957; Osler, Hawrisiak u. a., 1957). Diese Versuche sind jedoch deshalb kein Argument für die AT-Beteiligung an der Meerschweinchenanaphylaxie (und werden von Osler auch nicht in diesem Sinne gedeutet), weil die passive cutane Anaphylaxie an Ratten ausgelöst wurde. Das gilt auch für ähnliche Versuche von Rocha e Silva und Rothschild (1955), die Ratten mit Agar vorbehandelten und anschließend eine Abschwächung der cutanen Anaphylaxie sowie eine Verminderung des AT-Bildungsvermögens im Rattenblut beobachteten.

Am Meerschweinchen ist eine Beteiligung der Komplementkomponente C'3 am anaphylaktischen Schock fraglich, da Hyde (1932) an Tieren mit erblichem C'3-Mangel einen solchen Schock auslösen konnte.

Zirkulierende Antikörper sind für den anaphylaktischen Schock nicht erforderlich und können diesen unter Umständen sogar hemmen (vgl. Dale u. Kellaway, 1922; Ovary, Fudenberg u. Kunkel, 1960). Man muß daher, wenn man eine AT-Beteiligung am anaphylaktischen Schock annimmt, auch an eine Aktivierung des Plasmas durch zellständige Antigen-Antikörper-Komplexe denken. Eine AT-Bildung durch die Freisetzung von Glykogen, das für bestimmte anaphylaktische Erscheinungen beim Hund verantwortlich sein könnte (vgl. Inderbitzin, 1956), ist beim Meerschweinchen erst dann diskutabel, wenn eine solche Glykogenfreisetzung nachgewiesen ist.

Da die AT-Bildung in vitro mit einem Aufbrauch der an ihr beteiligten Serumfaktoren einhergeht, kann man ein Argument gegen die Beteiligung des AT an der Anaphylaxie darin erblicken, daß in vivo während des anaphylaktischen Schocks ein solcher Aufbrauch nicht nachweisbar ist (GIERTZ, HAHN, JURNA und LANGE, 1958). Die Beweiskraft dieses an sich negativen Befundes wird erhöht durch die Tatsache, daß bei einer anderen Schockform, nämlich dem Forssman-Schock des Meerschweinchens, ein deutlicher Schwund der Vorstufen der AT-Bildung im Serum nachweisbar ist (GIERTZ und HAHN, 1957a; GIERTZ, HAHN, JURNA und LANGE, 1958).

Mit dem gleichen Recht, mit dem man die Beteiligung des AT im anaphylaktischen Schock ablehnt, könnte man daher für den Forssman-Schock eine solche Beteiligung annehmen. Dafür spricht auch, daß dieser Schock nicht an isolierten Organen (HUMPHREY und MOTA, 1959; REDFERN, 1926) auslösbar ist. In unseren Versuchen am Herz-Lungen-Präparat ließ sich der Forssman-Schock nur bei Durchströmung mit Blut, nicht aber bei Verwendung einer plasmafreien Erythrocytensuspension auslösen. Als Parallele zwischen AT-Bildung und Forssman-Schock kann man anführen, daß beide durch Heparin (GIERTZ, 1959; GIERTZ, HAHN, JURNA und LANGE, 1958) und durch Glucocorticoide (ARBESMAN, NETER und BERTRAM, 1951; ARBESMAN, TERPLAN und NETER, 1955) hemmbar sind. Eine Bedeutung humoraler Faktoren für den Forssman-Schock ist insofern erwiesen, als dieser Schock an Tieren mit erblichem C′3-Mangel nicht auslösbar ist (HYDE, 1932) Der Plasmahistaminspiegel im Forssman-Schock ist auch erhöht, jedoch nur geringfügig (GIERTZ und HAHN, 1955; GIERTZ, HAHN, SCHMUTZLER und KOLLMEIER, 1964). Der Tod ist durch Antihistaminica nicht hemmbar (ARBESMAN, NETER und BECKER, 1950; HAHN und OBERDORF, 1950). Er ist also im Gegensatz zum anaphylaktischen Schock nicht durch Histamin bedingt. Das beweist jedoch nur, daß für den Tod im Forssman-Schock histaminunabhängige Mechanismen verantwortlich sind, und schließt eine Beteiligung des AT nicht aus.

Analogien zwischen AT-Bildung und anaphylaktischen Erscheinungen in vitro hinsichtlich ihrer Abhängigkeit von der Temperatur (MONGAR u. SCHILD, 1957b) und der Wasserstoffionenkonzentration (MONGAR u. SCHILD, 1958) kann man keine besondere Bedeutung beimessen, denn solche Abhängigkeiten zeigen viele Reaktionen, an denen Eiweißkörper beteiligt sind.

Gegen die Annahme, AT sei am echten anaphylaktischen Schock beteiligt, kann man mit größerem Gewicht einwenden, daß Heparin und Glucocorticoide zwar die AT-Bildung in vitro hemmen, in vivo aber den anaphylaktischen Schock des Meerschweinchens (im Gegensatz zum Forssman-Schock) wenig oder gar nicht beeinflussen (Lit. s.: GIERTZ, HAHN, JURNA und LANGE, 1958; HAHN und GIERTZ, 1960).

Eine Lösung des Problems der AT-Beteiligung am anaphylaktischen Schock ist ferner versucht worden, indem die Möglichkeit einer gegenseitigen Desensibilisierung zwischen AT-Schock und anaphylaktischem Schock geprüft wurde. Versuche am isolierten Organ sind hierzu wegen des Fehlens humoraler Faktoren nicht sehr geeignet. In allen derartigen Versuchen wurde durch Vorbehandlung mit AT keine Abschwächung einer nachfolgenden anaphylaktischen Reaktion erzielt (FRIEDBERG, ENGELHARDT und MEINEKE, 1963, 1964; GREEFF, BENFEY und BOKELMANN, 1959; GREEFF und BOKELMANN, 1959; GREISMAN, 1958).

Versuche am intakten Tier, bei dem im Gegensatz zum isolierten Organ die Teilnahme humoraler Faktoren an der Anaphylaxie möglich ist, führten zu unterschiedlichen Ergebnissen. Eine Reihe von Autoren konnte einen anaphylaktischen Schock auch dann auslösen, wenn das Tier durch AT-Vorbehandlung gegen erneute AT-Applikation völlig unempfindlich war (BESREDKA, 1920; BESREDKA,

Ströbel und Jupille, 1913a, b; Dewitzky, 1911; Friedberg, Engelhardt und Meineke, 1963, 1964; Friedberger, Szymanowski u. a., 1912)[1].

Andere Autoren fanden eine Abschwächung oder eine Unterdrückung des anaphylaktischen Schocks nach AT-Vorbehandlung (Dale und Kellaway, 1922; Frenger, Scheiffarth und Gemählich, 1958; Frick, Halpern und Liacopoulos, 1962; Frick, Liacopoulos und Halpern. 1961; Halpern, Liacopoulos und Briot, 1956b; Lumière und Couturier, 1925), und zwar vor allem dann, wenn das AT mehrfach hintereinander und über einen längeren Zeitraum vor der Antigenreinjektion gegeben wurde. Dieses Ergebnis kommt offenbar durch die Zerstörung der Gewebsmastzellen nach wiederholter AT-Applikation zustande (Frick u. Mitarb., 1961, 1962). Es spricht daher nicht für eine Beteiligung des AT, sondern nur für eine Beteiligung der Mastzellen und des Histamins an der Meerschweinchenanaphylaxie.

Untersuchungen über die AT-Wirkung an spezifisch desensibilisierten Tieren ergaben ebenfalls keinen Hinweis auf eine AT-Beteiligung an der Anaphylaxie. Die spezifische Desensibilisierung beruht z. T. auf einer Absättigung der sessilen und einer Vermehrung der zirkulierenden Antikörper und braucht daher die AT-Wirkung selbst dann nicht abzuschwächen, wenn das AT eine Rolle spielen sollte. Tritt aber eine Abschwächung auf, so könnte diese auf einer Entleerung der Histamindepots beruhen. Am spezifisch desensibilisierten Tier wurde gelegentlich eine Abschwächung der AT-Wirkung beobachtet (Bessau, 1911; Lumière u. Couturier, 1925; Tchernoroutzky, 1913), in anderen Fällen und in allen Versuchen am isolierten Organ fehlte sie jedoch (Besredka, 1920; Dale u. Kellaway, 1922; Friedberger, Szymanowski u. a., 1912; Greeff, Benfey u. Bokelmann, 1959; Greeff u. Bokelmann, 1959; Greisman, 1958).

Diese Betrachtung schließt nicht aus, daß irgend eine gemeinsame letzte Strecke bei der AT-bedingten und der anaphylaktischen Histaminfreisetzung existiert. Bei beiden Schockformen wird das Histamin überwiegend aus den Mastzellen freigesetzt. Die AT-Wirkung und die anaphylaktische Reaktion lassen sich durch eine Reihe von Eingriffen in den Zellstoffwechsel in gleicher Weise beeinflussen (Mota, 1959; Moussatché u. Danon, 1956; Rothschild u. Barreto, 1961; vgl. auch Mongar u. Schild, 1957a). Versuche, die eine Histaminfreisetzung durch AT aus Mitochondrien ergaben (Grossberg u. Garcia-Arocha, 1954), ließen sich später nicht bestätigen (MacIntosh, 1956) und fanden außerdem an Mitochondrien der Hundeleber statt. Aus der Mitochondrienfraktion der Meerschweinchenlunge ließ sich weder durch AT noch durch Antigen Histamin freisetzen, wohl aber aus Lungengewebsstückchen (Giertz, Reutter und Schmutzler, 1964b).

Unterschiede in den Bedingungen für die anaphylaktische und die AT-bedingte Mastzellzerstörung bestehen darin, daß Ca-Mangel oder Erhitzen des Präparates auf 45° C die anaphylaktische Reaktion im Gegensatz zur AT-Wirkung aufhebt (Mota, 1959).

b) *Ein der AT-Bildung und AT-Wirkung ähnliches Phänomen*

Der AT-Bildung und -Wirkung sehr ähnlich verhält sich die Aktivierung und Wirkung eines an Kaninchenthrombocyten wirksamen Histaminliberators. In Gegenwart von Kaninchenplasma sind Immunpräcipitate, Dextransulfat, Agar, Glykogen und Kaolin in der Lage, aus Kaninchenthrombocyten Histamin und Serotonin freizusetzen (Barbaro, 1957, 1961a, b; Haining, 1955, 1956b, c; Humphrey, 1959a, b; Humphrey und Jaques, 1953, 1955). Diese Histaminfreisetzung ist möglicherweise bedingt durch eine Aktivierung des Plasmas ähnlich der AT-Bildung, denn Haining (1956b) beobachtete die Histaminfreisetzung aus Thrombocyten auch durch Kaninchenplasma, aus dem die Immunpräcipitate nach der Inkubation wieder durch Abzentrifugieren entfernt waren. Wie die AT-Bildung ist die Histaminfreisetzung durch Immunpräcipitate oder Polysaccharide hemmbar durch Heparin, durch niedermolekulares Dextransulfat und durch Maltotriosesulfat (Haining, 1955, 1956b, c), und wie die AT-Wirkung wird sie durch Na-Salicylat und durch 3-Hydroxyphenylcinchoninsäure abgeschwächt

[1] Die Auslösbarkeit des anaphylaktischen Schocks an Tieren, die nach einer langdauernden Vorbehandlung gegen AT vollständig tachyphylaktisch sind, spricht unseres Erachtens nicht gegen eine Histaminbeteiligung am anaphylaktischen Schock (vgl. Friedberg, Engelhardt und Meineke, 1963, 1964); denn nach noch unveröffentlichten, gemeinsam mit Bernauer, Schmutzler und Seseke durchgeführten Versuchen in unserem Laboratorium stammt das im Anaphylatoxinschock liberierte Histamin vorwiegend aus extrapulmonalen, das bei der Anaphylaxie freigesetzte Histamin dagegen mehr aus endopulmonalen Quellen.

(HAINING, 1956b). Die Histaminfreisetzung durch Dextran und Dextransulfat aus Kaninchenthrombocyten geht nicht parallel mit einer Proteaseaktivierung (vgl. HAINING, 1956a). Sie ist nur insofern abhängig vom Molekulargewicht der verwendeten Dextranpräparate, als Dextran oder Dextransulfat unter einem Molekulargewicht von 10000 kein Histamin freisetzt (HAINING, 1955, 1956c). Die Beteiligung des Komplements an der Histaminfreisetzung durch Immunpräcipitate ist nach BARBARO (1957, 1961a, b) fraglich. GIERTZ, REUTTER und SCHMUTZLER (1964a) wiesen eine Aktivierung des AT-ähnlichen Faktors in Kaninchenplasma durch Agar auch dann nach, wenn sie Plasma von hereditär C'3-defekten Kaninchen verwandten.

Unterschiede zwischen dem AT und dem Histaminliberator aus Kaninchenserum bestehen vor allem darin, daß sich letzterer, allerdings in abgeschwächtem Maße, auch in Serum bildet, das vor der Zugabe der Immunpräcipitate für 30 min auf 64° C erhitzt wurde (BARBARO. 1961b) und daß die Wirksamkeit des aktivierten Faktors nur vorübergehend nachweisbar ist (HUMPHREY und JAQUES, 1955).

Wie zwischen der AT-Bildung und -Wirkung und anaphylaktischen Vorgängen, so gibt es auch Übereinstimmungen zwischen der anaphylaktischen Histaminfreisetzung und der Histaminliberation durch Immunpräcipitate oder Polysaccharide aus Kaninchenthrombocyten. Beide Vorgänge werden durch Heparin gehemmt (DRAGSTEDT, WELLS und ROCHA E SILVA, 1942; HAINING, 1955, 1956b; MCINTIRE, ROTH und RICHARDS, 1949). Eine Hemmung der anaphylaktischen Histaminfreisetzung aus Kaninchenblutzellen durch Salicylat wurde zwar nicht gefunden, aber in diesen Versuchen kamen sehr kleine Salicylatkonzentrationen zur Anwendung (MCINTIRE, RICHARDS und ROTH, 1957). Es ist auch schon länger bekannt, daß die anaphylaktischen Schocksymptome des Kaninchens durch Salicylate gehemmt werden (LEPPER, CALDWELL u. a., 1950). Die Histaminliberation aus Kaninchenthrombocyten durch den AT-ähnlichen Faktor in Kaninchenplasma wird wie die anaphylaktische Histaminfreisetzung aus Kaninchenthrombocyten und wie die Histaminliberation aus Meerschweinchenlungengewebe durch Ratten-AT in Gegenwart von Dinitrophenol bei Abwesenheit von Glucose gehemmt (ROTHSCHILD und GARCIA LIMA, 1963). Wie für die Aktivierung und Wirkung des histaminliberierenden Stoffes aus Kaninchenplasma ist eine Beteiligung von Proteasen an der anaphylaktischen Histaminfreisetzung aus Kaninchenthrombocyten sehr fraglich (MCINTIRE, 1956; MCINTIRE, ROTH und SPROULL, 1950, 1952).

Literatur

ACKERMANN, H., E. EICHENBERGER, F. HUNZIKER, H. LAUENER u. J. SCHMUTZ: Über ein chemisch neuartiges, starkwirksames Antihistaminikum. Med. exp. (Basel) **6**, 205—212 (1962).

ADAMKIEWICZ, L. M., and V. W. ADAMKIEWICZ: Glucagon, insulin and anaphylactoid inflammation. J. Physiol. (Lond.) **145**, 667—670 (1959a).

— V. W., and L. M. ADAMKIEWICZ: Alloxan diabetes and dextran anaphylactoid inflammation. Amer. J. Physiol. **197**, 377—379 (1959b).

— — Glucose and the dextran anaphylactoid inflammation. Amer. J. Physiol. **198**, 51—53 (1960).

—, and J. E. BATA: Insulin and the distribution of U-C^{14}-glucose and U-C^{14}-dextran in rats. Fed. Proc. **21**, 201 (1962).

— R. J. FITKO and A. A. FORTIER: Hypoglycemic drugs and the dextran anaphylactoid inflammation. Canad. J. Biochem. **38**, 823—827 (1960).

—, and Y. LANGLOIS: Sensitization by insulin to the dextran anaphylactoid reaction. Rev. canad. Biol. **15**, 231 (1956).

— — Sensitization by insulin to the dextran anaphylactoid reaction. Canad. J. Biochem. **35**, 251—256 (1957).

— — Insulin, mast cell components, and anaphylactoid inflammation. Canad. J. Biochem. **36**, 483—489 (1958).

— — and L. J. POIRIER: Sensitization by insulin to dextran anaphylactoid inflammation in spinal rats. Amer. J. Physiol. **195**, 635—638 (1958).

ADAMKIEWICZ, V. W., W. B. RICE and J. D. MCCOLL: Antiphlogistic effect of trypsin in normal and in adrenalectomized rats. Canad. J. Biochem. **33**, 332—339 (1955).
—, and P. J. SACRA: Passive transfer of dextran anaphylactoid reaction in rats. Amer. J. Physiol. **205**, 357—359 (1963).
ADANT, M.: L'action des anaphylatoxines sur les organes isolés. C. R. Soc. Biol. (Paris) **144**, 1295—1296 (1950).
— Quelques effets de l'injection intraveineuse de dextran et de polyvinylpyrrolidone au chien normal ou hépatectomisé. Bull. Acad. roy. Méd. Belg., Sér. **6**, 19, 264—298 (1954).
ALMON, L., and H. T. PARSONS: The lack of correlation between hypersensitivity to egg white and symptoms of injury. J. Allergy **8**, 547—559 (1937).
ANTWEILER, H.: Über die Beeinflussung des Dextranödems der Rattenpfote durch gelöste Oligo- und Poly-Kieselsäure (Versuche zur Pathogenese der Silikose). Arch. Hyg. (Berl.) **139**, 341—348 (1955).
— Histamine liberation by cotton dust extracts: evidence against its causation by bacterial endotoxins. Brit. J. industr. Med. **18**, 130—132 (1961).
ARBESMAN, C. E., E. NETER and C. F. BECKER: The effect of pyribenzamine, neohetramine, and rutin on reversed anaphylaxis in guinea pigs. J. Allergy **21**, 25—33 (1950).
— E. NETER and L. F. BERTRAM: The effect of ACTH and cortisone on certain immunologic mechanisms including reversed anaphylaxis. J. Allergy **22**, 340—349 (1951).
— K. L. TERPLAN and E. NETER: The effects of ACTH and cortisone on the pathology of reversed anaphylaxis in the guinea pig. J. Allergy **26**, 123—132 (1955).
ARCHER, G. T.: Release of histamine from rat mast cells by blood treated with dextran. Nature (Lond.) **184**, 1151—1152 (1959a).
— The release of histamine from the mast cells of the rat. Aust. J. exp. Biol. med. Sci. **37**, 383—389 (1959b).
ARRIGONI-MARTELLI, E., e M. KRAMER: Significato della liberazione di serotonina da dextran, ovomucoide, ovalbumina nella cute del ratto per la patogenesi dell'edema provocato. Boll. Soc. ital. Biol. sper. **34**, 1130—1132 (1958).
ASBOE-HANSEN, G.: The mast cell an object of cortisone action on connective tissue. Proc. Soc. exp. Biol. (N. Y.) **80**, 677—679 (1952).
— The mast cell. Int. Rev. Cytol. **3**, 399—431 (1954).
— Hormonal effects on connective tissue. Physiol. Rev. **38**, 446—462 (1958).
— Endocrine control of connective tissue. Amer. J. Med. **26**, 470—481 (1959).
AUER, J., and P. A. LEWIS: The physiology of the immediate reaction of anaphylaxis in the guinea-pig. J. exp. Med. **12**, 151—175 (1910).
AUSTEN, K. F., and W. E. BROCKLEHURST: The influence of ionic strength on the anaphylactic reaction in guinea-pig lung. J. Physiol. (Lond.) **153**, 66P—67P (1960).
BAEHR, G., u. E. P. PICK: Pharmakologische Studien an der Bronchialmuskulatur der überlebenden Meerschweinchenlunge. Naunyn-Schmiedebergs Arch. exp. Path. Pharmak. **74**, 41—64 (1913).
BARBARO, J. F.: Release of histamine from rabbit blood by means of antigen-antibody precipitates. Fed. Proc. **16**, 405 (1957).
— The release of histamine from rabbit platelets by means of antigen-antibody precipitates. I. The participation of the immune complex in histamine release. J. Immunol. **86**, 369—376 (1961a).
— The release of histamine from rabbit platelets by means of antigen-antibody precipitates. II. The role of plasma in the release of histamine. J. Immunol. **86**, 377—381 (1961b).
BARTLET, A. L., and M. F. LOCKETT: Effect of adrenalectomy on tissue histamine in rats. J. Physiol. (Lond.) **147**, 51—57 (1959).
BAUER, J.: Über die Herkunft des Anaphylatoxins. Berl. klin. Wschr. **49**, 344—345 (1912).
BEACH, V. L., and B. G. STEINETZ: Quantitative measurement of Evans Blue space in the tissues of the rat: influence of 5-hydroxytryptamine antagonists and phenelzine on experimental inflammation. J. Pharmacol. exp. Ther. **131**, 400—406 (1961).
BECKER, E. L.: In vitro models for the allergic reaction. In: Mechanisms of hypersensitivity. S. 305—314. Boston: Little, Brown and Co. (1959).
— The possible significance of a particular group of serine esterases in pathological permeability changes. In: Mechanism of cell and tissue damage produced by immune reactions, p. 37—50. Basel: Benno Schwabe & Co. 1962.
BEHRMANN, V. G., and F. W. HARTMANN: Mechanism of reduced capillary resistance produced by macromolecular infusions. Fed. Proc. **14**, 11 (1955).
BEILER, J., R. BRENDEL and G. J. MARTIN: Action of parenteral trypsin on experimentally-induced edemas of different types in rats. Proc. Soc. exp. Biol. (N. Y.) **89**, 274—276 (1955).
BENDITT, E. P., S. BADER and M. ARASE: Anaphylaxis versus the anaphylactoid reaction produced by testis extract and ovomucoid in rats. Fed. Proc. **12**, 384—385 (1953).

BENDITT, E. P., S. BADER, M. ARASE, C. CORLEY and K. B. LAM: Relationship of mast cells and histamine to mechanism of edema production by ovomucoid in rats. Fed. Proc. **13**, 422—423 (1954).

— — and K. B. LAM: Studies of the mechanism of acute vascular reactions to injury. I. The relationship of mast cells and histamine to the production of edema by ovomucoid in rats. Arch. Path. **60**, 104—115 (1955).

—, and D. A. ROWLEY: Antagonism of 5-hydroxytryptamine by chlorpromazine. Science **123**, 24 (1956).

— R. L. WONG, M. ARASE and E. ROEPER: 5-Hydroxytryptamine in mast cells. Proc. Soc. exp. Biol. (N. Y.) **90**, 303—304 (1955).

BENOS, S. A.: Action protectrice de la cortisone à l'égard de la vasoparalysie provoquée par le dextran chez le rat surrénalectomisé. Arch. int. Pharmacodyn. **97**, 115—123 (1954).

BERALDO, W. T., W. DIAS DA SILVA and A. D. LEMOS FERNANDES: Inhibitory effects of carbohydrates on histamine release and mast cell disruption by dextran. Brit. J. Pharmacol. **19**, 405—413 (1962).

BERNAUER, W., H. GIERTZ, F. HAHN, W. SCHMUTZLER, G. SESEKE u. B. U. SIEVERS: Zum Mechanismus der Histaminaseaktivierung im anaphylaktischen Schock. Naturwissenschaften **51**, 412—413 (1964).

BESREDKA, A.: Anaphylatoxine et anaphylaxie. Ann. Inst. Pasteur **34**, 334—342 (1920).

—, et H. STRÖBEL: De l'anaphylatoxine typhique. C. R. Soc. Biol. (Paris) **71**, 413—415 (1911 a).

— — De la nature des anaphylatoxines. C. R. Soc. Biol. (Paris) **71**, 599—600 (1911 b).

— — et F. JUPILLE: Microbes peptonés et apeptonés. C. R. Soc. Biol. (Paris) **71**, 691—693 (1911).

— — — Anaphylatoxin, Peptotoxin und Pepton in ihren Beziehungen zur Anaphylaxie. Z. Immun-Forsch. **16**, 249—267 (1913 a).

— — — Anaphylatoxine, peptotoxine et peptone dans leurs rapports avec l'anaphylaxie. Ann. Inst. Pasteur **27**, 185—203 (1913 b).

BESSAU, G.: Über das Wesen der Antianaphylaxie. Zbl. Bakt. I. Orig. **60**, 637—651 (1911).

BESSE, J. H., et R. PATAY: A propos de l'action hypotensive de la polyvinylpyrrolidone chez le Chien. C. R. Soc. Biol. (Paris) **147**, 1721—1722 (1953).

BHATTACHARYA, B. K., and G. P. LEWIS: The release of 5-hydroxytryptamine by histamine liberators. Brit. J. Pharmacol. **11**, 202—208 (1956).

BICKHARDT, R., u. H. J. HEITE: Vergleichende Untersuchungen über die exsudationshemmende Wirkung von Calcium und Strontium am Eiweißödem der Rattenpfote. Naunyn-Schmiedebergs Arch. exp. Path. Pharmak. **221**, 393—398 (1954).

BIEDL, A., u. R. KRAUS: Experimentelle Studien über Anaphylaxie. 4. Mitteilung. Zur Charakteristik des anaphylaktischen Schocks. Z. Immun-Forsch. **7**, 205—222 (1910a).

— — Über die Giftigkeit heterologer Sera und Kriterien der Anaphylaxie. Z. Immun-Forsch. **7**, 408—414 (1910b).

BIER, O.: Sur le rôle de l'alexine dans la genèse d'anaphylatoxine. C. R. Soc. Biol. (Paris) **106**, 569—570 (1931).

— M. SIQUEIRA and A. G. OSLER: Studies on the mechanism of hypersensitivity phenomena. I. The effect of in vivo antigen-antibody reactions on passive cutaneous anaphylaxis in the rat. Int. Arch. Allergy **7**, 1—9 (1955).

BINET, L., et M. BURSTEIN: Passage dans la circulation d'une substance vasodilatatrice au cours du choc par la polyvinylpyrrolidone chez le Chien. C. R. Soc. Biol. (Paris) **143**, 808—809 (1949).

—, et D. QUIVY: Sur la mobilisation de l'histamine cutanée chez le Rat, sous l'action de diverses substances injectées localement. C. R. Soc. Biol. (Paris) **150**, 655—656 (1956).

— — Sur la mise en évidence d'une déplétion locale d'histamine chez le Rat. C. R. Soc. Biol. (Paris) **151**, 1292—1293 (1957).

— — Le salicylate de sodium modifie-t-il chez le Rat l'histamino-libération de l'oedème anaphylactoide? C. R. Soc. Biol. (Paris) **152**, 1319—1321 (1958a).

— — Sur la libération d'histamine, determinée chez le Rat par l'injection locale de 5-hydroxytryptamine, dans diverses conditions expérimentales. C. R. Acad. Sci. (Paris) **247**, 1153 à 1155 (1958 b).

BLISS, J. Q., D. G. JOHNS and A. S. BURGEN: Transfusion reactions due to plasma incompatibility in dogs. Circulat. Res. **7**, 79—85 (1959).

—, and P. B. STEWART: The selective response of skin to autologous and non-autologous plasma in non-sensitized subjects. Canad. J. med. Ass. **76**, 847—852 (1957).

— — and J. L. FULLER: The selective cutaneous response to autologous and non-autologous plasma in dogs: observations on the effects of inbreeding and of immaturity. Brit. J. exp. Path. **39**, 30—36 (1958).

—, and J. D. WALKER: Histamine release by homologous plasma in the dog. Canad. J. Biochem. **37**, 371—375 (1959).

BLOOM, W. L., and M. L. WILLCOX: Determination of dextran in blood and urine. Proc. Soc. exp. Biol. (N. Y.) **76**, 3—4 (1951).
BLUDAU, W., u. H. J. HEITE: Untersuchungen über die Bedeutung des Anions bei vergleichender Prüfung der exsudationshemmenden Wirkung verschiedener Erdalkalisalze am Eiweißödem der Rattenpfote. Arzneimittel-Forsch. **4**, 639—643 (1954).
BOEHNCKE, K. E.: Über die Abspaltung des Anaphylatoxins aus Meningokokken. Z. Hyg. Infekt.-Kr. **72**, 305—315 (1912).
—, u. K. BIERBAUM: Über den Einfluß der Kälte und über die Erschöpfung des Antigens bei der Darstellung des Anaphylatoxins. Z. Immun-Forsch. **14**, 130—136 (1912).
BOHNSTEDT, R. M., u. W. LANZ: Einwirkung des Megaphens auf allergische Phänomene im Tierexperiment. Naunyn-Schmiedebergs Arch. exp. Path. Pharmak. **227**, 488—496 (1956).
BOIS, P., and H. SELYE: Production of anaphylactoid inflammation and gastric ulcers with 5-hydroxytryptamine. Rev. canad. Biol. **15**, 238—239 (1956).
BONACCORSI, A., and G. B. WEST: Absence of capillary permeability response in rats to dextran and egg-white. J. Pharm. Pharmacol. **15**, 372—378 (1963).
BORDET, J.: Le mécanisme de l'anaphylaxie. C. R. Soc. Biol. (Paris) **74**, 225—227 (1913a).
— Gélose et anaphylatoxine. C. R. Soc. Biol. (Paris) **74**, 877—878 (1913b).
— L'origine sérique de l'anaphylatoxine et l'antianaphylaxie. Bull. Acad. Méd. Belg. **29**, 635—639 (1919).
— The present views on anaphylaxis. Bull. Johns Hopk. Hosp. **32**, 269—275 (1921).
— Les théories actuelles de l'anaphylaxie. C. R. Acad. Sci. (Paris) **179**, 243—249 (1924).
— Remarques sur la note de M. M. AUGUSTE LUMIÈRE et HENRI COUTURIER, intitulée Sur la toxicité du sérum gélosé. Arch. int. Pharmacodyn. **30**, 353—354 (1925).
— Traité de l'immunité dans les maladies infectieuses. Paris: Masson 1939.
—, et E. B. MCKINLEY: Sur la toxicité des globulines du sérum normal. C. R. Soc. Biol. (Paris) **92**, 762—764 (1925).
—, et E. ZUNZ: Production d'anaphylatoxine dans le sérum traité par de l'agar épuré de son azote (pararabine). Z. Immun-Forsch. **23**, 42—48 (1915a).
— — Le sérum traité par l'agar épuré de son azote (pararabine) se proteolyse-t-il ? Z. Immun-Forsch. **23**, 49—60 (1915b).
BOVET, D., S. COURVOISIER et M. R. DUCROT: Activité de la polyvinylpyrrolidone dans le choc traumatique expérimental et sur les accidents provoqués par certaines toxines microbiennes. C. R. Acad. Sci. (Paris) **224**, 70—72 (1947).
BRIOT, M., et B. N. HALPERN: Symptomatologie et pathogénie du syndrome oedémateux produit par le dextran chez le rat. C. R. Soc. Biol. (Paris) **146**, 15—20 (1952a).
— — Action inhibitrice de la prométhazine (phenergan) et de l'adrénaline sur l'oedème du rat par le dextran. C. R. Soc. Biol. (Paris) **146**, 21—24 (1952b).
BROCKLEHURST, W. E.: The release of histamine and formation of a slow-reacting substance (SRS-A) during anaphylactic shock. J. Physiol. (Lond.) **151**, 416—435 (1960).
BRONFENBRENNER, J.: The nature of anaphylatoxin. Studies on immunity. II. J. exp. Med. **21**, 480—492 (1915).
BRUGNATELLI, E.: Über die Bildung des Streptokokkenanaphylatoxins. Z. Immun.-Forsch. **16**, 342—347 (1913).
BÜCH, O., u. T. WAGNER-JAUREGG: Hemmung des Polyvinylpyrrolidon-Ödems der Rattenpfote durch intraperitoneale Injektion Ödem erzeugender Substanzen. Arzneimittel-Forsch. **12**, 639—640 (1962).
BUSHBY, S. R. M., and A. F. GREEN: The release of histamine by polymyxin B and polymyxin E. Brit. J. Pharmacol. **10**, 215—219 (1955).
BUSQUET, H., et C. VISCHNIAC: Gomme arabique et tachyphylaxie. Rapport du phénomène avec l'état colloidal et l'incoagulabilité du sang. C. R. Soc. Biol. (Paris) **100**, 642—643 (1929).
BUTTLE, G. A. H., P. F. D'ARCY, E. M. HOWARD and D. N. KELLETT: Plethysmometric measurement of swelling in the feet of small laboratory animals. Nature (Lond.) **179**, 629 (1957).
CASS, R., and P. B. MARSHALL: Effects of adrenocortical hormones on tissue histamine and 5-hydroxytryptamine in the rat. Arch. int. Pharmacodyn. **136**, 311—332 (1962).
CAVALLERO, C., and C. BRACCINI: Effect of cortisone on the mast cells of the rat. Proc. Soc. exp. Biol. (N. Y.) **78**, 141—143 (1951).
CHEN, G., and A. WICKEL: Protective effect of steroids against acute egg-white toxicity in adrenalectomized rats. Endocrinology **51**, 21—25 (1952).
CÎRSTEA, M., et G. SUHACIU: Evaluation du role de l'histamine dans la production de l'hypotension anaphylactique chez le chien. J. Physiol. (Paris) **53**, 719—731 (1961a).
— — Effets d'un choc anaphylactique préalable et du traitement à la polyvinylpyrrolidone sur la réaction anaphylactique chez le chien. J. Physiol. (Paris) **53**, 781—792 (1961b).

CÎRSTEA, M., and G. SUHACIU: Tweens and anaphylactic shock in dogs. Arch. int. Pharmacodyn. **147**, 156—165 (1964).
CITRON, J.: Kritisches zur Anaphylaxiefrage. Folia serol. **7**, 352—366 (1911).
CLARK, W. G., and E. M. MACKAY: Effect of l-epinephrine and l-arterenol on egg white edema in the rat. Proc. Soc. exp. Biol. (N. Y.) **71**, 86—87 (1949a).
— — Effect of epinephrine, antihistaminics and adrenergic blockade on egg white edema in adrenal insufficient rats. Proc. Soc. exp. Biol. (N. Y.) **72**, 510—515 (1949).
CODE, C. F., D. T. CODY, M. HURN, H. C. KENNEDY and M. J. STRICKLAND: The simultaneous release of histamine and a histamine-destroying factor during anaphylaxis in rats. J. Physiol. (Lond.) **156**, 207—216 (1961a).
— — and J. C. KENNEDY: Studies on the mechanism of anaphylaxis in the rat. J. Physiol. (Lond.) **159**, 61P—62P (1961b).
CODY, D. T., C. F. CODE and J. C. KENNEDY: Studies on the mechanism of anaphylaxis in the rat. J. Allergy **34**, 26—34 (1963).
COHEN, H., M. GRAFF and W. KLEINBERG: Inhibition of dextran edema by proteolytic enzymes. Proc. Soc. exp. Biol. (N. Y.) **88**, 517—519 (1955).
COHEN, Y., et F. BOISMARE: Propriétés antiinflammatoires de quelques dérivés de la diamidine étudiées sur l'oedème de la patte du rat. C. R. Acad. Sci. (Paris) **253**, 2161—2163 (1961).
COMSA, J.: Influence of the thymus upon the egg-white allergy in the rat. Nature (Lond.) **184**, 1726—1727 (1959).
CONARD, V., et W. MUTSAARS: Effet antagoniste des colorants basiques sur la genèse de l'anaphylatoxine. C. R. Soc. Biol. (Paris) **143**, 129—130 (1949).
CORBASCIO, A. N.: Effects of injected dextran on connective tissue mast-cells and on cells of the afferent glomerular artery of the rat kidney. Fed. Proc. **17**, 29 (1958).
COULSON, E. J., and H. STEVENS: Some observations on the immunochemistry of dextrans. J. Immunol. **86**, 241—252 (1961).
COURVOISIER, S., et R. DUCROT: Action de la chlorpromazine (4.560 R.P.) sur le syndrome oedémateux provoqué par le dextrane ches le rat. Arch. int. Pharmacodyn. **102**, 33-54 (1955).
— J. FOURNEL, R. DUCROT, M. KOLSKY et P. KOETSCHET: Propriétés pharmacodynamiques du chlorhydrate de chloro-3 (diméthylamino-3′ propyl)-10 phénothiazine (4.560 R.P.). Etude expérimentale d'un nouveau corps utilisé dans l'anesthésie potentialisée et dans l'hibernation artificielle. Arch. int. Pharmacodyn. **92**, 305—361 (1953).
CRAPS, L.: Contribution à la pathogénie de l'anaphylaxie cutanée chez le rat. Int. Arch. Allergy **20**, Suppl. 2.
—, et T. INDERBITZIN: L'exosérose cutanée anaphylactoide et anaphylactique chez le rat. Int. Arch. Allergy **18**, 268—285 (1961).
CRIVELLARI, C. A.: Sensibilité des rats décapsulés à l'égard de la nicotine, décylamine, de l'acétylcholine et de l'histamine. C. R. Soc. Biol. (Paris) **96**, 223 (1927a).
— Sensitiveness of adrenalectomized rats to certain toxic substances. Amer. J. Physiol. **81**, 414—421 (1927b).
CRONHEIM, G. E., and I. M. TOEKES: The effect of 2-dimethylaminoethanol (deanol) on anaphylactoid edema in rats. J. Pharmacol. exp. Ther. **127**, 167—170 (1959).
CUNY, L., et D. QUIVY: Influence nulle de la polyvinylpyrrolidone sur la vitesse d'élimination de l'héparine injectée chez le Chien par voie veineuse. C. R. Soc. Biol. (Paris) **142**, 1399—1402 (1948).
DA COSTA CRUZ, J.: Formation d'anaphylatoxine au dépens de sérum inactivé par la chaleur. C. R. Soc. Biol. (Paris) **127**, 715—717 (1938).
DALE, H. H.: The anaphylactic reaction of plain muscle in the guinea-pig. J. Pharmacol. exp. Ther. **4**, 167—223 (1913).
— Some chemical factors in the control of the circulation. Lecture III. Local vasodilator reactions. — Histamine (cont.). — Acetylcholine. — Conclusion. Lancet **1929 I**, 1285—1290.
— Antihistamine substances. Brit. med. J. **1948 II**, 281—283.
—, and C. H. KELLAWAY: Anaphylaxis and anaphylatoxins. Phil. Trans. B **211**, 273—315 (1922).
—, and P. P. LAIDLAW: The physiological action of β-iminazolylethylamine. J. Physiol. (Lond.) **41**, 318—344 (1910).
DAVIES, G. E., and J. S. LOWE: A permeability factor released from guinea-pig serum by antigen-antibody precipitates. Brit. J. exp. Path. **41**, 335—344 (1960).
— — The effects of guinea-pig gamma globulins on capillary permeability and serum complement. Immunology **4**, 289—300 (1961).
— — Further studies on a permeability factor released from guinea-pig serum by antigen-antibody precipitates: relationship to serum complement. Int. Arch. Allergy **20**, 235—250 (1962a).
— — Chemical mediators of inflammation in guinea-pig skin. Transact. St. John's Dermatol. Soc., Winter 1962b, p. 157—162.

De Kruif, P. H., and W. M. German: Anaphylatoxin and anaphylaxis. X. Anaphylatoxin and amino-nitrogen. J. infect. Dis. **20**, 833—854 (1917).
Devitt, J. E., W. J. Pirozynski and P. B. Samuels: Mast cell resistance to hormonal influence. Proc. Soc. exp. Biol. (N. Y.) **83**, 335—337 (1953).
Dewitzky, W.: Contribution à l'étude de l'anaphylaxie. C. R. Soc. Biol. (Paris) **70**, 134—136 (1911).
Dews, P. B., A. L. Wnuck, R. V. Fanelli, A. E. Light, J. A. Tornaben, S. Norton, C. H. Ellis and E. J. De Beer: The pharmacology of No. 48—80, a long-acting vasodepressor drug. J. Pharmacol. exp. Ther. **107**, 1—11 (1953).
Doepfner, W., u. A. Cerletti: Über den Serotonin-Antagonismus einiger Antihistaminika unter Berücksichtigung ihrer chemischen Struktur. Int. Arch. Allergy **10**, 348—354 (1957).
— — Comparison of lysergic acid derivatives and antihistamines as inhibitors of the edema provoked in the rat's paw by serotonin. Int. Arch. Allergy **12**, 89—97 (1958).
Doerr, R.: Allergie und Anaphylaxie. Handb. pathogen. Mikroorganism. 3. Aufl. Bd. 1, 2. S. 759—1008. Jena, Berlin und Wien: Gustav Fischer und Urban & Schwarzenberg 1929.
— Die Immunitätsforschung. Ergebnisse und Probleme in Einzeldarstellungen. Band VI. Die Anaphylaxie. Band VII. Die Anaphylaxie II. Band VIII. Allergie. Wien: Springer 1950 bis 1951.
—, u. V. K. Russ: Darstellung von Anaphylaxiegiften in vitro ohne Komplement. Zbl. Bakt. I. Orig. **63**, 243—256 (1912).
Dold, H.: Anaphylatoxin, charakterisiert durch eine eigenartige Flockungs-Phase der Serum-Globuline. Arch. Hyg. (Berl.) **89**, 101—129 (1920a).
— Über das seroskopische Verhalten der Sera nach Einsaat von Kaolin, Agar, Inulin und Stärke. Arch. Hyg. (Berl.) **89**, 373—382 (1920b).
— Über die Entstehung anaphylatoxinartiger (serotoxinartiger) Eigenschaften im Serum durch Schütteln. Klin. Wschr. **5**, 1281 (1926a).
— Über die Entstehung anaphylatoxinartiger (serotoxinartiger) Eigenschaften im Meerschweinchenserum durch längere Lagerung (Lagerungs-Serotoxin). Klin. Wschr. **5**, 1472 (1926b).
—, u. K. Aoki: Weitere Studien über das Bakterienanaphylatoxin. Z. Immun-Forsch. **15**, 171—179 (1912).
—, u. M. Bürger: Über die Wirkung des sogenannten Anaphylatoxins sowie arteigenen Serums auf den isolierten Darm. Z. Hyg. Infekt.-Kr. **78**, 169—187 (1914).
Domenjoz, R.: Die Wirkung von Isonikotinsäurehydrazid auf die Formalinentzündung und das Dextranödem. Schweiz. med. Wschr. **82**, 1023—1025 (1952).
— Pharmacological evaluation of anti-inflammatory agents, a contribution to the pharmacology of phenylbutazone (Butazolidine T. M.). Ann. Univ. Sarav. **1**, 317—344 (1953).
— Pharmakotherapeutische Weiterentwicklung der Antipyretica-Analgetica. Naunyn-Schmiedebergs Arch. exp. Path. Pharmak. **225**, 14—42 (1955).
— The pharmacology of phenylbutazone analogues. Ann. N. Y. Acad. Sci. **86**, 263—291 (1960).
— K. Mörsdorf, E. G. Stenger u. W. Theobald: Zur entzündungshemmenden Wirkung von Natriumsalicylat. Ann. Univ. Sarav. **3**, 302—312 (1955).
— — — — Der Einfluß der Narkose auf die Wirkung von Natriumsalicylat und Phenylbutazon (Butazolidin Geigy) am experimentellen Pfotenödem der Ratte. Naunyn-Schmiedebergs Arch. exp. Path. Pharmak. **230**, 325—327 (1957).
— W. Theobald u. K. Mörsdorf: Die Beeinflussung der an der Ratte gleichzeitig gesetzten Formalin- und Dextranentzündung. Arzneimittel-Forsch. **5**, 488—489 (1955).
Dragstedt, C. A., J. A. Wells and M. Rocha e Silva: Inhibitory effect of heparin upon histamine release by trypsin, antigen, and proteose. Proc. Soc. exp. Biol. (N. Y.) **51**, 191—192 (1942).
Duričić, I., V. Savić, I. Spužić et V. Savić: L'apport de l'histamine dans le choc anaphylactique chez les chiens. Acta med. jugosl. **13**, 399—405 (1959).
Ecker, E. E., J. Kovacs and L. Pillemer: Complement in anaphylactic shock. Enzymologia **7**, 305—306 (1939).
Edlund, T., B. Löfgren and L. Väli: Toxicity of dextran in rats. Nature (Lond.) **170**, 125 (1952).
Eichenberger, E., M. Schmidhauser u. G. Rufener: Beiträge zur Pathogenese des Eiweißödems der Ratte. Helv. physiol. pharmacol. Acta **10**, 505—511 (1952).
Erspamer, V., and A. Ottolenghi: Pharmacological studies on enteramine. VIII. Action of enteramine on the diuresis and renal circulation of the rat. Arch. int. Pharmacodyn. **93**, 177—201 (1953).
Fabinyi-Szebehely, M., L. Hahn and J. Szebehely: Investigation in vivo of new inhibitors of hyaluronidase. Brit. J. Pharmacol. **8**, 30—33 (1953).
Feldberg, W., and M. Schachter: Histamine release by horse serum from skin of the sensitized dog and non-sensitized cat. J. Physiol. (Lond.) **118**, 124—134 (1952).

FELDBERG, W., and J. TALESNIK: Reduction of tissue histamine by compound 48/80. J. Physiol. (Lond.) **120**, 550—568 (1953).
FERLUGA, J.: Die Wirkung des durch Polysaccharide aktivierten Rattenblutserums auf den isolierten Darm und Uterus der Ratte. Allergie u. Asthma **6**, 229—232 (1960).
— Permeabilitätserhöhung der Kapillaren durch Anaphylatoxin-Aktivatoren bei der Ratte. Naturwissenschaften **48**, 459 (1961).
FISCHER, R., u. J. FREY: Über die Wirkung verschiedener Antihistaminica und von Novocain auf die Eiweißhyperergie der Ratte. Naunyn-Schmiedebergs Arch. exp. Path. Pharmak. **213**, 392—394 (1951).
FLANDRE, O., M. DA ON, J. L. FERRAN, F. FRANÇOIS et J. J. WEISBUCH: Activité anti-inflammatoire de la 9-alpha-fluoro-16-béta-méthyl-prednisolone (béta-méthasone). Thérapie **18**, 1227—1235 (1963).
FORMANEK, K., u. H. HÖLLER: Über ein experimentell erzeugtes Ödem der Rattenpfote durch Injektion von homologem Serum. Naunyn-Schmiedebergs Arch. exp. Path. Pharmak. **237**, 430—437 (1959).
— — u. E. STOKLASKA: Das Verhalten der Eiweißkörper im Serum und in der Ödemflüssigkeit bei Ratten mit Pfotenödemen. Naunyn-Schmiedebergs Arch. exp. Path. Pharmak. **242**, 228—237 (1961).
FRANK, E.: Über den entzündungshemmenden Effekt verschiedener Substanzen am Dextranödem der Rattenpfote. Influence de différentes substances pharmacologiques sur l'oedème de la patte du rat provoqué par le dextran. Ann. Univ. Sarav. **3**, 267—287 (1955).
FRENGER, W., F. SCHEIFFARTH u. M. GEMÄHLICH: Untersuchungen zum Wirkungsmechanismus des Anaphylatoxins. II. Mitteilung. Der Einfluß der Prednisonvorbehandlung und des Anaphylatoxinschockes auf den Ablauf der passiven Anaphylaxie beim Meerschweinchen. Z. Immun.-Forsch. **115**, 367—372 (1958).
FREY, J., u. R. FISCHER: Der Einfluß von Hypophysenvorderlappenextrakten auf die Eiweißhyperergie der Ratte im Vergleich zu dem von ACTH und Cortison. Naunyn-Schmiedebergs Arch. exp. Path. Pharmak. **214**, 423—426 (1956).
FRICK, O. L., B. N. HALPERN and P. LIACOPOULOS: The mechanism of protection from anaphylactic shock in the guinea-pig by pre-treatment with anaphylatoxin. J. Physiol. (Lond.) **163**, 191—199 (1962).
— P. LIACOPOULOS and B. N. HALPERN: Mechanism of refractoriness to anaphylactic shock in guinea-pigs treated with anaphylatoxin. Excerpta med. (Amst., Int. Congr. Ser. No. **42**, 129 (1961).
FRIEDBERG, K. D., G. ENGELHARDT u. F. MEINEKE: Über die Tachyphylaxie der Anaphylatoxinreaktion und ihre Bedeutung für die Anaphylaxie. Int. Arch. Allergy **22**, 166—169 (1963).
— — — Untersuchungen über die Anaphylatoxin-Tachyphylaxie und über ihre Bedeutung für den Ablauf echter anaphylaktischer Reaktionen. Int. Arch. Allergy **25**, 154—181 (1964).
—, u. L. LENDLE: Zur Frage anaphylaxieartiger Reaktionen bei Einwirkung von Quarz und Kieselsäureverbindungen auf Serum und Gesamtorganismus. Beitr. Silikose-Forsch. **41**, 1—17 (1955).
— H. STEGEMANN u. W. VOGT: Anreicherung von Anaphylatoxin durch Gelfiltration. Naturwissenschaften **50**, 423 (1963).
FRIEDBERGER, E.: Weitere Untersuchungen über Eiweißanaphylaxie. IV. Mitteilung. Z. Immun.-Forsch. **4**, 636—689 (1910a).
— Weitere Mitteilungen über die Beziehungen zwischen Überempfindlichkeit und Infektion. Berl. klin. Wschr. **47**, 1922—1924 (1910b).
—, u. S. GIRGOLAFF: Über Anaphylaxie. XXII. Mitteilung. Weitere Versuche über die Bedeutung der Bakterienmenge für die Anaphylatoxinbildung in vitro. Z. Immun.-Forsch. **11**, 479—484 (1911).
— E. GOLDSCHMID, Z. SZYMANOWSKI, A. SCHÜTZE u. E. NATHAN: Über Anaphylaxie. XII. bis XV. Mitteilung. Beiträge zur Frage der Bildung des Anaphylatoxins aus Mikroorganismen. Z. Immun.-Forsch. **9**, 369—450 (1911).
—, u. T. ITO: Über Anaphylaxie. XXI. Mitteilung. Näheres über den Mechanismus der Komplementwirkung bei der Anaphylatoxinbildung in vitro. Z. Immun.-Forsch. **11**, 471—478 (1911).
—, u. E. JERUSALEM: Über Anaphylaxie. IX. Mitteilung. Das Verhalten des Anaphylatoxins gegenüber einigen physikalischen und chemischen Einflüssen. Z. Immun.-Forsch. **7**, 748—761 (1910).
—, u. G. JOACHIMOGLU: Über Anaphylaxie. 58. Mitteilung. Über die vermeintliche Anaphylatoxinbildung aus Stärke. Z. Hyg. Infekt.-Kr. **84**, 336—368 (1917).
—, u. G. KAPSENBERG: Über Anaphylaxie. XXXIII. Mitteilung. Die Anaphylatoxinbildung aus tierischen Bacillen und durch Plasma an Stelle von Serum. Z. Immun.-Forsch. **16**, 152—159 (1913).

FRIEDBERGER, E., u. P. KONITZER: Über Anaphylaxie. LXII. Mitteilung. Die Filtrationsfähigkeit des Anaphylatoxins durch keimdichte Filter (Berkefeldkerzen und Membranfilter de Haen). Z. Immun.-Forsch. **31**, 293—300 (1921).
—, u. T. KUMAGAI: Über Anaphylaxie. L. Mitteilung. Beiträge zur Wirkung von Eiweißgiften auf isolierte Organe. A. Die Einwirkung von Anaphylatoxin auf den isolierten Darm, nebst einigen Versuchen über die Einwirkung des homologen Antigens auf den isolierten Uterus präparierter Meerschweinchen. Z. Immun.-Forsch. **22**, 269—305 (1914).
— A. LURÀ, O. A. CEDERBERG u. G. CASTELLI: Über Anaphylaxie. XXXVII.—XLII. Mitteilung. Neuere Untersuchungen über den Mechanismus der anaphylaktischen Vergiftung mit besonderer Berücksichtigung der Anaphylatoxinvergiftung. Z. Immun.-Forsch. **18**, 227—330 (1913).
—, u. S. MITA: Über Anaphylaxie. XIX. Mitteilung. Die Anaphylaxie des Frosches und die Einwirkung des Anaphylatoxins auf das isolierte Froschherz. Z. Immun.-Forsch. **10**, 362—387 (1911).
— — u. T. KUMAGAI: Über Anaphylaxie. XXXIV. Mitteilung. Die Bildung eines akut wirkenden Giftes (Anaphylatoxin) aus Toxinen (Tetanus, Diphtherie, Schlangengift). Z. Immun.-Forsch. **17**, 506—538 (1913).
—, u. A. MORESCHI: Über Anaphylatoxin. Berl. klin. Wschr. **49**, 741—744 (1912).
—, u. E. NATHAN: Über Anaphylaxie. XVI. Mitteilung. Die Anaphylatoxinbildung aus Eiweiß im Reagenzglas durch normale Sera. Z. Immun.-Forsch. **9**, 567—574 (1911).
—, u. E. PUTTER: Bestehen Beziehungen zwischen der Anaphylatoxinbildung in vitro und der Änderung der Oberflächenspannung? Z. Immun.-Forsch. **36**, 215—232 (1923).
— Z. SZYMANOWSKI, T. KUMAGAI, ODAIRA u. A. LURÀ: Die Spezifität der Antianaphylaxie und ihre Beziehungen zur Resistenz bei einigen der Anaphylaxie ähnlichen Vergiftungen. (Über Anaphylaxie. XXIX. Mitteilung.) Z. Immun.-Forsch. **14**, 371—411 (1912).
—, u. C. VALLARDI: Über Anaphylaxie. VIII. Mitteilung. Die quantitativen Beziehungen bei der Anaphylatoxinbildung. Z. Immun.-Forsch. **7**, 94—157 (1910).
FRIEDEMANN, U.: Weitere Untersuchungen über den Mechanismus der Anaphylaxie. Z. Immun.-Forsch. **2**, 591—641 (1909).
FRIEDLAENDER, S., S. FEINBERG and A. FEINBERG: Histamine antagonists. VI. Comparative antihistaminic activity of some ethylenediamine drugs in the guinea pig. J. Lab. clin. Med. **32**, 47—50 (1947).
FRIES, B.: Effect of polyphloretin phosphate (PPP) on capillary permeability. Acta pharmacol. (Kbh.) **14**, 378—384 (1958).
GADDUM, J. H., and K. A. HAMEED: Drugs which antagonize 5-hydroxytryptamine. Brit. J. Pharmacol. **9**, 240—248 (1954).
GARATTINI, S., L. LAMESTA, A. MORTARI, V. PALMA and L. VALZELLI: Pharmacological and biochemical effects of 5-hydroxytryptamine in adrenalectomized rats. J. Pharm. Pharmacol. **13**, 385—388 (1961).
GASPAR-NEMETH, U., u. B. ISSEKUTZ: Beiträge zum Wirkungsmechanismus des Azulenols. Acta physiol. Acad. Sci. hung. **4**, 301—305 (1953).
GEIGER, W. B.: Protease activation in immune reactions. J. Immunol. **68**, 11—18 (1952).
GELFAND, M. D., and G. B. WEST: Experimental studies with the butanolamide and propanolamide of 1-methyl-lysergic acid. Int. Arch. Allergy **18**, 286—291 (1961).
GEMÄHLICH, M., W. FRENGER u. F. SCHEIFFARTH: Untersuchungen zur Morphologie der Mastzellen im Anaphylatoxinschock beim Meerschweinchen. Int. Arch. Allergy **13**, 370—376 (1958).
GEORGES, G., et M. HEROLD: Influence de la sérotonine sur l'oedème plantaire au dextran chez le rat. C. R. Soc. Biol. (Paris) **151**, 695—698 (1957).
— — et J. CAHN: Recherches sur l'oedème plantaire à la sérotonine et au dextran chez le rat intact et le rat myélotomisé. C. R. Soc. Biol. (Paris) **152**, 1666—1670 (1958).
GIBERTINI, G., R. VECCHATI e A. GIBERTI: Proprietà antiedema di farmaci ad attività antireumatica. Atti Soc. lombarda Sci. Med.-biol. **6**, 206—211 (1951).
GIERTZ, H.: Anaphylatoxin und Anaphylaxie. Habilitationsschrift, Düsseldorf 1959.
— Wirkstoffbeteiligung an allergischen Reaktionen. Int. Arch. Allergy **22**, 170—186 (1963).
—, u. F. HAHN: Die inverse Anaphylaxie vom Standpunkt der Histamintheorie der Anaphylaxie. Int. Arch. Allergy **6**, 23—44 (1955).
— — Über das Anaphylatoxinbildungsvermögen des Serums im invers-anaphylaktischen Schock. Naturwissenschaften **44**, 264—265 (1957a).
— — Über die Reaktionsbedingungen der Anaphylatoxinbildung. Naturwissenschaften **44**, 467 (1957b).
— — Über den heutigen Stand der Anaphylatoxinforschung. Allergie u. Asthma **4**, 38—44 (1958).
— — Weitere Untersuchungen über die Bildung und die Natur des Anaphylatoxins. Int. Arch. Allergy **19**, 94—111 (1961).

GIERTZ, H., F. HAHN, H. HAHN u. W. SCHMUTZLER: Über den Plasmahistamingehalt bei der Meerschweinchenanaphylaxie. Klin. Wschr. **40**, 598—600 (1962).
— — I. JURNA u. A. LANGE: Zur Frage der Beteiligung des Anaphylatoxins im anaphylaktischen Schock. Int. Arch. Allergy **13**, 201—212 (1958).
— — — u. W. SCHMUTZLER: Vergleichende Untersuchungen über den anaphylaktischen Schock und den Anaphylatoxinschock am intakten Meerschweinchen. Naunyn-Schmiedebergs Arch. exp. Path. Pharmak. **242**, 65—75 (1961).
— — u. A. LANGE: Zum Mechanismus der Anaphylatoxinbildung. Naturwissenschaften **43**, 329 (1956a).
— — — Über die Natur und Bildung von Rattenserumanaphylatoxin. Naunyn-Schmiedebergs Arch. exp. Path. Pharmak. **229**, 366—373 (1956b).
— — W. OPFERKUCH u. W. SCHMUTZLER: Vergleichende Untersuchungen über den anaphylaktischen Schock und den Anaphylatoxinschock an der isolierten Meerschweinchenlunge. Naunyn-Schmiedebergs Arch. exp. Path. Pharmak. **242**, 42—64 (1961).
— — u. W. SCHMUTZLER: Über die Aktivität der Plasmahistaminase bei verschiedenen Schockformen des Meerschweinchens. Int. Arch. Allergy **25**, 343—359 (1964).
— — — u. J. KOLLMEIER: Plasma- und Bluthistamin bei verschiedenen Schockformen des Meerschweinchens. Int. Arch. Allergy **25**, 26—45 (1964).
— W. REUTTER and W. SCHMUTZLER: Histamine release from rabbit blood cells by an anaphylatoxin-like substance formed in normal and C'3 defect rabbit plasma. Nature (Lond.) **202**, 1346 (1964a).
— — — Zur Frage der Histaminfreisetzung durch Anaphylatoxin aus intrazellulären Partikeln. In Vorbereitung (1964b).
—, u. W. SCHMUTZLER: Über die Freisetzung von Wirkstoffen aus der isolierten Meerschweinchenlunge im anaphylaktischen und Anaphylatoxin-Schock. Naunyn-Schmiedebergs Arch. exp. Path. Pharmak. **238**, 103—104 (1960).
GOTH, A.: Inhibition of anaphylactoid edema in the rat by 2-deoxyglucose. Amer. J. Physiol. **197**, 1056—1058 (1959).
— Probable mechanism of histamine release by dextran. Fed. Proc. **20**, 257 (1961).
— R. M. ALLMAN, B. C. MERRITT and J. HOLMAN: Effect of cortisone on histamine liberation induced by Tween in the dog. Proc. Soc. exp. Biol. (N. Y.) **78**, 848—852 (1951).
— J. HOLMAN and J. H. COPENHAVER: Mechanism of action of cortisone in experimental hypersensitivity. Fed. Proc. **11**, 349 (1952).
— W. L. NASH, M. NAGLER and J. HOLMAN: Inhibition of histamine release in experimental diabetes. Amer. J. Physiol. **191**, 25—28 (1957).
GOTZL, F. R., and C. A. DRAGSTEDT: Effect of thyroidectomy and of experimental hyperthyroidism upon histamine content of rat tissues. Proc. Soc. exp. Biol. (N. Y.) **45**, 688—689 (1940).
GÖZSY, B., and L. KÁTÓ: Changes in permeability of the skin capillaries of rats after histamine depletion with 48/80, dextran or egg white. J. Physiol. (Lond.) **139**, 1—9 (1957a).
— — Action of reticulo-endothelial-system stimulators on the histamine depleted rats. Arch. int. Pharmacodyn. **112**, 235—246 (1957b).
— — Behaviour of capillary endothelium during dextran induced oedema. Experientia (Basel) **15**, 391—392 (1959a).
— — Histamine and antihistamines in capillary response to injury. Rev. canad. Biol. **18**, 310—336 (1959b).
— — Maximal edema induced in rats by minute amounts of dextran. Rev. canad. Biol. **19**, 425—433 (1960a).
— — Capillary response in serotonin and histamine depleted rats. Ind. J. med. Res. **48**, 115—120 (1960b).
— — Investigations into the mechanism of action of neuroleptic drugs. Arch. int. Pharmacodyn. **128**, 75—81 (1960c).
— — Investigations into the mechanism of dextran-induced edema in rats. Canad. J. Biochem. **41**, 1855—1863 (1963).
GRAETZ, F.: Die Bedeutung der Lungenblähung als Kriterium der Anaphylaxie. Z. Immun.-Forsch. **8**, 740—780 (1911).
GREEFF, K., B. G. BENFEY u. A. BOKELMANN: Anaphylaktische Reaktionen am isolierten Herzvorhofpräparat des Meerschweinchens und ihre Beeinflussung durch Antihistaminica, BOL, Dihydroergotamin und Reserpin. Naunyn-Schmiedebergs Arch. exp. Path. Pharmak. **236**, 421—434 (1959).
—, u. A. BOKELMANN: Anaphylaktische Reaktionen am isolierten Meerschweinchenherzen. Verh. dtsch. Ges. Kreisl.-Forsch. **25**, 298—302 (1959).
—, u. C. CONTZEN: Über den Mechanismus der diuresehemmenden Wirkung des Dextrans bei Ratten. Naunyn-Schmiedebergs Arch. exp. Path. Pharmak. **239**, 35—53 (1960).

GREISMAN, S. E.: The role of anaphylatoxin during in vitro anaphylaxis. J. Immunol. **81**, 214—219 (1958).
— Activation of histamine-releasing factor in normal rat plasma by E. coli endotoxin. Proc. Soc. exp. Biol. (N. Y.) **103**, 628—632 (1960).
GRÖNWALL, A.: Dextran and its use in colloidal infusion solutions. Stockholm and New York, 1957.
GROSS, F.: Zur Auslösung und Beeinflussung der Ödembildung nach Injektion von Hühnereiweiß an der Ratte. Naunyn-Schmiedebergs Arch. exp. Path. Pharmak. **211**, 421—426 (1950a).
— Unspezifische Beeinflussung entzündlicher Reaktionen. Schweiz. med. Wschr. **80**, 697—701 (1950b).
GROSSBERG, A. L., and H. GARCIA-AROCHA: Histamine liberation in vitro and mode of binding of histamine in tissues. Science **120**, 762—763 (1954).
GROSSMAN, M. I., and C. R. ROBERTSON: Stimulation of gastric secretion by urticariogenic wetting agent (Tween 20) and its inhibition by benadryl. Proc. Soc. exp. Biol. (N. Y.) **68**, 550—552 (1948).
GUTH, P. S., J. W. BYRON and J. L. AMBRUS: Histamine releasers and histamine sensitivity. J. Pharm. Pharmacol. **13**, 254—256 (1961).
GYERMEK, L., I. LÁZÁR u. A. Z. CSÁK: The antiserotonin action of chlorpromazine and some other phenothiazine derivatives. Arch. int. Pharmacodyn. **108**, 62—74 (1956).
HAAS, H., E. HOHAGEN u. G. KOLLMANNSPERGER: Vergleichende Untersuchungen mit Analgeticis. Arzneimittel-Forsch. **3**, 238—247 (1953).
HAHN, F.: Zur Anaphylatoxinfrage. Naturwissenschaften **41**, 465—470 (1954a).
— Toxicity of dextran in rats and the formation of anaphylactic toxins. J. Pharmacol. exp. Ther. **110**, 24 (1954b).
— Anaphylaktoide Reaktionen durch künstliche Plasmaersatzstoffe. Verh. dtsch. Ges. inn. Med. **60**, 719—721 (1954c).
— On anaphylatoxin. Int. Arch. Allergy **11**, 119—128 (1957).
— Anaphylatoxin: formation, actions and rôle in anaphylaxis. In: Polypeptides which affect smooth muscles and blood vessels. p. 275—292. London: Pergamon Press 1960.
— Zur Pharmakologie und Toxikologie körperfremder kolloidaler Blutersatzmittel. Ber. 9. Tag. dtsch. Ges. Bluttransf., Braunschweig 1960. Bibl. haemat. (Basel) **12**, 137—172 (1961).
—, u. H. GIERTZ: Die theoretischen Grundlagen der Allergie. Arch. Ohr.-Nas. u. Kehlk.-Heilk. **176**, 1—81 (1960).
— — u. W. SCHMUTZLER: Studien über die anaphylaktische und anaphylaktoide Histaminfreisetzung in der Meerschweinchenlunge. Int. Arch. Allergy **18**, 62—74 (1961).
—, u. A. LANGE: Versuche zur Isolierung von Rattenserum-Anaphylatoxin. Naunyn-Schmiedebergs Arch. exp. Path. Pharmak. **227**, 12—22 (1955).
— — Das Anaphylatoxin. Eine alte Theorie der Anaphylaxie in neuer Sicht. Dtsch. med. Wschr. **81**, 1269—1274 (1956).
— — u. H. GIERTZ: Anaphylaktoide Reaktionen durch künstliche Blutersatzstoffe. Naunyn-Schmiedebergs Arch. exp. Path. Pharmak. **222**, 603—614 (1954).
—, u. A. OBERDORF: Antihistaminica und anaphylaktoide Reaktionen. Z. Immun.-Forsch. **107**, 528—538 (1950).
—, u. A. WELLMANN: Experimentelle Untersuchungen über Histaminfreisetzung durch künstliche Blutersatzmittel. Klin. Wschr. **30**, 998—999 (1952).
HAHN, H. jr.: Über den Plasmahistamingehalt bei der Meerschweinchenanaphylaxie. Inaugural-Dissertation, Freiburg 1964.
HAINING, C. G.: Histamine release in rabbit blood by dextran and dextran sulphate. Brit. J. Pharmacol. **10**, 87—94 (1955).
— Activation of rabbit serum protease by dextran sulphate. Brit. J. Pharmacol. **11**, 107—110 (1956a).
— Inhibition of histamine release by sodium salicylate and other compounds. Brit. J. Pharmacol. **11**, 357—363 (1956b).
— The release of cellular histamine in rabbit blood by dextran and dextran sulphate. In: "Histamine" Ciba-Found. Symp. p. 160—166. London: Churchill 1956.
HALPERN, B. N.: Sur le mécanisme d'action des antihistaminiques de synthèse. Presse méd. **57**, 949—951 (1949a).
— Action des substances modificatrices de la perméabilité capillaire et notamment du rutoside et de l'adrénaline sur l'oedème du rat provoqué par l'ovalbumine. C. R. Soc. Biol. (Paris) **143**, 825—827 (1949b).
— Histamine release by long chain molecules. In: "Histamine" Ciba-Found. Symp. p. 92—123. London: Churchill 1956.
— Substances histamino-libératrices et processus de libération de l'histamine endogène. Actualités pharmacol. Série **13**, 109—129 (1960a).

HALPERN, B. N.: Histamine and processes of histamine liberation. In: Fundamentals of Modern Allergy. p. 27—42. New York, Toronto, London: McGraw-Hill Book Co. 1960b.
— G. BIOZZI, M. BRIOT et B. BENACERRAF: Modalités de la recharge des tissus en histamine après sa déplétion par une substance libératrice d'histamine et action empêchante de la cortisone sur cette recharge. C. R. Soc. Biol. (Paris) **147**, 1180—1184 (1953).
—, et M. BRIOT: Rôle de la perméabilité capillaire dans le déterminisme de l'oedème produit chez le rat par l'ovalbumine et action des antihistaminiques de synthèse sur ce syndrome. C. R. Soc. Biol. (Paris) **143**, 822—824 (1949).
— — Étude pathogénique et thérapeutique du syndrome oedémateux provoqué chez le rat par l'ovalbumine. Arch. int. Pharmacodyn. **82**, 247—296 (1950).
— — Libération d'histamine par la peau de rat sous l'effet du contact avec le dextran, in vitro. C. R. Soc. Biol. (Paris) **146**, 1552—1555 (1952a).
— — Action inhibitrice de la prométhazine sur l'oedème provoqué par l'ovalbumine et le dextran chez le rat surrénalectomisé. Arch. int. Pharmacodyn. **91**, 291—302 (1952b).
— — Mécanisme histaminique de l'action de la polyvinylpyrrolidone chez le chien. C. R. Soc. Biol. (Paris) **147**, 643—647 (1953a).
— — Mécanisme histaminique de l'action de certains polymères. Acta allerg. (Kbh.) Suppl. III, p. 168—169 (1953b).
— — Modalités de la déplétion de l'histamine cutanée par le dextran chez le rat. C. R. Soc. Biol. (Paris) **148**, 959—963 (1954a).
— — Hyperhistaminémie provoquée par l'injection du dextran chez le rat. C. R. Soc. Biol. (Paris) **148**, 1046—1049 (1954b).
— — D. MOUTON et J. TRUFFERT: Corrélation entre la libération de l'histamine et du potassium cellulaire. C. R. Soc. Biol. (Paris) **149**, 1223—1229 (1955).
— — et T. NEVEU: Dextran et anaphylatoxine. C. R. Soc. Biol. (Paris) **148**, 308—312 (1954a).
— — — Dextran et anaphylatoxine. Presse méd. **62**, 389 (1954b).
— P. LIACOPOULOS et M. BRIOT: Aspects qualitatifs et quantitatifs de l'antagonisme des antihistaminiques de synthèse à l'égard de l'histamine, des substances histamino-libératrices et de la réaction anaphylactique. C. R. Soc. Biol. (Paris) **150**, 313—316 (1956a).
— — — Mécanisme de protection du cobaye contre le choc anaphylactique mortel par l'anaphylatoxine. Acta allerg. (Kbh.) **10**, 9—14 (1956b).
— — et M. LIACOPOULOS-BRIOT: Libération de 5-hydroxytryptamine chez le rat sous l'influence de substances histamino-libératrices. C. R. Soc. Biol. (Paris) **151**, 1692—1696 (1957).
— — — Recherches sur les substances exogènes et endogènes agissant sur la perméabilité capillaire et leurs antagonistes. Arch. int. Pharmacodyn. **119**, 56—101 (1959).
— M. LIACOPOULOS-BRIOT et P. LIACOPOULOS: Recherches sur les modalités de la protection croisée exercée par les diverses substances histamino-libératrices chez le rat albinos. C. R. Soc. Biol. (Paris) **152**, 285—291 (1958).
— T. NEVEU et A. BRANELLEC: Modalités de libération d'histamine par diverses substances histamino-libératrices en hypothermie profonde. C. R. Soc. Biol. (Paris) **153**, 14—18 (1959).
—, et C. STIFFEL: Modifications de la température cutanée après injection intraveineuse de polyvinylpyrrolidone (PVP) chez le chien et ses rélations avec la libération d'histamine. C. R. Soc. Biol. (Paris) **149**, 35—39 (1955).
— — M. LIACOPOULOS-BRIOT et L. CONOVICI: Recherches expérimentales sur un nouvel antihistaminique de synthèse, la cinnarazine. Arch. int. Pharmacodyn. **142**, 170—184 (1963).
HANNA, C. H., and L. H. MARSHALL: Effect of ether and barbiturate anesthesia on the reaction of rats to dextran and of dogs to polyvinylpyrrolidone. Amer. J. Physiol. **191**, 615—620 (1957).
HANZLIK, P. J., and H. T. KARSNER: Anaphylactoid phenomena from the intravenous administration of various colloids, arsenicals and other agents. J. Pharmacol. exp. Ther. **14**, 379—423 (1920).
— — Further observations on anaphylactoid phenomena from various agents injected intravenously. J. Pharmacol. exp. Ther. **23**, 173—235 (1924a).
— — Treatment of anaphylactoid phenomena from some agents by hypertonic sugar and salt solutions. J. Pharmacol. exp. Ther. **23**, 237—242 (1924b).
— — Effects from the intraperitoneal injection of various agents causing anaphylactoid phenomena. J. Pharmacol. exp. Ther. **23**, 243—260 (1924c).
— — and J. FETTERMAN: Anaphylactoid phenomena from thromboplastic agents. J. Pharmacol. exp. Ther. **14**, 229—242 (1920).
HARRIS, J. M.: Rats resistant to dextran and egg-white. Int. Arch. Allergy **22**, 109—111 (1963).
— H. KALMUS and G. B. WEST: Genetical control of the anaphylactoid reaction in rats. Genet. Res., **4**, 346—355 (1963).
—, and P. S. J. SPENCER: A modified plethysmographic apparatus for recording volume changes in the rat paw. J. Pharm. Pharmacol. **14**, 464—466 (1962).

HARRIS, J. M., and G. B. WEST: Anaphylactoid reaction in rats. Nature (Lond.) **191**, 399—400 (1961).
— — Rats resistant to the dextran anaphylactoid reaction. Brit. J. Pharmacol. **20**, 550—562 (1963).
HARVEY, J. A.: Modification of histamine sensitivity after 48/80 treatment. J. Pharm. Pharmacol. **13**, 61—62 (1961).
HASHIMOTO, H.: Über die Einwirkung des Bakterienanaphylatoxins auf das isolierte Gefäßpräparat des Meerschweinchens und der Ratte. Z. Immun.-Forsch. **56**, 271—275 (1928).
HECHT, G., u. H. WEESE: Periston, ein neuer Blutflüssigkeitsersatz. Münch. med. Wschr. **90**, 11—15 (1943).
HEILMEYER, L., J. FREY u. R. FISCHER: Einwirkung von TBI (Conteben) auf die Eiweißhyperergie der Ratte. Naunyn-Schmiedebergs Arch. exp. Path. Pharmak. **213**, 387-391 (1951).
— — — Über Wirkungen von adrenotropem Hypophysenvorderlappenhormon, 11-Dehydro- und 11-Desoxy-Corticosteron im Modellversuch am Tier. Naunyn-Schmiedebergs Arch. exp. Path. Pharmak. **214**, 416—422 (1952).
HEITE, H. J., u. H. HÖLAND: Untersuchungen am Rattenpfotenödem über die Einflußgröße des peripheren Nervensystems auf Entzündungsvorgänge. Acta neuroveg. (Wien) **13**, 217—233 (1956).
HEKTOEN, L., and A. G. COLE: The proteins of egg white. The proteins in egg white and their relationship to the blood proteins of the domestic fowl as determined by the precipitin reaction. J. infect. Dis. **42**, 1—24 (1928).
HERSHBERGER, L. G., and L. M. HANSEN: Effect of hydrocortisone on activation and activity of anaphylatoxin in vitro. Proc. Soc. exp. Biol. (N. Y.) **98**, 150—153 (1958).
HERTTING, G., u. E. STOKLASKA: Zur Beeinflussung des Rattenpfotenödems durch die Narkose. Naunyn-Schmiedebergs Arch. exp. Path. Pharmak. **231**, 562—567 (1957).
— — Über den Einfluß nervöser Faktoren auf das Dextranödem der Rattenpfote und auf die ödemhemmende Wirkung von Chlorpromazin. Naunyn-Schmiedebergs Arch. exp. Path. Pharmak. **237**, 423—429 (1959).
HICKS, R., and G. B. WEST: Adrenal cortical hormones and the formation of histamine and 5-hydroxytryptamine. Nature (Lond.) **181**, 1342—1343 (1958a).
— — Adrenalectomy and tissue amines. Nature (Lond.) **182**, 401—402 (1958b).
HILDEBRAND, G.: Zur Analyse der Anaphylaktoiden Reaktion. 4. Mitteilung: Giftbildung in vivo und in vitro. Arzneimittel-Forsch. **8**, 36—39 (1958a).
— Zur Analyse der Anaphylaktoiden Reaktion. 5. Mitteilung (Schluß): Anaphylaktischer Schock und Anaphylaktoide Reaktion. Arzneimittel-Forsch. **8**, 656—662 (1958b).
HILLEBRECHT, J.: Zur routinemäßigen Prüfung antiphlogistischer Substanzen im Rattenpfotentest. Arzneimittel-Forsch. **4**, 607—614 (1954).
— Über die Wirksamkeit des 2-(β-Chloräthyl)-2,3-dihydro-4-oxo(benzo-1,3-oxazins), gemessen am Kaolin-, Hühnereiweiß- und Serotonin-Ödem der Rattenpfote. (Zugleich ein Beitrag zur Frage des Pathomechanismus des Kaolin- und Hühnereiweißödems). Arzneimittel-Forsch. **9**, 623—628 (1959).
HIRSCHFELD, L., u. R. KLINGER: Gerinnungsphänomene und Anaphylatoxinbildung. Zbl. Bakt. I. Abt. Ref. **57**, Beiheft S. 231—235 (1913).
— — Über das Wesen der Inaktivierung und der Komplementbindung. Z. Immun.-Forsch. **21**, 40—76 (1914).
HOENE, R.: Acquisition of topical resistance to thermal injury. Proc. Soc. exp. Biol. (N. Y.) **85**, 56—61 (1954).
— P. LABBÉ and H. SELYE: A phenomenon of topical protection against hyperergic inflammation by a preceding local inflammation. Proc. Soc. exp. Biol. (N. Y.) **79**, 65—68 (1952).
HOFFMAN, R. A.: Influence of the adrenal gland on hypothermic response of the rat to chlorpromazine, reserpine, and serotonin. Amer. J. Physiol. **196**, 876—880 (1959).
HUMPHREY, J. H.: Cellular components involved in the immediate allergic reactions. In: Immunopathology. p. 215—224. Basel: Benno Schwabe u. Co. 1959a.
— Biochemical aspects of reactions in hypersensitive responses. In: Cellular and humoral aspects of the hypersensitive states. p. 1—35. New York: P. B. Hoeber Inc. 1959b.
—, and R. JAQUES: Liberation of histamine and serotonin from platelets by antigen-antibody reactions in vitro. J. Physiol. (Lond.) **119**, 43 P (1953).
— — The release of histamine and 5-hydroxytryptamine (serotonin) from platelets by antigen-antibody reactions (in vitro). J. Physiol. (Lond.) **128**, 9—27 (1955).
—, and I. MOTA: The mechanism of anaphylaxis: Specificity of antigen-induced mast cell damage in anaphylaxis in the guinea pig. Immunology **2**, 31—43 (1959).
HYDE, R. R.: The complement deficient guinea pig: a study of an inheritable factor in immunity. Amer. J. Hyg. **15**, 824—836 (1932).
INDERBITZIN, T.: Das Problem der allergischen Reaktionsmechanismen. (Eine analytische Studie.) Int. Arch. Allergy **9**, 146—188 (1956).

IRINO, S.: Effect of histamine releasers and of anti-inflammatory drugs on the egg-white edema of rat hind paws in relation to skin histamine. Acta med. Okayama **12**, 93—111 (1958).
ISHIZAKA, K.: Gamma globulin and molecular mechanisms in hypersensitivity reactions. Progr. Allergy **7**, 32—106 (1963).
—, and T. ISHIZAKA: Biologic activity of aggregated γ-globulin. II. A study of various methods for aggregation and species differences. J. Immunol. **85**, 163—171 (1960).
— — and T. SUGAHARA: Biological activity of aggregated γ-globulin. III. Production of arthus-like reactions. J. Immunol. **86**, 220—227 (1961).
— — Biological activities of aggregated γ-globulin. I. Skin reactive and complement fixing properties of heat denatured γ-globulin. Proc. Soc. exp. Biol. (N. Y.) **101**, 845—850 (1959)
JANCSÓ, N.: Histamine as a physiological activator of the reticulo-endothelial system.Nature (Lond.) **160**, 227—228 (1947).
— Inflammation and the inflammatory mechanisms. J. Pharm. Pharmacol. **13**, 577—594 (1961).
JAQUES, R.: The anaphylatoxin-forming capacity of rat serum as influenced by proteus polysaccharides. Further pharmacodynamic differentiation of anti-allergic polysaccharides and steroids. Int. Arch. Allergy **18**, 75—84 (1961).
—, u. R. DOMENJOZ: Histamin-antagonistische Wirkung bei Pyrazolen und Antihistaminen. Naunyn-Schmiedebergs Arch. exp. Path. Pharmak. **212**, 124—125 (1950/51).
JASMIN, G.: Étude de l'inflammation anaphylactoide. Rev. canad. Biol. **15**, 107—185 (1956a).
— Die anaphylaktoide Entzündungsreaktion. Allergie u. Asthma **2**, 208—212 (1956b).
— Étude sur les propriétés anti-inflammatoires de la chlorpromazine. Arch. int. Pharmacodyn. **112**, 1—7 (1957).
— Effect of histamine liberators on urinary excretion of 5-hydroxyindoleacetic acid. Proc. Soc. exp. Biol. (N. Y.) **105**, 581—583 (1960).
—, et P. BOIS: Étude sur la pathogenèse de l'oedème au dextrane chez le rat. Experientia (Basel) **14**, 101 (1958).
— — Effect of insulin, fasting and tolbutamide on dextran edema in rats. Proc. Soc. exp. Biol. (N. Y.) **101**, 656—658 (1959).
— — and M. S. SU: Sensitivity of the rat to increasing doses of dextran. Canad. J. Biochem. **40**, 697—702 (1962).
JOACHIMOGLU, G.: Über Anaphylaxie. XXVIII. Mitteilung. Weiteres über Anaphylatoxinbildung aus Bakterien von peptonfreien Nährböden, zugleich ein Beitrag zur Frage der quantitativen Verhältnisse bei der Giftbildung. Z. Immun.-Forsch. **14**, 280—284 (1912).
JOBLING, J. W., and W. PETERSEN: Serotoxin. Studies on ferment action XIV. J. exp. Med. **19**, 480—500 (1914a).
— — The mechanism of anaphylatoxin formation. Studies on ferment action XV. J. exp. Med. **20**, 37—51 (1914b).
JONES, J. H.: Studies on the activation of anaphylatoxin. Int. Arch. Allergy **17**, 99—105 (1960).
JORI, A., A. P. BENTIVOGLIO and S. GARATTINI: The mechanism of the local inflammatory reaction induced by compound 48/80 and dextran in rats. J. Pharm. Pharmacol. **13**, 617—619 (1961).
KABAT, E. A.: Heterogeneity in extent of the combining regions of human antidextran. J. Immunol. **77**, 377—385 (1956).
— Études immuno-chimiques sur les dextranes et les substances des groupes sanguins. Rev. Hémat. **12**, 606—624 (1957).
— Immunchemische Untersuchungen an Dextranen und Blutgruppensubstanzen. Behringwerk-Mitt. **34**, 39—71 (1958).
— The upper limit for the size of the human antidextran combining site. J. Immunol. **84**, 82—85 (1960).
—, and A. E. BEZER: The effect of variation in molecular weight on the antigenicity of dextran in man. Arch. Biochem. **78**, 306—318 (1958).
KADATZ, R.: Pharmakologische Eigenschaften des 2-(β-Chloräthyl)-2,3-dihydro-4-oxo-(benzo-1,3-oxazin), eines neuen Antiphlogisticum. Arzneimittel-Forsch. **7**, 651—653 (1957).
KALBHEN, D. A.: Bestimmung der freien Aminosäuren im gesunden und entzündeten Pfotengewebe der Ratte. Arch. int. Pharmacodyn. **143**, 337—361 (1963a).
— Qualitative und quantitative Bestimmung der Nukleotide und Glycolysephosphate im gesunden und entzündeten Pfotengewebe. Arch. int. Pharmacodyn. **143**, 362—376 (1963b).
KARADY, S., B. ROSE and J. S. L. BROWNE: Decrease of histaminase in tissue by adrenalectomy and its restoration by cortico-adrenal extract. Amer. J. Physiol. **130**, 539—542 (1940).
KÁTÓ, L., and B. GÖZSY: Role of histamine and leucotaxin in function of cellular defense mechanism. Amer. J. Physiol. **184**, 296—300 (1956).
— — Effect of phenothiazine derivatives on dextran-induced edema. J. Pharmacol. exp. Ther. **129**, 231—236 (1960a).

Kátó, L., and B. Gözsy: Kinetics of edema formation in rats as influenced by critical doses of dextran. Amer. J. Physiol. **199**, 657—660 (1960b).
— — Quantitative evaluation of antihistaminic effects. Toxicol. appl. Pharmacol. **2**, 144—150 (1960).
— — Improved method for quantitative evaluation of drug effects on dextran edema in the rat. Toxicol. appl. Pharmacol. **3**, 145—152 (1961a).
— — Quantitative interaction between dextran and antihistamines in the rat. Fed. Proc. **20**, 256 (1961b).
— — Le rôle des mastocytes dans la réaction anaphylactoide provoquée par le dextran. J. Physiol. (Paris) **54**, 619—624 (1962).
Kawamoto, S.: Effects of peptone, sinomenine, polyvinylpyrrolidone, and corbicula extract on the tissue mast cells in the dog. Okayama-Igakkai-Zasshi **70**, 3803—3812 (1958).
Keller, R.: Veränderungen an den Gewebemastzellen der Ratte im Schock. Helv. physiol. pharmacol. Acta **15**, C20 (1957a).
— Tissue mast cells in anaphylactic shock and anaphylactoid reactions. Int. Arch. Allergy **11**, 328—341 (1957b).
—, and I. Beeger: Das Verhalten isolierter sensibilisierter Mastzellen nach Einwirkung des Antigens unter verschiedenen Versuchsbedingungen. Med. exp. **4**, 51—58 (1961).
Kemper, F., u. G. Amelin: Eine neue elektrische Methode zur Messung von Volumina, Drucken und anderen sowie ein Beispiel ihrer Anwendung. Z. ges. exp. Med. **131**, 407—411 (1959).
Kitchin, H. W., W. Y. Smith, G. L. Wallace jr., M. Perkins and J. L. Morrison: Studies with dextran in the albino rat. Arch. int. Pharmacodyn. **99**, 17—31 (1954).
Klein, H.: Zur Phasenbestimmung der lokalen Hühnereiweiß-Entzündung: Ödemtest nach Selye. Klin. Wschr. **29**, 548—549 (1951).
Kondo, K.: Studies on urinary excretion of histamine in the rat. Part 2. Actions on the urinary excretion of histamine, of the histamine releasers of different classes and of the substances affecting histamine release. Okayama-Igakkai-Zasshi **71**, 3289—3299 (1959).
Königsfeld, H.: Anaphylaxie-Versuche am isolierten Froschherzen. Z. ges. exp. Med. **44**, 723—728 (1925).
Kopaczewski, W.: Le rôle des phénomènes physiques dans la production du choc anaphylatoxique. C. R. Soc. Biol. (Paris) **82**, 590—593 (1919).
—, et Z. Gruzewska: La toxicité sérique et les propriétés physiques des gels colloidaux. C. R. Acad. Sci. (Paris) **170**, 133—135 (1920).
—, et S. Mutermilch: Sur l'origine des anaphylatoxines. Z. Immun.-Forsch. **22**, 539—549 (1914).
Kramer, M.: Entzündungshemmung durch Eisenpräparate. Naunyn-Schmiedebergs Arch. exp. Path. Pharmak. **220**, 391—397 (1953).
— Biochemische und pharmakologische Differenzierung der Wirkung ödemerzeugender Substanzen. Naunyn-Schmiedebergs Arch. exp. Path. Pharmak. **225**, 82—84 (1955).
— Pharmakologische Differenzierung des Eiklar- und Dextranödems der Ratte. Naunyn-Schmiedebergs Arch. exp. Path. Pharmak. **228**, 302—306 (1956a).
— Die Bedeutung der Histaminfreisetzung durch Compound 48/80, Dextran und Eiereiweiß für die Ödementstehung bei der Ratte. Naunyn-Schmiedebergs Arch. exp. Path. Pharmak. **228**, 340—346 (1956b).
— Aktivierung proteolytischer Fermente bei Entzündungsreaktionen. Naunyn-Schmiedebergs Arch. exp. Path. Pharmak. **234**, 432—438 (1958).
—, e E. Arrigoni-Martelli: Significato dell'attività antiserotoninica e sedativa centrale di derivati fenotiazinici per la loro azione inibitrice sull'edema da dextran nel ratto. Boll. Soc. ital. Biol. sper. **34**, 1128—1130 (1958).
Krantz, J. C., C. J. Carr, J. G. Bird and S. Cook: Sugar alcohols. XXVI. Pharmacodynamic studies of polyoxyalkylene derivatives of hexitol anhydride partial fatty acid esters. J. Pharmacol. exp. Ther. **93**, 188—195 (1948).
Krantz, J. C. jr., C. J. Carr, H. M. Bubert and J. G. Bird: Sugar alcohols. XXVII. Drug allergy in the canine family. J. Pharmacol. exp. Ther. **97**, 125—128 (1949).
Kraus, R.,, u. P. Kirschbaum: Zur Frage der anaphylaktischen Vergiftung. Wien. klin. Wschr. **26**, 783—785 (1913).
Küchle, H. J., u. H. Wegener: Quantitative Untersuchungen über Wirksamkeit und Wirkungsstärke entzündungshemmender Substanzen. Z. ges. exp. Med. **118**, 136—142 (1952).
Kumagai, T.: Über Anaphylaxie. XXXVI. Mitteilung. Die Lungenblähung bei der Anaphylatoxinvergiftung und bei einigen ähnlich wirkenden Giften. Z. Immun.-Forsch. **17**, 607—638 (1913).
Lagunoff, D., and E. P. Benditt: Mast cell degranulation and histamine release observed in a new in vitro system. J. exp. Med. **112**, 571—580 (1960).

LECOMTE, J.: 5-hydroxytryptamine et membrane nictitante du chat. Arch. int. Pharmacodyn. **100**, 457—464 (1955).
— Absence d'activité histamino-libératrice de certains polymères, étudiés in vitro, chez le rat. C. R. Soc. Biol. (Paris) **151**, 1281—1283 (1957),
— Action de deux dérivés de l'adrénochrome sur l'oedème au dextran chez le rat. C. R. Soc. Biol. (Paris) **152**, 1409—1410 (1958).
—, et M. L. BEAUMARIAGE: Libérateurs d'histamine et choc anaphylactique du coq. C. R. Soc. Biol. (Paris) **150**, 1028—1030 (1956).
— A. DRESSE et H. VAN CAUWENBERGE: Médullo-surrénale et résistance du rat à l'oedème anaphylactoide. Arch. int. Physiol. **68**, 618—622 (1960).
—, et H. VAN CAUWENBERGE: Libérateurs d'histamine et oedème atopique du rat. C. R. Soc. Biol. (Paris) **149**, 2274—2276 (1955).
— — et M. VLIERS: Oedème au dextran et médications anti-inflammatoires. Arch. int. Pharmacodyn. **121**, 65—70 (1959).
LEFEBVRE, P., et H. VAN CAUWENBERGE: Glucagon et réactions oedémateuses du rat. Arch. int. Pharmacodyn. **138**, 222—229 (1962).
LÉGER, J., and G. MASSON: Effect of antihistaminic substances on the edema produced by egg white in the rat. Amer. J. med. Sci. **214**, 305—307 (1947).
— — Studies on eggwhite sensitivity in the rat. Influence of the endocrine glands. Ann. Allergy **6**, 131—143 (1948).
— — and J. L. PRADO: Factors influencing an anaphylactoid reaction in the rat. Fed. Proc. **6**, 150—151 (1947 a).
— — — Réaction oedemateuse chez le rat. Influence des substances anti-histaminiques. Rev. canad. Biol. **6**, 359—361 (1947 b).
— — — Hypersensitivity to egg white in the rat. Proc. Soc. exp. Biol. (N. Y.) **64**, 366—370 (1947 c).
LENDLE, L., u. U. WEISSER: Anaphylaktoide Reaktionen von Hühnereiweiß und Dextran an isolierten Organen von Ratten. Int. Arch. Allergy **20**, 143—173 (1962).
LENFELD, J., u. B. STOJAN: Beitrag zur Frage der neurohumoralen Regulation der Entzündungen. Naunyn-Schmiedebergs Arch. exp. Path. Pharmak. **241**, 162—163 (1961).
LEPOW, I. H.: Nonspecific factors in immunity and hypersensitivity. J. Allergy **28**, 52—61 (1957).
— Complement: a review. (Including esterase activity). In: Mechanisms of hypersensitivity. p. 267—279. Boston: Little, Brown and Co. 1959.
LEPPER, M. H., E. R. CALDWELL, P. K. SMITH and B. F. MILLER: Effects on anaphylactic shock of salicylates, aminopyrine and other chemically and pharmacologically related compounds. Proc. Soc. exp. Biol. (N. Y.) **74**, 254—258 (1950).
LEVINSON, S. O., F. NEUWELT and H. NECHELES: Human serum as blood substitute in treatment of hemorrhage and shock. J. Amer. med. Ass. **114**, 455—461 (1960).
LEVY, S. W., and G. DE VAILLANCOURT: Effects of inflammation on proteins and enzymes in rat plasma. Canad. J. Biochem. **38**, 575—584 (1960).
LEWIS, G. P.: Active polypeptides derived from plasma proteins. Physiol. Rev. **40**, 647—676 (1960).
LIACOPOULOS, P., B. N. HALPERN et M. LIACOPOULOS-BRIOT: Modalités de l'inhibition des effets de l'histamine des substances histamino-libératrices et de la 5-hydroxytryptamine sur la perméabilité capillaire par leurs antagonistes. C. R. Soc. Biol. (Paris) **151**, 1661—1666 (1957).
LINDNER, E.: Ein Beitrag zur atopischen Reaktion des Hundes gegen polymere Stoffe. Z. ges. exp. Med. **121**, 32—43 (1953).
LOEWIT, M.: Anaphylaxiestudien. 4. Mitteilung. Die anaphylaktische und anaphylaktoide Vergiftung beim Meerschweinchen. Naunyn-Schmiedebergs Arch. exp. Path. Pharmak. **73**, 1—32 (1913).
—, u. G. BAYER: Anaphylaxiestudien. 6. Mitteilung. Die Abspaltung von Anaphylatoxin aus Agar nach BORDET. Naunyn-Schmiedebergs Arch. exp. Path. Pharmak. **74**, 164—180(1913).
LOUBATIÈRES, A.: L'injection de polyvinylpyrrolidone déclenche ches le chien un choc grave prolongé. C. R. Soc. Biol. (Paris) **142**, 1340—1342 (1948).
LUMIÈRE, A.: Le problème de l'anaphylaxie. Paris: Doin 1924.
—, et H. COUTURIER: Sur la toxicité du sérum gélosé. Arch. int. Pharmacodyn. **30**, 151—155 (1925).
— — Conditions sur la toxicité du sérum gélosé. Arch. int. Pharmacodyn. **31**, 335—338 (1926).
— et P. MEYER: Caractéristiques colloidales du sérum après contact avec l'amidon. C. R. Soc. Biol. (Paris) **118**, 884—885 (1935 a).
— — Kolloidik des mit Stärke behandelten Serums. Klin. Wschr. **14**, 382 (1935 b).
— — Über das durch Kaolin oder Stärke erzeugte sogenannte „Anaphylatoxin“. Klin. Wschr. **14**, 1251—1252 (1935 c).

MacIntosh, F. C.: Histamine and intracellular particles. In: Histamine. Ciba Found. Symp. p. 20—35. London: Churchill 1956.
Manwaring, W. H., and Y. Kusama: Analysis of the anaphylactic and immune reactions by means of the isolated guinea-pig lungs. J. Immunol. **2**, 157—165 (1917).
Marmorston-Gottesman, J., and J. Gottesman: The use of histamine as a standard test for diminished resistance in suprarenalectomized rats. J. exp. Med. **47**, 503—514 (1928).
Marshall, L. H., and C. H. Hanna: Circulatory reaction of tolerant and nontolerant dogs to polyvinylpyrrolidone and of rats to dextran. Amer. J. Physiol. **189**, 209—213 (1957).
— — Circulatory reactions of dogs and rats to polyvinylpyrrolidone or dextran after 48/80. Proc. Soc. exp. Biol. (N. Y.) **97**, 587—590 (1958).
Marshall, P. B.: The influence of adrenal cortical deficiency on the histamine content of rat tissues. J. Physiol. (Lond.) **102**, 180—190 (1943).
Martin, G. J.: Anti-inflammatory effect of trypsin. Ann. N. Y. Acad. Sci. **68**, 70—87 (1957).
—, R. Brendel and J. M. Beiler: Effects of parenterally administered trypsin and phosphorylated hesperidin. Arch. int. Pharmacodyn. **96**, 124—129 (1953).
— — — Inhibition of egg-white edema by proteolytic enzymes. Proc. Soc. exp. Biol. (N. Y.) **86**, 636—638 (1954).
Masson, G. M. C., A. C. Corcoran and S. Franco-Browder: Mechanism of arterial pressure response to histamine-liberators. Amer. J. Physiol. **195**, 407—411 (1958).
McIntire, F. C.: The mechanism of histamine release. In: Histamine. Ciba Found. Symp. p. 416—430. London: Churchill 1956.
— R. K. Richards and L. W. Roth: Histamine release inhibition in vitro and anti-anaphylactic effects in vivo of some chemical compounds. Brit. J. Pharmacol. **12**, 39—43 (1957).
— L. W. Roth and R. K. Richards: The in vitro release of histamine from the blood cells of sensitized rabbits: relationship to blood coagulation mechanisms. Amer. J. Physiol. **159**, 332—336 (1949).
— — and M. Sproull: In vitro histamine release from sensitized rabbit blood cells. Evidence against participation of fibrinolysin. Proc. Soc. exp. Biol. (N. Y.) **73**, 605—609 (1950).
— — — Mechanism of anaphylaxis in the rabbit. Further evidence against plasma protease mechanism. Proc. Soc. exp. Biol. (N. Y.) **81**, 691—692 (1952).
Medaković, M.: Egg white reaction in rats and 5 hydroxytryptamine. Arch. int. Physiol. **67**, 294—305 (1959).
—, and I. Spužić: 5-Hydroxytryptamine in blood during experimental traumatic shock in rats. Nature (Lond.) **183**, 1685 (1959).
Meidinger, F.: La polyvinylpyrrolidone (P.V.P.) colloïde protecteur de synthèse in vitro et in vivo. Bull. Soc. Chim. biol. (Paris) **29**, 411—416 (1947).
Meier, R., F. Gross u. P. Desaulles: Über die Bedeutung der Nebennieren und der Nebennierenrindensteroide für den Ablauf entzündlicher Reaktionen. Klin. Wschr. **29**, 653—663 (1951).
Menkin, V.: The role of inflammation in immunity. Physiol. Rev. **18**, 366—418 (1938).
Meyer, M.: Über die Wirkung von Alkoholen auf das Dextranödem der Ratten. Inaugural-Dissertation, Freiburg 1963.
Miles, A. A., and D. L. Wilhelm: Enzyme-like globulins from serum reproducing the vascular phenomena of inflammation. I. An active permeability factor and its inhibitor in guinea-pig serum. Brit. J. exp. Path. **36**, 71—81 (1955).
Misch, W.: Untersuchungen über den Abbau von Bakterien durch Abwehrfermente. (Abderhaldensches Dialysierverfahren.) Z. Hyg. Infekt-Kr. **89**, 211—222 (1919).
Moeller, J.: Überempfindlichkeit gegen Dextran bei renalem Hochdruck. Dtsch. med. Wschr. **80**, 561—564 (1955).
Molomut, N.: The effect of hypophysectomy on immunity and hypersensitivity in rats with a brief description of the operative technic. J. Immunol. **37**, 113—131 (1939).
Mongar, J. L., and H. O. Schild: Inhibition of the anaphylactic reaction. J. Physiol. (Lond.) **135**, 301—319 (1957a).
— — Effect of temperature on the anaphylactic reaction. J. Physiol. (Lond.) **135**, 320—338 (1957b).
— — The effect of calcium and pH on the anaphylactic reaction. J. Physiol. (Lond.) **140**, 272—284 (1958).
Moran, N. C., and B. Westerholm: The influence of reserpine on 5-hydroxytryptamine and histamine content of rat mast cells and of some rat tissues. Acta physiol. scand. **58**, 20—29 (1963).
Moreschi, C., u. C. Vallardi: Über die Wirkung der Normal- und Immunantikörper bei der Anaphylatoxinbildung im Reagenzglase. Z. Immun.-Forsch. **11**, 31—57 (1911).
Morrison jr., A. E., J. S. Lundy and H. E. Essex: An evaluation of replacement fluids in laboratory animals following control hemorrhage. Circulation **5**, 208—214 (1952).

MORRISON, J. L., W. L. BLOOM and A. P. RICHARDSON: Effect of dextran on the rat. J. Pharmacol. exp. Ther. **101**, 27—28 (1951).
— A. P. RICHARDSON and W. L. BLOOM: The effects of antihistaminic agents on the reaction of the rat to dextran. Arch. int. Pharmacodyn. **88**, 98—105 (1951).
MÖRSDORF, K.: Spektrofluorometrische Bestimmung des 5-Hydroxytryptamin-Gehaltes der Rattenpfote bei experimentellen Entzündungen. Med. exp. **1**, 87—90 (1959a).
— Zur Frage einer möglichen Bedeutung des 5-Hydroxytryptamin (5-HT) bei der experimentellen Entzündung. Naunyn-Schmiedebergs Arch. exp. Path. Pharmak. **236**, 46—49 (1959b).
— Serum-Glutamat-Oxalacetat-Transaminase bei lokaler Gewebsschädigung. Naunyn-Schmiedebergs Arch. exp. Path. Pharmak. **238**, 125—127 (1960).
— Die Ödembereitschaft der Rattenpfote in Abhängigkeit ihres Gehaltes an 5-Hydroxytryptamin (5-HT). Naunyn-Schmiedebergs Arch. exp. Path. Pharmak. **240**, 29—30 (1960/61).
— Die serotoninfreisetzende Wirkung einiger zur Auslösung experimenteller Entzündungen verwendeter Stoffe in vitro. Med. exp. **4**, 293—297 (1961a).
— Der Zusammenhang zwischen Dextranschwellung und Serotoninfreisetzung. Med. exp. **4**, 345—348 (1961b).
—, u. H. H. BODE: Zur Beeinflussung der permeabilitätssteigernden Wirkung des Serotonins durch verschiedenartige Pharmaka. Arch. int. Pharmacodyn. **118**, 292—297 (1959).
—, u. L. FEHRES: 5-Hydroxytryptamin (5-HT) und hyperergische Reaktion. Med. exp. **1**, 58–63 (1959).
MÖSER, L.: Über den Eiweißgehalt der Stärke und eine Methode der Herstellung eiweißfreier Stärkepräparate. Z. Hyg. Infekt.-Kr. **83**, 113—116 (1917).
MOTA, I.: Action of anaphylactic shock and anaphylatoxin on mast cells and histamine in rats. Brit. J. Pharmacol. **12**, 453—456 (1957).
— Mast cell and histamine in rat anaphylaxis: the effect of Haemophilus pertussis. Nature (Lond.) **182**, 1021—1022 (1958).
— The mechanism of action of anaphylatoxin. Its effect on guinea pig mast cells. Immunology **2**, 403—413 (1959).
MOUSSATCHÉ, H., and A. P. DANON: Inhibition by sulphydril blocking agents of the guinea-pig gut reaction to anaphylaxis and to anaphylatoxin. Naturwissenschaften **43**, 227 (1956).
MUTERMILCH, S.: Rôle des phénomènes d'adsorption dans la production de l'anaphylatoxine. C. R. Soc. Biol. (Paris) **73**, 56—58 (1912).
NATHAN, E.: Über Anaphylatoxinbildung durch Agar. Z. Immun.-Forsch. **17**, 478—486 (1913a).
— Über Anaphylatoxinbildung durch Stärke. Z. Immun.-Forsch. **18**, 636—650 (1913b).
— Über Anaphylatoxinbildung durch Inulin (zugleich ein Beitrag über die Bedeutung des physikalischen Zustandes für die Anaphylatoxinbildung. Z. Immun.-Forsch. **23**, 204—220 (1915).
NETZER, W., u. W. VOGT: Über Anaphylatoxinbildung. Naunyn-Schmiedebergs Arch. exp. Path. Pharmak. **243**, 363 (1962).
— — Anaphylatoxinbildung durch pyrogenes Lipopolysaccharid. Naunyn-Schmiedebergs Arch. exp. Path. Pharmak., **248**, 261—268 (1964).
NEUZIL, E., R. PAUTRIZEL et J. MARQUEVIELLE: Action des polymères hydrosolubles sur la réaction de précipitation spécifique. Action de la polyvinylpyrrolidone. C. R. Soc. Biol. (Paris) **143**, 1185—1187 (1949).
NISHIYAMA, R., K. TASAKA and S. IRINO: The sites of action of some histamine-releasing substances in the dog. Acta Med. Okayama **11**, 133—144 (1957).
NOVY, F. G., and P. H. DE KRUIF: Anaphylatoxin and anaphylaxis. II. Agar anaphylatoxin: guinea-pig serum. J. infect. Dis. **20**, 536—565 (1917a).
— — Anaphylatoxin and anaphylaxis. III. Agar anaphylatoxin: rabbit serum. J. infect. Dis. **20**, 566—588 (1917b).
— — Anaphylatoxin and anaphylaxis. IV. Agar anaphylatoxin: rat serum. J. infect. Dis. **20**, 589—617 (1917c).
— — Anaphylatoxin and anaphylaxis. V. Effect of multiple doses of anaphylatoxin. J. infect. Dis. **20**, 618—628 (1917d).
— — Anaphylatoxin and anaphylaxis. IX. Specific anaphylactic shock. J. infect. Dis. **20**, 776—832 (1917e).
— — and F. O. NOVY: Anaphylatoxin and anaphylaxis. VII. Peptone anaphylatoxin. J. infect. Dis. **20**, 657—716 (1917).
— — and R. L. NOVY: Anaphylatoxin and anaphylaxis. I. Trypanosome anaphylatoxin. J. infect. Dis. **20**, 499—535 (1917).
ODA, T., T. MURANO and S. YOSHIMOTO: Pharmacological aspects of dioxo-9.9(methyl-2-dimethyl-amino-3-propyl-)10-phenothiazine (dysedon). Osaka Cy. med. J. **7**, 33—42 (1961).
OLESEN, E. S.: Effect of acid polysaccharides on the fibrinolytic system in guinea pig serum. Acta pharmacol. (Kbh.) **15**, 307—318 (1959).

Osler, A. G.: The role of complement in the mediation of tissue injury induced by allergic reactions of the immediate type. In: Immunopathology. p. 227—236. Basel: Benno Schwabe u. Co. 1959.
— M. M. Hawrisiak and Z. Ovary: Mechanism of passive cutaneous anaphylaxis. Fed. Proc. **16**, 428 1957.
— — — M. Siqueira and O. G. Bier: Studies on the mechanism of hypersensitivity phenomena. II. The participation of complement in passive cutaneous anaphylaxis of the albino rat. J. exp. Med. **106**, 811—834 (1957).
— H. G. Randall, B. M. Hill and Z. Ovary: Studies on the mechanism of hypersensitivity phenomena. III. The participation of complement in the formation of anaphylatoxin. J. exp. Med. **110**, 311—339 (1959a).
— — — — Some relationships between complement, passive cutaneous anaphylaxis, and anaphylatoxin. In: Mechanisms of hypersensitivity. p. 281—304. Boston: Little, Brown and Co. 1959b.
Ovary, Z., H. Fudenberg and H. G. Kunkel: Anaphylactic reactions in the skin of the guinea pig with high and low molecular weight antibodies and γ-globulins. J. exp. Med. **112**, 953—961 (1960).
Parker, J. T., and F. Parker jr.: Anaphylaxis in the white rat. J. med. Res. **44**, 263—287 (1924).
Parratt, J. R.: Thyroxine and histamine release in the rat. J. Physiol. (Lond.) **138**, 51 P—52 P (1957).
—, and G. B. West: Oedema producing substances in the rat. J. Physiol. (Lond.) **135**, 10 P to 11 P (1957a).
— — Inhibition of oedema production in the rat. J. Physiol. (Lond.) **135**, 24 P—25 P (1957b).
— — 5-Hydroxytryptamine and tissue mast cells. J. Physiol. (Lond.) **137**, 169—178 (1957c).
— — Release of 5-hydroxytryptamine and histamine from tissues of the rat. J. Physiol. (Lond.) **137**, 179—192 (1957d).
— — 5-Hydroxytryptamine and the anaphylactoid reaction in the rat. J. Physiol. (Lond.) **139**, 27—41 (1957e).
— — Inhibition by various substances of oedema formation in the hind-paw of the rat induced by 5-hydroxytryptamine, histamine, dextran, eggwhite and compound 48/80. Brit. J. Pharmacol. **13**, 65—70 (1958).
— — Hypersensitivity and the thyroid gland. Int. Arch. Allergy **16**, 288—302 (1960).
Parrot, J.-L., et C. Laborde: Inhibition de l'histidine-décarboxylase par la cortisone et par le salicylate de sodium. J. Physiol. (Paris) **53**, 441—442 (1961).
Pautrizel, R., et A. Pautrizel-Bezian: Etudes sur le mécanisme de production de l'anaphylaxie. Action de la polyvinyl pyrrolidone. C. R. Soc. Biol. (Paris) **144**, 1167—1169 (1950).
Perla, D., and J. Marmorston-Gottesman: Effect of injections of cortin on resistance of suprarenalectomized rats to histamine poisoning. Proc. Soc. exp. Biol. (N. Y.) **28**, 650—653 (1931).
Perlmutt, J. H., W. M. Parkins and H. M. Vars: Response of dogs to intravenous administration of polyvinylpyrrolidone and its monomer. Proc. Soc. exp. Biol. (N. Y.) **83**, 146—150 (1953).
Pfeiffer, H., u. S. Mita: Experimentelle Beiträge zur Kenntnis der Eiweiß-Antieiweißreaktion. Z. Immun.-Forsch. **6**, 18—87 (1910).
Pillemer, L., L. Blum, I. H. Lepow, O. A. Ross, E. W. Todd and A. C. Wardlaw: The properdin system and immunity. I. Demonstration and isolation of a new serum protein, properdin, and its role in immune phenomena. Science **120**, 279—285 (1954).
— M. D. Schoenberg, L. Blum and L. Wurz: Properdin system and immunity. II. Interaction of the properdin system with polysaccharides. Science **122**, 545—549 (1955).
Ponder, E., and R. V. Ponder: The interaction of dextran with serum albumin, γ-globulin, and fibrinogen. J. gen. Physiol. **43**, 753—758 (1960).
Pratt, H. N.: Studies of anaphylaxis in the albino rat with reference to diet and histamine. J. Immunol. **29**, 301—317 (1935).
Quivy, D.: La coagulation sanguine chez le chien au cours de divers chocs libérateurs d'héparine ou d'histamine. Arch. int. Pharmacodyn. **105**, 429—437 (1956).
Randall, H. G., S. L. Talbot, H. C. Neu and A. G. Osler: Studies on the mechanism of hypersensitivity phenomena. IV. An isometric smooth muscle assay system. Immunology **4**, 388—400 (1961).
Ravin, H. A., A. M. Seligman and J. Fine: Polyvinylpyrrolidone as a plasma expander. New Engl. J. Med. **247**, 921—929 (1952).
Rédei, A.: Investigations on the mechanism of dextran induced oedema in rats. Med. exp. **6**, 73—78 (1962).
— S. Nagy and S. Karády: Insulin and the dextran anaphylactoid reaction. Naturwissenschaften **48**, 380—381 (1961).

REDFERN, W. W.: A study of the primary toxicity of heterophile immune rabbit serum for guinea-pigs, and its apparent relation to the phenomenon of anaphylaxis. Amer. J. Hyg. **6**, 276—310 (1926).
REPPE, W.: Polyvinylpyrrolidon. Monographien zur Angewandte Chemie und Chemie-Ingenieur-Technik, 1954, Nr. 66.
RICE, C. E.: An investigation of some of the factors determining the decrease in complement activity in anaphylactic shock. J. Immunol. **75**, 85—95 (1955).
RICKETTS, C. R.: Interaction of dextran and fibrinogen. Nature (Lond.) **169**, 970 (1952).
RIECHERT, W., u. H. BARGHORN: Beeinflussung des Rattenpfotenödems und des Lungenödems nach doppelseitiger Vagotomie durch Mutterkornalkaloide, durch Narkose (Avertin) und deren Charakterisierung durch Trypanblau. Naunyn-Schmiedebergs Arch. exp. Path. Pharmak. **221**, 489—496 (1954).
—, u. O. ESCHBACH: Die Beeinflussung des Hühnereiweiß-Rattenpfotenödems durch Reserpin. Arzneimittel-Forsch. **5**, 295—296 (1955).
—, u. H. KLEIN: Zur Beeinflussung der Ödemphase der Hühnereiweißentzündung der Ratte durch Ergotamin, Dihydroergotamin (DHE) und Hydergin (CCK). Naunyn-Schmiedebergs Arch. exp. Path. Pharmak. **213**, 425—428 (1951).
RILEY, J. F.: The effects of histamine-liberators on the mast cells of the rat. J. Path. Bact. **65**, 471—479 (1953).
RITZ, H.: Über die Rolle hypertonischer Salzlösungen bei der Anaphylaxie. Z. Immun.-Forsch. **12**, 644—656 (1912).
—, u. H. SACHS: Über das Anaphylatoxin. Berl. klin. Wschr. **48**, 987—992 (1911).
— — Über Komplementinaktivierung durch Bakterien. (Ein Beitrag zur biologischen Bedeutung physikalischer Serumveränderungen mit Bemerkungen zur Frage der Entstehung des Anaphylatoxins.) Z. Immun.-Forsch. **26**, 483—502 (1917).
— — Die physikalische Theorie der Anaphylatoxinbildung. (Bemerkungen zu der Arbeit von E. FRIEDBERGER und G. JOACHIMOGLU: „Über die vermeintliche Anaphylatoxinbildung aus Stärke.") Z. Hyg. Infekt.-Kr. **86**, 235—244 (1918).
ROCHA E SILVA, M.: Beiträge zur Pharmakologie des Trypsins. I. Wirkung des Trypsins auf die glatten Muskeln des Dünndarms und die Gebärmutter von Säugetieren. Die Freisetzung von Histamin nach Durchströmung der Meerschweinchenlunge mit Trypsin. Naunyn-Schmiedebergs Arch. exp. Path. Pharmak. **194**, 335—350 (1940a).
— Beiträge zur Pharmakologie des Trypsins. II. Wirkung des Trypsins auf den Blutkreislauf bei Katze, Kaninchen und Hund. Naunyn-Schmiedebergs Arch. exp. Path. Pharmak. **194**, 351—361 (1940b).
— Concerning the mechanism of anaphylaxis and allergy. Brit. med. J. **1952 I**, 779—784.
— Anaphylatoxin and histamine release. Quart. Rev. Allergy 8, 220—238 (1954).
— Histamine. Its role in anaphylaxis and allergy. Springfield: Charles C. Thomas 1955.
— Histamine release by naturally occurring substances. In: "Histamine" Ciba-Found. Symp. p. 124—138. London: Churchill 1956.
— Meccanismo della liberazione dell'istamina e sua importanza per la biologia e la medicina. Terapia (Milano) **43**, 163—171 (1958).
— Discussion. In: Polypeptides which affect smooth muscles and blood vessels. p. 321. London: Pergamon Press 1960.
—, and M. ARONSON: Histamine release from the perfused lung of the guinea pig by serotoxin (anaphylatoxin). Brit. J. exp. Path. **33**, 577—586 (1952).
— O. BIER and M. ARONSON: Histamine release by anaphylatoxin. Nature (Lond.) **168**, 465—466 (1951).
—, and A. M. ROTHSCHILD: Anaphylatoxin, histamine depletion and skin reactions in the rat. Nature (Lond.) **175**, 987—988 (1955).
— — Experimental design for bioassay of a material inducing strong tachyphylactic effect (anaphylatoxin). Brit. J. Pharmacol. **11**, 252—262 (1956).
ROSE, B., and J. S. L. BROWNE: The effect of adrenalectomy on the histamine content of the tissues of the rat. Amer. J. Physiol. **131**, 589—594 (1941).
ROTHLIN, E., and A. CERLETTI: Pharmacologic studies on a new antihistamine and its combination with calcium. Ann. Allergy **13**, 80—89 (1955).
ROTHSCHILD, A. M., and J. U. BARRETO: Effect of metabolic inhibitors on the release of histamine by anaphylatoxin and by antigen in vitro. Experientia (Basel) **17**, 555—556 (1961).
—, and E. GARCIA LIMA: Effect of dinitrophenol and glucose on amine release from isolated rabbit blood platelets. Experientia (Basel) **19**, 19 (1963).
—, and M. ROCHA E SILVA: Activation of a histamine-releasing agent (anaphylatoxin) in normal rat plasma. Brit. J. exp. Path. **35**, 507—518 (1954).
ROWLEY, D. A., and E. P. BENDITT: 5-Hydroxytryptamine and histamine as mediators of the vascular injury produced by agents which damage mast cells in rats. J. exp. Med. **103**, 399—412 (1956).

RYLANT, P.: L'anaphylaxie cardiaque. C. R. Soc. Biol. (Paris) 88, 1208—1211 (1923).

SACHS, H.: Zur physikalischen Theorie der Anaphylatoxinbildung. (Historische Bemerkungen zu der Arbeit von H. DOLD: „Anaphylatoxin, charakterisiert durch eine eigenartige Flockungs-Phase der Serumglobuline".) Arch. Hyg. (Berl.) **89**, 322—326 (1920).

—, u. E. STILLING: Über die Vermittelung hämolytischer Serumwirkungen durch Inulin. Z. Immun.-Forsch. **26**, 530—544 (1917).

SAITO, N.: Effects of histamine and of histamine releasers on the granulopexy and permeability of the vascular endothelium of the skin. Fol. pharmacol. jap. **54**, 1268—1281 (1958).

SANYAL, R. K.: Splenectomy and the anaphylactoid reaction in the rat. Allergie u. Asthma **6**, 52—56 (1960a).

— The effect of insulin on hypersensitivity reactions in the rat. Allergie u. Asthma **6**, 317—320 (1960b).

— P. S. J. SPENCER and G. B. WEST: Insulin and hypersensitivity. Nature (Lond.) **184**, 2020 (1959).

—, and G. B. WEST: Anaphylactic shock in the albino rat. J. Physiol. (Lond.) **142**, 571—584 (1958).

SCHACHTER, M., and J. TALESNIK: The release of histamine by egg-white in non-sensitized animals. J. Physiol. (Lond.) **118**, 258—263 (1952).

SCHAYER, R. W.: Binding and release of histamine. Fed. Proc. **14**, 275—276 (1955).

— The origin and fate of histamine in the body. In: "Histamine" Ciba Found. Symp. p. 183 to 188. London: Churchill 1956.

— Formation and binding of histamine by rat tissues in vitro. Amer. J. Physiol. **187**, 63—65 (1956b).

— Histidine decarboxylase of rat stomach and other mammalian tissues. Amer. J. Physiol. **189**, 533—536 (1957).

— K. J. DAVIS and R. L. SMILEY: Binding of histamine in vitro and its inhibition by cortisone. Amer. J. Physiol. **182**, 54—56 (1955).

— Z. ROTHSCHILD and P. BIZONY: Increase in histidine decarboxylase activity of rat skin following treatment with compound 48/80. Amer. J. Physiol. **196**, 295—298 (1959).

—, and R. L. SMILEY: Binding and release of radioactive histamine in intact rats. Amer. J. Physiol. **177**, 401—404 (1954).

— — and K. J. DAVIS: Inhibition by cortisone (adrenocortical preparation) of binding of new histamine in rat tissues. Proc. Soc. exp. Biol. (N. Y.) **87**, 590—592 (1955).

— — — Formation and binding of histamine by rat tissues in vitro. Amer. J. Physiol. **187**, 63—65 (1956).

SCHEIFFARTH, F., u. G. BERG: Zur Verwertbarkeit der Eiklarhyperergie als Testmethode bei der Prüfung entzündungshemmender Stoffe. Arzneimittel-Forsch. **2**, 304—307 (1952).

— W. FRENGER u. M. GEMÄHLICH: Untersuchungen über den Wirkungsmechanismus des Anaphylatoxins. I. Mitteilung. Das Verhalten des Meerschweinchens im Anaphylatoxinschock nach vorausgehender Verabreichung einer histaminliberierenden Substanz. Z. Immun.-Forsch. **115**, 224—227 (1958).

— — L. R. TRABULSI u. M. GEMÄHLICH: Der Ablauf des Anaphylatoxinschockes unter Erhöhung des Serumproperdins und nach Verabfolgung von Prednison. Z. Immun.-Forsch. **115**, 277—283 (1958).

— M. GEMÄHLICH, L. ZICHA u. W. FRENGER: Untersuchungen über den Wirkungsmechanismus des Anaphylatoxins. III. Mitteilung. Vitalmikroskopische Untersuchungen der Gefäßreaktionen des Meerschweinchens und der Ratte nach lokaler Applikation von Anaphylatoxin, Histamin und Serotonin. Z. Immun.-Forsch. **115**, 373—379 (1958).

SCHMID, E., L. ZICHA, F. SCHEIFFARTH u. O. BÜTTNER: Untersuchungen über den Antagonismus von Antihistaminen gegen Serotonin. Arzneimittel-Forsch. **9**, 474—476 (1959).

SCHMIDT, J.: Die Beeinflussung des Serotonin-Ödems der Rattenpfote durch Noradrenalin und Adrenalin. Acta biol. med. germ. **10**, 194—196 (1963).

SCHMIDT, P.: Studien zur Frage der Entstehung des anaphylaktischen Anfalls. Z. Hyg. Infekt.-Kr. **83**, 89—112 (1917).

—, u. W. SCHÜRMANN: Zur Frage der Stärkekleisteranaphylaxie. (Erwiderung auf die Arbeit von E. FRIEDBERGER und G. JOACHIMOGLU: „Über die vermeintliche Anaphylatoxinbildung aus Stärke".) Z. Hyg. Infekt-Kr. **86**, 195—212 (1918).

SCHMUTZLER, W., u. H. GIERTZ: Der Einfluß von Polyvinylpyrrolidon auf den anaphylaktischen Schock des Meerschweinchens und anaphylaktoide PVP-Wirkungen am Hund. Naunyn-Schmiedebergs Arch. exp. Path. Pharmak. **243**, 363—364 (1962).

— — u. F. HAHN: Neue Untersuchungen über die Rolle des Histamins bei der Meerschweinchenanaphylaxie. Int. Arch. Allergy **22**, 69—76 (1963).

SCHOCH, E. P., and D. GLICK: The effect of cold, stress, ACTH, cortisone, pyrogen, and nitrogen mustard on tissue mast cells in the skin and subcutaneous tissues of the rat. J. invest. Derm. **20**, 119—123 (1953).

SCHULTZ, W. H.: Physiological studies in anaphylaxis. I. The reaction of smooth muscle of the guinea-pig sensitized with horse serum. J. Pharmacol. exp. Ther. **1**, 549—567 (1910).
SCOTT, W. J. M.: The effect of histamine in sublethal suprarenal insufficiency. Arch. Path. Lab. Med. **4**, 491 (1927).
— The influence of the adrenal glands on resistance. III. Susceptibility to histamine as a test of adrenal deficiency. J. exp. Med. **47**, 185—191 (1928).
SCROGGIE, A. E., and L. B. JAQUES: The release of histamine and heparin by antigen from the isolated perfused liver of the sensitized dog. J. Immunol. **62**, 103—116 (1949).
SEELICH, F.: Die physikalisch-chemischen Vorgänge bei der Antigen-Antikörperreaktion und deren Beziehung zu den anaphylaktischen Erscheinungen. Wien. klin. Wschr. **60**, 709—713 (1948).
SEITZ, A.: Über Bakterienanaphylaxie. Z. Immun.-Forsch. **11**, 588—608 (1911).
SELYE, H.: Studies on adaptation. Endocrinology **21**, 169—188 (1937).
— Effect of ACTH and cortisone upon an "anaphylactoid reaction". Canad. med. Ass. J. **61**, 553—556 (1949).
— Influence of inoculation site upon the course of the "anaphylactoid reaction" to dextran. J. Allergy **25**, 97—103 (1954).
— Empfindlichkeit gegen Dextran bei totalnephrektomierten Ratten. Z. Immun.-Forsch. **112**, 363—368 (1955).
— E. BAJUSZ u. M. NADASDI: Kann die „anaphylaktoide Entzündung" durch Glukocorticoide verhindert werden? Allergie u. Asthma **4**, 262—264 (1958).
SETNIKAR, I., M. SALVATERRA and O. TEMELCOU: Antiphlogistic activity of iproniazid. Brit. J. Pharmacol. **14**, 484—487 (1959).
SLOMKA, M. B., and A. GOTH: Some observations on development of tolerance to histamine liberation. J. Pharmacol. exp. Ther. **116**, 52—53 (1956a).
— — Some observations on nature of refractoriness to histamine liberators. Proc. Soc. exp. Biol. (N. Y.) **93**, 30—32 (1956b).
SMITH, D. E., and Y. S. LEWIS: Influence of hypophysis and adrenal cortex upon tissue mast cell of the rat. Proc. Soc. exp. Biol. (N. Y.) **87**, 515—518 (1954).
SPARROW, E. M., and D. L. WILHELM: Species differences in susceptibility to capillary permeability factors: histamine, 5-hydroxytryptamine, and compound 48/80. J. Physiol. (Lond.) **137**, 51—65 (1957).
SPENCER, P. S. J., and G. B. WEST: Sensitivity of the hyperthyroid and hypothyroid mouse to histamine and 5-hydroxytryptamine. Brit. J. Pharmacol. **17**, 137—143 (1961).
— — Further observations on the relationship between the thyroid gland and the anaphylactoid reaction in rats. Int. Arch. Allergy **20**, 321—343 (1962).
— — Thyroid-adrenocortical antagonism and histamine metabolism. Nature (Lond.) **199**, 1298—1299 (1963).
SQUIRE, J. R., J. P. BULL, W. d'A. MAYCOCK and C. R. RICKETTS: Dextran — Its properties and use in medicine. Oxford 1955.
STEGEMANN, H., W. VOGT u. K. D. FRIEDBERG: Über die Natur des Anaphylatoxins. Hoppe Seylers Z. physiol. Chem. **337**, 269—276 (1964).
STENGER, E. G.: Zur Frage des Entstehungsmechanismus der experimentellen Dextran-Schwellung der Rattenpfote. Arzneimittel-Forsch. **8**, 693—694 (1958).
— Prüfung der pro- und antiphlogistischen Wirkung von Monojodessigsäure, Natriumfluorid, Kaliumcyanid und 2,4-Dinitrophenol an der Ratte. Arch. int. Pharmacodyn. **120**, 39—47 (1959).
STERN, P., u. R. MILIN: Die antiallergische Wirkung der Azulene. Arzneimittel-Forsch. **6**, 445—450 (1956).
STONE, C. A., H. C. WENGER, C. T. LUDDEN, J. M. STAVORSKI and C. A. ROSS: Antiserotonin-antihistaminic properties of cyproheptadine. J. Pharmacol. exp. Ther. **131**, 73—84 (1961).
STUCKI, J. C., and C. R. THOMPSON: A screening procedure for substances which inhibit dextran edema in the rat. Amer. J. Physiol. **193**, 275—282 (1958).
SUKIENNIKOWA, N.: Ein experimenteller Beitrag zur „Anaphylatoxin"-Frage. Z. Immun.-Forsch. **17**, 304—313 (1913).
SUPEK, Z., M. JOVIĆ u. S. KECKES: Der 5-Hydroxytryptamin-Gehalt der Haut der Ratte bei experimenteller Entzündung. Arzneimittel-Forsch. **11**, 132 (1961).
SWINGLE, W. W., E. J. FEDOR, M. BEN, R. MAXWELL and C. BAKER: Protection afforded by aqueous-alcohol solutions of cortisone against dextran. Proc. Soc. exp. Biol. (N. Y.) **84**, 63—65 (1953).
— — R. MAXWELL, M. BEN and G. BARLOW: Cortisone-fore treatment of adrenalectomized rats infused with globin and dextran. Amer. J. Physiol. **172**, 527—534 (1953).
SZYMANOWSKI, Z.: Anaphylaktische Studien. II. Zur Frage des Bakterienanaphylatoxins. Z. Immun.-Forsch. **16**, 13—16 (1913).
TCHERNOROUTZKY, M.: Sur l'anaphylatoxine de BORDET. C. R. Soc. Biol. (Paris) **74**, 1213—1214 (1913).

TELFORD, J. M.: Effect of adrenalectomy on histamine metabilism in the rat. Nature (Lond.) **197**, 600 (1963).
—, and G. B. WEST: The effects of corticosteroids and related compounds on the histamine and 5-hydroxytryptamine content of rat tissues. Brit. J. Pharmacol. **15**, 532—539 (1960).
— — Some effects of corticosteroids on the metabolism of histamine and 5-hydroxytryptamine in the rat. Brit. J. Pharmacol. **16**, 360—368 (1961a).
— — The action of adrenal cortical hormones on histamine metabolism. Biochem. Pharmacol. **8**, 152—153 (1961b).
— — Some aspects of experimental allergy. Part I. Int. Arch. Allergy **22**, 11—30 (1963a).
— — Some aspects of experimental allergy. Part II. Int. Arch. Allergy **23**, 29—58 (1963b).
THEOBALD, W., u. R. DOMENJOZ: Das Serotonin-Ödem der Ratte und seine Beeinflussung durch Antiphlogistica. Arzneimittel-Forsch. **8**, 18—19 (1958).
UDA, T.: The mode of inhibitory actions of guaiazulene and some other anti-inflammatory agents on the anaphylactoid edema. Fol. pharmacol. jap. **56**, 1151—1163 (1960).
UNGAR, G.: Biochemical mechanism of the allergic reaction. Int. Arch. Allergy **4**, 258—281 (1953).
— Mechanism of histamine release. In: "Histamine" Ciba-Found. Symp. p. 431—442. London: Churchill 1956.
—, and E. DAMGAARD: Tissue reactions to anaphylactic and anaphylactoid stimuli, proteolysis and release of histamine and heparin. J. exp. Med. **101**, 1—15 (1955).
— — and F. P. HUMMEL: Action of salicylates and related drugs on inflammation. Amer. J. Physiol. **171**, 545—553 (1952).
— — — Activation of profibrinolysin by antigen-antibody reaction and by anaphylactoid agents; its relation to complement. J. exp. Med. **98**, 291—303 (1953).
—, and H. HAYASHI: Enzymatic mechanisms in allergy. Ann. Allergy **16**, 542—581 (1958).
—, and S. H. MIST: Observations on the release of serum fibrinolysin by specific antigen, peptone, and certain polysaccharides. J. exp. Med. **90**, 39—51 (1949).
— T. YAMURA, J. B. ISOLA and S. KOBRIN: Further studies on the role of proteases in the allergic reaction. J. exp. Med. **113**, 359—380 (1961).
VAN CAUWENBERGE, H., C. LAPIÈRE, F. HALKIN et J. LECOMTE: Modifications pharmacodynamiques et humorales de l'oedème provoqué chez le rat par l'histamine. C. R. Soc. Biol. (Paris) **153**, 514—516 (1959).
— — J. LECOMTE et J. RENSON: Modifications pharmacodynamiques et hormonales de l'augmentation de la perméabilité vasculaire provoquée par la 5-hydroxytryptamine. C. R. Soc. Biol. (Paris) **152**, 1848—1851 (1958).
—, et J. LECOMTE: Réactions cortico-surrénaliennes après administration parentérale de blanc d'oeuf au rat albinos. Rev. franç. clin. biol. **4**, 128—137 (1959).
— — J. GOBLET and M. VLIERS: Egg white edema in rats and adrenal activity. J. Allergy **24**, 479—482 (1953).
— — et C. LAPIÈRE: Influence de la chloroquine sur l'oedème à l'ovalbumine ou au dextran, et sur le test d'AMBROSE et de EDS chez le rat. C. R. Soc. Biol. (Paris) **152**, 1405—1408 (1958).
— — et M. VLIERS: Etude de l'activité cortico-surrénalienne au cours d'administrations successives de blanc d'oeuf chez le rat albinos. Acta allerg. (Kbh.) **11**, 109—114 (1957).
VARGA, F., J. MÉHES, A. PÁR u. E. RÓNAI: Beiträge zur Prüfung entzündungshemmender Substanzen. Acta physiol. Acad. Sci. hung. **23**, 69—78 (1963).
VAUGHAN, V. C., V. C. VAUGHAN JR. and J. H. WRIGHT: The ferment produced in protein sensitization. Z. Immun.-Forsch. **11**, 673—682 (1911).
—, and S. M. WHEELER: The effects of egg-white and its split products on animals; a study of susceptibility and immunity. J. infect. Dis. **4**, 476—508 (1907).
VEILLEUX, R.: Anaphylactoid oedema produced in rats by certain dextrins. Brit. J. Pharmacol. **21**, 235—237 (1963).
VIAUD, P.: Les amines dérivées de la phénothiazine. J. Pharm. Pharmacol. **6**, 361—389 (1954).
VOEGTLIN, C., and H. A. DYER: Natural resistance of albino rats and mice to histamine, pituitary and certain other poisons. J. Pharmacol. exp. Ther. **24**, 101—117 (1925).
VOGEL, G., u. M. L. MAREK: Über die Hemmung verschiedener Rattenpfoten-Ödeme durch Serotonin-Antagonisten. Arzneimittel-Forsch. **11**, 1051—1054 (1961).
VOGT, W.: Anaphylatoxinbildung durch ein Metallferment. Naunyn-Schmiedebergs Arch. exp. Path. Pharmak. **246**, 31—32 (1963a).
— Einfluß von Fermenten des Blutes und von divalenten Kationen auf die Anaphylatoxinbildung. Int. Arch. Allergy **22**, 144—149 (1963b).
— Weitere Untersuchungen zur Fermentnatur der Anaphylatoxinentstehung. Naunyn-Schmiedebergs Arch. exp. Path. Pharmak. **247**, 327 (1964).
—, u. G. SCHMIDT: Abtrennung des anaphylatoxinbildenden Prinzips aus Cobragift von anderen Giftkomponenten. Experientia (Basel) **20**, 207—208 (1964).

VOGT, W., u. N. ZEMANN: Analyse der erregenden Wirkung von Anaphylatoxin auf glatte Muskulatur. Naunyn-Schmiedebergs Arch. exp. Path. Pharmak. **247**, 328—329 (1964).
VON GONZENBACH u. HIRSCHFELD: Untersuchungen über die Rolle des Komplementes bei der Anaphylatoxinbildung. Z. Immun.-Forsch. **15**, 350—369 (1912).
VON WORZIKOWSKY-KUNDRATITZ, K. R.: Über Muskelveränderungen bei der anaphylaktischen und der anaphylaktoiden Vergiftung des Meerschweinchens. Naunyn-Schmiedebergs Arch. exp. Path. Pharmak. **73**, 33—48 (1913).
VOORHEES, A. B., H. J. BAKER and E. J. PULASKI: Reactions of albino rats to injections of dextran. Proc. Soc. exp. Biol. (N. Y.) **76**, 254—256 (1951).
VUGMAN, I., and A. M. ROTHSCHILD: Effect of glucose and insulin on the histamine release by compound 48/80 from alloxan diabetic rats. Acta physiol. lat.-amer. **11**, 108 (1961).
VUKOBRATOVIĆ, S.: Action de l'hypothermie et des hormones sur l'histamine endogène. Allergie u. Asthma **4**, 271—275 (1958).
— Protection par les substances histamino-libératrices chez les animaux sensibilisés au choc anaphylactique. Acta med. jugoslav. **13**, 393—397 (1959a).
— Mécanisme de protection des substances histamino-libératrices dans le choc anaphylactique. Acta allergol. (Kbh.) **14**, 397—407 (1959b).
— Les modifications cardio-vasculaires en euthermie et en hypothermie profonde, provoquées par la libération de l'histamine endogène. Allergie u. Asthma **7**, 278—284 (1961).
—, et A. BATA: Hypothermie expérimentale et allergie. Presse. méd. **65**, 7—8 (1957).
WAALKES, T. P., and H. COBURN: Comparative effects of glycogen and antigen-antibody reactions on serotonin and histamine in the rabbit. Proc. Soc. exp. Biol. (N. Y.) **101**, 122—125 (1959).
— — Studies on the relationship of the release of serotonin and histamine, by chemical means, to anaphylaxis in the rabbit. J. Allergy **31**, 395—405 (1960).
WALTON, K. W., and C. R. RICKETTS: Anaphylactoid response in guinea pigs to the parenteral administration of sulphate esters of high molecular weight of dextran. Nature (Lond.) **173**, 31 (1954).
— J. A. RICHARDSON and W. L. THOMPSON: Hypotension and histamine release following intravenous injection of plasma substitutes. J. Pharmacol. exp. Ther. **127**, 39—45 (1959).
WASSERMANN, M., u. F. KEYSSER: Über Toxopeptide. Folia serol. **7**, 243—251 (1911).
WEBB, R. L.: Peritoneal reactions in the white rat with special reference to the mast cells. Amer. J. Anat. **49**, 283—334 (1931).
WELTMAN, A. S., and A. M. SACKLER: Effects of thymectomy on the resistance of rats to drowning and histamine stress. Nature (Lond.) **192**, 460—461 (1961).
WEST, G. B.: 5-hydroxytryptamine, tissue mast cells and skin oedema. Int. Arch. Allergy **10**, 257—275 (1957a).
— Oedema and 5-hydroxytryptamine in the rat. In: 5-Hydroxytryptamine. p. 168—171. Edited by G. P. LEWIS. London, New York, Paris, Los Angeles: Pergamon Press 1957.
— Chemical nature and possible role of mediators in allergic reactions. Int. Arch. Allergy **18**, 56—61 (1961a).
— The action of dextran in rats. Biochem. Pharmacol. 8, 153 (1961b).
WILHELM, D. L., A. A. MILES and M. E. MACKAY: Enzyme-like globulins from serum reproducing the vascular phenomena of inflammation. II. Isolation and properties of the permeability factor and its inhibitor. Brit. J. exp. Path. **36**, 82—104 (1955).
— P. J. MILL and A. A. MILES: Enzyme-like globulins from serum reproducing the vascular phenomena of inflammation. III. Further observations on the permeability factor and its inhibitor in guinea-pig serum. Brit. J. exp. Path. **38**, 446—461 (1957).
WILHELMI, G.: Über die pharmakologischen Eigenschaften von Irgapyrin, einem neuen Präparat aus der Pyrazolreihe. Schweiz. med. Wschr. **79**, 577—582 (1949).
— Über die enztündungshemmende Wirkung von Cortison, ACTH, Pyrazolen und anderen Antiphlogistica. Medizinische **1952 II**, 1591—1595.
—, u. R. DOMENJOZ: Vergleichende Untersuchungen über die Wirkung von Pyrazolen und Antihistaminen bei verschiedenen Arten der experimentellen Entzündung. Naunyn-Schmiedebergs Arch. exp. Path. Pharmak. **212**, 125—127 (1950/51).
— — Vergleichende Untersuchungen über die Wirkung von Pyrazolen und Antihistaminen bei verschiedenen Arten der experimentellen Entzündung. Arch. int. Pharmacodyn. **85**, 129—143 (1951a).
— — Die Beeinflussung des Hühnereiweiß-Ödems an der Rattenpfote durch Pyrazole sowie Cortison und ACTH. Arzneimittel-Forsch. **1**, 151—154 (1951b).
—, u. R. PULVER: Untersuchungen zur Frage eines peripheren Angriffspunktes der Pyrazole bei der antiphlogistischen Wirkung. Arzneimittel-Forsch. **5**, 221—224 (1955).
WILLIAMS, F.: Plasma volume changes in egg-white injected rats. Effect of cortisone. Proc. Soc. exp. Biol. (N. Y.) **86**, 77—81 (1954).

WILSON, A.: The effect of adrenalectomy on the blood histamine of rabbits. J. Physiol. (Lond.) **99**, 241—245 (1941).

WINDER, C. V., J. WAX and M. A. BEEN: Rapid foot volume measurements on unanesthetized rats, and the question of a phenylbutazone effect on anaphylactoid edema. Arch. int. Pharmacodyn. **112**, 174—187 (1957).

WINTER, C. A., E. A. RISLEY and G. W. NUSS: Carrageenin-induced edema in hind paw of the rat as an assay for antiinflammatory drugs. Proc. Soc. exp. Biol. (N. Y.) **111**, 544—547 (1962).

WYMAN, L. C.: Studies on suprarenal insufficiency. III. The effect of thyroidectomy and of forcing fluid on suprarenal insufficiency in rats. Amer. J. Physiol. **87**, 42—50 (1928).

YAMASAKI, H., S. IRINO, T. UDA, K. UCHIDA, H. OHNO, N. SAITO, K. KONDO, K. JINZENJI and T. YAMAMOTO: Pharmacology of guaiazulene, with special reference to anti-inflammatory effect due to histamine-release inhibition. Fol. pharmacol. jap. **54**, 362—377 (1958).

— K. KONDO and T. UDA: Anti-inflammatory effect and histamine-release inhibitory effect of some derivatives of acetanilide and pyrazolone. Okayama-Igakkai-Zasshi **72**, 1091—1096 (1960).

— — — T. YAMAMOTO and K. ENDO: Pharmacological studies of lumisantonin derivatives, with special reference to anti-inflammatory effect and to histamine-release inhibitory action. Fol. pharmacol. jap. **56**, 1249—1262 (1960); Acta Med. Okayama **15**, 347–366 (1961).

ZEMPLÉNYI, J. F., and Z. LOJDA: Mast cell histamine and the accumulation of colloid particles in the vascular endothelium. Quart. J. exp. Physiol. **45**, 50—54 (1960).

ZUNZ, E.: Recherches sur l'anaphylaxie. Contribution à l'étude des effects de l'injection intraveineuse de sérum traité par l'agar ou la pararabine chez les cobayes neufs. J. Physiol. (Paris) **17**, 470—483 (1917/18).

—, et M. GELAT: Des effets de l'injection intraveineuse de sérum traité par l'agar chez les lapins neufs. C. R. Soc. Biol. (Paris) **78**, 428—429 (1915).

—, et C. MOHILEVITCH: Des effets de l'injection intraveineuse de sérum traité par la pararabine chez les lapins neufs. C. R. Soc. Biol. (Paris) **79**, 601—602 (1916).

Section F

Release of Histamine from Mast Cells

By

IVAN MOTA

With 25 Figures

I. Introduction

The mast cells are connective tissue cells characterized morphologically by the presence in their cytoplasm of numerous metachromatic granules and biochemically by their high content of heparin and histamine. The relationship between mast cells and histamine was firmly established by the fundamental papers of RILEY, WEST and co-workers (RILEY, 1953a, b; RILEY and WEST, 1953; CASS, RILEY, WEST, HEAD and STROUD, 1954) and is dealt with in detail by RILEY and WEST in this volume. Besides heparin and histamine, BENDITT, WONG, ARASE and ROEPER (1955) showed that the mast cells contain also 5-hydroxytryptamine and BHATTACHARYA and LEWIS (1956) showed that 5-hydroxytryptamine is released from rat tissues perfused with compound 48—80. It seems of interest to call attention to the fact that the role of histamine, heparin and 5-hydroxytryptamine is, up to now, completely unknown and that there is not yet any evidence that the mast cells deliver to the blood or tissues any of these substances under normal conditions. Notwithstanding, the papers referred to above, which suggest that the mast cells can act as a source of heparin, histamine and 5-hydroxytryptamine, have opened a wide field of approach to the study of mast cell physiology. In the present chapter, an attempt will be made to gather and analyze the many papers that have been published in the last years concerning the phenomenon of histamine liberation from the mast cells, with emphasis on the behavior of these cells in anaphylaxis. As we are concerned more with experimental details than with ideas, references will preferentially be made to original work rather than to reviews.

The physiological activity of many cells can be reflected by their morphology. For instance, the appearance, formation and extrusion of the secretory granules reflect the physiological activity of the pancreatic acinar cells. Usually glandular cells at the height of their secretory activity are crowded with granules that are finally discharged at the free end of the cell. In this respect, if one considers the mast cell as a connective tissue unicellular gland, it looks rather like a ready-made cell for granule extrusion. Indeed, scattering of mast cell granules outside the cell bodies in normal tissues have frequently been interpreted as proof of physiological secretory activity. However, mast cells are very fragile cells and in ordinary histological preparations, granule scattering due to artificial rupture of the cell body is very frequent. One must be very careful when evaluating this as evidence of secretory activity. The first definite demonstration of mast cell alteration that could be attributed to a probable release of a pharmacologically active substance was that of WILANDER (1938) who described degranulation and loss of metachromasia of dog liver mast cells after peptone shock and related these alterations to heparin liberation.

More recently, the development of drugs which were specifically able to release histamine from the tissues, made possible a new approach to mast cell physiology and the determination of whether histamine, besides heparin, could also arise from mast cells. RILEY (1953a) was the first to show that injection of histamine liberators in rats was followed by damage to the mast cells. From then on, many other papers showed that histamine release is usually accompanied by mast cell damage. However, it must be pointed out here that the expression "histamine liberation from the mast cells" is, correctly speaking, only a presumption that is problaby valid for those cases in which most of the histamine content of a tissue is correlated with its mast cell population and is only truly valid when one works with free, isolated mast cells. Notwithstanding, since up to now, all the experimental data obtained have strongly suggested that histamine release is usually concommitant with mast cell alterations, these alterations will be considered here as reliable morphological evidence of histamine liberation.

We shall confine our discussion to those histamine-releasing compounds whose effect on mast cells has been specifically studied. Before starting our discussion, we would like to define certain terms and make some general remarks on the problem of mast cell fixation which is a very important one in the study of these cells and which has not always been properly considered by all the authors. With the increasing interest of physiologists, pharmacologists, biochemists and immunologists in mast cell physiology it seems worthwhile to call attention to certain histological peculiarities of these cells. Indeed, there would be no problem in mast cell fixation if it were not that many authors continually fail to remember that the mast cell granules of many species are soluble in water and that to preserve them, tissues must be fixed in alcoholic solutions, as stated many years ago by EHRLICH (1877). Furthermore the large variation amongst species, the fact that in rats and mice, two very common laboratory animals, the mast cell granules are exceptionally resistant to almost any fixative including the aqueous one, has certainly contributed to this attitude. However, in most species, the mast cell granules are poorly fixed, or not fixed at all by the large majority of the fixatives usually employed in histological techniques. In 1937, HOLMGREN and WILANDER using the observation that lead subacetate precipitates heparin, successfully employed a 4% aqueous solution of lead subacetate to fix mast cells. Indeed, aqueous lead subacetate solution, contrary to other aqueous fixatives, is able to fix mast cells in such a way as to render these cells resistant to paraffin embedding and staining in aqueous solutions. In our studies on the behavior of dog and guinea-pig mast cells in peptone and anaphylactic shock, we felt it necessary to improve the fixative power of this mixture and tried a 1 or 4% solution of lead subacetate in 50% ethanol containing 1% acetic acid (MOTA, JUNQUEIRA, BERALDO and FERRI, 1954; MOTA and VUGMAN, 1956). A much better fixation was obtained with this mixture than by using the original aqueous HOLMGREEN and WILANDER solution. A careful comparative study of this fixative mixture was made by FERRI (1955) who found it superior to all the other fixative mixtures he tried [HELLY, ZENKER BOUIN, GENDRE, DUBOSCQ-BRASIL, neutral formaldehyde, SUSA, CARNOY, EHRLICH, HOLMGREN and WILANDER, and the modification of the last as used by LECOMTE and BAECKELAND (1953)]. An interesting observation was made by FERRI (1955) that the mast cell's resistance to different fixatives varies not only from species to species but also from organ to organ in a same species. For instance, in the dog, most of the skin mast cells can be fixed with a 10% solution of neutral formaldehyde while in the liver, these cells are completely washed away by the same fixative. Besides, it is our experience that in order to fix the mast cells properly, it is very important not only to use an adequate fixative but also to speed the fixation process by injecting the fixative through the vessels. For instance, in dog liver and guinea-pig lung, these cells are only properly fixed when fixation is performed by injecting the fixative through the vessels or bronchi: fixation by immersion of these tissues in the fixative being insufficient to preserve the fine cytological details of these cells. Furthermore, in some organs like guinea-pig uterus and ileum, a good fixation of the mast cells can only be obtained by injecting the fixative under pressure into the lumen. Here, the pressure will speed up the penetration of the fixative resulting in a much better fixation of the mast cells than is obtained by direct immersion of these organs in the fixative. Actually there are many other similar cases in which, to achieve a proper fixation, a device has to be improvised. Furthermore a good fixation must not only preserve the mast cells but also fix these cells. that is, it must not only prevent the action of autolytic enzymes but also modify these cells in such a way that they can endure subsequent histological treatments. For instance, as long ago as 1923, MICHELS observed that in some species, preservation of the mast cells with alcohol does not render these cells resistant to paraffin embedding. Thus, embedded material of whitefish and carp revealed no mast cells, whereas frozen sections properly treated, showed a large number of mast cells. Probably the temperature used in the embedding process accounts for this fact. We also had a similar finding when working with guinea-pig lung tissue, a fact that explains the not surprising observations of SMITH (1959) who was not able to find mast cells in guinea-pig lung after fixation in absolute ethyl alcohol and embedding in paraffin. Indeed, it is our belief that in many other instances the conspicuous mast cell population of the guinea-pig lung has not been observed due to ignorance of a proper histological technique. Furthermore, it is our experience that mast cell morphology is much better preserved in frozen sections than in paraffin embedding which frequently causes distortion of these cells and sometimes even disappearance of the mast cell granules. Obviously, fixation of the mast cells in tissue spreads or membranes such as the pleura or mesentery is much easier since these tissues do not have to be embedded and cut. In this respect, we consider the mesentery a very suitable preparation in which to study the mast cells. In this serous membrane there is a large number of mast cells uniformly distributed between two very thin sheets of mesothelial cells allowing a direct microscopical observation without the necessity of embedding and cutting the material. Unlike the pleura, this tissue does not need to be detached from adjacent tissues, a procedure which usually induces disruption of the cells by stretching; and being very thin it allows, not only an almost immediate contact with drugs whose effect on the mast cells is to be studied, but also a very rapid penetration of the fixative into the tissue, a condition essential for an efficient fixation of the mast cells.

In conclusion, to study properly mast cell cytological detail, one must choose a fixative taking into consideration not only the animal species under observation but also the organs to be fixed and the subsequent histological procedures to which the tissue will be later submitted. For instance, it must be noted that although the lead subacetate mixture is an excellent fixative for mast cells, it is a very poor fixative for all the other cells. Therefore, in the case of rat and mouse mast cells which are resistant to practically all fixatives it is preferable to use a fixative mixture able to fix not only the mast cells but the other cells too. Thus, in this chapter, unless otherwise stated, the term fixative implies a 4% solution of lead subacetate in 50% ethanol containing 1% acetic acid when dog or guinea-pig tissues are concerned, or a 50% aqueous ethanol solution containing 10% formaldehyde and 5% acetic acid when rat or mouse tissues are concerned.

The morphological change of the mast cell connected with histamine release is highly variable, varying not only with the nature of the histamine-releasing agent used, but also with the species studied. Therefore, it is convenient to use more than one term when describing these different changes. The terms disruption, degranulation and fusion include all the mast cell alterations related to histamine release so far described. The term *disruption* has been largely used to indicate extrusion of the mast cell granules which in properly treated tissue sections can be found scattered in the neighborhood of these cells. Rat mast cell damage induced by antigen or compound 48—80 is a typical example of this type of mast cell alteration. Disruption also implies a loss of granules or degranulation, but we have reserved the latter term for the damage presented by guinea-pig mast cells in anaphylaxis, in which no granule scattering is observed. Octylamine, peptone, stilbamidine, protamine sulphate, d-tubocurarine, dextran, antihistamines and many other substances also induce rat mast cell disruption, which seems to be the only known rat mast cell change in response to histamine releasing agents. The term does not imply a rupture of the cellular membrane and as defined here cannot be used in reference to dog or guinea-pig mast cells, since their mast cells do not respond to any known histamine-releasing agent by granule scattering. On the other hand, in sensitized guinea-pig tissues, antigen induces mast cell damage characterized by a partial or total disappearance of the mast cell granules, which are never found scattered around the cell. We have called this phenomenon *degranulation*. As defined here, this term cannot be used in reference to rat mast cells since in this species the granules do not disappear but are always found in the tissue around the cells. A third type of mast cell damage is observed when guinea-pig tissues are incubated with some histamine releasers such as octylamine or compound 48—80. In this case, mast cell changes are represented by an apparent loss of granule limit and fusion of the metachromatic material in which some basophilic granules can sometimes be observed. In the final stage of this change the cell looks like a metachromatic blot and apparently disappears by a total loss of its contents through dissolution. We have called this phenomenon *fusion* although this term does not give a clear idea of the change to which it is attached.

II. Mast cell damage and histamine release

A. By naturally occurring substances

Histamine-releasing agents of natural origin are amongst the first substances known to release histamine. The histamine releasing ability of peptone, some animal venoms, bacterial toxins, proteases, Ascaris extract and lecithin has been known for a long time. More recently the histamine releasing activities of d-tubocurarine, lichenformin, protamine, atropine, quinine and the antibiotics polymyxin B and E have been reported. When these substances were tried on the mast cells it was observed that they produced definite changes in these cells, peptone being the first to be tried. Mast cells changes induced by peptone were first described in the dog by WILANDER (1938) and later in mice and rats by MOTA and YONEDA (1952). Observing these cells in liver, spleen, lung, intestine, kidney and ovary of dogs submitted to peptone shock, WILANDER (1938) described mast cell alterations characterized by degranulation and decrease in the metachromasia of the remaining granules. This author related these alterations to heparin liberation and believed that liver mast cells emptied their granule content into the blood. He also noted that only in the liver did the mast cells present conspicuous alterations. On the other hand, in mice and rats it was observed that mast cell damage induced by peptone was rather generalized and not restricted to any particular organ (MOTA and YONEDA, 1952; MOTA, 1953). Later on, in collaboration with JUNQUEIRA, BERALDO and FERRI (MOTA, JUNQUEIRA, BERALDO and FERRI, 1954; MOTA, FERRI and JUNQUEIRA, 1956), we did some experiments to find out why the mast cell alterations were confined to the liver when peptone was injected into dogs. A freshly prepared 20% solution of peptone in 0.85% sodium chloride was used after being shaken with permutit and filtered. Peptone was injected at the dosage level of 0.5 g/kg of body weight through the femoral or portal vein or lingual artery. Liver biopsies were made before and after the shock. The abdomen was opened and small pieces of liver, collected from two or more lobes, were reduced to 2 mm thick slices and immersed in the fixative. This procedure was found quite useful for later mast cell counts. However, to observe the qualitative alterations of these cells, an entire hepatic lobe was excised after ligature of its pedicle and immediately fixed by perfusion of the fixative through the branches of the portal vein. Following the peptone injection, samples of the liver were taken either immediately or 15—20 min after the shock. Furthermore, in all dogs the tongue was fixed by perfusion of the fixative through the lingual artery. For mast cells counts, 10 μg thick paraffin sections of the liver stained with toluidine blue were used and the number of metachromatic granule containing cells determined in one hundred 6400 μ^2 areas with the aid of a square-ruled ocular micrometer. For observation of the mast cell morphology, frozen sections 50 μ thick

Table 1. *Mast cell and histamine content of the liver and histamine content of the tongue, before and after peptone shock*

Dog	Peptone injected through	Mast cells[1] Liver		Histamine γ/g Liver		Histamine γ/g Tongue	
		Before	After	Before	After	Before	After
1	Femoral v.	15.4	13.3	13	8.6	—	—
2	Femoral v.	36.7	2.2	47	20	—	—
3	Femoral v.	34.0	11.2	33	26	—	—
4	Femoral v.	43.8	22.0	108	83	—	—
5	Portal v.	14.0	6.0	13	1.6	3.6	3.3
6	Portal v.	24.0	14.0	20	20	7.6	6.3
7	Portal v.	24.0	2.0	33	16	10.0	6.3
8	Ling. art.	20.4	14.5	—	—	5.3	2.0
9	Ling. art.	—	—	—	—	8.6	6.3
10	Ling. art.	—	—	—	—	10.6	5.3

[1] Average of three 0.64 mm² areas of 10 μ thick sections.

stained with toluidine blue were used. To study the histamine content, tongue and liver samples were taken before and after peptone shock, and histamine extracted according to the method of CODE (1937). In the above conditions, we observed that mast cell alterations were present in both the liver and the tongue but were more numerous in the latter when the peptone solution was injected directly into the lingual artery. Therefore, we suggested that the restriction of dog mast cell damage almost exclusively to the liver was due to the anatomical and physiological peculiarities of this organ in the dog (BAUER, DALE, POULSSON and RICHARDS, 1932; AREY, 1941), that promotes blood stasis during the shock allowing a greater and more delayed contact of the peptone with its cells than with those of other organs. This conclusion would also explain why in mice and rats, in which peptone is not particularly concentrated in the liver, the mast cell changes were found to be generalized (Mota and Yoneda, 1952; Mota, 1953). Furthermore by making tongue and liver biopsies before and after the injection of the peptone, we were able to observe a parallel decrease in the histamine content and mast cell population of both these organs. These findings are illustrated in Table 1 and Fig. 1 Mast cell damage induced by peptone in dog tongue was also observed by Arvy

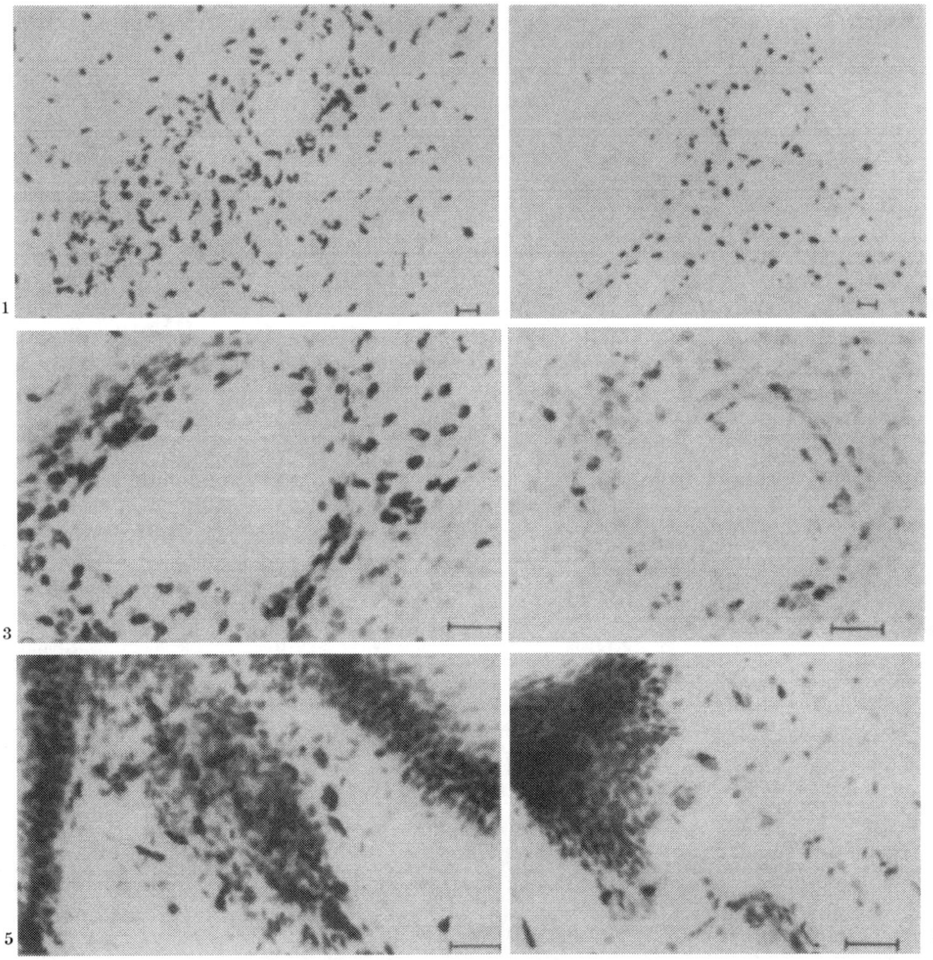

Fig. 1. Tongue and liver of a dog, fixed in lead subacetate-ethanol-acetic acid. The scales represent 3 μ. *1 and 2:* Mast cells around throttle vein in dog liver, 1 from control biopsy, 2 from biopsy after peptone shock (dog 4). Note evident decrease in the mast cell number. *3 and 4:* Mast cells around central vein in dog liver, 3 from control biopsy, note cells rich in intense metachromatic granules; 4 from biopsy after peptone schock, note cells poor in granules and reduction of metachromasia of remaining ones. *5 and 6:* Mast cells in the lamina propria of tongue, 5 from control animal, 6 from dog injected with peptone

and Quivy (1955). The active agent in peptone is not known; but according to Eldridge and Paton (1957), a histamine-releasing activity of a low order is present throughout its constituents.

In 1947 Schild and Gregory showed that d-tubocurarine was able to release histamine from skeletal muscle; and in 1953 Riley, in his paper on the effects of histamine-liberators on rat mast cells, observed that d-tubocurarine is one of the most active disintegrators of rat mast cells. Thus, according to Riley (1953a), after a slow intravenous injection of 5 mg of d-tubocurarine into rats of about 200 g body weight, most of the mesenteric mast cells disappear.

Some of the side-effects of polymyxin B and E in man and laboratory animals led BUSHBY and GREEN (1955) to suspect that these antibiotics probably caused release of histamine. This proved to be the case; and these investigators showed that local or intravenous injections of polymyxins B and E into rats, guinea-pigs, dogs or cats produced signs characteristic of histamine release. These authors also observed the effect of these antibiotics on rat mast cells. They reported that, when 5 mg/kg of either polymyxin was injected subcutaneously or intraperitoneally into rats, disruption of the mesenteric mast cells occurred. The *in vitro* effect of polymyxin B on rat mast cells was studied by NORTON and DE BEER (1955). These authors quantitatively studying rat mast cell disruption, found that a solution of polymyxin B containing 0.4 μg/ml produced disruption of 50% of the mesenteric mast cells. Later on, PARRATT and WEST (1957) showed that polymyxin B releases histamine almost selectively from rat mast cells, little serotonin being released.

The shock condition produced by injection of ascaris extracts was first reported by LEROY (1910) and confirmed by SHIMAMURA and FUJI (1917), EMERY and HERRICK (1930), MACHEBOEUF and MANDOUL (1939) and MANDOUL (1939). These authors studied the effect of ascaris extract injected into cats, dogs and guinea-pigs and showed that a picture very similar to anaphylaxis was produced mainly in the dogs and guinea-pigs, then followed by desensitization to further injections if the animal survived the first injection. Contraction of the isolated intestine of the cat, rat, rabbit and guinea-pig produced by ascaris extract was reported by EMERY and HERRICK (1928), and ESSEX, MARKOWITZ and MANN (1931) showed that when ascaris extract was applied intradermally into human skin, it produced a typical wheal and flare reaction. Although the above authors noted that many of the symptoms presented by the injected animals could be attributed to histamine, they concluded that these symptoms were not due to the histamine sometimes already present in ascaris extract. Thus, MACHEBOEUF and MANDOUL (1939) were able to kill guinea-pigs two or three minutes after injecting a dyalized histamine-free ascaris extract with a typical anaphylactic picture. It remained for ROCHA E SILVA and GRAÑA (1946a, b) to demonstrate that injection of ascaris extract produced histamine release and noncoagulability of the blood from heparin in dogs and increase in blood histamine in guinea-pigs. Release of histamine from the perfused guinea-pig lung was first observed by BIER (1946) and confirmed by ROCHA E SILVA and GRAÑA (1946a, b). These authors noticed that the shock produced in dogs and guinea-pigs by ascaris extract differs from true anaphylaxis only in that the animals have not been prepared by previous injections of the extract. However, the authors suggested that the animals may have been sensitized due to previous contact with intestinal parasitic worms. Indeed according to BERALDO and his colleagues (BERALDO and DIAS DA SILVA, 1960; GAZZINELLI, PUDLES, GUIA and ALMEIDA NEVES, 1960; GAZZINELLI, GUIA, NEVES, PUDLES, BERALDO and DIAS DA SILVA, 1961; DIAS DA SILVA, BERALDO and PUDLES, 1961), the shock induced in guinea-pigs by ascaris extract is true anaphylaxis due to a natural sensitization of this species to an antigenic fraction (a glycoprotein) present in *Ascaris lumbricoides*. They based their conclusion on the following facts: a) a purified fraction they obtained from ascaris extract was active in very low concentration similar to that of antigen; b) ascaris fraction induced contraction of the isolated guinea-pig ileum followed by desensitization to further additions; c) ascaris fraction induced guinea-pig mast cell damage very similar to those produced by antigen in sensitized tissues; d) non-sensitized guinea-pig ileum could be passively sensitized by incubation with guinea-pig serum or with extract of spleens taken from sensitized guinea-pigs; e) the several agents that inhibit histamine release and mast cell damage in guinea-pig anaphylaxis (metabolic inhibitors, calcium lack, antipyretics, nicotinamide, antihistamines, etc.) also inhibit histamine release and mast cell damage induced by ascaris fraction. Furthermore, previous heating of a piece of ileum at 45° C completely abolished the contraction induced by ascaris fraction. However, according to UVNÄS and his colleagues (UVNÄS, DIAMANT, HÖGBERG and THON, 1960), ascaris extract contains a naturally occurring histamine liberator, active on rat mast cells.

B. By long chain molecules

It is known that many natural and synthetic polymers are able to release histamine from the tissues of certain species. A curious and yet unexplained fact is that the histamine-releasing activity of each polymer is specific for a determined species. Thus, ovomucoid is harmful when injected into rats but harmless for almost all other animal species; and likewise polyvinylpyrrolidone is harmful only to dogs. The histamine-releasing properties of ovomucoid, dextran, polyvinylpyrrolidone and tweens are well known. Although only ovomucoid and dextran are known to cause damage to the mast cells, the other two polymers probably also act by damaging the mast cells. The release of histamine by ovomucoid from rat skin was first shown by SCHACHTER and TALESNIK (1953) who also observed that ovomucoid did not release histamine from cat or dog skin. That the histamine-releasing activity of ovomucoid was accompanied by mast cell damage was shown by BENDITT and his colleagues (BENDITT, BADER, ARASE, CORLEY and LAM, 1954; BENDITT, BADER and LAM, 1955). These authors demonstrated that 3 mg of ovomucoid injected intravenously into rats of about 200 g produced a degree of hyperemia and increased vascular permeability that correlated with the density of the mast cell population in the tissue, and that the ovomucoid disrupted the mast cells producing histamine release both *in vivo* and *in vitro*. The observation of FELDBERG and TALESNIK (1953) that rats depleted of their mast cells by repeated injections of compound 48—80 are no longer sensitive to ovomucoid, suggests that ovomucoid might act specifically on the mast cells.

In 1951, VOORHEES et al., described a curious condition produced by dextrans of several molecular weights when injected into rats. The condition was characterized by weakness, dyspnea and edema of the snout and paws. Analyzing this phenomenon, HALPERN and BRIOT (1952) were able to show that dextran released histamine from rat skin *in vitro*. Disruption of rat mast cells after intravenous injection of dextran was first reported by ROWLEY and BENDITT (1956) who concluded that this polymer releases both histamine and 5-hydroxytryptamine from mast cells but that the edema associated with mast cell damage is due largely to 5-hydroxytryptamine.

When studying the effect of dextran and ovomucoid on rat mast cells *in vitro*, we observed that besides their species-specificity, dextran and ovomucoid also present some tissue specificity (unpublished results). Thus, we have found that when rat diaphragm, mesentery and skin are incubated with Tyrode solution containing dextran 150 (12 mg/ml) or crystalline ovomucoid (3 mg/ml), for 15 min at 37° C, mast cell disruption and histamine release occurred only in the skin but neither of these phenomena were produced in the diaphragm or mesentery. The addition of 10% fresh rat serum to the incubating medium did not modify the results. Thinking that some *in vivo* factor or condition might be required for mast cell damage in the mesentery, some experiments were performed in which rats of about 200 g were injected intraperitoneally with 20 ml of a Tyrode solution containing 5 mg dextran per ml. The animals, when sacrificed two hours later, presented pronounced edema of the paw and snout. The mesentery was fixed and stained by injecting into the peritoneal cavity a solution of 1% toluidine blue containing 1% acetic acid and 10% formaldehyde. However, even in this condition no change in the mesenteric mast cells were observed. Recently, LAGUNOFF and BENDITT (1960) observed that dextran and ovomucoid have no discernible effect on isolated mast cells obtained from rat peritoneal cavity. However, this might be expected since dextran has no effect on non-isolated mesenteric mast cells anyhow.

C. By histamine liberators

In this section will be studied a group of many different substances characterized by their strong histamine-releasing action. Their effect on the mast cells was first described by RILEY (1953a) and by MOTA (1953) and MOTA, BERALDO and JUNQUEIRA (1953). RILEY (1953a) was able to show that many histamine liberators such as stilbamidine, propamidine, diaminoheptane, d-tubocurarine and peptone produced disruption of the mast cells when injected intravenously into rats. Taking advantage of the fluorescent property of stilbamidine, Riley performed very interesting experiments in which he followed this drug after it had been injected intravenously into rats. Thus, after an intravenous and rapid (5 sec) injection of 1 ml of saline containing 25 mg stilbamidine into rats, fresh peritoneal spreads were prepared and examined microscopically under direct ultraviolet light. In this way, bright and sharply defined fluorescent spots situated predominantly near small blood vessels could be seen against a dark background. When, following this, a 1% toluidine blue solution was run onto the preparation and visual light transmitted through the specimen, the fluorescent spots could easily be recognized as mast cells, thus showing that the stilbamidine was rapidly and selectively taken up by these cells. An entirely different picture was seen when the mast cells were observed after a slow (30—60 sec) injection. Instead of the sharply defined fluorescence of the mast cells in the peritoneal spreads, there were pools of fluorescent material around some of the vessels and counterstaining with toluidine blue, revealed a widespread disruption of the mast cells. These observations showed that stilbamidine, and probably other histamine-liberators, are selectively concentrated in the mast cells after which these cells disrupt.

Compound 48—80, a condensation product of paramethoxyphenethylmethylamine with formaldehyde (BALTZLY, BUCK, DE BEER and WEBB, 1949), is selected here as a prototype of the substances that PATON (1955) has classified as histamine liberators. It will particularly be discussed here, not only because it is a very efficient histamine liberator and mast cell destroyer but also because it is the most well studied of these compounds. PATON (1951), FELDBERG and PATON (1951), and FELDBERG and SCHACHTER (1952) were the first to show that the depressor activity of compound 48—80 was due to its strong histamine-releasing property. They showed that it produced a rise in plasma histamine when injected into cats and dogs and that it released histamine from perfused cat and dog skin. The disruptive effect of compound 48—80 on rat mast cells was first described by MOTA (1953) and MOTA, BERALDO and JUNQUEIRA (1953). These authors observed that when injected intravenously into rats, compound 48—80 produced a pronounced fall in the blood pressure, considerable increase in plasma histamine, and generalized mast cell damage. Disruption of the mast cells was observed in the skin, tongue, submaxillary glands, lymphatic glands, thymus, mesentery and spleen. They also observed that, contrary to what happens in dogs, the disruption of rat mast cells induced by compound 48—80 was not associated with heparin release, and suggested that in rats heparin could be bound to the cytoplasmic constituents of mast cells in a more stable linkage than in dog mast cells. The disruptive effect of compound 48—80 was also shown in *in vitro* experiments, performed by immersing fragments of rat mesentery in saline (sodium chloride 0.85%) containing different concentrations of compound 48—80 (from 1/1000 to 1/20,000). This disruptive effect could also be observed under phase contrast microscopy as a rapid bubbling of the mast cell surface during a few seconds (see Fig. 2). These results were then interpreted as suggestive of a direct effect of compound 48—80 on the mast cells.

Later on, FAWCETT (1954) studied the histamine-releasing and disruptive effect of compound 48—80 on mast cells by injecting this compound dissolved in Tyrode

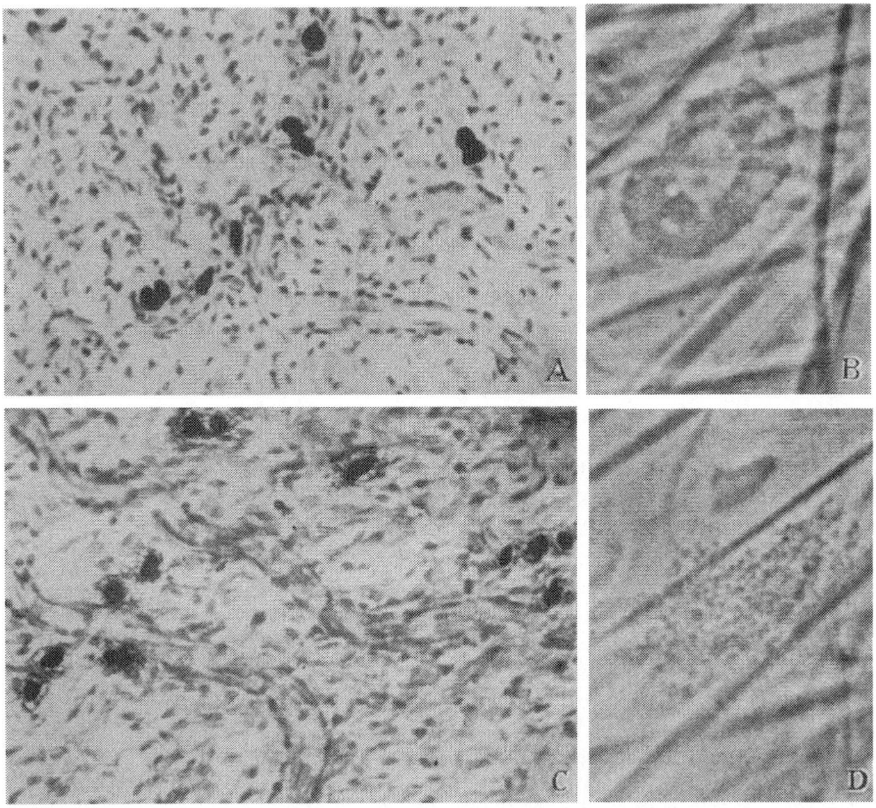

Fig. 2. Mast cells of rat mesentery. A and C toluidine blue stained (×400). B and D phase contrast (×1300). A and B from control animal. C and D compound 48/80 injected animal

solution into the peritoneal cavity of rats. He observed that a series of increasing doses of compound 48—80 had a graded disruptive effect on the mast cells and resulted in a graded increase in the amount of histamine that appeared in the peritoneal fluid and concluded that the histamine set free by this compound originated from the mast cells. Furthermore, FAWCETT (1955) also studied the regeneration of the mast cell population after its destruction by compound 48—80. After injecting into the peritoneal cavity 20 ml of Tyrode solution containing 500 to 1000 μg 48—80, this author observed that almost all the mesenteric mast cells had been destroyed by this treatment but that a fair number apparently survived the release of most of their granules. Regeneration of the mast cell population was performed by cell division and by differentiation from non-granular precursors present in the adventitia of small blood vessels as well as in avascular areas of the mesentery. Ten days after the injection of compound 48—80 the number of mast cells was as great as before and the cells were approaching normal size but they were still more vacuolated than usual, and there was a greater than normal variation in the size of the granules. Rather similar findings were later reported by RILEY and WEST (1955) who made a parallel study of the tissue histamine recovery after injecting compound 48—80. They concluded that there was a close correlation between the fall and subsequent recovery of the tissue histamine on the one hand and the disruption and restoration of the mast cells on the other. NORTON (1954) using the technique for the *in vitro* observation of mast cell disruption induced by compound 48—80 described by MOTA, BERALDO and JUNQUEIRA (1953) made a careful study of this phenomenon. She rapidly dissected

Table 2. *Disruption of mast cells by different batches of 48/80*

Batch No.	Expt. No.	Percentage disruption					ED 50 (μg/ml)	Fiducial limits (P = 0.95)
		concn. of 48/80 (μg/ml)						
		0	0.1	0.2	0.4	0.8		
NS 280	1	10		28	76	92	0.27	0.23—0.32
	2	6		26	68	90	0.30	0.26—0.35
	3	8		54	66	86	0.20	0.12—0.31
	4	2	28	68	76		0.16	0.12—0.19
	5	6	12	48	70		0.22	0.19—0.26
AE 92	3			56	82	86	0.13	0.07—0.26
AE 2	1			40	88	100	0.23	0.20—0.26
	2			4	68	100	0.33	0.28—0.39
GD 78	3			40	64	72	0.26	0.19—0.35
VI 64	1			44	54	62	0.30	0.16—0.56
VI 53	3			6	28	90	0.47	0.42—0.53
VI 65	3			12	36	64	0.57	0.45—0.70

pieces of rat mesentery and incubated them in Ringer-Locke solution containing different concentrations of compound 48—80 for 30 min at room temperature. The pieces were then removed to 4% formaldehyde solution containing 0.1% toluidine blue then transferred through acetone and xylene and mounted on slides. From those pieces, five microscopical fields were selected at random from widely separated areas of the mesentery. In each field, using a 430 x magnification, the first 10 mast cells were examined, starting from the left-hand side of the field and proceeding clockwise. For each drug concentration 50 cells were counted and the percentage of disrupted cells obtained. In these conditions, it was observed that the percentage of mast cells which became disrupted was graded according to the concentration of compound 48—80. Based on this finding, NORTON developed a method to assay the activity of compound 48—80 by counting the number of disrupted mast cells in standard conditions (see Table 2). Furthermore, having observed that dilution of the Ringer-Locke solution in which the mast cells were bathed, inhibited the disruption of these cells by compound 48—80, this author suggested that this compound could make the mast cell membrane more permeable to extracellular ions thereby causing disruption of these cells. A different approach to the mechanism of action of compound 48—80 was presented by JUNQUEIRA and BEIGUELMAN (1955). These authors studied the influence of temperature, pH, lack of oxygen and several metabolic inhibitors on the disruptive effect of compound 48—80 on rat mast cells. The experiments were performed *in vitro* incubating pieces of rat mesentery in 0.9% sodium chloride plus 10% phosphate buffer (0.15 M pH 7.4) containing the substances or in the conditions to be studied. To study the effect of pH and temperature, pieces of mesentery were previously incubated at different temperatures or pH for 10 min after which compound 48—80 was added (final concentration 0.1 mg/ml). The influence of oxygen lack was observed, incubating pieces of mesentery in WARBURG's flasks in nitrogen atmosphere and in the presence of red phosphorus for 10 min after which compound 48—80 was added. To study the effect of the metabolic inhibitors, these substances were dissolved in different concentrations in the buffered saline and the mesentery incubated in them for 10 min after which compound 48—80 was added. To observe the mast cells, the mesentery was fixed and stained in a 10% formaldehyde solution containing 1% toluidine blue and 0.1% acetic acid. These experiments showed that the disruptive effect of compound 48—80 was temperature and pH dependent and was inhibited in the absence of oxygen. Table 3 shows the effect and concentration of the different metabolic inhibitors

Table 3. *Influence of metabolic inhibitors on the action of compound 48/80 on rat mast-cells "in vitro."* Mesentery fragments were incubated in the inhibitor dissolved in saline-buffer solution during 15 min at 37° C, and compound 48/80 added (1/20,000 final concentration), for another 10 min. Fixation and staining as described in text

Inhibitor	Concentrations used		Granules extrusion
	Maximal	Minimal	
p-Cl Hg benzoate	0.33×10^{-2} M	1×10^{-3} M	Absent
o-Iodosobenzoate	0.33×10^{-2} M	1×10^{-3} M	Absent
Iodoacetate	0.33×10^{-2} M	0.16×10^{-2} M	Absent
2,4-Dinitrophenol	0.33×10^{-2} M	0.12×10^{-3} M	Absent
Arsenite	0.33×10^{-2} M	1×10^{-3} M	Absent
Cyanide	0.33×10^{-2} M	1×10^{-3} M	Absent
Malonate	0.33×10^{-2} M	—	Present
Fluoride	0.33×10^{-2} M	—	Present
Urethane	0.06 M	—	Absent
Uranil nitrate	1×10^{-3} M	0.5×10^{-3} M	Absent

used. It was observed that p-chloromercuribenzoate, o-iodosobenzoate, iodoacetate, 2-4 dinitrophenol, arsenite, cyanide, urethane and uracyl nitrate inhibited the extrusion of mast cell granules induced by compound 48—80. The authors also observed that glutathione was able to revert the inhibition produced by p-chloromercuribenzoate, iodoacetate and o-iodosobenzoate, all of which are SH blocking substances, and concluded that —SH groups present in structural proteins or enzymes participate in the disruptive effect of compound 48—80. Similar conclusions were later drawn by HÖGBERG and UVNÄS (1957) who using these and other inhibitors, and a larger range of temperature, concluded that the effect of 48—80 could be blocked by several enzyme inhibitors and was dependent on the temperature. They observed as well that the inhibition produced by temperatures above 45° C was irreversible, a fact also observed by MONGAR and SCHILD (1955) in relation to the anaphylactic release of histamine in guinea-pigs. The probable dependence of compound 48—80 on enzymes containing essential —SH groups was also suggested by HÖGBERG and UVNÄS (1958). FELDBERG and TALESNIK (1953) were the first to succeed in depleting rat tissues of most of their histamine and to study how long it takes for the tissue to recover its original histamine level. They observed that after repeated intraperitoneal injections of increasing doses of compound 48—80, there was a reduction of about 90% of the skin and skeletal and cardiac muscle histamine which recovered very slowly in the course of weeks. They also made the curious observation that the histamine content in the liver and in the wall of the stomach and duodenum was not reduced by compound 48—80. Trying to find an explanation for FELDBERG and TALESNIK's observations, MOTA, BERALDO, FERRI and JUNQUEIRA (1956) studied simultaneously the effect of 48—80 on the mast cell population and the histamine content of rat tissues. Thus, rats weighing 100—250 g, weren given daily intraperitoneal injections of increasing doses of compound 48—80, beginning with 100 μg and increasing by 100 μg daily up to 500 μg. Twenty four hours after the last injection the animals were killed and adjacent pieces were taken for histamine assay and for observation of the mast cells from the following tissues: skin, tongue, oesophagus, cardiac and fundic region of stomach, duodenum, ileum, rectum and liver. The results of these experiments, as can be seen in Table 4, showed a positive correlation between the mast cell population and the histamine content for skin, tongue, oesophagus and cardia but not for the lower segments of the gastrointestinal tract and liver. Thus in skin and tongue, a high histamine content was associated with an abundance of mast cells; in oesophagus and forestomach, a medium histamine content was associated with a less dense mast cell population; while in the fundic region of the stomach and duodenum, a relatively high content histamine was not associated with a dense mast cell population. Confirming FELDBERG and TALESNIK's (1953) findings, it was observed that treatment with compound 48—80 greatly reduced the histamine content of the skin, tongue, oesophagus and forestomach but did not reduce the histamine in the wall of the fundic region of the stomach, duodenum, ileum and liver. In skin, tongue, oesophagus and cardia, in which the histamine content showed a positive correlation to the mast cell population, the reduction of histamine by 48—80 was associated with a corresponding reduction or disappearance of the mast cell population. On the other hand, compound 48—80 had no effect on the histamine content of those tissues which contain few or no mast cells as in the wall of the fundus or duodenum (see Table 4). The authors concluded that the histamine of the mast cells was very susceptible to compound 48—80 and that the inability of this compound to release histamine of some tissues was due to the fact that in these, the histamine was not of mast cell origin as it happens in the lower digestive tract of the rat.

Table 4. *Histamine content (μg/g) and mast cell density of various tissues from control and 48/80 injected rats. The mast cell content is recorded on relative scale of 0 to + + + +*

Tissues	Control rats		48/80 injected rats	
	Histamine	Mast cells	Histamine	Mast cells
Skin (foot)	61.0	+ + + +	8.6	+
Skin (dorsum)	27.9	+ + +	5.4	+
Tongue	14.5	+ + +	2.9	+
Oesophagus	4.5	+ +	1.9	0
Cardia	3.0	+	1.0	0
Fundus	15.1	+	14.8	0
Duodenum	14.8	0	14.2	0
Ileum	5.5	0	5.4	0
Rectum	2.5	0	2.8	0
Liver	0.5	+	0.4	0

The effect of compound 48—80 on rat isolated mast cells was observed by UVNÄS and THON (1959). These authors showed that rat mast cells isolated by differential centrifugation in Ficoll (a polysaccharide of high molecular weight) and resuspended in a buffered (pH 7) isotonic salt solution were still able to respond to compound 48—80, provided that cat serum had been added to the isolating medium. We have also observed that compound 48—80 is able to act on isolated mast cells (unpublished results). Rat mast cells were isolated by differential centrifugation in a 30% solution of bovine serum albumin and the cells resuspended in Tyrode solution. Addition of compound 48—80 reproduced exactly the same mast cell response as induced when compound 48—80 was allowed to act on isolated pieces of rat mesentery (Mota, Beraldo and Junqueira, 1953). However, in our conditions this phenomenon was observed with washed mast cells resuspended in Tyrode solution without any added serum. Lagunoff and Benditt (1960) working with isolated mast cells deposited on the surface of a Millipore filter, were also able to observe rat mast cell disruption by compound 48—80 without adding serum. This discrepancy may be explained if mast cells isolated with Ficoll are less susceptible to the effect of compound 48—80 than when isolated by other techniques.

All the papers quoted above have suggested very strongly that compound 48—80 is a very efficient agent to release histamine from rat mast cells, either *in vivo* or *in vitro*. However, in the guinea-pig, compound 48—80 is not so efficient

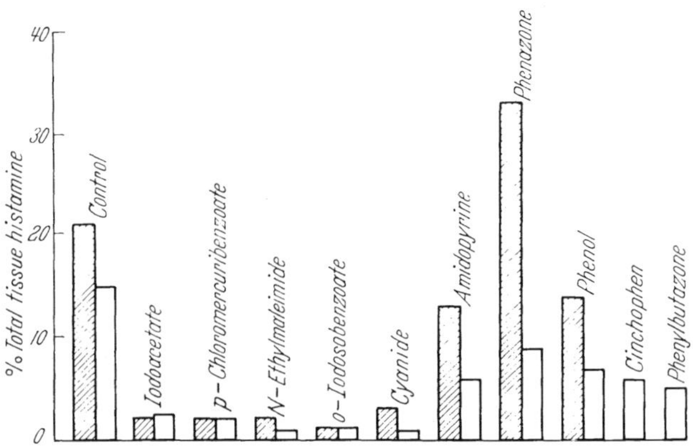

Fig. 3. Effect of metabolic inhibitors and antipyretics on histamine release by antigen (white columns) or compound 48/80 (black columns) from rat skin

a histamine-releasing agent as it could be assumed from its activity when acting on rat tissues. Indeed, as pointed out by Mongar (1956), the activity of histamine releasers is very variable depending upon the species, the tissue and method used for determining the activity. Furthermore, the mechanism of action of compound 48—80 must be different when acting on rat and guinea-pig mast cells, since all the agents that inhibit rat mast cell disruption by 48—80 will potentiate, instead of inhibiting, the damage to guinea-pig mast cells induced by this compound (Mota, 1959a, b; Mota and Ishii, 1960). For instance, it has been observed (Mota, 1959b; Mota and Ishii, 1960) that several metabolic inhibitors (iodoacetate, o-iodosobenzoate, p-chloromercuribenzoate, N-ethylmaleimide and cyanide), antipyretics, previous heating at 45° C and calcium lack, which produce inhibition of mast cell damage and histamine release from rat tissues (see Fig. 3), will potentiate, instead of inhibiting, mast cell damage and histamine release from guinea-pig tissues. The same results were also obtained when rat and guinea pig tissues were submitted to compound 48—80 after having been previously incubated with antihistamines (Mota and Dias da Silva, 1960a). These results have suggested that compound 48—80 acts probably through a different mechanism on guinea-pig and rat mast cells and that in the latter species the histamine-releasing mechanism of compound 48—80 is very similar to that of anaphylaxis (Mota, 1959a; Mota and Ishii, 1960). This same conclusion was also drawn by Chakravarty (1960) studying the mechanism of histamine release in anaphylaxis in rats and guinea-pigs. An explanation for the different mechanism of action of compound 48—80 when acting on guinea-pig and rat mast cells is not yet known. According to Boreus (1960a) who made a parallel study of the effect of several histamine liberators on the mesenteric mast cells of rats, guinea-pigs and hamsters, compound 48—80 would act through a non-enzymatic lytic mechanism when acting on guinea-pig mast cells. In this respect it would act by a mechanism similar to that of octylamine, and indeed, guinea-pig mast cell damage induced by compound 48—80 is morphologically undistinguishable from that induced by octylamine. The difference in the action of compound 48—80 when acting on rat and guinea-pig tissues seems to be more evident when this compound is used in the living animal. In fact, the syndrome produced by compound 48—80 when injected into guinea-pigs is not the one which is usually associated with histamine release in this species. Thus, the asthma and lung emphysema that occur after the injection of antigen, anaphylatoxin, peptone and ascaris extract, all of which are known to release histamine in this species, are not present in guinea-pigs submitted to lethal doses of compound 48—80. FEINBERG and STERNBERGER (1955) were the first to call the attention to this fact. They administered to guinea-pigs lethal, or near lethal doses, of this compound (3 or 4 mg/kg) and observed scratching, weakness, prostration and at times embarrassment in respiration, but no typical asthmatic symptoms. Autopsy of the animals receiving fatal doses always showed hemorrhagic and collapsed lungs. It was also observed that daily intraperitoneal injections of compound 48—80 failed to render the animals refractory to further action of the compound and that doses of antihistamines several times larger than those required to protect against histamine, failed to prevent against fatal reaction induced by 48—80. The authors concluded that in the living guinea-pig this compound is not an efficient histamine liberator and that other toxic effects are responsible for the lethal effect of 48—80 when acting in this species. Later on, MOTA and VUGMAN (1956c) confirmed these findings and studied the effect of compound 48—80, when injected into the intact animal, on the histamine content and the mast cell population of guinea-pig tissues. To study the effect of compound 48—80 on the mast cells and histamine content of guinea-pig lung, a cannula was tied into the trachea of the animal and connected to a respiratory pump. The thorax was opened and lung samples were collected before, and 2 to 15 min after the intracardiac injection of 0.5 mg compound 48—80 in 1 ml saline. The lung samples were either extracted for histamine assay or fixed for mast cell observation. To fix the mast cells, the fixative was injected into the lung through a bronchial branch. Histamine was extracted by reducing the lung samples to small pieces and boiling with N HCl, and assayed on the guinea-pig ileum, after neutralization with NaOH. Seven out of fourteen animals presented respiratory disturbances as shown by diminution in the amplitude of the respiratory movements and respiratory stoppage with collapsed lungs. However, no difference was observed either in the mast cell population or in the histamine content of the lung after the injection of compound 48—80. This result was in contrast to the decrease in histamine content and mast cell population observed when antigen was injected into sensitized guinea-pigs (MOTA and VUGMAN, 1956a, b). The plasma histamine level was also assayed before and after the intracardiac injection of 0.5 mg 48—80, having presented no significant increase although the dose of 48—80 had been enough to kill all the injected animals. In contrast, similar experiments with rats showed an increase in plasma histamine ranging from 0.0—0.1 up to 8 to 10 μg/ml. Furthermore, the histamine content and mast cell population of the guinea-pig mesentery and skin (from symmetrical sites in the foreleg, paw and the lateral regions of the head), were observed after repeated intraperitoneal injections of compound 48—80. Guinea-pigs were injected intraperitoneally daily with increasing doses of 48—80 according to the following schedule: 100, 200, 200, 300, 300, 400, 400, 500, 500, 600, 800, 1,000, 1,000, 1,500 and 1,500 μg. At the first 500 μg, the animals became uneasy, pawing of the snout and intense scratching being the most frequent signs. Half an hour after the injection of the first 1,500 μg of 48—80, the animals remained in lateral decubitus, with paralysis of the hindlegs, tremors, and apparent respiratory disturbances. Circulatory changes characterized by ischaemia altering with hyperaemia were frequently seen in the vessels of the ear. All the signs subsided after 3 hours. After the second injection of 1,500 μg of 48—80, the animals presented the same signs and all of them died within a period of 2 hours. At autopsy the lungs were collapsed and cyanotic. The observation of the mast cell population and histamine content of the mesentery and skin showed that, in spite of the repeated injections of large doses of 48—80, there was no difference between the histamine and mast cell content of the control and injected animals.This fact is in striking contrast to what happens in rats receiving repeated injections of 48—80. It was concluded, therefore, that the main effect of compound 48—80 when injected into guinea-pigs was not due to histamine liberation, and that the mast cells and the tissue histamine in this species were less susceptible to compound 48—80 than those of other species. In this same paper the authors were not able to observe mast cell damage when pieces of guinea-pig mesentery were incubated with isotonic sucrose containing compound 48—80. However, it was later observed that when guinea-pig tissues were incubated *in vitro* with compound 48—80 dissolved in Tyrode solution, mast cell damage occurred very similar to that induced by octylamine in guinea-pig tissues (MOTA, 1959a). Actually, there is a large individual variation in the sensitivity of guinea-pigs to compound 48—80 and while in some individuals, the mast cells disappear almost completely after incubation of the tissue with compound 48—80 (1 mg/ml), in others only qualitative alterations are produced. Probably in their first *in vitro* experiments to see the effect of compound 48—80 on guinea-pig mast cells, the authors failed to observe the qualitative mast cell alterations which were certainly present. This may, perhaps,explain the more recent results of BOREUS (1960a) who also did not observe mast cell damage when guinea-pig mesentery was incubated with compound 48—80. However, since in the intact guinea-pig, even after repeated doses of this compound there is not a reduction in the histamine content and mast cell population of the tissues, it is reasonable to admit that for some unknown reason this compound does not act as an efficient mast cell destroyer in the living guinea-pig.

The reason why compound 48—80 acts so differently on rat and guinea-pig tissues is of considerable theoretical interest and must be explained by any hypothesis concerned with the mechanism of action of this compound. The observations of JUNQUEIRA and BEIGUELMAN (1955) showing that the disruptive effect of compound 48—80 on rat tissues is pH, oxygen and temperature dependent and can be inhibited by many metabolic and enzyme inhibitors, led HÖGBERG and UVNÄS (1957) to try the effect of several enzymes on rat mast cells. Out of 30 enzymes tested, only one, lecithinase A was found to be active in disrupting rat mast cells. This observation suggested to the authors that a lytic enzyme might be activated by compound 48—80 and, when a comparative study was made of the effect of lecithinase A and compound 48—80, the disruptive effect of these substances were found to be inhibited alike by the same agents, but for the effect of heating to 45° C, which blocked compound 48—80 whereas lecithinase was still active at 60° C. The authors suggested that compound 48—80 exerts its effect by activating an enzyme which acts upon lecithin and related compounds. Since lecithinase has two active amino groups, the authors postulated that the mast cell has an enzyme with two active amino groups, one of which being anchored to its membrane (A, in Fig. 4), while the other was thought to be blocked with a negatively charged inhibitor. They admitted that 48—80 interacts with this inhibitor (B, in Fig. 4) activating an enzyme which would cause extrusion of the mast cell granules. However, since 48—80 also releases histamine from isolated rat mast cell granules (MOTA, JUNQUEIRA, BERALDO and FERRI, 1954) to reinforce this theory one has to admit either the existence of a similar enzyme located on the mast cell granules or that the histamine-releasing mechanism of 48—80 on the intact cell is different from that effective on the isolated granules. Furthermore, these authors were also able to render rat mast cells resistant to the disruptive effect of compound P 3010aa (with substances reacting with primary and secondary amines, they used, instead of 48—80, a corresponding tertiary amine, the P 3010 aa) by incubating these cells with this compound in presence of 1,3-diphosphoimidazole which inactivates, by phosphorylation, enzymes with essential amino groups including lecithinase; they were also able to restore the sensitivity of the mast cells by dephosphorylation with phospho amidase. To explain these results, they admitted that on reaction with the liberator the amino-containing enzyme is activated by removal of the normally occurring inhibitor. However, if this occurs in the presence of diphosphoimidazole, the essential amino groups of the enzyme become phosphorylated as soon as the inhibitor is removed by the liberator and inactivation of the enzyme occurs. Nevertheless, the same authors showed that the amino groups could be phosphorylated even before removal of the naturally occurring inhibitor since, if mast cells were treated with diphosphoimidazole and then washed, the disruptive effect of compound 48—80 was still blocked due to previous phosphorylation.

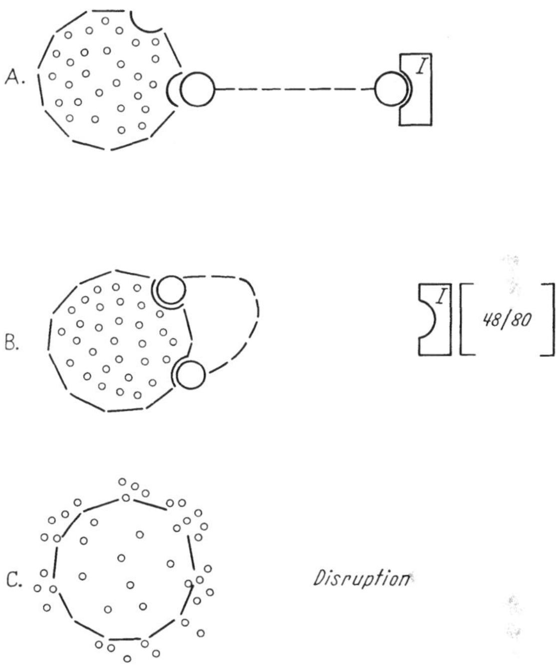

Fig. 4. Hypothesis to explain the fragmentation of mast cells produced by 48/80

D. By antihistamines

In 1946, PELLERAT and MURAT reported the curious observation that an increase in blood histamine occurred when antihistamines were injected into human beings. An explanation for this finding was presented by ARUNLAKSHANA (1953a) who showed that diphenhydramine and antazoline were able to release histamine from human and guinea-pig lung. She incubated human and guinea-pig lung tissue with these antihistamines and assayed the released histamine on the guinea-pig ileum after destruction of the antihistamines; diphenhydramine was destroyed by autoclaving the incubation fluid at 2 atm for 2 hours and antazoline by boiling it at atmospheric pressure for 4 hours. The histamine-releasing activity of diphenhydramine was found very intense at a concentration of 10^{-3} but negligible at 10^{-5}. Later on, TASAKA (1957) also observed that Benadryl and Neo-antergan were able to release histamine from chopped dog skin and that a subcutaneous injection of 25 mg Benadryl/kg released $^1/_3$ of rat skin histamine. Recently, DIAS DA SILVA (1960) and MOTA and DIAS DA SILVA (1960a) have confirmed the histamine-releasing effect of many antihistamines and studied their effect on rat and guinea-pig mast cells. They used the following antihistamines: antazoline hydrochloride, chlorpheniramine maleate, diphenhydramine hydrochloride, bromodiphenhydramine hydrochloride, isothipendyl hydrochloride, mepyramine hydrogen maleate,

Table 5. *Mast cell content of guinea-pig mesentery incubated at 37° for 15 min in Tyrode solution with and without added antihistamine.* Each figure is the mean count of 30 microscopical fields (magnification 130) in each of 2 experiments

Antihistamine	Concentration µg/ml	Number of mast cells in: Tyrode alone	Number of mast cells in: Tyrode with antihistamine	% Reduction
Chlorpheniramine maleate	50	12	13	0
	100	12	2	83
Bromodiphenhydramine hydrochloride	12.5	15	14	0
	25	15	3	78
Isothipendyl hydrochloride	25	19	20	0
	50	19	1	94
Antazoline hydrochloride	25	21	21	0
	50	21	4	81
Diphenhydramine hydrochloride	50	14	14	0
	100	14	1	93
Methapyrilene hydrochloride	100	17	18	0
	200	17	2	88
Mepyramine hydrogen maleate	200	24	25	0
	500	24	6	75
Promethazine hydrochloride	6.25	11	11	0
	12.50	11	3	73
Chlorpheniramine hydrochloride	100	31	31	0
	200	31	2	94
Tripelennamine hydrochloride	100	13	13	0
	200	13	3	77
Phenindamine hydrogen tartrate	25	27	29	0
	50	27	10	63

methapyrilene hydrochloride, phenindamine hydrogen tartrate, promethazine hydrochloride and tripelennamine hydrochloride. Taking advantage of the observation that bromodiphenhydrazine, diphenhydrazine and mepyramine lose their antihistamine activity after boiling for 10 min with 20% hydrochlorid acid, these antihistamines were used in the experiments concerning histamine release while the effect on the mast cells was studied with all the antihistamines. To study the effect of the antihistamines on the mast cells and tissue histamine, samples of rat and guinea-g tissues were incubapited for a standard time of 15 min at 37° C in 4 ml Tyrode solution containing different concentrations of the antihistamines, after which the tissues were transferred, either to 20% hydrochloric acid for histamine extraction and destruction of the antihistamines, or to a fixative for mast cell observation. In these conditions it was observed that all the antihistamines used produced damage to both rat and guinea-pig mast cells. Rat mast cell damage was very similar to that described with compound 48—80(MOTA, BERALDO and JUNQUEIRA, 1953) while guinea-pig mast cell damage was characterized by fusion of the metachromatic material similar to that described with octylamine and compound 48—80 (MOTA, 1959a). The effect of the antihistamines on guinea-pig mesenteric mast cells is illustrated in Table 5 and Fig. 5. Using phase contrast microscopy and isolated rat peritoneal mast cells, it was observed that these cells responded to antihistamines by the sudden appearance of intracellular vacuoles, transient swelling of the cell and extrusion of granules.

The antihistamines were able to release considerable quantity of histamine from various rat and guinea-pig tissues but very little from the stomach and

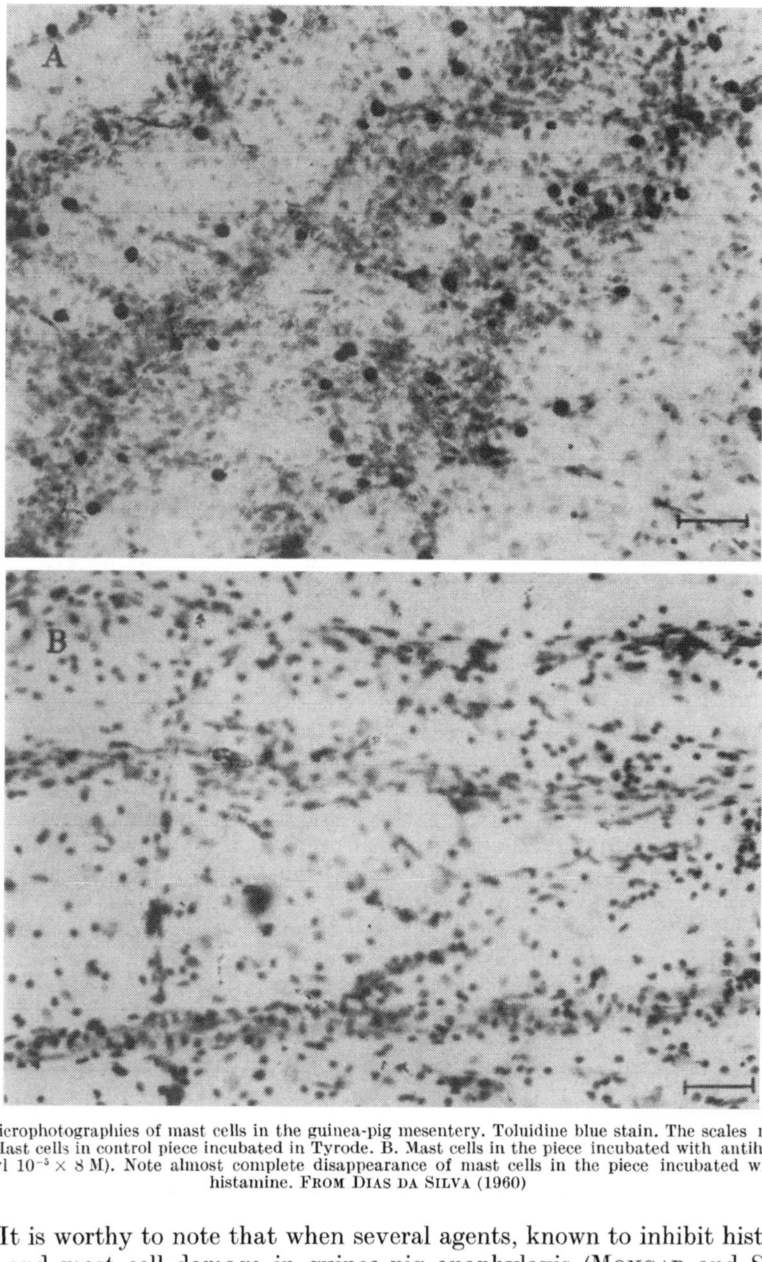

Fig. 5. Microphotographies of mast cells in the guinea-pig mesentery. Toluidine blue stain. The scales represent 50 μ. A. Mast cells in control piece incubated in Tyrode. B. Mast cells in the piece incubated with antihistamine (Ambodryl $10^{-5} \times 8$ M). Note almost complete disappearance of mast cells in the piece incubated with antihistamine. From Dias da Silva (1960)

ileum. It is worthy to note that when several agents, known to inhibit histamine release and mast cell damage in guinea-pig anaphylaxis (Mongar and Schild 1957a, b; Mota, 1958a, 1959b), were tried on histamine release and mast cell damage by antihistamines, it was observed that these agents potentiated mast cell damage and histamine release by antihistamines in guinea-pig tissues but inhibited these same phenomena in rat tissues. The authors studied also the effect of time of contact, concentration, pH and temperature on the histamine-releasing property of the antihistamines. Having observed that the effects of the antihistamines on the mast cells and tissue histamine increased with concentration, pH and temperature, and that the effects of these drugs were potentiated, in guinea-pig tissues by pre-treatment with metabolic inhibitors like those of octylamine and compound 48—80, the authors concluded that the antihistamines behave as typical histamine liberators. More recently we have observed that some tranquilizers such as promazine, are also very efficient mast cell destroyers. Indeed, this property is shared by many other phenothiazine derivatives (MOTA, unpublished). In their paper, MOTA and DIAS DA SILVA (1960a) have suggested that the histamine releasing effect of the antihistamines could be explained if one admits that these drugs compete with histamine, not only at its site of action, the histamine receptor, but also at its site of storage in the cell. However, no experimental evidence of this has yet been produced.

E. By anaphylatoxin

In 1951, ROCHA E SILVA, BIER and ARONSON showed that anaphylatoxin releases large quantities of histamine when perfused through the isolated guinea-pig lung. This finding presented an explanation for the anaphylactoid picture produced when guinea-pigs were injected with anaphylatoxin; a fact observed many years ago by FRIEDBERGER (1910). Since then, the old theory of the participation of anaphylatoxin as a mediator in the mechanism of anaphylaxis has been very much discussed and it has been questioned whether anaphylatoxin releases histamine from the same site as does antigen in anaphylaxis. The observation that the histamine released in anaphylaxis comes from the mast cells (MOTA, 1953; MOTA and VUGMAN, 1956a; MOTA, 1957, 1958a, b, 1959a; HUMPHREY and MOTA, 1959a, b) led MOTA (1959c) to find out whether anaphylatoxin causes also damage to mast cells. In my first experiments (MOTA, 1957), anaphylatoxin was tried on rat mast cells, since we had previously observed that these cells were disrupted when sensitized rat tissues contacted antigen. However, anaphylatoxin either injected intravenously into the intact rat or incubated *in vitro* with rat tissues did not produce any mast cell damage or histamine release, although under the same conditions, the same anaphylatoxin preparation induces conspicuous damage to guinea-pig mast cells. RILEY (1953a) in an attempt to relate mast cells and anaphylaxis, injected anaphylatoxin intravenously into rats and despite the minimal clinical evidence of shock, he found that the appearances in the peritoneal spreads closely resembled those seen after the use of histamine liberators. Thus, many of the mesenteric mast cells were swollen and in process of vacuolation or degranulation. However, I have not been able to confirm RILEY's findings and even when 10 ml of rat serum anaphylatoxin, very active on the guinea-pig ileum, were injected into the peritoneal cavity of rats and the animals sacrificed one hour later, no damage to the mast cells could be observed in the mesentery. Therefore, as the guinea-pig is the only species in which anaphylatoxin releases histamine and causes an anaphylactoid shock (ROCHA E SILVA, 1955), this animal was chosen as a suitable species to study the effect of anaphyltoxin on the mast cells. Since antigen causes histamine release and mast cell damage in sensitized guinea-pig mesentery (MOTA, 1958a, 1959c), and we had previously observed that anaphylatoxin caused damage to mesenteric guinea-pig mast cells (MOTA, 1957), this tissue was used to study the effect of anaphylatoxin on the mast cells.

Anaphylatoxin was prepared by incubating rat serum or heparinized plasma with agar (1 mg/ml) at 37° C for 30 min after which the agar was removed by centrifugation and the supernatant dialyzed against cold saline for 24 hours. The activity of this preparation was tested on the isolated guinea-pig ileum and the activated serum or plasma kept at 4° C until use. Pieces of guinea-pig mesentery were then incubated with anaphylatoxin or with non-activated rat serum for 15 min at

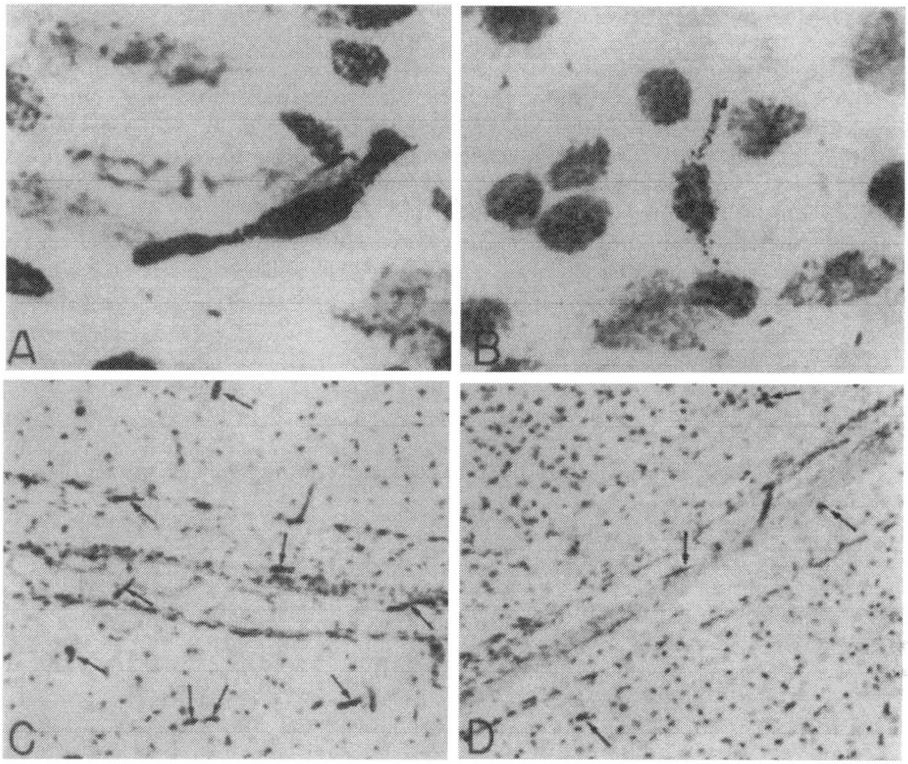

Fig. 6. Photomicrographs of whole-mount guinea pig mesentery after fixation in lead subacetate-ethanol-acetic acid and staining in toluidine blue. (A) Mast cell in guinea pig mesentery incubated in Tyrode solution. Observe cell crowded with granules. × 1000. (B) Mast cell in guinea pig mesentery incubated with anaphylatoxin. Observe that the cell has lost most of its granules. × 1000. (C) Mast cells in mesentery incubated in Tyrode solution. Observe several mast cells (arrows), some of them following the vessels. × 250. (D) Mast cells in guinea pig mesentery incubated with anaphylatoxin. Observe reduction in mast cell number. × 250

37° C and transferred to fixative for mast cell observation. As can be seen in Fig. 6 these experiments showed that anaphylatoxin produces mast cell alterations which were very similar to that induced by antigen in guinea-pig anaphylaxis and quite different from that produced by octylamine or compound 48—80. These results suggested that the histamine released by antigen and anaphylatoxin had at least one common origin, the mast cell. Furthermore, when the several agents known to inhibit mast cell damage by antigen (Mota, 1958a, 1959a) were tried to see whether they would inhibit mast cell damage by anaphylatoxin, it was observed that there were points of similarity and discrepancy. Thus, when iodoacetate (0.001 M), p-chloromercuribenzoate (0.001 M) or phenol (0.01 M) were left in contact with pieces of mesentery at 37° C for 15 min before the addition of anaphylatoxin, the destruction of mast cells by anaphylatoxin was greatly reduced. Since these substances are known to inhibit the mast cell degranulation induced by antigen on one hand and to potentiate the mast cell damage produced by histamine-liberators on the other hand, it was concluded that the histamine-releasing mechanism of anaphylatoxin is nearer to that of antigen in anaphylaxis than to that of the histamine-liberators. Actually the fact that iodoacetate and p-chloromercuribenzoate inhibited mast cell destruction by anaphylatoxin, agrees with previous results of ROTHSCHILD and ROCHA E SILVA (1956) showing that these substances inhibit histamine release by anaphylatoxin and with results of MOUSSATCHÉ and DANON (1956) who showed that sulphydryl blocking agents inhibit the response of the guinea-pig ileum to anaphylaxis and anaphylatoxin. Furthermore it was observed that cold (15° C) and phenol also abolished the mast cell damage induced by anaphylatoxin, and that a previous contact of the mesentery with anaphylatoxin in the cold, almost completely abolished the mast cell damage when the same piece of mesentery was later incubated with anaphylatoxin at 37° C. Since phenol is known to inhibit the mast cell damage induced by antigen without inhibiting desensitization (MOTA, 1959a), experiments were done to test whether phenol would also inhibit mast cell degranulation by anaphylatoxin without preventing desensitization to a further dose of anaphylatoxin. Thus, pieces of mesentery were incubated for 15 min with phenol (0.01 M) in Tyrode solution. Phenol was then removed, the mesentery washed in Tyrode solution and transferred to anaphylatoxin. In other experiments, anaphylatoxin was added to mesentery in the presence of phenol, after 15 min the mesentery was washed in Tyrode containing phenol to remove anaphylatoxin, then in Tyrode solution to remove phenol, and finally a second dose of anaphylatoxin was added. The results of these experiments were as follows: a) Prior contact of mesentery with phenol did not prevent mast cell degranulation on subsequent incubation with anaphylatoxin; b) when a first dose of anaphylatoxin was added in the presence of phenol and a second dose in the absence of phenol, there was no reduction in mast cell number. This showed that contact of the tissue with anaphylatoxin in the presence of phenol inhibited mast cell degranulation without inhibiting desensitization and suggested that anaphylatoxin acts indirectly by activating some transient intermediate substance, which may be an enzyme.

On the other hand, when lack of calcium and previous heating of the tissue at 45° C, which inhibit the antigen-induced mast cell damage, were tested in experiments with anaphylatoxin, it was observed that both these treatments did not prevent mast cell damage by anaphylatoxin. However, these discrepancies were considered to be more apparent than real. Indeed, the failure of calcium to prevent mast cell damage by anaphylatoxin agreed with previous experiments by ROCHA E SILVA (1954) showing that calcium, although necessary for anaphylatoxin formation, is not necessary for anaphylatoxin action. Therefore, anaphylatoxin formation could be secondary to antigen-antibody combination and a factor in the production of the anaphylactic reaction, and yet absence of calcium could inhibit histamine release and mast cell destruction by antigen. As regards the effect of heating at 45° C, it seems reasonable to suppose that such treatment might not prevent the action of preformed anaphylatoxin, and yet destroy some factor necessary for the sequence of events leading to the formation of anaphylatoxin in anaphylaxis. However, it must be pointed out here that although these findings, as a whole, indicate that anaphylatoxin shares with antigen part of the pathway leading to histamine release, they do not prove that anaphylatoxin is implicated in the histamine releasing mechanism of anaphylaxis. Indeed, the fact that a piece of ileum can be completely desensitized to anaphylatoxin and still present a maximal anaphylactic response (GREISMAN, 1958; MOTA, 1959c) suggests that anaphylatoxin probably is not implicated in the anaphylactic release of histamine.

III. The anaphylactic release of histamine from the mast cells

The first reference to mast cell damage in anaphylaxis is that of JAQUES and WATERS (1941) who in their paper on the origin of the anticoagulant of anaphylactic shock in the dog, stated they had been able to confirm the mast cell alterations described by WILANDER (1938) in peptone shock and extended them to anaphylactic shock. However, no description of the mast cell alterations as induced by antigen was presented by the authors. Later, STUART (1952) in a communication to the American Association of Anatomists, reported the response to anaphylaxis of rabbit, guinea-pig, dog and mouse mast cells using hen's egg albumin as antigen. He observed that the mast cells showed great response to anaphylaxis, reflected mostly in rupture and disappearance of cells and extra-cellular dispersion of granules. He stated to believe that a correlation exists between mast cell number, distribution and response to anaphylaxis, and the reactivity of susceptible tissues in various species. Unfortunately, the author did not refer to the way he used to sensitize the animals, what fixative he used and described the mast cell damage conjointly without discriminating the various species studied. Some authors have quoted KELLER's paper (1957) as if it were on anaphylaxis without note that there is no anaphylaxis in this paper but in the title. The same is true of WEGELIUS, HJELMMAN and WASASTJERNA's paper (1955) which also does not concern anaphylaxis. Both these papers are concerned with the effect on the mast cells of an anti-connective tissue rabbit antiserum. The effect of a specific rabbit antiserum prepared with isolated rat mast cells on these cells was recently studied by SMITH (1959) and SMITH and LEWIS (1961). Interesting as these papers are, they do not concern anaphylaxis.

Our own interest on the behavior of mast cells in anaphylaxis arose from the old observation that heparin released by peptone is originated from the mast cells (WILANDER, 1938) and from my own observations in collaboration with BERALDO and JUNQUEIRA (MOTA, 1953; MOTA, BERALDO and JUNQUEIRA, 1953) showing that most of the substances known to release histamine, cause damage to the mast cells. Indeed, in my first experiments on rat anaphylaxis, definite mast cell damage induced by antigen was observed (MOTA, 1953). Thus, it seemed rather reasonable to expect that the histamine released by antigen in anaphylaxis could also be originated from the mast cells. However, as logical as this could be, and in spite of the observations of mast cell damage in anaphylaxis already reported, the fact that the histamine released by antigen in anaphylaxis is originated from the mast cell was not easily accepted by everybody, these cells being considered as a source only for the histamine released by the chemical histamine liberators. This would imply, for instance, that while the histamine released from dog liver by peptone or from rat skin by compound 48—80 would be originated from the mast cells, the histamine released by antigen from these same organs would not be originated from the mast cells. Presently, due to the many experimental data so far produced there is little room for doubt that most – although certainly not all – of the histamine released by antigen from sensitized tissues, comes from the mast cells in most of the species. Of course, we known that in rabbits most of the histamine released from blood by antigen does not come from the mast cells but very probably from the platelets (HUMPHREY and JAQUES, 1954, 1955). However, even in this species, it is possible that the histamine released by antigen from other tissues, as it was shown to occur by SCHACHTER (1953), might come from the mast cells.

Due to the fact that each species has its own peculiarities, the release of histamine from mast cells in anaphylaxis will be considered separately in each species.

A. In guinea-pig anaphylaxis

The first description of mast cell damage induced by antigen in guinea-pig anaphylaxis was that by VUGMAN and myself working with actively sensitized intact guinea-pigs (MOTA and VUGMAN, 1956a, b). This finding was later extended to isolated tissues taken either from actively or passively sensitized guinea-pigs (MOTA, 1958a, 1959a; HUMPHREY and MOTA, 1959a, b). Recently, the antigen-induced mast cell damage in sensitized guinea-pig tissues has been confirmed by BOREUS (1960b, c) and BOREUS and CHAKRAVARTY (1960a, b) and related to the anaphylactic formation of slow reacting substance which, according to these authors, is also originated from the mast cells.

1. Correlation between histamine and mast cells in guinea-pig lung

The fact that the guinea-pig is very sensitive to anaphylaxis and that most of the classical work on the anaphylactic release of histamine has been performed in this species, prompted us to study the behavior of the mast cell in the anaphylactic reaction in this species. However, as a search in the literature available at that time showed no data on the relationship between mast cells and histamine in guinea-pig tissues, it was decided to find out whether the histamine content and the mast cell population of the guinea-pig lung were correlated. As a preliminary step, experiments were performed to investigate whether the mast cell population as well as the histamine content of each lobe of a symmetrical pair of pulmonary lobes were similar. Thus, the inferior pulmonary pair of lobes were excised and either fixed for mast cell count or cut into HCl and boiled for histamine extraction and assay. The pulmonary lobes were fixed by injecting the fixative through a bronchial branch. Fixation was allowed to proceed overnight and frozen sections 50 μ thick were stained by acidified toluidine blue. The number of mast cells was

Table 6. *Mast cell number*[1] *in guinea-pig inferior pulmonary lobes*

Right	Left
81	89
68	76
56	41
151	162
162	173
33	31
75	86
88	98
101	87
82	84
35	39

[1] The *cells* were counted under a magnification of 250 ×. Each figure is mean of 100 fields. Difference between the means of the two lobes nonsignificant ($P > 0.05$).

Table 7. *Histamine content* ($\mu g/g$) *in guinea-pig inferior pulmonary lobes*

Right	Left
20	18
33	37
30	28
17	19
39	37
28	28
30	35
95	93
21	21
26	20
19	20

Difference between the means of the two lobes nonsignificant ($P > 0.05$).

determined in one hundred randomly chosen 0.1364 mm^2 areas with the aid of a square ruled ocular micrometer, the magnification being 250 x, while histamine was assayed on the guinea-pig ileum and expressed as $\mu g/g$ of tissues. As it is shown in Tables 6 and 7, the histamine content and the mast cell population of symmetrical guinea-pig pulmonary lobes were found to be closely related. This established, the correlation between the mast cell population and the histamine content of the guinea-pig lung was investigated by taking from each pair of inferior pulmonary lobe, one lobe for histamine extraction and the other one for mast cell count. The values so obtained were statistically analyzed and a high positive correlation between mast cells and histamine was found (r 0.90). Furthermore, the values were plotted on a graph and a line of regression obtained. As it is shown in Fig. 7, there is a close correlation between the mast cell population and the histamine content of the guinea-pig lung. Similar finding was reported by Boreus and Chakravarty (1960a) who extended it to other guinea-pig tissues and calculated the average histamine content in each mast cell, from the histamine value and mast cell count per g of tissue. The weight of the counted sections was estimated from their area, thickness and specific gravity. From these data, four different guinea-pig tissues showed 21 to 34 $\mu\mu$g histamine base per mast cell, these values being of about the same order as those obtained by Graham, Lowry, Wahl and Priebat (1955) in the parenchyma and capsule of beef liver.

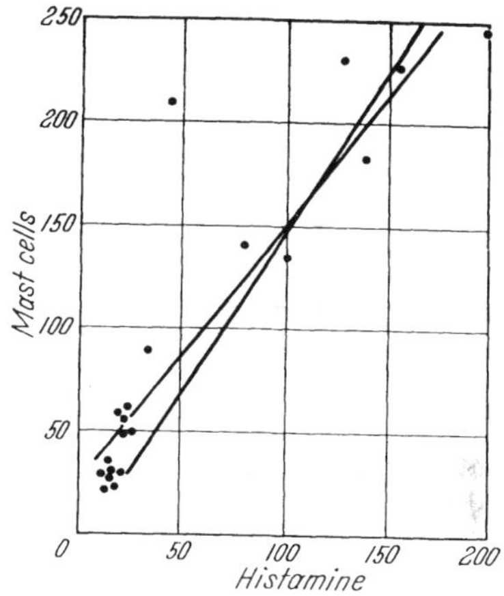

Fig. 7. Correlation between mast cells and histamine in the guinea-pig lung

2. Antigen-induced mast cell damage and histamine release in the intact guinea-pig

The effect of antigen on the mast cell population and the histamine content of the guinea-pig lung was then investigated. The animals were sensitized by injecting 100 mg of egg albumin intraperitoneally and 100 mg subcutaneously and were used after 3 weeks of the sensitization. In the first experiments, 2 groups of sensitized guinea-pigs were injected with either egg albumin or histamine. The histamine-injected group was used to obtain control lungs in conditions similar to those found in the animals dying in acute anaphylaxis. Mast cells were then counted in frozen lung sections obtained from both groups and a significantly smaller number of these cells was found in the animals submitted to anaphylaxis (Mota and Vugman, 1956a). Later on, these experiments were duplicated by making biopsies of the lung before and after the injection of antigen into sensitized guinea-pigs (Mota and Vugman, 1956b). The animals were anaesthetized and a cannula was tied into the trachea and connected to a respiration pump. The thorax was opened and the left or right inferior pulmonary lobe was ligated and excised, after which antigen (1 mg egg albumin in 0.5 ml sodium chloride) was injected directly into the right ventricle. A few seconds after the injection of antigen, the lungs were immobilized in inspiration, although the heart continued beating. Three to 5 min later, the remaining opposite lobe was ligated and excised. The extirpated lobes were either extracted with HCl for histamine assay or fixed for mast cell observation. The results of these experiments showed that anaphylaxis produced a significant reduction in the number of mast cells and in the histamine content of the lung (see Tables 8 and 9). The diminution in the number of recognizable mast cells seemed to be due chiefly to loss of granules from the cells located in the walls of the alveoli (see Fig. 8). The antigen-induced mast cell alterations were characterized by a disappearance of the mast cell granules (degranulation) without any morphological evidence of their fate. No granules were found outside the cells and those remaining inside the cells kept their usual aspect. Indeed, we have never observed any other visible guinea-pig mast cell damage by antigen but degranulation. Diminution in the number of these cells was clearly due to total loss of their granular content.

Table 8. *Mast cell number*[1] *in guinea-pig inferior pulmonary lobes before and after anaphylaxis*

G.P.	Before	After	G.P.	Before	After
1	162	87	12	249	152
2	114	96	13	91	77
3	139	98	14	137	55
4	103	92	15	75	94
5	234	225	16	84	83
6	115	62	17	75	73
7	169	159	18	197	68
8	92	73	19	191	110
9	115	91	20	88	73
10	93	68	21	171	127
11	90	84	22	55	31

[1] The cells were counted under a magnification of 250 ×. Each figure is mean of 100 fields. Difference between the means of the two lobes highly significant ($P < 0.01$).

Table 9. *Histamine content (μg/g) in guinea-pig inferior pulmonary lobes before and after anaphylaxis*

Before	After
20	9
28	12
11	9
32	15
21	11
19	17
26	20
29	25
32	17
28	18
40	21
15	15
36	25

Difference between the means of the two lobes highly significant ($P < 0.01$).

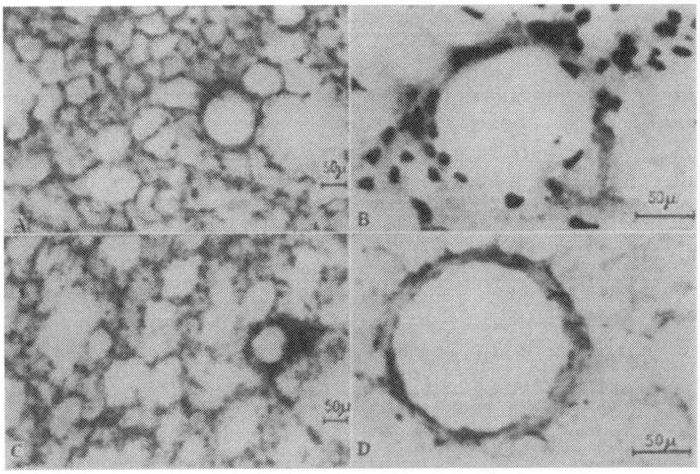

Fig. 8. Frozen sections from guinea pig lung after lead subacetate-ethanol-acetic acid fixation, stained with toluidine blue (pH about 4). (*A*) and (*B*). Lung from sensitized animal injected with histamine (group II); numerous mast cells in the walls of alveoli and around bronchioles. (*C*) and (*D*). Lung after anaphylactic shock (group I); note reduction in the number of mast cells

3. Antigen-induced mast cell damage and histamine release in isolated tissues

The above mentioned experiments, however, were carried out in the intact guinea-pig and the occurrence of oedema during anaphylaxis couid have accounted for the reduction in the mast cell population and in the histamine content of the lung. Thus, it was decided to carry out corresponding experiments with isolated tissues *in vitro*, under conditions in which oedema formation could be excluded. The behavior of mast cells in the anaphylactic release of histamine induced by antigen from isolated sensitized guinea-pig lung was then studied using the technique developed by MONGAR and SCHILD (1953). Lung tissue was chopped with a McIlwain tissue chopper (MCILWAIN and BUDDLE, 1953) into rods of 0.8 × 0.8 mm cross-section. A series of uniform samples of equal volume (0.2 ml) were prepared and incubated in 10 ml beakers at 37° C for 15 min with Tyrode solution or Tyrode solution containing 1 mg/ml egg albumin. After incubation the samples were used either for histamine extraction or for mast cell observation. For microscopical observation and counts of the mast cells, the chopped lung tissue was fixed, cut and stained as in the preceeding *in vivo* experiments. As can be seen in Fig. 9, antigen induced a diminution in both mast cell population and histamine content of the chopped lung tissue and there is a correlation between histamine release and mast cell reduction. Thus, in 5 experiments in which a substantial histamine release occurred, there was also a substantial reduction in the mast cell number; whereas in the 3 experiments in which histamine release was less than 30%, there was only a small decrease in mast cell number although many mast cells were degranulated. This experiment was then duplicated by taking pieces of mesentery from guinea-pigs sensitized to different antigens and incubating the pieces at 37° C for 15 min in Tyrode solution containing the specific antigen. The results of these experiments showed that incubation of sensitized mesenteries with the corresponding antigen resulted in each case in alterations of the mast cells represented by partial or total loss of granules with a consequent reduction in the numbers of cells containing metachromatic granules. Under similar conditions, mesenteries taken from control unsensitized animals showed no alteration. As can be seen in Table 10, there was a large variation in mast cell response to antigen, the reduction in the number of these cells varying from a 75% decrease to none at all. However, even when there was no overall reduction in their number, typical degranulation of mast cells was always present. In fact, it was always possible to recognize intermediate steps of the degranulation process represented by cells which had lost either a small part of their granular content, or about half of their granules or other cells which had lost almost all their granular content and could be recognized only by containing a few remaining

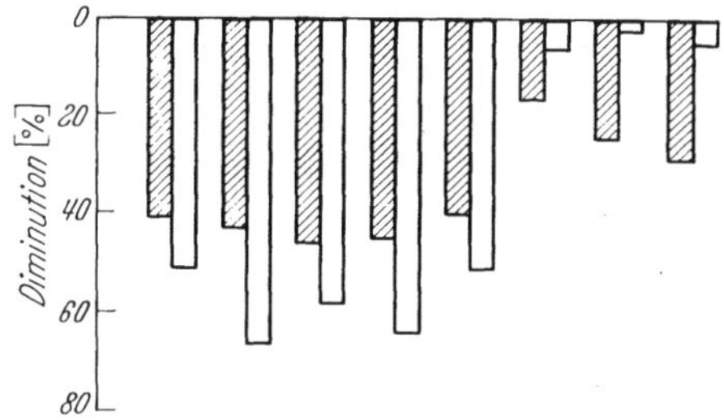

Fig. 9. Diminution of histamine content (▨) and mast cell number (□) of chopped sensitized guinea-pig lung in anaphylaxis

Table 10. *Reduction in mast cell number*[1] *in guinea-pig mesentery incubated at 37° C for 15 min with antigen*

Guinea-pig	Sensitized to	N° of mast cells in		% Reduction
		Tyrode	Antigen	
1	Ovalbumin	30	25	16
2	Ovalbumin	18	6	66
3	Ovalbumin	26	16	38
4	Human serum albumin	30	26	16
5	Human serum albumin	17	7	59
6	Human serum albumin	28	28	0
7	Bovine serum albumin	20	5	75
8	Bovine serum albumin	35	20	45
9	Bovine serum albumin	19	15	21
10	Horse serum	30	14	52
11	Horse serum	22	11	50
12	Horse serum	28	20	28

[1] Means of thirty microscopical fields at a magnification of 80 ×.

metachromatic granules in their cytoplasm. These partially degranulated mast cells were more easily observed in tissues that had contacted antigen for a few seconds or in tissues in which antigen had induced only a small or no reduction in the number of these cells (MOTA, 1958a, 1959a).

4. Mast cell response to increased concentrations of antigen

Experiments were then performed to see whether the reduction in mast cell number induced by antigen would increase with the concentration of antigen. Thus, pieces of sensitized mesentery were incubated with different concentrations of antigen for 15 min at 37° C and afterwards fixed. These experiments showed that antigen produces mast cell damage in very low concentration of the order of 10^{-6}, and that the decrease in mast cell number is related to the concentration of antigen (MOTA, 1958a, 1959a).

5. Mast cell response to time of contact with antigen

To see the effect of time of contact with antigen on the mast cell damage, pieces of sensitized mesentery were incubated with antigen for periods of 15 sec up to 15 min. A significant decrease (50—70%) in mast cell number was detected as early as one minute after incubation and degranulation was seen to occur after 15 sec. To test whether histamine release would also occur within 15 sec, pieces of mesentery were incubated for 15 sec in 1 ml of Tyrode solution and afterwards transferred to 1 ml of a 0.1% solution of antigen in Tyrode for the same period. Both control and antigen solutions in which the mesentery had been incubated were then tested for histamine content. In each of 7 experiments a detectable amount of histamine was released after 15 sec contact of the tissue with antigen. The very short time in which detectable morphological alterations of mast cell and histamine release can be produced in the mesentery is possibly explained by the thinness of this tissue and the high velocity of the antigen-antibody reaction (MOTA, 1958a, 1959a).

6. Effect of low temperature on mast cell damage by antigen

To test the effect of low temperature, pieces of sensitized mesentery were incubated with antigen at 15° C; some of the pieces were then immediately transferred to fixative and others to antigen solution at 37° C, kept there for 15 min and fixed afterwards. Microscopical observation of the mesentery showed that mast cell degranulation was absent in the pieces of mesentery that had been fixed immediately after contact with antigen at 15° C, but present in those that were fixed after warming to 37° C. However, the diminution in mast cell number in the pieces of mesentery that had been in contact with antigen at 15° C and were subsequently brought to 37° C was smaller than in control pieces from the same mesentery in which antigen was added in the first instance at 37° C (MOTA, 1959a; HUMPHREY and MOTA, 1959a).

7. Mast cell response to antigen in sensitized tissues, stored in cold

It has been known for many years that sensitized tissues can be kept in cold Tyrode solution overnight and remain able to respond to antigen with an anaphylactic contraction. In order to observe the behavior of mast cells in guinea-pig tissues under these condition, samples of mesentery taken from the same guinea-pig were either immediately incubated with antigen or kept in Tyrode solution at 4° C for 24 hours and then incubated with antigen. Although the number and morphology of the mast cells were not affected by keeping the tissue in the cold, the response to antigen was smaller in the samples kept in the cold than in those incubated immediately with antigen. For instance, in a typical experiment, the reduction in mast cell number in the samples placed in contact with antigen immediately after removal from the animal was 61% while in another sample kept in the cold overnight the reduction was only 18%. Actually, in experiments in which samples of mesentery taken from guinea-pig passively sensitized with ^{131}I-labelled antibodies were kept overnight in the cold, it was observed that 90% of the antibodies originally fixed in the tissue were lost during this time. However, the 10% left were enough to produce mast cell degranulation by antigen. These experiments showed that the mast cells are well preserved when tissues are kept overnight in cold Tyrode solution and that these cells are still able to react with antigen in these conditions (HUMPHREY and MOTA, 1959a).

8. Guinea-pig mast cell damage compared with mast cell damage by chemical histamine liberators

Contrasting with rat mast cells that respond to antigen or to chemical histamine liberators in a very similar way (MOTA, 1953, 1957), guinea-pig mast cells respond to antigen and to chemical histamine releasers in a way that is quite different (MOTA, 1958a, 1959a). Thus when pieces of guinea-pig lung or mesentery are incubated with octylamine or compound 48—80 in Tyrode solution at 37°C damage to the mast cells occurs, as is shown by reduction in the number of these cells. As with antigen in anaphylaxis, this reduction is proportional to the concentration of the substance. Therefore, both antigen and octylamine produce conspicuous alterations of the same cell. However, cytologically the alterations induced by octylamine or compound 48—80 are different from those induced by antigen. The first visible change induced by octylamine or compound 48—80 is an apparent loss of the granule limit, as if a diffusion of the metachromatic material from the granules had taken place. When this phenomenon progresses, the cell looks like a metachromatic blot in which some basophilic granules can sometimes be noticed. In the final stages, these metachromatic blots present an irregular contour and a faint metachromasia and the cell is apparently in a state of dissolution. Thus, while the antigen-induced mast cell damage in the guinea-pig is characterized by a total or partial loss of granules without fusion of the metachromatic material, the octylamine-induced mast cell alterations are characterized by an apparent fusion of the metachromatic material without any loss of granules. This morphological difference was thought to reflect a difference in the mechanism of action of these agents on the mast cell, although both produce histamine release. Indeed, this agreed with the conclusion by MONGAR and SCHILD (1957a, b) that in the guinea-pig the histamine-releasing mechanism of the antigen-antibody reaction is different from that of chemical histamine releasers as well as with the fact that sodium iodoacetate, phenol, lack of calcium or heating to 45° C, although producing a partial or total inhibition of mast cell damage by antigen, do not block the mast cell destruction by octylamine or compound 48—80 (MOTA, 1958a, 1959a).

9. Passive sensitization of the mast cell

Since isolated tissues can be sensitized by incubation with antibodies *in vitro* (DALE, 1913) it seemed likely that mast cells could also be sensitized in this way. To test this possibility, guinea-pig mesentery was incubated for half an hour with rabbit anti-ovalbumin serum, washed in Tyrode solution and then incubated with antigen. Under these conditions similar alterations of mast cells were produced as in mesentery of actively sensitized guinea-pigs. Similar experiments were done with guinea-pig uterus and ileum. Two horns of the uterus or two segments of the ileum were used. One piece of each organ was incubated for half an hour with rabbit anti-ovalbumin serum diluted at a ratio of 1 : 5 with Tyrode solution and the other was used as a control and incubated in plain Tyrode solution and 15 min later the antigen (ovalbumin 1 mg/ml) was added. Only the organs which had been incubated with the antiserum showed an anaphylactic contraction whereas the

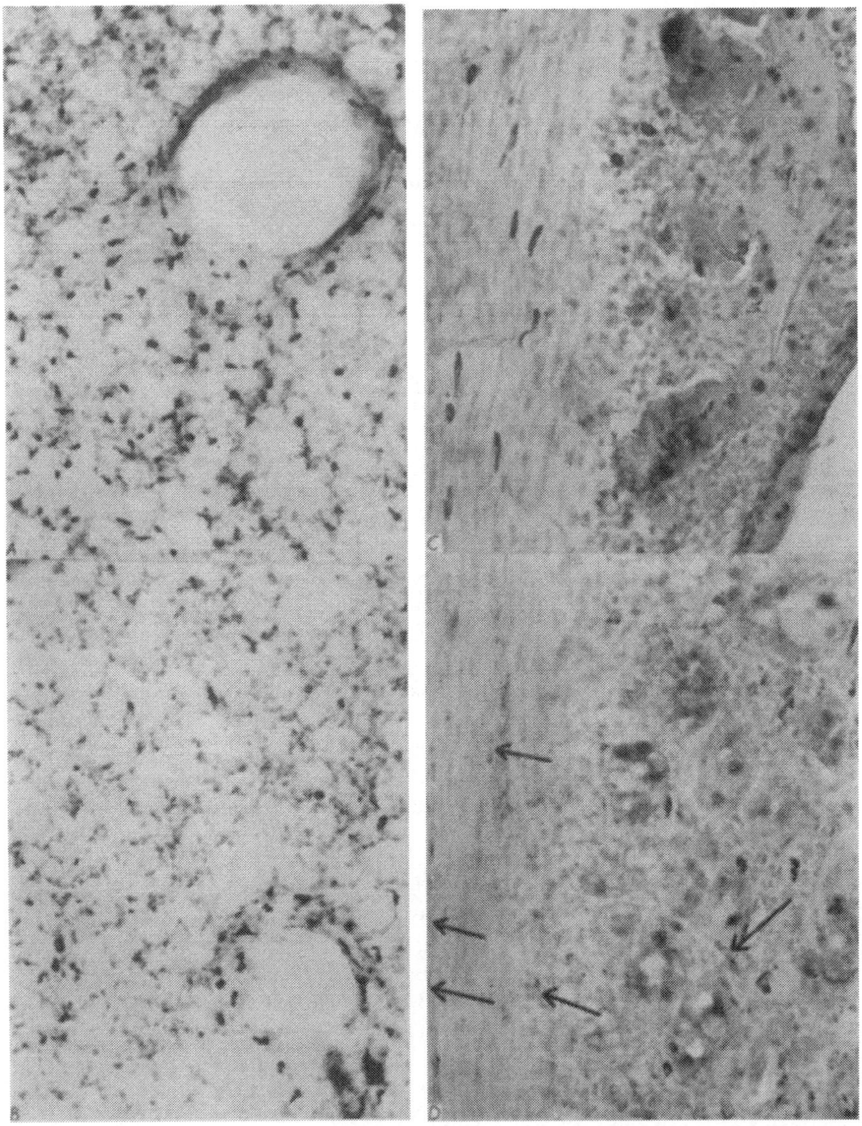

Fig. 10. *A*. Mast cells in sensitized guinea-pig lung incubated with Tyrode solution, approx. × 110. Note numerous mast cells distributed through the pulmonary tissue and concentrated around the bronchioles. *B*. Mast cells in sensitized guinea-pig lung after contact with ovalbumin, approx. × 110. Note diminution in mast cell number. *C*. Mast cells in non-sensitized guinea-pig ileum after contact with ovalbumin, approx. × 160. Note mast cells crowded with granules in the mucosa and muscular layer. *D*. Mast cells in sensitized guinea-pig ileum after contact with ovalbumin, approx. × 160. Note degranulated mast cells in the mucosa and in the muscle layer

controls gave no reaction. After 30 min of contact with antigen, the pieces were removed and fixed. The mesentery was fixed by immersion while the uterus and ileum were fixed by injecting the fixative under pressure into the lumen. These organs were then ligated at both ends and immersed in the fixative for 20—24 hours. Frozen section 50 μ thick were then stained with toluidine blue and examined. Both sensitized uterus and ileum showed typical degranulation of the mast cells present in the mucosa and amongst the muscle fibres, while the control pieces showed no visible mast cell damage. Degranulation of mast cells in the ileum can be seen in Fig. 10 (MOTA, 1958a, 1959a).

10. Effect of different amounts of antibodies on mast cell damage

It seemed likely that the large variation in the mast cell response observed in actively sensitized guinea-pigs was due to the well-recognized individual variations in antibody response. Passive sensitization was therefore used, in order to test whether the effect of antigen on mast cells would be correlated with the amount of antibody injected. Thus, three groups of guinea-pigs were passively sensitized by injecting them with different amounts of rabbit anti-ovalbumin, namely 0.008 mg, 0.3 mg and 3.0 mg antibody/100 g body weight. The animals were killed 48 hours later, the mesenteries dissected and incubated as already described and the number of mast cells determined. As can be seen in Fig. 11, the results of this experiment showed that in passively sensitized guinea-pigs, the mast cell response to antigen was rather uniform and graded with the dose of antibody below a certain level, suggesting that the large variation observed in actively sensitized animals was due to variation in the relatively small amounts of antibodies produced by them (HUMPHREY and MOTA, 1959a).

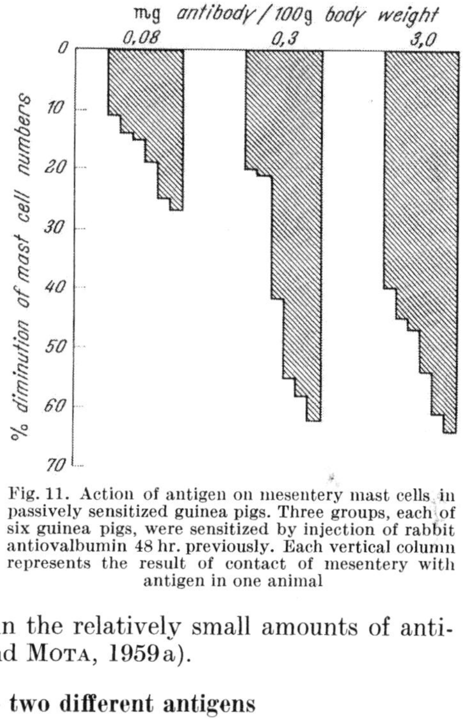

Fig. 11. Action of antigen on mesentery mast cells in passively sensitized guinea pigs. Three groups, each of six guinea pigs, were sensitized by injection of rabbit antiovalbumin 48 hr. previously. Each vertical column represents the result of contact of mesentery with antigen in one animal

11. Mast cell response to two different antigens

It was shown by DALE (1913) that guinea-pig tissues could be sensitized to more than one antigen and that desensitization to one antigen does not result in desensitization to the other. Thus, if anaphylactic response of the tissue were due to mast cells, these cells should still be able to respond to a second antigen after having been in contact with a first one. To test this, guinea-pigs were injected with a rabbit anti-serum containing 5 mg antibodies to ovalbumin and 3 mg antibodies to SSSIII. Forty-eight hours afterwards, the animals were killed and samples of mesentery were examined after the following treatment: incubation with ovalbumin alone; incubation with ovalbumin followed by SSSIII; incubation with SSSIII alone; incubation with SSSIII and ovalbumin simultaneously. After incubation, all samples were fixed and mast cell counts made. The results of these experiments are summarized in Fig. 12. As can be seen there, incubation with a second antigen resulted in a further decrease in the number of mast cells but some cells remained apparently intact. It can also be observed that incubation with two antigens at the same time was not more effective than the most effective of the antigens alone, and that even after consecutive applications of the two different antigens some of the mast cells remained intact. This experiment suggested that the multiple anaphylactic response of tissues may be explained in terms of cumulative mast cell damage (HUMPHREY and MOTA, 1959a).

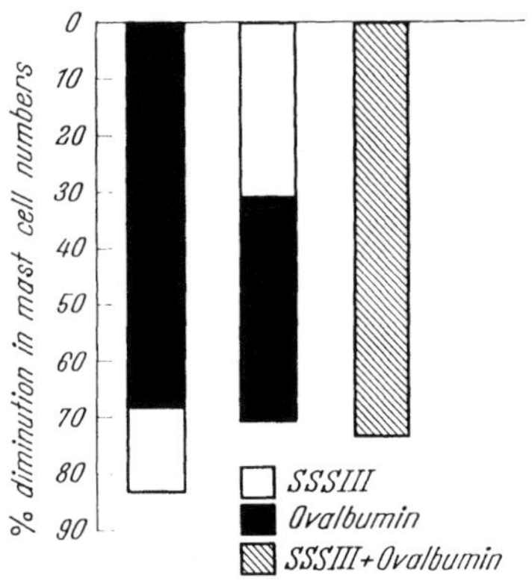

Fig. 12. Effect on mast cells of adding different antigens successively or simultaneously. Guinea pigs were sensitized with anti-ovalbumin and anti-SSSIII. Portions of mesentery were examined after contact with each antigen alone, or with each successively, or with both together □ SSSIII ■ Ovalbumin ▨ SSSIII + Ovalbumin

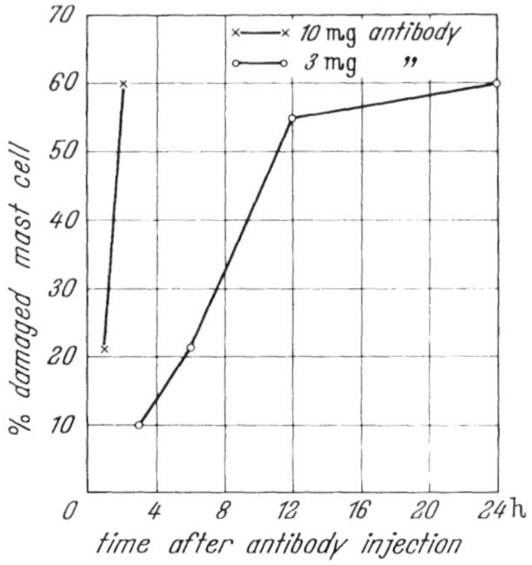

Fig. 13. Development of susceptibility of mesentery mast cells to antigen. Groups of guinea pigs received 3 or 10 mg anti-ovalbumin intravenously, and the susceptibility of mesentery mast cells to contact with antigen was measured after various intervals of time. ×——× 10 mg antibody, ○——○ 3 mg antibody

12. Latent period for the production of mast cell damage

It is an old observation that in passive sensitization, unless very large amounts of antibodies are used (and in this case formation of antigen-antibody complexes might be implicated) some time must elapse before a typical anaphylactic shock can be obtained on intravenous injection of antigen (BENACERRAF and KABAT, 1949). Thus we investigated whether a similar latent period would also be necessary for the production of mast cell damage (HUMPHREY and MOTA, 1959a). Two groups of eight guinea-pigs were injected intravenously with rabbit anti-ovalbumin, one group receiving 3 mg and the other 10 mg antibody per animal. Afterwards, the guinea-pigs were killed at different time intervals. The mesenteries were dissected out, incubated immediately with antigen and fixed and stained for microscopical observation of the mast cells. The number of degranulated mast cells was counted and calculated as a percentage of the total (200 cells being counted). As may be seen in Fig. 13, before any mast cell degranulation was elicited, there was a latent period which was shorter in the group injected with the larger amount of antibodies. The percentage of degranulated mast cells after two hours was not determined in the group receiving the larger amount of antibodies because by then the reduction in the total number of mast cells was so great as to make the count very difficult. Perhaps not surprisingly, the earliest observable degranulated mast cells were located along the capillary walls. This phenomenon was most evident in the group injected with the smaller amount of antibodies. These results are in agreement with the previous observations of BENACERRAF and KABAT (1949) showing that a latent period is necessary for the production of passive anaphylaxis in the guinea-pig and that such latent period is inversely proportional to the dose of antibodies. Probably this time is necessary for the antibodies to leave the blood stream and to become in some way attached to the mast cell membrane. This is also supported by the observation that the first mast cells to show degranulation *in vitro* (in response to antigen added externally) are those around the capillaries. Actually, SCHILD (1936) had already shown that the amount of histamine released by antigen from passively sensitized guinea-pig tissues increased with time during the first 48 hours after administration of the antiserum. The fact that it is possible to obtain a reaction similar to anaphylaxis without a latent period by using a large amount of antibodies does not necessarily invalidate these ideas if it is accepted that reaction of antigen with sufficient antibody free in the blood stream can activate some mechanism which is relatively inefficient compared with reaction between antigen and absorbed antibody, and, while producing the same symptoms would not be true anaphylaxis (HUMPHREY and MOTA, 1959a). Indeed it is probable that the anaphylactic picture obtained in this case is due to the formation of soluble antigen-antibody since GERMUTH and MCKINNON (1957) have shown that preformed soluble antigen-antibody complexes when injected into giunea-pigs produce an anaphylactic-like condition. However, that the underlying mechanism operating in this condition is not equal to that working in active or passive anaphylaxis after the latent period is suggested by the observation that antigen-antibody complexes do not duplicate the mast cell damage and histamine release occurring in anaphylaxis (MOTA, 1961).

13. Time required for passive sensitization of mast cells in vitro

The latent period is often interpreted as the time necessary for antibodies to pass from the circulation to the tissue spaces and for "fixation" of antibodies on or in the cells. Since *in vitro* antibody may be brought into immediate contact with the tissue surface and the mesentery is extremely thin, it might be expected that sensitization would occur with a shorter latent period than in the intact animal. To test this, pieces of sensitized mesentery were incubated at 37° C with rabbit antiserum containing 50 μg per ml of anti-ovalbumin and after 5, 10 and 15 min of incubation, one of the pieces of mesentery was taken out of the serum, rinsed briefly in Tyrode solution, incubated with the antigen and fixed for observation of the mast cell morphology. Microscopical observation of the mesentery showed that after 10 min incubation in the presence of this concentration of antibodies there was a 50% reduction in the total number of mast cells when the tissue was subsequently incubated with antigen. Even 5 min contact with antibody was enough to produce 26% of typical degranulated mast cells (HUMPHREY and MOTA, 1959a).

14. Effect of non-sensitizing antibodies

To test whether the mast cell damage induced by antigen in sensitized guinea-pig tissues could be due to the interaction of antibody with antigen in the tissues, without necessarily being related with the production of the complete picture of anaphylaxis, experiments were performed with antisera produced by species whose antibodies do not passively sensitize guinea-pig so as to produce anaphylaxis (horse, fowl, rat and goat antibody). In fact, mast cell damage due to interaction of antibody and its specific antigen in the tissues, but unrelated to anaphylaxis, might be expected to occur after passive transfer of antibodies from the above-mentioned species and subsequent contact of the tissue with antigen. However, when guinea-pigs were injected with fowl anti-rabbit γ-globulin (1—5 mg), goat anti-rabbit albumin (2—16 mg), rat anti-ovalbumin or anti-human serum albumin (1.5—7 mg), or horse anti-diphtheria toxoid (400—1600 i.u. antitoxin) neither anaphylactic shock, contraction of the isolated ileum nor mast cell damage occured on subsequent contact with the corresponding antigen. Thus, fowl, goat, horse and rat antibodies, which are ineffective in producing passive anaphylaxis in guinea-pigs do not sensitize the mast cells to antigen (Humphrey and Mota, 1959a).

15. Effect of reversed passive sensitization

It has been known for some time that when heterologous serum is injected into guinea-pigs, followed after an interval by the specific rabbit antiserum, typical anaphylaxis results, and this phenomenon is known as reversal passive anaphylaxis. However, this phenomenon occurs only when the antigen consists wholly or partly of γ-globulin, and experiments were performed to test whether mast cell damage would occur in reversed passive anaphylaxis induced by injecting γ-globulin or albumin as the antigen. Thus, each of one group of guinea-pig was injected intravenously with 10 mg of human serum albumin and each of another group with 10 mg of human γ-globulin. Forty-eight hours later, some animals from each group were injected intravenously with 5 mg of the corresponding antiserum. The result was typical anaphylaxis in all the guinea-pigs injected with human globulin, but in none of those receiving human albumin. The mesenteries of the remaining guinea-pigs in each group were dissected out and incubated with rabbit anti-human serum albumin or anti-human serum γ-globulin. Microscopical observation of the mesenteries showed that mast cell damage similar to that produced by antigen in sensitized tissues occurred only in the mesenteries of the animals injected with human γ-globulin and subsequently incubated with anti-human γ-globulin (Humphrey and Mota, 1959a).

16. Effect of antibodies against guinea-pig γ-globulin or guinea-pig albumin

The results of the previous experiments were compatible with the hypothesis that γ-globulin is normally reversibly adsorbed on to tissues, and that anaphylaxis results when the adsorbed γ-globulin is involved in an immunological reaction, irrespective of whether the adsorbed γ-globulin is acting as the antigen or as the antibody-provided that both the γ-globulins come from a suitable species. If this hypothesis is correct, injection of rabbit antibodies against guinea-pig γ-globulin should cause anaphylaxis, whereas rabbit antibodies against guinea-pig albumin should not. Normal guinea-pigs were accordingly injected with 0.5 ml of rabbit serum containing 1.8 mg/ml of antibodies against guinea-pig γ-globulin or 3 mg/ml of antibodies against guinea-pig albumin. Furthermore the activity of these antisera was also tested on the isolated ileum and on the mesenteric mast cells.The results of these experiments showed that only rabbit antibodies against guinea-pig γ-globulin shocked the animals, produced contraction of the isolated ileum and degranulation of the mast cells (Humphrey and Mota, 1959a). Similar damage to mouse mast cells was also obtained by using rabbit antibodies against mouse γ-globulin. These results have been more recently extended to rat mast cells by Austen and Humphrey (1961) and Keller (1962).

17. Effect of Forssman antibodies

It is known that injection of serum of rabbits immunized with sheep red cells into guinea-pigs produces death with symptoms resembling those of anaphylaxis (Friedberger, 1910). There are, however, differences between the typical symptoms of anaphylactic shock and those which occur after injection of Forssman antibodies. It was interesting, therefore, to test whether Forssman antibodies would cause mast cell degranulation similar to that observed in anaphylaxis. When 0.4 ml rabbit anti-Forssman antiserum was injected intravenously into 350 g guinea-pigs, they died within 2—3 min, and post-mortem examination revealed marked emphysema and even more marked oedema of the lungs. However, blood taken from heart just before death, contained no detectable histamine when tested immediately on the isolated guinea-pig ileum. Furthermore, incubation of guinea-pig mesentery with Forssman antibodies did not produce any mast cell damage (HUMPHREY and MOTA, 1959a). The implication of these results with the probable location of antibodies responsible for histamine release in anaphylaxis will be discussed later.

B. In rat anaphylaxis

The rat was the first species in which mast cell damage by antigen was unequivocally observed and described under specified conditions of sensitization (MOTA, 1953). Furthermore, as it had already been demonstrated to occur in other species, plasma histamine increase was observed to occur after injection of antigen into sensitized rats and release of histamine from the mast cells was observed when sensitized rat tissues contact antigen *in vitro* (MOTA, 1957, 1958b, 1959b; MOTA and ISHII, 1960; CHAKRAVARTY, 1959; GARCIA-AROCHA, 1961a). The anaphylactic release of histamine in *pertussis*-treated sensitized rats was recently confirmed and studied in detail by CODE and his colleagues (1961). It is known that rats are not easy to sensitize as compared to guinea-pigs, and present a large individual variation in their susceptibility to anaphylaxis. Thus, some special device has to be used to sensitize these animals in order to obtain a strong anaphylactic response when they are later challenged with antigen. Although this resistance to sensitization can be overcome by repeated injections of antigen (HALPERN, LIACOUPOULOS and CASTILLO, 1955), by using FREUND's adjuvant (LIPTON, STONE and FREUND, 1956) or alum-precipitated antigen (MOTA, 1957) it is our experience that these animals present a more uniform and high degree of sensitization when they are injected with *B. pertussis* organisms along with the sensitizing dose of antigen as first observed by MALKIEL and HARGIS (1952a). In fact, in anaphylaxis of pertussis-treated rats, mast cell damage and histamine release are easily detected, provided that adequate histological and pharmacological techniques are used.

1. Antigen-induced mast cell damage and histamine release in the intact rat

In my first experiments on the behavior of mast cells in rat anaphylaxis (MOTA, 1953), rats were sensitized by injecting intraperitoneally 3 ml of horse serum three times, with an interval of 2 days between each injection and challenged fifteen days later. The animals were anaesthetized with sodium barbital and as a criterium of anaphylactic shock the blood pressure was recorded. In these conditions a poor degree of sensitization was obtained as estimated by the blood pressure. Thus, only 3 out of 10 sensitized rats presented a rapid fall in blood pressure when 1 ml of horse serum was injected into the femural vein, all the others having presented a slight or no change in their blood pressure. The microscopical observation of the tissues showed that definite mast cell damage characterized by granule scattering, was present only in those rats that had presented a fall in blood pressure. Furthermore, it was also observed that only rats presenting a conspicuous clinical anaphylactic syndrome presented mast cell damage. This was thought as a strong suggestion that visible mast cell damage would be produced only in well sensitized rats. Indeed, it was later observed (MOTA, 1957) that rats sensitized with alum-precipitated horse serum presented more intense anaphylaxis, as well as more generalized mast cell alterations and histamine release than those sensitized with plain horse serum. In these experiments, rats were sensitized with 1 ml of alum-precipitated horse serum intraperitoneally, given for 3 days, and challenged 18—30 days later with 1 ml/100 g of body weight horse serum intravenously. In these conditions, it was observed that although some mast cells kept their usual morphology and the number of altered mast cells varied from animal to animal, microscopical examination of the tissues showed constant and

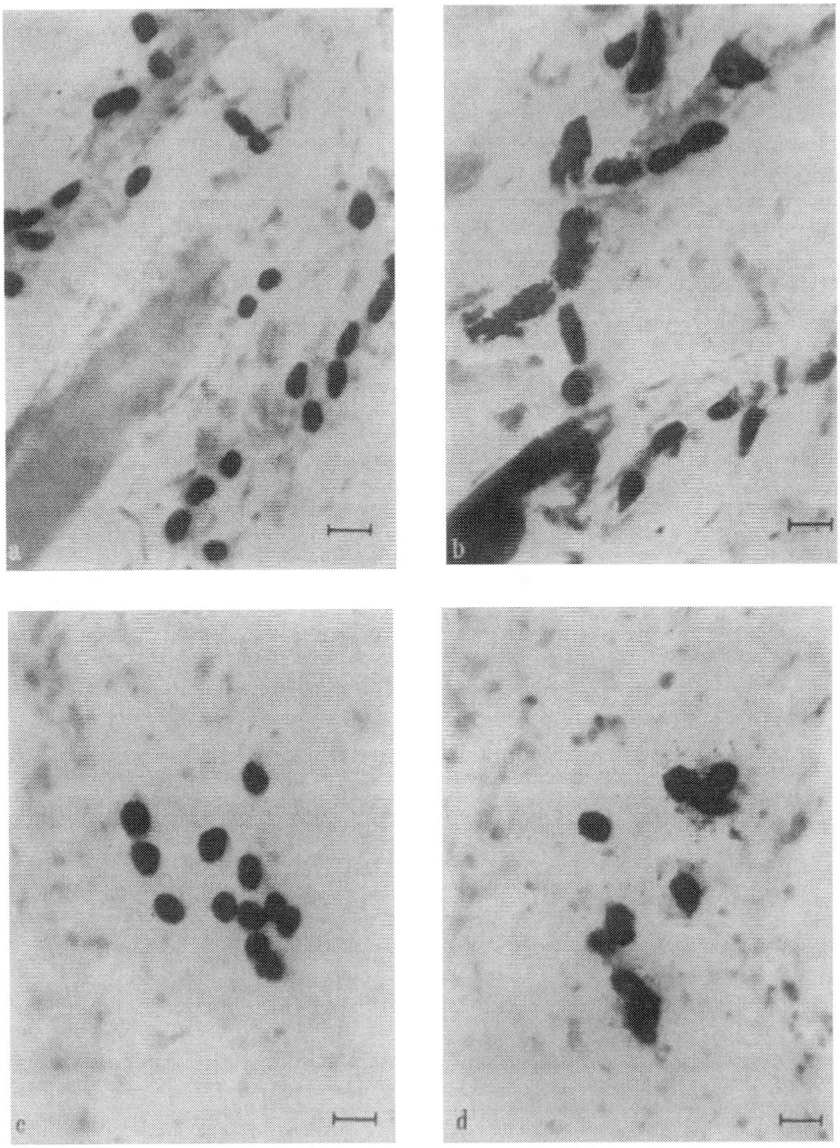

Fig. 14. (*a*) Skin of a non-sensitized rat injected with horse serum showing normal mast cells. (*b*) Skin of a sensitized rat injected with horse serum showing disrupted mast cells. (*c*) Mesentery of a non-sensitized rat incubated with horse serum showing normal mast cells. (*d*) Mesentery of a sensitized rat incubated with horse serum showing disrupted mast cells. Scale in all photomicrographs = 20 μ

definite alterations of these cells, represented by granule extrusions very similar to those promoted by the injection of compound 48—80 (see Fig. 14). Mast cell damage was present only in tissues of the shocked rats, absent from the control ones injected with horse serum and was easily distinguishable from artifacts.

Furthermore, when plasma was taken from shocked rats at several times after the injection of antigen, a variable but definite increase in plasma histamine was observed reaching a maximum in about 5 min and then declining so that no histamine could be detected twenty minutes later. Furthermore, no histamine could be detected in plasma of sensitized rats that had been previously depleted by compound 48—80 of the histamine bound to the mast cells and then shocked.

These results were then interpreted as suggesting that most, if not all, the histamine released in rat anaphylaxis would come from the mast cells – a fact that has been repeatedly confirmed since then – and that histamine would be responsible for the major part of the anaphylactic syndrome in rats, a fact that has not been confirmed by later findings, as we shall see.

2. The effect of Bordetella pertussis on the anaphylactic release of histamine from rat mast cells

The well established fact that mice as well as rats present a much more severe anaphylaxis when *B. pertussis* is administered along with the sensitizing dose of antigen (Malkiel and Hargis, 1952a, b) seemed to us as an excellent opportunity to check whether mast cell damage and the consequent increase in plasma histamine was indeed correlated with severity of the anaphylactic picture in the rat. Rats of both sexes weighing 200—250 g were sensitized by injecting intraperitoneally 1 ml of horse serum or 1 ml of horse serum plus 1 ml of *B. pertussis* vaccine containing 20,000 million organisms, and used from ten days on after sensitization. An equal number of non-treated and pertussis-treated rats were then submitted to various treatments. A first group was injected into the tail vein with 1 ml horse serum. All the pertussis-treated rats presented a very intense shock as shown by difficulty in breathing, weakness, severe prostration, cyanosis and convulsions. Death usually occurred within half an hour but sometimes it took as long as 4 hours for the rats to die. On the other hand, non-treated rats presented slight or no sign of shock and were killed with ether 4 hours after the injection of antigen. Pieces of the following organs were fixed immediately after the death of the animals for mast cell observation: skin, tongue, thymus, lymphatic glands, diaphragm, submaxillary gland, mesentery, heart and abdominal muscle. The microscopical observation of the tissues showed that mast cell damage characterized

Table 11. *Mast cell damage in organs of rats submitted to anaphylaxis*

Rat	Skin (snout)	Tongue	Thymus	Lymph gland	Sub-maxillary gland	Diaphragm	Heart	Mesentery	Abdominal muscle
1	+	+	+	+	+	+	+	+	+
2	+	+	0	0	0	+	0	+	+
3	+	+	0	—	+	—	0	0	0
4	+	+	0	0	0	0	—	0	—
5	+	0	0	0	0	0	0	0	0
6	+	+	+	+	+	+	+	+	+
7	+	+	—	0	0	+	0	+	+
8	+	0	+	+	+	+	+	+	+
9	+	+	+	+	+	+	0	+	+
10	+	0	0	0	+	+	0	0	0
11	+	+	0	+	0	0	0	0	0
12	+	+	+	+	+	+	0	+	+
13	+	+	+	—	0	+	+	+	0
14	+	+	0	+	0	+	+	0	+
15	+	+	—	0	0	+	+	0	+

+ Present, 0 Absent, — Not observed.

by granules scattering was present only in pertussis-treated rats. As can be seen in Table 11, disrupted mast cells were always present in the skin, although not always present in the other organs, in all the rats. A second group of rats was similarly injected under light ether anaesthesia. Five minutes later, about 2 ml of blood was obtained by punction of the vena cava in a syringe containing heparin, the plasma immediately obtained by centrifugation at 0° C, and histamine assayed directly on the guinea-pig ileum. In this experiment also, only the pertussis-treated rats responded to antigen, shown by appearance of histamine in plasma, as can be seen in Table 12. Keeping in mind that a strict comparison cannot be made between our results and those obtained by CODE (1939) in blood of dogs and guinea-pigs during anaphylaxis, the methods used being different, the quantities of histamine we have found in rat plasma (MOTA, 1958b, 1959b) were higher than those he found in guinea-pigs and of about the same value of those he found in dogs.

Table 12. *Plasma histamine concentration (μg/ml) in anaphylaxis of untreated and B. pertussis-treated rats*

Rat	Untreated	Treated
1	< 0.03	1.9
2	< 0.03	0.8
3	< 0.03	1.8
4	< 0.03	2.0
5	< 0.03	1.6
6	< 0.03	0.8
7	< 0.03	1.1
8	< 0.03	0.7
9	< 0.03	0.5
10	< 0.03	0.9
11	< 0.03	0.4
12	< 0.03	1.6
13	< 0.03	0.2

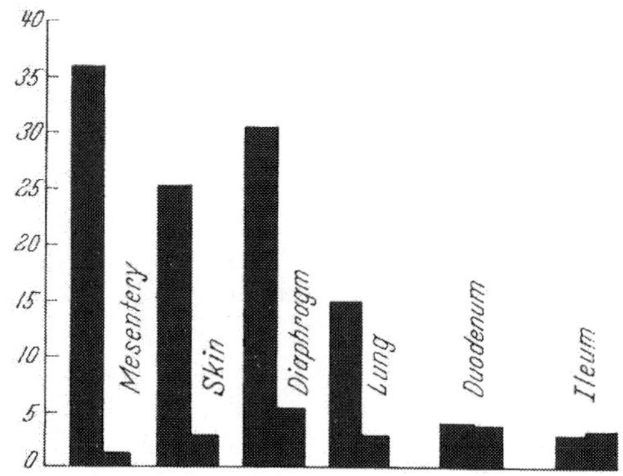

Fig. 15. *In vitro* histamine release by antigen (BSA) from organs of sensitized rats. First column histamine release by antigen, second column histamine diffused from control pieces. Ordinates: percentage histamine release by antigen

3. Antigen-induced mast cell damage and histamine release in isolated rat tissues

In a third group, the rats were beheaded under light ether anaesthesia and their skin, diaphragm, lung, mesentery, ileum and duodenum excised. To study histamine release by antigen, the tissue samples were incubated in 4 ml of Tyrode's solution 15 min at 37° C, then transferred to Tyrode solution containing 10% horse serum, incubated for a further 15 min, after which they were transferred to N-hydrochloric acid for histamine extraction. The histamine diffused from the tissues when incubated with Tyrode solution was assayed and subtracted from that released when the tissues were subsequently incubated with antigen, histamine release being expressed as a percentage of the total tissue histamine. The results of these experiments showed that antigen releases histamine from isolated sensitized rat tissues, but not from non-sensitized tissues, and that the percentage of released histamine was greater in the mesentery and diaphragm, less so in the lung and skin and absent in the duodenum and ileum. This same result was also obtained when bovine serum albumin (see Fig. 15) was used as antigen (MOTA, 1959b; MOTA and ISHII, 1960). Indeed histamine release and mast cell damage by antigen can be obtained with any antigen provided that the rats have been sensitized in such a way as to present a severe anaphylactic shock when injected with antigen.

4. Antigen-induced damage to isolated sensitized rat mast cells

All the above experiments were made with tissues containing not only mast cells but also a mixed cell population, and therefore it is not possible to know if damage to the mast cells is a direct consequence of an antigen-antibody reaction taking place on the mast cell or an indirect consequence of an antigen-antibody reaction taking place on other cells. To clear this up, experiments were performed in which the effect of the specific antigen was observed on isolated mast cells (MOTA and DIAS DA SILVA, 1960b). Wistar rats were sensitized by injecting 1 ml of horse serum plus 1 ml of *Haemophilus pertussis* vaccine containing 20,000 million organisms intraperitoneally and were used twenty-five days later. Evidence of sensitization was provided by testing whether the mesenteric mast cell presented extrusion of the granules in presence of the specific antigen; a tiny piece of mesentery was incubated with antigen and afterwards fixed and stained for mast cell observation. Animals whose mesentery did not present mast cell disruption on contact with antigen were discarded. Mast cells were isolated by a method similar to that described by PADAWER and GORDON (1955). The animals were bled under ether anaesthesia and 2 ml of saline (sodium chloride 0.85%) containing 50 μg heparin per ml were injected into the abdominal cavity and gentle massage of the gut through the abdominal wall was performed for about 1 min. The abdominal wall was then incised along the midventral line and the fluid from the abdominal cavity collected with a pipette. This was carefully layered over 1.5 ml of a 30% water solution of bovine serum albumin (fraction V, Armour) and centrifuged in an International refrigerated centrifuge model PR 1, at 90 r.p.m. for 2 min. The albumin solution was then removed with a pipette, avoiding contamination with interface cells, diluted to 20 ml with Tyrode solution and centrifuged at 1,000 r.p.m. for 5 min. This last operation was repeated once more and finally the deposit in the bottom of the tube was resuspended in 0.2—0.3 ml Tyrode solution This procedure resulted in a suspension containing 90—98% of mast cells most of which were well preserved. These cells were then studied by aid of phase contrast microscopy either under dry magnification (X 800) or with oil immersion objective (X 1000). A drop of the mast cell suspension was placed on a slide and covered with a square coverslip, two sides of which were sealed with melted paraffin. A small well of paraffin was then made at each free side of the coverslip in the same way as was described by STRANGEWAYS and CANTI (1927), the preparation kept in a warm stage 37° C, and a suitable group of well-preserved mast cells selected for observation. Horse serum heated at 37° C was then placed in one free side of the coverslip and sucked on to the cells with a piece of filter paper. Usually the mast cells stood still when the antigen was sucked through, although sometimes many were washed away. As a control to these experiments, the effect of horse serum on non-sensitized mast cells was also observed. In these conditions the effect of the antigen on sensitized mast cells was a very striking one. A few seconds after the antigen had been sucked on to the cells, there was a slight increase in cell size followed by a sudden appearance and disappearance of successive vacuoles which made the cell look as if it were bubbling. Sometimes it was possible to observe extrusion of the granules which occurred, so far as could be observed, without damage to the cellular membrane. This phenomenon was very rapid, but was slowed down by low temperature at which the phenomenon took as long as 1 min to be complete. When cell change was no longer seen, the cell had lost its regular contour, the granules had become more apparent and large empty spaces could be seen among them (Fig. 16). This phenomenon was very much like that produced by compound 48—80 when acting on mesenteric mast cells (MOTA,

BERALDO and JUNQUEIRA, 1953). UVNÄS and THON (1959) have independently obtained similar results. These authors isolated rat mast cells by differential centrifugation in Ficoll (a polysaccharide of high molecular weight) dissolved in isotonic salt solution and observed that antigen released both histamine and slow reacting substance from isolated sensitized mast cells. However, in their experiments, the response of the cells to antigen was dependent on the presence of cat

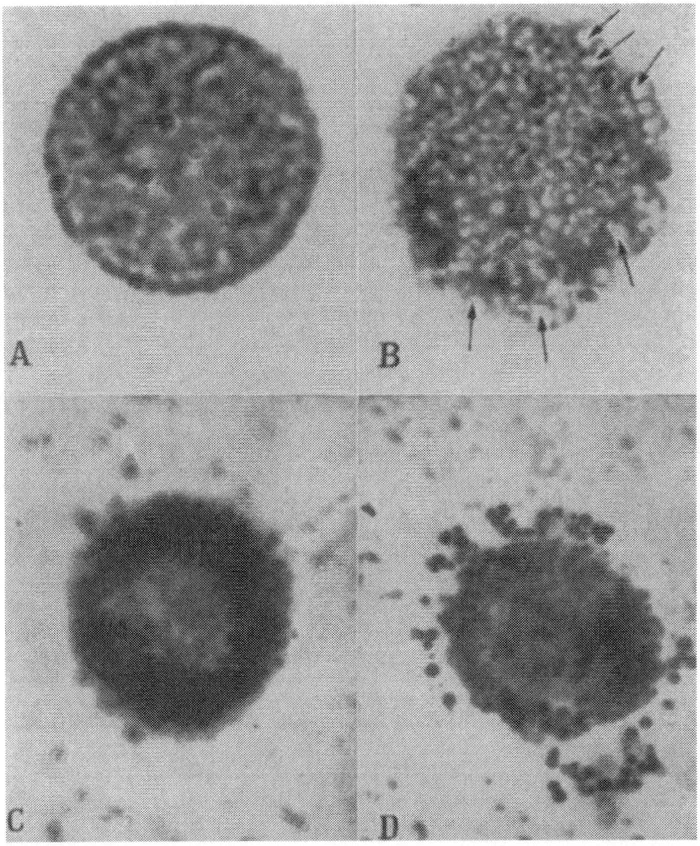

Fig. 16, (*A*) Isolated sensitized mast cell before contact with antigen. Phase contrast (× c. 666); (*B*) the same cell after contact with antigen. Arrows point to vacuoles (× c. 666). (*C*) Isolated mast cell after fixation with 1% formaldehyde and stained with toluidine blue (× c. 533). (*D*) Isolated mast cell after contact with antigen. Note granules outside the cell. Fixed and stained as stated above (× c. 533)

serum. AUSTEN and HUMPHREY (1961) have observed mast cell damage and histamine release by adding rabbit anti-rat γ-globulin to a suspension of isolated rat mast cells. They consider this phenomenon as a reversed anaphylaxis and observed that di-isopropyl phosphorofluoridate, salicylaldoxime, indol and calcium deficiency inhibited mast cell damage and histamine release caused by anti-rat γ-globulin. They noted that since washed peritoneal cells, treated with a purified anti-rat γ-globulin are still able to release histamine, it is evident that extrinsic serum factors cannot be involved in the reaction unless they are firmly bound on the cell surface. The effect of anti-rat γ-globulin on rat mast cells was more recently confirmed by KELLER (1962).

C. In mouse anaphylaxis

1. Antigen-induced mast cell damage in the intact mouse

Mouse mast cell damage in anaphylaxis was first described by CARTER, HIGGINBOTHAM and DOUGHERTY (1957). Mice were sensitized by a series of three subcutaneous injections of 0.1 ml horse serum given on alternate days. Three to 4 weeks after sensitization, the animals were injected subcutaneously on the dorsal surface with 1 ml of air to form an air pouch into which was injected 0.2 ml of 1 : 10 dilution of the appropriate antigen. At different time intervals thereafter, the enclosed bubble of connective tissue was dissected free from the surrounding tissues and a portion of it removed and spread on a glass microscopic slide. As controls, the authors used non-sensitized mice challenged with calf serum. In these conditions, it was observed that only a few of the mast cells shed their granules within a 5 min period in response to the local injection of antigen in the control mice while widespread mast cell disruption and concomitant dispersion of their granules into the surrounding ground substance followed the injection of antigen into sensitized mice.

2. The effect of Bordetella pertussis on the anaphylactic mast cell damage in mouse tissues

More recently we have been able to induce generalized mast cell damage by injecting antigen intravenously into sensitized mice (MOTA, 1962). Mice were sensitized by injecting 0.5 ml of horse serum plus 0.1 ml of *B. pertussis* vaccine containing 2,000 million organisms intraperitoneally and challenged 10 days later by injecting intravenously 0.3 ml of horse serum. In accord with the previous observations of MALKIEL and HARGIS (1952b), the animals presented very severe and fatal anaphylaxis. Mast cells were observed in frozen sections 50 μ thick, stained with toluidine blue, obtained from skin, tongue and diaphragm. The results of this experiment showed that generalized mast cell damage was present in shocked mice and absent from control non-sensitized mice injected with horse serum. The antigen-induced mouse mast cell alteration, very similar to that observed in rat anaphylaxis, was represented by extrusion of the mast granules which were kept in the vicinity of the mast cells, such as was previously described by CARTER, HIGGINBOTHAM and DOUGHERTY (1957). These experiments showed that mast cell damage by antigen occurs also in mouse anaphylaxis, and is enhanced when *B. pertussis* is injected along with the sensitizing dose of antigen, such as occurs in rat anaphylaxis.

3. Antigen-induced mast cell damage and histamine release in mouse tissues

It was thought of interest to find out whether mouse mast cell damage by antigen would also be induced under *in vitro* conditions. Thus, mice were sensitized by injecting 0.5 ml of horse serum plus 0.1 ml *Bordetella pertussis* containing 2,000 million organisms intraperitoneally. Ten to 15 days later, the animals were killed by decapitation and pieces of skin incubated for 15 min at 37° C with Tyrode solution containing 10% horse serum, after which the skin samples were transferred either to hydrochloric acid for histamine extraction or to fixative for mast cell observation. For microscopical observation of the mast cell the tissues were fixed and stained as in the preceeding *in vivo* experiments. In these conditions mast cell damage and histamine release were observed in 5 out of 11 mice used. Therefore, mast cell damage and histamine release in mouse anaphylaxis occur also in isolated tissues taken from sensitized mice.

D. In rat and mouse passive anaphylaxis

Since mast cell damage by antigen in the guinea-pig occurs not only after active sensitization but also after passive sensitization, experiments were performed to find out whether passive sensitization would also sensitize rats and mice so as to produce mast cell damage and histamine release on later contact with antigen (Mota, 1962). Wistar rats of both sexes weighing 200—300 g and albino mice of about 25 g were used in all experiments. For microscopical observation of the mast cells, rat and mouse tissues were fixed and stained as already described. Rabbit anti-bovine serum albumin and anti-ovalbumin serum were obtained after two intramuscular injections one week apart of ovalbumin or bovine serum albumin emulsified in Freund's adjuvant mixture (Freund and McDermott, 1942) followed by two or three intravenous injections of alum-precipitate ovalbumin or bovine serum albumin. The animals received 20 mg of each protein per injection. Rat anti-human serum albumin and anti-ovalbumin obtained by a similar schedule were kindly donated by Dr. J. H. Humphrey (National Institute for Medical Research, London).

1. Mast cell and histamine in rat passive anaphylaxis

Groups of 10 rats were injected intraperitoneally with 5 mg of rabbit anti-ovalbumin antibodies. Forty-eight hours later, one of the groups was injected intravenously with 10 mg of ovalbumin dissolved in 1 ml of saline. All the animals presented anaphylactic shock as showed by prostration and difficulty in breathing and recovered in about half hour. One hour later they were killed with ether and microscopical observation of their tissues, after fixation, showed no mast cell damage. From the other group blood was collected from the jugular vein in a syringe containing heparin 5 min after the injection of antigen and plasma obtained by centrifugation at 0° C and assayed for histamine. However, no increase in plasma histamine was detected. From a third group, the mesentery and the uterus were dissected out. The mesentery was incubated with Tyrode solution containing 1 mg per ml ovalbumin for 15 min at 37° C and fixed for mast cell observation, while the uterus was suspended in oxygenated De Jalon solution and 15 min later ovalbumin was added. Although the uterus contracted when in contact with antigen showing that the tissues had been sensitized, no mast cell damage or histamine release was observed in the mesentery.Some experiments were then performed with homologous antisera. Rats were injected with 2.4 mg of rat antibodies to ovalbumin and challenged 48 hours later by injecting intravenously 5 mg of ovalbumin. Although these animals presented signs of shock, no mast cell damage or increase in plasma histamine was observed. These experiments showed that in rats passive sensitization *in vivo* with heterologous or even homologous precipitating antibodies dōes not duplicate the mast cell damage observed after active anaphylaxis (Mota, 1962).

2. The effect of B. pertussis on mast cells and histamine in rat passive anaphylaxis

It is known that when *Bordetella pertussis* is injected along with the sensitizing dose of antigen, the histamine release and mast cell damage are very much increased in rat active anaphylaxis (Mota, 1958b) and it was thought necessary to find out whether the same result could be obtained in passively sensitized rats. Thus, a group of 10 rats was injected intraperitoneally with 1 ml of *B. pertussis* vaccine containing 20,000 million organisms and 48 hours later injected intravenously with 5 mg of rabbit anti-ovalbumin. Forty eight hours after the injection of antibodies, the animals were challenged by injecting 10 mg of ovalbumin intravenously. Surprisingly enough these animals presented a shock as mild as that presented by control rats sensitized only with ovalbumin without pertussis. Furthermore, neither plasma histamine increase nor mast cell damage was observed. This experiment was then duplicated but by injecting *B. pertussis* vaccine plus 1 ml of horse serum. Forty-eight hours later the animals were passively sensitized and shocked as already stated. Only mild shock with no increase in plasma histamine resulted. However, when 6 days later the same animals were injected with horse serum they presented very severe anaphylaxis, mast cell damage and histamine release, showing that the previous injection of pertussis vaccine had been effective in respect of active sensitization with horse serum. Furthermore, as it is known that pertussis-treated rats are only fully sensitized on the 10th day after the sensitizing injection, the effect of passive sensitization 10 days after inoculation with pertussis was tried. A group of 10 rats was injected intraperitoneally with *B. pertussis* plus 1 ml of horse serum and 8 days afterwards injected intravenously with 5 mg of rabbit anti-ovalbumin. Forty-eight hours later the animals were challenged by injecting 10 mg of ovalbumin intravenously. Only mild shock with no plasma histamine increase resulted. However, when the same animals were injected 48 hours later with horse serum, all of them presented severe anaphylaxis, mast cell damage and histamine release showing that the previous injection of *B. pertussis* had modified the sensitivity of the animals to active anaphylaxis but not to passive anaphylaxis.

3. The effect of adrenalectomy on mast cells and histamine in rat passive anaphylaxis

It is known that adrenalectomy increases the sensitivity of rats to active anaphylaxis (FLASHMAN, 1926) and we have observed that the number of disrupted mast cells in adrenalectomized rats after anaphylaxis is larger than in non-adrenalectomized ones (MOTA, 1957). Thus, it was considered of interest to study the effect of passive anaphylaxis on mast cells and histamine of adrenalectomized rats. The animals were subjected to one-stage adrenalectomy under ether anaesthesia and then given 0.85% sodium chloride as drinking water. Forty-eight hours after the adrenalectomy, groups of 10 rats each were injected intravenously with 1 mg of rabbit antibodies to bovine serum albumin, and then either immediately or 48 hours later injected intravenously with 5 mg of bovine serum albumin. The results of these experiments showed that although most of the rats in both groups presented signs of shock, this was definitely more severe in the group in which antibody and antigen were injected in rapid succession. In this group six rats died in about one hour and all of them presented severe intestinal congestion at autopsy. However, neither plasma histamine increase nor mast cell damage was observed, but for one animal in which a few disrupted mast cells were found.

4. The effect of antigen on rat mast cells and histamine after passive sensitization in vitro

Since passive sensitization performed in the intact rat failed to induce anaphylaxis with simultaneous mast cell damage and histamine release, it was decided to carry out corresponding experiments by incubating rat tissues *in vitro* with antiserum. Rat mesentery and diaphragm were dissected out from normal and pertussis-treated rats and incubated at 37° C in plain rabbit serum containing 1.3 mg anti-bovine serum albumin antibodies. The time of incubation with the antiserum varied from 30 min up to 3 hours and in some instances the tissues were incubated overnight at 4° C. Guinea-pig diaphragm and mesentery were simultaneously incubated with the same antiserum for comparison. Later transfer of these tissues to antigen solution led to mast cell damage and histamine release from guinea-pig tissues but neither occurred with rat tissues. It is our experience that horse serum is a better antigen than ovalbumin or bovine serum albumin for sensitizing rats and it was thought that mast cell damage and histamine release could be obtained if rat tissues were passively sensitized with antihorse serum rabbit serum. Thus, diaphragm and mesentery were incubated at 37° C for 3 hours with rabbit serum containing antibodies to horse serum, and then transferred to Tyrode solution containing 10% horse serum for 15 min at 37° C. However, no mast cell damage or histamine release was observed, although incubation of guinea-pig tissues with this same antiserum led to mast cell damage and histamine release on later contact with antigen. Some experiments were then carried out with homologous antiserum. Rat mesentery was incubated with rat antiserum containing 2.9 mg per ml of antibodies to human serum albumin or 4.8 mg to ovalbumin for one up to three hours at 37° C and then transferred to Tyrode solution containing 1 mg per ml human serum albumin or ovalbumin. Even so no mast cell damage or histamine release was observed.

5. Mast cell behaviour in mouse passive anaphylaxis

It is known that pre-treatment with *B. pertussis* greatly increases the severity of passive anaphylaxis in mice (Kind, 1953; Pittman and Germuth, 1958; Muñoz, Schuchardt and Verwey, 1954) and the behaviour of mast cells was studied in non-treated and pertussis-treated passively sensitized mice. A group of 10 mice was injected intraperitoneally with 0.1 ml of *B. pertussis* vaccine containing 2,000 million organisms while 10 control mice were injected with 0.1 ml saline. Four days later all the animals were injected intraperitoneally with 1.2 mg of rabbit anti-bovine serum albumin, and 6 hours later injected intravenously with 1 mg of bovine serum albumin in 0.5 ml of saline. These experiments confirmed that pre-treatment with pertussis increases the gravity of passive anaphylaxis in mice, all the pertussis-treated animals having died within 15—30 min after antigen injection. Nevertheless, the microscopical examination of the tissues of these mice showed no mast cell damage. Thus, contrary to what happens to actively sensitized mice, in which pre-treatment with *B. pertussis* increases very much the mast cell damage by antigen in anaphylaxis, pre-treatment with *B. pertussis*, although increasing the severity of anaphylaxis in passively sensitized mice, does not change the reactivity of the tissues of these animals so as to induce mast cell damage when they are later challenged with antigen (Mota, 1962). Possible reasons for this fact will be considered later.

IV. The effect of soluble antigen-antibody complexes on the mast cells and histamine

In 1957, Germuth and McKinnon made the important observation that soluble antigen-antibody complexes prepared in excess antigen produce anaphylactic shock when injected into unsensitized guinea-pigs. A syndrome similar to anaphylaxis was also obtained by injection of soluble complexes in mice by Tokuda and Weiser (1958) and in rats by Garcia-Arocha and McIlreath (1959). The observation that in the above mentioned species the character of the shock induced by soluble antigen-antibody complexes was very similar to that seen in anaphylaxis suggested that the sites of antigen-antibody action are the same regardless of whether anaphylaxis is induced by injection of antigen into an already sensitized animal or by injection of soluble preformed antigen-antibody complexes. If this were true, soluble complexes of antigen-antibody should duplicate all the cytological aspects of ordinary anaphylaxis including histamine release from the mast cells. Thus, some experiments were carried out to find out the effect of antigen-antibody complexes on the mast cells of guinea-pigs, rats and mice (MOTA, 1961). To prepare the soluble complexes, antigen was added to antiserum at equivalence, the mixture incubated at 37° C for half an hour and kept for 24 hours at 4° C. The precipitate was then washed three times with saline at 0° C to 1° C, re-suspended in Tyrode solution containing a total amount of bovine serum albumin ranging from 5 to 8 times that used to precipitate antibody at equivalence, stored at 4° C with occasional agitation for 48 hours and cleared by centrifugation. The antiserum was a pool of rabbit anti-bovine serum albumin containing 1.0 mg antibody N per milliliter, and crystalline bovine serum albumin was used as antigen. Twenty guinea-pigs of 250 g body weight were intravenously injected with 2 ml (2 mg Ab N) of this complexes preparation. Three out of these guinea-pigs died with emphysematous lungs, 10 presented severe shock and died overnight, 2 presented slight to moderate shock and 5 presented no effect at all. The emphysematous lungs were then fixed and stained for microscopical observation of the mast cells as already described. A microscopical inspection of many microscopical fields did not reveal any mast cell degranulation. However, it was considered that the amount of histamine released, although enough to induce emphysema could be very slight to produce any visible mast cell damage and we decided to perform *in vitro* experiments, in which the effect of the complexes on the mast cells could more easily be detected. Thus, 15 guinea-pigs were killed by breaking the neck, their lungs, ileum and mesentery dissected out, and the complexes preparation tried on these organs. The ileum was suspended in a Dale apparatus with 7 ml capacity and the activity of the complexes preparation tried by adding 0.4 ml (400 μg Ab N) of it to the bath. The lung was cut into slices 0.8 mm thick, washed in cold Tyrode solution and 10 to 12 of these slices used as samples. They were then shaken in beakers closed with parafilm caps for 15 min at 37° C in 4 ml (4 mg Ab N) of the complexes preparation or in 4 ml of Tyrode solution, after which the histamine content of the supernatants was assayed on the guinea-pig ileum. The mesentery was cut into pieces which were incubated with the complexes under the conditions described for the lung, and then transferred to a 4% solution of lead subacetate for fixation. The results showed that 6 out of the 15 ilea tried responded to the complexes with a definite contraction followed by desensitization as already reported by TRAPANI, GRAVEY and CAMPBELL (1958). However, no histamine release or mast cell damage could be detected when the lungs or mesentery of the same animals were incubated with the complexes. The same results were obtained when 1% fresh guinea-pig serum was added to the complexes. A group of 20 non-treated and 20 rats adrenalectomized 48 hours before were then injected with 2 ml (2 mg Ab N) of the complexes preparation. All the animals presented moderate to severe shock and 12 of the adrenalectomized rats died showing generalized intestinal congestion at autopsy. However, no mast cell damage was observed but for one adrenalectomized rat in which generalized mast cell damage was found. This experiment was duplicated with a group of 12 adrenalectomized rats from which blood was collected 5 min after injecting the complexes and the plasma histamine assayed on the ileum. Although all the animals presented severe shock no increase in plasma histamine was found but for one rat in which 0.5 μg/ml of histamine was found. Twenty mice were then injected with 0.5 ml (0.5 mg Ab N) of the complexes preparation. All the animals presented moderate to severe shock and 9 of them died within 10 min. However, microscopical examination of their tissues did not reveal any mast cell damage. Since pre-treatment with *B. pertussis* aggravates the shock induced by soluble antigen-antibody complexes in mice (TOKUDA and WEISER, 1958), 20 pertussis-treated mice were injected with 0.5 ml of the complexes.

Although 18 of these mice presented severe shock and died within 20 min, no mast cell damage could be observed in their tissues. Thus, it was concluded that soluble antigen-antibody complexes do not duplicate the mast cell damage and histamine release observed in active and passive anaphylaxis of guinea-pigs. In this respect we consider strongly suggestive the results showing that neither histamine release nor mast cell damage occur, when guinea-pig lung or mesentery are incubated with soluble antigen-antibody complexes, under conditions in which both, mast cell damage and histamine release are promptly produced when antigen contacts sensitized tissues. However, under the more complex conditions in the intact animal, the complexes may release histamine, although the failure in observing mast cell degranulation in lungs of guinea-pigs dying of acute shock induced by soluble complexes suggested that, if there is histamine release *in vivo* this must be very small. In addition these results suggested that the complexes do not act as a histamine releaser or by sensitizing the tissues and reproducing passive anaphylaxis. Also the possibility that anaphylatoxin could have been formed by reaction between antigen-antibody complexes and serum proteins was ruled out as anaphylatoxin induces guinea-pig mast cell damage similar to that produced by antigen-antibody reaction in anaphylaxis (MOTA, 1959c). In rats and mice these results were not surprising as we had observed that passive sensitization of rats and mice does not produce mast cell damage when these animals are challenged with antigen (MOTA, 1962). Actually, the fact that rats and mice are more susceptible to passive anaphylaxis when antigen and antibody are injected in rapid succession, suggests that formation of soluble antigen-antibody complexes may be very important in rat and mouse passive anaphylaxis.

V. Inhibition of mast cell damage and histamine release in anaphylaxis

The many substances used as inhibitors of histamine release and mast cell damage by antigen can be divided into six principal groups: metabolic inhibitors (MONGAR and SCHILD, 1957a); antipyretic and related compounds (MONGAR and SCHILD, 1957a); nicotinic and isonicotinic acid derivatives (MOTA, DIAS DA SILVA and FERNANDES, 1960); antihistamines (MOTA and DIAS DA SILVA, 1960a); chymotrypsin substrates and inhibitors (AUSTEN and BROCKLEHURST, 1960, 1961).

The effect of several metabolic inhibitors and of some antipyretics and related substances on the anaphylactic release of histamine was studied by MONGAR and SCHILD (1955, 1957a). The effectiveness of the substances used by these authors as well as of other compounds in preventing the anaphylactic release of histamine has been confirmed and extended to the prevention of mast cell damage by antigen in anaphylaxis (MOTA, 1958a, 1959a, b; MOTA and ISHII, 1960; CHAKRAVARTY, 1960).

MONGAR and SCHILD (1957a) measured the anaphylactic release of histamine *in vitro* from guinea-pig lung, spleen and uterus tissue chopped into rods 0.8 mm × 0.8 mm in cross-section with the McIlwain tissue chopper. A series of samples of equal volume (0.2 ml) were obtained and incubated in 10 ml beakers for 15 min with 0.5 ml of the required concentration of the inhibitor. After this treatment 0.5 ml of antigen solution (2 mg/ml egg albumin) was added and a further 15 min period at 37° C was allowed for the histamine release process to take place. The incubation fluid was then removed from the tissue particles with a filter pipette and the histamine released assayed on the guinea-pig ileum. The histamine content of the tissues was determined by heating one sample in 10 ml Tyrode solution in a boiling water bath for 5 min. Under these conditions the authors observed that when monosodium iodoacetate (0.001 M), sodium chloromercuribenzoate

(0.001 M) and sodium cyanide (0.010 M) were previously incubated with sensitized tissues, the subsequent histamine release by antigen was greatly reduced. On the other hand, 2,4-dinitrophenol, fluoride and azide were practically without effect. The effect of antipyretics and some related compounds was also observed by MONGAR and SCHILD (1957 a). They found that all the antipyretics tried inhibited the release of histamine by antigen from sensitized guinea-pig lung and that the most active, phenylbutazone, produced 50% inhibition in 4 mM concentration, whereas the least active, salicylate, produced 50% inhibition in 70 mM concentration. The authors called the attention to the fact that the most active compounds, phenylbutazone, antipyrine, amidopyrine and cinchophen, were potent antipyretics and antirheumatics.

In the group of related compounds, phenol was the most active producing a 50% inhibition of histamine release in anaphylaxis in 0.004 M concentration. Furthermore, phenol in 0.010 M concentration almost completely abolished the anaphylactic contraction of the guinea-pig ileum. This concentration of phenol reduced also the sensitivity of the ileum to histamine to about one-fifth, but it was seen that its main effect lain in inhibiting histamine release. By treating sensitized tissues with phenol, washing the phenol away with Tyrode solution and then adding the specific antigen, the authors obtained an answer similar to that presented by untreated tissues and concluded that phenol did not cause damage to tissue antibodies. Alternatively the possibility was considered that phenol could combine reversibly with antibody and in this way prevent the antigen-antibody reaction. In this case, phenol would prevent desensitization and a later addition of antigen after removal of phenol would produce histamine release and an anaphylactic contraction. However, when a sensitized guinea-pig ileum was treated with antigen in presence of phenol the anaphylactic contraction was inhibited but nevertheless, when phenol was later washed out, the muscle was desensitized. Similarly, when sensitized lung was treated with antigen in the presence of phenol it failed to release histamine but if phenol was washed out, the tissue was desensitized (see Fig. 17). Thus, phenol neither inactivates antibody nor prevents desensitization. Furthermore, it was observed that if phenol is removed soon after addition of antigen, some histamine is still released though less than in a control experiment without phenol. To explain these facts, the authors assumed that combination of antigen with cellular antibody results in the activation of a short-lived enzyme system which catalizes the reactions leading to histamine release and the other manifestations of anaphylaxis. An inhibitory substance like phenol would interfere with the actions but not with inactivation of the enzyme, so that, in the presence of phenol, histamine release would be inhibited but after removal of phenol no enzyme would be left to complete the reaction. Later on, these experiments were duplicated to see if phenol would inhibit the mast cell damage by antigen without inhibiting desensitization (MOTA, 1959 a). A preliminary test was made to see whether phenol denatured antibody. Sensitized mesentery was

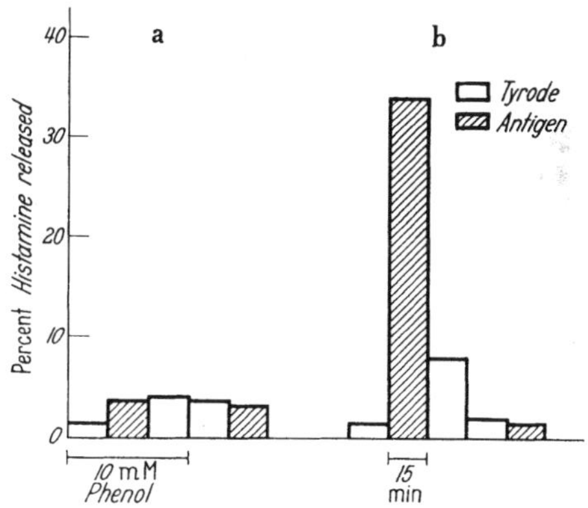

Fig. 17. Effect of phenol on histamine release and desensitization in chopped, sensitized guinea pig lung. (*a*) Phenol treated sample; (*b*) control. Phenol reduces the histamine release by antigen from 34 to 4%, but it does not prevent desensitization, as shown by the absence of histamine release with a second dose of antigen after removal of the phenol

incubated for 15 min with 0.010 M phenol in Tyrode solution and then transferred to Tyrode solution containing no phenol. Addition of antigen now produced the usual degranulation of the mast cells, showing that antibody was not denatured. The next test was whether phenol prevented desensitization. Addition of antigen in presence of 0.010 M phenol did not produce mast cell degranulation. Furthermore, when the mesentery was washed in 0.010 M phenol to remove antigen, then in Tyrode solution to remove phenol and a second dose of antigen was added, this also failed to produce mast cell degranulation. Thus, phenol inhibited mast cell degranulation without interfering with desensitization. In agreement with Mongar and Schild's observations these experiments showed that it is possible to interrupt the sequence of events which followed the reaction of antigen with antibody and produced histamine release from the mast cells. It seems possible that the inhibitory effect of phenol is due to its anti-chymotrypsin property (Austen and Brocklehurst, 1961). Contrasting with the metabolic inhibitors and antipyretics so far used, other agents were observed to produce not a partial but total inhibition of histamine release and mast cell damage by antigen. For instance, when guinea-pig lung tissue or mesentery were incubated with calcium-free Tyrode solution containing 0.01% versene for 15 min at 37° C, no mast cell damage or histamine release occurred on subsequent contact with antigen. The effect of versene could be reversed by adding calcium and was shown to depend

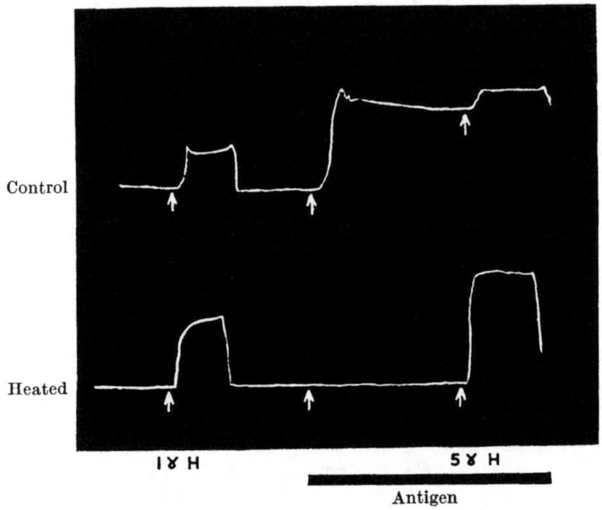

Fig. 18. Two segments of ileum from same sensitized guinea pig in Tyrode solution, at 37° C. Absence of anaphylactic reaction in segment which was heated to 45° C for 5 minutes three hours before the experiment

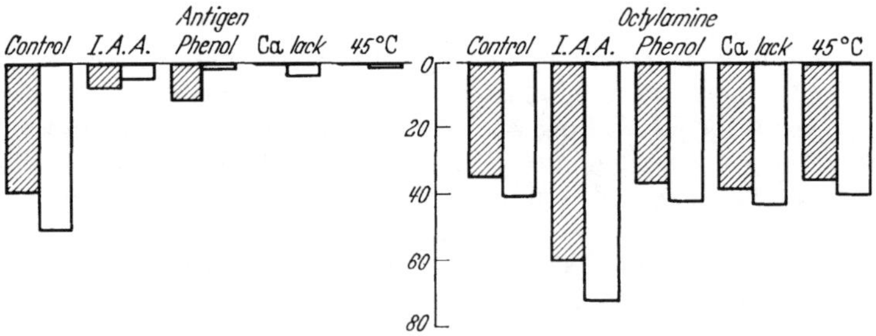

Fig. 19 Effect of various inhibitors on histamine release (□) and mast cell decrease (▨) in chopped sensitized guinea-pig lung by antigen or by octylamine. Figures represent percentage diminution

on the pH (Mongar and Schild, 1957c, 1958; Mota, 1958a, 1959a). Furthermore, Mongar and Schild (1957b) also made the interesting observation that heating of a tissue at 45° C for 15 min produced a complete and irreversible inhibition of histamine release by antigen. Heat also inactivated the mechanism responsible for the anaphylactic contraction of the isolated sensitized guinea-pig muscle. In a typical experiment two pieces of ileum taken from a sensitized guinea-pig were suspended in a large isolated organ bath at 37° C, one of them having been heated to 45° C, for 15 min, 10 hours previously. Both preparations were well sensitive to histamine but only the piece that had not been heated to 45° C responded to antigen as it is shown in Fig. 18. Similarly, when sensitized guinea-pig tissues were previously heated to 45° C, the subsequent mast cell damage by antigen was completely and irreversibly prevented (MOTA, 1958a, 1959a). These observations suggested that a heat-labile factor is required in the anaphylactic reaction and it could be shown that this factor is not antibody but a constituent of normal tissue. The evidence for this was provided by performing passive sensitization *in vitro*, which showed that although normal guinea-pig lung could be easily passively sensitized, lung which had been heated to 45° C could no longer be sensitized in this way (MONGAR and SCHILD, 1957b). The effect of iodoacetate, phenol, lack of calcium and previous heating at 45° C, on the histamine release and mast cell damage by antigen is shown in Fig. 19. In this same figure, it can be observed that the same agents that inhibit the anaphylactic release of histamine from the mast cells, potentiate the histamine release and mast cell damage by octylamine. However, when the effects of these several agents were studied in the rat, it was clearly observed that, in this species, the release of histamine and mast cell damage either by antigen or by chemical releasers were simultaneously inhibited. Thus when sensitized rat skin or mesentery was incubated for 15 min at 37° C with sodium monoiodoacetate (0.001 M), sodium p-chloromercuribenzoate (0.001 M), sodium cyanide (0.005 M), and several antipyretics, the subsequent histamine release by either antigen or compound 48—80 was greatly reduced as can be seen in Fig. 3. However, as can also be seen there, phenazone was exceptional in reducing histamine release by antigen and increasing histamine release by compound 48—80. Furthermore, when sensitized rat tissues were previously heated to 45° C for 15 min or incubated for the same period of time in calcium-free Tyrode solution containing 0.01% sodium dihydrogen edetate, the subsequent histamine release and mast cell damage by antigen or compound 48—80 was completely prevented by these agents (see Fig. 20). Therefore, while in the guinea-pig the release of histamine from the mast cells by antigen or chemical histamine liberators can be easily distinguished by its morphological aspect and response to different inhibitory agents, the mast cell damage induced by antigen or compound 48—80 in the rat is morphologically very alike and the histamine-releasing mechanism of the two agents is simultaneously inhibited by various substances and conditions (MOTA, 1958a, 1959a, b; MOTA and ISHII, 1960). Rather similar conclusions were drawn by CHAKRAVARTY (1959, 1960) who, studying the anaphylactic release of histamine in rats and guinea-pigs, also observed that the release of histamine either by antigen or compound 48—80 from rat tissues was simultaneously inhibited by many substances and conditions. For instance, polyphloretin phosphate (0.02 M), 2,4-dinitrofluorobenzene (0.02 M), iodoacetate (0.001 M), ethyl alcohol

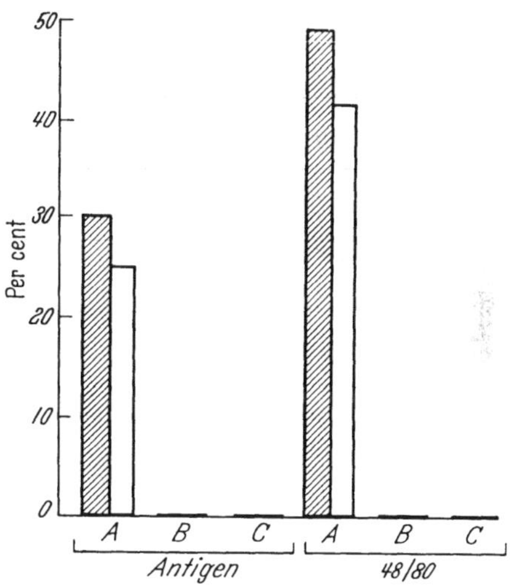

Fig. 20. Effect of Tyrode solution (A), calcium lack (B) or previous heating of the tissue at 45° C (C) on histamine release (black columns) and mast cell disruption (white columns) induced by antigen or compound 48/80 in sensitized rat mesentery

(0.01 M) and many azo dyes inhibited histamine release from rat tissues by either antigen or compound 48—80. Thus, while the results obtained in the guinea-pig seem to suggest that the histamine-releasing mechanism of antigen and chemical releasers are quite different, the results obtained in rats suggest that this conclusion probably does not apply to all species since, at least in the rat, there is a very close similarity between the histamine release mechanism of antigen and compound 48—80. This is not to say that the mechanism of action of these two agents is necessarily identical in this species. For instance, if all inhibitors act on one step of the histamine release mechanism common to antigen and compound 48—80 both these agents could be inhibited in the same way, and yet other stages in their mechanism of action could be quite different. This common step may well be the activation of a cellular enzyme as suggested by ROCHA e SILVA (1944).

In 1958, ALIVISATOS reported the synthesis and isolation of a dinucleotide of histamine. The structure of this compound is that of diphosphopyridine nucleotide (DPN) in which histamine replaced the nicotinamide moiety. Its biosynthesis involves a simple exchange reaction between free histamine and the nicotinamide of DPN. The author suggested that the exchange reaction of DPN with histamine could be involved in the mechanism of anaphylaxis. The fact that this reaction takes place in the presence of diphosphopyridine nucleotidase (DPNase) prompted us to investigate the effect of various compounds known to inhibit the activity of this enzyme on the anaphylactic mast cell damage and histamine release. Furthermore, the effect of these compounds on the mast cell damage and histamine release by compound 48—80 was also investigated (MOTA, DIAS DA SILVA and FERNANDES, 1960). Pyridine and the following DPNase inhibitors were used: nicotinamide, nicotinic acid, isonicotinic acid, isonicotinic acid hydrazide and diethylnicotinamide. These substances were dissolved in Tyrode solution and when necessary the pH was adjusted to 7.8 with sodium hydroxide or hydrochloric acid. Histamine release was measured in rat skin or guinea-pig lung, and the mast cells observed in the mesentery. To study the effect of these compounds on mast cell damage and histamine release by antigen or compound 48—80, rat or guinea-pig tissue samples were incubated for 15 min at 37° C in 4 ml Tyrode solution containing different concentrations of the substances to be tested. After this treatment either antigen or compound 48—80 was added and the tissues incubated for a further period of 15 min at 37° C after which the mesentery was transferred to fixative for mast cell observations while the skin and lung samples were transferred to N hydrochloric acid for histamine extraction. The incubation fluids were acidified with one drop of concentrated hydrochloric acid, boiled and kept at 0° C until assayed. At the end of the experiment, the tested compound was added to the incubation fluids so that all contained the same concentration of the compound. This was done to eliminate any possible interference of the tested compounds with the response of the ileum to histamine during the assay. The results of these experiments showed that mast cell damage and histamine release by antigen from rat or guinea-pig tissues were inhibited alike by all the compounds tested and, on the other hand, the mast cell damage and histamine release by compound 48—80 was inhibited in rat tissues and potentiated in guinea-pig tissues by these same compounds. Diethylnicotinamide was the most effective inhibitor of mast cell damage and histamine release by antigen, followed closely by nicotinamide, while isonicotinic acid hydrazide was the weakest inhibitor of all. The inhibitory effect of these compounds was directly proportional to their concentration as can be seen in Fig. 21. ALIVISATOS (1958) suggested that histamine released in anaphylaxis would combine with DPN, in presence of DPNase, displacing nicotinamide. Thus, it was expected that in presence of nicotinamide, which inhibits this exchange reaction, less histamine would combine with DPN and consequently more histamine would be found in the incubation fluid. However, the above results showed that in presence of nicotinamide much less histamine was released. Actually, it could be speculated that histamine could be ligated to the tissues in such a way that requires the activity of DPNases for its release. However, this hypothesis is complicated by the observation that histamine release by compound 48—80 from guinea-pig tissues is potentiated instead of inhibited. Furthermore, before going deeper into this question and try an explanation for the inhibitory effect of these compounds on the anaphylactic release of histamine, we thought it necessary to find out whether this inhibitory effect was specific to histamine. Thus, we decided to investigate whether the formation of slow reacting substance in anaphylaxis would also be inhibited by several nicotinic and isonicotinic acid derivatives. The experiments concerning slow reacting substance (SRS) were performed like those for histamine release, with the difference, that after incubation, the incubation fluids were removed, kept at 0° C, and SRS immediately assayed. The assay for SRS was carried out on the guinea-pig ileum in the presence of mepyramine 10^{-6} M. The values for SRS are expressed in arbitrary units, referring to a standard sample of Bradykinin. As depicted in

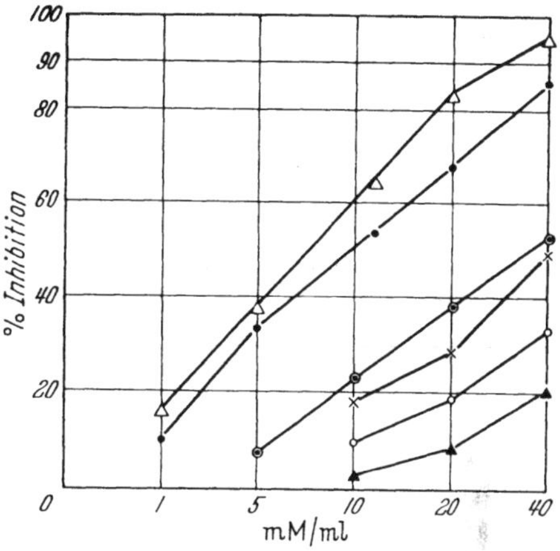

Fig. 21. Effect of different concentrations of pyridine (○——○) and DPN-ase inhibitors (nicotinamide ●——●, nicotinic acid ×——×, diethylnicotinamide △——△, isonicotinic acid hydrazide ▲——▲, isonicotinic acid ⊙——⊙) on histamine release by antigen from guinea-pig lung. Ordinates: % Inhibition was calculated from the difference between the amount of histamine released by antigen plus inhibitor and that released by antigen alone. Abscissae: concentration of inhibitor. Each point is mean of 2 experiments

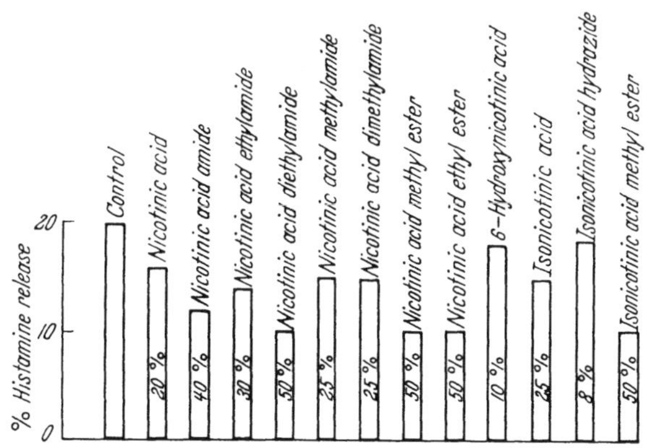

Fig. 22

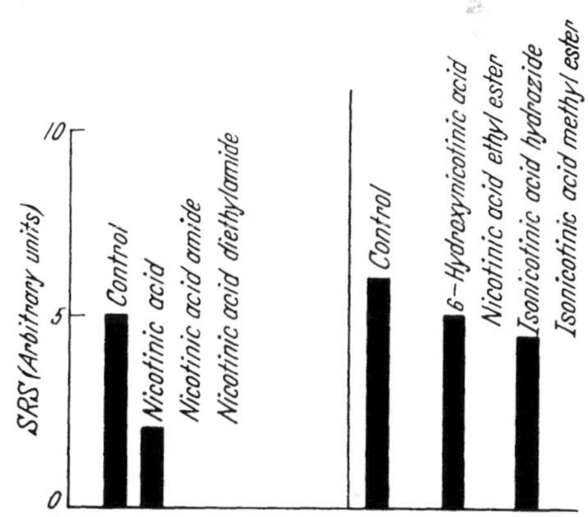

Fig. 23

Fig. 22. Effect of nicotinic acid derivatives on histamine release by antigen from guinea-pig lung

Fig. 23. Effect of nicotinic acid derivatives on formation of SRS induced by antigen-antibody reaction in sensitized guinea-pig lung

Fig. 22 and 23, the results of these experiments showed that all the compounds used inhibited both the release of histamine and the formation of SRS. This fact suggested that the inhibition of the anaphylactic release of histamine by these compounds is not specific to histamine and that these compounds seem to inhibit histamine release in anaphylaxis in a nonspecific manner (MOTA and DIAS DA SILVA, unpublished results). Indeed, according to MOUSSATCHÉ and DANON (1961), nicotinamide and nicotinic acid interfere with the mitochondrial pyridine nucleotides and probably inhibit histamine release in anaphylaxis by affecting cellular metabolism.

During our studies on the release of histamine from the mast cells by antihistamines, it was observed that according to their concentration, these compounds were able to inhibit the anaphylactic mast cell damage and histamine release induced by antigen (MOTA and DIAS DA SILVA, 1960a). In these experiments, sensitized rat or guinea-pig tissues were first incubated for 15 min at 37° C in Tyrode solution containing the antihistamine, washed for 5 min in Tyrode solution and then transferred to Tyrode solution containing antigen. In the experiments with guinea-pig tissues, ovalbumin was added to give a final concentration of 1 mg/ml, and in the experiments with rat tissues, horse serum was added to produce a 10% solution. The tissues were then incubated for a further period of

Table 13. *Effect of antihistamines on histamine release by antigen or compound 48/80.* Sensitized lung tissue was previously incubated with antihistamine, washed in Tyrode solution and transferred to antigen (1 mg/ml) or to compound 48/80 (1 mg/ml). Each figure is the mean of 2 experiments

Antihistamine	Concentration µg/ml	% Histamine release by		% Inhibition
		Antihistamine	antigen	
Bromodiphenhydramine hydrochloride	0	—	36	—
	5	0	34	0
	10	0	37	0
	15	0	31	14
	25	11	25	30
	30	21	23	36
Diphenhydramine hydrochloride	0	—	28	—
	25	0	30	0
	50	0	25	10
	100	11	6	78
	150	39	0	100
	200	49	0	100
Mepyramine hydrogen maleate	0	—	32	—
	25	0	31	0
	50	0	33	0
	100	0	20	38
	200	0	9.5	66
	250	0	0	100
	500	25	0	100
	800	55	0	100
			48/80	% Potentiation
Bromodiphenhydramine hydrochloride	0	—	14	—
	15	9	19	35
	30	26	25	78
Diphenhydramine hydrochloride	0	—	16	—
	100	9	20	25
	150	20	40	150
Mepyramine hydrogen maleate	0	—	16	—
	250	0	25	56
	500	20	28	75

15 min and transferred to hydrochloric acid solution for histamine extraction or to fixative for mast cell observation. At the end of the experiments, histamine was assayed in all the incubation fluids. By means of these control samples, the histamine release by the antihistamine itself, and the histamine released by antigen after previous contact of the tissue with the antihistamine could be determined. The results of these experiments showed that previous contact of sensitized guinea-pig or rat tissues with antihistamines prevents histamine release and mast cell damage induced by later contact with antigen. As can be seen in Table 13, the concentration of antihistamines necessary to produce a total inhibition of histamine release by antigen was very near to the concentration which itself released histamine and the concentration of diphenhydramine and mepyramine able to release histamine by themselves always produced a total inhibition of histamine release by antigen. However, a complete inhibition of histamine release in anaphylaxis with bromodiphenhydramine was never obtained. The minimal concentrations of antihistamines necessary to produce a total inhibition of mast cell reduction by antigen are shown in Table 14. As can be observed there, the concentration of antihistamine necessary for complete prevention of mast cell decrease by antigen was frequently smaller than the concentration necessary for complete

Table 14. *Effect of antihistamines on mast cell damage by antigen or compound 48/80.* Sensitized guinea-pig mesentery was previously incubated with antihistamine, washed in Tyrode solution and transferred to antigen or to compound 48/80

Antihistamine	Concentration μg/ml	% Mast cell diminution by antigen	% Inhibition
Chlorpheniramine maleate	0	50[1]	—
	50	0	100
Bromodiphenhydramine hydrochloride	0	37	—
	12.5	0	100
Isothiopendyl hydrochloride	0	60	—
	25	0	100
Antazoline hydrochloride	0	50	—
	25	0	100
Diphenhydramine hydrochloride	0	37	—
	50	0	100
Methapyrilene hydrochloride	0	68	—
	100	0	100
Mepyramine hydrogen maleate	0	37	—
	200	0	100
Promethazine hydrochloride	0	68	—
	6.25	0	100
Tripelennamine hydrochloride	0	50	—
	100	0	100
Phenindamine hydrogen tartrate	0	68	—
	25	0	100
		% Mast cell diminution by 48/80	**% Potentiation**
Bromodiphenhydramine hydrochloride	0	28	—
	12.5	64	127
Diphenhydramine hydrochloride	0	32	—
	50	76	137
Mepyramine hydrogen maleate	0	48	—
	200	92	91

[1] Mean of 2 experiments.

inhibition of histamine release. For example, 100 μg/ml mepyramine completely prevented a mast cell decrease by antigen but produced only a partial reduction of histamine release. This discrepancy may be due to qualitative alterations of mast cells which were not considered in our measurements, and also to the possible release of histamine from mast cells before any visible morphological change occurs (SMITH, 1958).

As a matter of fact the inhibitory effect of antihistamines on histamine release in anaphylaxis had already been observed by ARUNLAKSHANA (1953b) who considered that the inhibition was due to the release by the antihistamine of a large proportion of the available tissue histamine, and therefore that the residue left for release by antigen was considerably diminished. Our findings, however, suggest that this cannot be the whole explanation. For instance, the histological evidence showing that mast cells fail to be degranulated by the specific antigen after pre-treatment with an antihistamine demonstrates that a true protection is being exerted. Furthermore, there is no evidence that the histamine-releasing property of antihistamines and their property of preventing histamine effects in anaphylaxis are correlated. For example, bromodiphenhydramine in a concentration that released histamine by itself did not completely inhibit histamine release in anaphylaxis, whereas mepyramine completely blocked histamine release by antigen in concentrations which did not by themselves release histamine. Furthermore, compound 48—80 in a concentration which released a small amount of histamine does not inhibit but, on the contrary, potentiates an anaphylactic histamine release (MONGAR and SCHILD, 1952). The mechanism of the inhibitory effect of antihistamines on the anaphylactic mast cell damage and histamine release is not yet known. It is possible that antihistamine molecules in a critical concentration near to that required for histamine release become attached to the mast cell membrane and interfere with the antigen-antibody reaction. Alternatively they may inhibit the enzymatic system required in the anaphylactic reaction (MONGAR and SCHILD, 1957a). The inhibition of histamine release in anaphylaxis by antihistamines may help to explain the protective effect of these drugs in anaphylaxis. In some cases, at least, the protection may be due more to inhibition of cellular damage than to competition at the receptor site. This, however, probably does not apply to the protective effect exerted by antihistamines in the anaphylactic shock of the intact guinea-pig, as concentrations of antihistamines necessary to inhibit histamine release *in vitro* are much higher than those likely to be obtained by protective doses of antihistamines *in vivo*. On the other hand it is possible that the reduction in passive cutaneous anaphylaxis by high doses of antihistamines in rats (BROCKLEHURST, HUMPHREY and PERRY, 1955) may be due in part to the anti-anaphylactic effect of such doses of antihistamines. The inhibition of histamine release may possibly be attended by a simultaneous inhibition of the release of other pharmacologically active substances, since BROCKLEHURST (1958) and CHAKRAVARTY (1959, 1960) have shown that inhibition of histamine release in anaphylaxis is usually accompanied by inhibition of SRS formation. The so-called unspecific effects of antihistamines in isolated tissues (HAWKINS and ROSA, 1956) may also be explained, at least partially, by their anti-anaphylactic effect.

As a protective agent in anaphylaxis, mepyramine seems to be safer than bromodiphenhydramine or diphenhydramine as the ratio between its protective concentration and the concentration that releases histamine is greater. Mepyramine may owe its strong anti-anaphylactic effect to the pyridine nucleus in its molecule. Indeed, since many pyridine derivatives are able to inhibit histamine release by antigen without releasing histamine by themselves (MOTA, DIAS DA SILVA and

FERNANDES, 1960), it may be possible to produce an antihistamine molecule able to inhibit anaphylaxis without being a histamine releaser. This would be a safer antihistamine than the present ones.

The inhibition of the anaphylactic release of histamine from chopped guinea-pig lung by chymotrypsin substrates and inhibitors was recently studied by AUSTEN and BROCKLEHURST (1960, 1961). The authors used sensitized guinea-pig lung chopped into rods 0.4 × 0.4 × 50 mm, washed with Tyrode solution at 23° C and divided in samples of approximately 100 mg wet weight. These were incubated in Tyrode solution at 37° C for 45 min with continuous agitation and then washed twice with Tyrode solution at 37° C. Washing was carried out by removing the supernatant fluid through a filter formed by nylon tuft and replacing it with fresh warm Tyrode solution. Immediately after the second wash each sample of tissue was immersed in 3.0 ml warm Tyrode solution with or without the potential inhibitor. Ten seconds later the antigen, 1.0 mg ovalbumin or 3.0 mg bovine gamma globulin per ml reaction mixture was added. After rocking for 15 min at 37° C, the supernatant fluid was removed from the tissues and kept at 0° C until assayed on the same day using the isolated guinea-pig ileum. Under these conditions, the authors observed that the anaphylactic release of histamine in the guinea-pig is prevented by chymotrypsin inhibitors and substrates but not by trypsin, carboxypeptidase or leucine aminopeptidase substrates and concluded that activation of a chymotrypsinlike enzyme is a necessary condition for the anaphylactic release of histamine. In the light of these observations, it is worthwhile to recall that probably most of the histamine released in anaphylaxis comes from the mast cells (MOTA and VUGMAN, 1956a, b) and that rat mast cells are very rich in a chymotrypsin-like enzyme that is inhibited by diisopropylfluorophosphate (BENDITT and ARASE, 1959). Therefore it is possible that, at least some of the inhibitors used by these authors were interfering with the enzymatic equipment of the mast cells. Unfortunately it is not yet known whether guinea-pig mast cells, like rat mast cells, contain a chymotrypsin-like enzyme too.

VI. The mechanism of the anaphylactic release of histamine from the mast cells

It is well known that the anaphylactic phenomenon can be considered as a sequence of reactions starting by the union of antigen with antibody and having as one of its many consequences the release of histamine. In this respect it is closely related with the response of sensitized mast cells to antigen in most of the species. Nothwithstanding a great volume of research in the field there is not yet a comprehensive explanation for the mechanism of histamine release by antigen. Although anaphylaxis can be considered as depending primarily upon the specific interaction between antigen and antibody it is certainly in the area of the biochemical changes following the reaction of antigen with antibody where the mechanism of histamine release is likely to be found. In the investigation of the mechanism of histamine release it was thought that the study of the inhibition of histamine release by chemical compounds of known properties could possibly contribute to clear up this issue. However, it was soon observed that inhibition of histamine release could be obtained with a large number of unrelated substances and that most of the substances able to inhibit histamine release in anaphylaxis depressed the cellular functions in a general way, and so, only indirectly the histamine-releasing mechanism. In this respect a clear distinction between the specific and the non-specific inhibitors of the anaphylactic phenomenon leading to histamine release is needed. However, the investigations on the inhibition of the anaphylactic release of histamine, have contributed to reveal certain aspects of these phenomena. For instance, the experiments with phenol showed that the release of histamine from the mast cells by antigen is not a direct consequence of the antigen-antibody reaction but that the union of antigen with antibody only triggers off a complexe series of events leading to mast cell damage and histamine release (MONGAR and SCHILD, 1957a, b; MOTA, 1959a). On the other hand some substances able to inhibit histamine release from the mast cells, as N-ethylmaleimide (MOTA, 1959b; MOTA and ISHII, 1960) probably is not acting on an antigen-antibody activated enzyme as even when the tissue is washed repeatedly after contact with this substance the anaphylactic release of histamine is still prevented (AUSTEN and BROCKLEHURST, 1961).

Furthermore, the inhibition of the anaphylactic release of histamine from the mast cells by various metabolic inhibitors and its dependence on pH and temperature (MONGAR and SCHILD, 1957a, b; MOTA, 1958a, 1959a, b; MOTA and ISHII, 1960; CHAKRAVARTY, 1959, 1960) strongly suggested the existence of an enzymatic mechanism in this phenomenon. Actually, as far back as 1914, JOBLING and PETERSEN advanced the hypothesis that a proteolytic enzyme was activated and that this activated enzyme caused the cellular damage. Since then this hypothesis have been backed up by other workers (ROCHA e SILVA, 1941; UNGAR, 1953). Indeed, as stated by UNGAR and HAYASHI (1958) it is almost a platitude to assume that enzymes must play a role in allergic phenomena since the rate of chemical processes in living matter is controlled by enzymes. The same seems to hold true for the mast cell damage by antigen. The difficult thing here is to determine the precise nature of these enzymes and how they are triggered off by the antigen-antibody reaction. For instance, it is known that the mast cell granules are of a lipidic-proteic nature (HEDBOM and SNELLMAN, 1955) and their quick disappearance subsequent and consequent to the antigen-antibody reaction is strongly suggestive of an enzymatic reaction (MOTA, 1958a, 1959a). However, the clearing up of this problem depends largely on the advance of our biochemical knowledge of how is histamine bound to the tissues, particularly to mast cell granules. In this respect the findings of BENDITT and ARASE (1959) are very suggestive. These authors working with isolated mast cells demonstrated the presence in these cells of an enzymatic activity showing a striking similarity to that of alpha-chymotrypsin. Thus, both chymotrypsin and the mast cell enzyme were able to split the synthetic substrate 3-chloroacetoxy-2-naphthoic acid anilide and hydrolyzed the N-acetylated ethyl esters of tryptophan and tyrosine, which are typical chymotrypsin substrates. Furthermore, they also observed that both enzymes were inhibited to the same extent by several different concentrations of diisopropylfluorophosphate. Actually, the mast cell chymotrypsin-like enzyme had already been histochemically demonstrated in the mast cells of the rat, mouse, rabbit, dog and man by GOMORI (1953). The probable implication of this enzyme in the anaphylactic release of histamine from the mast cells is suggested by the more recent observations of AUSTEN and BROCKLEHURST (1961) showing that chymotrypsin inhibitors and substrates inhibit the anaphylactic release of histamine. However, the mechanism leading to the anaphylactic release of histamine from the mast cells is possibly multiple and involving the activation of more than one enzyme. For instance, the discovery of a heat-labile factor in the tissues, probably a pro-enzyme that requires calcium for its activation (MONGAR and SCHILD, 1957b, 1958) and is necessary for the anaphylactic release of histamine, suggested the participation of complement in this phenomenon. Further suggestion to this was the observation that diisopropylfluorophosphate, that inhibits the hemolytic activity of complement (LEVINE, 1955; BECKER, 1956) is also capable of inhibiting the anaphylactic release of histamine (AUSTEN and BROCKLEHURST, 1961). However, in spite of observations in favour of the participation of complement in anaphylaxis (see for instance, BECKER, 1957, 1959) there is not yet evidence that complement is necessary for the anaphylactic release of histamine from the mast cells. The fact that complement may be necessary for the anaphylactic release of histamine from rabbit platelets (HUMPHREY and JAQUES, 1955) or for the production of passive cutaneous anaphylaxis in rats (OSLER, HAWRISIAK, OVARY, SIQUEIRA and BIER, 1957) does not imply that complement is necessarily involved in the anaphylactic release of histamine from the mast cells since these cells are not involved in those conditions. Thus, in spite of some similarity between the anaphylactic release of histamine from mast cells and leakage of hemoglobin from red cells in immune hemolysis the two processes do not seem to be alike. According to AUSTEN and BROCKLEHURST (1961) there are at least six points of difference between anaphylaxis (that is, histamine release) in guinea-pig lung and immune hemolysis;

1) Thiols such as cysteine, thioglycollic acid and reduced glutathione inhibit immune hemolysis and the esterase activity of the first component of complement but do not inhibit anaphylaxis;

2) Iodoacetate does not inhibit immune hemolysis but iodoacetate and several thiol oxidizing agents produce irreversible changes which prevent anaphylaxis (iodoacetate also inhibits guinea-pig mast cell damage by antigen (MOTA, 1959a);

3) Esters of basic amino acids such as arginine and lysine inhibit immune hemolysis, but do not inhibit anaphylaxis;

4) Peptides with a terminal aromatic amino acid exhibiting a free carboxyl group, i.e. carboxypeptidase substrates, inhibit immune hemolysis but do not prevent anaphylaxis;

5) Potassium cyanide does not prevent immune hemolysis but does inhibit the anaphylactic release of histamine;

6) Phenylacetic acid does not inhibit immune hemolysis but inhibits the antigen-induced histamine release.

Another factor necessary for the anaphylactic release of histamine is cellular integrity. Indeed, as shown by COPENHAVER, NAGLER and GOTH (1953), MONGAR and SCHILD (1956), and MACINTOSH (1956), histamine release from intracellular particles can be demonstrated only when antigen is applied to intact cells, but not when it is added to isolated intracellular particles. Noteworthy too is the fact that these authors failed to passively sensitize intracellular particles showing that cellular integrity is also necessary for sensitization. Damage to the cellular membrane may be the principal factor responsible for this fact. In fact we have observed that when sensitized guinea-pig mesentery is stretched producing mast cell disruption, the disrupted mast cells do not respond to later contact with antigen. Furthermore, the fact that desensitization of the mast cells occurs on contact with antigen in the cold (MOTA, 1959a; HUMPHREY and MOTA, 1959a), implies that active uptake of antigen-antibody reaction occurs since large molecules would not diffuse into a living cell. Thus, attachment of antibodies to the cells and their union with the specific antigen must then occur on the cellular membrane. However, it is known that histamine is located in the mast cell granules (MOTA, BERALDO, FERRI and JUNQUEIRA, 1954; WEST, 1955; HAGEN, BARRNETT and FU-LI LEE, 1959) and therefore, the union of antigen with antibody on the mast cell membrane must trigger off an enzymatic mechanism able to release histamine from the intracellular mast granules. Actually the existence of a lytic enzyme on the mast cell membrane has been postulated by HÖGBERG and UVNÄS (1957, 1960). That the cell surface is an important regulator of enzymic processes occurring within the cell is well known (see for instance, Best, 1960), however the manner through which the regulation is accomplished is not yet known. Probably both membrane and intracellular enzymes are involved in the anaphylactic release of histamine from the mast cells. Furthermore, the probability cannot be ruled out that pinocytosis can be involved in the anaphylactic damage to mast cells. In fact, many different types of cells, and probably the mast cells, present very active membranous movements that produce invaginations which frequently pinch off inside the cell to form vesicles. Thus, antigen-antibody aggregates formed on the cell surface may, by this way, enter the cells.

A. Type and location of antibodies involved in mast cell damage by antigen

The experiments described here have shown that mast cell damage by antigen invariably occurs in those circumstances in which an anaphylactic release of histamine is produced in actively sensitized rats, mice and guinea-pigs. On the other hand, while these same phenomena are easily duplicated in anaphylaxis of passively sensitized guinea-pigs, they are hardly observed in anaphylaxis of passively sensitized rats and mice. The observation that in passively sensitized guinea-pigs the mast cell reaction to antigen was rather uniform and graded with the dose of antibody (Humphrey and Mota, 1959a) suggested that the large variation observed in actively sensitized guinea-pigs could be due to variation in the relatively small amount of antibodies produced by them. Alternatively, some variation in the quality of antibody was considered, e.g. a difference between precipitating and non-precipitating antibody. However, the studies of Kabat and Boldt (1944) and of Kabat and Benacerraf (1949) showed that precipitating and non-precipitating antibodies were equally efficient to passively sensitize guinea-pigs. To the same conclusion pointed out our experiments on the behaviour of guinea-pig mast cells in passive anaphylaxis (Humphrey and Mota, 1959a). However, our experiments with rats (Mota, 1961, 1962) strongly suggested that passive sensitization of rats with rabbit or even with homologous *precipitating antibodies* obtained after multiple antigen injections does not duplicate the full picture of active anaphylaxis, in this species, especially when *B. pertussis* is used as adjuvant. Thus, after passive sensitization *in vivo* or *in vitro*, contact of rat tissues with the specific antigen did not lead to mast cell damage or histamine release such as occurs in actively sensitized rats, and the same was also observed when mice were passively sensitized with rabbit antibodies. Furthermore, passive anaphylaxis failed to produce mast cell damage or histamine release even in rats that had been actively sensitized to a separate antigen together with *B. pertussis* and whose tissues were able to respond with mast cell damage and histamine release on contact with this antigen. In this respect it is worth noticing the fact that passive sensitization of rats with rabbit antiserum sensitizes their tissues so that the uterus will present an anaphylactic contraction when in contact with antigen but no mast cell damage or histamine release occur when other tissues of the same animal are incubated with antigen. These results are in striking contrast with what happens in passively sensitized guinea-pigs in which contact with antigen duplicates the mast cell damage as seen in active anaphylaxis. However, there is no doubt that passively sensitized rats and mice present symptoms resembling those of actively sensitized animals when challenged with antigen. Furthermore it must be emphasized that although *pertussis*-treated mice and adrenalectomized rats can present fatal passive anaphylaxis, the picture differs from fatal active anaphylaxis in that mast cell damage and histamine release is only very exceptionally found in the former, while both phenomena are a constant finding in the latter. To sum up, all those findings have suggested that in active sensitization in rats there must be some operative factor or condition, not reproducible in passive sensitization with rabbit or rat precipitating antibodies. An easy explanation for this fact would be to invoke the production by actively sensitized rats and mice of a non-precipitating type of antibodies responsible for mast cell lysis and histamine release on reaction with antigen. For instance while on one hand, mast cell damage and histamine release are very much increased in anaphylaxis of *pertussis*-treated rats which produce very little precipitating antibodies, on the other hand both these phenomena may be very reduced in rats chronically immunized with FREUND's adjuvant having considerable amount of circulating precipitating antibodies. Actually, rats sensitized with FREUND's adjuvant seem to be able to produce both types of antibodies since some of these animals present marked mast cell damage and histamine release when challenged with antigen while others do not. However, this seems to keep no relation with the amount of precipitating antibodies produced by the animal. Thus, there is a dissociation between the amount of precipitating antibodies produced by immunized rats and the induction of mast cell damage by antigen in anaphylaxis. Therefore, as a provisory working-hypothesis we think that rat anaphylaxis is brought about by two different antigen-antibody reactions: a) the reaction of antigen with the usual type of precipitating antibodies found in serum after repeated injections of antigen – that do not cause mast cell damage – and b) the reaction of antigen with "mast cell lytic antibodies" which are responsible for the anaphylactic release of histamine. It seems that rats will produce normally both types of antibodies and that depending upon the condition of immunization each one of these types of antibody would predominate over the other. Thus, rats immunized with multiple injections of antigen in FREUND's adjuvant would produce predominantly antibodies unable to produce mast cell damage on later reaction with antigen, while rats injected with *B. pertussis* along with the sensitizing dose of antigen would produce predominantly "mast cell lytic antibodies." However, one has to postulate that the "mast cell lytic antibodies" would not always attain an adequate concentration in the serum to produce passive sensitization for explaining the repeated failure of serum taken from fully sensitized *pertussis*-treated rats to passively sensitive rat tissues either in vivo or in vitro (MOTA, 1962). However, it should be expected that mast cell damage and histamine release could possibly be obtained in passively sensitized rats provided the "mast cell lytic antibodies" could be used for inducing passive sensitization. Indeed, very recently I have succeeded in obtaining sera from immunized rats which are able to passively sensitize rat mast cells, although I have not yet been able to determine the conditions needed for the appearance of the "mast cell lytic antibodies" in serum of immunized rats. So far, it seems that these antibodies appear very early in the course of immunization and then disappear or lose their property of causing mast cell damage and histamine release on reaction with antigen. They are probably different from serum precipitating antibodies obtained after repeated injections of antigen in FREUND's adjuvant since rat antibodies obtained in that way do not sensitize rat mast cells so as to induce histamine release on later contact with antigen. Furthermore I have observed that the "mast cell lytic antibodies" are destroyed by heating at 56 C., a fact that suggests that these antibodies may be similar to human reagins which are also thermolabile antibodies. Another similarity to human reagins is suggested by the observation that when intradermally injected into rat skin these antibodies will remain at the injection site for at least 30 days, a fact in striking contrast with the behavior of rabbit or rat precipitating antibodies which do not stay in the injection site for more than 24 hours (MOTA, 1963).

It is a matter of considerable interest to know whether the "mast cell lytic antibody" is specific to these cells. So far there is no theoretical basis to support this possibility. However, we have observed that when "mast cell lytic antibody" is injected into several rat tissues (subcutaneous, splenic, hepatic, renal, intestinal and in the lingual or abdominal muscle) fixation of this antibody, as revealed by a later local anaphylactic reaction, occurs only in those tissues containing mast cells. This, it seems quite probable that rat anaphylaxis is brought about by two different species of antibodies, one of which, here provisionally called "mast cell lytic antibodies," is much more effective in causing anaphylactic cell damage than the other.

Since mast cells are so regularly damaged in all circumstances in which histamine is released in anaphylaxis, it is a matter of considerable interest to know where in a tissue the antigen-antibody reaction must take place to produce this effect. The very conspicuous alterations presented by the mast cell in rat anaphylaxis led us to propose the hypothesis that mast cells might contain antibodies (Mota, 1957) and later on Humphrey and Mota (1959a) produced more convincing arguments suggesting that the union of antigen with antibody must take place in, or very near to, the mast cells. In the first place, the experiments with Forssman antibody showed that combination of antigen with antibody on or in cells, under circumstances in which cell damage is undoubtedly produced, does not necessarily cause mast cell degranulation. In this case, owing to the restricted localization of the antigen (Tanaka and Leduc, 1956) the antigen-antibody reaction must have occurred preferentially at the endothelial cells of blood vessels, and yet no changes occurred in the mast cell, even though many of these were situated only a few micra away. In the second place was considered the observation that antibodies against normal guinea-pig gamma-globulin cause mast cell alterations similar to those induced by antigen in sensitized guinea-pigs. These results were interpreted as strongly suggestive that antibodies were adsorbed on the mast cells. Our later results showing that washed isolated mast cells taken from sensitized animals were still able to respond to the specific antigen (Mota and Dias da Silva, 1960b) showed that mast cells contain antibodies and that damage induced to these cells in anaphylaxis is the consequence of an antigen-antibody reaction occurring in the mast cell itself.

B. Role of mast cells in anaphylaxis

The anaphylactic phenomenon is very probably the result of antigen-antibody reactions involving different sensitized cells and causing multiple responses according to the types of cells involved in the reaction. There should exist then for each type of cell a specific anaphylactic response depending upon the physiological characteristic of the cell hit by the antigen-antibody reaction. In this sense a sensitized muscle fiber will contract on reaction with antigen and a mast cell will release its stores of pharmacologically active substances. To consider properly the role of mast cells in anaphylaxis one has firstly to define the criterium by which anaphylaxis is been judged. For instance, when anaphylaxis is judged by histamine release, it is quite probable that one is studying the mast cell response to antigen. Indeed, the histamine released by antigen from most tissues is probably originated from the mast cells in most species but the known exception of rabbit blood, in which histamine is probably originated from platelets (Humphrey and Jaques, 1954, 1955). The contribution of the basophils, which are the richest histamine-containing blood cells (Graham et al., 1952) to the anaphylactic release of histamine from rabbit blood is still to be determined. On the other hand when one considers the generalized anaphylactic syndrome evoked by injection of antigen into circulation of a sensitized animal, the role of the mast cell in this phenomenon, will depend upon the sensitivity of the tissues of the species concerned to the pharmacologically active substances released from these cells. In this case there seems to be a great difference in the role played by the mast cells in the several species, particularly between guinea-pigs and rats. In guinea-pig anaphylaxis, due to the high sensitivity of this species to histamine, mast cells probably play a role as important as histamine does. However, this is not to say that direct damage to other cells cannot also be responsible for anaphylaxis in guinea-pigs. Unfortunately, since there is not yet a mean of depleting guinea-pigs of their tissue mast cell population, no definitive experiment could be done to see whether guinea-pigs depleted of their mast cell population and histamine would present anaphylaxis. However, the fact that Forssman antibody which produces an antigen-antibody reaction not leading to mast cell damage and histamine release is by itself capable of killing guinea-pigs, suggests that well sensitized guinea-pigs would probably suffer anaphylaxis even in absence of mast cells and histamine. In normal guinea-pigs, however, these cells are probably important due to the high sensitivity of the bronchial muscles of this species to histamine.

In 1957 (Mota, 1957), having observed that antigen induced mast cell damage and plasma histamine increase in sensitized rats, and that antihistamines and pre-treatment with compound 48—80 protected rats against anaphylaxis, we concluded that mast cells and histamine played an important role in rat anaphylaxis. However, the protection then observed was probably due to the fact the animals used in those experiments were poorly sensitized. Indeed, later on, Sanyal and West (1958) working with fully sensitized *pertussis*-treated rats did not observe any protection against anaphylaxis either by pre-treatment with mepyramine, BOL-148, both these substances together, or by depletion of tissue histamine and 5-hydroxytryptamine by polymyxin B or reserpine. In fact, we have duplicated and confirmed these results as well as our previous observation that there is generalized mast cell disruption and histamine release in rat anaphylaxis. Thus, we have observed that in *pertussis*-treated rats neither antihistamines, nor antagonists of 5-hydroxytryptamine, nor both together, nor depletion of the mast cell population by repeacted injections of compound 48—80 was able to protect rats from death caused by anaphylaxis. However, it must be pointed out that while the control non-treated shocked rats became prostrated in 3—6 min after antigen injection and died within half an hour to 4 hours, the animals receiving antihistamines or antagonists of 5-hydroxytryptamine became prostrated only half an hour after antigen injection and died within 5 hours or overnight. Thus it seems as if pre-treatment with mepyramine and BOL-148 has protected these animals against a first immediate stage of the anaphylactic reaction but not against a second later. More recently when studying active cutaneous anaphylaxis in *pertussis*-treated sensitized rats we have observed that such animals respond to intradermically injected antigen with a two-stage reaction. A first stage represented by a transient immediate reaction that can be abolished by pretreatment with antihistamines and anti-5-hydrotryptamines and a second stage represented by a later reaction on which antagonists of histamine and 5-hydroxytryptamine have no effect. The first stage can be reproduced by injection of antiserum containing "mast cell lytic antibody" but the same antiserum does not duplicate the second stage. These results suggest that anaphylaxis in rats sensitized with *pertussis* plus antigen is probably a mixture of two reactions represented by an immediate and a delayed type of hypersensitivity. Indeed the presence of a delayed type of hypersensitivity in rats injected with *B. pertussis* subcutaneously in the footpad have already been reported by ROWLEY et al. (1959). Whether there is any association between the production of "mast cell lytic antibody and the production of a delayed hypersensitivity is now being investigated. Recently, GARCIA-AROCHA (1961a, b) observed that 5-hydroxytryptamine and histamine are released when antigen is added to peritoneal cell suspensions or to the fluid perfusing the small intestine or the hindquarters of sensitized rats (see Figs. 24 and 25). Contrarily to ours and WEST's results, this author observed that treatment with either the combination of mepyramine with BOL-148 or with chlorpromazine resulted in substancially complete protection of 25% of the animals and partial protection of 75% of the other. However, this author observed the animals for a period of only 3 hours and this fact may explain his results. He concluded that white the possibility cannot be excluded that factors other than 5-hydroxytryptamine participate in rat anaphylaxis, the evidence strongly favors the conclusion that each of these amines plays an important role. Actually, the existence of other factors, besides histamine and 5-hydroxytryptamine, responsible for the anaphylactic reaction in rats had been strongly suggested by the previous papers of ROCHA E SILVA and ROTHSCHILD (1955) and BROCKLEHURST, HUMPHREY and PERRY (1955, 1960). These authors observed that rats deplected of skin histamine and 5-hydroxytryptamine and pretreated with mepyramine and dibromolysergic acid diethylamide, still showed a strongly positive passive cutaneous anaphylaxis. ROCHA E SILVA and ROTHSCHILD (1955) stated that either one has to postulated different mechanisms for the release of histamine by histamine liberators and by the antigen-antibody reaction or some other substance is released in rat skin under the action of the anaphylactic reaction. In fact, it is possible that while compound 48—80 acts chiefly through liberation of histamine and 5-hydroxytryptamine from mast cells, the reaction of antigen with antibody in rat passive cutaneous anaphylaxis does not involve release of histamine or 5-hydroxytryptamine as we have observed that there is no mast cell damage in passive cutaneous anaphylaxis in rats (MOTA, unpublished). There is no wonder in this since rabbit or rat precipitating antibodies do not cause mast cell damage on reaction with antigen (MOTA, 1962). It is, perhaps, possible that direct damage to endothelial cells can account for the increased capillary permeability in passive cutaneous anaphylaxis. On the other hand, we have observed

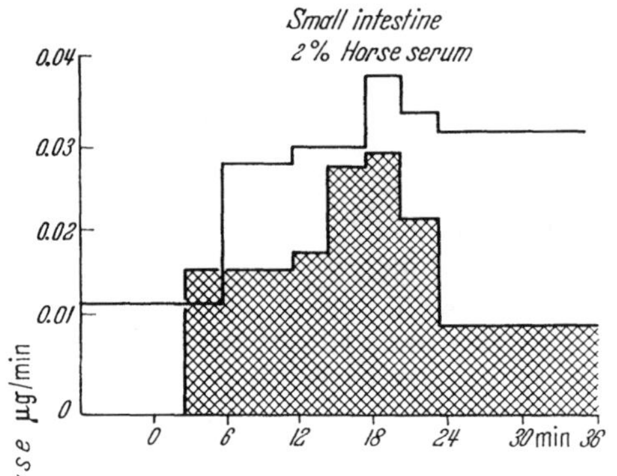

Fig. 24

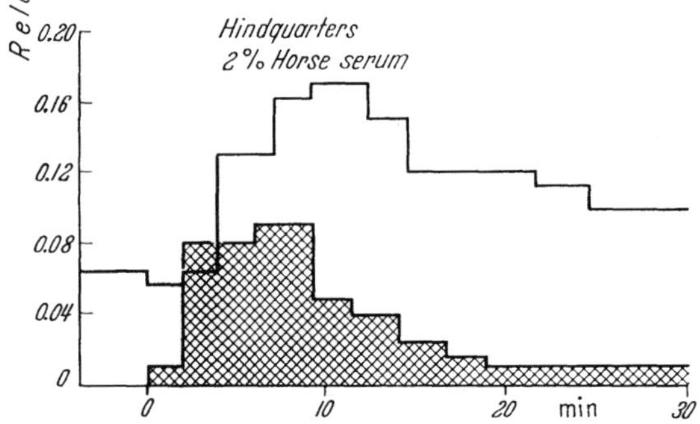

Fig. 25

Fig. 24. Small intestine from sensitized rat. At 0 time perfusion was transferred from Locke's solution to Locke's solution containing 2% horse serum. The discharge of 5-HT preceded that of histamine. Open blocks = histamine; shaded blocks = 5-HT

Fig. 25. Hindquarters from sensitized rat. At 0 time perfusion was transferred from Locke's solution to Locke's solution containing 2% horse serum. Output of 5-HT started before that of histamine. Open blocks = histamine; shaded blocks = 5-HT generalized mast cell damage in active cutaneous anaphylaxis in both rats and guinea-pigs (MOTA, unpublished), where histamine and other substances released from mast cells probably contribute somehow to the reaction. Indeed I have observed that the role played by histamine and 5-hydroxytryptamine in a cutaneous antigen-antibody reaction seems to be dependent upon the type of antibody involved in this reaction, since while passive cutaneous anaphylaxis induced with precipitating antibody is not modified by mepyramine and BOL-148, passive cutaneous anaphylaxis induced with "mast cell lytic antibody" can be completely prevented by pre-treatment with mepyramine and BOL-148. It may be worthwhile to mention that it is our experience that only rats sensitized so as to show mast cell disruption and histamine release on contact with antigen present severe anaphylaxis. It seems, therefore, that the conditions necessary to induce an effective sensitization in rats, so as to produce a severe and frequently fatal anaphylaxis, are the same, or at least are coexistent with, those conditions leading to mast cell damage. This means that mast cell damage by antigen can be used as criterium of effectiveness of active sensitization in rats, although these cells by themselves may not play an important role in anaphylaxis of this species. In conclusion, so far as we can judge from evidence which is by no means yet so complete as we would like it to be, the mast cells play a very important role in guinea-pig anaphylaxis, due to the known high sensitivity of this species to histamine, but probably an insignificant role in rat anaphylaxis due to the low sensitivity of this species to histamine and 5-hydroxytryptamine. Nevertheless, in both species the reaction of antigen with antibodies fixed on the mast cells will induce damage to these cells which by an yet unknown mechanism causes histamine liberation.

References

ALIVISATOS, S. G. A.: Formation of histamine-containing dinucleotides by enzymatic interaction of histamine and coenzyme I. Nature (Lond.) **181**, 271 (1958).

AREY, L. B.: Throttling veins in the liver of certain mammals. Anat. Rec. **81**, 21 (1941).

ARUNLAKSHANA, O.: Histamine release by antihistamines. J. Physiol. (Lond.) **119**, 47 P (1953a).

— Studies of the release, potentiation and antagonism of histamine. Ph. D. Thesis: University of London (1953b).

ARVY, L., et D. QUIVY: Taux des labrocytes et coagulabilité sanguine chez le chien au cours de divers chocs. C. R. Soc. Biol. (Paris) **149**, 481 (1955).

AUSTEN, K. F., and W. E. BROCKLEHURST: Inhibition of the anaphylactic release of histamine from chopped guinea- pig lung by chymotrypsin substrates and inhibitors. Nature (Lond.) **186**, 866 (1960).

— — Anaphylaxis in chopped guinea-pig lung. I. Effect of peptidase substrates and inhibitors. J. exp. Med. **113**, 521 (1961).

—, and J. H. HUMPHREY: Release of histamine from rat peritoneal mast cell by antibody against rat γ-globulin. J. Physiol. (Lond.) **158**, 36 P (1961).

BALTZLY, R., J. S. BUCK, E. J. DE BEER and F. J. WEBB: A family of long acting depressors. J. Amer. chem. Soc. **71**, 1301 (1949).

BAUER, W., H. H. DALE, L. T. POULSSON and D. W. RICHARDS: The control of circulation through the liver. J. Physiol. (Lond.) **74**, 343 (1932).

BECKER, E. L.: Concerning the mechanism of complement action. I. Inhibition of complement activity by diisopropylfluorophosphate. J. Immunol. **77**, 462 (1956).

— Hypersensitivity. J. cell. comp. Physiol. **50**, 303 (1957).

— *In vitro* models for the allergic reaction. In Mechanisms of hypersensitivity. Boston: Little, Brown & Company 1959.

BENACERRAF, B., and E. A. KABAT: A quantitative study of passive anaphylaxis. V. The latent period in passive anaphylaxis and its relation to the dose of rabbit antiovalbumin. J. Immunol. **62**, 517 (1949).

BENDITT, E. P., and M. ARASE: An enzyme in mast cells with properties like chymotrypsin. J. exp. Med. **110**, 451 (1959).

— — S. BADER, C. CORLEY and K. B. LAM: Relationship of mast cells and histamine to mechanism of edema production by ovomucoid in rats. Fed. Proc. **13**, 422 (1954).

BENDITT, E. P. and S. BADER and K. B. LAM: Studies of the mechanism of acute vascular reactions to injury. I. The relationship of mast cells and histamine to the production of edema by ovomucoid in rats. Arch. Path. **60**, 104 (1955).
— R. L. WONG, M. ARASE and E. ROEPER: 5-Hydroxytryptamine in mast cells. Proc. Soc. exp. Biol. (N. Y.) **90**, 303 (1955).
BERALDO, W. T., and W. DIAS DA SILVA: Histamine release and mast cell damage induced by a purified fraction obtained from Ascaris extract. Cienc. e Cult. **12**, 100 (1960).
BEST, J. B.: Enzymic processes in cells. Int. Rev. Cytol. **9**, 129 (1960).
BHATTACHARYA, B. K., and G. P. LEWIS: The release of 5-hydroxytryptamine by histamine liberators. Brit. J. Pharmacol. **11**, 202 (1956).
BIER, O. G.: Cited in ROCHA E SILVA and GRAÑA (1946a).
BOREUS, L. O.: A comparison of mast cell reactions in the rat, hamster and guinea-pig. Acta physiol. scand. **49**, 251 (1960a).
— A study of the anaphylactic mast cell reaction *in vivo* following desensitization of sensitized guinea-pigs. Acta physiol. scand. **50**, 375 (1960b).
— Quantitative studies on the anaphylactic mast cell reaction *in vivo* in the guinea-pig. Acta physiol. scand. **48**, 431 (1960c).
—, and N. CHAKRAVARTY: The histamine content of guinea-pig mast cells. Experientia (Basel) **16**, 192 (1960a).
— — Tissue mast cells, histamine and "slow reacting substance" in anaphylactic reaction in guinea-pig. Acta physiol. scand. **48**, 315 (1960b).
BROCKLEHURST, W. E.: Histamine and other mediators in hypersensitivity reactions. IIIrd International Congress of Allergology. Paris: Flammarion 1958.
— J. H. HUMPHREY and W. L. M. PERRY: The role of histamine in cutaneous antigen-antibody reactions in the rat. J. Physiol. (Lond.) **129**, 205 (1955).
— — — Cutaneous antigen-antibody reactions in the rat. J. Physiol. (Lond.) **150**, 489 (1960).
BUSHBY, S. R., and A. F. GREEN: The release of histamine by polymyxin B and polymyxin E. Brit. J. Pharmacol. **10**, 215 (1955).
CARTER, P. B., R. D. HIGGINBOTHAM and R. D. DOUGHERTY: The local response of tissue mast cell to antigen in sensitized mice. J. Immunol. **79**, 259 (1957).
CASS, R., J. F. RILEY, G. B. WEST, K. W. HEAD and S. W. STROUD: Heparin and histamine in mast cell tumours from dogs. Nature. (Lond.) **174**, 318 (1954).
CHAKRAVARTY, N.: Observations on histamine release and formation of a lipid-soluble smooth-muscle stimulating principle (SRS) by antigen-antibody reaction and compound 48—80. Thesis, Karolinska Institutet, Stockholm, Sweden (1959).
— The mechanism of histamine release in anaphylactic reaction in guinea-pig and rat. Acta physiol. scand. **48**, 146 (1960).
CODE, C. F.: The quantitative estimation of histamine in the blood. J. Physiol. (Lond.) **89**, 257 (1937).
— The histamine content of the blood of guinea-pig and dogs during anaphylactic shock. Amer. J. Physiol. **127**, 78 (1939).
— D. T. CODY, M. HURN, J. C. KENNEDY and M. J. STRICKLAND: The simultaneous release of histamine and a histamine-destroying factor during anaphylaxis in rats. J. Physiol. (Lond.) **156**, 207 (1961).
COPENHAVER, J. H., M. E. NAGLER and A. GOTH: The intracellular distribution of histamine. J. Pharmacol. **109**, 401 (1953).
DALE, H. H.: The anaphylactic reaction of plain muscle in the guinea-pig. J. Pharmacol. **4**, 167 (1913).
DIAS DA SILVA, W.: The behaviour of mast cell in guinea-pig anaphylaxis: the effect of anti-histamines. M. D. Thesis, Universidade de Minas Gerais, Brasil (1960).
— W. T. BERALDO and J. PUDLES: Histamine release and mast cell damage by purified Ascaris fraction *in vitro*. Its mechanism of action. Brit. J. Pharmacol. **17**, 236 (1961).
EHRLICH, P.: 1877. Cited in MICHELS, N. A., The mast cells. In, H. DOWNEY, Handbook of Haematology **1**, 232 (1938).
ELDRIDGE, E., and W. D. M. PATON: In, PATON, W. D. M.; Histamine release by compounds of simple chemical structure. Pharmacol. Rev. **9**, 269 (1957).
EMERY, F. E., and C. A. HERRICK: Changes in the tonicity of smooth muscle produced by toxins of *Ascaris lumbricoides*. Amer. J. Physiol. **85**, 366 (1928).
— — The effects of *Ascaris* extracts on circulation and respiration. Amer. J. Physiol. **91**, 143 (1930).
ESSEX, H. E., J. MARKOWITZ and F. C. MANN: Physiological responses and immune reactions to extracts of certain intestinal parasites. Amer. J. Physiol. **98**, 18 (1931).
FAWCETT, D. W.: Cytological and pharmacological observations on the release of histamine by mast cells. J. exp. Med. **100**, 217 (1954).
— An experimental study of mast cell degranulation and regeneration. Anat. Rec. **121**, 29 (1955).

FEINBERG, S. M., and L. A. STERNBERGER: Action of histamine liberator compound 48—80 in the guinea-pig. J. Allergy **26**, 170 (1955).
FELDBERG, W., and W. D. M. PATON: Release of histamine from skin and muscle in the cat by opium alkaloids and other histamine liberators. J. Physiol. (Lond.) **114**, 490 (1951).
—, and M. SCHACHTER: Histamine release by horse serum from skin of the sensitized dog and the non-sensitized cat. J. Physiol. (Lond.) **118**, 124 (1952).
—, and J. TALESNIK: Reduction of tissue histamine by compound 48—80. J. Physiol. (Lond.) **120**, 550 (1953).
FERRI, A. G.: Contribution to the study of mast cell physiology. Thesis, Universidade de Sao Paulo, Brasil (1955).
FLASHMAN, D. H.: The effect of suprarenalectomy on active anaphylactic shock in the white rat. J. infect. Dis. **33**, 461 (1926).
FREUND, J., and K. McDERMOTT: Sensibilization to horse serum by means of adjuvants. Proc. Soc. exp. Biol. (N. Y.) **49**, 548 (1942).
FRIEDBERGER, E.: Die aktiven Stoffe in der Anaphylaxie. Z. Immun.-Forsch. **4**, 636 (1910).
GARCIA-AROCHA, H.: Release of histamine and 5-hydroxytryptamine from cells of the peritoneal fluid of rats. Canad. J. Biochem. **39**, 395 (1961a).
— Liberation of 5-hydroxytryptamine and histamine in the anaphylactic reaction of the rat. J. Biochem. Physiol. **39**, 403 (1961b).
—, and F. J. McILREATH: Production of anaphylaxis *in vivo* and *in vitro* by soluble antigen-antibody complexes. XXI. Internat. Congress of Physiol. Buenos Aires: Amorrortu e Hijos 1959.
GAZZINELLI, G., M. M. GUIA, A. G. A. NEVES, J. PUDLES, W. T. BERALDO and W. DIAS DA SILVA: Purification of the toxic fraction from *Ascaris lumbricoides* and their effect on the guinea-pig. Nature (Lond.) **190**, 813 (1961).
— J. PUDLES, M. M. GUIA and A. G. ALMEIDA NEVES: Purification of the toxic fractions from *Ascaris lumbricoides.* Ciênc. e Cult. **12**, 101 (1960).
GERMUTH, F. G., and G. E. MCKINNON: Studies on the biological properties of antigen-antibody complexes. I. Anaphylactic shock induced by soluble antigen-antibody complexes in unsensitized normal guinea-pigs. Bull. Johns Hopk. Hosp. **101**, 13 (1957).
GOMORI, G.: Chloroacetyl esters as histochemical substrates. J. Histochem. Cytochem. **1**, 469 (1953).
GRAHAM, H. T., O. H. LOWRY, N. WAHL and M. K. PRIEBAT: Mast cells as sources of tissue histamine. J. exp. Med. **102**, 307 (1955).
— F. WHEELWRIGHT, H. H. PARISH, A. R. MARKS and O. H. LOWRY: Distribution of histamine among blood elements. Fed. Proc. **11**, 350 (1952).
GREISMAN, S. E.: The role of anaphylatoxin during *in vitro* anaphylaxis. J. Immunol. **81**, 214 (1958).
HAGEN, P., R. J. BARRNETT and FU-LI LEE: Biochemical and electron microscopic study of particles isolated from mastocytoma cells. J. Pharmacol. **126**, 91 (1959).
HALPERN, B. N., et M. BRIOT: Libération d'histamine par la peau du rat sous l'effect de contact avec le dextran in vitro. C. R. Soc. Biol. (Paris) **146**, 1552 (1952).
— P. LIACOPOULOS et C. P. CASTILLO: L'anaphylaxie expérimentale chez le rat albine. C. R. Soc. Biol. (Paris) **149**, 314 (1955).
HAWKINS, D. F., and L. M. ROSA: Some discrepancies in the histamine theory of anaphylaxis in smooth muscle. Ciba Symposium on Histamine. London: Churchill 1956.
HEDBOM, A., and O. SNELLMAN: Isolation and analysis of the large cytoplasmic granules of tissue mast cells. Exp. cell. Res. **9**, 148 (1955).
HÖGBERG, B., and B. UVNÄS: The mechanism of the disruption of mast cells produced by compound 48—80. Acta physiol. scand. **41**, 345 (1957).
— — Inhibitory action of allicin on degranulation of mast cells produced by compound 48—80, histamine liberator from *Ascaris,* lecithinase A, and antigen. Acta physiol. scand. **44**, 157 (1958).
— — Further observations on the disruption of rat mesentery mast cells caused by compound 48—80, antigen-antibody reaction, lecithinase A and decylamine. Acta physiol. scand. **48**, 133 (1960).
HOLMGREN, H., u. O. WILANDER: Beitrag zur Kenntnis der Chemie und Funktion der Ehrlichschen Mastzellen. Z. mikr.-anat. Forsch. **42**, 242 (1937).
HUMPHREY, J. H., and R. JAQUES: The histamine and serotonin content of the platelets and polymorphonuclear leucocytes of various species. J. Physiol. (Lond.) **124**, 305 (1954).
— — The release of histamine and 5-hydroxytryptamine (serotonin) from platelets by antigen-antibody reactions *(in vitro).* J. Physiol. (Lond.) **128**, 9 (1955).
—, and I. MOTA: The mechanism of anaphylaxis: specificity of antigen-induced mast cell damage in anaphylaxis in the guinea-pig. Immunology **2**, 31 (1959a).

HUMPHREY, J. H., and I. MOTA: The mechanism of anaphylaxis: observations on the failure of anti-bodies from certain species to sensitize guinea-pigs in direct and reversed passive anaphylaxis. Immunology **2**, 19 (1959b).

JAQUES, L. B., and E. T. WATERS: The identity and origin of the anticoagulant of anaphylactic shock in the dog. J. Physiol. (Lond.) **99**, 454 (1941).

JOBLING, J. W., and W. PETERSEN: The mechanism of anaphylatoxin formation. XV. Studies on ferment action. J. exp. Med. **20**, 37 (1914).

JUNQUEIRA, L. C. U., and B. BEIGUELMAN: Studies on the *in vitro* action of compound 48—80, a formaldehyde condensation product, on rat mast cells. Tex. Rep. Biol. Med. **13**, 69 (1955).

KABAT, E. A., and B. BENACERRAF: A quantitative study of passive anaphylaxis in the guinea-pig. IV. Passive sensitization with non-precipitable or univalent rabbit anti-ovalbumin. J. Immunol. **62**, 97 (1949).

—, and M. H. BOLDT: A quantitative study of passive anaphylaxis in the guinea-pig. J. Immunol. **48**, 181 (1944).

KELLER, R.: Tissue mast cells in anaphylaxis shock and anaphylactoid reactions. Int. Arch. Allergy **11**, 328 (1957).

— Effect of antibodies against rat γ-globulin or rat albumin on isolated peritoneal mast cells. Nature (Lond.) **193**, 282 (1962).

KIND, L. S.: The altered reactivity of mice after immunization with *Haemophilus pertussis*. J. Immunol. **79**, 411 (1953).

LAGUNOFF, D., and E. P. BENDITT: Mast cell degranulation and histamine release observed in a new *in vitro* system. J. exp. Med. **112**, 571 (1960).

LECOMTE, J., et E. BAECKELAND: Les mastocites hépatiques du chien au cours du choc peptonique. Acta haemat. (Basel) **10**, 165 (1953).

LEROY, A.: Sur la toxicité du liquide perientérique d'*Ascaris megalocephala*. Arch. int. Physiol. **9**, 276 (1910).

LEVINE, L.: Inhibition of immune hemolysis by diisopropylfluorophosphate. Biochim. biophys. Acta (Amst.) **18**, 283 (1955).

LIPTON, M. M., J. H. STONE and J. FREUND: Systemic and local anaphylaxis in the albino rat. J. Immunol. **77**, 453 (1956).

MACINTOSH, F. C.: Histamine and intracellular particles. Ciba Symposium on Histamine. London: Churchill 1956.

MACHEBOEUF, M., et R. MANDOUL: A propos de la toxicité des extraits d'*Ascaris*. C. R. Soc. Biol. (Paris) **130**, 1032 (1939).

MALKIEL, S., and B. J. HARGIS: Histamine sensitivity and anaphylaxis in the pertussis vaccinated rat. Proc. Soc. exp. Biol. (N. Y.) **81**, 689 (1952a).

— — Anaphylactic shock in the pertussis vaccinated mouse. Proc. Soc. exp. Biol. (N. Y.) **80**, 122 (1952b).

MANDOUL, R.: Étude comparative de la toxicité des extraits d'Ascaris. C. R. Soc. Biol. (Paris) **130**, 1035 (1939).

MCILWAIN, H., and H. L. BUDDLE: A mechanical tissue chopper. Biochem. J. **53**, 412 (1953).

MICHELS, N. A.: The mast cell in the lower vertebrates. Cellule **33**, 339 (1923).

— The mast cells. Handbook of Haematology. New York: Hoeber 1938.

MONGAR, J. L.: Measurement of histamine-releasing activity. Ciba Symposium on Histamine. London: Churchill 1956.

—, and H. O. SCHILD: A comparison of the effects of anaphylactic shock and of chemical histamine releasers. J. Physiol. (Lond.) **118**, 461 (1952).

— — Quantitative measurement of the histamine-releasing activity of a series of mono-alkylamines using minced guinea-pig lung. Brit. J. Pharmacol. **8**, 103 (1953).

— — Inhibition of anaphylaxis. J. Physiol. (Lond.) **130**, 40 (1955).

— — Effect of antigen and organic bases on intracellular histamine in guinea-pig lung. J. Physiol. (Lond.) **131**, 207 (1956).

— — Inhibition of the anaphylactic reaction. J. Physiol. (Lond.) **135**, 301 (1957a).

— — Effect of temperature on the anaphylactic reaction. J. Physiol. (Lond.) **135**, 320 (1957b).

— — The need for calcium in the anaphylactic reaction. J. Physiol. (Lond.) **136**, 31 P (1957c).

— — The effect of calcium and pH on the anaphylactic reaction. J. Physiol. (Lond.) **140**, 272 (1958).

MOTA, I.: Mast cell damage by anaphylaxis, peptone shock and compound 48—80. Thesis. Universidade de Sao Paulo. Brasil (1953).

— Action of anaphylactic shock and anaphylatoxin on mast cells and histamine in rats. Brit. J. Pharmacol. **12**, 453 (1957).

— Mast cells and anaphylaxis. J. Physiol. (Lond.) **140**, 6 P (1958a).

— Mast cell and histamine in rat anaphylaxis: the effect of *Haemophilus pertussis*. Nature (Lond.) **182**, 1021 (1958b).

— Effect of antigen and octylamine on mast cells and histamine content of sensitized guinea-pig tissues. J. Physiol. (Lond.) **147**, 425 (1959a).

MOTA, I.: Inhibition of mast cell damage and histamine release in rat anaphylaxis. Symposium on Histamine. Sao Paulo, Brasil (1959b).
— The mechanism of action of anaphylatoxin. Its effect on guinea-pig mast cells. Immunology **2**, 403 (1959c).
— The mechanism of action of antigen-antibody complexes. The effect on the mast cells. Nature (Lond.) **191**, 572 (1961).
— Failure of rat and rabbit antiserum to passively sensitized normal and pertussis-treated rats and mice so as to induce mast cell damage and histamine release on later contact with antigen. Immunology **5**, 11 (1962).
— Biological characterization of "mast cell sensitizing" antibodies. Life Sciences **1**, 465 (1963).
— W. T. BERALDO, A. G. FERRI and L. C. U. JUNQUEIRA: Intracellular distribution of his-histamine. Nature (Lond.) **174**, 698 (1954).
— — — — Action of 48—80 on the mast cell population and histamine content of the wall of the gastro-intestinal tract of the rat. Ciba Symposium on Histamine. London: Churchill 1956.
— — and L. C. U. JUNQUEIRA: Protamine- like property of compound 48—80 and stilbamidine and their action on the mast cells. Proc. Soc. exp. Biol. (N. Y.) **83**, 455 (1953).
—, and W. DIAS DA SILVA: The anti-anaphylactic and histamine-releasing properties of the antihistamines. Their effect on the mast cells. Brit. J. Pharmacol. **15**, 396 (1960a).
— — The antigen-induced damage to isolated sensitized mast cells. Nature (Lond.) **186**, 245 (1960b).
— — and J. F. FERNANDES: The inhibition of mast cell damage and histamine release in anaphylaxis by pyridine and diphosphopyridine nucleotidase inhibitors. Comparison with compound 48—80. Brit. J. Pharmacol. **15**, 405 (1960).
— A. G. FERRI and L. C. U. JUNQUEIRA: Action of peptone on the mast cells and histamine content of dog tissues. Acta haemat. (Basel) **15**, 409 (1956).
—, and T. ISHII: Inhibition of mast cell disruption and histamine release in rat anaphylaxis in vitro. Comparison with compound 48—80. Brit. J. Pharmacol. **15**, 82 (1960).
— L. C. U. JUNQUEIRA, W. T. BERALDO and A. G. FERRI: Action of peptone on mast cells of the dog. Nature (Lond.) **173**, 547 (1954).
—, and I. VUGMAN: Effect of anaphylactic shock and compound 48—80 on the mast cells of the guinea-pig lung. Nature (Lond.) **177**, 427 (1956a).
— — Effects of compound 48—80 and anaphylaxis on mast cells and histamine content of guinea-pig tissues. Cien. e Cult. **8**, 42 (1956b).
— — Action of compound 48—80 on the mast cells and histamine contents of guinea-pig tissues. Brit. J. Pharmacol. **11**, 304 (1956c).
—, and S. YONEDA: Mast cell behaviour in peptone shock. Paper presented at the Soc. Bras. de Anatomia, Sao Paulo, Brasil (1952).
MOUSSATCHÉ, H., and A. P. DANON: Inhibition by sulphydryl blocking agents of the guinea-pig gut reaction to anaphylaxis and to anaphylatoxin. Naturwissenschaften **10**, 227 (1956).
— — Inhibition by nicotinamide and nicotinic acid of the histamine release in the anaphylactic reaction in vitro. Influence of some metabolites. An. Acad. Bras. Cienc. **33**, 173 (1961).
MUÑOZ, J., L. F. SCHUCHARDT and W. F. VERWEY: Passive anaphylaxis in *H. pertussis* treated mice. Fed. Proc. **13**, 507 (1954).
— — — Anaphylaxis in *Haemophilus pertussis*-treated mice. J. Immunol. **80**, 77 (1954).
NORTON, S.: Quantitative determination of mast cell fragmentation by compound 48—80. Brit. J. Pharmacol. **9**, 494 (1954).
—, and E. J. DE BEER: Effect of some antibiotics on rats cells in vitro. Arch. int. Pharmacodyn. **102**, 352 (1955).
OSLER, A. G., M. M. HAWRISIAK, Z. OVARY, M. SIQUEIRA and O. G. BIER: Studies on the mechanism of hypersensitivity phenomena. II. The participation of complement in passive cutaneous anaphylaxis of the albino rat. J. exp. Med. **106**, 811 (1957).
PADAWER, J., and A. S. GORDON: Isolation of mast cells from other cellular elements of rat peritoneal fluid. Proc. Soc. exp. Biol. (N. Y.) **88**, 29 (1955).
PATON, W. D. M.: Compound 48—80: a potent histamine liberator. Brit. J. Pharmacol. **6**, 499 (1951).
— Histamine metabolism. Int. Arch. Allergy **6**, 203 (1955).
PARRATT, J. R., and G. B. WEST: Release of 5-hydroxytryptamine and histamine from tissue of the rat. J. Physiol. (Lond.) **137**, 179 (1957).
PELLERAT, J., et M. MURAT: Action des antihistaminiques de synthèse sur l'histamine. C. R. Soc. Biol. (Paris) **140**, 297 (1946).
PITTMAN, M., and F. G. GERMUTH: Some quantitative aspects of passive anaphylaxis in pertussis-vaccinated mice. Proc. Soc. exp. Biol. (N. Y.) **87**, 425 (1958).
RILEY, J. F.: The effects of histamine liberators on the mast cells of the rat. J. Path. Bact. **65**, 471 (1953a).

RILEY, J. F.: Histamine in tissue mast cells. Science **118**, 332 (1953b).
—, and G. B. WEST: The presence of histamine in tissue mast cells. J. Physiol. **210**, 528 (1953).
— — Tissue mast cells studies with a histamine-liberator of low toxicity (compound 48—80) J. Path. Bact. **69**, 269 (1955).
ROCHA E SILVA, M.: Concerning the mechanism of anaphylactic and tryptic shock. J. Immunol. **40**, 399 (1941).
— Recent advances concerning the histamine problem. J. Allergy **15**, 399 (1944).
— Anaphylatoxin and histamine release. Quart. Rev. Allergy 8, 220 (1954).
— Histamine. Its role in anaphylaxis and allergy. Springfield: Charles C. Thomas 1955.
— O. G. BIER and M. ARONSON: Histamine release by anaphylatoxin. Nature (Lond.) **168**, 465 (1951).
—, and A. GRAÑA: Anaphylaxis-like reactions produced by *Ascaris* extracts. I. The changes in the histamine content and the coagulability of the blood in guinea-pigs and in dogs. Arch. Surg. **52**, 523 (1946a).
— — Anaphylaxis-like reactions produced by *Ascaris* extracts. II. The mechanism of the shock induced in dogs. Arch. Surg. **52**, 713 (1946b).
—, and A. M. ROTHSCHILD: Anaphylatoxin, histamine depletion and skin reactions in therat. Nature (Lond.) **175**, 987 (1955).
ROTHSCHILD, A. M., and M. ROCHA E SILVA: Mechanism of histamine release by anaphylatoxin, compound 48—80 and hypotonic solutions. Cien. e Cult. 8, 180 (1956).
ROWLEY, D. A., and E. P. BENDITT: 5-Hydroxytryptamine and histamine as mediator of the vascular injury produced by agents which damage mast cells in rats. J. exp. Med. **103**, 399 (1956).
— J. CHUTKOW and C. ATTIG: Severe active cutaneous hypersensitivity in the rat produced by hemophilus pertussis vaccine. J. Exp. Med. **110**, 751 (1959).
SANYAL, R. K., and G. B. WEST: The relationship of histamine and 5-hydroxytryptamine to anaphylactic shock in different species. J. Physiol. (Lond.) **144**, 525 (1958).
SCHACHTER, M.: Anaphylaxis and histamine release in the rabbit. Brit. J. Pharmacol. 8, 412 (1953).
—, and J. TALESNIK: Anaphylaxis and histamine release in the rabbit. Brit. J. Pharmacol. 8, 412 (1953).
SCHILD, H. O.: Histamine release and anaphylactic shock in isolated lungs of guinea-pigs. Quart. J. exp. Physiol. **26**, 165 (1936).
—, and R. A. GREGORY: Liberation of histamine from striated muscle by curarine, strychnine and related substances. Abstr. Comm. XVII. Internat. Physiol. Congress, Oxford (1947).
SHIMAMURA, T., and N. FUJI: Cited by ESSEX, MARKOWITZ and MANN (1917).
SMITH, D. E.: Nature of the secretory activity of the mast cell. Amer. J. Physiol. **193**, 573 (1958).
— An immunological approach to the study of mast cell function. XXI. International Congress of Physiological Sciences. Buenos Aires: Amorrortu e Hijos 1959.
—, and Y. S. LEWIS: Preparation and effects of an anti-mast cell serum. J. exp. Med. **113**, 683 (1961).
SMITH, W. G.: Mast cell population of lung of the guinea-pig and other tissues. Nature(Lond.) **184**, 1154 (1959).
STRANGEWAYS, T. S. P., and R. J. CANTI: The living cell *in vitro* as shown by darkground illumination and the changes induced in such cells by fixing reagents. Quart. J. micr. Sci. **71**, 1 (1927).
STUART, E. G.: Mast cell responses to anaphylaxis. Anat. Rec. **112**, 394 (1952).
TANAKA, N., and E. LEDUC: A study of the cellular distribution of Forssman antigen in various species. J. Immunol. **77**, 198 (1956).
TASAKA, K.: Histamine release and its inhibition by antihistamines. Folia pharmacol. jap. **53**, 1029 (1957).
TOKUDA, S., and R. S. WEISER: Production of anaphylaxis in the white mouse with soluble antigen-antibody complexes. Science **127**, 1237 (1958).
TRAPANI, I. L., J. S. GRAVEY and D. H. CAMPBELL: Stimulating action of soluble antigen-antibody complexes on normal guinea-pig smooth muscle. Science **127**, 700 (1958).
UNGAR, G.: Biochemical mechanism of the allergy reaction. Int. Arch. Allergy **4**, 258 (1953).
—, and H. HAYASHI: Enzymatic mechanism in allergy. Ann. Allergy **16**, 542 (1958).
UVNÄS, B., and I. THON: Isolation of biologically intact mast cells. Exp. Cell. Res. **18**, 512 (1959).
— B. DIAMANT, B. HÖGBERG and I. L. THON: Mechanism of mast-cell disruption induced by a principle extracted from *Ascaris suis*. Amer. J. Physiol. **199**, 575 (1960).
VOORHEES, A. B., H. J. BAKER and E. J. PULASKI: Reactions of albino rats to injections of dextran. Proc. Soc. exp. Biol. (N. Y.) **76**, 254 (1951).
WEGELIUS, O., G. HJELMMAN and C. WASASTJERNA: Morphological changes caused by anti-hamster serum in the mast cells of the hamster. Acta path. microbiol. scand. **36**, 309 (1955).
WEST, G. B.: Histamine in mast cell granules. J. Pharmacol. 7, 80 (1955).
WILANDER, O.: Studien über Heparin. Skand. Arch. Physiol. **81**, Suppl. 15 (1938).

Section G

Interaction of Mast Cells with Cationic Histamine Releasers

By

R. D. HIGGINBOTHAM

With 2 Figures

Mast cells are characteristic elements of the connective tissues and appear to serve as cellular sites for storage and release of both heparin and histamine in the tissues. These cells respond to various kinds of injurious stimuli by shedding their histamine- and heparin-containing granules into the ground substance where their biologically-active substances may influence subsequent tissue responses. A great deal of interest has been focussed on the possibility that these cells may play an important role in the development of allergic and other types of inflammatory lesions of the connective tissues. An important aspect of research in this area has been concerned with the release of histamine from mast cells in response to administration of histamine releaser drugs (RILEY, 1959). It is of interest that amongst the various speculations on the mechanisms involved in histamine release is the suggestion that this cellular response to cationic histamine releasers may be effected through an ion exchange mechanism in the mast cell granules in which histamine is competitively displaced by the releaser agent and heparin serves as the cation exchanger (GREEN, 1962; KÜTTNER, 1961). The following discussion will be concerned with the role of heparin in the interaction of mast cells and histamine releaser drugs and, for the sake of brevity, will not attempt to consider the importance of histamine in this reaction.

Heparin, a mucopolysaccharide of a highly acidic nature by virtue of its carboxylic and sulfuric acid groups, has a relatively strong affinity for a variety of cationic substances (WALTON, 1955; HIGGINBOTHAM, 1959a). This macromolecule is present in significant amounts in the mast cell granules and confers its acidic character upon the granules as evidenced by their strong metachromatic reaction with certain basic dyes, such as toluidine blue. The direct interaction of mast cells with histamine releaser drugs is indicated by the observations of RILEY (1953) and of SMITH (1958) that following injection of toluidine blue or stilbamidine, the cytoplasmic granules of mast cells can be observed to concentrate these drugs from the extracellular fluids. A further observation of RILEY (1959) that granules of mast cells intravitally stained with toluidine blue will readily exchange this cationic dye for another cation, stilbamidine, would support the idea that the heparin-containing granules of mast cells may serve as cation exchangers. Mast cell granules may thus interact with various cationic substances in the tissues such as those arising from metabolic processes within the cell [histamine formation (HAGEN, 1961)] or substances such as toluidine blue or stilbamidine which can traverse the cell membrane (RILEY, 1953; SMITH, 1958) (assimilation, pinocytosis, etc.). The sequestration of a toxic cationic substance by the granules of the mast cells with the concomitant formation of an acid-base complex between the heparin constituent of the granules and the cation would seemingly result in a reduction of the pharmacologically active concentration of the latter substance in the tissues and thereby enhance tolerance of the organism to a given dose of the injurious agent. As working hypothesis, it has been considered that the uptake of cationic substances by mast cells represents a fundamental mechanism for the inactivation of various pharmacologically active cationic substances in the tissues (HIGGINBOTHAM, 1959a). The interaction of mast cells with certain histamine releaser drugs has been considered as an example of this function and its significance is therefore additional to that of the mobilization of histamine.

I. Binding of histamine releasers

In our investigation of the above hypothesis, it was found that treatment of mice with heparin markedly enhanced their resistance to the lethal effects of various toxic cationic substances. Compound 48/80 (a low polymer of p-methoxy-N-methylphenylethylamine nuclei) was selected for our initial studies (HIGGINBOTHAM and DOUGHERTY, 1956) on this problem since this synthetic substance can readily initiate the degranulation of mast cells (MOTA et al., 1953), is a potent releaser of histamine (GREEN, 1962), has a protamine-like inhibitory effect on heparin (MOTA et al., 1953), and produces a lethal intoxication in the mouse and other species of laboratory animals (PAPACOSTAS et al., 1959). In this study, it was found that the lethal effects of intraperitoneally administered compound 48/80 were completely inhibited by pretreatment of the experimental animals with adequate amounts of heparin by the same route (HIGGINBOTHAM and DOUGHERTY, 1956). This protective effect of heparin is seemingly dependent on the direct interaction of this acidic mucopolysaccharide with the noxious cationic substance in the tissues. Results of dose response studies indicated that the amount of heparin required for protection was directly proportional to the amount of compound 48/80 employed for a challenge dose. Moreover, untreated mice challenged with an otherwise lethal dose of compound 48/80 and showing symptoms of acute intoxication could be revived if treated immediately by the intravenous route with large doses of heparin. These animals usually recovered and survived with little to no apparent residual effects. This would suggest that the injected heparin could complex and neutralize a significant proportion of the challenge agent under *in vivo* conditions.

Inasmuch as mast cells contain approximately 3% heparin (PADAWER, 1957), the rapid release of this protective mucopolysaccharide from these cells in response to local administration of compound 48/80 or other noxious cationic drugs may significantly influence the injurious effects of these agents in the tissues. Recalculation of results published elsewhere concerning the quantitative relationships between heparin and various toxic agents capable of initiating mast cell degranulation are shown in Table 1 and illustrate the generalized nature of this protective effect of heparin (HIGGINBOTHAM, 1958a, 1962). The 50% protective dose of heparin (PD_{50}) was determined by challenging groups of mice by the intravenous route with a uniform lethal dose of one of the challenge agents in mixture with one of a series of graded amounts of heparin. The PD_{50} of heparin is, of course, the dose of heparin which will neutralize that amount of the challenge dose which is in excess of the LD_{50} of this latter drug. Since the various challenge agents differ considerably with regard to their LD_{50}'s and their respective heparin PD_{50}'s, the relative effectiveness of heparin has been compared on the basis of a "neutralization index" which represents the ratio of the amount of the challenge dose in excess of the LD_{50} to the amount of heparin required for a PD_{50}. Although compound 48/80, polymyxin B and clupein differ quite widely with regard to their chemical natures and relative lethal activities, it appears that heparin can neutralize similar amounts of each of these substances. This is of interest since the relative affinity of heparin for each of these substances under *in vitro* conditions is also quite similar (HIGGINBOTHAM, 1958a). The venom of Russell's Viper is a crude mixture of various substances; it may produce an anaphylactic-like shock (ROCHA E SILVA, 1955), is very active in initiating degranulation of mast cells (HIGGINBOTHAM, 1959a), and will complex heparin *in vitro*. Although heparin appears to be somewhat less effective in neutralizing Russell's Viper venom than the other agents, the neutralization index of heparin for the active constituent of the venom may very well be comparable to that obtained with the other drugs.

Table 1. *Neutralization of various histamine releasers by heparin*[1]

Challenge agent	Drug LD_{50}	Challenge dose	Heparin PD_{50}	Heparin neutralization Index[2]
		(μg/gm)		
Compound 48/80	2.2	2.67	0.36	1.3
Polymyxin B	4.3	5.0	0.56	1.3
Clupein	42.3	50.0	7.13	1.08
Russell's Viper venom	0.15	0.25	0.5	0.2

[1] Groups of mice given single i. v. injection of standard dose of challenge agent containing one of a series of graded doses of heparin.

[2] Neutralization index: $\frac{\text{Challenge Dose} - LD_{50}}{\text{Heparin } PD_{50}}$.

Under conditions in which heparin has an equivalent affinity for various toxic agents, as shown in Table 1, a given amount of heparin can more effectively inhibit the activity of a standard lethal dose of one of the more potent agents, such as compound 48/80, than one of a lesser toxicity, such as clupein. On the other hand, if the neutralizing effect of heparin is dependent on its capacity to bind the lethal agent, it would be expected that relatively small amounts of a substance of low toxicity can exhaust the capacity of a limited amount of heparin to neutralize the toxicity of a more potent agent. In terms of the postulated protective function of mast cells, this can be of importance since various cationic substances in the tissues could reduce the capacity of mast cell granules to complex various toxic agents. It has been observed, for example, that either toluidine blue or protamine can enhance the toxicity of compound 48/80. While it may be argued that this enhancement is due to the fact that each of the agents can also serve as a histamine releaser, it was observed in another study that ACTH (which also forms complexes with heparin, but is relatively non-toxic) can potentiate the lethal effects of an otherwise sublethal dose of polymyxin B (HIGGINBOTHAM and DOUGHERTY, 1957). This enhancing effect was found to be directly proportional to the amount of ACTH employed and could be reproduced with other agents having an affinity for heparin such as toluidine blue, protamine or neomycin. It is thus conceivable that the functional state of mast cells may be markedly impaired by various cationic substances which form poorly dissociable complexes with the heparin constituent of their granules and thereby reduce their capacity for sequestering other and perhaps more toxic cationic substances from the surrounding ground substance of the connective tissue.

If the heparin constituent of mast cell granules functions as a cationic exchanger, it is inevitable that the function of a given amount of heparin becomes impaired unless regenerated. One may speculate that elution of various cations that have been sequestered by the granules and formed poorly dissociable complexes with the heparin constituent may be accomplished by physiologic processes of the cell involving sodium, histamine and/or some other appropriate cation (Higginbotham, 1959a). The equilibrium of such a reaction would be governed by the relative concentration of the various cations as well as by the dissociation constants of their respective heparin complexes. Such interactions of heparin with various cationic substances have been considered in greater detail by Jaques (1943). In this manner, even highly toxic agents could be slowly released and subsequently detoxified by the metabolic processes of other cells without subjecting the organism to the pharmacologic effects of the bound substance that would otherwise occur if released more rapidly. In this regard, studies with heparin and neomycin have suggested that toxic amounts of this latter cation can be released from complex with heparin at a rate sufficiently slow as to not exceed the tolerance of the tissues for this substance (Higginbotham, 1960). On the other hand, since both sulfate and glucuronic acid are present in the mast cell as characteristic components of the heparin molecule (Walton, 1955), detoxification processes of this nature might also be carried out by this cell.

When minimal amounts of a toxic substance are involved, disposal of the sequestered agent would not necessarily involve any marked morphologic change in the mast cells and would represent a physiologic function of these cells. However, the interaction of mast cells with cationic agents oftentimes leads to a swelling of the granules. This change in the granules is analogous, in some respects, to the swelling of ion exchange resins during hydration or, with weakly cross-linked resins, during conversion from one salt form to another (Kitchener, 1957). With small amounts of a given agent, the swelling of the mast cell granules may be reversible, as noted by Smith (1958). With larger amounts of the agent, the swelling may progressively increase until the capacity of the cell to contain them is exceeded and the granules are then rapidly released into the surrounding ground substance (Dougherty and Schneebeli, 1958). In effect, this swelling would increase availability of ion active groups in the interior of the granule for complexing the provocative cation. Moreover, following cell rupture, the ionic environment of these granules would no longer be restricted by functions of an intervening cell membrane and thus dissemination of the granules would allow for direct interaction with the cation at concentrations present in the ground substance.

II. Cellular ingestion of complexes

These shed granules may then be rapidly ingested by local connective tissue cells such as fibroblasts and histiocytes which can then deal with them according to their respective metabolic capacities. This rather remarkable example of transfer of a biologically active substance, heparin, from mast cells to other cells of the connective tissue has been carefully studied and the observation confirmed by the use of mast cell granules labeled *in vivo* with radioactive sulfate and whose fate in the tissues was determined by means of radioautographic techniques (Higginbotham et al., 1956). The ingestion of shed granules occurs whether the stimulus for their secretion by mast cells is very mild (e.g., injection of saline) or severe (local anaphylaxis, venom) as shown in Fig. 1. Smith and Lewis (1958) have reported that this process occurs during various types of stressful situations and, according to Burton (1959), it can even be visualized in tissue culture preparations. The significance of this process is undoubtedly dependent on the nature of the particular situation at hand. In the case of compound 48/80, etc., it would appear to be the means for sequestering and transporting this noxious agent, in a neutralized form, from one cell to another. Since many cells can participate in removing the granular debris secreted by a single mast cell (Fig. 1), the capacity for detoxification of substances bound by the granules would be increased manyfold.

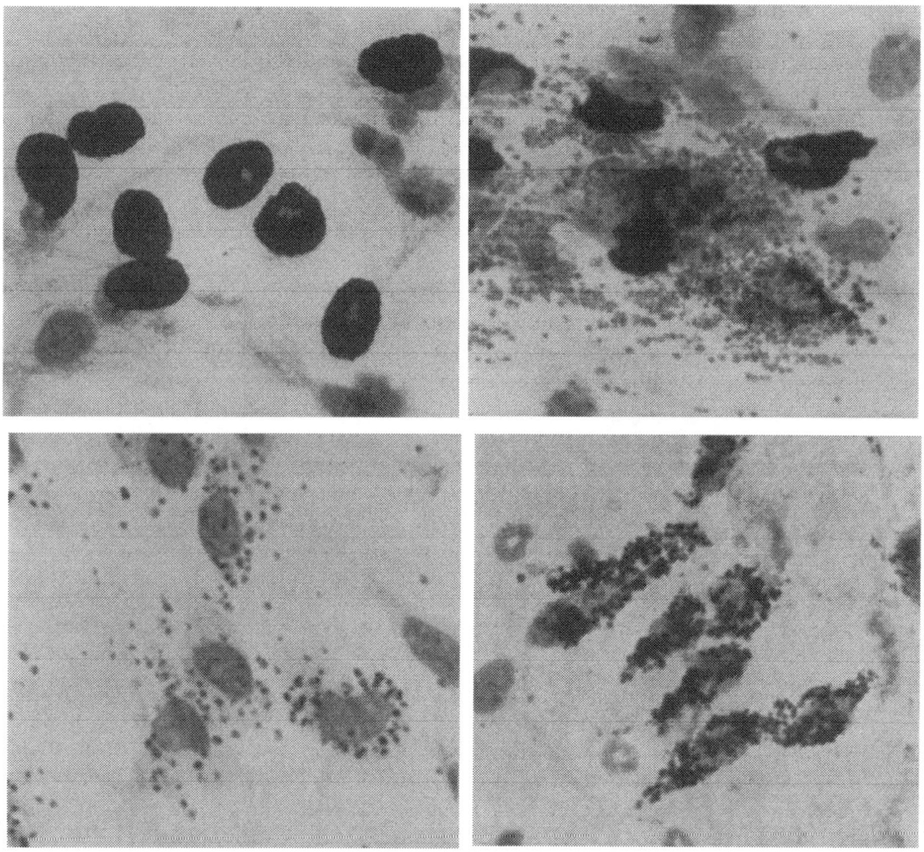

A B C D

Fig. 1, A to D. Air dried spreads of loose subcutaneous connective tissue of mice. May Gruenwald-Giemsa ($\times$ 640) A. Normal mast cells prior to exposure to noxious agent. B. Disruption of mast cells in response to local injection of 0.5 μg Russell's Viper venom 5 minutes previously. Shed granules exhibit a reddish metachromasia ("free" heparin) in contrast to more darkly-staining granules in cells. C. Uptake of shed granules by local connective tissue cells 15 to 45 minutes after venom injection. Ingested granules are now more basophilic suggesting that heparin constituent has formed complex with venom or tissue constituents. D. Numerous darkly-staining granules of a compound 48/80-heparin complex appearing in cells within 30 minutes after local injection of this mixture

When mixtures of heparin and compound 48/80 are injected subcutaneously into mice, the majority of the local fibroblasts rapidly accumulate the compound 48/80-heparin complex and deposit this material in their cytoplasm as metachromatic granules (HIGGINBOTHAM and DOUGHERTY, 1956) (Fig. 1D). Although heparin alone can also be ingested by these cells, the granules formed can be readily differentiated from those formed with the compound 48/80-heparin complex. Compound 48/80 appears to greatly increase both the rate and the amount of material ingested (HIGGINBOTHAM, 1958a). Other agents, such as polymyxin and clupein, also appear to enhance this uptake of heparin by fibroblasts, but the granules formed in each case are characteristic of the cation incorporated in the complex (HIGGINBOTHAM, 1958a). These granules tend to disappear from the cytoplasm within 24 to 48 hours after their formation which suggests that they have been metabolized by the cell.

As a consequence of the ingestion of mast cell granules or injected mucopolysaccharide complexes these cells possess numerous metachromatic granules in their cytoplasms and have been designated as "quasi-mast cells" to denote their resemblance to and to differentiate them from naturally occurring mast cells (HIGGINBOTHAM, 1958a). In this regard, it was observed by EDER and SCHAUER (1961) that compound 48/80-heparin granules in fibroblasts and histiocytes exhibited a strong ATP-ase activity as did granules of normal mast cells, but unlike the latter cells, the "quasi-mast cells" did not appear to have a measureable leucyl-aminopeptidase activity. In view of the similarity and differences between mast cells and "quasi-mast cells" it is obvious that additional information concerning mast cells and their functions might be obtained by further studies on the formation and activity of "quasi-mast cells".

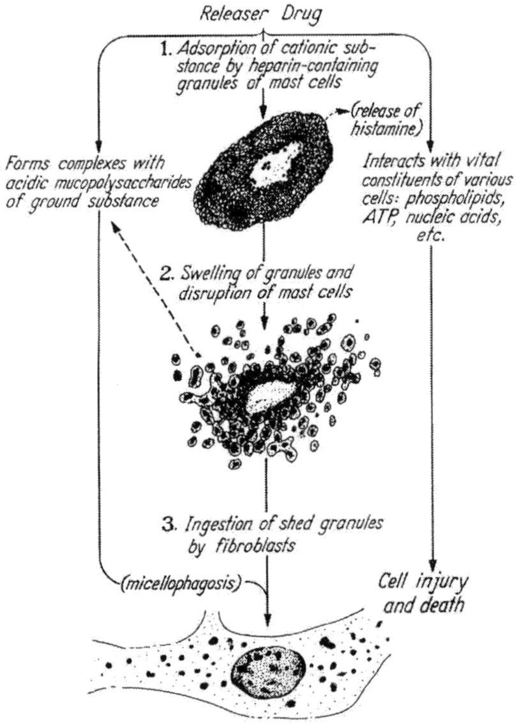

Fig. 2. General scheme illustrating proposed role of mast cells in resistance of tissues to toxic cationic agents. The sequestration of noxious agent by heparin-containing granules of mast cells and acidic mucopolysaccharides of ground substance reduces amount of injurious agent available to interact with more vital constituents of the tissues. Toxic substance in complex with heparin disposed of by local connective tissue cells

III. Summary

The protective aspects of the interaction of mast cells with certain histamine releasers such as compound 48/80, or polymyxin B have been summarized as a sequence of events which are schematically illustrated in Fig. 2. It can be seen that the acidic mucopolysaccharides of the ground substance (e.g., chondroitin sulfate B) or of the mast cell granules (e.g., heparin, heparin monosulfate) may adsorb the noxious agents by a cation exchange reaction which involves the release of histamine and possibly other cationic substances. The formation of acid-base complexes between the sulfated polysaccharides and the injurious agents reduces the amount of the latter substances free to produce their primary toxic effects possibly through interaction with more vital constituents of cells such as phospholipids (HARRIS et al., 1961), ATP (DARLOW, 1956), nucleic acids (HIGGINBOTHAM, 1958b), etc., elsewhere in the tissues. This sequestration of the toxic drug by the polysaccharides is therefore essentially a protective phenomenon. The significance of the associated release of histamine undoubtedly depends on the functional state of the tissue at the time of release. On one hand, histamine may initiate an increased vascular permeability leading to a local dilution of the injurious agent in the tissue and consequent diminution of its effects. On the other hand, this amine may be exceedingly injurious since compound 48/80 can markedly enhance the sensitivity of mice to either histamine or serotonin (Higginbotham, 1959b).

The secretion of heparin-containing granules by mast cells in response to releaser drugs and the subsequent ingestion of the shed granules by local fibroblasts and histiocytes allows for a localization of the injurious agent in an inactive form to await disposal by the metabolic processes of the phagocytic cells. It has been postulated that a similar process occurs which involves the mucopolysaccharides of the ground substance and is concerned with the maintenance of the physiologic state of the connective tissue and has been called "micellophagosis" (Higginbotham, 1959a). Under normal conditions, this latter process is sufficient to deal with the various cationic substances diffusing through the ground substance between the blood and parenchymal tissues. However, when the binding capacity of the ground substance is exceeded, the unbound cations are available for interaction with mast cells and can thereby initiate their secretory activity. By secreting their heparin-containing granules into the ground substance, mast cells supplement the exhausted mucopolysaccharides of the ground substance with a more highly acidic macromolecule. Mast cells can thus serve as a reserve source of mucopolysaccharide for reducing the injurious concentrations of various substances in the tissues. It is important to note that the interaction of heparin with noxious substances is not restricted by the high degree of specificity generally associated with toxin-antitoxin systems, and may thus bind and neutralize toxic agents of such diverse natures as a synthetic polyamine (compound 48/80, a bacterial polypeptide (polymyxin B), a nuclear protein (clupein) or a crude mixture of biologically active substances (Russell's Viper venom).

These observations concerning the interaction of mast cells with histamine releasers strongly suggest that these cells have an important role in the detoxification processes in the tissues.

Acknowledgements

Studies supported in part by USPH Grant A-3407 Rl.

References

Burton, A. L.: Observations préliminaires sur le sort des mast cells du fluide péritonéal de rat en cultures de tissus. Rev. canad. Biol. **18**, 103 (1959).

Darlow, G.: Reaction between histamine liberators and phosphates. J. Physiol. (Lond.) **131**, 13P (1956).

Dougherty, T. F., and G. Schneebeli: Microcinematographic demonstration of mast cell disintegration in living isolated loose connective tissue of mice (motion picture). Fed. Proc. **17**, 37 (1958).

Eder, M., u. A. Schauer: Fermenthistochemische und experimentelle Untersuchungen an Gewebsmastzellen. Beitr. path. Anat. **124**, 251 (1961).

Green, J. P.: Binding of some biogenic amines in tissues. Advanc. Pharmacol. **1**, 349 (1962).

Hagen, P.: Biosynthesis and storage of histamine, heparin and 5-hydroxytryptamine in the mast cell. Canad. J. Biochem. **39**, 639 (1961).

Harris, A. F., A. Saifer and S. K. Weintraub: Interaction of compound 48/80 and stilbamidine with strandin. Proc. Soc. exp. Biol. (N. Y.) **107**, 35 (1961).

Higginbotham, R. D.: Studies on the functional interrelationship of fibroblasts and ground substance mucopolysaccharides. Ann. N. Y. Acad. Sci. **73**, 186 (1958a).

— Mast cells, heparin and toxic agents. Fed. Proc. **17**, 516 (1958b).

— On the participation of micellophagosis in the resistance of tissues to injurious agents. Int. Arch. Allergy **15**, 195 (1959a).

— Effect of compound 48/80 on toxicity of histamine and of serotonin in mice. Proc. Soc. exp. Biol. (N. Y.) **102**, 4 (1959b).

— Effect of heparin on neomycin. Tex. Rep. Biol. Med. **18**, 408 (1960).

— Sulfated polysaccharides and resistance to Russell's viper venom. Proc. Soc. exp. Biol. (N. Y.) **110**, 135 (1962).

HIGGINBOTHAM, R. D. and T. F. DOUGHERTY: Mechanism of heparin protection against a histamine releaser (48/80). Proc. Soc. exp. Biol. (N. Y.) **92**, 493 (1956).

— — Potentiation of polymyxin B toxicity by ACTH. Proc. Soc. exp. Biol. (N. Y.) **96**, 466 (1957).

— —, and W. S. S. JEE: The fate of shed mast cell granules. Proc. Soc. exp. Biol. (N. Y.) **92**, 256 (1956).

JAQUES, L. B.: Reaction of heparin with proteins and complex bases. Biochem. J. **37**, 189 (1943).

KITCHENER, J. A.: Properties and behavior: swelling and equilibria. *In:* Ion Exchangers in Organic and Biochemistry. New York: Interscience Publishers 1957.

KÜTTNER, K.: Ionenaustausch biologisch wichtiger Amine an synthetischen und natürlichen Austauschern als Modell für die pharmakologische Histaminliberation. Inaugural-Dissertation, University of Bern, Switzerland (1961).

MOTA, I., W. T. BERALDO, and L. C. U. JUNQUEIRA: Protamine-like property of compound 48/80 and stilbamidine and their action on mast cells. Proc. Soc. exp. Biol. (N. Y.) **83**, 455 (1953).

PADAWER, J.: Studies on mammalian mast cells. Trans. N. Y. Acad. Sci. **19**, 690 (1957).

PAPACOSTAS, C. A., E. R. LOEW, and G. B. WEST: Studies on the toxicology of a histamine liberator, compound 48/80. Arch. int. Pharmacodyn. **120**, 353 (1959).

RILEY, J. F.: The effects of histamine liberators on the mast cells of the rat. J. Path. Bact. **65**, 471 (1953).

— The Mast Cells. Edinburgh, Scotland: E. & S. Livingstone, Ltd. 1959.

ROCHA E SILVA, M.: Histamine. Its Role in Anaphylaxis and Allergy. Springfield, Illinois: Charles C. Thomas 1955.

SMITH, D. E.: Dynamics of release of histamine from tissue mast cells. Science **128**, 207 (1958).

—, and Y. LEWIS: Phagocytosis of granules from disrupted mast cells. Anat. Rec. **132**, 93 (1958).

WALTON, K. W.: Chemistry and mode of action of heparin and related compounds. Brit. med. Bull. **11**, 62 (1955).

Section H

Release of Histamine in Relation to Phosphorylation and Respiration

By

H. Moussatché

With 1 Figure

Although a few papers published several years ago led to the conclusion that a close relationship existed between histamine release and cell metabolism, it was not until recently that this connection could be well established.

The concept prevailing in the two last decades, largely accepted after Rocha e Silva's experiments with trypsin (Rocha e Silva, 1938, 56; Rocha e Silva et al., 1946), and confirmed by other authors (Ungar, 1956), postulated that a proteolytic enzyme activation with ensuing break of the peptide linkage by which histamine would be bound to the tissues, occurred. Criticism of this theory was presented by McIntire (1956).

The first experiments suggesting a relationship between cell metabolism and histamine release were made by Parrot (1942-44), who showed that histamine is not released by the antigen from sensitized guinea-pig tissues in the absence of oxygen.

Experiments carried out by several research workers in the last years using metabolites or inhibitors of the enzymes of the aerobic and anaerobic cycles, definitely demonstrated a close connection between histamine and cell respiration.

At present there is a growing literature showing that enzymatic processes are involved in the release of histamine in anaphylaxis or by drugs which mobilize the amine bound to the tissue (histamine releasing compounds). However, the complexity of the experimental evidences does not allow at present an unitary view of both phenomena, since there are indications of differences in the mechanisms of release. Notwithstanding the efforts done by several investigators in this direction, some difficulties have to be overcome.

I. Release by Anaphylaxis

A. Experiments in guinea-pigs. Influence of oxygen and some metabolites

Most of the experiments showing the importance of the oxidation-reduction enzymes in the release of histamine during the anaphylactic reaction were performed in guinea-pig tissues.

As pointed out above, the experiments of Parrot on sensitized guinea-pig lungs showed that molecular oxygen was necessary for histamine release by antigen. Mongar and Schild (1957), Chakravarty (1960), and Moussatché and Prouvost-Danon (1960), carried out experiments confirming and extending these facts, opening a new way for the understanding of the mechanism of histamine release as an energy requiring phenomenon. That the inhibitory action of oxygen lack was not due to an irreversible damage to the tissue, was shown by the release of histamine from tissue slices under oxygen after pre-incubation in anaerobiosis (MOUSSATCHÉ and PROUVOST-DANON, 1960).

Normal release of histamine occurs by lowering the oxygen concentration, inhibition being observed only in lung slices kept under oxygen tension lower than 10% (MOUSSATCHÉ and PROUVOST-DANON, 1960). Similar results were obtained by other authors (CHAKRAVARTY, 1962; EDMAN, MONGAR and SCHILD, 1964).

The importance of oxygen for the chain reactions of anaphylaxis was also studied by measuring oxygen uptake following the addition of antigen to the sensitized tissue placed in Warburg flasks. BÜNGELER (1931), was one of the first to study the subject, observing either a decrease or an increase in oxygen uptake. The experiments were carried out on whole animals or spleen, kidney, liver, intestine and urinary bladder slices, the results depending on the level of sensitization and amount of antigen injected. Since no quantitative figures are given by BÜNGELER, it is difficult to know what he meant by "level of sensitization." BÖSTRÖM (1934), also carried out experiments on this problem, observing changes in aerobic and anaerobic glycolysis of liver and skin of guinea-pigs during anaphylaxis. Similar changes were obtained by the author when the higher doses of the antigen were added to normal tissues. However, it should be observed that such reactions were obtained in the liver and it is not known whether histamine can be released from guinea-pig liver slices *in vitro* by antigen. FOLLIS (1953) could not detect any difference in the oxygen consumption of various sensitized tissues when the antigen was added *in vitro*. SONAK (1958) also measured the oxygen uptake and carbon dioxide output of liver, lung and brain of guinea-pigs submitted to severe anaphylactic shock, observing no significant difference in the oxygen consumption but an increase in the carbon dioxide output under conditions of anaerobic glycolysis.

BENDA et al. (1954) and LOCKER and KÖLB (1954) studied the respiration of liver slices during anaphylaxis, observing a decrease of oxygen uptake and glucose utilization in dog's, but no significant change in rabbit's liver. The experiments were done on animals previously shocked by intravenous injection of the antigen, pieces of liver being taken some minutes thereafter, and sliced for respiration studies. Decrease in tissue respiration was related to a decrease in the coenzymes and energy-rich phosphate compounds.

It must be pointed out however, that although the liver is the *shock organ* of the dog, antigen does not release histamine easily by *in vitro* perfusion (ROCHA E SILVA et al., 1947) or after slicing and incubation of the organ in Warburg flasks (MOUSSATCHÉ and PROUVOST-DANON, unpublished). This makes the study of histamine release and its relationship to respiration difficult in this animal species, because of the interference of factors which may come into play after the onset of the *in vivo* shock and which might influence the *in vitro* oxygen uptake.

Experiments designed to compare rates of oxygen consumption of paired normal and sensitized guinea-pig lungs during the first and second thirty minute intervals of respiration in Warburg flasks showed a statistically significant increase in the oxygen uptake during anaphylaxis (MOUSSATCHÉ and PROUVOST-DANON, 1956a, 1961b). This increase cannot be attributed to the action of the released histamine on the plain muscle of the bronchiolar tree or its oxidation by diamine oxidase, since control experiments gave negative results.

These experiments have been confirmed by MONGAR in unpublished observations (MONGAR and SCHILD, 1962). However, using the CUNNINGHAM and KIRK differential capillary respirometer, MONGAR and PERERA (1964) did not observe increase in oxygen consumption of sensitized mast cells treated with antigen (MONGAR and PERERA, 1964).

B. Influence of metabolites

From the standpoint of more specific information on the enzymatic steps involved in the anaphylactic reaction, the study of the influence of metabolites is perhaps more conclusive than that of enzyme inhibitors, since these substances only occasionally inhibit one enzyme alone in the multienzyme system represented by the cell. Metabolites, as specific substrates for enzymes, can inform which of them is playing a role during anaphylaxis.

The increase in oxygen uptake observed during *in vitro* anaphylaxis led to the investigation of the influence of metabolites on this process. For this purpose, metabolites must be selected which, according to previous knowledge, are consumed by the tissues under the conditions of the experiments (BARRON, 1941). Using standard manometric methods, MOUSSATCHÉ and PROUVOST-DANON (1957a, 58) measured oxygen uptake and the release of histamine from sensitized guinea-pig lung slices after the addition of several metabolites plus antigen to the incubation media. Succinate, alpha-ketoglutarate, acetate, lactate were assayed (MOUSSATCHÉ and PROUVOST-DANON, 1957b). All of them, excepting lactate, increased the amount of histamine released, as can be seen in Table I; similar results with succinate were obtained by other workers (AUSTEN and BROCKLEHURST, 1961a; YAMASAKI et al., 1960).

Table 1. *Influence of some metabolites on histamine release from sensitized guinea-pig lung slices during the anaphylactic reaction*

Metabolite	QO_2	%	Histamine release (microgr./g. w.w.)	%
Control	6.55 ± 0.28 (4)[1]	100	3.5 ± 0.17 (4)	100
Succinate 0.01 M	11.02 ± 0.17 (4)	168	9.0 ± 0.78 (4)	257
Control	4.23 ± 0.08 (4)	100	1.2 ± 0.25 (4)	100
Ketoglutarate 0.01 M . . .	5.08 ± 0.15 (4)	120	4.3 ± 0.38 (4)	358
Control	6.79 ± 0.14 (4)	100	3.8 ± 0.40 (4)	100
Malate 0.01 M	7.97 ± 0.25 (4)	117	7.8 ± 0.70 (4)	205
Control	4.37 ± 0.34 (4)	100	12.4 ± 0.70 (4)	100
Acetate 0.04 M.	5.32 ± 0.59 (4)	122	24.6 ± 2.40 (4)	198
Control	4.13 ± 0.37 (4)	100	4.1 ± 0.13 (4)	100
Lactate 0.04 M.	5.70 ± 0.08 (4)	138	3.4 ± 0.59 (4)	83

[1] Mean and standard error with number of Warburg flasks in parentheses.

In order for succinate to be able to increase the amount of histamine released it must be present at the moment or added not later than 15 minutes after the antigen-antibody reaction has set in.

A number of other substrates and metabolites assayed to investigate enhancement of the anaphylactic reaction *in vitro* were studied by AUSTEN and BROCKLEHURST (1961b). Besides succinic acid, other dibasic acids and intermediates of the Krebs cycle were investigated. Succinic, alpha-ketoglutaric and maleic acids increased the anaphylactic histamine release by about 100%. Lower values were obtained with malonic, adipic and pimelic acids while citric, fumaric and malic acids were not effective. The authors believe that the enhancement produced by some of the substances assayed was probably due to potentiation of any of the chain reactions activated by the antigen-antibody interaction.

The influence of glucose was investigated recently by several workers (DIAMANT, 1961; PROUVOST-DANON and MOUSSATCHÉ, 1961a; ROTHSCHILD et al., 1961); since it can be metabolized both under anaerobic and aerobic conditions, it gives more information about the metabolic pathways involved in the mechanism of histamine release. In guinea-pig lungs, glucose enhanced histamine release under oxygen (DIAMANT, 1962a) and reversed the inhibitory action of oxygen lack (DIAMANT, 1961; PROUVOST-DANON and MOUSSATCHÉ 1961a; ROTHSCHILD, 1961). Optimal enhancement of the histamine release was found when glucose was present in the phosphate buffer incubation media at 5.6 mM concentration. Some experiments made by DIAMANT (1962a) on the reverting action of glucose in guinea-pig tissues shall be referred to later, in connection with observations in rat tissues.

C. Influence of enzyme inhibitors

The relationship between histamine and cell metabolism can also be demonstrated in experiments with enzyme inhibitors. MONGAR and SCHILD (1955, 57) showed that several substances, some of them well known enzyme poisons, inhibit histamine release. Thus, 10^{-3} M iodoacetate and N-ethyl-maleimide, produce almost complete inhibition. p-Chloromercuribenzoate, a more specific blocking agent for SH-groups than the two former compounds, inhibits histamine release from minced guinea-pig lungs (MONGAR and SCHILD, 1957) as well as the release from sensitized guinea-pig ileum by antigen and anaphylatoxin (MOUSSATCHÉ and PROUVOST-DANON, 1956b). The effect on lung tissue was in part reverted by cysteine (MONGAR and SCHILD, 1962). Thioglycolate, reduced glutathione and cysteine, substances which reduce S-S bonds, potentiate histamine release at 10 mM concentration and inhibit it at a higher concentration (50 mM) (EDMAN and MONGAR, 1961). EDMAN and MONGAR concluded that both free SH and S-S groups play a role in anaphylactic histamine release as can be inferred from the inhibitory action of sulfhydryl blocking reagents and the potentiation by S-S reducing substances. High concentrations of SH reagents might have inhibitory action by splitting S-S bonds of some essential protein. The inhibition induced by thioglycolate, reduced glutathione and sodium sulphite was reversed by washing the tissue with Tyrode solution (EDMAN and MONGAR, 1961).

A large number of different compounds were assayed in the anaphylactic reaction (MONGAR and SCHILD, 1962). Since their action as metabolic inhibitors in many cases has been scarcely studied or is relatively unspecific, the results obtained cannot contribute to a more thorough knowledge on the importance of oxidative metabolism in histamine release before more about their site of action is known.

There are several compounds whose properties as enzyme inhibitors and concentration range for specific action have been well established. Malonate, one of the classical examples of a specific competitive inhibitor of succinic dehydrogenase (QUASTEL and WOOLDRIDGE, 1928; DIXON and WEBB, 1958), showed significant inhibitory action on histamine release (MOUSSATCHÉ and PROUVOST-DANON, 1957a, 58; YAMASAKI et al., 1960) from sensitized lung slices by antigen. The inhibitory action was observed with or without addition of succinate to the media, being significant even at the 0.01 M level, a concentration which inhibits almost specifically succinic dehydrogenase (KREBS, 1949). These results did agree with those obtained by AUSTEN and BROCKLEHURST (1961b) and CHAKRAVARTY (1960).

In order to try other selective competitive inhibitors, some of them obtained by synthesis, AUSTEN and BROCKLEHURST (1961a) assayed several amino acids and aminoesters not split by common peptidases, with negative results. Only chymotrypsin substrates and inhibitors showed inhibitory action on the release of histamine and slow-reacting substance during anaphylaxis, leading the authors to the conclusion that activation of a chymotrypsin-like enzyme is a necessary step in the release of histamine.

Cyanide, one of the most useful inhibitors of heavy metal catalysis, employed at 10 mM concentration, decreased histamine release by antigen to 22 % of the control value (MONGAR and SCHILD, 1957). Even lower concentration (1 mM) produced almost complete inhibition of histamine release by antigen (ROTHSCHILD, 1961; AUSTEN and BROCKLEHURST, 1961c), anaphylatoxin (ROTHSCHILD, 1961) and 48/80 (ROTHSCHILD et al., 1961), these effects being reversed by glucose. Experiments with low concentration of cyanide on tissues incubated in open reaction flasks, showed a progressive reversal of inhibition, partially explained by loss of HCN (AUSTEN and BROCKLEHURST, 1961c). Since cyanide inhibits many of the iron and copper containing enzymes and others which do not involve heavy metals (DIXON and WEBB, 1958), it is an unspecific inhibitor, giving little insight into the enzymatic mechanisms involved in histamine release.

The study of the uncouplers of the oxidative phosphorylation deserves a special place. The coupling of respiration and phosphorylation is the aerobic mechanism by which chemical energy, set free during the oxidative reactions, is preserved in the cell as phosphate energy-rich compounds (adenosine di- and triphosphate, phosphocreatine and others), before becoming available for any energy requiring reactions. It is now well established that phosphorylation and energy-rich compound formation occur at least on three sites of the respiratory chain (BARRON, 1941; LEHNINGER, 1951): first on phosphorylation occuring between diphosphopyridine nucleotide and flavoprotein; second, between cytochromes *b* and *c*, and the third occurring between cytochromes *c* and *a* or between *a* and a_3 (cytochrome oxidase). During the anaerobic glycolytic cycle there is formation of one molecule of adenosine triphosphate at the site of oxidation of D-phosphoglyceraldehyde to 1,3-phosphoglyceric acid, the only oxidative step in this series of glycolytic reactions. Each molecule of glucose utilized yields two energy rich phosphate compounds.

There are at present many chemicals which uncouple oxidative phosphorylation. Uncouplers inhibit phosphate uptake and formation of energy-rich compounds by mitochondria leaving the oxygen uptake by the cell unaltered. Three of the most powerful uncouplers of oxidative phosphorylation, 2,4-dinitrophenol, pentachlorophenol and sodium azide (LEHNINGER, 1951) were assayed on sensitized guinea-pig lung slices. They showed high inhibitory action on histamine release without inducing, a significant decrease in the oxygen consumption of the tissues. Dinitrophenol, which at the concentration of 10^{-4} M is known as an uncoupler of oxidative phosphorylation in cells (CROSS et al., 1949; KREBS, 1954), inhibited histamine release almost completely, while oxygen consumption remained normal or even increased. The same happened with pentachlorophenol and sodium azide, both substances known to act like dinitrophenol (MOUSSATCHÉ and PROUVOST-DANON, 1958a). The decrease in oxygen uptake observed in the experiments with sodium azide cannot explain the lowering in histamine release, since low tensions of oxygen can decrease oxygen consumption to 50 % of that of control experiments (at pure oxygen 760 mm tension), without decreasing the histamine release (MOUSSATCHÉ and PROUVOST-DANON, 1960).

Dinitrophenol inhibited the enhancement of histamine release induced by succinate and alpha-ketoglutarate (MOUSSATCHÉ and PROUVOST-DANON, 1958), notwithstanding the stimulation of oxygen uptake produced by these metabolites (LEHNINGER, 1951).

ROTHSCHILD (1961) confirmed these results showing that dinitrophenol blocked histamine release by antigen from sensitized rat diaphragm and by anaphylatoxin from guinea-pig lung. Inhibition of histamine release by dinitrophenol (10^{-4}M concentration) from sensitized guinea-pig lung slices incubated with or without succinate was confirmed by YAMASAKI et al. (1961). Working with compound 48/80, a chemical histamine releaser, ROTHSCHILD et al. (1961) and DIAMANT and UVNÄS (1961) obtained inhibition of histamine release by dinitrophenol, in the diaphragm and lung of the rat.

Dinitrophenol has no inhibitory action on the anaerobic release of histamine during anaphylaxis, in media containing glucose (PROUVOST-DANON and MOUSSATCHÉ, 1961b). This result agrees with the biochemical observations that 2,4-dinitrophenol has no uncoupling effect on anaerobic phosphorylation (STICKLAND, 1956). Anaerobic glycolysis supplies the energy required through the phosphate energy-rich bond formation, even in the presence of dinitrophenol. The reversal by glucose of the inhibitory action of cyanide and dinitrophenol in aerobic conditions (ROTHSCHILD, 1961) became clear; anaerobic glycolysis furnishes the energy required for histamine release, since 2,4-dinitrophenol does not uncouple anaerobic phosphorylation and cyanide, in spite of its very unspecific enzyme inhibitory action, has no inhibitory effect on phosphoglyceraldehyde dehydrogenase (DIXON and WEBB, 1958), an enzyme involved in the generation of the energy-rich bond by oxidation of 3-phosphoglyceraldehyde. On the other hand, SH groups essential for maintaining enzymatic activity, can be readily blocked by iodoacetate. Fluoride and iodoacetate inhibited the anaerobic reversal of histamine release by glucose (PROUVOST-DANON and MOUSSATCHÉ, 1961b). Some authors did not observe inhibitory action of dinitrophenol on histamine release at concentrations inhibiting oxidative phosphorylation (MONGAR and SCHILD, 1957, 62).

The fundamental importance of the enzymes of the respiratory chain, for the maintenance of the steady state of cell metabolism under aerobic conditions, and their efficiency in energy generation, led to the investigation of the action of highly specific respiratory enzyme inhibitors. Two of them, antimycin A, an inhibitor of electron transfer between cytochromes *b* and *c*, acting on a component of the respiratory chain, referred to as "Slater factor" (POTTER and REIF, 1952; AHMED et al., 1951), and carbon monoxide, which combines with the prosthetic group of cytochrome oxidase (cytochrome a_3), were investigated.

A schematic representation of the respiratory chain, its components and inhibitors, is given in Fig. 1.

An amount of antimycin A as low as 1.7 μg/g of tissue was enough to decrease the amount of histamine released, to 50% of the control values (MOUSSATCHÉ and PROUVOST-DANON, 1962a). This figure for antimycin A is very similar to that employed in inhibition studies of oxidative systems by other authors, suggesting a similar mode of action. Metabolites such as succinate and alpha-ketoglutarate which enhance the release of histamine in anaphylaxis were not effective when antimycin A was present in the incubation media. This result might be expected since antimycin A inhibits a factor in the electron transport necessary for the oxidation of such metabolites and oxidative phosphorylation operating via the Krebs cycle (POTTER and REIF, 1952).

On the basis of the classical experiments of HALDANE and SMITH on the photochemical dissociation of the carbon monoxide-iron compound, WARBURG (1926) demonstrated that carbon monoxide inhibits the respiration of living cells in the dark, this inhibition being abolished by light. MOUSSATCHÉ and PROUVOST-DANON (1962a) showed that carbon monoxide at a concentration higher than 75% significantly inhibited histamine release and oxygen consumption by tissues in the dark. Light reversed both inhibitory effects.

It should be noted that CO does not combine with most of the cytochromes, combination with cytochromes a_2 and a_3 (cytochrome oxidase) being exceptional. AUSTEN and BROCKLEHURST (1961c) also studied the effect of CO on histamine release from chopped and whole perfused guinea-pig lungs and failed to show inhibition during anaphylaxis. To explain these contradictory results, one has to analyze thoroughly the conditions of the experiments. Perhaps the presence of glucose, a normal constituent of Tyrode solution, may explain AUSTEN and BROCKLEHURST's results.

Inhibition by a metabolic analog was recently reported by CHAKRAVARTY (1962), who showed that 2-deoxyglucose inhibits histamine release by antigen from sensitized guinea-pig lung. KIPNIS and CORI (1959) observed in the rat

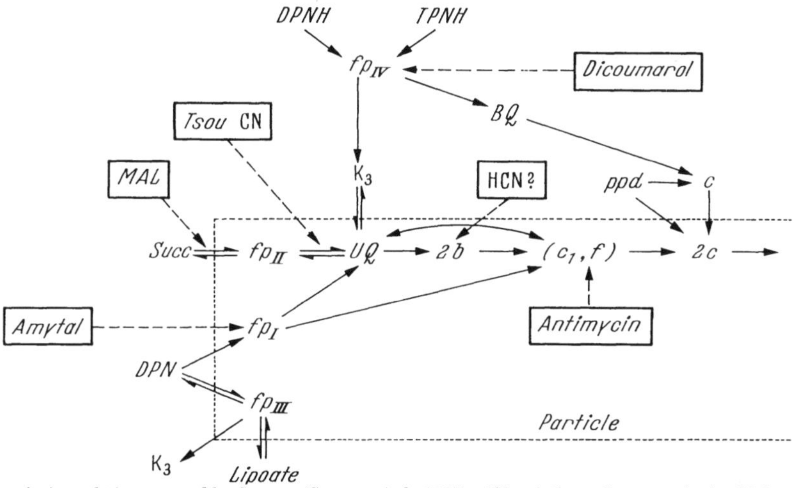

Fig. 1. Respiratory chain proposed by SLATER (SLATER et al., 1961). *Abbreviations:* Succ, succinate; Mal, malonate; DPNH, Reduced diphosphopyridine nucleotide; TPNH, Reduced triphosphopyridine nucleotide; b, c_1, c, a, a_3 Cytochromes; f, Antimycin and 2,3-dimercaptopropanol sensitive factor; ppd, p-phenylenediamine; fp_I, Mahler flavoprotein; fp_{II}, Singer Tsou flavoprotein; fp_{III}, Straub Massey flavoprotein; fp_{IV}, Ernester-Ljunggren-Danielson flavoproteine (DT diaphorase); K_3, Menadione; BQ, Benzoquinol. The dotted boundary refers to the components of the respiratory chain within mitochondria

diaphragm that 2-deoxyglucose was phosphorylated by hexokinase but accumulated inside the cell blocking the glycolytic pathway and glucose penetration. In anaerobiosis, 2-deoxyglucose inhibited the reversal by glucose of the anaphylactic histamine release, probably by inhibition of glucose penetration. Under oxygen, 2-deoxyglucose inhibited histamine release from tissues, when incubated in a substrate-free medium. Addition of substrates which are metabolized by the oxidative cycle (pyruvate, acetate) restored the histamine releasing process by antigen. The anaphylactoid oedema of rats caused by dextran was also inhibited by 2-deoxyglucose which was ineffective in histamine release provoked by compound 48/80.

Following ALIVISATOS's suggestion (1959) about the role of histamine in cellular damaging mechanisms, experiments were performed in order to analyze the action of nicotinamide and analogs on histamine release. The reaction of histamine with the ribose moiety of diphospyridine nucleotide is catalyzed by a purified beef spleen diphosphopyridine nucleotidase (DPNase), histamine replacing nicotinamide (ALIVISATOS, 1958). Histamine released from tissues can be bound by DPN through the DPNase of the glucosidase type, widely found in animal tissues, forming a histamine adenine nucleotide, without coenzyme function and leading to asphyxiation. Isolation and identification of an imidazoleacetic acid riboside (KARJALA, 1955; TABOR and HAYASHI, 1955) from rat urine supported this suggestion. Nicotinamide, an inhibitor of DPNase, was investigated both on histamine release by antigen (MOTA et al., 1960; MOUSSATCHÉ and PROUVOST-DANON, 1961a; YAMASAKI et al., 1961) and by compound 48/80. The results showed that nicotinamide inhibited histamine release by antigen but potentiated the mast cell damage and histamine release by 48/80 (MOTA et al., 1960) in the guinea pig. Some analogs of nicotinic and isonicotinic acid, isonicotinic acid hydrazide, diethylnicotinamide and pyridine were tried with similar results. Succinate (MOUSSATCHÉ and PROUVOST-DANON, 1961 a, YAMASAKI et al., 1961) and alphaketoglutarate (MOUSSATCHÉ and PROUVOST-DANON, 1961 a) reverted the inhibitory action of nicotinamide and nicotinic acid.

These experiments did not give support to ALIVISATOS's suggestion, since the inhibition of DPNase should yield more free histamine. MOTA and ISHII (1960) suggested that DPNase is required to release histamine from its linkage to the tissues. However, YAMASAKI's et al. (1961) experiments showed that DPNase does not increase the *in vitro* histamine release from chopped guinea-pig lungs or sub-cellular large granules of dog liver. They admitted the hypothesis of a blocking action of nicotinamide on intermediary chemical stimuli arising from the antigen-antibody combination.

A more direct influence of nicotinamide and nicotinic acid on the respiratory chain was suggested by MOUSSATCHÉ and PROUVOST-DANON (1961a): nicotinic acid does not inhibit DPNase (MANN and QUASTEL, 1941; MCILWAIN, 1950), and experiments of BIRT and BARTLEY (1960) indicate that nicotinamide decreases the endogenous respiration and capacity of mitochondria to maintain the original levels of oxidized and reduced coenzymes, the ratio of reduced to oxidized pyridine nucleotides being greatly diminished. BIRT and BARTLEY (1960) also showed that addition of succinate to a nicotinamide containing medium partially altered the ratio of reduced to oxidized coenzymes, a greater amount of reduced pyridine nycleotides being observed. This should be in agreement with CHANCE and WILLIAMS's suggestion (1956), that reduced nucleotides are involved in the mechanism of energy rich compound formation during oxidative phosphorylation. Since histamine release is an energy requiring process, nicotinamide, as well as other substances not yet investigated for effects on the respiratory chain but known to inhibit histamine release may, by changing the ratio of reduced/oxidized pyridine nucleotides and, accordingly, the amount of energy rich compounds available, lead to the inhibition of histamine release.

Recent progress in the biochemistry of the respiratory chain (GREEN, 1961; SLATER et al., 1961) showed the importance of benzo-and naphthoquinone coenzymes in electron transport and oxidative phosphorylation in the cell. The study of the role of these factors in the mechanism of histamine release is restricted to some preliminary experimental observations. Thus, WOSILAIT (1961) showed that "pyridine nucleotide vitamin K_1 reductase," an enzyme widely spread in bacteria, higher plants and mammalian tissues, catalyzed the reduction of vitamin K_1 by pyridine nucleotides. The ease with which quinones undergo oxidation led to investigate the fate of reduced vitamin K_1. A "vitamin K_1 cytochrome - *c* reductase" was found in liver mitochondria of rats. WOSILAIT showed that salicylate as well as other anticoagulants inhibited "pyridine nucleotide vitamine K_1 reductase", a correlation being found between the inhibitory potency of anticoagulants (dicoumarol, tromexan and salicylate) in respect to the enzyme activity and depression of respiration. These results are interesting for the explanation of the inhibitory action of salicylates on histamine release observed by HAINING (1956) and ROTHSCHILD et al. (1961). "Vitamine K_1H^2 cytochrome - *c* reductase" was less sensitive to anticoagulants than "vitamin K_1 reductase" but was very sensitive to antimycin A, 0.1 μg/ml reducing the enzymatic activity to 15%. Both enzymes are involved in the mechanism of oxidative phosphorylation.

D. Experiments with "aged" tissues

KIELLEY and KIELLEY (1951), and WADKINS and LEHNINGER (1958), showed that mitochondria allowed to stand for a few hours at room temperature or a few days at 2° C completely lost the phosphorylative coupling activity. On the grounds that oxidative phosphorylation is essential for histamine release during anaphylaxis, experiments were done with sensitized guinea-pig lung slices "aged" at 2° C in the icebox for 24 to 96 hours (MOUSSATCHÉ and PROUVOST-DANON, 1962b). When tissue slices were incubated in Warburg flasks at 37° C after standing 48 hours at 2°C, a decrease in oxygen uptake could be observed, but antigen addition was almost completely ineffective. Succinate increased the oxygen uptake but did not reverse the inhibitory effect on the histamine release. Glucose (5.6 mM) and adenosine (1 mM) reversed both oxygen uptake and histamine release inhibition.

Recent investigations on the biochemical composition and behaviour of mitochondria and submitochondrial fragments allow some speculations on the mechanism by which "ageing" can inhibit histamine release. HÜLSMAN et al. (1958) extracted from aged cytochrome (mitochrome) by iso-octane an unsaturated fatty acid with uncoupling properties. Fresh cytochrome contains much less uncoupling material. Ageing releases a naturally occurring uncoupler normally bound to mitochrome or cytochromes.

It is not yet possible to understand the role played by these new respiratory components in the control of cell metabolism in its relation to anaphylaxis but it is conceivable that changes in the steady state of cell respiration and oxidative phosphorylation induced by antigens, chemical releasers, metabolites or enzyme inhibitors can interfere with histamine release. It can be expected that here an important physiological, pharmacological and pathological field might be opened.

E. Experiments in species other than the guinea-pig

CHAKRAVARTY (1960) studied the effect of anoxia on rat lung fragments but did not find any influence of oxygen lack on histamine release by antigen; this suggests that endogenous anaerobic metabolism was furnishing the energy required. These results are at variance with those of PROUVOST-DANON and MOUSSATCHÉ (1961a) and DIAMANT (1962a) who had found that there was no histamine release by antigen from rat lung tissue in anaerobiosis, except when glucose was present in the incubation medium.

DIAMANT (1962a) thoroughly investigated the influence of factors like carbon dioxide, glucose and pH of the incubating media on the amount of histamine released from rat lungs in Tyrode and phosphate media and found that, as in the guinea-pig, glucose reversed the inhibitory action of anoxia, the release of histamine increasing with glucose concentrations up to 2.8 mM.

In the isolated sensitized rat diaphragm, ROTHSCHILD (1961) observed that histamine release by antigen was abolished by dinitrophenol, but that glucose reversed the inhibitory effect and produced significant potentiation of the histamine release by the antigen under oxygen.

DIAMANT (1962b) reported further observations on the relationship between preexposure of rat and guinea-pig tissues to anoxia and the influence of glucose on the subsequent release of histamine by 48/80 or antigen under oxygen. Rat lung tissue, pre-exposed for thirty minutes to anoxia in glucose-free medium, cannot recover the histamine releasing capacity by 48/80 even after prolonged subsequent contact with glucose. When pre-exposure took place in presence of glucose, the histamine releasing capacity was preserved. The author admits that pre-exposure to nitrogen anoxia in a glucose-free medium exhausted the endogenous carbohydrate store leading to a deficit of ATP. This lack of ATP can inhibit the phosphorylating reactions involved in the first steps of glycolysis and impair the metabolism of the added glucose. The different results obtained previously (MOUSSATCHÉ and PROUVOST-DANON, 1960) might be explained by assuming that the Krebs cycle could start again under oxygen when endogenous metabolites did not reach a very low level, as suggested by the consumption of oxygen.

II. Experiments with chemical releasers

Some observations on the interrelation between enzyme inhibitors and histamine release by chemical compounds were presented above.

The enzymatic interpretation of the mechanism involved in histamine release elicited by chemical compounds presents difficulties hardly ever found when antigen is used. The specificity of the antigen-antibody reaction leads to a greater simplification of the subsequent chain of reactions. Chemical releasers can interact with several enzymes, producing side effects not sufficiently understood from a biochemical point of view to allow a correct working hypothesis on their mechanism of action. Thus, it has been shown that compound 48/80 inhibited oxygen uptake of guinea-pig lung at concentrations which were able to release histamine (MOUSSATCHÉ and DANON, unpublished observations).

On the other hand, advantage was taken of a few facts observed with histamine releasers to build up a theory on their mode of action, as for example the displacement theory (PATON, 1957, 58).

The large group of the chemical histamine releasers is not a homogenous one and includes many different kinds of compounds such as carbohydrate polymers, organic and inorganic bases, etc., possessing definite differences in their mechanism of action. Since it has not been shown that histamine release by amines is influenced by oxido-reduction mechanisms, no reference to papers dealing with them will be made.

The first observations on chemical releasers were started by ANREP and coworkers who showed that curarine, a complex mixture obtainable from curare, was able to release histamine. ROCHA E SILVA and SCHILD (1949), obtained similar results and the rat diaphragm using a definite compound, D-tubocurarine and MCINTOSH and PATON (1949) showed that a very wide range of organic bases, useful in medical practice such as morphine, strychnine, codeine, were good histamine releasers.

Up to now there is no general theory to explain the contradictory results obtained when different methods for histamine release were used. While there are good evidences for an enzymatic participation in the release induced by 48/80 and similar compounds in the rat, amines such as octylamine, do not seem to be dependent on this mechanism; incidentally, in the guinea-pig, histamine release by 48/80 is unaffected by enzymatic inhibitors (MONGAR and SCHILD, 1957) nor is it enhanced by the presence of substrates (MOUSSATCHÉ and PROUVOST-DANON, 1957c). Perhaps polymers like 48/80 and other macromolecules act by a mechanism more similar to that of antigen and in a manner not followed by small molecular weight amines and other organic compounds.

The mechanism of the histamine releasing activity of chemical compounds was investigated by many research workers using 48/80, a particularly powerful releasing polymer, obtained by condensation of formaldehyde and p-methoxyphenethyl-methylamine. 48/80 is a very active histamine liberator in the rat, cat and dog. Large number of the experiments were carried out on fragments of the rat's mesentery, diaphragm or skin which contain mast cells as well as on the mast cells isolated from the rat's peritoneal cavity.

A. Experiments in rats with compound 48/80. Influence of oxygen and enzyme inhibitors

MOTA et al. (1953) showed that 48/80 promotes a vigorous extrusion of rat mast cell granules, and these were used as test object by JUNQUEIRA and BEIGUELMAN (1955), for the assay of the action of several metabolic inhibitors, pH, oxygen lack and temperature. An inhibitory effect was observed at temperatures below 25°C and pH below 6.26. Inhibitors of sulfhydryl groups such as p-chloromercuri-benzoate, o-iodosobenzoate and iodoacetate as well as cyanide, urethane, uranyl nitrate, arsenite and 2,4-dinitrophenol, enzyme inhibitors with different points of action, inhibited the extrusion of mast cell granules. Glutathione reverted the inhibitory action of sulfhydryl blocking agents but adenosinetriphosphate did not revert the effect of oxidative phosphorylation uncouplers like arsenite and 2,4-dinitrophenol. Lack of permeability to ATP may be a factor to be considered in these experiments. Malonate and fluoride were inactive. Attention must be paid to the correlation between granule extrusion and histamine release since the latter can occur without gross visible changes in the mast cell (WEST, 1959; SMITH, 1958).

MOTA and ISHII (1960), confirmed the results for sulfhydryl blocking agents, and extended the observations to rat skin, showing the analogy between mast cell damage induced by 48/80 and by antigen. ROTHSCHILD et al. (1961), showed that dinitrophenol blocked histamine release by compound 48/80 from isolated rat diaphragm, and that glucose markedly decreased this inhibitory effect. Succinate, fumarate, pyruvate and D-xylose could not substitute glucose. Inhibitory effects of cyanide, salicylate, thiopental and sodium oleate were also counteracted by glucose. Independently, at the same time, DIAMANT and UVNÄS (1961) tested the influence of enzyme inhibitors showing that, like that due to antigen-antibody reaction, histamine release by compound 48/80 from isolated rat lung tissue was inhibited by 2,4-dinitrophenol, sodium azide, thyroxine, cyanide, ninhydrin, Pb^{++}, Zn^{++} and Cu^{++} ions. Glucose counteracted the blocking action of the first three compounds but was unable to influence the inhibition due to the other agents. Out of 6 mono- and dissacharides assayed, glucose alone had restaurative action, fructose, lactose and sucrose being ineffective; the small influence of galactose and maltose was attributed to contamination with glucose.

From the point of view of the role of oxidative metabolism it is important to investigate the influence of oxygen on the process. The above workers studied the influence of oxygen lack and showed that under anaerobiosis, compound 48/80 lost its histamine releasing activity to a marked extent, but that anoxia had a significantly smaller effect when glucose was added to the incubation media.

As specified above, CHAKRAVARTY (1959) did not observe any influence of oxygen lack on histamine release by antigen and 48/80 from rat tissues. The author accepted however, that probably, the same mechanism was involved in histamine release by the antigen and the chemicals, since enzyme inhibitors, calcium lack and ethyl alcohol had the same effect on both acting on rat and guinea-pig tissues.

B. Experiments in the cat

Evidences for an enzymatic mechanism involved in histamine release by 48/80 from cat's paw were presented by CHAKRAVARTY (1959).

Heating the perfused paw to 45° C completely inhibited histamine release by 48/80. Other enzyme inhibitors such as iodoacetate (10^{-3}M), allicin (extracted from *Allium sativum)* which reacts with sulfhydryl groups, as well as several polymers caused inhibition of histamine release, the amount released being 1 to 37 % of the control. As in the rat, CHAKRAVARTY did not obtain inhibition by anoxia.

More recently, WESTERHOLM (1960a, b) succeeded in showing that in chopped cat skin, histamine release by 48/80 was inhibited by anoxia or 2,4-dinitrophenol, this inhibition being abolished by glucose.

C. Experiments with other histamine releasers

It has been known for a long time that there are tissue extracts from animals belonging to the several branches of the phylum, which induce toxic effects in other animals. Some of these extracts showed histamine releasing properties.

Extracts from *Ascaris lumbricoides* and *Ascaris megalocephala* were investigated (SHINAMURA and FUJI, 1917; MACHEBOEUF and MANDOUL, 1939; BIER, 1946; ROCHA E SILVA and GRAÑA, 1946) and shown to produce anaphylactic-like symptoms of shock in guinea-pigs and dogs. An active complex substance was isolated from *A. lumbricoides* extracts by GAZZINELLI et al. (1961), which contained carbohydrate and protein components and produced anaphylactic-like reactions in the guinea pig (BERALDO et al., 1961) with mast cell alterations very similar to those observed by MOTA and VUGMAN (1956) with antigen and by MOTA (1957) with anaphylatoxin. However, the active fraction did not act through anaphylatoxin formation.

Similar observations were made by HÖGBERG et al. (1956), with *Ascaris* extracts purified by the authors. Some experiments were done with extracts from *Ascaris suum*, zoologically synonim of *Ascaris lumbricoides*. The results led to the conclusion that a respiratory enzymatic process was involved (UVNÄS et al. 1960), since sulfhydryl blocking reagents, uncouplers of the oxidative phosphorylation and anoxia inhibited histamine release while glucose reverted the inhibitory effect and enhanced the releasing potency under oxygen.

Quite identical results were obtained with extracts from *Cyanea capillata*, a jellyfish from the Swedish coast (UVNÄS, 1960) tested on the cat skin and isolated rat mast cells.

Sinomenine, a convulsant drug related to morphine, extracted from *Sinomenium acutum*, Rehd. et Wilson, is a histamine releaser studied by YAMASAKI and coworkers (YAMASAKI, 1961). For its action it showed respiratory metabolism dependence, oxygen lack and respiratory inhibitors inhibiting its effects on cat skin.

References

AHMED, K., H. G. SCHNEIDER, and F. M. STRONG: Studies on the biological action of Antimycin A. Arch. Biochem. **28**, 281—288 (1951).

ALIVISATOS, S. G. A.: Formation of histamine-containing dinucleotides by enzymatic interaction of histamine and coenzyme. Nature (Lond.) **181**, 271 (1958).

— In: H. O. SCHILD. Mechanism of the anaphylactic reaction as studied by means of inhibitors. Edited by J. H. SCHAFFER, G. A. LOGRIPPO and M. W. CHASE. "Mechamism of hypersensitivity" 1959. p. 259—264. Henry Ford International Symposium. Little, Brown, Co. Boston, Toronto.

AUSTEN, K. F., and W. D. BROCKLEHURST: Anaphylaxis in chopped guinea pig lung. I. Effect of peptidase substrates and inhibitors. J. exp. Med. **113**, 521—540 (1961a).

Austen, K. F., and W. D. Brocklehurst: Anaphylaxis in chopped guinea-pig lung. II. Enhancement of the anaphylactic release of histamine and slow reacting substance by certain dibasic aliphatic acids and inhibition by monobasic fatty acids. J. exp. Med. **113**, 541—557 (1961b).

— — Anaphylaxis in chopped guinea-pig lung. III. Effect of carbon monoxide, cyanide, salicylaldoxime and ionic strength. J. exp. Med. **114**, 29—42 (1961c).

Barron, E. S. G.: Biological oxidations and reductions. Ann. Rev. Biochem. **10**, 1 (1941).

Benda, L., A. Locker u. E. Rissel: Zellstoffwechsel und Entzündung. V. Mitteilung. Die Gewebsatmung der Leber bei anaphylaktischem Schock. Z. ges. exp. Med. **124**, 189—200 (1954).

Beraldo, W. T., W. Dias da Silva, and J. Pudles: Antigenic properties of purified fractions from Ascaris lumbricoides Var. Suum on naturally sensitized guinea-pig. Brit. J. Pharmacol. **17**, 236—244 (1961).

Bier, O.: Cited in M. Rocha e Silva: Histamina e Anaphylaxia. São Paulo: Edigraf Ltda. 1946.

Birt, L. N., and W. Bartley: The pyridine nucleotide metabolism of mitochondria incubated with and without added substrates and metabolic inhibitors. Biochem. J. **76**, 427—438 (1960).

Boström, G.: Die anaphylaktische Stoffwechselreaktion des isolierten Gewebes. Klin. Wschr. **13**, 399—405 (1934).

Büngeler, W.: Die Gewebsatmung bei der Anaphylaxie. Z. ges. exp. Med. **75**, 223—262 (1931).

— Die Sauerstoffaufnahme des Gesamtkörpers bei der Anaphylaxie. Z. ges. exp. Med. **75**, 287—296 (1931).

Chakravarty, N.: Observations on histamine release and formation of a lipid-soluble smooth muscle stimulating principle ('SRS') by antigen-antibody reaction and compound 48/80. Karolinska Institutet, Thesis, Stockholm, 1—48 (1959).

— The mechanism of histamine release in anaphylactic reaction in guinea-pig and rat. Acta physiol. scand. **48**, 146—166 (1960).

— Inhibition of anaphylactic histamine release by 2-deoxyglucose. Nature (Lond.) **194**, 1182—1184 (1962a).

— Aerobic metabolism in anaphylactic reaction. Amer. J. Physiol. **203**, 1193 to 1198 (1962).

Chance, B., and G. R. Williams: Respiratory chain and oxidative phosphorylation. Advanc. Enzymol. **17**, 65 (1956).

Cross, J. R., J. V. Taggart, G. A. Covo, and D. E. Green: Studies on the cyclophorase system. VI. The coupling of oxidation and phosphorylation. J. biol. Chem. **117**, 655 (1949).

Diamant, B.: Histamine release elicited by extracts from ascaris suis. Influence of oxygen lack and glucose. Acta physiol. scand. **52**, 8—22 (1961).

— Comparison between the effects of glucose and sodium succinate on the in vitro release of histamine from guinea-pig and rat lung tissue. Acta physiol. scand. **56**, 103—111 (1962a).

— Observations on anaphylactic and compound 48/80 induced histamine release from guinea-pig and rat lung tissue in vitro. Acta physiol. scand. **55**, 11—25 (1962b).

—, and B. Uvnäs: Evidence for energy-requiring processes in histamine release and mast cell degranulation in rat tissues induced by compound 48/80. Acta physiol. scand. **53**, 315—329 (1961).

Dixon, M., and E. Webb: Enzymes. London, New York, Toronto: Longmans, Green and Co. 1958.

Edman, K. A. P., and J. L. Mongar: The essential role of SH and S-S groups in anaphylactic reaction. J. Physiol. (Lond.) **157**, 40 P (1961).

— — and H. O. Schild: The role of SH and S-S groups and oxygen in the anaphylactic reaction of chopped guinea-pig lung. J. Physiol. (Lond.) **170**, 124—137 (1964).

Follis, R. H.: The metabolism of tissue from anaphylactically hypersensitive animals when antigen is added in vitro. Bull. Johns Hopk. Hosp. **92**, 371 (1953).

Gazzinelli, G., M. M. Guia, A. G. A. Neves, and J. Pudles: Purification of the toxic fractions from Ascaris lumbricoides and their effect on the guinea-pig. Nature (Lond.) **190**, 813—814 (1961).

Green, D. E.: Coenzyme Q and electron transport. Quinones in Electron transport. Ciba Found. Symp., p. 130—160 (1961).

Haining, C. G.: Inhibition of histamine release by sodium salicylate and other compounds. Brit. J. Pharmacol. **11**, 357 (1956).

Högberg, B., G. Thufvesson, and B. Uvnäs: Histamine liberation produced in perfused paw of the cat by 48/80 and extracts from jelly fish (cyanea capillata) and eelworm (Ascaris lumbricoides from swine). Acta physiol. scand. **38**, 135 (1956).

Hülsman, W. C., W. B. Elliott, and H. Rudney: The nature and action of mitochrome. Biochim. biophys. Acta (Amst.) **27**, 664 (1958).

Junqueira, L. C. U., and B. Beiguelman: Studies on the in vitro action of compound 48/80, a formaldehyde condensation product, on rat mast cells. Tex. Rep. Biol. Med. **13**, 69—75 (1955).

Karjala, S. A.: The partial characterization of histamine metabolite from rat and mouse urine. J. Amer. chem. Soc. **77**, 504 (1955).

KIELLEY, W. W., and R. K. KIELLEY: Miokynase and adenosine triphosphatase in oxidative phosphorylation. J. biol. Chem. **191**, 485—500 (1951).
KIPNIS, D. M., and C. F. CORI: Penetration and phosphorylation of 2-deoxyglucose in rat diaphragm. J. biol. Chem. **234**, 171 (1959).
KREBS, H. A.: The tricarboxylic acid cycle. Harvey Lect. **49**, 165—199 (1949).
— The tricarboxilic acid cycle. In: Chemical Pathways of Metabolism, vol. **I**, 170 (1954).
LEHNINGER, A. L.: Oxidative phosphorylation in diphosphopyridine nucleotide-linked systems. Phosphorus Metabolism. Mc Elroy and Gall, Ed., p. 344—366 (1951).
LOCKER, A., u. H. KÖLB: Gehirnatmung und anaphylaktischer Schock. Z. ges. exp. Med. **124**, 170—175 (1954).
MACHEBOEUF, M., et R. MANDOUL: A propos de la toxicité des extraits d'Ascaris. C. R. Soc. Biol. (Paris) **130**, 1032—1035 (1939).
MANN, P. J. G., and J. H. QUASTEL: Nicotinamide cozymase and tissue metabolism. Biochem. J. **35**, 502—517 (1941).
MCILWAIN, H.: Properties of preparations from the central nervous system which degrade coenzymes I and II. Their connexion with carbohydrate metabolism. Biochem. J. **46**, 612 (1950).
MCINTIRE, F. C.: The mechanism of histamine release. Ciba Foundation Symp., p. 416-430(1956).
MCINTOSH, F. C., and W. D. M. PATON: The liberation of histamine by certain organic bases. J. Physiol. (Lond.) **109**, 190—219 (1949).
MONGAR, J. L., and B. A. V. PERERA: Oxygen consumption of isolated mast cells in the anaphylactic reaction. Nature (Lond.) **202**, 93 (1964).
—, and H. O. SCHILD: Inhibition of histamine release in anaphylaxis. Nature (Lond.) **176**, 163 (1955).
— — Inhibition of the anaphylactic reaction. J. Physiol. (Lond.) **135**, 301—319 (1957).
— — Cellular mechanisms in anaphylaxis. Physiol. Rev. **42**, 226—270 (1962).
MOTA, I.: Action of anaphylactic shock and anaphylatoxin on mast cells and histamine in rats. Brit. J. Pharmacol. **12**, 453 (1957).
— W. T. BERALDO, and L. C. U. JUNQUEIRA: Protamine-like property of compound 48/80 and stilbamidine and their action on mast cells. Proc. Soc. exp. Biol. (N. Y.) **83**, 455 (1953).
— W. DIAS DA SILVA, and J. FERREIRA FERNANDES: The inhibition of mast cell damage and histamine release in anaphylaxis by pyridine and diphosphopyridine nucleotidase inhibitors. Comparison with compound 48/80. Brit. J. Pharmacol. **15**, 405—409 (1960).
—, and T. ISHII: Inhibition of mast cell disruption and histamine release in rat anaphylaxis in vitro. Comparison with compound 48/80. Brit. J. Pharmacol. **15**, 82—87 (1960).
—, and I. VUGMAN: Effects of anaphylactic shock and compound 48/80 on the mast cells of the guinea-pig lung. Nature (Lond.) **177**, 427—429 (1956).
MOUSSATCHÉ, H., e A. PROUVOST-DANON: Consumo de oxigênio de alguns tecidos de cobaias submetidas a reação anafilática "in vitro". An. Acad. Bras. Cienc. **28**, XLVIII—XLIX (1956a).
— — Inhibition by sulfhydril blocking agents of the guinea-pig gut reaction to anaphylaxis and to anaphylatoxin. Naturwissenschaften **43**, 227—228 (1956b).
— — Histamina e metabolismo celular. I. Influência de alguns metabolitos sôbre a liberação de histamina na reação anafilática "in vitro". An. Acad. Bras. Cienc. **29**, XXX (1957a).
— — On the action of succinate and malonate upon the histamine release during the anaphylactic reaction in vitro. Naturwissenschaften **44**, 330—331 (1957b).
— — The effect of succinate and malonate on the chemical release of histamine from guinea-pig lung slices. Naturwissenschaften **44**, 637—638 (1957c).
— — Influence of sodium succinate and malonate on the histamine release in the anaphylactic reaction "in vitro". Arch. Biochem. **77**, 108—111 (1958).
— — Influence of oxidative phosphorylation inhibitors on the histamine release in the anaphylactic reaction "in vitro". Experientia (Basel) **14**, 414—418 (1958a).
— — Influence de l'anaérobiose et de différentes tensions d'oxygène sur la libération d'histamine dans la réaction anaphylactique *in vitro*. Experientia (Basel) **16**, 118—119 (1960).
— — Inhibition by nicotinamide and nicotinic acid of histamine release in anaphylactic reaction *in vitro*. Influence of some metabolites. An. Acad. Bras. Cienc. **33**, 173—178 (1961a).
— — Oxygen uptake by guinea-pig lung slices during anaphylactic reaction "in vitro". An. Acad. Bras. Cienc. **33**, 335—340 (1961b).
— — Influence of inhibitors of the respiratory chain in the histamine release during anaphylactic reaction in vitro. Action of antimycin A and carbon monoxide. Biochem. Pharmacol. **11**, 603—608 (1962a).
— — Histamina e metabolismo celular. VI. Influência do envelhecimento das fatias de tecido sensibilizado (longa permanencia em baixa temperatura) sôbre a liberação de histamina na reação anafilática in vitro. An. Acad. Bras. Cienc. **34**, V (1962b).
PARROT, J. L.: Sur la réaction cellulaire de l'anaphylaxie; son caractère aérobie. C. R. Soc. Biol. (Paris) **136**, 361—362 (1942).

PARROT, J. L., et G. RICHET, Action du cyanure de mercure sur les organes isolés du cobaye. Un nouveau type de libération de l'histamine. C. R. Soc. Biol. (Paris) **138**, 364—365 (1944).
PATON, W. D. M.: Histamine release by compounds of simple chemical structure. Pharmacol. Rev. **9**, 269—328 (1957).
— The release of histamine. Progr. Allergy **5**, 79—148 (1958).
POTTER, V. R., and A. E. REIF: Inhibition of an electron transport component by antimycin A. J. biol. Chem. **194**, 287—297 (1952).
PROUVOST-DANON, A., e H. MOUSSATCHÉ: Reação anafilática "in vitro" e metabolismo anaeróbico. IV. Reunião Associação Latino-Americana Ciências Fisiológicas. Comunicações, Julho, pg. 64 (1961a).
— — Influence of anaerobic glycolysis on the histamine release in the guinea-pig and rat anaphylactic reaction "in vitro". Nature (Lond.) **192**, 361—362 (1961b).
QUASTEL, J. H., and W. R. WOOLDRIDGE: Some properties of the dehydrogenating enzymes of bacteria. Biochem. J. **22**, 689 (1928).
ROCHA E SILVA, M.: Ação da tripsina sôbre o intestino e útero isolados de cobaia; libertação de histamina do pulmão, pela perfusão com soluções de tripsina. Arch. Inst. Biol. São Paulo **9**, 145—163 (1938).
— S. ANDRADE, and R. M. TEIXEIRA: Fibrinolysis in peptone and anaphylactic shock in the dog. Nature (Lond.) **157**, 801 (1946).
— Histamine release by naturally occurring substances. Histamine. Ciba Foundation Symp., p. 124—138 (1956).
—, and A. GRAÑA: Anaphylaxis-like reactions produced by Ascaris extracts. II. The mechanism of the shock induced in dogs. Arch. Surg. **52**, 523 (1946).
—, and H. O. SCHILD: The release of histamine by D-tubocurarine from the isolated diaphragm of the rat. J. Physiol. (Lond.) **109**, 448—458 (1949).
— A. E. SCROGGIE, E. FIDLAR, and L. B. JAQUES: Liberation of histamine and heparin by peptone from the isolated dog's liver. Proc. Soc. exp. Biol. (N. Y.) **64**, 141—146 (1947).
ROTHSCHILD, A. M.: Effect of metabolic inhibitors on the release of histamine by anaphylatoxin and by antigen in vitro. Experientia (Basel) **17**, 555—556 (1961).
— I. VUGMAN, and M. ROCHA E SILVA: Metabolic studies on the release of histamine by compound 48/80 in the rat diaphragm. Biochem. Pharmacol. **7**, 248 (1961).
SHINAMURA, K., and I. FUJI: Askaron, a toxin extracted from Ascaris lumbricoides (1916). Chem. Abstr. **11**, 2357—2359 (1917).
SLATER, E. C., J. P. COLPA-BOONSTRA, and J. LINKS: The oxidation of quinols by mitochondrial preparations. Quinones in Electron Transport. Ciba Foundation Symp., p. 161 (1961).
SMITH, D. E.: Dynamics of release of histamine from tissue mast cell. Science **128**, 207 (1958).
SONAK, R.: Tissue metabolism in sensitized guinea-pig: Folia biol. (Praha) **4**, 160 (1958).
STICKLAND, L. H.: Phosphorylations and dephosphorylations in yeast and their inhibition by various agents. Biochem. J. **64**, 515—523 (1956).
TABOR, H., and O. HAYASHI: The excretion of imidazoleacetic acid riboside following the administration of imidazoleacetic acid or histamine to rats. J. Amer. chem. Soc. **77**, 505 (1955).
UNGAR, G.: Mechanism of histamine release. Ciba Foundation Symp., p. 431—443 (1956).
UVNÄS, B.: Mechanism of action a histamine liberating principle in jelly fish (Cyanea Capillata). Ann. N. Y. Acad. Sci. **90**, 751—759 (1960).
— B. DIAMANT, B. HÖGBERG, and I. L. THON: Mechanism of mast-cell disruption induced by a principle extracted from Ascaris suis. Amer. J. Physiol. **199**, 575—578 (1960).
WADKINS, C. L., and A. L. LEHNINGER: Adenosine triphosphate exchange reaction of oxidative phosphorylation. J. biol. Chem. **233**, 1589—1597 (1958).
WARBURG, O.: Über die Wirkung des Kohlenoxyds auf den Stoffwechsel der Hefe. Biochem. Z. **177**, 471—488 (1926).
WEST, G. B.: Tissue mast cells and tissue amines. J. Pharm. Pharmacol. **11**, 513—534 (1959).
WESTERHOLM, B.: In vitro release of histamine from cat skin by compound 48/80. Acta physiol. scand. **50**, 41 (1960a).
— The influence of anoxia on 48/80-induced histamine release from cat skin. Acta physiol. scand. **50**, 300 (1960b).
WOSILAIT, W. D.: Role of vitamin K in electron transport. Fed. Proc. **20**, 1005—1011 (1961).
YAMASAKI, H.: Mechanism of histamine release by antigen and chemical substances as studied by means of inhibitors. Folia Farmac. Japon. **57**, 171—173, 1961 (Summary in: Contributions of Professor H. YAMASAKI and his associates from the Department of Pharmacology, p. 56 (1961).
— M. SABURE, and K. ENDO: Energy metabolic aspect of histamine release in anaphylaxis. Jap. J. Pharmacol. **10**, 21—29 (1960).
— S. MURAOKA, M. SUGIYAMA, and K. ENDO: Mechanism of histamine release inhibition by nicotinamide in "in vitro" antigen-antibody reaction. Jap. J. Pharmacol. **11**, 54—64 (1961).

Chapter 4

Metabolism of Histamine

Section A

L'excrétion de l'histamine

Par

JEAN-LOUIS PARROT et MADELEINE MORDELET-DAMBRINE

L'histamine est éliminée, soit libre, soit sous forme de métabolites formés par le foie, par le contenu de l'intestin, par les reins. Les voies d'élimination sont la bile, les fécès et l'urine.

L'injection d'histamine marquée a facilité l'étude de son excrétion; le tableau 1 mentionne les différents corps éliminés lors du catabolisme de l'histamine.

Dans d'autres parties du présent ouvrage sont traitées les questions suivantes:

1. L'absorption de l'histamine par l'appareil digestif.
2. Les enzymes qui assurent *in vivo* le métabolisme de l'histamine.
3. Le métabolisme de l'histamine *in vitro*.
4. La formation enzymatique de l'histamine à partir de l'histidine.
5. Le métabolisme de l'histamine chez l'homme.

Le présent chapitre se bornera donc à regrouper:

a) les voies chimiques de l'excrétion
b) les voies anatomiques de l'excrétion
c) quelques variations normales et pathologiques dans l'excrétion de l'histamine.

A. Voies chimiques de l'excrétion

I. Désamination oxydative

La désamination oxydative est la voie métabolique la plus anciennement connue: EUSTIS (1915), BEST et MCHENRY (1930) puis MCHENRY et GAVIN (1935) étudièrent l'inactivation de l'histamine par l'histaminase et plus récemment ZELLER (1942) et ZELLER et coll. (1957). Ces derniers auteurs considèrent que cette enzyme n'est pas spécifique et qu'il s'agit d'une diamino-oxydase. Pourtant KAPELLER-ADLER (1953) maintient le mot histaminase en fournissant des arguments en faveur de la spécifité de l'enzyme grâce à des techniques chromatographique, électrophorétique et spectrophotométrique (1962).

ZELLER, STERN et BLANKSMA (1956) font jouer un rôle à la monoamino-oxydase qui serait capable elle aussi de faire subir à l'histamine la désamination oxydative. Le catabolisme de l'histamine se poursuit après ce premier temps par l'action de la catalase et de l'aldéhyde-oxydase (ZELLER, 1942; TABOR, 1951) qui donnent lieu à l'apparition de l'acide imidazolacétique (MEHLER, TABOR et BAUER, 1952; TABOR, MEHLER et SCHAYER, 1953). Mais l'acide imidazolacétique peut être

Tableau 1. *Les métabolites de l'histamine*

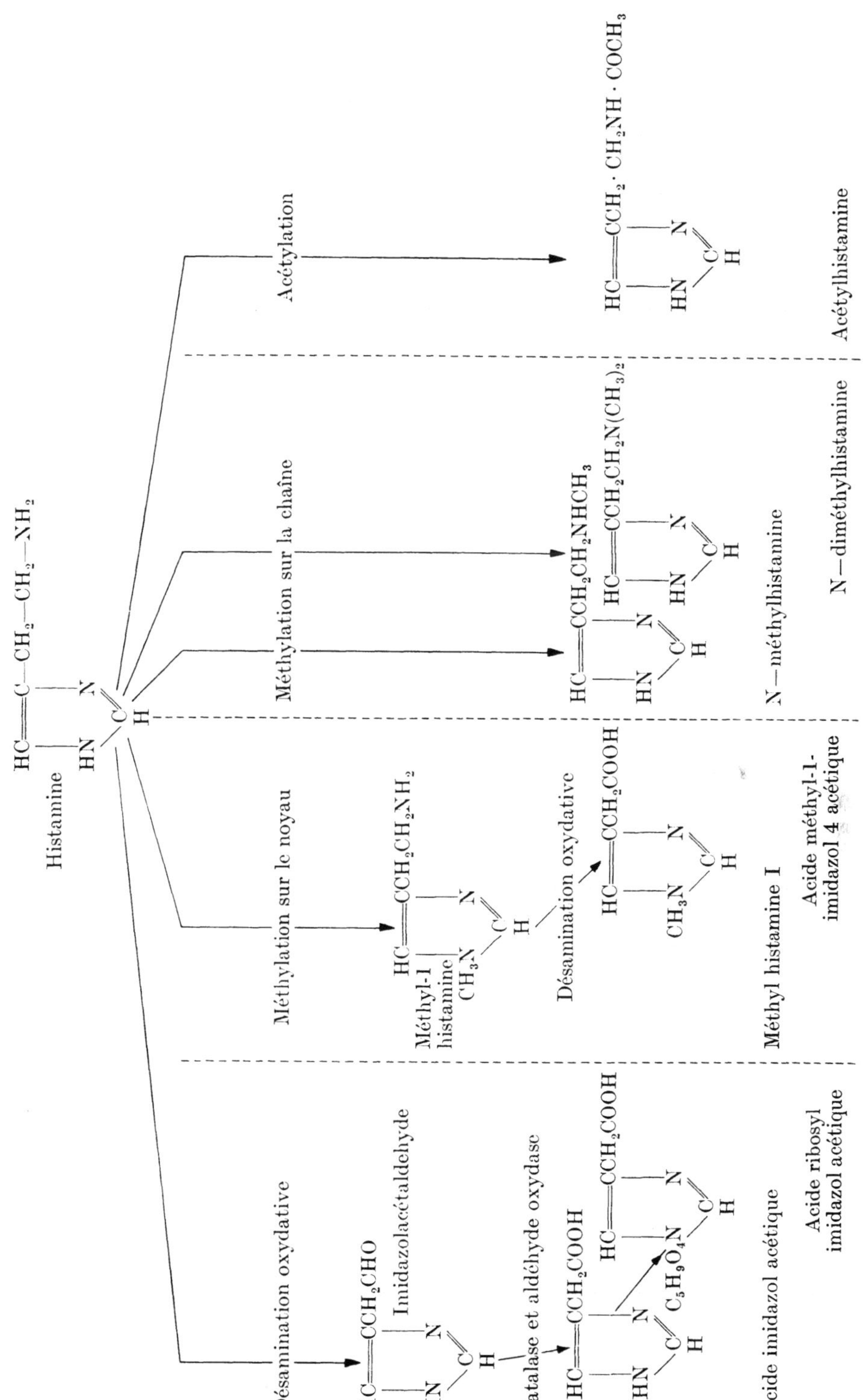

éliminé sous la forme de son riboside (Tabor et Hayaishi, 1955); c'est l'acide 1-ribosylimidazol-4-acétique (Karjala, 1955).

L'ensemble des réactions chimiques lors de la désamination oxydative peut se résumer ainsi ([1]):

a) $R—CH_2—CH_2NH_2 + O_2 + H_2O \longrightarrow R—CH_2CHO + H_2O_2 + NH_3$
Diamino-oxydase ou histaminase.

Cette réaction est inhibée par l'α-aminoguanidine et par l'iproniazide (Lindell et coll., 1960).

b) $H_2O_2 \longrightarrow {}^1/_2\, O_2 + H_2O$
Catalase.

c) $R—CH_2CHO + {}^1/_2\, O_2 \longrightarrow R—CH_2COOH$
aldéhyde-oxydase.

d'où la réaction globale:

$$R—CH_2—CH_2—NH_2 \longrightarrow R—CH_2—COOH + NH_3.$$

L'acide imidazolacétique est dépourvu d'activité pharmacologique.

II. Méthylation sur l'azote 1 du cycle

La méthylation sur l'azote 1 du cycle comme voie métabolique a été mise en évidence par Schayer (1952), Schayer, Kennedy et Smiley (1953).

Lindahl (1958a) indique que la formation de la 1-méthylhistamine nécessite la méthionine et un système générateur d'ATP; ceci conduit à penser que la S-adénosylméthionine fournit le groupement méthyl.

Par contre ce même auteur (1959) a montré l'action inhibitrice de l'acide *para*-chloromercuribenzoïque sur la méthylation de l'histamine à la concentration de 5×10^{-4} M tandis que le glutathion supprime cette inhibition. Il semble donc que les groupements SH soient nécessaires pour l'activité de l'enzyme méthylante.

L'iproniazide inhibe 50 p. 100 de la transformation de la méthylhistamine en acide méthylimidazolacétique (Lindell, Nilsson et coll., 1960). La 1-méthylhistamine et l'acide 1-méthylimidazol-4-acétique qui dérive du corps précédent par désamination oxydative ont été identifiés par Schayer et Karjala (1956), Karjala, Turnquest et Schayer (1956). Mais l'identité de l'enzyme responsable de cette oxydation est discutée; Kobayashi et Schayer (1956) pensent qu'il s'agit d'une monoamino-oxydase; Kapeller-Adler et Iggo (1957), d'une diamino-oxydase.

Karjala, Turnquest et Schayer (1956) considèrent la méthylation de l'anneau imidazole comme la principale voie du métabolisme de quantités «physiologiques» d'histamine. Dès 1911 Pyman avait indiqué que la méthylhistamine est quasiment inactive. White (1961) montre que le 1-méthyl-4-(β-aminoéthyl)-imidazole et l'acide-1-méthylimidazol-4-acétique n'exercent aucune action sur la pression artérielle du chat lorsque ces corps sont injectés dans un ventricule latéral du cerveau alors que l'histamine par la même voie détermine une réponse hypertensive.

III. Méthylation sur l'azote de la chaîne

La méthylation sur l'azote de la chaîne latérale donne des dérivés monométhylés et diméthylés. Ils ont été mis en évidence dans l'urine humaine normale par adsorption sur un échangeur d'ions suivie de chromatographie sur papier (Kapeller-Adler et Iggo, 1957). Les deux dérivés ont une activité du même

[1] R indique dans ces formules le noyau imidazole.

type que l'histamine. L'un et l'autre produisent sur la peau humaine la classique triade de Lewis. Le dérivé monométhylé est même deux fois plus actif que l'histamine sur les muscles lisses du cobaye (utérus). Sur la pression artérielle du chat ce dérivé a une activité deux fois plus faible que celle de l'histamine. Sur le bronchospasme du cobaye il est plus actif que l'histamine. La monométhylhistamine a une action égale à celle de l'histamine sur la sécrétion gastrique (SCHNEDORF et IVY, 1935). La diméthylhistamine possède une action sur les capillaires de l'homme égale à celle de l'histamine; sur la pression artérielle du chat, ce dérivé a une activité cinq à dix fois plus faible que l'histamine; sur l'utérus, trois fois plus faible et sur les bronches, cinq fois. Sur l'intestin isolé de cobaye, la diméthylhistamine exerce une activité qui est les trois quarts de celle de l'histamine (HUEBNER, TURNER et SCHOLZ, 1949). De plus ce dérivé a une faible action nicotinique.

Ces dérivés monométhylé et diméthylé ne sont pas attaqués par la diamino-oxydase et ils inhibent même la désamination oxydative de l'histamine (VARTIAINEN, 1935).

IV. Acétylation

L'acétylation est une voie métabolique dont l'importance varie suivant le régime alimentaire, carné ou végétarien. L'acétylation de l'histamine conduit au 4-(β-acétylaminoéthyl)-imidazole (ROSENTHAL et TABOR, 1948; URBACH, 1949; TABOR et MOSETTIG, 1949). Cette substance est dépourvue d'activité pharmacologique; elle inhibe la diamino-oxydase.

B. Voies anatomiques d'excrétion

I. Elimination rénale

C'est la voie la plus importante.

a) Histamine et acétylhistamine

Dès 1944, ANREP et coll. avaient décrit une méthode par adsorption sur charbon qui permit de concentrer l'histamine urinaire. Ces auteurs avaient trouvé que l'histamine urinaire est en partie libre et en partie conjuguée; cette dernière est inactive au point de vue pharmacologique, mais devient active après hydrolyse acide.

Quand l'histamine pure est administrée *per os* chez le chien, il apparaît de l'histamine conjuguée dans les urines; au contraire, quand l'histamine est injectée, elle est pour la plus grande part détruite ou fixée dans l'organisme; seule une faible quantité d'histamine apparaît dans les urines et il s'agit d'histamine libre. Les expériences montrent que le régime carné augmente le taux d'histamine conjuguée dans les urines. Chez les carnivores 98 à 100 p. 100 de l'histamine sont éliminés sous forme conjuguée.

La conjugaison se fait dans l'intestin lui-même (TABOR et MOSETTIG, 1949). On a pu montrer que le foie est capable d'acétyler *in vitro* l'histamine (MILLICAN, ROSENTHAL et TABOR, 1949; MILLICAN, 1953). Pourtant LIVINGSTON et CODE (1955) précisent que le foie est incapable d'acétyler l'histamine expérimentalement introduite dans la veine porte. D'après LINDAHL (1958b), il se formerait *in vitro*, par suite de la méthylation de l'histamine dans le foie de la souris, de l'acide 1-méthyl-imidazol-4-acétique. Ce dernier corps a été retrouvé dans l'urine de souris. Enfin, plus récemment LINDELL et SCHAYER (1958), LINDELL (1958), après injection lente d'histamine marquée dans une artère rénale, chez le chien anesthésié, ont pu constater l'excrétion par ce rein non seulement de méthylhistamine, mais aussi d'acide méthylimidazolacétique et d'acide imidazolacétique, ce qui montre le rôle du rein dans la «conjugaison» de l'histamine. Chez l'homme, HELANDER, LINDELL et WESTLING (1962) ont montré que le rein transforme les huit dixièmes de l'histamine prélevée dans le sang total après injection de cette amine radiomarquée. Par un mécanisme tubulaire le rein inactive l'histamine soit par oxydation soit par méthylation.

L'histamine libre éliminée par 24 heures chez l'homme est en moyenne de 12 μg mais l'élimination diurne est légèrement supérieure à l'élimination nocturne selon DUNÉR et PERNOW (1956a). Suivant ces mêmes auteurs, l'histamine conjuguée éliminée au cours du nycthémère est environ de 22 μg. L'élimination urinaire de l'histamine conjuguée est la même au cours de la journée et de la nuit. DUNÉR et PERNOW (1958b) indiquent qu'il existe une bonne corrélation entre l'élimination urinaire de l'histamine libre et de l'histaminémie plasmatique.

GADDUM (1951) fait remarquer que, chez l'homme, la concentration urinaire de l'histamine libre est moindre que celle du sang total mais plus élevée que celle du plasma. L'excrétion urinaire de l'histamine libre a été explorée chez quarante enfants sains. Elle est à peu près proportionnelle au poids du corps et varie de 0,30 à 0,42 μg/kg/24 heures (ADAM et MITCHELL, 1953). L'histamine libre des urines est peut-être partiellement fixée par la faible quantité de plasmapexine I que laisse passer le rein (PARROT et MORDELET-DAMBRINE, 1962).

b) Acide imidazolacétique et son dérivé ribosyl

Suivant KARJALA, TURNQUEST et SCHAYER (1956) l'urine contiendrait l'acide ribosylimidazol-4(5) acétique.

c) Méthylation sur le noyau

A la suite d'études faites chez la souris, KARJALA et coll. (1956) pensent que la méthylation de l'anneau imidazole est la voie principale du métabolisme, car on retrouve dans l'urine l'acide 1-méthylimidazol-4-acétique ou 1-méthylimidazol-5-acétique.

d) Méthylation sur la chaîne latérale

La méthylation sur l'azote de la chaîne latérale de l'histamine conduit à la présence dans l'urine humaine normale de dérivés monométhylé et diméthylé et représenterait une élimination de 15 à 20 p. 100 des dérivés de l'histamine.

II. Matières fécales

Les recherches d'URBACH (1949) montrent qu'après ingestion d'histamine il apparaît dans les matières fécales de l'histamine conjuguée identifiée comme étant l'acétyl-histamine ou 4-(β acétyl-aminoéthyl) imidazole. La flore bactérienne de l'intestin serait responsable de la formation de ce corps. Si le contenu intestinal est enrichi en histamine *in vitro*, il est capable d'acétyler cette amine. Cette transformation ne se produit pas si le contenu intestinal a été autoclavé. Des études ont montré que l'*Escherichia coli* et l'*Aerobacter aerogenes* sont capables d'acétyler l'histamine.

La diamino-oxydase de la muqueuse intestinale agit très lentement *in vivo* et *in vitro* sur l'histamine exogène (PARROT, 1948).

MYHRMAN et TOMENIUS (1939) et MYHRMAN (1943) ont fait le dosage de l'histamine totale dans les matières fécales par la technique de BARSOUM et GADDUM: la concentration moyenne chez l'homme normal est de 1,3 μg/cm^3.

III. Bile

Suivant UNGAR et POCOULÉ (1937) la bile contient 0,75 μg/l d'histamine chez le chien.

IV. Salive et sucs digestifs

BROWN et SMITH (1935) indiquent qu'une substance semblable à l'histamine est présente dans la salive humaine.

La présence d'histamine dans le suc gastrique a été mise en évidence en 1938 par MCINTOSH grâce à la technique de dosage de BARSOUM et GADDUM; elle fut confirmée par CODE et coll. (1942), EMMELIN et KAHLSON (1944) et de nombreux autres auteurs.

SMITH (1952) pense que la paroi pylorique constitue chez le chat un lieu de stockage de l'amine en vue de son excrétion dans le suc gastrique.

THOUVENOT et HARICHAUX (1961) mettent en évidence, après injection de chlorure d'acétylcholine, la présence d'histamine en concentration très élevée (de l'ordre de 3×10^{-6}) dans le suc sécrété à partir d'une préparation d'estomac isolé de porc et perfusé par le liquide de Tyrode. Ces valeurs sont plus élevées que celles que l'on trouve chez d'autres espèces, chez l'homme en particulier.

CODE et coll. (1947) ont mis en évidence chez le chien de fortes concentrations d'histamine dans le suc gastrique quand la concentration d'acide chlorhydrique est faible; inversement de fortes concentrations d'acide dans le suc gastrique sont associées à de basses concentrations d'histamine.

C. Quelques variations dans l'excrétion de l'histamine

I. Etat normal

a) Différence sexuelle

Il existe chez le rat une importante différence sexuelle dans l'éxcrétion urinaire de l'histamine (GUSTAFSSON, 1957; WESTLING, 1958). KIM (1959) a étudié l'excrétion urinaire de l'histamine chez le rat: les femelles éliminent 25 fois plus d'histamine endogène que les mâles; la différence entre les deux sexes concerne l'histamine libre et non l'histamine conjuguée. La castration du mâle augmente l'élimination urinaire de l'histamine, qui atteint alors la même valeur que chez la femelle normale. La castration de la femelle ne modifie aucunement l'élimination urinaire de l'histamine. Cette différence sexuelle porte sur le catabolisme de l'histamine et non sur sa biosynthèse car la même différence s'observe pour l'histamine exogène; les femelles en éliminent une plus grande proportion sous la forme libre; il en est de même pour les mâles castrés.

Cependant NETTER, COHN et SHORE (1961), étudiant chez le rat la diamino-oxydase et l'imidazol-N-méthyltransférase, n'ont pas trouvé de diférence sexuelle dans la distribution ni dans l'activité de ces deux enzymes. Il faut supposer, avec ces auteurs, qu'il existe chez les mâles une voie métabolique encore inconnue et que celle-ci fait défaut chez les femelles.

b) Gestation

Chez la femme, l'excrétion urinaire de l'histamine libre semble être normale durant la gestation ou légèrement augmentée à la fin avec un maximum de faible durée dans les quelques jours qui suivent la délivrance. Durant la grossesse, l'activité histaminolytique du plasma sanguin évaluée *in vitro* devient de 500 à 1000 fois plus grande. Il a été calculé que le plasma d'une femme enceinte entre le 5ème et le 9ème mois est capable de détruire 400 μg d'histamine par minute. L'augmentation de l'activité histaminolytique est seulement due à la désamination oxydative par l'histaminase. En 12 heures, 62 à 99 p. 100 de l'histamine marquée injectée est excrétée par l'urine. Il n'y a pas de différence dans l'excrétion de l'histamine marquée qu'il s'agisse de l'histamine urinaire elle-même ou de ses catabolites selon que la femme est enceinte ou non. Ces résultats sont surprenants quand on les compare à l'augmentation considérable de l'activité histaminasique démontrée *in vitro* dans le plasma de femme enceinte (Nilsson, Lindell et coll., 1959).

c) Fœtus

Il est probable que le fœtus humain est capable de former de l'histamine car l'expérience montre que la concentration d'histamine est plus élevée dans le sang fœtal que dans le sang maternel (Kahlson et coll., 1958).

Kahlson, Rosengren et Westling (1959) démontrent qu'il y a une forte augmentation dans la formation d'histamine qui se fixe dans les tissus du fœtus chez les animaux, en particulier dans le foie qui est riche en histidine-décarboxylase.

II. Pathologie

1. Allergie

La destinée de l'histamine exogène ne semble pas modifiée chez l'allergique: ainsi Adam et coll. (1950) établissent le pourcentage de l'histamine injectée qui est éliminé par les urines et n'observent pas de différence significative selon que le sujet est allergique ou non.

En ce qui concerne l'histamine endogène, l'élimination urinaire ne paraît pas non plus modifiée en dehors des crises; mais cette élimination peut s'élever quelque temps après une crise allergique.

a) Asthme bronchique

α) Urines. Au cours de crises d'asthme Parrot (1938) a dosé l'histamine totale des urines et du sang; les résultats obtenus dans une observation sont présentés dans le tableau 2.

Tableau 2. *Taux d'histamine urinaire et sanguine chez une femme asthmatique (âge: 34 ans)*

Temps		Histaminémie totale μg/ml	Histaminurie totale μg/ml
0	début d'une crise		
15 mn		200	< au seuil
45 mn	fin de la crise		
105 mn		60	120
le lendemain		50	< au seuil

Chez le sujet normal, le même auteur ne trouve pas une histaminurie totale qui dépasse le seuil de la technique employée. Notons que, aujourd'hui, cette histaminurie totale semble être de l'ordre de: 0,02 μg/ml.

Lorsqu'un malade allergique reçoit de la corticostimuline, l'histaminurie s'élève au profit de la fraction libre (Mitchell et coll., 1954).

Rose (1950) met en évidence une élimination élevée d'histamine urinaire chez les malades atteints d'asthme bronchique tandis que Mitchell, Logan et coll. (1954), ainsi que Dunér et Pernow (1958a) ne retrouvent pas d'histamine dans les urines lors de la crise mais au contraire après celle-ci, et les proportions d'histamine libre et d'histamine conjuguée ne diffèrent pas de celles d'un individu sain. Ces derniers auteurs ont mis en évidence, dans les trois cas, un facteur antihistaminique dans les urines lors des symptômes aigus de l'asthme bronchique.

β) Expectoration. Knott et Oriel (1930) ont décelé la présence de substances histaminiques dans les expectorations d'asthmatiques grâce au test de l'utérus isolé de cobaye. Aucune substance histaminique n'est décelée dans les expectorations de sujets non asthmatiques. Riesser (1937) conclut dans le même sens. Dans l'expectoration d'un asthmatique, le dosage de l'histamine a donné une valeur de 15 μg/litre (Parrot, 1938).

γ) Matières fécales. Une augmentation d'histamine est observée dans les matières fécales de malades atteints d'asthme bronchique selon Myhrman et Tomenius (1939). Les auteurs ont évalué le taux d'histamine fécale chez 24 malades atteints d'asthme, 8 d'entre eux présentaient des valeurs élevées, dans l'un de ces cas la valeur atteignait 250 μg/cm³; la quantité d'histamine fécale est en relation avec la gravité de l'asthme, dans les cas légers elle est peu abondante ou même indosable. Myhrman (1943) discute l'origine de cet excès d'histamine et il envisage le rôle des bactéries intestinales et l'excrétion de l'histamine par l'intestin.

b) Migraines

Le tableau 3 donne les résultats obtenus par Parrot (1938) au cours d'une crise de migraine typique observée chez un homme de 38 ans par ailleurs bien portant.

Tableau 3. *Taux d'histamine sanguine et urinaire chez un migraineux typique (homme, 38 ans)*

Temps		Histaminémie totale μg/l	Histaminurie totale μg/l
	quelques heures avant la crise	50	110
0	début de la crise		
30 mn		160	140
60 mn	amélioration	160	
65 mn	fin de la crise		50
le lendemain		90	

Entre les crises, mais pendant la même période de crises, l'histaminurie totale n'est pas descendue chez ce malade au-dessous de 25 microgrammes par litre.

c) Accidents sériques

Parrot (1938) dans deux cas a trouvé que l'histamine totale (c'est-à-dire après hydrolyse acide) des urines atteignait 80 microgrammes par litre; ce même chiffre a été observé dans un cas une dizaine d'heures après le début des accidents cutanés, et, dans l'autre, deux jours après la disparition des accidents sériques. Au cours même de ceux-ci l'histaminurie totale s'était montrée inférieure au seuil de la technique comme chez le sujet normal.

d) Allergie alimentaire

La diminution de l'excrétion urinaire de l'histamine lors des allergies alimentaires a été également observée. Après traitement par la prednisone l'excrétion de l'histamine revient à la normale (Dunér et Pernow, 1959).

e) Syndrome de Löffler

Dans le syndrome de Löffler avec infiltration d'éosinophiles dans les poumons et une éosinophilie sanguine modérée, une augmentation de l'excrétion urinaire de l'histamine libre a été démontrée (Dunér et Pernow, 1956b). La corticostimuline normalise l'excrétion de l'histamine. Il ne semble pas qu'il y ait de relation directe entre l'histamine éliminée dans les urines et le nombre d'éosinophiles dans le sang.

Ces auteurs sont amenés à imaginer deux types distincts d'allergie: celui où il y aurait une diminution de l'excrétion de l'histamine urinaire (asthme et allergie alimentaire) et un autre où il y aurait une augmentation de celle-ci (syndrome de LÖFFLER).

2. Brûlés

BIRKE, DUNÉR et coll. (1957) étudient l'excrétion de l'histamine chez les brûlés. La concentration d'histamine dans le sang et l'urine est augmentée durant les premières 24 heures après l'accident. Le taux d'histamine s'abaisse durant les quelques jours suivants pour revenir dans quelques cas à des valeurs subnormales.

3. Tumeurs

On observe une forte teneur histaminique dans les urines de sujets présentant une mastocytose (élimination accrue en particulier de l'histamine libre). Il est à remarquer que l'on trouve chez ces malades de fortes concentrations d'histamine dans différents organes tels que le foie, la rate, le cerveau (BLOOM, DUNÉR et coll., 1958).

Dans les carcinomes, l'excrétion urinaire de l'histamine est aussi augmentée dans un tiers des cas observés (PERNOW et WALDENSTRÖM, 1956).

4. Schizophrénie

L'histamine libre est dosée dans l'urine de 16 schizophrènes avant et après injection sous-cutanée d'histamine.

Les valeurs de l'excrétion de l'histamine et le pourcentage par rapport à la dose injectée ne sont pas significativement différentes de celles qui sont trouvées chez l'homme normal (ADAM et MITCHELL, 1957).

5. Insuffisance hépatique

Dans l'insuffisance hépatique l'élimination d'histamine est normale (JIMENEZ-DIAZ et LORENTE, 1946).

6. Insuffisance cardiaque

Dans les cas d'insuffisance cardiaque grave, l'histamine fécale peut être anormalement élevés: 5 fois sur 21 dosages concernant 16 malades (valeur allant de 6 à 220 $\mu g/cm^3$) (MYHRMAN, 1943).

D. Action hormonale sur l'excrétion de l'histamine

a) Les corticoïdes

ANGERVALL, BJURÖ et WESTLING (1961) ont étudié l'élimination de l'histamine urinaire chez les rats surrénalectomisés.

L'élimination de l'histamine urinaire chez les rats surrénalectomisés buvant de l'eau salée est augmentée progressivement dans les quatre jours qui suivent l'opération. Les rats buvant de l'eau ont une élimination urinaire inchangée jusqu'au huitième jour puis une augmentation apparaît.

La cortexone n'empêche pas l'augmentation de l'excrétion urinaire de l'histamine chez les rats surrénalectomisés buvant de l'eau salée. La cortisone et le cortisol provoquent une augmentation immédiate de l'histamine urinaire chez les rats surrénalectomisés ayant à boire de l'eau salée.

Une opération fictive provoque une augmentation faible et temporaire de l'histamine urinaire. La surrénalectomie provoque une diminution de l'activité de la diamino-oxydase.

b) Les oestrogènes et les androgènes

L'α-oestradiol chez le rat mâle, le propionate de testostérone chez la femelle, n'augmentent pas l'excrétion de l'histamine; cependant l'ovariectomie chez la ratte diminue l'excrétion urinaire de l'histamine.

La testostérone, injectée par voie sous-cutanée, diminue l'élimination urinaire de l'histamine libre chez le rat castré mâle ou femelle mais non chez la femelle normale; l'hormone testiculaire favorise la méthylation de l'histamine; les hormones ovariennes s'y opposent probablement (Westling et Wetterqvist, 1962).

E. Actions diverses

Leitch, Debley et Haley (1956) ont étudié l'effet de l'irradiation aux rayons X et du composé 48/80 sur l'excrétion de l'histamine.

a) L'irradiation du rat mâle aux rayons X augmente la quantité d'histamine urinaire endogène; l'excrétion de l'histamine endogène est 9 à 10 fois plus grande que normalement.

b) Quand le 48/80 est administré à des rattes, l'histamine urinaire est augmentée de trois fois tandis que chez le rat, l'augmentation est de huit fois. Cependant en valeur absolue, l'excrétion chez les femelles est alors trois fois plus grande que chez le mâle.

Conclusion

On peut considérer trois grandes modalités dans l'excrétion de l'histamine:

1) Excrétion de l'histamine en nature; c'est ainsi que l'on trouve normalement de l'histamine dans les urines.

2) Excrétion de métabolites dépourvus d'activité pharmacologique: ce sont

a) l'acétylhistamine
b) l'acide imidazolacétique
c) l'acide ribosylimidazolacétique
d) la 1-méthylhistamine
e) l'acide 1-méthylimidazolacétique.

3) Excrétion de métabolites doués d'activité pharmacologique. Il s'agit des dérivés méthylés sur la chaîne:

a) monométhylhistamine; ce corps, selon les tests, est aussi actif ou plus actif que l'histamine;

b) diméthylhistamine; ce corps, selon les tests, est aussi actif ou moins actif que l'histamine.

On remarquera d'autre part que trois métabolites de l'histamine sont capables d'inhiber l'histidine-décarboxylase. Ce sont l'acétylhistamine et les deux dérivés méthylés sur la chaîne.

Références bibliographiques

Adam, H. M., R. B. Hunter, and T. W. G. Kinnear: Observations on the urinary excretion of histamine in urticaria. Quart. J. exp. Physiol. **36**, 49 (1950).

—, and R. G. Mitchell: The urinary excretion of histamine in children. Arch. Dis. Child. **28**, 61 (1953).

Adam, J., and R. G. Mitchell: The urinary excretion of histamine in schizophrenia. J. Neurol. Neurosurg. Psychiat. **20**, 114 (1957).

Angervall, L., T. Bjurö, and H. Westling: The effect of adrenalectomy on the urinary excretion of histamine in the rat. Acta endocr. (Kbh.) **36**, 467 (1961).

Anrep, G. V., M. S. Ayadi, G. S. Barsoum, J. R. Smith, and M. M. Talaat: The excretion of histamine in urine. J. Physiol. (Lond.) **103**, 155 (1944).

Best, C. H., and E. W. McHenry: The inactivation of histamine. J. Physiol. (Lond.) **70**, 348 (1930).

Birke, G., H. Dunér, S. O. Liljedahl, B. Pernow, L. O. Plantin, and L. Troell: Histamine, catechol amines and adrenocortical steroids in burns. Acta chir. scand. **114**, 87 (1957).

Bloom, G., H. Dunér, B. Pernow, J. Winberg, and R. Zetterström: Spontaneous histamine shocks in urticaria pigmentosa. Acta paediat. (Uppsala) **47**, 152 (1958).

BROWN, C. L., and R. G. SMITH: A histamine-like substance in the gastric juice. Amer. J. Physiol. **113**, 455 (1935).
CODE, C. F., G. A. HALLENBECK, and R. A. GREGORY: The histamine content of gastric juice. Fed. Proc. **1** (part II.), 15 (1942).
— — — Histamine content of canine gastric juice. Amer. J. Physiol. **151**, 593 (1947).
DUNÉR, H., and B. PERNOW: Urinary excretion of histamine in healthy human subjects. Scand. J. clin. Lab. Invest. **8**, 296 (1956a).
— — The urinary excretion of histamine in a case of Loeffler's syndrome. Acta med. scand. **156**, 313 (1956b).
— — Urinary excretion of histamine in bronchial asthma. Acta med. scand. **161**, 361 (1958a).
— — The correlation between the occurrence of histamine in blood and urine. Scand. J. clin. Lab. Invest. **10**, 390 (1958b).
— — Histamine in man under physiological and pathological conditions. Acta med. scand. **168**, 307 (1959).
EMMELIN, N., and G. S. KAHLSON: Histamine as a physiological excitant of gastric secretion. Acta physiol. scand. **8**, 289 (1944).
EUSTIS, A. C.: The detoxicating effect of liver of Cathartes aura upon solutions of β imidazolylethylamine. Biochem. Bull. **4**, 97 (1915).
GADDUM, J. H.: The metabolism of histamine. Brit. med. J. **1951**, 987.
GUSTAFSSON, B. et coll.: 1957 cité d'après NETTER et coll. 1961.
HELANDER, C. G., S. E. LINDELL, and H. WESTLING: The elimination of C^{14} histamine in the human kidney. XXIIe Congrès international Physiol., Leyde, publication n° 690, 1962.
HUEBNER, C. F., R. A. TURNER, and C. R. SCHOLZ: Studies of imidazole compounds. IV. Derivatives of 4-ethylimidazole. J. Amer. chem. Soc. **71**, 3942 (1949).
JIMENEZ-DIAZ, C., et L. LORENTE: Elimination d'histamine dans les urines normales et pathologiques. Rev. clin. esp. **22**, 276 (1946).
— E. ARJONA, and J. PERIANES: Studies on histamine in allergic patients. Int. Arch. Allergy **6**, 243 (1955).
KAHLSON, G., E. ROSENGREN, and H. WESTLING: Increased formation of histamine in the pregnant rat. J. Physiol. (Lond.) **143**, 91 (1958).
— — — Formation of histamine by the foetus in the rat and man. J. Physiol. (Lond.) **145**, 30 (1959).
KAPELLER-ADLER, R.: Zur Kenntnis der Histaminase. Naunyn-Schmiedebergs Arch. exp. Path. Pharmak. **219**, 491 (1953).
— The enzymatic inactivation of histamine. Symposium de Varsovie, 1962 (à paraître).
—, and B. IGGO: Histamine and its derivatives in human urine. Biochim. biophys. Acta (Amst.) **25**, 394 (1957).
KARJALA, S. A.: The partial characterization of a histamine metabolite from rat and mouse urine. J. Amer. chem. Soc. **77**, 504 (1955).
— B. TURNQUEST, and R. W. SCHAYER: Urinary metabolites of radioactive histamine. J. biol. Chem. **219**, 9 (1956).
KIM, K. S.: Sex difference in histamine metabolism in rat. Amer. J. Physiol. **197**, 1255 (1959).
KNOTT, F. A., and G. H. ORIEL: Detection of histamine-like substances in asthmatic sputa and experiments on their possible bacteriological origin. J. Physiol. (Lond.) **70**, P. 31 (40) (1930).
KOBAYASHI, Y., and R. W. SCHAYER: In vitro demonstration of a new histamine-metabolizing enzyme. Arch. Biochem. **63**, 480 (1956).
LEITCH, J. L., V. G. DEBLEY, and T. J. HALEY: Endogenous histamine excretion in the rat as influenced by X-ray irradiation and compound 48/80. Amer. J. Physiol. **187**, 307 (1956).
LINDAHL, K. M.: On the biological methylation of histamine 3. Acta chem. scand. **12**, 2050 (1958a).
— Methylation of histamine by mouse liver in vitro. Acta physiol. scand. **43**, 254 (1958b).
— On the biological methylation of histamine 4. Acta chem. scand. **13**, 1476 (1959).
LINDELL, S. E.: Experiments on the inactivation of histamine in the kidney. Thèse. Lund: Berlingska Boktryckeriet 1958.
— K. NILSSON, B. E. ROOS, and H. WESTLING: The effect of enzyme inhibitors on histamine catabolism in man. Brit. J. Pharmacol. **15**, 351 (1960).
—, and R. W. SCHAYER: Formation of histamine in the kidney of the dog. Brit. J. Pharmacol. **13**, 89 (1958).
LIVINGSTON, R. H., and C. F. CODE: Role of the liver in the conjugation of histamine in intact animals. Amer. J. Physiol. **181**, 428 (1955).
MCHENRY, E. W., and G. GAVIN: Histaminase. IV: Further studies in purification. V: Source of the ammonia formed in the histamine-histaminase reaction. Biochem. J. **29**, 622 (1935).

McIntosh, F. C.: Histamine as a normal stimulant of gastric secretion. Quart. J. exp. Physiol. **28**, 87 (1938).
Mehler, A. H., H. Tabor, and H. Bauer: The oxydation of histamine to imidazoleacetic acid *in vivo*. J. biol. Chem. **197**, 275 (1952).
Millican, R. C.: The acetylation of histamine in normal and enterectomized rats. Arch. Biochem. **42**, 399 (1953).
— M. S. Rosenthal, and H. Tabor: On the metabolism of histamine. A: Urinary excretion following oral administration. B: Conjugation in vitro. J. Pharmacol. exp. Ther. **97**, 4 (1949).
Mitchell, R. G., G. B. Logan, G. A. Peters, and L. L. Henderson: Urinary excretion of histamine in patients having asthma and hay fever: observations on changes produced by administration of cortisone. J. Allergy **25**, 504 (1954).
Myhrman, G.: Continued investigations on histamine in faeces. Acta med. scand. **115**, 300 (1943).
—, u. J. Tomenius: Über das Vorkommen von Histamin in menschlichen Faeces. Naunyn-Schmiedebergs Arch. exp. Path. Pharmak. **193**, 14 (1939).
Netter, K. J., V. H. Cohn, and P. A. Shore: Sex difference in histamine metabolism in the rat. Amer. J. Physiol. **201**, 224 (1961).
Nilsson, K., S. E. Lindell, R. W. Schayer, and H. Westling: Metabolism of ^{14}C labelled histamine in pregnant and non-pregnant women. Clin. Sci. **18**, 313 (1959).
Parrot, J.-L.: Les manifestations de l'anaphylaxie et les substances histaminiques. Etude clinique expérimentale et thérapeutique. Thèse Méd. 1938. 1 vol. 112 p. Paris: Baillière éd.
— La fixation de l'histamine par les tissus du cobaye. Sa libération par une diamine. C. R. Soc. Biol. (Paris) **142**, 631 (1948).
—, et M. Mordelet-Dambrine: Captation de l'histamine par l'urine humaine. J. Physiol. (Paris) **54**, 387 (1962).
Pernow, B., and J. Waldenström: Increased urinary excretion of histamine in cases of carcinoid tumor. Abstr. XX. Int. Physiol. Congr. Brussels 718, 1956.
Pyman, F. L.: — CCXLV — Aminoalkylglyoxalines. J. chem. Soc. **99**, 2172 (1911).
Riesser, O.: 1937 cité d'après Myhrman 1943.
Rose, B.: Studies on the effect of ACTH on eosinophilia and bronchial asthma. Proc. I. Clin. ACTH Conf., U.R. Mote, Ed., Philadelphia, 491, (1950).
Rosenthal, S. M., and H. Tabor: An improved colorimetric method for the estimation of histamine. J. Pharmacol. exp. Ther. **92**, 425 (1948).
Schayer, R. W.: The metabolism of ring-labeled histamine. J. biol. Chem. **196**, 469 (1952).
—, and S. A. Karjala: Ring N-methylation; a major route of histamine metabolism. J. biol. Chem. **221**, 307 (1956).
— J. Kennedy, and R. L. Smiley: Studies on histamine-metabolizing enzymes in intact animals. J. biol. Chem. **205**, 739 (1953).
Schnedorf, J. G., and A. C. Ivy: Effect of methylhistamine and hydroxyethylglyoxaline on gastric secretion and blood pressure in the dog. Proc. Soc. exp. Biol. (N. Y.) **32**, 777 (1935).
Smith, A. N.: Compound 48/80 and acid gastric secretion. J. Physiol. (Lond.) **117**, 73 (1952).
Tabor, H.: Diamine oxydase. J. biol. Chem. **188**, 125 (1951).
—, and O. Hayaishi: The excretion of imidazoleacetic acid riboside following the administration of imidazoleacetic acid or histamine to rats. J. Amer. chem. Soc. **77**, 505 (1955).
— A. H. Mehler, and R. W. Schayer: Isotopic measurements on the oxydation of histamine to imidazoleacetic acid in vivo. J. biol. Chem. **200**, 605 (1953).
—, and E. Mosettig: Isolation of acetylhistamine from urine following oral administration of histamine. J. biol. Chem. **180**, 703 (1949).
Thouvenot, J., et P. Harichaux: Libération d'histamine par la muqueuse d'estomac isolé et perfusé de porc. C. R. Soc. Biol. (Paris) **155**, 603 (1961).
Ungar, G., et A. Pocoulé: Sur les voies d'élimination de l'histamine et son absence dans les urines normales. C. R. Soc. Biol. (Paris) **124**, 1204 (1937).
Urbach, K. F.: Nature and probable origin of conjugated histamine excreted after ingestion of histamine. Proc. Soc. exp. Biol. (N. Y.) **70**, 146 (1949).
Vartiainen, A.: The action of certain new histamine derivatives. J. Pharmacol. exp. Ther. **54**, 265 (1935).
Westling, H.: 1958 cité d'après Netter et coll. 1961.
—, and H. Wetterqvist: The sex difference in histamine methylation in the rat. XXII. Congrès int. Physiol. Leyde, publication n⁰ 691, 1962.
White, T.: Some effects of histamine and two histamine metabolites on the cat's brain. J. Physiol. (Lond.) **159**, 198 (1961).
Zeller, E. A.: Diamin-oxydase. Advanc. Enzymol. **2**, 93 (1942).
— J. R. Fouts, J. A. Carbon, J. C. Lazanas u. W. Voegtli: Über die Substratspezifität der Diaminooxydase. Helv. chim. Acta **39**, 1632 (1957).
— P. Stern, and L. A. Blanksma: Degradation of histamine by monoamine oxidase. Naturwissenschaften **43**, 157 (1956).

Section B

Catabolism of Histamine *in vivo*

By

RICHARD W. SCHAYER

With 1 figure

I. Introduction

The material covered in this chapter is limited to experiments in living mammals, excluding man, in which some evidence of catabolism of histamine has been presented. Studies in man are considered in Chapter 4, Section F; *in vitro* catabolism in Chapter 4, Section C; and absorption and excretion in Chapter 4, Section A.

II. Early studies

The earliest studies on histamine catabolism were limited to *in vitro* and perfusion experiments (Chapter 4, Section C). In this section the *in vivo* work preceding the introduction of isotopes is considered. In these early experiments it was usually essential to use large quantities of histamine; hence, the results are not necessarily valid for physiological situations.

DRAGSTEDT and MEAD (1935) found that after intravenous injection of 0.5 and 1.0 mg/kg doses of histamine into anesthetized dogs, histamine could still be detected in blood after 2 minutes but not after 5 minutes. BINET and MARQUIS (1935) showed that lung of living dogs either removed or inactivated histamine. ROSE and BROWNE (1938) found rapid disappearance of intravenously injected histamine in rats and its appearance in a number of tissues; particularly high concentrations were found in kidney. Adrenalectomy markedly retarded the disappearance of injected histamine from the tissues. The latter change is not apparent when very small doses of histamine are used (SCHAYER et al., 1952).

ALEXANDER (1944) observed that mice efficiently destroyed small amounts of injected histamine; after large doses, metabolism was retarded and large quantities could be recovered unchanged in the urine.

EMMELIN (1951) gave cats histamine intravenously in various concentrations over a period of several hours. The rapid decrease in arterial histamine concentration which was observed persisted even in eviscerated or nephrectomized cats. There was evidence of retention of histamine in kidney following large doses.

COHEN (1954) tied off loops of jejunen of anesthetized fasted rats and tested the fate of histamine under various conditions. In all cases there was little destruction since about 90% of the histamine could be recovered. Perfusion of rat small intestine *in situ* showed evidence of its ability to destroy histamine (VALETTE and COHEN, 1956).

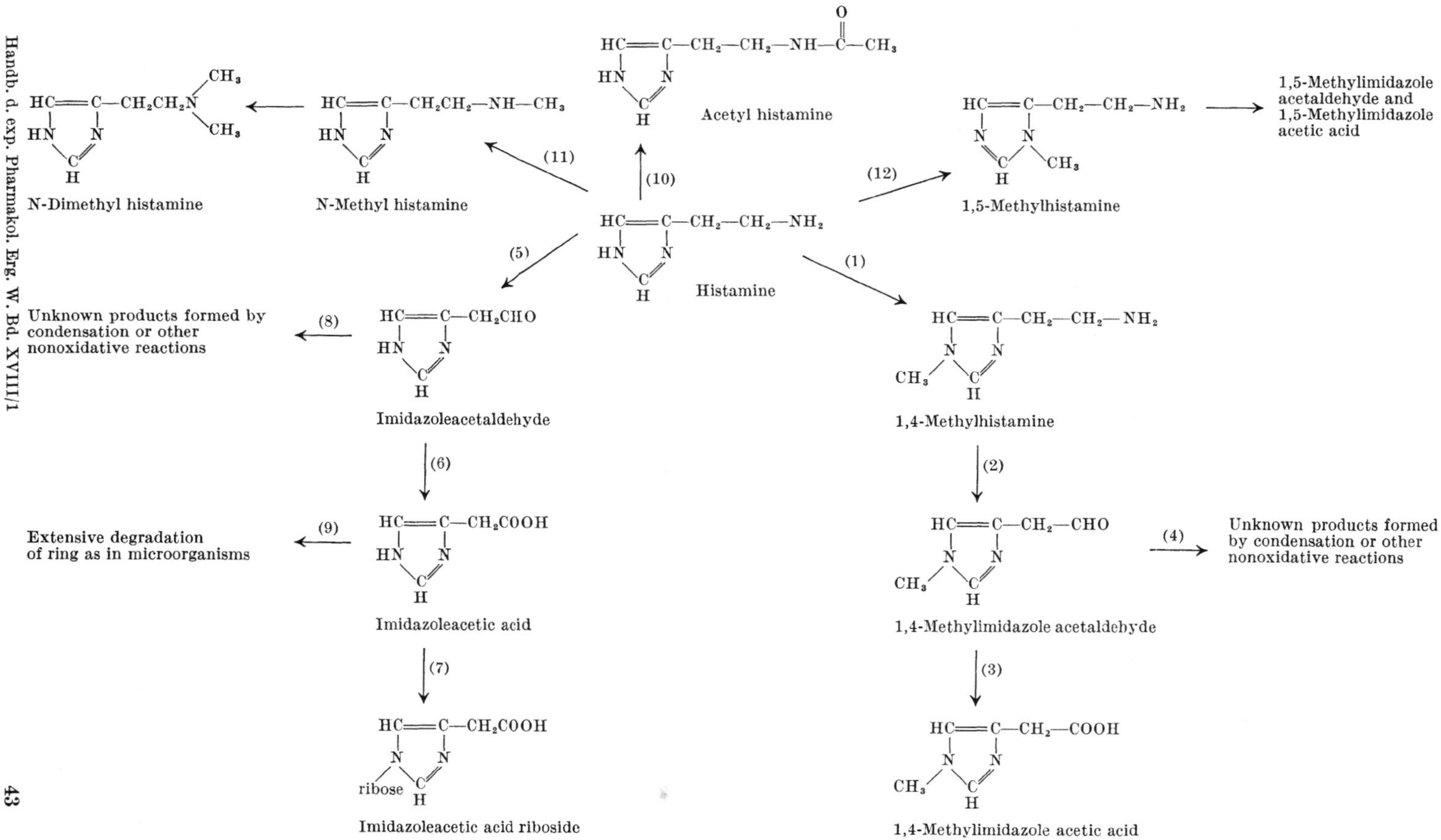

Fig. 1. *1.* The major pathway of inactivation in most mammalian species studied. *2.* Oxidation in vivo largely by a monoamine oxidase. *3.* Oxidation probably by an aldehyde dehydrogenase. *4.* Occurrence in vivo not proved. *5.* Catalyzed in vivo largely or entirely by diamine oxidase. *6.* Oxidation probably by an aldehyde dehydrogenase. *7.* Enzymatic synthesis in vitro reported (CROWLEY, 1960). *8.* Occrurence in vivo not proved. *9.* Occurs to a very small extent, if at all, in mammals. *10.* A minor pathway in animals. *11.* Occurrence in mammalian tissues not proved. *12.* Occurs only when large amounts of histamine are present

The early experiments did not define the means of destruction of histamine in the organism although it was considered likely that oxidation by histaminase (Chapter 4, Section C) or conjugation (Chapter 4, Section A) were involved. A number of other possible routes of catabolism of histamine have been established more recently; these are shown in Fig. 1 and are discussed in the next section.

III. Catabolic reactions of histamine

A. Oxidation by diamine oxidase or histaminase

On the basis of *in vitro* studies histaminase is identified by some workers with diamine oxidase (TABOR, 1954; ZELLER, 1938; ZELLER et al., 1953) while others maintain there are two distinct enzymes (KAPELLER-ADLER and RENWICK, 1956; BLASCHKO et al., 1958; and KOLB, 1956). Since in both cases the reaction product is the same, and since this pathway *in vivo* is blocked by diamine oxidase inhibitors, the two enzymes will be considered together.

From *in vitro* studies it has been known that histamine can be oxidized to imidazoleacetaldehyde, and then to imidazoleacetic acid (ZELLER, 1951). The first evidence of this pathway in living animals was the simultaneous and independent work of SCHAYER (1952) and of MEHLER et al. (1952). The former injected rats and guinea pigs with very small quantities of C^{14} histamine and found traces of C^{14}-imidazoleacetic acid in the urine; the latter injected large amounts of non-isotopic histamine into rats and were able to isolate imidazoleacetic acid in good yield. The large difference in yield was believed due to the size of the dose since MEHLER et al. (1952), had also found that recovery of injected imidazoleacetic acid was significant only with large doses. Evidence that imidazoleacetic acid is formed in high yield in rats under physiological conditions was obtained from an isotopic trapping experiment. Rats were injected with microgram quantities of C^{14} histamine plus a large amount of non-isotopic imidazoleacetic acid. A sufficient quantity of the latter was excreted so that isolation was possible; its degree of radioactivity indicated that imidazoleacetic acid is an intermediate in a major pathway of histamine catabolism in the rat (TABOR et al., 1953). BOUTHILLIER and GOLDNER (1953) confirmed these findings by demonstrating the presence of C^{14} imidazoleacetic acid in urine of rats given rather large doses of C^{14} histamine.

The proof of formation of imidazoleacetic acid from histamine in the rat does not identify the enzyme system involved since the end products of reactions catalyzed by diamine oxidase and monoamine oxidase are the same. The first evidence for the participation of diamine oxidase in the catabolism of physiological quantities of histamine *in vivo* was the demonstration in rats (SCHAYER, 1953) that *in vitro* inhibitors of diamine oxidase, isoniazid (ZELLER et al., 1952) and aminoguanidine (SCHULER, 1952) prevented the formation of a major metabolite, unidentified at that time. This metabolite of trace quantities of histamine was later identified by KARJALA et al. (1956), as 1-ribosylimidazole-4-acetic acid, following the independent discovery from two laboratories (KARJALA, 1955; TABOR and HAYAISHI, 1955) that this conjugate of ribose and imidazoleacetic acid is excreted in the urine of rats and mice following large doses of histamine or imidazoleacetic acid. The β-configuration of the ribosyl linkage has been proved by synthesis (BADDILEY et al., 1958).

Diamine oxidase seems to be involved in the metabolism of histamine in most species studied but is quantitatively most important in the rat.

The validity of basing inferences on behavior of diamine oxidase inhibitors *in vivo* has been substantiated by the fact that aminoguanidine and isoniazid prevent the *in vivo* oxidation of cadaverine, a model substrate for diamine oxidase (SCHAYER et al., 1954).

Imidazoleacetaldehyde has recently been obtained in crystalline form from the action of histaminase on histamine (KAPELLER-ADLER, 1960). It is quite unstable and it is probable that if conditions do not favor its rapid oxidation to imidazoleacetic acid, it might undergo some other type of reaction such as condensation. The writer believes that non-oxidative reactions of imidazoleacetaldehyde should be considered as a possible route to the formation of minor histamine metabolites.

B. Methylation of ring nitrogen

In early experiments on the fate of C^{14} histamine, chromatograms of urine of mice and cats showed the presence of a major metabolic product of histamine which was not formed by the action of diamine oxidase (SCHAYER, 1953; SCHAYER et al., 1953). Although diamine oxidase inhibitors such as aminoguanidine did not significantly affect the quantity of this compound excreted, iproniazid (1-isopropyl-2-isonicotinylhydrazine) almost completely blocked its formation. Iproniazid is an inhibitor of monoamine oxidase (ZELLER and BARSKY, 1952) but may inhibit other enzyme systems also. This enzyme system was tentatively named "histamine-metabolizing enzyme II."

The nature of "histamine-metabolizing enzyme II" was revealed following the isolation of a radioactive crystalline substance from the urine of mice which had been injected with large quantities of low-activity C^{14} histamine (KARJALA et al., 1956; KARJALA and TURNQUEST, 1955). This compound gave an elementary analysis consistent with that of a methylimidazoleacetic acid, suggesting that the precursor would be a methylated histamine. It was proved by isotope dilution assay that minute quantities of C^{14} histamine are methylated on the ring nitrogen remote from the side chain to form 1-methyl-4-(β-aminoethyl)imidazole. A portion of this compound is excreted unchanged in the urine but most is oxidized to 1-methylimidazole-4-acetic acid (SCHAYER and KARJALA, 1956). The probable intermediate is 1-methylimidazole-4-acetaldehyde. No methylation of the ring nitrogen adjacent to the side chain occurs when small quantities of histamine are injected. If mice are injected with large amounts of histamine, some of the abnormal isomers, 1,5-methylhistamine and 1,5-methylimidazoleacetic acid, may be formed (KARJALA and TURNQUEST, 1955). It is possible therefore that these compounds could be formed if massive release of tissue histamine occurred.

If mice, in which methylation is normally the principal route of catabolism of histamine, are injected with large quantities of histamine, diamine oxidase assumes the major role in detoxication (KARJALA et al., 1956).

No efficient *in vivo* inhibitors of the methylation of histamine have been reported.

Oxidation of the ring methylhistamine to methylimidazoleacetic acid is effected by an enzyme resembling monoamine oxidase. It is inhibited by iproniazid, and even more strongly by 1-isobutyl-2-isonicotinylhydrazine, but is virtually unaffected by aminoguanidine (ROTHSCHILD and SCHAYER, 1958). Thus, "histamine-metabolizing enzyme II" is a composite of a methylating enzyme and a monoamine oxidase-like enzyme.

Attempts to demonstrate formation of 1,4-methylimidazole acetic acid by direct methylation of imidazoleacetic acid have been unsuccessful (ROTHSCHILD and SCHAYER, 1958).

The possible formation of unidentified minor histamine metabolites by nonoxidative reactions of 1,4-methylimidazoleacetaldehyde should be considered.

The betaine corresponding to 1-methylimidazole-5-acetic acid, a compound bearing two methyl groups on the imidazole ring, has been isolated from the invertebrate *Anemonia sulcata* by ACKERMANN (1953) and synthesized by ACKERMANN and JANKA (1953).

C. Oxidation by monoamine oxidase

Histamine is oxidized *in vitro* by monoamine oxidase (ZELLER et al., 1956; KOBAYASHI, 1957). However, monoamine oxidase does not seem to be of importance in the first step of histamine catabolism *in vivo*, because aminoguanidine, which does not inhibit monoamine oxidase, largely blocks the formation of imidazoleacetic acid and imidazoleacetic acid riboside (SCHAYER et al., 1953). If monoamine oxidase has any effect on histamine catabolism *in vivo*, it is small.

D. Acetylation

Free and conjugated histamine in the urine of a large number of mammalian species was studied by ANREP et al. (1944). The conjugated form was identified as acetylhistamine by URBACH (1949) who demonstrated its synthesis by intestinal bacteria. TABOR and MOSETTIG (1949) isolated crystalline acetylhistamine after feeding a dog with a large quantity of histamine. The acetylation of histamine is largely bacterial since quantitative analyses of the urine of rats, guinea pigs, rabbits and cats injected with C^{14} histamine show little or no acetylation of the amino group of the side chain by mammalian tissue (SCHAYER, 1952 and 1956). LIVINGSTON and CODE (1955) infused histamine into the portal veins of dogs, monkeys and rats and measured the urinary excretion of free and conjugated histamine before, during and after the infusion. No evidence for acetylation of histamine was found in dogs and monkeys although a small increase in the conjugated form was found in rats. MILLICAN (1953) found increased acetylation of histamine in eviscerated rats, but it should be noted that the animals had been deprived of their most active histamine-destroying organ, the intestine.

E. Methylation of amino groups of side chain

KAPELLER-ADLER and IGGO (1957) report finding mono- and dimethylhistamine in human urine. It is not known whether this reaction can be carried out by mammalian tissue or whether bacteria are responsible.

IV. In vivo histamine catabolism in various mammalian species

A. Rats

Rats injected with histamine labeled with C^{14} in the 2-position of the imidazole ring respired a minute amount of $C^{14}O_2$. This may have originated from an impurity in the C^{14} histamine. No radioactivity was retained in the body for any appreciable period; the C^{14} was excreted in the urine (SCHAYER, 1952). No rigorous studies have been reported on rats, or any other species, to see if feces uncontaminated by urine are radioactive.

Isotope dilution assays have demonstrated large quantities of imidazoleacetic acid riboside but little free imidazoleacetic acid in rat urine. On the basis of evidence from paper chromatography, performed under conditions where histamine and methylhistamine were not separated (SCHAYER, 1952), it was concluded that methylation was unimportant in the rat. Later, WESTLING (1958) has found significant methylation by male rats.

There is a sex difference in histamine catabolism in rats. This was first suggested by the finding of Rose (1939) that blood histamine was much lower in male rats than in females. LEITCH et al. (1956) found that females excreted 9 to 10 times as much histamine in urine than did males. GUSTAFSSON et al. (1957) observed urinary histamine to be low in males, both germ-free or not germ-free, and mostly conjugated; in females it was high and largely in free form. WESTLING (1958) studied the difference in metabolism of injected C^{14} histamine; female rats excreted more unchanged C^{14} histamine while males showed a marked increase in the methylation route of inactivation.

KIM (1959) found urinary histamine in females to be about 25 times that of males; castration increased free histamine output of the latter but ovariectomy, or combined ovariectomy plus hysterectomy did not affect the output in females. Testosterone suppressed the increased output of urinary histamine in males but did not affect normal females. The author concluded that the difference was due to mode of breakdown rather than increased histamine production in females.

NETTER et al. (1961) confirmed the greater excretion of histamine in female rats but could detect no sex difference in the *in vitro* activity of the histamine-methylating enzyme, nor in the liver methionine-activating enzyme which synthesizes the coenzyme for histamine methylation. A combination of nephrectomy plus aminoguanidine (a histaminase inhibitor) markedly slowed histamine destruction in females but had less effect in males. The authors believe that this evidence may indicate the presence of an unidentified route of histamine inactivation in male rats. However, since this conclusion is based on *in vitro* enzyme assays it seems to the writer that WESTLING's *in vivo* demonstration of more extensive histamine methylation by male rats can account for the observed differences.

Evidence has been presented that the intestine is the site of the greatest *in vivo* histamine metabolizing activity in the rat (SCHAYER, 1953). This agreed with the *in vitro* findings of ZELLER et al. (1939). Antihistamines do not affect the pattern of urinary histamine metabolites in mice (SCHAYER, 1953 and 1958) or rats (GOLDNER and BOUTHILLIER, 1956).

HALPERN et al. (1959) used radioactive histamine to study various aspects of its distribution and fate in rats. A sufficient quantity of C^{14} histamine was given intravenously so that both the C^{14}, and the increase of biologically active histamine over the normal tissue content, could be measured simultaneously. From the changes in the ratio of biologically active histamine to total C^{14}, conclusions were drawn on the rate of metabolism in various tissues. This principle is the same as that used by SCHAYER (1953); however, the latter had two advantages. First, very small quantities of C^{14} histamine were injected and the ratio C^{14} histamine: total C^{14} determined; second, C^{14} histamine was determined by isotope dilution and no correction for endogenous histamine was needed.

From the rapidity of diffusion from the blood, it was concluded that injected C^{14} histamine entered cells of the tissues; the authors state this to be at variance with the views of SCHAYER (1956). The writer has intended to imply only that exogenous histamine cannot become bound in cells for significant periods, not that it cannot pass through cell walls. A confusing aspect of the paper by HALPERN and his coworkers is the frequent use of the term "C^{14} histamine" to what should be correctly called "total C^{14}".

B. Mice

The chromatographic pattern of radioactive urinary histamine metabolites from mice is markedly different from rats, and the principal excretory product is not diminished by diamine oxidase inhibitors. The principal route of histamine metabolism in mice is methylation; the methylhistamine is oxidized to methylimidazoleacetic acid by an enzyme having properties similar to monoamine oxidase, not diamine oxidase (ROTHSCHILD and SCHAYER, 1958). Evidence has been presented that liver is the site of greatest *in vivo* histamine-metabolizing activity in the mouse (SCHAYER, 1953). This agreed with *in vitro* findings of LINDAHL (1958). When mice were fed histamine, it was largely metabolized by oxidation, not methylation (SCHAYER, 1956).

C. Guinea pigs

In addition to analytical data in table 1, unpublished chromatographic evidence indicated that in many guinea pigs methylation and oxidation of histamine occurred to approximately the same extent. As in rats, there was no significant conversion of the 2-carbon of the ring of histamine to carbon dioxide, and there was no storage of exogenous histamine (SCHAYER, 1952).

D. Cats

Chromatograms of the urine of kittens injected with C^{14} histamine showed that methylation was the principal means of inactivation (SCHAYER et al., 1953). This was confirmed in mature cats by isotope dilution (SCHAYER, 1956). The oxidative mechanism is relatively unimportant *in vivo* despite the intense histaminase activity of cat kidney *in vitro* (HAEGER and KAHLSON, 1952). Fed histamine was metabolized by cats in about the same manner as injected histamine (SCHAYER, 1956).

E. Dogs

In this species methylation predominates. The dog is the only species tested in which none of the injected C^{14} histamine could be detected unchanged in urine. Dogs are also unique in that they do not seem to conjugate appreciable quantities of imidazoleacetic acid with ribose (SCHAYER, 1956). Dog kidney, which has strong *in vitro* diamine oxidase activity, shows this same activity *in vivo*; it also methylates *in vivo*. These and other experiments on the role of the canine kidney in histamine metabolism *in vivo* have been reported by LINDELL and SCHAYER (1958 and 1958a).

Quantitative analyses for the principal histamine metabolites in urine of various species given small concentrations of C^{14} histamine are shown in Table 1.

Table 1. *Quantitative analysis for histamine and its metabolic products in urine of various species given C^{14} histamine* (SCHAYER, 1959)

Species	Sex	Route	Per cent total Radioactivity in urine: Hist.	Me Hist.	Me ImAA	ImAA (total)	Acetyl Hist.	Reference
Rat	F	S.C.	12	4	6	51	3	SCHAYER, 1956
Rat	M	S.C.	1	16	7	51	2	WESTLING, 1958
Mouse	F	S.C.	—	19	32	21	1	SCHAYER and KARJALA, 1956
Mouse	F	Oral	—	—	8	65	—	SCHAYER, 1956
Rabbit	M	S.C.	—	—	41	40	0.5	SCHAYER, 1956
Guinea pig	F	S.C.	—	5	26	40—50	1—4	SCHAYER and KARJALA, 1956 SCHAYER, unpublished
Cat	M	S.C.	9	—	72	—	0	SCHAYER, 1956
Cat	F	Oral	0.3	0.6	77	9	—	SCHAYER, 1956
Dog	M	S.C.	0	7—9	61—66	21	0	SCHAYER, 1956

V. Evidence on in vivo catabolism of histamine by experiments on potentiation of histamine effects by enzyme inhibitors

Following the demonstration by MONGAR and SCHILD (1951) and ARUNLAKSHANA et al. (1954) that histaminase inhibitors potentiate the effects of histamine on isolated organs from guinea pigs, LINDELL and WESTLING tested the effect of inhibitors on the blood pressure response of anesthetized cats to histamine. A number of histaminase inhibitors potentiated the effects of histamine injected into the renal artery but were inactive when the histamine was injected into the femoral artery or vein. Similar results were obtained in dogs (LINDELL, 1957). These observations are in excellent accord with other evidence that histaminase activity of cats and dogs is largely in kidney but that in other tissues methylation is highly predominant (LINDELL and SCHAYER, 1958a; SCHAYER, 1956; LILJA and LINDELL, 1961).

ANGELAKOS and LOEW (1957) attempted to evaluate the role of histaminase in histamine destruction in living rats. They postulated that if the enzyme were active *in vivo*, diamine oxidase inhibitors should potentiate the toxicity of injected histamine. Since aminoguanidine and other potent inhibitors had no significant effect it was concluded that the enzyme was not active *in vivo;* alternate interpretations were also presented. An important factor not considered by these authors is the evidence that large quantities of injected histamine destroy the ability of rats to metabolize this compound (SCHAYER et al., 1953). Hence, at the toxic doses used by ANGELAKOS and LOEW, no further inhibition of *in vivo* histaminase activity would be possible. In experiments on intact mice (ANGELAKOS and LOEW, 1957) and cats (ANGELAKOS and LOEW, 1958) these authors again found no potentiation of histamine by inhibitors. This is probably because the diamine oxidase and monoamine oxidase inhibitors tested cannot block the major inactivation process of these species, methylation.

VI. Catabolism of histamine by individual tissues in vivo

This field has been investigated by two procedures; the first is in normal intact animals, the second in anesthetized animals subjected to surgery and perfusion.

A. Studies in intact animals

SCHAYER, 1953, introduced a technique for attempting to evaluate the histamine-metabolizing abilities of tissues by experiments in intact animals. The assumption was made that in a short period of time following intravenous injections of a minute quantity of C^{14} histamine, the ratio C^{14} histamine : total C^{14} in a tissue might provide a rough measure of its ability to destroy histamine. In kidneys, lung and muscle of rats killed 5 minutes after intravenous histamine, the radioactivity was mainly unchanged C^{14} histamine. However, in the small intestine, only about one-seventh to one-eighth of the total radioactivity was unchanged histamine. Liver was intermediate. Thus these experiments suggested that the intestine is the site of most active diamine oxidase in rats *in vivo*. This is in agreement with the *in vitro* findings of ZELLER et al. (1939) that the intestine is the only good source of diamine oxidase in the rat, although liver contained a small amount.

In the mouse, the same technique was used to locate the site of metabolism (now known to be methylation). The animals were pretreated with isoniazid to inhibit diamine oxidase so that only one enzyme would be measured. The results clearly suggest that liver is the principal site of methylation *in vivo*. This finding conforms to *in vitro* studies by LINDAHL (1958). A modification of this technique was later used by HALPERN et al. (1959) who apparently devised it independently. However, since they gave rather large doses of C^{14} histamine, and since they measured biologically active histamine and corrected for endogenous histamine, their results do not show where the destruction occurred.

B. Perfusion experiments

Perfusion experiments in which *in vivo* catabolism of histamine is followed have required adoption of radioisotope techniques by physiological laboratories and are therefore all quite recent.

1. Cat brain

WHITE (1960) perfused the cerebral ventricles of anesthetized cats with low concentrations of C^{14} histamine. In addition to unchanged C^{14} histamine, significant quantities of methylhistamine and methylimidazole acetic acid were found. Pretreatment with iproniazid subcutaneously prevented formation of the latter. Imidazoleacetic acid was found only in traces.

Perfusion of C^{14} L-histidine gave a much lower yield of C^{14} methylhistamine than that obtained from perfusion of C^{14} histamine. Although WHITE was unable to establish whether this difference might be due to greater protection of endogenous histamine, or to a difference in rate of oxidation to methylimidazole acetic acid, he suggested that the catabolism of newly-formed endogenous histamine of brain may differ from that of exogenous histamine.

2. Cat liver, lung and heart

LILJA and LINDELL (1961) studied metabolism of C^{14} histamine in cats using heart-lung-liver and heart-lung preparations. In the heart-lung-liver preparations, injected C^{14} histamine was very rapidly removed from the blood with large quantities of metabolites appearing in as little as 2 minutes. Thirty minutes after injection of C^{14} histamine the blood and tissues were assayed. There was a marked destruction of histamine, the appearance of methylhistamine and of a very large amount of methylimidazoleacetic acid. Only a small amount of imidazoleacetic acid, and no acetylhistamine were found. When the liver was removed, the heart-lung preparations removed injected histamine from the blood slowly. Histamine destruction was markedly retarded and although a large amount of methylhistamine was formed, oxidation to methylimidazoleacetic acid occurred to only a small extent. It was concluded that although the histamine-methylating enzyme in heart and lungs of cats is about as active as that in liver *in vitro*, the removal of liver has a profound effect on histamine destruction *in vivo*. The authors attribute this in part to the inability of tissues other than liver to oxidize significant quantities of methylhistamine to methylimidazole acetic acid. It may also be due to the dependence on liver for synthesis of S-adenosylmethionine, the cofactor of the methylating enzyme. In any event, liver is implicated as a major locus of inactivation of histamine in the cat.

Participation of the highly active monoamine oxidase of liver in the first step in histamine metabolism is excluded by the very low amount of imidazoleacetic acid formed.

3. Dog kidney

Anesthetized dogs were given small quantities of C^{14} histamine by steady infusion into one of the renal arteries and urine collected from both kidneys separately (LINDELL and SCHAYER, 1958a). It was assumed that the concentration of histamine metabolites in urine from the uninjected kidney would serve as a control and that the difference between this concentration and that found in urine from the injected kidney would convey information on the metabolism of histamine by renal tissue of living dogs. Strong evidence was obtained that kidney oxidizes the greater portion of histamine to imidazoleacetic acid, a finding consistent with the extremely high *in vitro* diamine oxidase activity of this tissue (WATON, 1956). However, a significant degree of methylation occurred, both methylhistamine and methylimidazoleacetic acid being detected. Since injection of histamine into dogs by other routes leads to a preponderance of methylated metabolites (SCHAYER, 1956; LINDELL and SCHAYER, 1958) it is probable that kidney is the most active source of *in vivo* diamine oxidase activity in the dog.

VII. Conclusion

The field of *in vivo* catabolism of histamine is probably the best understood, and least controversial, of any of the topics of this book. The major routes of catabolism are methylation and oxidation; there is no substantial evidence that any important pathway of *in vivo* histamine catabolism remains unidentified.

Footnote

Histamine metabolites are referred to as follows: (a) 1-methyl-4-(β-aminoethyl)imidazole may be called 1,4-methylhistamine; 1-methylimidazole-4-acetic may be called 1,4-methylimidazoleacetic acid or Me ImAA; imidazole-4(5)-acetic acid may be called imidazoleacetic acid or ImAA; 1-ribosylimidazole-4-acetic acid may be called imidazoleacetic acid riboside.

The author is indebted to Mrs. ELENA SESTOKAS for translations.

Bibliography

ACKERMANN, D., u. R. JANKA: Konstitution und Synthese des Anemonins. Hoppe-Seylers Z. physiol. Chem. **294**, 93 (1953).

— Über das Vorkommen von Homarin, Trigonellin und einer neuen Base Anemonin in der Anthozoe Anemonia sulcata. Hoppe-Seylers Z. physiol. Chem. **295**, 1 (1953).

ALEXANDER, F.: Metabolism of histamine. Quart. J. exp. Physiol. **33**, 71 (1944).

ANGELAKOS, E. T., and E. R. LOEW: Histamine toxicity in mice and rats following treatment with histaminase inhibitors. J. Pharmacol. exp. Ther. **119**, 444 (1957).

— — Influence of histaminase inhibitors on certain pharmacological effects of histamine. Arch. int. Pharmacodyn. **117**, 277 (1958).

ANREP, G. V., M. S. AYADI, G. S. BARSOUM, J. R. SMITH and M. M. TALAAT: The excretion of histamine in urine. J. Physiol. (Lond.) **103**, 155 (1944).

ARUNLAKSHANA, O., J. L. MONGAR and H. O. SCHILD: Potentiation of pharmacological effects of histamine by histaminase inhibitors. J. Physiol. (Lond.) **123**, 32 (1954).

BADDILEY, J., J. G. BUCHANAN, D. H. HAYES and P. A. SMITH: Synthesis of 1-β-D-ribofuranosyl-4(5)-glyoxalinylacetic acid, a metabolite of histamine. J. chem. Soc. **1958**, 3743.

BINET, L., and M. MARQUIS: Destruction of histamine by lung tissue. C. R. Soc. Biol. (Paris) **118**, 1285 (1935).

BLASCHKO, H., P. FRIEDMAN and K. NILSSON: Two kinds of histaminase. J. Physiol. (Lond.) **142**, 33 P (1958).

BOUTHILLIER, L. P., and M. GOLDNER: The metabolism of histamine-β-C^{14}. Arch. Biochem. **44**, 251 (1953).

COHEN, Y.: Fate of histamine in the small intestine of the rat in vivo. J. Physiol. (Paris) **46**, 305 (1954).

CROWLEY, G. M.: Enzymatic synthesis of imidazoleacetic acid ribotide. Fed. Proc. **19**, No. 1, Part I (1960).

DRAGSTEDT, C. A., and F. B. MEAD: Inactivation of histamine in vivo. Proc. Soc. exp. Biol. (N. Y.) **32**, 1435 (1935).
EMMELIN, N.: Disappearance of injected histamine from the blood stream. Acta physiol. scand. **22**, 379 (1951).
GOLDNER, M., and L. P. BOUTHILLIER: Effect of antihistamines on the metabolism of histamine in the intact rat. Canad. J. Biochem. Physiol. **34**, 116 (1956).
GUSTAFSSON, B., G. KAHLSON and E. ROSENGREN: Biogenesis of histamine studied by its distribution and urinary excretion in germ free reared and not germ free rats fed a histamine free diet. Acta physiol. scand. **41**, 217 (1957).
HAEGER, K., and G. KAHLSON: Disappearance of histamine from the whole body following adrenalectomy in cats. Acta physiol. scand. **23**, 255 (1952).
HALPERN, B. N., T. NEVEU and C. W. M. WILSON: The distribution and fate of radioactive histamine in the rat. J. Physiol. (Lond.) **147**, 437 (1959).
KAPELLER-ADLER, R.: The isolation of iminazole acetaldehyde as the only metabolite of the action in vitro of placental histaminase on histamine. Biochim. biophys. Acta (Amst.) **37**, 527 (1960).
—, and B. IGGO: Histamine and its derivatives in human urine. Biochim. biophys. Acta (Amst.) **25**, 394 (1957).
—, and R. RENWICK: On the enzymatic breakdown of histamine and cadaverine in human serum and urine. Clin. chim. Acta **1**, 197 (1956).
KARJALA, S. A.: The partial characterization of a histamine metabolite from rat and mouse urine. J. Amer. chem. Soc. **77**, 504 (1955).
—, and B. W. TURNQUEST: The characterization of two methylimidazoleacetic acids as radioactive histamine metabolites. J. Amer. chem. Soc. **77**, 6358 (1955).
— — and R. W. SCHAYER: Urinary metabolites of radioactive histamine. J. biol. Chem. **219**, 9 (1956).
KIM, K. S.: Sex difference in histamine metabolism in rats. Amer. J. Physiol. **197**, 1258 (1959).
KOBAYASHI, Y.: A histamine metabolizing enzyme system of mouse liver. Arch. Biochem. **71**, 352 (1957).
KOLB, E.: Histaminase and diamine oxidase in the serum of domestic animals (ruminant, pig, horse) and in Escherichia coli and Streptococcus faecalis. Zbl. Vet.-Med. **3**, 570 (1956).
LEITCH, J. L., V. G. DEBLEY and T. J. HALEY: Endogenous histamine excretion in the rat as influenced by x-ray irradiation and compound 48/80. Amer. J. Physiol. **187**, 307 (1956).
LILJA, B., and S. E. LINDELL: Metabolism of [C^{14}]-histamine in heart-lung-liver preparations of cats. Brit. J. Pharmacol. **16**, 203 (1961).
LINDAHL, K.: Methylation of histamine by mouse liver in vitro. Acta physiol. scand. **43**, 254 (1958).
LINDELL, S. E.: Effects of histaminase inhibitors on the blood pressure responses in dogs to histamine injected into the renal artery. Acta physiol. scand. **41**, 168 (1957).
—, and R. W. SCHAYER: Formation of histamine in the kidney of the dog. Brit. J. Pharmacol. **13**, 44 (1958).
— — Metabolism of injected C^{14} histamine in the kidney of the dog. Brit. J. Pharmacol. **13**, 52 (1958).
—, and H. WESTLING: Potentiation by histaminase inhibitors of the blood pressure responses to histamine in cats. Acta physiol. scand. **37**, 307 (1956).
LIVINGSTON, R. H., and C. F. CODE: Role of the liver in the conjugation of histamine in intact animals. Amer. J. Physiol. **181**, 428 (1955).
MEHLER, A. H., H. TABOR and H. BAUER: The oxidation of histamine to imidazoleacetic acid in vivo. J. biol. Chem. **197**, 475 (1952).
MILLICAN, R. C.: The acetylation of histamine in normal and enterectomized rats. Arch. Biochem. **42**, 399 (1953).
MONGAR, J. L., and H. O. SCHILD: Potentiation of the action of histamine by semicarbazide. Nature (Lond.) **167**, 232 (1951).
NETTER, K. J., V. H. COHN, JR. and P. A. SHORE: Sex difference in histamine metabolism in the rat. Amer. J. Physiol. **201**, 224 (1961).
ROSE, B.: Effect of cortin and desoxycorticosterone acetate on the ability of the adrenalectomized rat to inactivate histamine. Amer. J. Physiol. **127**, 780 (1939).
—, and J. S. L. BROWNE: The distribution and rate of disappearance of intravenously injected histamine in the rat. Amer. J. Physiol. **124**, 412 (1938).
ROTHSCHILD, Z., and R. W. SCHAYER: Synthesis and metabolism of a histamine metabolite, 1-methyl-4-(β-aminoethyl)-imidazole. Biochim. biophys. Acta (Amst.) **30**, 23 (1958).
SCHAYER, R. W.: The metabolism of ring-labeled histamine. J. biol. Chem. **196**, 469 (1952).
— Studies on histamine-metabolizing enzymes in intact animals. J. biol. Chem. **203**, 787 (1953).
— The metabolism of histamine in various species. Brit. J. Pharmacol. **11**, 472 (1956).

SCHAYER, R. W.: Histamine metabolism. Proceedings of the Third International Congress of Allergology, Paris (1958).
— Catabolism of physiological quantities of histamine in vivo. Physiol. Rev. **39**, 116 (1959).
—, and S. A. KARJALA: Ring N methylation; a major route of histamine metabolism. J. biol. Chem. **221**, 307 (1956).
—, J. KENNEDY and R. L. SMILEY: Studies on histamine metabolizing enzymes in intact animals. J. biol. Chem. **205**, 739 (1953).
—, R. L. SMILEY and J. KENNEDY: Effect of adrenalectomy on rate of metabolism of histamine in the mouse. Proc. Soc. exp. Biol. (N. Y.) **81**, 416 (1952).
— — — Diamine oxidase and cadaverine metabolism. J. biol. Chem. **206**, 461 (1954).
SCHULER, W.: Zur Hemmung der Diamino-oxydase (Histaminase). Experientia (Basel) **8**, 230 (1952).
TABOR, H.: Metabolic studies on histidine, histamine, and related imidazoles. Pharmacol. Rev. **6**, 299 (1954).
—, and O. HAYAISHI: The excretion of imidazoleacetic acid riboside following the administration of imidazoleacetic acid or histamine to rats. J. Amer. chem. Soc. **77**, 505 (1955).
— A. H. MEHLER and R. W. SCHAYER: Isotopic measurements on the oxidation of histamine to imidazoleacetic acid in vivo. J. biol. Chem. **200**, 605 (1953).
— — and E. R. STADTMAN: The enzymatic acetylation of amines. J. biol. Chem. **204**, 127 (1953).
—, and E. MOSETTIG: Isolation of acetyl histamine from urine following oral administration of histamine. J. biol. Chem. **180**, 703 (1949).
URBACH, K. F.: Nature and probable origin of conjugated histamine excreted after ingestion of histamine. Proc. Soc. exp. Biol. (N. Y.) **70**, 146 (1949).
VALETTE, G., and Y. COHEN: Inactivation of histamine perfused in the vascular system of the small intestine of the rat in situ. J. Physiol. (Paris) **48**, 732 (1956).
WATON, N. G.: Studies on mammalian histidine decarboxylase. Brit. J. Pharmacol. **11**, 119 (1956).
WESTLING, H.: The difference in the metabolism of injected [^{14}C]-histamine in male and female rats. Brit. J. Pharmacol. **13**, 498 (1958).
WHITE, T.: Formation and catabolism of histamine in cat brain in vivo. J. Physiol. (Lond.) **152**, 299 (1960).
ZELLER, E. A.: Über den enzymatischen Abbau von Histamin und Diaminen. Helvet. chim. Acta **21**, 880 (1938).
— In: The Enzymes, edited by J. B. SUMNER and K. MYRBACK, Vol. II, Part I. New York: Academic Press 1951.
—, and J. BARSKY: In vivo inhibition of liver and brain monoamine oxidase by 1-isonicotinyl-2-isopropyl hydrazine. Proc. Soc. exp. Biol. (N. Y.) **81**, 459 (1952).
— — J. R. FOUTS, W. F. KIRCHHEIMER and L. S. VAN ORDEN: Influence of isonicotinic acid hydrazide (INH) and 1-isonicotinyl-2-isopropyl hydrazide (IIH) on bacterial and mammalian enzymes. Experientia (Basel) **8**, 349 (1952).
—, H. BIRKHAUSER, H. MISLIN and M. WENK: Enzymic degradation of polyamines. V. The occurence of diamine oxidase in man, mammal and bird, with an appendix on the occurrence of cholinesterase in birds. Helvet. chim. Acta **22**, 1381 (1939).
—, J. R. FOUTS and W. VOEGTLI: On the identity of histaminase and diamine oxidase. Abstr. XIX Int. Physiol. Congress, p. 913 (1953).
— P. STERN and L. A. BLANKSMA: Degradation of histamine by monoamine oxidase. Naturwissenschaften **7**, 157 (1956).

Section C

In Vitro Metabolism of Histamine (Exclusive of Diamine Oxidase)

By

HERBERT TABOR

I. Acetylation of histamine

Following the oral administration of histamine to a variety of animals, acetylhistamine is excreted in the urine[1]. The conversion of histamine to acetylhistamine has also been demonstrated *in vitro* with rabbit liver slices, pigeon liver slices, or extracts of acetone powder of pigeon liver, in the presence of coenzyme A (MILLICAN et al., 1949).

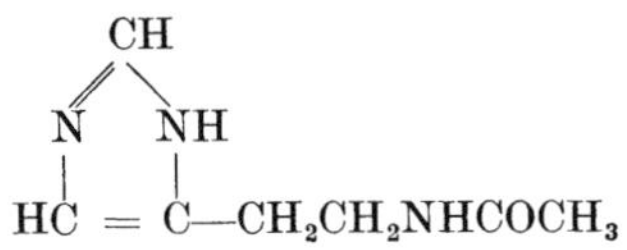

Acetylhistamine

The enzyme that catalyzes the acetylation of histamine has been purified from pigeon liver acetone powder (TABOR et al., 1953). During the purification procedure the enzyme that acetylates sulfanilamide, p-nitroaniline, and various other aromatic amines was also purified (KAPLAN and LIPMANN, 1948; CHOU and LIPMANN, 1952; BESSMAN and LIPMANN, 1953; TABOR et al., 1953). It is very likely that the same enzyme is responsible for the acetylation of these amines and for the acetylation of histamine, although the evidence is not conclusive.

The parallelism between histamine acetylation and aromatic amine acetylation permitted us to follow the reaction by a convenient spectrophotometric assay, based on the shift in the absorption spectrum of p-nitroaniline upon acetylation. The enzyme was purified 26-fold with this assay, and then tested for the acetylation of histamine.

A. Principle

(1) Generation of acetyl-CoA:

$$\text{Acetylphosphate} + \text{CoA} \xrightarrow{\text{transacetylase}} \text{Acetyl-CoA} + \text{phosphate}$$

(2) Acetylation of amine:

$$\text{R-NH}_2 + \text{Acetyl-CoA} \longrightarrow \text{RNH-Acetyl} + \text{CoA.}$$

B. Assay

p-Nitroaniline, which was used as the substrate, has an extinction coefficient of 6000 at 420 mμ (TABOR et al., 1953). At this wavelength, p-nitroacetanilide, the

[1] Refer to Chapter 4, Section B, by R. SCHAYER in this book for a review of the various *in vivo* studies on the metabolism of histamine.

acetylated derivative, has essentially no absorption. Thus the activity of the enzyme was measured by following the decrease in optical density at 420 mμ in the spectrophotometer.

The incubation mixture contained 40 μmoles of potassium phosphate buffer (pH 6.8), 5 μmoles of sodium thioglycolate, 12 μmoles of dilithium acetylphosphate, 4 units of transacetylase, 0.12 μmole of CoA, 0.1 μmole of p-nitroaniline, and enzyme in a total volume of 1.05 ml. A unit of enzyme was defined as the amount of enzyme causing a decrease of 0.001 unit of optical density per minute at 420 mμ.

C. Purification

The starting material for the purification procedure was an acetone powder of pigeon liver. This was extracted, and fractionated with acetone. Further purification was obtained by adsorption on alumina gel Cγ, and elution with phosphate buffer. For further details on the fractionation procedure and other properties of the enzyme, see TABOR et al., 1953.

D. Enzymatic acetylation with histamine as the substrate

The incubation mixture contained 2 μmoles of histamine, 300 μmoles of potassium pyrophosphate buffer, pH 9.3, 4 units of transacetylase, 10 μmoles of dilithium acetylphosphate, 0.1 μmole of CoA, 10 μmoles of sodium thioglycolate, 5 μmoles of disodium ethylenediaminetetraacetate, and 160 units of acetylating enzyme in a total volume of 1 ml. Under these conditions 50% of the histamine was acetylated in 30 min at 25° C.

The acetylation of histamine was measured by the disappearance of the ninhydrin-reacting material, using the method of MOORE and STEIN (1948), or by differential extraction into tertiary butanol at pH 8 (McINTIRE et al., 1947; MILLICAN, 1953). It is likely that other newer methods, such as the fluorometric assay for histamine could also be used for this purpose (SHORE et al., 1959; see also McINTIRE, Chapter 1, section C).

II. Methylation of histamine

Another pathway for the metabolism of histamine involves the methylation of the imidazole ring. An enzyme, imidazole-N-methyl transferase, which carries out this reaction *in vitro*, has been described in a variety of tissues by BROWN et al. (1959a, b), AXELROD et al., (1961) LINDAHL (1958/59/60) and WHITE (1959). The most active organ in the studies of BROWN et al. (1959b) was the guinea pig brain, which formed about 30 mμmoles of methylhistamine per 200 mg of whole tissue per hour.

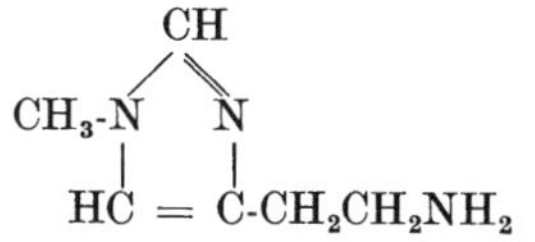

1,4-Methylhistamine
(1-Methyl-4 (β-aminoethyl)-imidazole)

The enzyme has been purified 30-fold from the soluble supernatant fraction of guinea pig brain (BROWN et al.,1959b). The methylating agent used was S-adenosylmethionine (LINDAHL 1958, 1959, 1960). The methylated histamine was detected by differential extraction into chloroform, and appeared to be the 1-methyl isomer. Other imidazoles were not substrates for the enzyme.

The purification procedure used by BROWN et al. (1959b) involved ammonium sulfate fractionation, adsorption of impurities with a calcium phosphate gel, and alumina gel Cγ adsorption and elution. For further details on this procedure see BROWN et al. (1959b).

The imidazole-N-methyl transferase was inhibited by low concentrations (5×10^{-7} M to 5×10^{-5} M) of chlorpromazine, 2-bromlysergic acid diethylamide, and serotonin (BROWN et al., 1959b).

A similar system has been partially purified from mouse liver by LINDAHL (1958, 1959, 1960).

The further metabolism of methylhistamine involves its oxidation to methylimidazole acetic acid. This activity has been shown *in vitro* in cat liver homogenates by KOBAYASHI (1958).

III. Formation of histamine ribotide

Following the demonstration that imidazole acetic acid could be converted *in vivo* to the corresponding riboside, CROWLEY (1960, 1964) demonstrated the conversion of imidazole acetic acid to the corresponding ribotide *in vitro*, using a purified rabbit liver preparation in a reaction requiring adenosine triphosphate and 1-pyrophosphoryl-ribose-5-phosphate. This work was confirmed and extended by FERNANDES et al. (1960), using a homogenate of the mucosa from dog small intestine. FERNANDES et al. found that their preparations formed the ribotide of histamine, as well as the ribotide of imidazole acetic acid. The ribotides formed could be converted to the corresponding ribosides by a snake venom nucleotidase.

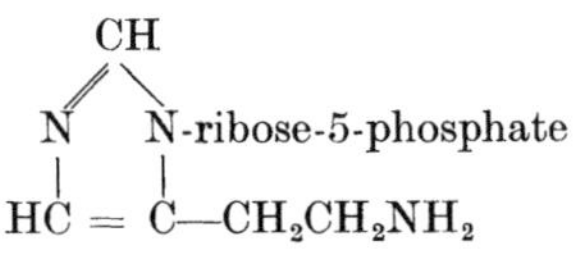

Histamine ribotide

IV. Formation of histamine dinucleotide

ALIVISATOS et al. (1960) have shown that histamine reacts with diphosphopyridine nucleotide in the presence of a soluble, purified beef spleen DPNase to form a dinucleotide, in which the nicotinamide moiety is replaced by histamine. This reaction proceeded fastest in the presence of high concentrations of histamine (1–3 M). These studies represent part of many studies carried out by ALIVISATOS et al. on various comparable reactions with various imidazoles (for references and further details, see ALIVISATOS et al., 1960).

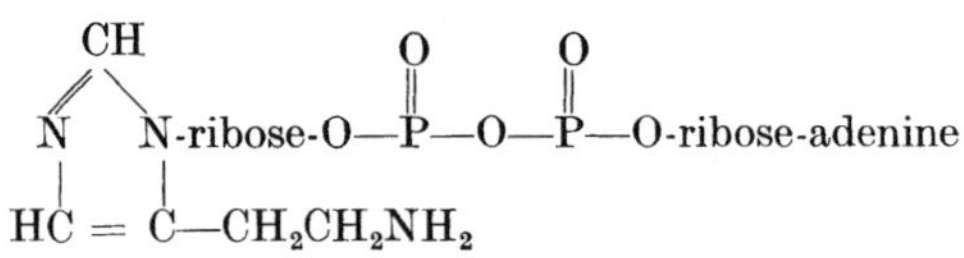

Histamine dinucleotide

Histamine dinucleotide could be converted to histamine ribotide by nucleotide pyrophosphatase (ALIVISATOS et al.., 1960) or by a phosphodiesterase preparation (MURAOKA et al, 1961). The ribotide could then be converted by 5′-nucleotidase, as above to the corresponding histamine riboside.

Recently, ABDEL-LATIF and ALIVISATOS (1961) have published an extension of these findings. In the presence of an enzyme from bull semen histamine reacted directly with either nicotinamide ribotide or nicotinamide riboside to form histamine ribotide and histamine riboside respectively. This enzyme also catalyzed the imidazololysis of the nicotinamide-ribose bond of DPN, as described above, and of TPN. For further details, see Chapter 4, section E.

References

ABDEL-LATIF, A. A., and S. G. A. ALIVISATOS: Alternative pathways of enzymic formation of ribotides and ribosides of histamine. Biochim. biophys. Acta (Amst.) **51**, 398 (1961).

ALIVISATOS, S. G. A., F. UNGAR, L. LUKACS and L. LAMANTIA: Imidazolytic processes. III. Enzymic conversion of coenzyme I to histamine dinucleotide. J. biol. Chem. **235**, 1742 (1960).

AXELROD, J., P. D. MACLEAN, R. W. ALBERS and H. WEISSBACH: Regional Neurochemistry, p. 307. Oxford: Pergamon Press 1961.

BESSMAN, S. P., and F. LIPMANN: Assay and distribution of coenzyme A. Arch. Biochem. **46**, 252 (1953).

BROWN, D. D., J. AXELROD and R. TOMCHICK: Enzymatic N-methylation of histamine. Nature (Lond.) **183**, 680 (1959).

— R. TOMCHICK and J. AXELROD: The distribution and properties of a histamine-methylating enzyme. J. biol. Chem. **234**, 2948 (1959).

CHOU, T. C., and F. LIPMANN: Separation of acetyl-transfer enzymes in pigeon-liver extract. J. biol. Chem. **196**, 89 (1952).

CROWLEY, G. M.: Enzymatic synthesis of imidazoleacetic acid ribotide. Fed. Proc. **19**, 309 (1960).

— The enzymatic synthesis of 5′, phosphoribosylimidazoleacetic acid. J. Biol. Chem. **239**, 2593 (1964).

FERNANDES, J. F., O. Y. CASTELLANI and M. PLESE: Biosynthesis of histamine ribotide and imidazoleacetate ribotide. Biochem. biophys. Res. Commun. **3**, 679 (1960).

KAPLAN, N. O., and F. LIPMANN: Assay and distribution of coenzyme A. J. biol. Chem. **174**, 37 (1948).

KOBAYASHI, Y.: Histamine catabolism by cat liver homogenates. Arch. Biochem. **77**, 275 (1958).

LINDAHL, K. M.: On the biological methylation of histamine. 3. Acta chem. scand. **12**, 2050 (1958); 4. Acta chem. scand. **13**, 1476 (1959).

— The histamine methylating enzyme system in liver. Acta physiol. scand. **49**, 114 (1960).

MCINTIRE, F. C., L. W. ROTH and J. L. SHAW: The purification of histamine for bioassay. J. biol. Chem. **170**, 537 (1947).

MILLICAN, R. C.: The acetylation of histamine in normal and enterectomized rats. Arch. Biochem. **42**, 399 (1953).

— S. M. ROSENTHAL and H. TABOR: On the metabolism of histamine; urinary excretion following oral administration: conjugation *in vitro*. J. Pharmacol. exp. Ther. **97**, 4 (1949).

MOORE, S., and W. STEIN: Photometric ninhydrin method for use in the chromatography of amino acids. J. biol. Chem. **176**, 367 (1948).

MURAOKA, S., M. INOUE and H. YAMASAKI: Enzymic formation of histamine ribotide from histamine dinucleotide. Nature (Lond.) **190**, 532 (1961).

SHORE, P. A., A. BURKHALTER and V. H. COHN JR.: A method for the fluorometric assay of histamine in tissues. J. Pharmacol. exp. Ther. **127**, 182 (1959).

TABOR, H., A. H. MEHLER and E. R. STADTMAN: The enzymatic acetylation of amines. J. biol. Chem. **204**, 127 (1953).

WHITE, T.: Formation and catabolism of histamine in brain tissue *in vitro*. J. Physiol. (Lond.) **149**, 34 (1959).

Section D

Enzymatic Formation of Histamine from Histidine

By

Richard W. Schayer

With 1 Figure

I. Introduction

This chapter includes only studies in mammals, excluding man; the latter is considered in Chapter 4, Section F.

Much of the early work in this field has been superseded and will not be presented in detail. Certain publications in Russian, Japanese and Hungarian were accessible only through abstracts; in some cases the material available was inadequate for a proper evaluation. It is regretted if any significant contribution has been overlooked for this reason.

II. Methods for the determination of histidine decarboxylase activity of mammalian tissues

Procedures used by several laboratories for preparation of enzyme and conditions for incubation of enzyme with substrate will be described. The subsequent assay for histamine by biological or chemical methods is given in Chapter 1, Sections C and D. The determination of histamine by the isotopic method is included in this section.

A. Method of Werle et al. (1955)

Experimental conditions. 3 cm³ kidney extract, 4 mg putrescine dihydrochloride dissolved in 2.5 cm³ H_2O (decomposition of histamine is competitively inhibited), 5 mg L-histidine base dissolved in 1 cm³ H_2O. Inhibitory substance is in 0.5 cm³ H_2O dissolved and added in the following molarities, as final concentration: 10^{-2}, 5×10^{-3}, 10^{-3}, 5×10^{-4}, 10^{-4}, 5×10^{-5} and 10^{-5}. Total volume 7 cm³. Time of incubation 3 hrs, temperature 37° C. Enzymic reaction is interrupted by adding 14 cm³ of 96 % ethyl alcohol and 1 cm³ of 1 N H_2SO_4. After standing 90 min or longer, the protein precipitate is filtered, washed 3 times, alcohol slowly evaporated and the mixture concentrated to 6 cm³. After neutralization with 1 N NaOH the mixture is made up to 7 cm³. Histamine formed from L-histidine is determined on an isolated, atropinized guinea pig ileum.

B. Method of Holtz and Westermann (1956) for histidine decarboxylase in nerve tissue

Sodium phosphate extract (M/15, pH 7.4) from bovine nerve and brain tissue (1:3) is incubated with 10 mg histidine per cm³ with added 100γ pyridoxal phosphate per cm³, under N_2 atmosphere and toluene for 24 hrs at 37° C. The amount of histamine is determined on isolated guinea pig intestine (20 cm³ Tyrode bath, atropine 10^{-7}). Similarly treated, histidine-free extract served as control, to which corresponding amount of histidine was added before the test.

C. Method of WATON (1956)

Formation of Histamine from Histidine by Mammalian Tissues

Rabbit kidneys, which are a rich source of histidine decarboxylase, were placed in 0.9% w/v NaCl, freed from all extraneous tissue, cut small and minced in a Latapie mincing machine. Where a tissue extract was required, the minced kidney was ground for 10 min. in a porcelain mortar with 1 g. silver sand and 10 ml. 0.9% w/v NaCl/g. tissue. This was centrifuged at 2,500 g for 10 min. and the supernatant fluid extract removed for incubation.

Generally 0.4 g minced tissue in 6 ml. Tyrode solution was used as a source of the enzyme. Occasionally this was replaced by 4 ml tissue extract plus 2 ml Tyrode solution. The mixture of tissue and Tyrode solution was placed in a 26 ml conical flask, 3 ml M/5-Na_2HPO_4 (pH 8.2) and 1 ml neutralized histidine (15 mg/ml) were added, and the mixture incubated at 38° C for 3 hr with mechanical agitation.

After incubation 1 N HCl was added from a microburette until a pH of 5.5–5.9 was obtained. The mixture was boiled for 1 min to coagulate proteins and prevent further enzyme action. After cooling, the contents of the flask were filtered through Whatman No. 1 paper.

The histamine content of the filtrate was assayed on the guinea-pig's isolated ileum suspended in a 2 ml bath of aerated Tyrode solution, with atropine, at 34° C.

Duplicate experiments were always carried out on each tissue mince or extract, and often the experiments were repeated with tissue from another animal. Blanks were carried out to estimate the histamine present in the incubation mixtures in the absence of the tissue, and again in the absence of the histidine solution.

D. Method of TELFORD and WEST (1961)

Formation of Histamine from Histidine by Rat Tissues

The method of WATON was first used. Values of enzyme activity in some tissues were found to be lower than those previously reported, but when the amount of tissue homogenate was doubled, consistent results were obtained. The following experiments refer to the increased amount of tissue homogenate.

Pooled tissue from freshly killed rats was cleaned and weighed, cut into small pieces, and ground in a glass mortar with a little sand and Tyrode solution (5 ml/g tissue). The resulting homogenate was allowed to stand and the supernatant fluid extract was removed for incubation. The composition of the incubation mixture was as follows.

Tissue homogenate (800 mg)	4.0 ml
Phosphate buffer (M/20-K_2HPO_4)	4.9 ml
L-Histidine (15 mg/ml, neutralised)	1.0 ml
Aminoguanidine (10 mg/ml, neutralised)	0.1 ml
Benzene (1 drop)	20 mg

The substrate (histidine) was always added last. The mixture was immediately shaken and incubated for 3 hr at 37°. The reaction was then stopped by reducing the pH of the solution to 4.0 with N HCl and by cooling to 4°. After neutralizing the mixture with N NaOH, its histamine content was determined. Mixtures containing boiled homogenate or no homogenate were similarly treated and assayed for histamine. In all experiments, mixtures without the substrate were also incubated and assayed for histamine. The final volume of the mixtures was maintained at 10 ml. The histamine content of the extract incubated in the presence of histidine less that of the extract incubated in the absence of histidine gives the amount of histamine formed from histidine during the incubation. This amount of formed histamine, when calculated per gram of tissue, was used as the index of histidine decarboxylase activity.

E. Method of Weissbach, Lovenberg and Udenfriend (1961)

An enzyme extract was prepared by homogenizing the tissue in 3 vol. of cold water followed by centrifugation at 78000 × *g*. The residue was discarded. Since enzyme activity was determined by assaying amine formation it was necessary to remove the endogenous histamine from the 78000 × *g* supernatant fraction. This was accomplished by dextran-gel filtration using Sephadex G-25. A 78000 × *g* supernatant fraction from guinea-pig kidney was used as the source of aromatic L-amino acid decarboxylase. Incubations with both enzymes were carried out in 20-ml beakers in air at 37° in a metabolic shaker. The incubation beakers contained enzyme, 7.10^{-5} *M* pyridoxal phosphate, 10^{-3} *M* iproniazid, L-histidine (2.10^{-3} *M* with the mast-cell enzyme and $1.6.10^{-2}$ *M* with the guinea-pig-kidney enzyme), 150 μmoles of phosphate buffer (pH 6.0) for the mast-cell enzyme and 250 μmoles Tris buffer (pH 9.0) for the guinea-pig-kidney enzyme. The final volume was 3.0 ml. At various time intervals 0.5 ml of the incubation mixture was transferred to a test tube containing 0.2 ml 5 % trichloroacetic acid and heated at 100° for 1 min. After cooling 1.5 ml of water were added and the precipitated protein was removed by centrifugation. The clear supernatant fraction was passed over a 0.5 × 3 cm Dowex-1 carbonate column to remove the histidine and the column was then washed with 1 ml of water. The effluent and washings were combined and assayed for histamine by the method of Shore et al.

F. Method of Mackay and Shepherd (1960)

Histidine. — It was necessary to prepare L-histidine zwitterion from commercial L-histidine monohydrochloride monohydrate to eliminate traces of histamine present. The hydrochloric acid was removed by adding excess silver carbonate to a warm concentrated aqueous solution of the monohydrochloride. After filtration, silverions were removed from the filtrate by passing in hydrogen sulphide. Filtration and subsequent concentration of the filtrate, under reduced pressure, gave a saturated solution of L-histidine zwitterion from which the latter was precipitated by addition of dehydrated alcohol.

Preparation of Histidine Decarboxylase. — Guinea-pig kidneys were used as the source of mammalian histidine decarboxylase. They were pulped with purified sand, approximately 3 ml of saline was then added/g of tissue, and the mixture was ground once more. The fluid was centrifuged at 15,000 *g* for 20 min, and the supernatant was used as a crude enzyme extract.

Incubation Experiments. — The incubation medium for the uninhibited reaction was prepared by pipetting into a centrifuge tube phosphate buffer of pH 8.0 (isotonic with blood), 2.0 ml; 0.9 % sodium chloride solution, 0.9 ml; L-histidine zwitterion solution (25.0 mg/ml saline), 1.0 ml; and 3×10^{-3} M aminoguanidine bicarbonate in saline, 0.1 ml. After the tubes and their contents had been left in the thermostat for about 15 min, 1.0 ml of enzyme extract was added, the tubes were stoppered, inverted to mix the solutions, and the time was noted. The final volume in each tube was 5.0 ml so that the final concentrations of L-histidine and aminoguanidine were respectively 32.2×10^{-3} M and 6×10^{-5} M. Aminoguanidine in the concentration used has been shown by Waton (1956) to inhibit completely any histaminase present; it was added as a routine precaution, though the histaminase activity of guinea-pig kidney extracts is very low. In order to measure the rate of the reaction in presence of decarboxylase inhibitor, the latter was added either in solid form or as a neutralized solution in saline, with the volume of pure saline added to the incubation medium correspondingly reduced. Inhibition was therefore studied at constant pH, temperature and substrate concentration. Since the enzyme concentration was constant only for a given extract at a given time, simultaneous studies on the inhibited and uninhibited reaction had to be carried out using the same extract.

The reaction was stopped by adding 0.20 ml of 2 N hydrochloric acid to the centrifuge tubes to make the media just acid, and boiling for 1 min to coagulate protein. The latter was centrifuged down, and the solutions were stored overnight at 4°. The histamine produced was estimated by the 4-point method on atropinized guinea-pig ileum at 34°, using an automatic assay apparatus. Control experiments were carried out to detect any histamine either in the reagents, or produced by interaction of enzyme with the inhibitors. The effect of inhibitors on the assay of histamine was checked, and the stability of histamine under the conditions used was also studied. No serious complications were encountered.

G. Method of SCHAYER et al. (1959) using radioisotopes

Minced tissue, or cell-free enzyme preparations, were incubated in 1–3 ml phosphate buffer pH 7.2 (containing 0.2% glucose) and 10–40γ C^{14} L-histidine under nitrogen for 3 hours at 37° C. After incubation 1 ml of a solution containing 66.4 mg histamine dihydrochloride carrier and 50 mg L-histidine monohydrochloride was added, mixed and about one third volume of 0.6 N perchloric acid added. After 30 minutes the precipitated protein was removed by filtration and washed with 0.2 N perchloric acid. The filtrate collected in a 37 × 200 mm test tube, was diluted to about 20 ml and then were added 10 ml saturated sodium sulfate solution, 8 gm anhydrous sodium sulfate, 10 drops of 10 N sodium hydroxide solution and 50 ml butanol. The mixture was shaken mechanically for 15 minutes, centrifuged and the clear butanol layer transferred to another tube. It was washed once by shaking for 15 minutes with 20 ml of an aqueous alkaline saturated solution of sodium sulfate containing 1 mg L-histidine monohydrochloride/ml. The butanol was shaken with 15 ml 1 N hydrochloric acid and the latter, containing the histamine carrier, evaporated to dryness on a steam bath in 25-ml Erlenmeyer flasks. Further removal of hydrochloric acid was made in a vacuum desiccator containing potassium hydroxide pellets.

The carrier histamine dihydrochloride samples were dissolved in 2 ml water, and then were added 3 ml of a solution of benzenesulfonylchloride in dioxane (60 mg benzenesulfonylchloride/ml dioxane) and about 0.3–0.4 gm of sodium bicarbonate. The reaction was allowed to proceed at room temperature for 30 minutes with gentle shaking. Water was added in small quantities over a period of 1–2 hours to a total of about 20 ml. The sides of the flask are scratched to help start crystallization. The crude dibenzenesulfonyl histamine (BSH) was collected and washed with cold 25% ethanol in water. Recrystallization was effected by dissolving in a few milliliters acetone, treating with charcoal, filtering through a 2-ml coarse sintered glass funnel containing filter-aid, and slow addition of small amounts of water, avoiding turbidity. The crystals of BSH were collected, dried and accurately weighed in vials suitable for liquid scintillation counting.

The BSH was dissolved in 5 ml dioxane with gentle warming and a solution of PPO and POPOP in 7 ml toluene added. The observed counts were corrected for background, for weight of sample and for blank (obtained by incubating boiled tissue or enzyme under the same conditions as the samples). Results are expressed as counts per minute per 100 mg of BSH.

Minor modifications may be made in the isotope procedure. Volumes of extraction fluids are not critical and may be altered to some extent; commercial C^{14} L-histidine is purified to remove traces of C^{14} histamine; various concentrations of C^{14} L-histidine may be used; nonisotopic histamine, usually 10 γ/ml incubate, may be added to reduce destruction of minute quantities of C^{14} histamine by methylation or other processes; aminoguanidine, 10 to 20 γ/ml incubate, should be used in extracts having significant diamine oxidase activity.

A method published by GRAHAM et al. (1956) was later found by these workers to be unreliable; an additive, sodium hydrosulfite, was causing a chemical decarboxylation of histidine. These authors have retracted the conclusions stated in the above reference.

III. Sources and properties of histidine decarboxylase

The tissues of various mammalian species, in which histidine decarboxylase activity has been reported, are listed in Table 1. The properties of enzyme from only a few of these sources have been studied in detail; some of the findings are shown in Table 2. The enzyme from all reported sources is soluble. At the present time, there appear to be at least two distinctly different enzymes which decarboxylate histidine *in vitro*. On one hand, enzyme from rat and mouse mast cells, rat stomach, rat fetal liver and rat hepatoma appears to be unequivocally specific for histidine, to have a high affinity for substrate molecules, to show maximum activity at a relatively low pH, to bind the coenzyme loosely, to be unaffected or inhibited by benzene, and to be unaffected by α-methyl DOPA. On the other hand, the enzyme from rabbit and guinea pig kidney has low affinity for substrate,

Table 1. *Sources of mammalian histidine decarboxylase.* (Numbers are references listed below)

	rabbit	guinea pig	rat	mouse	cat	dog	pig	hamster	ox	sheep
Kidney	1, 2, 3, 8, 9, 10	1, 2, 3, 8, 11, 12	2, 3, 8, 14	3, 8, 16	2		4, 5, 6	3	5	5
Liver	1, 2, 3	1, 2, 3, 6, 8, 16	2, 14	3, 8, 15	2, 5	24	3, 5, 6	3	5	5
Intestine	8	6, 8	14	8, 16						
Lung		3, 16, 21	17	15, 16, 18	8, 16	24				
Spleen				15						
Pancreas	3	1, 3						3		
Skin			13	18, 21						
Muscle			16	15, 21						
Stomach	8	6	8, 9, 14, 20	8, 23						
Nerv. syst.			17	16	22	12, 22	22		19	
Platelets	25		For other rat tissues see Table 2							

References: (1) WERLE and HERRMANN, 1937; (2) HOLTZ and HEISE, 1937; (3) WERLE and KRAUTZUN, 1938; (4) WERLE and HEITZER, 1938; (5) HOLTZ et al., 1938; (6) WERLE, 1940; (7) WERLE, 1942; (8) WATON, 1956; (9) SCHAYER, 1957; (10) GANROT et al., 1961; (11) WEISSBACH et al., 1961; (12) LOVENBERG et al., 1962; (13) SCHAYER et al., 1959; (14) TELFORD and WEST, 1961; (15) SCHAYER, 1960a; (16) SCHAYER, 1962; (17) SCHAYER, 1956; (18) SCHAYER, 1960; (19) HOLTZ and WESTERMANN, 1956; (20) KAHLSON et al., 1958; (21) SCHAYER, 1961a; (22) WHITE, 1960; (23) SCHAYER, unpublished; (24) BOROVSKAYA, 1940; (25) SCHAYER and KOBAYASHI, 1956.

Table 2. *Comparison of properties of histidine decarboxylase*
From several mammalian sources (Figures in parentheses are references)

Source	pH optimum	K_m*	Effect of dialysis on activity	Effect of benzene on activity	Presence of other amino acid decarboxylating activities	Inhibition by α-methyl DOPA
Rat peritoneal mast cells	ca. 7 (1)	—	strong loss	inhibitory	5 HTPD present (2) or weak (3)	—
Mouse mastocytoma (containing histamine but little 5 HT)	6.0 (4)	5×10^{-4}	—	none	5 HTPD undetectable	none
Mouse mastocytoma (containing both histamine and 5 HT)	7.0 (5)	—	loss if dialysis is prolonged	—	DOPA and 5 HTP decarboxylase activities present	weak (3)
Rat pyloric stomach	7.2 (6) 7.0 (7)	—	loss (3)	inhibits (6)	5 HTPD undetectable (4)	weak (3, 8)
Rat fetal liver	6.6 (9) 6.5 (10)	2×10^{-5} tested at pH 7.8 (11)	loss (3)	no effect (7)	5 HTPD undetectable (9)	weak (9, 11)
Rat hepatoma	ca. 7 (12) 6.5 (10)	8.7×10^{-4} (12)	—	inhibits (12) insignificant (10)	DOPA decarboxylase undetectable (12); 5 HTPD undetectable (12) or weak (10)	—
Guinea pig kidney	9.0—9.5 (4) ca. 9 (12)	ca. 5×10^{-2} (4, 12)	—	activates (4, 12, 13)	Numerous activities present (13, 14)	strong (4, 15, 16)
Rabbit kidney	8.6—9.0 (17) 8.0 (6)	ca. 10^{-1} (11)	insignificant loss (3, 17, 18)	activates (6, 19)	Numerous activities present (11, 20)	strong (11)

* K_m, the Michaelis constant, corresponds to the substrate concentration at which one-half the limiting velocity is reached, i.e. when one-half of the enzyme molecules are converted to the enzyme-substrate complex. A high value of K_m indicates a low affinity between enzyme and substrate (21).

References: (1) ROTHSCHILD and SCHAYER, 1959; (2) BENDITT, 1958; (3) SCHAYER, unpublished; (4) WEISSBACH et al., 1961; (5) HAGEN et al., 1960; (6) SCHAYER, 1957; (7) TELFORD and WEST, 1961; (8) CODE, personal communication; (9) BURKHALTER, 1962; (10) KAMESWAREN and WEST, 1961; (11) GANROT et al., 1961; (12) MACKAY et al., 1961 a; (13) LOVENBERG et al., 1962; (14) WERLE and AURES, 1959; (15) WERLE, 1961; (16) MACKAY and SHEPHERD, 1960; (17) WERLE and HERRMANN, 1937; (18) WERLE and KRAUTZUN, 1938; (19) WATON, 1956; (20) WERLE and HEITZER, 1938; (21) BALDWIN, 1957.

Table 3. *Inhibition of histidine decarboxylase from rabbit and guinea pig kidney*

Additive	Concentration (molarity unless otherwise indicated)	% Inhibition	Reference
Cu^{++}; Fe^{++}	—	marked	WERLE and HERRMANN (1937)
hydrogen cyanide	10^{-4}	20	WERLE and HERRMANN (1937)
potassium cyanide	10^{-3}	100	WERLE and KRAUTZUN (1938)
glutathione	5 mg/5.5 ml	55—63	WERLE and KRAUTZUN (1938)
ascorbic acid	5 mg/5.5 ml	48—66	WERLE and KRAUTZUN (1938)
hydrogen sulfide	saturated	37—100	WERLE and KRAUTZUN (1938)
carbon monoxide	saturated	19—26	WERLE and KRAUTZUN (1938)
sodium bisulfite	3×10^{-3}	76	WERLE and HEITZER (1938)
cysteine	4.2×10^{-3}	94	WERLE and HEITZER (1938)
cystine	5×10^{-3}	21	WERLE and HEITZER (1938)
tryptophan	3×10^{-3}	40	WERLE and HEITZER (1938)
L-DOPA	1.7×10^{-3}	100	WERLE and HEITZER (1938)
adenylpyrophosphoric acid	1.3×10^{-3}	50	WERLE and HEITZER (1938)
semicarbazide	10^{-4}	83	WERLE and HEITZER (1938)
hydroxylamine	10^{-4}	100	WERLE and HEITZER (1938)
pyruvic acid	10^{-2}	74	WERLE and HEITZER (1938)
hydrogen cyanide	10^{-4}	50	WERLE and HEITZER (1938)
glycine	8.9×10^{-3}	25	WERLE and HEITZER (1938)
glutamic acid	4.5×10^{-3}	10	WERLE and HEITZER (1938)
dimedon	10^{-2}	25—44	WERLE (1940)
Girard's reagents	10^{-2} to 10^{-3}	25—80	WERLE (1940)
phenylhydrazine	10^{-4}	100	WERLE (1940)
dinitrophenylhydrazine	10^{-3}	20	WERLE (1940)
germanin	10^{-3}	90	WERLE (1940)
trypan blue	10^{-3}	77	WERLE (1940)
imidazole	10 mg/ml	50—58	WERLE (1942)
D-histidine	10 mg/3 ml	80—98	WERLE (1942)
L-DOPA	0.2 mg/3 ml	26	WERLE (1942)
DL-DOPA	0.2 mg/3 ml	90	WERLE (1942)
D-DOPA	8.6×10^{-7}	20	WERLE (1942)
2-methyl-4-amino-5-bromomethyl pyrimidine hydrobromide	1.75 mg/3 ml	60	WERLE (1942)
4-methyl-5-oxyethyl-thiazole	1.3 mg/3 ml	60	WERLE (1942)
pyrocatechol	—	—	WERLE (1942)
hydroquinone	—	—	WERLE (1942)
resorcinol	—	—	WERLE (1942)
sodium fluoride	10^{-2}	50	WERLE (1942)
pyridoxal-3-phosphate	1.67 mg/ml	50	WERLE and KOCH (1949)
L-DOPA	2×10^{-3}	95	WERLE and KOCH (1949)
pyrocatechol	10^{-3}	87	WERLE and KOCH (1949)
pyrogallol	10^{-3}	82	WERLE and KOCH (1949)
hydroquinone	10^{-3}	65	WERLE and KOCH (1949)
resorcinol	10^{-3}	50	WERLE and KOCH (1949)
tryptophan	2×10^{-3}	26	WERLE and KOCH (1949)
indole	2×10^{-3}	21	WERLE and KOCH (1949)
alanine	2×10^{-1}	28	WERLE and KOCH (1949)
phenol	9×10^{-2}	30	WERLE and KOCH (1949)
tyrosine	9×10^{-2}	34	WERLE and KOCH (1949)
pyrogallol methyl ether	10^{-3}	11	WERLE and KOCH (1949)
adrenaline	—	strong	WERLE and KOCH (1949)
noradrenaline	—	strong	WERLE and KOCH (1949)
pyridoxine	10 mg/3 to 4 ml	78	WERLE and KOCH (1949)
aniline	7×10^{-2}	83	WERLE and KOCH (1949)
imidazole	10^{-1}	38	WERLE and KOCH (1949)
ascorbic acid	1 mg/ml	15	MARTIN et al. (1949)
quercitin	1 mg/ml	100	MARTIN et al. (1949)
homoeriodictyol	1 mg/ml	30	MARTIN et al. (1949)

Table 3 (cont'd.)

Additive	Concentration (molarity unless otherwise indicated)	% Inhibition	Reference
esculetin	1 mg/ml	30	MARTIN et al. (1949)
d-catechin	1 ml/mg	100	MARTIN et al. (1949)
hematoxylin	—	strong	GABOR et al. (1952)
hematin	—	strong	GABOR et al. (1952)
brazilin	—	strong	GABOR et al. (1952)
brazilein	—	strong	GABOR et al. (1952)
1-hydrazinophthalazine	6×10^{-5}	50	WERLE et al. (1955)
aminoguanidine	10^{-2}	50	WERLE et al. (1955)
isonicotinic acid hydrazide	7×10^{-4}	50	WERLE et al. (1955)
2,4-dihydrazinoquinazoline	3.3×10^{-5}	50	WERLE et al. (1955)
1-hydrazino-4-methyl-phthalazine	3×10^{-5}	50	WERLE et al. (1955)
1-hydrazinoisoquinoline	1.7×10^{-5}	50	WERLE et al. (1955)
5'-amino R[1]	10^{-5}	50	PARROT and LABORDE (1959)
3'-amino-4'-5'-6'-triethoxy-R[1]	10^{-5}	50	PARROT and LABORDE (1959)
6'-methoxy-5'-ethoxy-R[1]	10^{-5}	40	PARROT and LABORDE (1959)
4'-5'-6'-triethoxy-R[1]	10^{-5}	30	PARROT and LABORDE (1959)
narcotine camphosulfonate	10^{-5}	30	PARROT and LABORDE (1959)
narcotine	10^{-5}	20	PARROT and LABORDE (1959)

[1] R = 1-phthalidyl-2-methyl-6,7-methylenedioxy-8-methoxy-1,2,3,4-tetrahydroisoquinoleine.

shows maximum activity at a relatively high pH, binds coenzyme firmly, is activated by benzene and is strongly inhibited by α-methyl DOPA.

To some extent these differences may be attributable to the presence of different binding sites on the protein portion of the enzyme molecule. The group in the histidine decarboxylase of high affinity appears to be specific for the imidazole ring while that in kidney histidine decarboxylase appears to attract certain aromatic rings such as those of DOPA and 5-HTP more strongly than it does the ring of histidine.

Accordingly, the kidney enzyme is inhibited by α-methyl DOPA and other aromatic amino acids (Tables 2 and 3). On the other hand, the enzyme of high affinity is inhibited by these compounds only when the concentration is sufficiently high to react with the coenzyme, pyridoxal phosphate (ROTHSCHILD and SCHAYER, 1959; BURKHALTER, 1962).

IV. Histamine formation in vitro

A. Early studies

In this section the literature up to 1955—1956 will be reviewed. These dates were arbitrarily selected because of the introduction of new techniques for the study of histidine decarboxylase during this period. In some cases, discussion of material from the earlier papers has been postponed so that it might be included in a section on some specific topic.

Most of the data on sources and properties of the enzyme, and the inhibitory effect of compounds, has been deleted from the discussion of the individual papers and included in Tables 1, 2 and 3.

The first published evidence of conversion of histidine to histamine by an enzyme from a mammalian source was by WERLE (1936) and WERLE and HERRMANN (1937). It was shown that extracts of kidneys of rabbits or guinea pigs, when incubated with histidine in Tyrode solution at 37.5° C, under sterile or non-sterile conditions, produced a small quantity of a substance which had properties similar to those of histamine: it showed the same effect on atropinized guinea pig intestine, it lowered the blood pressure of atropinized dogs and cats to the same extent as the same amount of pure histamine, it was not inactivated by boiling for 90 minutes in 1 N hydrochloric acid, and was completely inactivated by dog kidney histaminase. No histamine formation was found in kidneys of beef, sheep, dog, rat, pig or cat; this was believed to be due, in some cases, to destruction of the amine by histaminase. Of the other rabbit tissues examined, only liver showed activity. In guinea pigs, liver and pancreas were active.

HOLTZ and HEISE (1937 and 1937a) independently made similar findings in guinea pig kidney and liver. In cat kidney, which has a very high histaminase activity, it was necessary to carry out the decarboxylation in the complete absence of oxygen in order to prevent destruction of the histamine formed.

The kidney enzyme was reported to be not very stable. It was not extractable with glycerine and its activity was rapidly destroyed by papain (WERLE and KRAUTZUN, 1938).

PARROT (1939) found that kidneys of sensitized and non-sensitized guinea pigs formed histamine at the same rate; he concluded that kidney histamine plays no part in anaphylactic shock.

WERLE and HEITZER (1938) made a 35-fold purification of the enzyme from rabbit kidney by treatment of aqueous extracts with kaolin followed by adsorption on aluminium hydroxide Cγ and elution. Their evidence indicated that tyrosine and tryptophan were also decarboxylated by an enzyme apparently identical with histidine decarboxylase. The enzyme is precipitated, and to some extent stabilized, by treatment of extracts with half-saturated ammonium sulfate.

From additional inhibitor studies WERLE (1940) concluded that the active center of the enzyme contained a carbonyl group but that its nature was in question. He found compounds which could inhibit histaminase to a much greater degree than histidine decarboxylase; these were useful in proving histamine formation since elimination of oxygen did not always completely prevent histamine destruction.

KUMAMOTO (1940) repeated and confirmed the *in vitro* work; he also found that perfusion of kidneys with Locke's solution containing 0.05 to 0.1% histidine resulted in histamine both in the outflow and in the transudate. He concluded that histamine formed in the kidney can enter the urine directly.

WERLE (1942) used putrescine, a substrate for diamine oxidase (histaminase), to prevent the destruction of histamine formed by tissue extracts; this technique permitted demonstration of histidine decarboxylase in pig kidney and intestine and the possible formation by human intestine.

Damage to kidney either by ureter stasis (WERLE et al., 1939) or by partial obstruction of the renal vein for 2 to 5 days (WERLE et al., 1940) reduced histidine decarboxylase activity. Blocking the renal artery of rabbits resulted in inactivation of histidine decarboxylase in 3 days; the enzyme was reactivated when the artery was opened. Enzyme activity was also reduced by decapsulation of the kidney or in nephrosis caused by salyrgan (WERLE and LELLMAN, 1945).

It has been reported that in rats, dogs and cats subjected to a blow on the head there was a sharp drop in histamine content of nerve tissue and a marked activation of histidine decarboxylase; these changes in nerve were not found after ether narcosis (KOSHTOYANTS et al., 1945). WERLE (1956) states that he did not confirm their findings on histamine changes. RYBKINA (1947) reported that stimulation of sciatic, phrenic and vagus nerves of several species for one minute liberates histamine and activates histidine decarboxylase.

B. Rabbit and guinea pig kidney histidine decarboxylase

There is general agreement that kidney histidine decarboxylase from the species usually studied, the rabbit and the guinea pig, as measured by *in vitro* techniques, differs in properties from those of the enzyme obtained from other extensively studied tissues (SCHAYER, 1957; MACKAY et al., 1961a; GANROT et al., 1961; WEISSBACH et al., 1961). Properties of histidine decarboxylase from various sources are shown in Table 2. It is worthy of mention that the variance is according to species as well as tissue since the kidney enzymes are from rabbit and guinea pig while all the other tabulated sources of active preparation are from rats or mice. Evidence from *in vitro* studies indicating a high rate of histamine synthesis in rabbit and guinea pig tissues should be regarded with greater than usual suspicion since these species, in contrast to rats and mice, are sensitive to histamine.

One important difference between enzyme types is the ability of kidney extracts to decarboxylate a large number of aromatic L-amino acids. Among these are DOPA, 5-HTP, tryptophan, tyrosine, o- and m-tyrosine, phenylalanine, dihydroxyphenylserine, 4-hydroxytryptophan, α-methyl DOPA and α-methyl 5-HTP (for references see Table 2). Aliphatic amino acids such as L-leucine and L-serine are not decarboxylated even when tested with tracer amounts of substrate (LOVENBERG et al., 1962).

GANROT et al. (1961) and LOVENBERG et al. (1962) have purified DOPA decarboxylase and found that the histidine decarboxylase activity accompanies it throughout a variety of procedures. Because of the parallel retention of both enzyme activities, and because the histidine decarboxylating action is blocked by DOPA decarboxylase inhibitors such as α-methyl DOPA, these laboratories suggested that the enzymes are identical. Both also found that the affinity of the purified enzyme for L-histidine was so low that its ability to produce histamine *in vivo* was questionable.

On the other hand, WERLE and AURES (1959) have reported complete separation of histidine decarboxylase from DOPA decarboxylase. Since the positive experiment, demonstrating separability, comes from the laboratory of a very experienced worker, it may be that the other groups failed to achieve proper conditions for separation. Another possible interpretation of this discrepancy is that under certain incubation conditions, purified DOPA decarboxylase can catalyze decarboxylation of histidine to a small extent, but that under the conditions used by WERLE and AURES, this did not occur. Formation of artifacts *in vitro* is discussed under „Interpretation of Findings of In Vitro Histidine Decarboxylase Assays."

LOVENBERG et al. (1962) found that benzene activated the histidine decarboxylating ability of a partially purified enzyme but reduced its DOPA decarboxylating power. This data does not support the view that the enzymes are identical. But since the mechanism of action of benzene is not known, and since the rates of decarboxylation of DOPA and histidine are markedly different, some reasonable explanation for this matter may be forthcoming.

In man, α-methyl DOPA, a powerful inhibitor of DOPA decarboxylase, decreases the urinary excretion of aromatic amines (OATES et al., 1960). WEISSBACH et al. (1961) cite these data and the unpublished findings by OATES and SJOERDSMA that α-methyl DOPA does not decrease urinary histamine in man, as evidence that *in vivo* histamine synthesis is not catalyzed to any significant extent by the enzyme with low affinity for L-histidine. This is not a very convincing argument since the affinity of tyrosine for the enzyme is also rather low (LOVENBERG et al., 1962) but the rate of its decarboxylation *in vivo* is markedly reduced by the inhibitor (OATES et al., 1960). α-Methyl DOPA also fails to affect histamine excretion in rats (WERLE, 1961). Neither human nor rat kidney histidine decarboxylase has been characterized with respect to substrate affinity or for susceptibility to inhibition by α-methyl DOPA.

When very small concentrations of C^{14} L-histidine are incubated with rabbit kidney extracts, the resulting histidine decarboxylase activity is not particularly impressive; in a comparative study, the enzyme from rat pyloric stomach was 15 times more active (SCHAYER, 1957). Regardless of the calculated affinities, kidney extracts can decarboxylate histidine *in vitro* when the concentration of the amino acid is less than that normally found free in plasma and when other amino acids are present. Any implication that a very low rate of *in vivo* histamine synthesis is of no significance to the organism is wholly unjustified.

HOLTZ and CREDNER (1944) have published evidence that guinea pig kidney converts histidine to histamine *in vivo* but of necessity used large amounts of histidine. Rigorous demonstration of formation of histamine from physiological concentrations of histidine in kidney of living guinea pigs or rabbits has not been attempted. Such experiments seem to have been done only with rats (SCHAYER et al., 1954a) and dogs (LINDELL and SCHAYER, 1958) and in both cases the evidence is very strong that the kidney of the living animal does decarboxylate histidine.

Some insight into the rate of histamine synthesis by kidney of living guinea pigs may be possible through consideration of the rate of urinary histamine excretion. The only known data which exclude dietary and bacterial sources show that the yield of urinary histamine from C^{14} L-histidine is about 0.015 % (SCHAYER, 1952). From this it can be roughly calculated that the guinea pig can form about 12γ of urinary histamine per day. On the basis of data from experiments with rats (SCHAYER et al., 1954a) and dogs (LINDELL and SCHAYER, 1958) it can be assumed with some confidence that a considerable amount of this histamine is formed in the kidney and excreted without entering the circulation, and that the kidney does not destroy a significant portion of the histamine which it synthesizes. Hence a reasonable, but very rough estimate of the rate of histamine formation in kidney of living guinea pigs, is of the order of 10γ per day. In contrast, guinea pig extracts, *in vitro*, can make very large quantities of histamine. WEISSBACH et al. (1961) report a rate of 48 γ histamine per gram tissue per hour, about 100 times the estimated *in vivo* rate.

On the basis of the best available evidence it seems likely that the high *in vitro* histamine forming capacity of rabbit and guinea pig kidney extracts is a gross exaggeration of the physiological rate.

In summary it is believed that the following possibilities exist for the mechanism of histamine formation from histidine by extracts, or purified enzyme, from rabbit and guinea pig kidney.

1) The reaction is catalyzed by a specific histidine decarboxylase having low affinity for substrate and having structure and properties similar to DOPA decarboxylase. α-Methyl DOPA could inhibit by attachment to groupings similar to those in DOPA decarboxylase and thus block accessibility of L-histidine to its specific binding site. Favoring this possibility is the claim of separation of histidine decarboxylase from DOPA decarboxylase by WERLE and AURES (1959).

2) The reaction is catalyzed by DOPA decarboxylase (or aromatic L-amino acid decarboxylase). L-histidine attaches to the same point on the protein as do other substrates and is decarboxylated in a like manner. This view raises a number of theoretical objections (see „Specificity of Histidine Decarboxylase") and cannot

be accepted without prior invalidation of the claim of separation of histidine decarboxylase and DOPA decarboxylase by WERLE and AURES.

3) The reaction is catalyzed by DOPA decarboxylase (or aromatic L-amino acid decarboxylase) but L-histidine attaches to the protein portion of the enzyme at a site suitable for an imidazole compound, but different from the site where aromatic amino acid substrate molecules attach. If the histidine molecule were properly oriented, and conditions were otherwise satisfactory, pyridoxal phosphate may catalyze the decarboxylation (see „Mechanism of Decarboxylation"). α-Methyl DOPA could efficiently inhibit this process if in its usual position of attachment it blocked accessibility of histidine to the imidazole-binding site.

4) The reaction can be catalyzed to a small extent by a specific histidine decarboxylase of high affinity; under the usual incubation conditions the existence of this process is obscured by other reactions.

None of these possibilities is proved, none is excluded, and more than one may be valid.

C. Histamine formation by mast cells

Mast cells contain a large percentage of the histamine bound in mammalian tissues (RILEY, 1959). SCHAYER, 1956a, showed that when suspensions of the free cells from the peritoneal cavity of rats were incubated with small concentrations of C^{14} L-histidine, C^{14} histamine was formed and bound in stable condition. Although only about 3 to 5 percent of the peritoneal cells were mast cells, their participation in the decarboxylation of L-histidine and binding of histamine was evident since the remaining cells, largely leucocytes, had no significant histamine forming power. When peritoneal cell suspensions were incubated with C^{14} L-histidine, the ratio of C^{14} histamine to non-isotopic, endogenous, histamine was the same in the intact cells and in the supernatant liquid; this finding suggested that the newly-formed C^{14} histamine was held in the same binding linkage as endogenous mast cell histamine. Formation of new histamine by intact mast cells was maximal at about pH 7.2 to 7.5. The possibility that free mast cells might bind exogenous histamine was tested. Peritoneal cell suspensions were incubated with C^{14} L-histidine either in the presence or absence of non-isotopic histamine. If exogenous histamine molecules were able to enter the binding sites, it would be expected that the amount of bound C^{14} histamine would be reduced. There was no effect. Rupture of the mast cell suspensions yielded soluble histidine decarboxylase of low activity.

With the availability of liquid scintillation counting, a more thorough study of the histidine decarboxylase activity of rat peritoneal mast cell was possible (ROTHSCHILD and SCHAYER, 1959). Attempts to separate mast cells from leucocytes using differential centrifugation in hypertonic sucrose solutions resulted in almost total loss of enzyme activity from the cells to the supernate. Although a complete separation of mast cells was never obtained, it was possible to enrich the mast cell count relative to the leucocyte count by centrifuging in balanced salt solution, and to show that the histidine decarboxylase activity was always proportional to the percentage of mast cells. The soluble enzyme gave no sharp pH maximum but was close to optimum in a range from pH 6.5 to 7.5. Pyridoxal phosphate could be clearly shown to be a coenzyme for this preparation (see „The Coenzyme of Histidine Decarboxylase"). Other properties are shown in Table 2.

Using a mouse mastocytoma ONO and HAGEN (1959) and HAGEN et al. (1960) demonstrated strong histidine decarboxylase activity and showed independently that mast cell histidine decarboxylase requires pyridoxal phosphate.

Dog mastocytoma also has a high histamine-forming capacity (LINDELL et al., 1959).

Schindler et al. (1959) found that a mouse mast cell tumor maintained in culture was able to maintain a high histamine level although the medium was virtually devoid of histamine. These cells were also able to concentrate exogenous histamine (Green and Day, 1961). It should be emphasized that the latter observation does not constitute an exception to the usual finding that the histamine bound in the tissues for significant periods of time arises from L-histidine and not exogenous histamine. Whatever may be the mechanism of "binding" of exogenous histamine by the mastocytoma cells in cultures, it is not the same as physiological binding; the authors report that the endogenous and exogenous histamine in these cells differed in rate of turnover and in conditions of release.

Weissbach et al. (1961), using a mast cell tumor which contained large quantities of histamine but only small amounts of serotonin, studied the characteristics of the histidine decarboxylase; findings are listed in Table 2. Endogenous histamine was removed from the mast cell extract by dextran-gel filtration using Sephadex G-25.

D. Rat stomach histidine decarboxylase

The extremely high histidine decarboxylase activity of the pyloric portion of rat stomach was reported by Schayer (1957) and confirmed by several groups (Kahlson et al., 1958; Telford and West, 1961; Weissbach et al., 1961). Some of the properties are shown in Table 2. The enzyme appears to be specific for histidine. The high affinity for substrate is evident since following removal of endogenous histidine, the enzyme efficiently decarboxylates C^{14} L-histidine even at concentrations of 0.25 γ per ml (Schayer, unpublished).

The enzyme of rat stomach is associated with at least two types of cell. One type contains a binding mechanism and is responsible for the retention of C^{14} histamine in stomach which follows injection of C^{14} L-histidine (Schayer, 1958, 1959). There is considerable evidence that histamine released from the bound state in stomach is involved in gastric secretion in many species (Code, 1956) including rats (Schayer and Ivy, 1957 and 1958).

Most of the histidine decarboxylase activity of stomach appears to be of the inducible type and unrelated to bound histamine (see „Inducible Form of Histidine Decarboxylase"). The inducible nature of rat stomach histidine decarboxylase is apparent since placing rats in a warm environment, 37° C, reduced stomach enzyme activity to less than 10 percent of its „normal" value in 4 hours. The enzyme is fully reactivated by returning the animals to room temperature for 16 hours. Code and Hallenbeck (1961) have recently published a preliminary report which shows that rat stomach histidine decarboxylase activity is markedly elevated during pregnancy.

E. Rabbit platelet histidine decarboxylase

Rabbit platelets, when incubated with C^{14} L-histidine, form C^{14} histamine and bind it in stable condition (Schayer and Kobayashi, 1956). The extractable histidine decarboxylase is of high activity; this *in vitro* finding has a physiological counterpart, the high histamine content of rabbit platelets (Code, 1952).

The rabbit platelet enzyme is of particular interest for several reasons. First, it is the only histidine decarboxylase known to be from a non-cellular source. Second, maximum activity occurs at pH 7.2 to 7.4; it appears to be the only reported case of histidine decarboxylase from a species other than rats or mice having optimal activity in this range. Third, the platelet enzyme does not lose significant activity during dialysis (Schayer, 1959a); this firmness of binding of pyridoxal phosphate is a property of rabbit and guinea pig kidney enzymes rather than those from rats and mice. Thus the platelet enzyme shares properties of both enzyme types shown in Table 2.

The affinity of the rabbit platelet enzyme has not been studied by conventional methods. But since the soluble enzyme forms histamine from minute concentrations of L-histidine with efficiency comparable to that of intact platelets, it is likely that the affinity is high.

The enzyme appears to be specific since rabbit platelets do not seem to synthesize the serotonin which they contain (UDENFRIEND, 1958).

F. Rat liver histidine decarboxylase

1. Fetus

The increased urinary histamine of pregnant rats (see "In Vivo Histamine Formation") provided KAHLSON et al. (1957, 1958a) with a clue which led to the discovery of an extraordinarily high histidine decarboxylase activity in fetal liver. Since the histamine content of the liver tissue was low and since it did not bind significant quantities of the histamine which it synthesized, it was concluded that the rate of turnover of histamine in this tissue is high. Activity was maximal on or about the 19th or 20th days of pregnancy, dropped markedly on the day before parturition, and was very low in the young rats. Lungs and gastrointestinal tract behaved similarly although activities were much lower. TELFORD and WEST (1961b) confirmed these observations on liver. BURKHALTER (1962) has studied this enzyme using a fluorometric assay. Some of the properties are shown in Table 2.

2. Adult

When rat liver preparations are incubated with L-histidine, very little histamine is formed (WATON, 1956; KAHLSON et al., 1958a; MACKAY et al., 1960; TELFORD and WEST, 1961). Addition of a trace of benzene increases activity (TELFORD and WEST, 1961). These workers have implied that rat liver histidine decarboxylase activity, as measured in the presence of benzene, reflects the histamine-forming capacity *in vivo*; however, they have given no evidence to support this assumption. One test of histamine synthesis by rat liver *in vivo* has led to inconclusive results; KAHLSON (1960) reported that surgical removal of a large portion of liver increases urinary histamine but TELFORD and WEST have reported a decrease under these circumstances. Neither has published data to this time. Evidence that there is no *in vivo* counterpart to the high *in vitro* histamine forming activity of liver incubated with benzene is presented in the section on "The Effect of Adrenal Steroids and Other Hormones on Histamine Formation" and "Recent Hypotheses on the Significance of Histidine Decarboxylase".

The data of TELFORD and WEST (1961b) show that during the first few days following birth of rats, the liver histidine decarboxylase undergoes a change in properties from those of the fetal form (Table 2) to those of the adult form, with optimal activity at pH 8 in the presence of benzene. TELFORD and WEST also state that on organ basis, adult rat liver can form about as much histamine as a fetal liver.

3. Hepatoma

Following the finding by KAHLSON and his coworkers that during pregnancy, urinary histamine excretion is increased and fetal liver histidine decarboxylase activity becomes very high, MACKAY et al. (1960) tested another type of rapidly growing liver tissue, a transplantable hepatoma (F-Hep), which can grow subcutaneously in rats of the August strain. In female rats bearing this tumor, urinary histamine rose steeply to very high levels but dropped to normal when the tumor was removed. The hepatoma was found to have histidine decarboxylase activity, which was increased tenfold after addition of pyridoxal phosphate.

The enzyme from hepatoma differed markedly from that of guinea pig kidney (Table 2) and was not associated with other decarboxylases. Urinary excretion of 5-HIAA in hepatoma-bearing rats was within the normal range.

These findings were confirmed by KAMESWAREN and WEST (1961). They report that histidine decarboxylase activity is even higher when the tumor becomes necrotic, about 20 days after implantation; this is cited as evidence opposing the growth hypothesis of KAHLSON (see "Recent Hypotheses on the Significance of Histidine Decarboxylase").

Some tumors activate the reticuloendothelial system (OLD et al., 1960); since this process is often associated with increased histidine decarboxylase in spleen, lymph nodes, liver and lung (SCHAYER, 1961), these tissues should be considered as potential contributors to urinary histamine in tumor-bearing animals.

G. Histidine decarboxylase of nerve tissue

HOLTZ and WESTERMANN (1956; 1956a) tested various portions of bovine nervous tissue for histamine forming ability. Highest activity was found in splenic nerves and sympathetic ganglia, less in phrenic nerve and vagus, and low activity in spinal cord, brain-stem and cerebral cortex. The distribution of DOPA decarboxylase was similar. In splenic nerve the high enzyme activity is associated with a high histamine content, about 100 γ per gram (EULER, 1956).

Rat and mouse brain contain the enzyme (Table 1) as does rat sciatic nerve (SCHAYER, 1962).

WHITE (1959) investigated minced brain tissue from cats, dogs and pigs using the isotope method. The highest rate of histamine formation occurred in the hypothalamus; definite activity was also found in the cerebral cortex and the area postrema. In one experiment using the pooled tissue from 5 pigs, high activity was detected in the median eminence. Since the surviving tissues used in these studies were able to methylate a significant percentage of the histamine which they formed, the values obtained are lower than the actual rate of histamine synthesis.

The relevance of these studies to events in the brain of living animals was indicated by demonstration of C^{14} histamine formation during ventricular perfusion of anesthetized cats with C^{14} L-histidine (WHITE, 1960).

LOVENBERG et al. (1962) purified the non-specific aromatic L-amino acid decarboxylase from dog brain-stem. The relative rates of decarboxylation of amino acids were similar to those obtained with the kidney enzyme; histidine was also decarboxylated.

V. Histamine formation in vivo

BLOCH and PINÖSCH (1936) reported that after subcutaneous injection of guinea pigs with 100 mg histidine monohydrochloride per 100 g body weight, the histamine content of lung was nearly doubled. Corresponding increases were not found in other tissues. EDLBACHER et al. (1940) obtained similar results but confirmation could not be made by MACKAY (1938), HOLTZ and CREDNER (1944) or ROCHA E SILVA (1955). In view of the later findings with isotopes (SCHAYER, 1952) that conversion of L-histidine to histamine occurs to only a small extent in the guinea pig, there is probably some explanation of the observations of BLOCH and PINÖSCH other than new synthesis of histamine.

Holtz and Credner (1941 and 1944) identified histamine in the urine of guinea pigs given large doses of histidine parenterally.

There have been a number of reports on increased histamine in tissues following injury; in some cases the levels were so high that new formation has seemed more likely than redistribution. Dekanski (1945) found that 10 minutes after an extensive cutaneous burn, skin histamine of mice was about double the normal concentration. This experiment was repeated by Ballani et al. (1959) who failed to find any rapid effect of burns on skin histamine. The latter also refer to unpublished work in rats in which burns produced no significant rapid increase of skin histamine. Later, Ballani et al. (1959a) found that 14 to 21 days after the burn, there was an increase in skin histamine; they attributed this to infiltrating leucocytes. Dekanski's findings appear to be inexplicable by any known mechanism for new histamine formation.

After injury to guinea pig skin either by contact dermatitis or the tuberculin reaction, Inderbitzin (1955; 1956) observed a local increase of histamine which became apparent three hours after challenge and reached a maximum, about four to seven times normal, in 48 to 72 hours. He felt that the increased histamine was due either to local neo-synthesis or to import in leucocytes. Fisher and Cooke (1958) reinvestigated Inderbitzin's work and found considerably higher local histamine levels in allergic dermatitis than in toxic dermatitis. Since the former condition, but not the latter, was characterized by a massive influx of mononuclear leucocytes, these cells were believed to be responsible for the increased histamine, either by increased formation, reduced synthesis or both. Injection of germanin, an *in vitro* inhibitor of kidney histidine decarboxylase but not histaminase (Werle, 1940) prevented the increase in histamine at the site of the allergic lesion. The significance of this obervation seems to be difficult to interpret clearly. Germanin has never been shown to inhibit histidine decarboxylase *in vivo*; also, the large dose used, a total of 500 mg per animal, may have caused some redistribution of mononuclear cells, may have released some of their histamine, or may have interfered with the chemical method of histamine assay.

Somewhat more convincing, because of theoretical support, are the increased histamine levels seen in animals poisoned by endotoxin. Kun (1947) found large quantities of histamine in the liver and muscle of rabbits immediately after death from meningococcal endotoxin; the loss of histamine from blood was insufficient to account for the increase. Hinshaw et al. (1961; 1961a) found an increase in blood histamine of dogs and monkeys given lethal doses of E. coli endotoxin. The early rise in blood histamine can be readily explained by release, but the persistent elevation of blood levels is consistent with the new synthesis. Since endotoxin can activate histidine decarboxylase and increase the rate of *in vivo* histamine synthesis (Schayer, 1960a) it is possible that a significant accumulation of histamine might occur in dying animals if there were some depletion of available S-adenosylmethionine, the cofactor of the principal histamine-destroying enzyme of most species (Schayer, 1956; Lindahl, 1958, 1960; Brown et al., 1959).

Following the finding that D-catechin was an *in vitro* inhibitor of kidney histidine decarboxylase (Martin et al., 1949), this compound was tested for effect *in vivo* (Moss et al., 1950). It was reported that prolonged treatment of guinea pigs with D-catechin rendered them insusceptible to anaphylactic shock but not histamine shock. The results were considered consistent with blocking of histamine synthesis in lung; however, the effect of the drug on lung histamine levels was not given. Malkiel and Werle (1951) found no effect of D-catechin on anaphylaxis. Schayer (1953) found no significant effect of D-catechin on formation and binding of C^{14} histamine in intact mice.

Parrot (1961) and Parrot and Laborde (1956, 1959) claim that certain derivatives of benzyl-1-isoquinoline, which appear to be useful in the treatment of allergy in man, act through inhibition of histidine decarboxylase *in vivo*. The evidence is as follows: (a) the substances inhibit guinea pig histidine decarboxylase activity *in vitro*; also, kidney histidine decarboxylase of guinea pigs sacrificed 3 to 4.5 hours after ingestion of 100 mg of drug showed only about one-half the normal activity, (b) the histamine content of liver, kidney and ileum was below normal within 2.5 to 4.5 hours following a dose of the drug, (c) ileum of treated animals failed to show the Schultz-Dale phenomenon and was insensitive to anaphylatoxin, (d) the drugs protected guinea pigs from histamine aerosol, maximum protection occurring at the time of minimum endogenous histamine levels, (e) the compounds showed no antihistamine action and did not affect the rate of destruction of histamine *in vitro*.

As stated elsewhere in this chapter, it is probable that the non-isotopic assay for kidney histidine decarboxylase activity gives results which have little relevance to the rate of histamine synthesis in living animals. Reduced enzyme activity in kidneys of animals dosed orally with drugs a few hours earlier is not satisfactory evidence for *in vivo* activity since the inhibition may be due entirely to unmetabolized drug entering the incubation mixture, (b) the rapid reduction of tissue histamine reported is not easily reconciled with the evidence from isotopic experiments which indicates that the rate of turnover of bound histamine in animal tissues is slow. The possibility that the drop of histamine levels might be due to release seems to have been inadequately excluded. Even though serum histamine was slightly reduced the difficulties in obtaining meaningful serum histamine levels are well known. Furthermore, the rate of *in vivo* histamine destruction was not determined and cannot be reliably predicted from *in vitro* tests, (c) failure to obtain a Schultz-Dale reaction could also be explained by histamine release, (d) the protection by these drugs against histamine aerosols is not convincingly explained by the postulate that tissues with low histamine content trap more exogenous histamine than normal tissues. In the writer's opinion stronger experimental support will be required for acceptance of the contention that the drugs studied by Parrot's group act through histidine decarboxylase inhibition *in vivo*.

Introduction of the use of radioisotope techniques has materially advanced knowledge of histamine formation *in vivo*. Schayer (1952) injected small quantities of C^{14} L-histidine, 2 mg/kg, into guinea pigs. C^{14} histamine was found in some tissues at the earliest interval tested, 6 hours, and thereafter to the longest interval tested, 56 days. C^{14} histamine was also found in urine for about one week after injection but with a rapidly decreasing rate from a maximum on the first day. After injection of C^{14} histamine, none of this substance could be detected in blood, liver, lung, kidney or intestine after 4 hours. Furthermore, tissue histamine was not synthesized from 1-carbon fragments. These results showed that in the guinea pig, the source of histamine bound for significant periods (more than 4 to 5 hours) is L-histidine, not exogenous histamine. This same finding has been made in all the other species investigated, mice, rats and cats (Schayer, 1953 and 1956; Schayer and Smiley, 1954). There is no valid evidence known to the writer to oppose this conclusion. From the C^{14} histamine assays of tissues and urine from guinea pigs injected with C^{14} L-histidine it can be estimated, very roughly, that the conversion of L-histidine to histamine is of the order of 0.05 % in this species. The statement in a review by Van Arsdel and Beall (1960) that less than 10 % of injected histidine is converted to histamine, while true, gives the wrong impression on the possible extent of conversion; this may have been a typographical error.

The half-life of histamine bound in several pooled guinea pig tissues was estimated to be roughly 50 days; later studies in rats showed that the duration of binding of histamine varies greatly from one tissue to another, the turnover being very fast in lung and liver, slow in skin and muscle, and intermediate in stomach and intestine (SCHAYER, 1959).

The view of *in vivo* histamine formation from the earliest isotopic study (SCHAYER, 1952) was that decarboxylation of L-histidine occurred at two principal sites. First were cells containing a mechanism for binding; here the resulting histamine could be retained for long periods. Second were cells possessing no binding mechanism; histamine produced by these cells was rapidly destroyed or excreted. There has been no reason to the present time to alter these views on the dichotomous mode of histamine production *in vivo.*

Injection of C^{14} L-histidine also results in histamine formation and binding in mice, rats and cats (SCHAYER, 1956b). In mice (SCHAYER, 1953), the bound C^{14} histamine is largely in skin; treatment of mice with two *in vitro* histidine decarboxylase inhibitors, D-catechin and 3,4-dihydroxychalcone, did not materially affect the formation and binding of C^{14} histamine. In rats, the newly bound C^{14} histamine in skin can be released *in vivo* by Compound 48/80 (SCHAYER and SMILEY, 1954). In rats with skin histamine depleted by repeated doses of Compound 48/80, the rate of binding of new skin histamine was not materially different from normal.

Small female rats, injected with a minute quantity of C^{14} L-histidine, and given aminoguanidine to reduce histamine destruction, excreted in urine the equivalent of about 0.15% of the injected dose as C^{14} histamine. Assuming the daily dietary intake of histidine to be about 40 mg (rats do not synthesize histidine) about 60 γ urinary histamine per day should result. This calculated value checks well with the observation by KAHLSON et al. (1957) that three female rats, presumably somewhat larger than those used in the isotopic study, fed a synthetic, histamine-free diet, and given aminoguanidine, excreted an average of 76, 86 and 104 γ histamine per 24 hours. Since some C^{14} histamine is bound in the tissues, and since there is some destruction by methylation, acetylation and by incompletely inhibited diamine oxidase, a conversion of histidine to histamine in the rat is probably roughly 0.2%.

An important source of urinary histamine in rats is decarboxylation of histidine in kidney from which histamine can be excreted into the urine without entering the circulation. This conclusion was inferred from the observation that although aminoguanidine, a diamine oxidase inhibitor, efficiently protects circulating histamine from destruction, it had little effect on urinary C^{14} histamine resulting from injected C^{14} L-histidine (SCHAYER et al., 1954a). This observation also suggests that rat kidney does not destroy any significant portion of the histamine which it synthesizes. A similar conclusion was reached from data obtained from experiments on anesthetized dogs (LINDELL and SCHAYER, 1958). C^{14} L-histidine, in very low concentrations, was slowly infused into one renal artery and urine collected from both kidneys separately. There was considerably more C^{14} histamine in the urine from the injected kidney than from the control kidney. Furthermore, no C^{14} methylhistamine could be detected in the urine. Since C^{14} methylhistamine is excreted in the urine after injection of C^{14} histamine into the blood stream (LINDELL and SCHAYER, 1958a) it is apparent that no large amount of histamine formed by the kidney entered the circulation.

From the percent conversion of injected C^{14} L-histidine to bound C^{14} histamine in rat skin, it can be calculated that roughly 2 γ of new histamine is added to each gram of abdominal skin per day (SCHAYER et al., 1954). Presumably, since there is an equilibrium, approximately this same amount would be lost each day through release, or through destruction of mast cells.

White (1960) perfused the cerebral ventricles of anesthetized dogs with C^{14} L-histidine and was able to show *in vivo* histamine synthesis by brain tissue.

A number of studies have appeared recently in which urinary histamine excretion is used as a measure of the rate of synthesis of this substance by mammalian tissues. All employ female rats since this is the only known experimental animal in which a high degree of inhibition of histamine destruction can be achieved (Schayer, 1959b). Controls for histamine formed by bacteria, or taken in the diet, are needed.

Gustafsson et al. (1957) found histamine in the urine of germ-free rats fed a histamine-free diet; obviously this was of mammalian origin. Since there was no definite difference between germ-free and not germ-free rats fed on the synthetic diet, it was considered feasible to use the latter for future work. During pregnancy, histamine excretion remained essentially normal until about the 15th day; then it rose rapidly to a peak 1 or 2 days before parturition, and then dropped precipitously (Kahlson et al., 1958a). The amount of histamine excreted was roughly proportional to the number of young in the litter; this suggested that the fetus was the site of synthesis. Similar results were obtained in pregnant rats by injecting C^{14} L-histidine and measuring C^{14} histamine in urine. Fetal liver was identified as a source of highly active histidine decarboxylase (see "Rat Liver Histidine Decarboxylase").

To test the theory that increased histamine synthesis is necessary for fetal development, Kahlson and Rosengren (1959; 1959a) reduced the availability of pyridoxal phosphate, the coenzyme of histidine decarboxylase, by feeding pregnant rats a pyridoxin deficient diet and injecting a pyridoxal-trapping agent, semicarbazide. Under these conditions histamine excretion was reduced to about 15 % of normal and the fetuses did not develop. The authors acknowledge the lack of specificity of this treatment which undoubtedly affects a large number of pyridoxal phosphate-dependent enzymes. Also, rats repeatedly injected with a toxic substance and offered a deficient diet would have a markedly reduced food intake. Since rats do not synthesize histidine this could reduce the substrate concentration and contribute to the decreased histamine formation.

The possibility that histamine production might be related to rapid growth led Kahlson's group to test rats with regenerating livers; increased urinary histamine was found (Kahlson and Rosengren, 1959a). On the other hand, Kameswaren et al. (1961), in a preliminary communication, state that urinary histamine is decreased during liver regeneration.

A third type of rapid growth, healing of skin wounds, was associated with a rapid activation of histidine decarboxylase at the site of the wound, and with a slowly-developing increase in histidine decarboxylase activity parallel to the formation of granulation tissue; according to Kahlson (personal communication) the latter is not due to mast cells. An increased output of urinary histamine as measured by both isotopic and non-isotopic methods (Kahlson et al., 1960) could be shown to accompany these changes.

Since these results were compatible with a role for newly-synthesized histamine in wound healing, this group experimentally lowered or raised the histamine forming capacity of rat skin to test the effect on the rate of tissue repair. One experiment employed pyridoxin deficient diet plus semicarbazide; under these conditions wound healing was markedly retarded. As previously mentioned, this probably produces a marked reduction in available pyridoxal phosphate and cannot be cited as convincing evidence of a role for histamine in wound healing. On discontinuing semicarbazide and restoring pyridoxin to the diet, histamine excretion rose to normal and in some cases exceeded it. This was called the ,,overshooting" phase; during this period the rate of wound healing was found to be more rapid than normal. To some extent this "overshoot" may be due to the abnormally high food consumption by starved rats offered a normal diet.

A third procedure made use of on observation by SCHAYER et al. (1959) and SCHAYER and GANLEY (1959) that repeated injections of rats with the histamine releasers, Compound 48/80 and polymyxin B, increase the rate of synthesis of free histamine by rat skin. After confirming these effects, KAHLSON's group found that pretreatment of rats with these histamine liberators augmented the rate of healing.

The reviewer believes that an interpretation of these results is complicated by the generally unrecognized multiplicity of actions of Compound 48/80. Thus in addition to disrupting mast cells and liberating amines in some species, Compound 48/80 treatment also increases rat skin histidine decarboxylase (SCHAYER et al., 1959), increases rat adrenal weight (BARTLET and LOCKETT, 1959), activates the reticuloendothelial system (ZWEIFACH, 1960), renders rats tolerant to various vasotoxic substances, to microtrauma, and to severe trauma (ZWEIFACH, 1961) and probably produces a large number of other alterations not recognized at present.

MACKAY et al. (1960 and 1961), testing KAHLSON's idea that histamine may be related to rapid growth, found that urine of female August rats in which a transplantable hepatoma (F-Hep) was growing subcutaneously, excreted large quantities of histamine in urine. Urinary 5-HIAA was within the normal range.

There has been a recent claim that histidine decarboxylase activity of kidney is greatly elevated in pregnant mice, but not rats (ROSENGREN and STEINHARDT, 1961).

VI. Specificity of histidine decarboxylase

The histidine decarboxylase having optimum activity near pH 7 and high affinity for L-histidine is generally accepted as specific; it does not appear to decarboxylate DOPA or 5-HTP (Table 2). Only for the enzyme from rabbit and guinea pig kidney is there a basis for controversy on specificity.

The claim that 5-HTP was decarboxylated by a specific enzyme, distinct from DOPA decarboxylase (CLARK et al., 1954), led several laboratories to purify DOPA decarboxylase. Two of these groups reported that histidine decarboxylating activity is retained during purification of kidney DOPA decarboxylase and have proposed that a single enzyme decarboxylates several amino acids including histidine (GANROT et al., 1961; LOVENBERG et al., 1962). This subject is discussed in more detail under "Rabbit and Guinea Pig Kidney Histidine Decarboxylase".

Although the kidney histidine decarboxylase differs in properties from the high affinity enzyme, it is probably structurally similar to DOPA decarboxylase; hence the difficulty in separation. But there is a considerable amount of evidence opposing the concept that DOPA decarboxylase and histidine decarboxylase of kidney are identical.

First, there are theoretical objections. Histidine is the only compound of a large number of alleged substrates for DOPA decarboxylase which is not aromatic. The imidazole ring of histidine is slightly basic; in contrast, the substituent groups of the aromatic amino acid substrates are weakly acidic. It seems unlikely that both acidic and basic groups would attach to the same position on the surface of a protein. Even if such an attachment did occur it is questionable that the spatial relationships required for decarboxylation of benzenoid amino acids could be satisfied by an amino acid having a five-membered ring (see "Mechanism of

Decarboxylation"). The influence of the imidazole ring on other biological phenomena is pronounced; whereas the amines formed by decarboxylation of aromatic amino acids are pressor substances and substrates of monoamine oxidase, histamine is a dilator and a substrate of diamine oxidase.

According to the mechanism proposed by METZLER et al. (1954) histidine might be decarboxylated by any pyridoxal protein provided the α-amino group were suitably oriented with respect to the aldehyde group of pyridoxal phosphate (see "Mechanism of Decarboxylation"). Attachment of L-histidine to DOPA decarboxylase, in a position permitting decarboxylation, might occur under some conditions. But if histidine were attached to a point on the protein different from the point of attachment of DOPA and other aromatic amino acids, it could not be considered as a typical substrate.

The earlier literature indicated a number of differences between the enzymes. For example, DOPA decarboxylase activity of guinea pig kidney is about five times that of rabbit kidney (HOLTZ et al., 1938a) yet their histidine decarboxylase activities are about the same (HOLTZ et al., 1939). Although a number of inhibitors affect the two activities similarly, in some cases there are marked differences. Histidine decarboxylase is strongly inhibited by D-DOPA which does not materially affect DOPA decarboxylase (WERLE, 1940). 1-Hydrazinisoquinoline gave 50% inhibition of guinea pig kidney histidine decarboxylase at 1.7×10^{-5} M; more than 100 times this concentration, 2×10^{-3} M, was required for 50% inhibition of DOPA decarboxylase (WERLE et al., 1955).

Although none of the foregoing is proof of specificity, it remains that purified kidney DOPA decarboxylase has been prepared which is free of demonstrable histidine decarboxylating activity (WERLE and AURES, 1959). The proponents of the opposite view have, at the present time, made no attempt to explain this finding. Unless it can be shown that there is some error in the work of WERLE and AURES, the non-identity of DOPA decarboxylase and histidine decarboxylase must be tentatively considered to be established.

VII. Effect of benzene and other organic solvents on histidine decarboxylase activity

WATON (1956) observed that addition of a drop of chloroform to incubates of kidney extract with histidine increased the yield of histamine. On further investigation it was found that many organic solvents could cause this change but that benzene was the most active. Under optimal conditions, saturation of the aqueous portion of the incubate, benzene produced five- to ten-fold increases in histamine formation (WATON, 1956a). Time studies showed that 3 to 7 hour incubations produced histamine maximally. The benzene-induced activation of rabbit kidney histidine decarboxylase could be reversed by freeze-drying, but the freeze-dried enzyme could still be re-activated by addition of more benzene. WATON suggested that the effect of benzene might be due to some change in the physical state of the enzyme, such as a break-up of micelles, so that additional active groups could come in contact with substrate.

This potentiating effect has been confirmed in several laboratories (SCHAYER, 1957; MACKAY et al., 1961a; LOVENBERG et al., 1962) and extended to liver and kidney of rats (TELFORD and WEST, 1961; SCHAYER, unpublished) and to liver and kidney of mice (SCHAYER, unpublished). There is either no effect, or inhibition, of histidine decarboxylase activity from some of the sources listed in Table 2.

A partially purified (about ten-fold) enzyme from kidney had its ability to decarboxylate histidine and tyrosine increased by benzene, but its ability to decarboxylate DOPA and 5-HTP decreased (LOVENBERG et al., 1962). If this is a single non-specific enzyme as the authors propose, the data would not appear to support WATON's conjecture that benzene increases the number of active enzyme surfaces. On the other hand, if WATON is correct, these data support the claim of WERLE and AURES (1959) that kidney histidine decarboxylase and DOPA decarboxylase are non-identical.

MACKAY et al. (1961a) suggest that the mechanism of action may involve an increased rate of breakdown of the enzyme-substrate complex.

Also possible is that benzene triggers the same mechanism *in vitro* that leads to activation of histidine decarboxylase *in vivo* (see "Inducible Form of Histidine Decarboxylase").The fact that these two rather unusual types of activation are associated with histamine formation may be purely a coincidence. Yet they are not dissimilar in time of activation and in reversibility. Benzene fails to increase activity in some tissues known to contain the inducible form of the enzyme; however, this could be due to improper conditions. Obviously the mechanism of both phenomena merits study.

Finally, some organic solvents such as chloroform so profoundly alter the configuration of proteins that they can be used as deproteinizing agents. A low concentration or organic solvent might cause a mild modification in enzyme configuration which would enhance the opportunities for attachment of histidine molecules, or facilitate orientation of the α-amino group with the aldehyde group of the coenzyme (see "Mechanism of Decarboxylation").

VIII. The coenzyme of histidine decarboxylase

Pyridoxal-5-phosphate is the coenzyme of histidine decarboxylase. In the earlier studies this was not easily demonstrable since the kidney enzymes used firmly bind the coenzyme. WERLE and KOCH (1949) obtained a small potentiation of activity by addition of pyridoxal phosphate. However, contemporary workers in the field of amino acid decarboxylases, perhaps influenced by the unique difficulty in showing the pyridoxal requirement for bacterial histidine decarboxylase, apparently did not consider the evidence of WERLE and KOCH as adequate (SCHALES, 1951; GALE, 1953).

As interest turned to mast cells as a source of histamine, identification of the coenzyme became easy. ROTHSCHILD and SCHAYER (1958, 1959), using histidine decarboxylase from rat peritoneal mast cells, found a large loss of activity after dialysis which could be raised to a level above normal by addition of pyridoxal phosphate. Rat stomach and mouse mastocytoma histidine decarboxylase behaved similarly (SCHAYER, 1959a). Tissues of B_6 deficient rats were low in histidine decarboxylase activity; this could be increased either by feeding pyridoxin, or by adding pyridoxal phosphate to the *in vitro* incubations. Injections of C^{14} L-histidine into B_6-deficient rats resulted in an abnormally low urinary C^{14} histamine.

Similar evidence of the pyridoxal phosphate requirement of mouse mastocytoma histidine decarboxylase were published somewhat later by ONO and HAGEN (1959) and HAGEN et al. (1960). This group was evidently unaware of the earlier work of ROTHSCHILD and SCHAYER, since they claimed to have made the first successful demonstration of the coenzyme requirement of histidine decarboxylase. MACKAY et al. (1960) state that pyridoxal phosphate caused a ten-fold increase in the activity of rat hepatoma enzyme.

IX. Mechanism of decarboxylation

The most extensive studies on the mechanism of decarboxylation are based principally on data from rabbit and guinea pig kidney, liver and intestine (WERLE and KOCH, 1949). Since the enzyme from kidney has different properties from the other sources listed in Table 2, and shows a different pattern of inhibition, the conclusions from these studies are not necessarily valid in all respects for the histidine decarboxylase of high affinity.

WERLE and KOCH proposed that substrate molecules bound to an active surface on the protein portion of the enzyme can become oriented so that the α-amino group reacts with the aldehyde group of the coenzyme, pyridoxal phosphate, to form a SCHIFF base; then a migration of double bonds produces an unstable configuration which readily loses carbon dioxide. The resulting structure breaks down, yielding the free amine and the enzyme-coenzyme in its original form.

A general mechanism for all reactions catalyzed by pyridoxal phosphate enzymes has been proposed by METZLER et al. (1954). Since most of these enzymatic reactions can be duplicated by non-enzymatic model reactions in which pyridoxal and a suitable metal salt serve as catalysts, these workers believe that the catalytic potentialities of pyridoxal phosphate enzymes are, to an exaggerated degree, those of the prosthetic group, and that the non-enzymatic reactions proceed by a closely similar mechanism. According to this mechanism, after reaction of the α-amino group of the amino acid with the aldehyde group of pyridoxal phosphate to form a SCHIFF base, decarboxylation results from the electronic changes shown in Fig. 1.

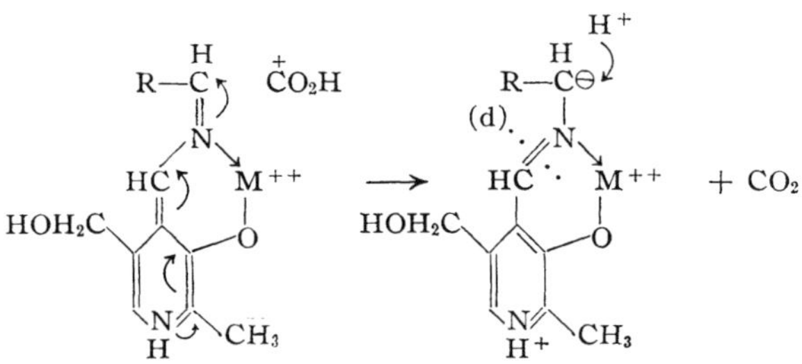

Fig. 1. Electronic changes leading to decarboxylation of α-amino acids (see text)

This non-enzymatic reaction involves a metal ion and a requirement for ions has not been shown by histidine decarboxylase. METZLER et al. (1954) believe that if a metal ion requirement for enzymatic decarboxylation cannot be found, a portion of the enzyme protein may fill this role. WERLE and KOCH (1949) have demonstrated non-enzymatic decarboxylation of L-histidine by pyridoxal phosphate alone.

From the preceding discussion it seems probable that the sequence of events leading to decarboxylation is basically the same for histidine decarboxylase from all sources.

X. Inhibition of histidine decarboxylase activity

Most studies on histidine decarboxylase inhibition have used enzyme from rabbit or guinea pig kidney. Since it is not known with certainty whether the measurements were made on DOPA decarboxylase or on a specific histidine decarboxylase of low affinity, or whether in either case the enzyme is concerned with histamine formation *in vivo*, the significance of the results is questionable (see "Rabbit and Guinea Pig Kidney Histidine Decarboxylase").

It is generally agreed that α-methyl DOPA is one of the most powerful *in vitro* inhibitors of the kidney enzyme (UDENFRIEND et al., 1960; WERLE, 1961; MACKAY and SHEPHERD, 1960; GANROT et al., 1961; WEISSBACH et al., 1961). Yet all available evidence indicates that this substance has no pronounced effect on histamine formation *in vivo* (WERLE 1961; OATES and SJOERDSMA, 1962; SCHAYER, unpublished; KAHLSON, unpublished).

Theories on the structural requirements for inhibition of the kidney enzyme have been published (WERLE and KOCH, 1949; MACKAY and SHEPHERD, 1960). Inhibitors, excluding carbonyl reagents, probably act principally by attachment to the protein and block entry of substrate. It is unlikely that the more active inhibitors of kidney histidine decarboxylase, e. g. α-methyl DOPA, operate through interaction with pyridoxal phosphate to any significant extent, since they do not inhibit the histidine decarboxylase of high affinity.

The efficacy of inhibitors varies according to the conditions used. Some of the results of studies on inhibition of kidney histidine decarboxylase activity are shown in Table 3; those of MACKAY and SHEPHERD (1960) are shown in Table 4.

There is very little data on inhibition of the histidine decarboxylase of high affinity. All carbonyl reagents tested, e. g. hydroxylamine and semicarbazide, inhibit by trapping pyridoxal phosphate. WEISSBACH et al. (1961) report that α-methylhistidine does not inhibit enzyme from a mouse mastocytoma. However, when low concentrations of C^{14} L-histidine are used as substrate, α-methylhistidine is a powerful inhibitor of histidine decarboxylase from mouse mastocytoma and rat stomach (SCHAYER, unpublished). The inhibitory effect is probably due to attachment of the imidazole ring of α-methylhistidine to the site on the protein at which L-histidine is bound. α-Methyl DOPA is a very poor inhibitor under these conditions so it is unlikely that pyridoxal phosphate interaction is involved. The reason for the discrepancy in the results of WEISSBACH et al. and SCHAYER may be that under the conditions used by the former, there were many more molecules of enzyme and substrate per molecule inhibitor than in the isotopic studies. α-Methylhistidine does inhibit histamine formation *in vivo* in normal mice (SCHAYER, unpublished) and in rats (KAHLSON et al., 1962a).

XI. Effect of adrenal steroids and other hormones on histamine formation

The earliest studies relating the adrenal corticosteroids to histamine formation (ROSE and BROWNE, 1938) indicated that histamine levels of certain tissues were increased in adrenalectomized rats. This effect was accentuated if the animals were maintained on water rather than saline. Similar findings have been reported by MARSHALL (1943). HICKS and WEST (1958) found little difference in tissue histamine levels of adrenalectomized and sham-operated rats but confirmed the marked increase in animals maintained on water rather than saline. BARTLET and LOCKETT (1959) in addition to showing an increase in tissue histamine in adrenalectomized rats, found that restoration of skin histamine following depletion by Compound 48/80 was accelerated by adrenalectomy.

BJURÖ and WESTLING (1959) and ANGERVALL et al. (1961) have extended these studies by following urinary excretion of histamine in adrenalectomized or sham-operated female rats. Adrenalectomized rats maintained on saline show increased urinary histamine from the 4th postoperative day; if the rats are given water, the increase does not occur until the 8th day. If adrenalectomized rats maintained on saline are transferred to water, the high urinary histamine level is reduced. These effects are not due to changes in histaminase activity since they occur in rats in which this enzyme is inhibited by aminoguanidine. These authors also observed that adrenalectomized rats given cortisone or cortisol had increased urinary histamine and consider this finding to be anomalous. However, it is known that a higher percentage of injected histamine is excreted unchanged in cortisone-treated mice than in normal ones (SCHAYER et al., 1953) and that histamine excretion is increased in man given cortisone (MITCHELL and CODE, 1954). The data from these several papers suggest that the changes in tissue or urinary histamine in adrenalectomized rats may be due in part to an increased rate of formation (SCHAYER, 1956); they also show that there is a pronounced effect of salt on histamine retention. Whatever may be the mechanism by which lack of salt enhances histamine retention, it is an abnormal process; adrenalectomized rats given water are dying animals.

Interest in the effect of cortisone on histamine formation was engendered by a publication by GOTH et al. (1951). Injection of Tween 20 into dogs resulted in a drop in blood pressure presumably due to released histamine; a second injection 24 to 48 hours later still produced a significant hypotensive effect. But if the dogs were pretreated with cortisone, only the first injection of Tween 20 was effective; the second was not. The authors postulated that cortisone had prevented the reaccumulation of histamine. GOTH (personal communication, 1961) now has reservations about the original interpretation since similar actions of cortisone are not found in dogs given compound 48/80 or other histamine releasers.

HALPERN and his coworkers (HALPERN, 1956; HALPERN and BRIOT, 1956) studied the effect of cortisone on the rate of replenishement of skin histamine of rats after depletion by histamine liberators. Several techniques were used; one involved evaluation of local capillary permeability changes following intradermal injection of dextran. The second measured total skin histamine and another the rate of replacement of releasable histamine. Although cortisone blocked the return of skin sensitivity to dextran, it caused only a small retardation in reaccumulation of total skin histamine which was not statistically significant. In attempt at an explanation of this discrepancy, HALPERN proposed that only the replenishment of "physiologically active histamine" was reduced by cortisone. This concept may be valid if "physiologically active histamine" of rat skin can be identified with newly-bound histamine; the latter is strongly influenced by cortisone (SCHAYER et al., 1954). On the other hand, it has been shown since HALPERN'S work that factors such as serotonin may be of great importance in certain permeability reactions in rat skin (ROWLEY and BENDITT, 1956). Furthermore, since HALPERN'S work was concerned principally with skin in which histamine is largely in mast cells, and since cortisone can cause morphological changes in these cells (ASBOE-HANSEN, 1952; TELFORD and WEST, 1961) the observations on histamine may be secondary to alterations in mast cell function.

Cortisone and other steroids markedly suppressed the rate of binding of new C^{14} histamine in skin of rats injected with tracer quantities of C^{14} L-histidine (SCHAYER et al., 1954; SCHAYER, 1959). This effect was also shown *in vitro* (SCHAYER et al., 1955). Segments of rat abdominal skin, when incubated with C^{14} L-histidine, formed C^{14} histamine; roughly 70% was retained by the skin segments despite thorough washing. Pretreatment of animals with cortisone reduced the amount of bound C^{14} histamine to about one-fourth the normal value. Adrenalectomy increased the amount of formation and binding of C^{14} histamine in rat skin. ACTH and desoxycorticosterone had no effect under the conditions employed.

The inhibitory effect of glucocorticoids on formation of C^{14} histamine was extended to other rat tissues. Histamine formation by rat lung was reduced by cortisone and increased by adrenalectomy (SCHAYER, 1956); in lung this is due to an effect on histidine decarboxylase activity. More potent steroids such as prednisone and prednisolone reduce rat lung histidine decarboxylase activity to very low levels. Since rat lung was later found not to retain C^{14} histamine *in vivo* (SCHAYER, 1959), it seems in retrospect that the term "binding" was used loosely in these early papers since it failed to distinguish between C^{14} histamine held in the natural binding linkage and that held by other means. In the earlier papers the term "*in vitro* binding" is probably valid for skin, mast cells (SCHAYER, 1956a) and rabbit platelets (SCHAYER and KOBAYASHI, 1956) but of questionable significance for other tissues. Rat pyloric stomach is unique in that corticoids increase histamine formation *in vitro* (SCHAYER, 1956) and *in vivo* (SCHAYER, 1959). *In vivo* results in hypophysectomized animals are much like those from adrenalectomized animals (SCHAYER, 1959).

The conclusions drawn from this work were that the adrenal cortex has a marked influence on the rate of formation and binding of new histamine in rat tissues; only for lung, and possibly muscle, could the effect be attributed to changes in activity of histidine decarboxylase. In mice reduction of lung histidine decarboxylase activity can be effected by large doses of prednisone, but to a much smaller extent than in rats; after similar treatment of guinea pigs, lung histidine decarboxylase was not significantly changed (SCHAYER, 1963). No definite effect of cortisone on *in vivo* histamine formation and binding in mice has been observed (SCHAYER et al., 1953). In the case of rat skin, the action of corticoids may be at any point in the complex chain of events which follows the entry of free histidine molecules into the circulation of the skin and culminates in its decarboxylation and binding, usually, if not invariably, in a mast cell.

These studies showed clearly that there was no correlation between histidine decarboxylase, histamine content, or mast cell population of a tissue. This conclusion has been restated by other laboratories (KAHLSON et al., 1960; TELFORD and WEST, 1961).

Work in this field has recently been undertaken by WEST and his co-workers. A number of corticoids, and some sex hormones, were injected into rats for periods of 4 to 9 days. Histamine content of skin and small intestine was markedly reduced while that of stomach was increased; the extent of this effect was roughly proportional to the glucocorticoid activity. Sex hormones had a weak effect while desoxycorticosterone and ACTH were inactive (HICKS and WEST, 1958; TELFORD and WEST, 1960). These authors acknowledge that steroids may affect tissue histamine content by means other than rate of formation; for example, they appear to cause changes in mast cells (ASBOE-HANSEN, 1952; TELFORD and WEST, 1961). This could result in a marked impairment of the ability of certain tissues to retain histamine.

TELFORD and WEST (1961) then studied the action of corticoids in histidine decarboxylase of rat tissues; only liver and stomach were tested since little or no activity could be found in other tissues by their method. Liver histidine decarboxylase activity (as measured in the presence of benzene) was suppressed while that of pyloric stomach was increased. Effects of released corticoids in two conditions of stress were tested. Exposure of rats to cold produced a reduction in liver histidine decarboxylase activity and an increase of that in stomach. Treatment of rats with the histamine liberators Compound 48/80 and polymyxin B decreased enzyme activity in liver but had little if any effect on the stomach enzyme. The authors report inability to detect histidine decarboxylase activity in rat skin after repeated injections of Compound 48/80.

Some of the findings and conclusions of TELFORD and WEST (1961) are in real or apparent conflict with some of those published earlier by the writer; hence an attempt at resolution will be made.

It is agreed that suppression of histidine decarboxylase activity of some rat tissues may occur in moderate stress; this is probably attributable to glucocorticoid release and reflects the pronounced response of this species to these hormones. For example, the writer has observed that moderate cold does reduce histidine decarboxylase activity of rat lung to a value below normal, whereas in guinea pigs under similar conditions, lung histidine decarboxylase activity is increased (SCHAYER, 1963). Cold increased enzyme activity in mouse skin (SCHAYER, 1960). But rats do not constitute an exception to the writer's findings on increased histamine synthesis in severe stress. In tissues of rats dying from shock due either to trauma or endotoxin, histidine decarboxylase activity of tissues, including liver, is elevated to many times the normal value (SCHAYER, 1962 and unpublished). TELFORD and WEST suggest that suppression of liver histidine decarboxylase by released corticoids may account in part for the slow replenishment of skin histamine in 48/80-treated animals. If this proposal were valid, it would be expected that urinary histamine in depleted rats would be abnormally low. On the contrary, injection of such rats with C^{14} L-histidine results in an abnormally large output of C^{14} histamine in the urine (SCHAYER et al., 1959). WILSON found histamine excretion to be higher in Compound 48/80-treated rats than in normals; furthermore there was no evidence for uptake of injected or fed histamine by depleted skin (WILSON, 1963).

The failure of TELFORD and WEST to find increased histidine decarboxylase activity in rat skin following treatment with Compound 48/80 is probably due to the low sensitivity of their method. This effect has been shown repeatedly in the writer's laboratory in both *in vitro* and *in vivo* experiments and it has been confirmed by KAHLSON et al. (1960). There is a large amount of evidence that rat skin decarboxylates histidine *in vivo* (see "Interpretation of Findings of In Vitro Histidine Decarboxylase Assays").

The effects of corticoids on histamine formation has been shown to occur in only one species other than the rat. In this species, the mouse, the effect is small and large doses of steroids are required to demonstrate it. Since merely placing rats and mice in a warm environment, 37° C, lowers histidine decarboxylase activity of lung and muscle (SCHAYER, 1962) it is possible that the effect of corticoids on histidine decarboxylase activity is secondary to circulatory changes. In the guinea pig, in which lung histidine decarboxylase may be almost entirely in mast cells, neither the response to warmth nor to glucocorticoids is significant. With the present evidence, there is no substantial basis for assuming that the effect on histamine formation provides insight into that fundamental mode of action of glucocorticoids which appears to be basically similar in all species.

The only endocrine glands, other than the adrenal, which have been shown to affect histamine formation are the pituitary and the thyroid.

Certain pituitary actions appear to be mediated by the adrenal cortex since hypophysectomy and adrenalectomy produce similar effects on *in vivo* formation and binding of C^{14} histamine (SCHAYER, 1959). However, hypophysectomy, but not adrenalectomy, results in a marked drop in histidine decarboxylase activity of rat stomach (SCHAYER, 1957).

A possible role of the thyroid in histamine formation was indicated by the findings that skin histamine was elevated in hyperthyroid states and low in myxodema (GOTZL and DRAGSTEDT, 1940; FELDBERG and LOESER, 1954). PARRATT and WEST (1960) found normal histamine levels in tissues of rats treated with thyroxine, but did observe a pronounced increase in urinary histamine.

BJURÖ et al. (1961) also found increased urinary excretion of histamine in rats treated with thyroxine or triiodothyronine as well as increased excretion of C^{14} histamine after injection of C^{14} L-histidine. Since rats treated with these drugs showed no change in histamine catabolism, and had elevated stomach histidine decarboxylase activity, an effect of the thyroid gland on histamine formation in the rat was strongly indicated.

Injection of adrenaline and noradrenaline can activate the inducible form of histidine decarboxylase in some tissues (see "Inducible Form of Histidine Decarboxylase").

XII. Interpretation of findings of in vitro histidine decarboxylase assays

Since results from *in vitro* studies of enzymes are obtained under artificial conditions, their relationship to reality is always questionable until there is evidence that similar changes occur in the living organism. The problem with histidine decarboxylase is particularly difficult because of its extremely low activity.

In vivo, histidine decarboxylase produces very small quantities of histamine. This may be due to a low concentration of enzyme molecules. In the rat, the yield of histamine from L-histidine has been estimated as roughly 0.2 %; the yield is probably even less in histamine-sensitive species. In contrast, enzymes involved in major pathways of metabolism of proteins, carbohydrates and fats probably convert thousands or millions of times more molecules per unit time than does histidine decarboxylase.

Plasma concentrations of free L-histidine in a number of species is roughly 10 γ per ml. For some *in vitro* assays it is necessary to use 1 to 10 mg L-histidine per ml in order to obtain sufficient histamine to measure.

Since conventional *in vitro* techniques must attempt to assay enzyme with extremely low *in vivo* activity using substrate concentrations 100 to 1000 times that found in plasma, the chances for error are great and care in interpretation is essential. The two most extreme errors are (a) failure to detect enzyme which functions *in vivo* and (b) detection of "enzyme" which does not function *in vivo*. There is less chance of error with the isotope method since low substrate concentrations can be used.

For comparing the ability of *in vitro* methods to reflect conditions in the living animal, rat skin will be used as an example. There is probably more evidence that rat skin has histidine decarboxylase activity *in vivo* than for any other tissue. Some of this evidence is:

1. Injection of small amounts of C^{14} L-histidine produces C^{14} histamine bound in skin for many weeks (SCHAYER, 1959). Synthesis is slow; addition of new histamine to rat abdominal skin has been estimated to occur at a rate of roughly 2 γ per gram per day (SCHAYER et al., 1954).

2. Attempts to demonstrate *in vivo* binding of exogenous C^{14} histamine in rat skin and other mammalian tissues have failed (SCHAYER, 1952; SCHAYER and SMILEY, 1954; SCHAYER, 1956).

3. Surviving skin tissue, with cells intact, forms C^{14} histamine and binds it (SCHAYER et al., 1955a).

4. Following depletion of rat skin by Compound 48/80, several weeks are required to restore the normal histamine content (FELDBERG and TALESNIK,

1953); depleted skin does not bind exogenous histamine *in vivo* (SCHAYER and SMILEY, 1954).

5. The histamine of rat skin is largely in mast cells (RILEY, 1959); intact mast cells have been shown by a variety of procedures to convert histidine to histamine (see "Histamine Formation in Mast Cells").

The only known attempts to find histidine decarboxylase in rat skin by non-isotopic procedures have failed (WATON, 1956; TELFORD and WEST, 1961 a). With the isotope technique, the enzyme is readily detectable although it is of low activity (SCHAYER et al., 1959; KAHLSON et al., 1960; BJURÖ et al., 1961). The fact that histidine decarboxylase activity of rat skin is low does not indicate a lack of importance; on the contrary, it indicates agreement with *in vivo* data.

In addition to failing to measure histidine decarboxylase which is present in tissues, some *in vitro* methods might measure "histidine decarboxylase" which is not present *in vivo*. Conversion of histidine to histamine in very small yields occurs rather easily by non-enzymatic processes; pyridoxal phosphate alone can catalyze the reaction at a somewhat elevated temperature (WERLE and KOCH, 1949). It is therefore possible that a pyridoxal enzyme not involved in histamine formation in the body could, under certain *in vitro* circumstances, particularly in the presence of a very high concentration of L-histidine, catalyze the decarboxylation of a minute fraction of the histidine molecules and be called histidine decarboxylase erroneously.

The following suggestions are offered relative to interpretation of *in vitro* findings on histamine formation.

1. Failure to detect histidine decarboxylase in a tissue does not necessarily mean its absence; this failure could be due to one or more of a large number of factors. This statement which is frequently seen in the literature, that histidine decarboxylase does not occur in certain tissues, is almost never justified. Recognition should be given to the difficulty of proving a negative proposition (BEVERIDGE, 1951).

2. It is a fallacy to conclude that tissues which apparently do not produce histamine *in vitro* either do not need it, or get it from some exogenous source.

3. It is unjustified to assume that rate of formation of histamine *in vivo* is comparable to that measured *in vitro*.

4. It is of questionable validity to conclude that a tissue with a high histamine-forming power *in vitro* requires it for some special function, qualitatively different from the function of histamine elsewhere. The number of functions proposed for histamine is large; so is the number of these which are unsupportable.

5. The high *in vitro* histamine forming power of some tissues might be an artifact. Cases in which a high rate of histamine formation is found should be even more suspect than usual pending *in vivo* justification. This is particularly true when high concentrations of substrate, and non-physiological additives such as benzene, are used.

6. Expression of histidine decarboxylase activity as "amount of histamine formed per unit time per unit weight of tissue" should not be used as an invitation to experimentation or speculation of the pharmacological effects a comparable amount of injected histamine might have. Such a process could easily lead to fallacious conclusions on physiological functions of histamine, or more likely, its lack of function.

7. Histidine decarboxylase can exist in an inducible form; its activity may be increased or decreased in certain tissues as a response to various environmental changes. For example, as determined by the isotopic method *in vitro*, histidine

decarboxylase activity of stomachs of rats and mice kept at 22° is high, but in stomachs of animals kept at 37°, it is low. The adaptive nature of the activity must be considered in interpreting results.

XIII. Recent hypotheses on the significance of histidine decarboxylase

The writer has suggested that there are two types of histidine decarboxylase with respect to *in vivo* function (SCHAYER, 1960). The first is located in cells containing a binding mechanism and is the source of the histamine bound by these cells. The second type is not related to bound histamine; it produces free histamine, and is believed to be concerned with circulatory homeostasis (see "Inducible Form of Histidine Decarboxylase"). The writer knows of no case in which histidine decarboxylase cannot reasonably be relegated to one or the other of these two categories.

KAHLSON's hypothesis that newly-synthesized histamine is concerned with rapid growth was based on observations made on animals during pregnancy, wound healing and liver regeneration (KAHLSON, 1960). Since that time he and his co-workers have provided additional supporting evidence, for example the marked increase in histidine decarboxylase during the growth of transplanted rat mammary carcinoma (HÅKANSSON, 1961). This hypothesis, however, obviously cannot include the numerous cases where histidine decarboxylase undergoes a relatively rapid activation in response to various stresses or to injection of catechol amines (SCHAYER, 1960). Therefore, if KAHLSON's theory is correct, there are at least two important functions for newly-synthesized, unbound histamine. Recently workers from KAHLSON's laboratory have found marked activation of histidine decarboxylase in kidneys of pregnant mice, a situation where there is no apparent relationship to rapid growth. The concepts of KAHLSON and SCHAYER may be capable of unification in terms of the microcirculatory adjustments occurring in some cases of rapid growth. KAHLSON et al. (1962) have recently shown that in the LANDSCHÜTZ I tumor, growing in the mouse peritoneal cavity as single free cells, histidine decarboxylase correlated with the number of cells in mitosis, not with the total number of cells. In this instance a relationship to the microcirculation is not possible but changes in peritoneal mast cells might confuse the interpretation. TELFORD and WEST (1960a) and MACKAY et al. (1961) have cited data which they believe opposes KAHLSON's growth theory. But since their opposition depends to a considerable degree on inability to find activation of histidine decarboxylase in growth situations, and since both groups use methods which are of low sensitivity, the validity of their criticism is questionable.

WEST's group has suggested several functions for histidine decarboxylase from rat tissues, none of which is related to growth. They propose that the histamine formed in stomach may function as a local stimulus for gastric secretion; that formed in fetal liver increases fetal and placental blood supply and inhibits the mother's uterine movements; that formed in adult liver is used for storage and utilization in various other tissues; that formed in the hepatoma increases the blood supply to the tumor.

Insofar as these proposals involve regulation of blood supply, the writer is in agreement. Otherwise there are reasons to doubt their validity.

In rat stomach it is conceded that bound histamine may be related to gastric secretion (SCHAYER and IVY, 1957 and 1958). But the greater part of the histidine decarboxylase of stomach appears to be of the inducible type and hence not concerned with synthesis of bound histamine (see "Histidine Decarboxylase of Rat Stomach").

If the fetal liver enzyme is concerned with providing histamine to inhibit the mother's uterine movement, it implies a function specific for rats. In most other species tested, histamine contracts uterine smooth muscle (ROCHA E SILVA, 1955). KAHLSON et al. (1958b) and LINDELL (personal communication) have found evidence for increased histamine production by the human fetus.

TELFORD and WEST (1961) proposed that adult rat liver provides histamine for storage and use in other tissues. Even though the authors do not mean to imply that long-term binding of exogenous histamine occurs (WEST, personal communication, 1961) there are serious obstacles to the acceptance of this view. First, a high histamine forming power of rat liver *in vivo* under normal conditions has not been demonstrated; the need for use of a non-physiological additive, benzene, to produce significant *in vitro* activity indicates that the proposal is insubstantially founded. Second, the extremely rapid inactivation of exogenous histamine has been shown by many laboratories. Third, if other rat tissues need blood-borne histamine, antihistamines should markedly affect their function; this is not observed in normal animals. Fourth, injected C^{14} histamine disappears from the blood in about 5 minutes; if at this point Compound 48/80 is injected, large amounts of histamine are released into the blood but it is devoid of demonstrable radioactivity (NEVEU, 1960). Fifth, according to TELFORD and WEST (1961a) liver is the principal source of histamine synthesis in the adult rat and its rate of synthesis is suppressed following a series of injections with Compound 48/80. If, so Compound 48/80-treated rats should excrete less histamine in the urine than normals; however, the opposite occurs (SCHAYER et al., 1959; WILSON, 1963).

XIV. The inducible form of histidine decarboxylase

In previous sections a number of instances have been mentioned in which a pronounced increase in histidine decarboxylase activity has been observed. Examples are skin after repeated dosing of rats with Compound 48/80 (SCHAYER et al., 1959), rat fetal liver, healing wounds, and a rat hepatoma. There is evidence that the increased activity in the first case is associated with the development of new mast cells. In the other cases there is an association of increased enzyme activity with a rapid proliferation of cells. Hence these examples do not rigorously demonstrate the inducible characteristics of histidine decarboxylase even though in some cases the inducible form of the enzyme may be involved.

Activation of histidine decarboxylase has also been observed many times under conditions which cannot be related to development of new cells. The stimuli which elicit this response are either local irritants, or systemic stresses which lead to release of catechol amines and to vasoconstriction (SCHAYER, 1960, 1960a, 1961, 1961a and 1962).

The inducible form of histidine decarboxylase from mouse liver or from guinea pig lung efficiently decarboxylates minute quantities of C^{14} L-histidine; it is strongly inhibited by α-methylhistidine, slightly inhibited by α-methyl DOPA, and unaffected by L-tryptophan. These findings suggest that the inducible enzyme is specific and has a high affinity for substrate molecules (SCHAYER, 1963).

The histamine synthesized by the inducible enzyme is called induced histamine to distinguish it from the bound histamine of tissues. Because of the differences in mechanism and rate of mobilization, there are important differences in the manifestations of induced histamine and released histamine (SCHAYER, 1961).

Most of the studies in this field have used mice; however, the inducibility of histidine decarboxylase in rats, guinea pigs and cats has been shown (SCHAYER, 1961a and 1962); these are the only species tested.

At the time of preparation of this Chapter, confirmation of the existence of the inducible form of histidine decarboxylase has not been reported. It is not known if non-isotopic procedures can detect it. Since this work is entirely from one laboratory, only a brief statement of the findings, in table form, will be made.

Table 4. *Inducible histidine decarboxylase activity and microcirculatory behavior*

Stimulus	Observed circulatory or other biological change	Observed change in histidine decarboxylase activity	Interpretation
Local irritation (1, 2)	Slow phase of inflammation (3)	Gradual increase at site of irritation; rate of increase parallel to rate of development of histamine-reproducible microcirculatory changes (2)	Newly-synthesized histamine provides increased local blood supply to remove irritant
Systemic stimuli causing release of catechol amines (4, 5)	Rapidly-developing vasoconstriction due to catechol amines; subsequent gradual re-opening of capillary bed (6)	Gradual increase in muscle, lung and skin and to a smaller extent in other tissues; rate of increase parallel to the rate of diminution of vasoconstriction. Activity gradually returns to normal when stimulus is removed	Newly-synthesized histamine opposes catechol amine action and prevents prolonged closing of capillary beds
Lethal trauma, e.g. tourniquet shock (7)	Early loss of fluids; vasoconstriction; subsequent gradual re-opening of capillary bed; dilatation in small vessels progresses until circulatory failure occurs (8)	Gradual increase in many tissues; activity is maximal when animals are dying	A rate of histamine synthesis which would normally serve a homeostatic function is excessive for animal with a reduced blood volume
Lethal dose of endotoxin (5)	Rapidly developing vasoconstriction; subsequent gradual re-opening of capillary bed continues until circulatory failure and endothelial damage occur (9)	Gradual increase to very high levels in all tissues tested; much higher activities in liver, spleen, lymph nodes and lung than found in traumatic chock. Activity is maximal when animals are dying	The rate of histamine synthesis becomes so rapid that circulatory failure may occur in animals with normal blood volume
Infection, early phase (2)	Increased phagocytic activity in liver, spleen, lymph nodes and lung	Increase in liver, spleen, lymph nodes and lung, but not in muscle	Locally-synthesized histamine provides an increased blood supply to RES cells and contributes to increased phagocytic activity (10, 11)
Infection, terminal phase (2, 12)	Circulatory failure (13)	Increase to very high levels in all tissues tested	The rate of histamine synthesis becomes so rapid that circulatory failure may occur in animals with normal blood volume
Freund's adjuvant (2, 14)	Slow development of inflammatory lesions in spleen, liver, lymph nodes and lung (15)	Slow increase in spleen, liver, lymph nodes and lung	Newly-synthesized histamine mediates early microcirculatory changes of inflammatory reaction
Pertussis vaccine (mice) (14)	Slow development of sensitivity to histamine, 5-HT, and anaphylaxis	Increase in lung during period corresponding closely to time of sensitization	Prolonged exposure of microvascular endothelial and smooth muscle cells to newly-synthesized histamine renders them susceptible to irreversible damage

Table 4 (Cont'd.)

Stimulus	Observed circulatory or other biological change	Observed change in histidine decarboxylase activity	Interpretation
Endotoxin plus epinephrine (under certain conditions of dosage and timing) (5, 12)	Rapidly-developing vasoconstriction which persists until damage or death occurs (16)	No significant change; normal activation does not occur	The rate of histamine synthesis is inadequate for reopening capillary bed
Warmth (37°C) (2)	Dilatation of larger blood vessels; increased blood volume (17)	Gradual reduction of activity to levels below normal	Reduction in rate of histamine synthesis opposes flooding of capillary bed and maintains homeostasis

References: (1) Schayer, 1961a; (2) Schayer, 1962; (3) Zweifach, 1953; (4) Schayer, 1960; (5) Schayer, 1960a; (6) Zweifach, 1961; (7) Schayer, 1962a; (8) Chambers et al., 1944; (9) Zweifach et al., 1957; (10) Halpern, 1959; (11) Schayer, 1961; (12) Schayer, 1961b; (13) Robinson, 1960; (14) Schayer and Ganley, 1961; (15) Stoerk, 1959; (16) Zweifach and Thomas, 1957; (17) Best and Taylor, 1961.

The material of Table 4 shows the correlation between changes in histidine decarboxylase activity and circulatory changes which follow a number of diverse stimuli. In all cases, the facts are consistent with the hypothesis that the inducible form of histidine decarboxylase is located in or near vascular endothelial cells, and that by alterations in activity in response to environmental changes, it synthesizes histamine at a rate required to maintain circulatory homeostasis.

XV. Conclusion

In vitro histidine decarboxylase assays may be of the greatest importance for elucidating the significance of histamine in the organism. Ideally, these assays may reflect the ability of a tissue to synthesize histamine and may supersede assays for histamine content of tissues as the fundamental measurement in histamine research.

However, it is apparent that results of *in vitro* histidine decarboxylase assays are frequently of questionable relevance to events in the living animal. The recent findings of high enzyme activities in tissues of rats and mice is a healthy trend since in these histamine-insensitive species an *in vivo* counterpart is reasonable. When studies are extended to histamine-sensitive species, including man, the need for methods of the highest sensitivity may be essential. The writer can see little possibility that non-isotopic methods for histidine decarboxylase will serve more than a very limited function in future research in this field.

Abbreviations used are DOPA for 3,4-dihydroxyphenylalanine, 5-HT for 5-hydroxytryptamine, 5-HTP for 5-hydroxytryptophan, 5-HTPD for 5-hydroxytryptophan decarboxylase, and 5-HIAA for 5-hydroxyindoleacetic acid.

The author is indebted to Mrs. Elena Sestokas for translations.

Bibliography

Angervall, L., T. Bjurö and H. Westling: The effect of adrenalectomy on the urinary excretion of histamine in the rat. Acta endocr. (Kbh.) **36**, 467 (1961).

Asboe-Hansen, G.: The mast cell. Cortisone action on connective tissue. Proc. Soc. exp. Biol. **80**, 677 (1952).

Baldwin, E.: Dynamic aspects of biochemistry, p. 30. Cambridge, England: Cambridge University Press 1957.

BALLANI, G. K., Y. K. SINHA and R. K. SANYAL: Effect of cutaneous burn on histamine and 5-hydroxytryptamine in mice. J. Pharm. Pharmacol. **11**, 192 (1959a).
— C. D. THA and R. K. SANYAL: Histamine and 5-hydroxytryptamine after cutaneous burn in mice and rats. J. Pharm. Pharmacol. **11**, 512 (1959).
BARTLET, A. L., and M. F. LOCKETT: Effect of adrenalectomy on tissue histamine in rats. J. Physiol. (Lond.) **147**, 51 (1959).
BENDITT, E. P.: 5-Hydroxytryptamine and 5-hydroxytryptophan decarboxylase in rat mast cells. 5-Hydroxytryptamine, p. 32. New York: Pergamon Press 1958.
BEST, C. H., and N. B. TAYLOR: The physiological basis of medical practice. Baltimore: Williams & Wilkins 7th Ed., 1961, p. 886.
BEVERIDGE, W. I. B.: The art of scientific investigation, p. 25. New York: W. W. Norton & Co. 1951.
BJURÖ, T., and H. WESTLING: Sodium chloride intake and urinary histamine in adrenalectomized rats. Nature (Lond.) **184**, 1241 Suppl. 16 (1959).
— — and H. WETTERQVIST: The effect of thyroid hormones on histamine formation in the rat. Brit. J. Pharmacol. **17**, 479 (1961).
BLOCH, W., u. H. PINÖSCH: Die Umwandlung von Histidin in Histamin im tierischen Organismus. Hoppe-Seylers Z. physiol. Chem. **239**, 236 (1936).
BOROVSKAYA, V. M.: Origin of histamine in the animal body. J. Physiol. U.S.S.R. **29**, 96 (1940).
BROWN, D. D., R. TOMCHICK and J. AXELROD: The distribution and properties of a histamine-methylating enzyme. J. biol. Chem. **234**, 2948 (1959).
BURKHALTER, A.: Histamine formation by fetal rat liver. Biochem. Pharmacol. **11**, 315 (1962).
CHAMBERS, R., B. W. ZWEIFACH and B. E. LOWENSTEIN: The peripheral circulation during the tourniquet shock syndrome in the rat. Ann. Surg. **120**, 791 (1944).
CLARK, C. T., H. WEISSBACH and S. UDENFRIEND: 5-Hydroxytryptophan decarboxylase: preparation and properties. J. biol. Chem. **210**, 139 (1954).
CODE, C. F.: Histamine in blood. Physiol. Rev. **32**, 47 (1952).
— Histamine and gastric secretion. Ciba Foundation Symposium on Histamine, p. 189. London: Churchill 1956.
—, and G. A. HALLENBECK: Effect of pregnancy on the histidine decarboxylase activity of the rat's stomach. J. Physiol. (Lond.) **159**, 66 P (1961).
DEKANSKI, J.: The effect of cutaneous burns on histamine in mice. J. Physiol. (Lond.) **104**, 151 (1945).
EDLBACHER, S., M. SIMON u. M. BECKER: Über den Abbau des D-Histidins beim Meerschweinchen. Naturwissenschaften **28**, 411 (1940).
EULER, VON U. S.: Noradrenaline, p. 139. Springfield, Illinois: Charles C Thomas 1956.
FELDBERG, W., and A. A. LOESER: Histamine content of human skin in different clinical disorders. J. Physiol. (Lond.) **126**, 286 (1954).
—, and J. TALESNIK: Reduction of tissue histamine by compound 48—80. J. Physiol. (Lond.) **120**, 550 (1953).
FISHER, J. P., and R. A. COOKE: Experimental toxic and allergic contact dermatitis. J. Allergy **29**, 396 (1958).
GÁBOR, M., I. SZÓRÁDY and Z. DIRNER: Inhibiting effect of the members of the hematoxilia group on the action of histidine decarboxylase. Acta physiol. Acad. Sci. hung. **3**, 595 (1952).
GALE, E. F.: Amino acid decarboxylases. Brit. med. Bull. **9**, 135 (1953).
GANROT, P. O., A. M. ROSENGREN and E. ROSENGREN: On the presence of different histidine decarboxylating enzymes in mammalian tissues. Experientia (Basel) **17**, 263 (1961).
GOTH, A., R. M. ALLMAN, B. C. MERRITT and J. HOLMAN: Effect of cortisone on histamine liberation induced by Tween in the dog. Proc. Soc. exp. Biol. (N. Y.) **78**, 848 (1951).
GOTZL, F. R., and C. A. DRAGSTEDT: Effect of thyroidectomy and of experimental hyperthyroidism upon histamine content of rat tissues. Proc. Soc. exp. Biol. (N. Y.) **45**, 688 (1940).
GRAHAM, H. T., T. W. HANNEGAN and C. M. NOURSE: Dependence of tissue histamine content on local histidine decarboxylase activity. Biochim. biophys. Acta **20**, 243 (1956).
GREEN, J. P., and S. M. DAY: Uptake and metabolism of amines by mast cells in culture. Fed. Proc. **20**, No. 1, Part I, 136 (1961).
GUSTAFFSSON, B., G. KAHLSON and E. ROSENGREN: Biogenesis of histamine studied by its distribution and urinary excretion in germ free reared and not germ free rats fed a histamine free diet. Acta physiol. scand. **41**, 217 (1957).
HAGEN, P., N. WEINER, S. ONO and FU-LI LEE: Amino acid decarboxylases of mouse mastocytoma tissue. J. Pharmacol. exp. Ther. **130**, 9 (1960).
HÅKANSSON, R.: Formation of histamine in transplants from a rat mammary carcinoma. Experientia (Basel) **17**, 402 (1961).

HALPERN, B. N.: Histamine release by long chain molecules. Ciba Foundation Symposium on Histamine, p. 92. London: Churchill 1956.
— The role and function of the reticulo-endothelial system in immunological processes. J. Pharm. Pharmacol. **11**, 321 (1959).
—, et M. BRIOT: Action des hormones cortico-surrénaliennes sur le métabolisme de l'histamine endogène. Rev. franç. Étud. clin. Biol. **1**, 151 (1956).
HICKS, R., and G. B. WEST: Adrenalectomy and tissue amines. Nature (Lond.) **182**, 401 (1958).
HINSHAW, L. B., M. M. JORDAN and J. A. VICK: Mechanism of histamine release in endotoxin shock. Amer. J. Physiol. **200**, 987 (1961).
— — — Histamine release and endotoxin shock in the primate. J. clin. Invest. **40**, 1631 (1961a).
HOLTZ, P., u. K. CREDNER: Decarboxylierung von Dioxyphenylalanin (Dopa) und Histidin in vivo. Naturwissenschaften **29**, 649 (1941).
— — Histaminausscheidung nach Belastung mit Histidin. Hoppe-Seylers Z. physiol. Chem. **280**, 1 (1944).
— — u. H. WALTER: Über die Spezifität der Aminosäuredecarboxylasen. Hoppe-Seylers Z. physiol. Chem. **262**, 111 (1939).
—, and R. HEISE: Formation of histamine in the organism. Naturwissenschaften **25**, 201 (1937).
— — Über Histaminbildung im Organismus. Naunyn-Schmiedeberg's Arch. exp. Path. Pharmak. **186**, 377 (1937a).
— — and K. LÜDTKE: Enzymatic destruction of 1-dihydroxyphenylalanine (dopa) by the kidney. Naunyn-Schmiedeberg's Arch. exp. Path. Pharmak. **292**, 87 (1938a).
— — u. W. SPREYER: Fermentative Bildung und Zerstörung von Histamin und Tyramin. Naunyn-Schmiedeberg's Arch. exp. Path. Pharmak. **188**, 580 (1938).
—, u. E. WESTERMANN: Über die Histidindecarboxylase der Nerven. Naturwissenschaften **43**, 37 (1956).
— — Über die Dopa-Decarboxylase und Histidindecarboxylase des Nervengewebes. Naunyn-Schmiedeberg's Arch. exp. Path. Pharmak. **227**, 538 (1956a).
INDERBITZIN, T.: The effect of acute and delayed cutaneous allergic reactions on the amount of histamine in the skin. Int. Arch. Allergy **7**, 140 (1955).
— The relationship of lymphocytes, delayed cutaneous allergic reactions and histamine. Int. Arch. Allergy **8**, 150 (1956).
KAHLSON, G.: A place for histamine in normal physiology. Lancet **1960 I**, 67.
— K. NILSSON, E. ROSENGREN and B. ZEDERFELDT: Wound healing as dependent on rate of histamine formation. Lancet **1960 II**, 230.
—, and E. ROSENGREN: Inhibition of histamine formation and some of its consequences. J. Physiol. (Lond.) **149**, 66 P (1959).
— — Prevention of fetal development by enzyme inhibition. Nature (Lond.) **184**, 1238 (1959a).
— — and C. STEINHARDT: Activation of histidine decarboxylase in tumor cells of mice. Nature, (Lond.) **194**, 380 (1962).
— — and S. E. SVENSSON: Inhibition of histamine formation in vivo. Nature (Lond.) **194**, 876 (1962).
— — and H. WESTLING: Urinary excretion of histamine in pregnant rats. J. Physiol. (Lond.) **140**, 12 P (1957).
— — — and T. WHITE: The site of increased histamine formation in rat pregnancy. J. Physiol. (Lond.) **142**, 37 P (1958).
— — — — The site of increased formation of histamine in the pregnant rat. J. Physiol. (Lond.) **144**, 337 (1958a).
— — and T. WHITE: Formation of histamine by the foetus in the rat and man. J. Physiol. (Lond.) **145**, 30 P (1958b).
KAMESWAREN, L., J. M. TELFORD and G. B. WEST: Histamine formation in the rat. J. Physiol. (Lond.) **157**, 23 P (1961).
—, and G. B. WEST: Histidine decarboxylase in rat hepatoma. J. Pharm. Pharmacol. **13**, 191 (1961).
KOSHTOYANTS, K., D. E. RYBKINA and R. L. MITROPOLITANSKAYA: The system histamine-histidine decarboxylase-histaminase in the nerve tissue of homiothermal animals subjected to different conditions. Compt. Rend. Acad. Sci. U.S.S.R. **49**, 381 (1945).
KUMAMOTO, K.: The formation of histamine from histidine by animal tissue. Hukuoka Acta. Med. **33**, 80 (1940).
KUN, E.: Effect of meningococcal endotoxin on histamine content of blood and tissue of rabbits. Proc. Soc. exp. Biol. (N. Y.) **66**, 197 (1947).
LINDAHL, K.: On the biological methylation of histamine. 3. Acta chem. scand. **12**, 2050 (1958).
— The histamine methylating enzyme system in liver. Acta physiol. scand. **49**, 1 (1960).
LINDELL, S.-E., H. RORSMAN and H. WESTLING: Formation of histamine in a canine mastocytoma. Experientia (Basel) **15**, 31 (1959).

LINDELL, S.-E., and R. W. SCHAYER: Formation of histamine in the kidney of the dog. Brit. J. Pharmacol. **13**, 89 (1958).
— — Metabolism of injected [14 C] histamine in the kidney of the dog. Brit. J. Pharmacol. **13**, 52 (1958a).
LOVENBERG, W., H. WEISSBACH and S. UDENFRIEND: Aromatic-L-amino acid decarboxylase. J. biol. Chem. **237**, 89 (1962).
MACKAY, D., P. B. MARSHALL and J. F. RILEY: Histidine decarboxylase activity in a malignant rat hepatoma. J. Physiol. (Lond.) **153**, 31 P (1960).
— J. D. REID and D. M. SHEPHERD: Histidine Decarboxylase and growth. Nature (Lond.) **191**, 1311 (1961).
— J. F. RILEY and D. M. SHEPHERD: Amino-acid decarboxylase activities in rat hepatoma. J. Pharm. Pharmacol. **13**, 257 (1961a).
—, and D. M. SHEPHERD: A study of potential histidine decarboxylase inhibitors. Brit. J. Pharmacol. **15**, 552 (1960).
MACKAY, M.: Effect of histidine on the histamine content of the lungs and on histamine reactions. Aust. J. exp. Biol. med. Sci. **16**, 137 (1938).
MALKIEL, S., and M. D. WERLE: D-catechol and antihistaminogenesis. Science **114**, 98 (1951).
MARSHALL, P. B.: The influence of adrenal cortical deficiency on the histamine content of rat tissues. J. Physiol. (Lond.) **102**, 180 (1943).
MARTIN, G. J., M. GRAFF, R. BRENDEL and J. M. BEILER: Effect of vitamin P compounds on action of histidine decarboxylase. Arch. Biochem. **21**, 177 (1949).
METZLER, D. E., M. IKAWA and E. E. SNELL: A general mechanism for vitamin B_6-catalyzed reactions. J. Amer. chem. Soc. **76**, 648 (1954).
MITCHELL, R. G., and C. F. CODE: Urinary excretion of histamine after administration of cortisone. J. clin. Endocr. **14**, 707 (1954).
MOSS, J. N., J. M. BEILER and G. J. MARTIN: Inhibition of anaphylaxis in guinea pigs by D-catechin. Science **112**, 16 (1950).
NEVEU, T.: Contribution a l'étude du métabolisme de l'histamine. J. Physiol. (Paris) **52**, 6 (1960).
OATES, J. A., L. GILLESPIE, S. UDENFRIEND and A. SJOERDSMA: Decarboxylase inhibition and blood pressure reduction by α-methyl-3,4-dihydroxy-DL-phenylalanine. Science **131**, 1890 (1960).
—, and A. SJOERDSMA: A unique syndrome associated with secretion of 5-hydroxytryptophan by metastatic gastric carcinoids. Amer. J. Med. **32**, 333 (1962).
OLD, L. J., D. A. CLARKE, B. BENACERRAF and M. GOLDSMITH: The reticuloendothelial system and the neoplastic process. Ann. N. Y. Acad. Sci. **88**, 264 (1960).
ONO, S., and P. HAGEN: Pyridoxal phosphate: a coenzyme for histidine decarboxylase. Nature (Lond.) **184**, 1143 Suppl. 15 (1959).
PARRATT, J. R., and G. B. WEST: Hypersensitivity and the thyroid gland. Int. Arch. Allergy **16**, 288 (1960).
PARROT, J.-L.: Inhibition de l'histidine decarboxylase *in vivo*. Thérapie **16**, 472 (1961).
— Choc anaphylatique des organes isolée. Absence de variation dans le pouvoir décarboxylant du rein de cobaye à l'égard de la l-histidine. C. R. Soc. Biol. (Paris) **130**, 334 (1939).
—, and C. LABORDE: Inhibition of histidine decarboxylase in vivo by derivatives of benzyl-l-isoquinoline. Ciba Foundation Symposium on Histamine, p. 57. London: Churchill 1956.
— — Inhibition de l'histidine-décarboxylase in vivo par certains dérivés de la benzyl-l-isoquinoléine. J. Physiol. (Paris) **51**, 546 (1959).
RILEY, J. F.: The mast cells. London, E. S. Livingstone (1959).
ROBINSON, H. J.: Adrenal steroids and resistance to infection. Antibiot. and Chemother. **7**, 199 (1960).
ROCHA e SILVA, M.: Histamine. Its role in anaphylaxis and allergy. Springfield, Illinois: Charles C Thomas 1955.
ROSE, B., and G. S. L. BROWNE: The distribution and rate of disappearance of intravenously injected histamine in the rat. Amer. J. Physiol. **124**, 412 (1938).
ROSENGREN, E., and C. STEINHARDT: Elevated histidine decarboxylase activity in the kidney of the pregnant mouse. Experientia, Basel, **17**, 1 (1961).
ROTHSCHILD, A. M., and R. W. SCHAYER: Histidine decarboxylase from rat peritoneal fluid mast cells. Fed. Proc. **17**, No. 1, Part I (1958).
— — Characterization of histidine decarboxylase from rat peritoneal fluid mast cells. Biochim. biophys. Acta **34**, 392 (1959).
ROWLEY, D. A., and E. P. BENDITT: 5-Hydroxytryptamine and histamine as mediators of the vascular injury produced by agents which damage mast cells in rats. J. exp. Med. **103**, 399 (1956).
RYBKINA, D. E.: Comparative study of the acetylcholine content and the system histidine decarboxylase-histaminase in nerves during stimulation. Bull. exptl. Biol. Med. (U.S.S.R.) **24**, 53 (1947).

SCHALES, O.: Amino acid decarboxylases. The Enzymes, Vol. 2. New York: Academic Press 1951.
SCHAYER, R. W.: Biogenesis of histamine. J. biol. Chem. **199**, 245 (1952).
— Studies on histamine-metabolizing enzymes in intact animals. J. biol. Chem. **203**, 787 (1953).
— Formation and binding of histamine by rat tissue in vitro. Amer. J. Physiol. **187**, 63 (1956).
— Formation and binding of histamine by free mast cells of rat peritoneal fluid. Amer. J. Physiol. **186**, 199 (1956a).
— The metabolism of histamine in various species. Brit. J. Pharmacol. **11**, 472 (1956b).
— Histidine decarboxylase of rat stomach and other mammalian tissues. Amer. J. Physiol. **189**, 533 (1957).
— Histamine metabolism. Proceedings IIIrd International Congress of Allergology, Paris (1958).
— Histamine metabolism in the mammalian organism. From Henry Ford Hospital International Symposium on "Mechanisms of Hypersensitivity". Boston: Little, Brown & Co. 1959.
— Further evidence that pyridoxal phosphate is the coenzyme of mammalian histidine decarboxylase. Fed. Proc. **18**, No. 1, Part I, 1256 (1959a).
— Catabolism of physiological quantities of histamine in vivo. Physiol. Rev. **39**, 116 (1959b).
— Relationship of stress-induced histidine decarboxylase to circulatory homeostasis and shock. Science **131**, 226 (1960).
— Relationship of induced histidine decarboxylase activity and histamine synthesis to shock from stress and from endotoxin. Amer. J. Physiol. **198**, 1187 (1960a).
— Significance of induced synthesis of histamine in physiology and pathology. Chemotherapia **3**, 128 (1961).
— Proceedings of a conference on recent progress and present problems in the field of shock. Fed. Proc. **20**, No. 2, Part III, 154 (1961a).
— Proceedings of a conference on recent progress and present problems in the field of shock. Fed. Proc. **20**, No. 2, Part III, 207 (1961b).
— Evidence that induced histamine is an intrinsic regulator of the microcirculatory system. Amer. J. Physiol. **202**, 66 (1962).
— Role of induced histamine and tourniquet shock in mice. Amer. J. Physiol. **203**, 412 (1962a).
— Histidine decarboxylase in mast cells. Ann. N. Y. Acad. Sci. **103**, Art. 1, 164 (1963).
— K. J. DAVIS and R. L. SMILEY: Binding of histamine in vitro and its inhibition by cortisone. Amer. J. Physiol. **182**, 54 (1955).
—, and O. GANLEY: Adaptive increase in mammalian histidine decarboxylase activity in response to nonspecific stress. Amer. J. Physiol. **197**, 721 (1959).
— — Relationship of increased histidine decarboxylase activity to Bordetella pertussis vaccine sensitization of mice. J. Allergy **32**, 204 (1961).
—, and A. C. IVY: Evidence that histamine is a gastric secretory hormone in the rat. Amer. J. Physiol. **189**, 369 (1957).
— — Release of C^{14}-histamine from stomach and intestine on feeding. Amer. J. Physiol. **193**, 400 (1958).
— J. KENNEDY and R. L. SMILEY: Studies on histamine metabolizing enzymes in intact animals. II. J. biol. Chem. **205**, 739 (1953).
—, and Y. KOBAYASHI: Histidine decarboxylase and histamine binding in rabbit platelets. Proc. Soc. exp. Biol. (N. Y.) **92**, 653 (1956).
— Z. ROTHSCHILD and P. BIZONY: Increase in histidine decarboxylase activity of rat skin following treatment with compound 48/80. Amer. J. Physiol. **196**, 295 (1959).
—, and R. L. SMILEY: Binding and release of radioactive histamine in intact rats. Amer. J. Physiol. **177**, 401 (1954).
— — and K. J. DAVIS: Inhibition by cortisone of the binding of new histamine in rat tissues. Proc. Soc. exp. Biol. (N. Y.) **87**, 590 (1954).
— K. Y. T. WU and R. L. SMILEY: Sources of urinary histamine in the rat. Amer. J. Physiol. **179**, 481 (1954a).
SCHINDLER, R., M. DAY and G. A. FISCHER: Culture of neoplastic mast cells and their synthesis of 5-hydroxytryptamine and histamine in vitro. Cancer Res. **19**, 47 (1959).
STOERK, H. C.: The role of mycobacteria in allergic reactions. In the Henry Ford Hospital International Symposium on Mechanisms of Hypersensitivity, p. 635. Boston: Little, Brown & Co. 1959.
TELFORD, J. M., and G. B. WEST: The effects of corticosteroids and related compounds on the histamine and 5-hydroxytryptamine content of rat tissues. Brit. J. Pharmacol. **15**, 532 (1960).
— — Studies with histidine decarboxylase. J. Physiol. (Lond.) **155**, 16 P (1960a).
— — The formation of histamine in the rat. J. Pharm. Pharmacol. **13**, 75 (1961).

TELFORD, J. M., and G. B. WEST: Some effects of corticosteroids on the metabolism of histamine and 5-hydroxytryptamine in the rat. Brit. J. Pharmacol. **16**, 360 (1961a).
— — The effect of age on the formation of histamine in the rat. J. Physiol. (Lond.) **157**, 306 (1961b).
UDENFRIEND, S.: 5-Hydroxytryptamine, p. 48. London: Pergamon Press 1958.
— W. M. LOVENBERG and H. WEISSBACH: L-Amino acid decarboxylase activity in mammalian tissues and its inhibition by α-methyl-DOPA. Fed. Proc. **19**, No. 1, Part I, 7 (1960).
VAN ARSDEL, JR., P. P. and G. N. BEALL: The metabolism and functions of histamine. Arch. int. Med. **106**, 714 (1960).
WATON, N. G.: Studies on mammalian histidine decarboxylase. Brit. J. Pharmacol. **11**, 119 (1956).
— Effect of organic solvents on mammalian histidine decarboxylase. Biochem. J. **64**, 318 (1956a).
WEISSBACH, H., W. LOVENBERG and S. UDENFRIEND: Characteristics of mammalian histidine decarboxylating enzymes. Biochim. biophys. Acta **50**, 177 (1961).
WERLE, E.: Über die Bildung von Histamin aus Histidin durch tierisches Gewebe. Biochem. Z. **288**, 292 (1936).
— Zur Kenntnis der Histidin-decarboxylase und der Histaminase. Biochem. Z. **304**, 201 (1940).
— Zur Kenntnis der Aminosäuredecarboxylasen und der Histaminase. Biochem. Z. **311**, 270 (1942).
— In General Discussion, Ciba Foundation Symposium on Histamine, p. 451. London: Churchill 1956.
— Hemmung der Histidin-Decarboxylase durch α-Methyldopa. Naturwissenschaften **48**, 54 (1961).
—, u. D. AURES: Über die Reinigung und Spezifität der DOPA-Decarboxylase. Hoppe-Seylers Z. physiol. Chem. **316**, 45 (1959).
—, u. K. HEITZER: Zur Kenntnis der Histidindecarboxylase. Biochem. Z. **299**, 420 (1938).
—, u. H. HERRMANN: Über die Bildung von Histamin aus Histidin durch tierisches Gewebe. Biochem. Z. **291**, 105 (1937).
—, u. W. KOCH: Zur Kenntnis der Aminosäuredecarboxylasen und ihres Wirkungsmechanismus. Biochem. Z. **319**, 305 (1949).
—, u. K. KRAUTZUN: Über die Bildung von Histamin aus Histidin durch tierische Gewebe. Biochem. Z. **296**, 315 (1938).
—, u. G. LELLMANN: Verhalten der Histidindecarboxylase und der Histaminase bei Nierenschädigungen. Z. ges. exp. Med. **114**, 674 (1945).
— M. J. MADLENER u. H. HERRMANN: Über das Verhalten der Histidindecarboxylase und Histaminase bei Nierenschädigungen; Harnleiterstauung bei Meerschweinchen. Z. ges. exp. Med. **106**, 105 (1939).
— — — Histidinedecarboxylase activity in kidneys after obstruction of blood flow. Z. ges. exp. Med. **107**, 252 (1940).
— A. SCHAUER u. G. HARTUNG: Einfluß von Hydrazin- und Guanylhydrazonderivaten auf die Aktivität der Monoaminoxydase, Dopadecarboxylase und Histidindecarboxylase. Klin. Wschr. **33**, 562 (1955).
WHITE, T.: Formation and catabolism of histamine in brain tissue in vitro. J. Physiol. (Lond.) **149**, 34 (1959).
— Formation and catabolism of histamine in cat brain in vivo. J. Physiol. (Lond.) **152**, 299 (1960).
WILSON, C. W. M.: Metabolism of histamine after administration of compound 48/80. Int. Arch. Allergy **22**, 102 (1963).
ZWEIFACH, B. W.: Mechanism of inflammation. Montreal, Acta, Inc. (1953).
— The contribution of the reticuloendothelial system to the development of tolerance. Ann. N. Y. Acad. Sci. **88**, 203 (1960).
— Functional behavior of the microcirculation. Springfield, Illinois: Charles C Thomas 1961.
— B. BENACERRAF and L. THOMAS: The relationship between the vascular manifestations of shock produced by endotoxin, trauma and hemorrhage. II. The possible role of the reticuloendothelial system in resistance to each type of shock. J. exp. Med. **106**, 403 (1957).
—, and L. THOMAS: The relationship between the vascular manifestations of shock produced by endotoxin, trauma and hemorrhage. I. Certain similarities between the reactions in normal and endotoxin-tolerant rats. J. exp. Med. **106**, 385 (1957).

Section E

Histamine — Pyridine Coenzyme Interactions

By

S. G. A. Alivisatos

With 1 Figure

Certain enzyme catalyzed interactions of histamine with either diphosphopyridine nucleotide (coenzyme I, abbreviated DPN^+) (Alivisatos, 1958a, b; Alivisatos et al., 1960) or triphosphopyridine nucleotide (coenzyme II, abbreviated TPN^+) (Alivisatos and Abdel-Latif, 1960; Abdel-Latif and Alivisatos, 1961a) lead to displacement products in which the nicotinamide moiety of pyridine coenzymes is irreversibly replaced by histamine. The sequence of reactions, as catalyzed *in vitro* by the enzyme (diphosphopyridine nucleotidase, abbreviated DPNase), is as follows (Alivisatos, 1959):

$$\text{Nicotinamide}^+ \cdot \text{R} + \text{Enzyme} \leftrightarrows \text{Enzyme}^+ \cdot \text{R} + \text{Nicotinamide} \qquad (\text{I})$$

$$\text{Enzyme}^+ \cdot \text{R} + \text{H} \cdot \text{OH} \rightarrow \text{HO} \cdot \text{R} + \text{Enzyme} + \text{H}^+ \qquad (\text{IIa})$$

$$\text{Enzyme}^+ \cdot \text{R} + \text{Histamine} \rightarrow \text{Histamine} \cdot \text{R} + \text{Enzyme} + \text{H}^+ \qquad (\text{IIb})$$

In these equations $\text{Nicotinamide}^+ \cdot \text{R}$ denotes pyridine coenzymes. Reaction (I) represents a reversible exchange of the nicotinamide moiety of pyridine coenzymes with the enzyme (Zatman et al., 1953). The exchange-product (enzyme intermediate) is labile. In the presence of suitable nucleophiles [i. e., water (IIa) or an imidazole like histamine (IIb)] it dissociates irreversibly (Alivisatos, 1959). In *in vitro* studies reactions (IIa) (hydrolysis) and (IIb) [imidazolysis (Alivisatos, 1959; Alivisatos et al., 1958) or histaminolysis (Alivisatos, 1958a, b; Alivisatos et al., 1960)] are interchangable. Histamine, however, is approximately 50 times more efficient than water as a participant in the above reactions (Alivisatos, 1958a, b; Alivisatos et al., 1960). Thus in the presence of an excess of histamine, histaminolysis [reaction (IIb)] proceeds to completion (Figure 1). Nicotinamide and its analogues (e.g., isonicotinic acid hydrazide, etc.) are potent inhibitors of the hydrolysis (Zatman et al., 1954) and imidazolysis (Alivisatos, 1958a, b; Alivisatos et al., 1960) of pyridine coenzymes. Reaction (I) provides an explanation for this inhibitory effect (Zatman et al., 1953).

Preliminary studies (Alivisatos, in press) indicate that diphosphohistamine nucleotide may be formed *in vivo*. Thus, 13 μmoles (approx. 1.5 mg) of 2 (ring)-C^{14}-labeled histamine were administered intraperitonealy to a guinea pig (500 g body weight). Immediately after death the animal body was immersed in liquid nitrogen and pulverized in the frozen state. Diphosphohistamine nucleotide (approx. 2×10^{-7} moles) was isolated from the trichloroacetic acid extract of this powder after addition of carrier (non-radioactive) dinucleotide. These studies are still in progress.

The enzymic degradation of histamine dinucleotides *in vitro* proceeds as follows: In the presence of nucleotide pyrophosphatases (Kornberg and Pricer, 1950) both diphosphohistamine nucleotide (Alivisatos, 1958a, b; Alivisatos et al., 1960) and triphosphohistamine nucleotide (ALIVISATOS and ABDEL-LATIF, 1960; ABDEL-LATIF and ALIVISATOS, 1961a) hydrolyze to 5′-adenylic acid (AMP) or 5′, 2′-diphosphoadenosine (abbreviated 2′, 5′-ADP) and to histamine ribonucleotide. Further hydrolysis of the latter, in the presence of 5′-nucleotidases [phosphatases (HEPPEL and HILMOE, 1951)] leads to histamine ribonucleoside (ALIVISATOS, 1958a, b; ALIVISATOS et al., 1960; ALIVISATOS and ABDEL-LATIF, 1960; ABDEL-LATIF and ALIVISATOS, 1961a; MURAOKA et al., 1961). Preliminary studies (ALIVISATOS and ABDEL-LATIF, unpublished observations) indicate that histamine ribonucleoside may be oxidatively deaminated to imidazoleacetic acid ribonucleoside. This sequence of degradations for triphosphohistamine nucleotide may be written as follows:

$$H_2O + \text{Histamine} \cdot \text{ribose} \cdot \text{pyrophosphate} \cdot (2'\text{-phosphoribose}) \cdot \text{adenine} \xrightarrow[\text{pyrophosphatase}]{\text{nucleotide}} \text{Histamine} \cdot \text{ribose} \cdot \text{phosphate} + 2', 5'\text{-ADP} \quad \text{(III)}$$

$$\text{Histamine} \cdot \text{ribose} \cdot \text{phosphate} + H_2O \xrightarrow{5'\text{-nucleotidase}} \text{Histamine ribonucleoside} + \text{inorganic phosphate} \quad \text{(IV)}$$

$$\text{Histamine ribonucleoside} \xrightarrow[\text{(ZELLER et al., 1956; KOBAYASHI, 1957)}]{\text{(monoamine oxidase-like enzymes ?)}} \text{imidazoleacetic acid ribonucleoside} \quad \text{(V)}$$

The possible occurrence of reaction (V) is still under study (ALIVISATOS and ABDEL-LATIF, unpublished observations). The catabolic fate of histamine dinucleotides after their *in vivo* administration is also under study (ALIVISATOS and ABDEL-LATIF, unpublished observations). However, an obvious limitation of such studies is imposed by the doubtful permeability of the dinucleotides through cell membranes. Information provided by such studies is most probably related to the extracellular degradation of these compounds.

Of the above mentioned catabolic products, imidazoleacetic acid ribonucleoside was isolated several years ago as a urinary metabolite of histamine, after administration of small doses of the C^{14}-labeled drug to rats (KARJALA, 1955). It may also be formed by interaction of imidazoleacetic acid and 5′-phosphoribosyl-1′-pyrophosphate (CROWLEY, 1960). Hydrolysis of the resulting ribonucleotide in the presence of 5′-nucleotidases (phosphatases) would lead to the ribonucleoside. Probably, this reaction sequence also occurs *in vivo*. This may be surmised from the lack of reactivity of imidazolacetic acid with the pyridine coenzymes (see below) and from experiments in which large doses of imidazoleacetic acid were administered to rats with subsequent isolation of the ribonucleoside from the urine (TABOR and HAYAISHI, 1955). Preliminary evidence indicates that a similar pathway involving histamine and 5′-phosphoribosyl-1′-pyrophosphate may also exist (FERNANDES et al., 1960) but this awaits more rigorous verification (ALIVISATOS, in press). Two recently uncovered alternative pathways for the formation of histamine ribonucleoside (ABDEL-LATIF and ALIVISATOS, 1961b, 1962) involve interaction of histamine with either nicotinamide ribonucleotide or nicotinamide ribonucleoside. The enzyme is a ribonucleosidase present in semen as an extracellular soluble constituent (LEONE and BONADUCE, 1959).

The observation that histamine interacts with respiratory coenzymes which are inactivated in the process, is suggestive of an involvement of such interactions in certain phases of the mechanism of hypersensitive phenomena (ALIVISATOS et al., 1959). If this were true, a notable prerequisite would be the presence of the enzyme (diphosphopyridine nucleotidase) in the cells concerned. The peculiar and somewhat erratic distribution of diphosphopyridine nucleotidase in various organs and tissues of different species might thus explain differences in sensitivity towards histamine (ALIVISATOS et al., 1959).

In the vast majority of cases this enzyme is firmly bound with the insoluble structural material of cells. Thus it is almost absent from human erythrocytes (ABDEL-LATIF and ALIVISATOS, 1961b, 1962; GROSSMAN and KAPLAN, 1958). In contrast to this, rabbit red cells are rich in diphosphopyridine nucleotidase (ALIVISATOS and DENSTEDT, 1951). It is found in the stromata and interestingly, it is confined on the outer surface of the erythrocytes (ALIVISATOS and DENSTEDT, 1951). In other cells (liver, kidney, brain) it is found in the microsomal fraction (KAPLAN et al., 1960). The present status of this subject was recently reviewed briefly by KAPLAN et al. (1960). Guinea pig lungs are a good source of the enzyme (S. G. A. ALIVISATOS and F. UNGAR, unpublished observations).

In animals relatively non-sensitive to histamine (for example, mice and rats) it would be expected that when small doses of the drug are administered, routes of detoxication (SCHAYER, 1959) would prevail. Those would include, among others (SCHAYER, 1959), oxidative deamination to imidazole acetic acid and the above mentioned interactions of the latter as well as of histamine with 5′-phosphoribose-1′-pyrophosphate. However, since imidazoleacetic acid ribonucleoside would be a common excretion product of such detoxication processes and of reaction sequences commencing with the histaminolysis of pyridine coenzymes (see above), it would be difficult at present to correlate the sensitivity of a given animal species with the pattern of excretion products of histamine detected in the urine (see, for example, SCHAYER, 1959). More promising would be the isolation and quantitative comparison of histamine dinucleotides from sacrificed animals, in the pattern outlined above for guinea pigs (ALIVISATOS, in press). Utilization of blocking agents (SCHAYER, 1959) would also be of value in this respect. Again, in interpreting results of this type of experiments it should be considered that certain inhibitors, like iproniazid, etc., besides their well recognized action (ZELLER and BARSKY, 1952) may block the activity of diphosphopyridine nucleotidases.

In the last few years the hypothesis of an involvement of histamine-pyridine coenzyme interactions in *in vivo* hypersensitive phenomena received support from a number of observations. Most important was the above mentioned demonstration of the occurrence of histamine dinucleotides after in vivo administration of histamine (ALIVISATOS, in press). It was also found that L-histidine (ALIVISATOS, 1958b) and imidazoleacetic acid (ALIVISATOS and LAMANTIA, 1960; ALIVISATOS et al., 1962) are both unreactive in the pyridine coenzyme-DPNase system. Both compounds are devoid of *in vivo* histamine-like activities. Apparently, the presence of a free carboxyl in the side chain of the imidazole is incompatible with participation in reactions catalyzed by diphosphopyridine nucleotidases. Esterification of the carboxyl (as in imidazoleacetic acid ethylester) partially restores reactivity with the coenzymes (ALIVISATOS et al., 1962).

As mentioned above, nicotinamide is a potent inhibitor of diphosphopyridine nucleotidase catalyzed interactions (ALIVISATOS, 1959; ZATMAN et al., 1953). Nicotinamide, at the same time, is a well known *in vivo* inhibitor of the effects of histamine both in humans (DAÏNOW, 1944; BUTTURINI, 1946) and in experimental animals (HALPERN and DAÏNOW, 1944; ALECHINSKY, 1947). Equally suggestive but more difficult to interpret are certain *in vitro* observations of MOTA, et al. In these experiments, mast cells obtained from the peritoneal cavity of sensitized animals were observed under the microscope. Upon addition of the sensitizing agent they suffered extensive morphological alterations accompanied by histamine release (MOTA and DIAS DA SILVA, 1960a). In the presence of nicotinamide these phenomena were largely prevented (MOTA et al., 1960). A possible interpretation of this effect (ALIVISATOS et al., 1961 b) could be that the primary damage inflicted upon the cells as a result of an antigen antibody reaction was the inactivation of their pyridine coenzymes following intracellular histamine liberation. Subsequent lysis of the cells and liberation of the excess histamine in the surrounding could have been the result of metabolic failure of the mast cells due to deprivation of respiratory coenzymes. In this manner the effect of nicotinamide could be understood. The prerequisites for such an interpretation, i.e., presence of DPNase, DPN^+ and histamine, the latter at quantities at least 10 times as those of DPN^+, were demonstrated in mast cells (F. UNGAR and S. G. A. ALIVISATOS, unpublished observations). Unfortunately, considering the multitude of substances qualifying as protecting agents (MOTA et al., 1960; MOTA and DIAS DA SILVA, 1960b) a non specific effect of nicotinamide upon the mast cells cannot be excluded with certainty (M. ROCHA E SILVA, personal communication).

Another point of interest is that equations (IIa) and (IIb), occurring within the pH range of activity of the diphosphopyridine nucleotidase (pH 6.0 to pH 9.0), are accompanied by the ejection of a hydrogen ion (ALIVISATOS, 1960). This observation, together with the well known effects of histamine upon the secretion of hydrogen ions from the stomach mucosa led recently to the following proposal (ALIVISATOS, 1960): An "onium" structure (similar to those present in pyridine coenzymes or S-adenosyl methionine) involving either nitrogen or sulfur, may constitute the so called "hydrogen ion pump", i.e. the structure whose hydrolysis or, alternatively, imidazolysis, would yield the necessary hydrogen ions. This "onium" structure could be an integral part of either a relatively small molecule or a large entity, possibly a lipoprotein embeded in the mosaic of the cell membrane of the secretory cells. A similar intracellular distribution could also apply to the enzyme responsible for the catalysis of the postulated processes. In view of the large quantities of hydrogen ions secreted in the stomach, these processes should be reversible, provided that the required energy from aerobic or glycolytic metabolic sources would be available. However, in view of the irreversibility of the hydrolytic or imidazolytic degradation of "onium" structures (ALIVISATOS, 1959), restoration would probably proceed through phosphorolytic pathways involving ribonucleoside triphosphates (ALIVISATOS, 1960).

Experimental

In *in vitro* studies of the histaminolysis of pyridine coenzymes (ALIVISATOS, 1958a, b; ALIVISATOS et al., 1960) the enzyme was a solubilized and purified preparation from beef spleen (ALIVISATOS and WOOLLEY, 1956). However, well washed homogenates (ALIVISATOS and WOOLLEY, 1956) from various organs, including beef spleen and guinea pig lung may also be utilized for qualitative studies.

Tissues either freshly obtained or stored at —20°C for up to a year's period are cut into small pieces. An approximately equal volume of cold 0.05 M Tris (hydroxymethyl)-aminomethane-HCl buffer (abbreviated Tris), pH 7.5 is added and the mixture is homogenized in the cold, in a Waring Blender for 4 minutes. The homogenate is then passed through cheese cloth to remove larger particles which are discarded. Soluble proteins are removed by washing the particles 3 times on the centrifuge (16.000 $\times$ *g* for 30 minutes) with cold 0.9% NaCl buffered with 0.05 M Tris. Stored at —20°C such homogenates retain their activity for several months. Methods for the solubilization and partial purification of the enzyme from washed particles have been described (ALIVISATOS and WOOLLEY, 1956; HOFMANN, 1957; WALLENFELS et al., 1960).

The enzymic activity of various preparations is expressed in terms of units. A unit is defined (ZATMAN et al., 1953; ABDEL-LATIF and ALIVISATOS, 1961 b, 1962) as the amount of enzymic protein catalyzing the hydrolysis of one μmole of DPN^+ per hour under standard conditions (i.e., 0.7 μmoles of DPN^+ in a total volume of one ml, buffered with 0.1 M tris at pH 8.0; the quantity of enzyme (DPNase) to be included in the test should cause during incubation (15 min at 38°C) split of approximately one third of the DPN^+ originally present. The reaction is stopped by addition of 6 ml 2 M cyanide. Spectrophotometric readings of the cyanoderivative in one cm. lightpath quartz cuvettes at 327 mμ against a sample from which DPN^+ was omitted. Molar extinction coefficient 6.000 M^{-1} cm^{-1}; results are extrapolated to one hour incubation).

In small scale histaminolytic experiments designed for the detection of histaminolysis in a given tissue, or for studies of the influence of the concentration of the reactants (Figure 1), or of the pH upon the yield of diphosphohistamine nucleotide the mixture (0.5 ml) contains 5 μmoles DPN^+, 10 units of DPNase and histamine (0 to 500 μmoles). In order to avoid large buffer concentrations, the desired quantities of histamine are usually composed from free base histamine and from the dihydrochloride of histamine. The ratio of the two forms is chosen so as to obtain the desired pH value (ALIVISATOS et al., 1960).

Further buffering is achieved by addition of 0.025 M acetate, phosphate, tris, or pyrophosphate, according to the desired pH. Most studies are performed at pH 8.1, with tris. The progress of histaminolysis is conveniently followed by the

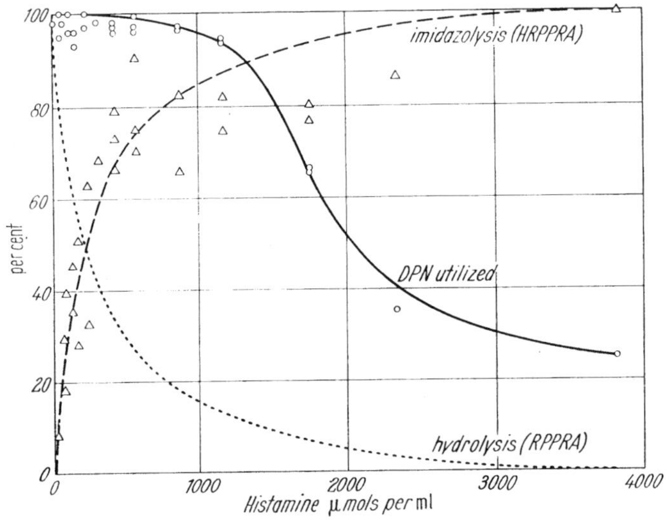

Fig. 1. Dependence of yield of diphosphohistamine nucleotide on concentration of histamine. The reaction mixture (0.505 ml) contained 0.25 ml of 0.1 M (with respect to pyrophosphate) sodium pyrophosphate-phosphoric acid buffer, pH 8.35; 5 μmoles of DPN^+; 11.5 units of DPNase; and histamine at quantities indicated in the abscissa. The ratio of histamine-free base to its dihydrochloride was 1.08, in all cases. The pH of the mixtures at zero time was 8.20 and remained almost constant during the experimental period (4 hr, 38°). Appropriate controls (omission of DPN, DPNase, or histamine) accompanied the experimentals at all histamine concentrations. The reaction was stopped by addition of 1 N HCl to pH 1.0 at 0° C. Yields of diphosphohistamine nucleotide (HRPPRA) and of diphosphoribose nucleotide (RPPRA) were calculated on the basis of total DPN^+ utilization (alcohol dehydrogenase) from the apparent decrease of ribose initially detectable by orcinol. (From J. biol. Chem. **235**, 1742, 1960) (ALIVISATOS et al., 1960)

apparent decrease of ribose, as determined by the orcinol procedure (MEJBAUM, 1939) in aliquots taken at various time intervals from the incubation mixture (ALIVISATOS, 1958a, b; ALIVISATOS et al., 1960). This apparent decrease is due to the formation of the histamine-ribose bond, which, under the conditions of the test (ALIVISATOS and LAMANTIA, 1960), is resistent to acid hydrolysis.

Preparative experiments are designed so as to achieve maximum histaminolytic utilization of the coenzyme (DPN^+ or TPN^+). Main factors to be considered are the inhibitory action of nicotinamide which is generated during reaction (I) and the competition between histamine and H_2O [reactions (II) and (III)]. The former is overcome by utilization of relatively large enzyme concentrations (approximately two units for every μmole of the coenzymes). The latter imposes high histamine concentrations (1 to 2 M) in the reaction medium. When histamine analogues of the coenzymes labeled with C^{14} or N^{15} at the histamine moiety are desired, an additional limitation should be considered: the content of labeled atoms per mole of the product will depend on the dilution of labeled histamine by non-labeled compound. Since at least 1 M histamine concentrations are required (see above), the total volume of incubation should be held at a minimum.

In a typical preparation 522 μmoles of previously neutralized DPN^+, 1007 μmoles (100 μcuries) 2(ring)C^{14}-labeled histamine (pH 8.1) 2570 units DPNase, 340 μmoles sodium pyrophosphate, pH 8.4 and 1050 μmoles Tris, pH 8.3 were incubated in a volume of 2.5 ml at 38° C. Complete utilization of the DPN^+ originally present was achieved in 8 hours (alcohol dehydrogenase). The mixture was then immersed in boiling water bath for 90 seconds, insoluble proteins were removed by centrifugation, and the supernatant was separated on a Dowex 50 hydrogen form column (ALIVISATOS, 1958a, b; ALIVISATOS et al., 1960). The eluate obtained with 0.666 N HCl contained the dinucleotide. It was lyophilized to dryness, the residue was redissolved in a small volume of water and filtered. Ten volumes of ethyl alcohol and 600 μmoles of barium acetate were added to the filtrate and it was left overnight at 4° C. The barium salt of the dinucleotide (152 μmoles, 55,000 counts per minute per μmole in a windowless flow counter) was obtained as a white precipitate. In ionophoretic studies (ALIVISATOS, 1958a, b; ALIVISATOS et al., 1960) it moved as a single spot, covering the expected relative distances at the right directions in 3 different pH values.

Summary

Histamine interacts irreversibly with coenzymes I and II. The products, diphosphohistamine nucleotide and triphosphohistamine nucleotide, were isolated and their properties were studied. There are indications that interactions of this nature may occur *in vivo* and that they might be involved in certain phases of histaminic biologic reactions.

Acknowledgment

Research described in this contribution was partly supported by grants from the National Science Foundation (GB306), the U.S. National Institutes of Health (GM-10981), the American Cancer Society (P241) and its Illinois Section, and a contract with the U.S. Atomic Energy Commission [AT(11-1)1221].

Addendum in press

It was recently demonstrated that when 2(ring, histamine)C^{14}-labeled histamine-adenine dinucleotide phosphate (i.e., the histamine analogue of coenzyme II) is administered to experimental animals (mice or guinea pigs), it is converted almost exclusively to histamine ribonucleoside (ALIVISATOS et al., 1963). It was also demonstrated in *in vivo* experiments that histamine ribonucleoside cannot be oxidized to imidazoleacetic acid ribonucleoside (ALIVISATOS et al., 1963). Preliminary evidence indicates that histamine ribonucleoside is found among the urinary excretion products after administration of 2 C^{14}-labeled histamine to experimental animals (S. G. A. ALIVISATOS, in press).

In other experiments, it was recently demonstrated (ALIVISATOS et al., 1964) that histamine (50 mM) and serotonin (10 mM) *in vitro* uncouple oxidative phosphorylation in mitochondria. In view of the probable involvement of protein-bound phosphohistidine as an intermediate in oxidative phosphorylation (PETER et al., 1963) it is probable that histamine or serotonin interfere with the activation process leading to the formation of the phosphohistidine intermediate. According to a proposal (ESTABROOK et al., 1963), pyridine coenzymes are involved in this activation. If this is correct, it is probable that uncoupling occurs by virtue of charge transfer complexing (ALIVISATOS et al., 1961; VAN EYS, 1958). Most recently it was found that serotonin may serve as a mediator of the nonenzymic oxidation of DPN^+ by cytochrome *c* (ALIVISATOS and WILLIAMS-ASHMAN, 1964) and this might explain, partially, the effect of certain hydroxylated indoles in oxidative phosphorylation. With respect to the mechanism of action of DPNase, KOSOWER (KOSOWER, 1962) recently proposed that electrostatic interactions leading to "intimate ion pair" formation rather than covalent bonding (ALIVISATOS, 1959) between the adenosine-diphosphoribose radical and the enzyme might better explain the action of this enzyme in transfer, etc., reactions.

Nomenclature: Since this review was written, the terminology of pyridine coenzymes changed (Report of the Commission of Enzymes of the International Union of Biochemistry, Pergamon Press, Oxford 1961, p. 16) as follows: Diphosphopyridine nucleotide was renamed *nicotinamide-adenine dinucleotide*, abbreviated *NAD*; triphosphopyridine nucleotide was renamed *nicotinamide-adenine dinucleotide phosphate (NADP)*. Accordingly, histamine analogues of these coenzymes are termed: *Histamine-adenine dinucleotide (HAD)* and *histamine-adenine dinucleotide phosphate (HADP)*. Diphosphopyridine nucleotidase is now termed *nicotinamideadenine dinucleotidase (NADase)* or *NAD-glycohydrolase*.

References

ABDEL-LATIF, A. A., and S. G. A. ALIVISATOS: Imidazolytic processes. IV. Enzymic formation of triphosphohistamine nucleotide. J. biol. Chem. **236**, 2710 (1961a).

— — Alternative pathways of enzymic formation of ribotides and ribosides of histamine. Biochim. biophys. Acta (Amst.) **51**, 398 (1961b).

— — Purification and properties of pyridine nucleosidase (Glycosidase) from bull semen. J. biol. Chem. **237**, 500 (1962).

ALECHINSKY, A.: Nicotinamide et choc histaminique. C. R. Soc. Biol. (Paris) **141**, 524 (1947).

ALIVISATOS, S. G. A.: Formation of histamine containing dinucleotides by enzymatic interaction of histamine and coenzyme I. Nature (Lond.) **181**, 271 (1958a).

— Enzymatic interaction of histamine and coenzyme I with formation of a new dinucleotide. Fed. Proc. **17**, 180 (1958b).

— The mechanism of action of diphosphopyridine nucleotidases. Nature (Lond.) **183**, 1034 (1959).

— Mechanism of the gastric secretion of hydrogen ions. Nature (Lond.) **186**, 368 (1960).

— Histamine-Pyridine Coenzyme Interactions. In a Symposium of the Histamine Club, Chicago, April 1964. Edited by G. UNGAR. Fed. Proc. In Press.

—, and A. A. ABDEL-LATIF: Enzymic interaction of TPN with histamine. Proc. 138th Nat. Meet. Amer. Chem. Soc., p. 26c (1960).

— — unpublished observations.

— — F. UNGAR, and G. A. MOURKIDES: *In vivo* degradation of histamine-adenine dinucleotide phosphate to histamine ribonucleoside. Nature **199**, 907 (1963).

—, and O. F. DENSTEDT: Lactic dehydrogenase and DPNase activity of blood. Science **114**, 281 (1951).

—, and L. LAMANTIA: Resistance to acid hydrolysis of N-ribosyl derivatives of various substituted imidazoles and pyrimidine imidazoles (purines). Biochem. biophys. Res. Commun. **2**, 164 (1960).

— —, and B. MATIJEVITCH: Imidazolytic processes. V. Enzymically catalyzed reactivity of certain imidazoles with coenzyme I. Biochim. biophys. Acta (Amst). **58**, 201 (1962).

— — F. UNGAR, and B. SAVICH: Enzymic formation of inosinic-adenylic pyrophosphate. Biochim. biophys. Acta (Amst.) **30**, 660 (1958).

— In: J. H. SHAFFER, G. A. LOGRIPPO, and M. W. CHASE: (Editors), "Mechanisms of Hypersensitivity", p. 259. Boston: Little, Brown & Co. 1959.

— — A. JIBRIL, and G. A. MOURKIDES: Non-enzymic reactions of indoles with pyridine coenzymes and related structures. Biochim. biophys. Acta (Amst.) **51**, 361 (1961).

— F. UNGAR, O. CALLAGHAN, and C. BIAVA: Effect of indoles and imidazoles, including serotonin and histamine, on the morphology and oxidative phosphorylation of guinea pig liver mitochondria. Nature **201**, 47 (1964).

— —, and L. LUKACS: On the mechanism of biologic histaminic reactions, p. 387. Vth International Congress of Biochemistry, Moscow, August 1961b. London: Pergamon Press 1961.

— — —, and L. LAMANTIA: Imidazolytic processes. III. Enzymic conversion of coenzyme I to histamine dinucleotide. J. biol. Chem. **235**, 1742 (1960).

—, and H. G. WILLIAMS-ASHMAN: Serotonin-mediated oxidation of dihydronico-tinamide derivatives by cytochrome *c*. Biochim. biophys. Acta (Amst.) **86**, 392 (1964).

—, and D. W. WOOLLEY: Solubilization and purification of the diphosphopyridine nucleotidase from beef spleen. J. biol. Chem. **219**, 823 (1956).

BUTTURINI, U.: Sull'azione antiistamica ed antiallergica dell'amide nicotinica; ricerche cliniche e sperimentali. G. Clin. med. **27**, 681 (1946).

CROWLEY, G. M.: Enzymatic synthesis of imidazoleacetic acid ribotide. Fed. Proc. **19**, 309 (1960).

DAINOW, I.: Recherches cliniques sur certaines propriétés anti-allergiques de la nicotinamide. Z. Vitaminforsch. **15**, 245 (1944).

ESTABROOK, R. W., J. GONZE, and S. P. NISSLEY: A possible role for pyridine nucleotide in coupling mechanism of oxidative phosphorylation. Fed. Proc. **22**, 1071 (1963).

EYS, J. VAN: The reaction of quarternary pyridine derivatives with imidazoles. J. biol. Chem. **233**, 1203 (1958).

FERNANDES, J. F., O. CASTELLANI, and M. PLESE: Biosynthesis of histamine ribotide and imidazoleacetate ribotide. Biochem. biophys. Res. Commun. **3**, 679 (1960).

GROSSMAN, L., and N. O. KAPLAN: Nicotinamide riboside phosphorylase from human erythrocytes. I. Phosphorolytic activity. J. biol. Chem. **231**, 717 (1958).

HALPERN, B. N., et I. DAÏNOW: Recherches expérimentales sur une nouvelle propriété pharmacodynamique de l'amide nicotinique: action antagoniste vis-à-vis de certain effets de l'histamine. Z. Vitaminforsch. **15**, 250 (1944).

HEPPEL, L. A., and R. J. HILMOE: Purification and properties of 5-nucleotidase. J. biol. Chem. **188**, 665 (1951).

HOFMANN, E. C. G.: DPN- und TPN-spezifische Nucleosidasen in Erythrocyten. I. Spezifität und Reinigung der Enzyme. Biochem. Z. **329**, 428 (1957).
KAPLAN, N. O.: In: P. D. BOYER, H. LARDY, and K. MYRBÄCK (Editors), "The Enzymes" Vol. 3, p. 166. New York and London: Academic Press 1960.
KARJALA, S. A.: The partial characterization of a histamine metabolite from rat and mouse urine. J. Amer. chem. Soc. **77**, 504 (1955).
KOBAYASHI, Y.: A histamine metabolizing enzyme system of mouse liver. Arch. Biochem. **71**, 352 (1957).
KORNBERG, A., and W. E. PRICER, JR.: Nucleotide pyrophosphatase. J. biol. Chem. **182**, 763 (1950).
KOSOWER, E. M.: "Molecular Biochemistry" pp. 109, 250. New York: McGraw-Hill 1962.
LEONE, E., and L. BONADUCE: Soluble pyridine nucleotide nucleosidase from seminal vesicles. Biochim. biophys. Acta (Amst.) **31**, 292 (1959).
MEJBAUM, W.: Über die Bestimmung kleiner Pentosemengen insbesondere in Derivaten der Adenylsäure. Hoppe-Seylers Z. physiol. Chem. **258**, 117 (1939).
MOTA, I., and W. DIAS DA SILVA: Antigen-induced damage to isolated sensitized mast cells. Nature (Lond.) **186**, 245 (1960a).
— — The anti-anaphylactic and histamine releasing properties of the antihistamines. Their effect on the mast cells. Brit. J. Pharmacol. **15**, 396 (1960b).
— —, and J. FERREIRA FERNANDES: The inhibition of mast cell damage and histamine release in anaphylaxis by pyridine and diphosphopyridine nucleotidase inhibitors. Comparison with compound 48/80. Brit. J. Pharmacol. **15**, 405 (1960).
MURAOKA, S., M. INOUE, and H. YAMASAKI: Enzymic formation of histamine ribotide from histamine dinucleotide. Nature (Lond.) **190**, 532 (1961).
PETER, J. V., D. E. HULTQUIST, M. DELUCA, G. KREIL, and P. D. BOYER: Bound phosphohistidine as an intermediate in a phosphorylation reaction of oxidative phosphorylation catalyzed by mitochondrial extracts. J. biol. Chem. **238**, PC 1182 (1963).
SCHAYER, R. W.: Catabolism of physiological quantities of histamine *in vivo*. Physiol. Rev. **39**, 116 (1959).
TABOR, H., and O. HAYAISHI: The excretion of imidazoleacetic acid riboside following the administration of imidazoleacetic acid or histamine to rats. J. Amer. chem. Soc. **77**, 505 (1955).
WALLENFELS, K., D. STATHAKOS, and H. DIEKMANN: A new procedure for the solubilization of beef spleen diphosphopyridine nucleotidase. Biochem. biophys. Res. Commun. **3**, 632 (1960).
ZATMAN, L. J., N. O. KAPLAN, and S. P. COLOWICK: Inhibition of spleen diphosphopyridine nucleotidase by nicotinamide, an exchange reaction. J. biol. Chem. **200**, 197 (1953).
— — —, and M. M. CIOTTI: Effect of isonicotinic acid hydrazide on diphosphopyridine nucleotidases. J. biol. Chem. **209**, 453 (1954).
ZELLER, E. A., and J. BARSKY: *In vivo* inhibition of liver and brain monoamine oxidase by 1-isonicotinyl-2-isopropyl hydrazine. Proc. Soc. exp. Biol. (N. Y.) **81**, 459 (1952).
— P. STERN, and L. A. BLANKSMA: Degradation of histamine by monoamine oxidase. Naturwissenschaften **43**, 157 (1956).

Section F

Histamine Metabolism in Man*[1]

By

S. E. LINDELL and H. WESTLING

With 7 Figures

It has been shown that there are considerable differences between the species as regards the catabolism of histamine both in vitro (BLASCHKO, FRIEDMAN, HAWES and NILSSON, 1959) and in vivo (SCHAYER, 1956, 1959). Such differences have also been found in studies of histamine formation (WATON, 1956; SCHAYER, see Chapter 4, Section D). Besides, it is well known, that some species are more sensitive to histamine than others and that man has a comparatively high sensitivity. For these reasons alone a separate discussion of histamine metabolism in man seems warranted. Furthermore histamine metabolism in man has been studied not only in healthy subjects but also in patients with various diseases. The abundant literature on the occurrence of histamine in various tissues, blood and urine from man has recently been reviewed by VAN ARSDEL and BEALL (1960) and by DUNÉR and PERNOW (1960).

In the present review of the metabolism of histamine in man the subject will be divided into 7 parts, of which the first will deal with *the formation of histamine*. The second part will be entitled *the catabolism of histamine in man*. Then will follow data on the *occurrence of histamine in tissues, blood and urine* in health and disease. Finally we shall discuss some of these observations in the light of the present knowledge of formation and catabolism of histamine in man. In doing so we shall point out some methodological difficulties and limitations.

I. Histamine formation in man

A. General remarks

Opinion has been divided over the origin of histamine in the body. One view is that man cannot synthesize histamine himself but has to rely on other manufacturers, e.g. intestinal bacteria for his supply of histamine. This view has been eloquently expressed by GADDUM (1956), who referred to histamine as a vitamin. The basis for this theory is found in WATON's experiments (1956). WATON studied the decarboxylation of histidine in various species, including man. There was no demonstrable histamine formation from L-histidine incubated with human, canine or feline tissues, while tissues from rodents such as rabbit, rat and guinea pig showed a considerable decarboxylation of histidine attributed to an enzyme called histidine decarboxylase.

GADDUM's hypothesis is supported by the observation that bacteria, some of which are normally present in the human intestine (EGGERTH, 1939; WERLE, 1941) can decarboxylate histidine which is a normal constituent of our food.

* Supported by United States Public Health Service (Grant E 3379).

[1] This review attempts to cover the literature up to December 1961.

It has also been shown that when L-histidine (4–5 g) was given by mouth the urinary excretion of free and conjugated histamine increased (IRVINE et al., 1959). Pretreatment with succinylsulphathiazole prevented this increased excretion of histamine almost completely and for this reason it seems likely that most of the increase in urinary histamine was due to histamine formed by intestinal bacteria. However, DUNÉR et al. (1961) found no increase in the urinary excretion of free and conjugated histamine after ingestion of 5 g L-histidine by 4 healthy subjects.

Additional support for GADDUM's theory might be taken from experiments published by DEMIS and BROWN (1961). These authors gave 14 mg L-histidine labelled with C^{14} (10 μC) orally to 11 healthy subjects, two patients with urticaria pigmentosa and one patient with chronic urticaria and found no radioactive histamine or known histamine metabolites in the urine.

It should be mentioned here that very large doses of histamine (133 mg) have been given orally to man without any significant increase in urinary free histamine (ADAM, 1949). This should mean that less than 2 mg histamine reached the circulating blood (ADAM, CARD, RIDDELL, ROBERTS and STRONG, 1954) and indicates that histamine in the intestine is fairly efficiently metabolized before it is absorbed by the blood, if it is absorbed.

The idea that human tissues take up and store histamine of exogenous origin is not easy to reconcile with the results of the studies made by SCHAYER and his co-workers. SCHAYER and COOPER (1956) injected histamine labelled with C^{14} in the 2-position of the imidazole ring intradermally in 3 healthy subjects. All the injected C^{14} was excreted in the urine within 48 hours, and most of it within 6–12 hours. Similar results have later been obtained by others (NILSSON et al., 1959), who have given C^{14}-histamine subcutaneously or intravenously.

Studies on the fate of C^{14}-labelled histamine given by mouth are limited to one subject (SCHAYER, 1956). From these it is impossible to exclude the possibility that some of the injected histamine was retained in the body. It seems, however, very unlikely that histamine absorbed into the blood from the intestine should be treated differently from histamine absorbed from the subcutaneous tissue or injected directly intravenously.

To summarize the evidence from experiments in intact man it may be said that there is little to show that the human body can form histamine from L-histidine. But there is also no evidence that man can take up and store histamine, on the contrary there is strong evidence that any histamine absorbed from the intestine is efficiently metabolized before reaching the systemic circulation. In the opinion of the present authors, it seems rather likely that man like other animals (SCHAYER, Chapter 4, Section D) produces its own histamine and does not store exogenous histamine.

B. Formation of histamine in vitro

In animals the formation of labelled histamine from L-histidine labelled with C^{14} in the imidazole ring has been repeatedly demonstrated by SCHAYER (see Chapter 4, Section D). It might be expected that SCHAYER's technique could be used with advantage also in studies of histidine decarboxylase in human tissue. In this way LILJA, LINDELL and SALDEEN (1960) demonstrated decarboxylation of histidine in *human lung tissue* in the absence of bacteria. DEMIS and BROWN (1961) and LINDELL et al. (1961 a) found histamine formation from L-histidine incubated with *skin from subjects with urticaria pigmentosa. Blood from subjects with chronic myelogenous leukemia* has been found to decarboxylate histidine under sterile conditions (HARTMAN, CLARK and CYR, 1961). The authors attributed this decarboxylation to the basophil cells. This finding was confirmed by LINDELL, RORSMAN and WESTLING (1961b), who also demonstrated histamine formation from C^{14}-histidine in blood from healthy subjects and patients with polycythemia vera. The capacity of the blood samples to form histamine correlated well with the number of basophils.

Table 1. *Formation of C^{14}-histamine by human stomach in vitro*[1]

The figures refer to amounts of C^{14}-histamine formed from C^{14}-L-histidine by 1 g of tissue during 3 hours and are expressed as counts per minute above background (cpm)/g. 1 μg histamine formed from this histidine is calculated to give 5100 cpm under the standardized conditions of assay used. The experimental condition in exp. 1—4 were different from those in exp. 5—8.

Case no. and diagnosis	Mucosa		Muscularis + submucosa	
	corpus	antrum	corpus	antrum
1. Peptic ulcer	77	19	0	—
2. Peptic ulcer	45	—	0	—
3. Peptic ulcer	25	13	1	9
4. Achlorhydria. Gastric cancer	21	—	3	—
5. Peptic ulcer	133	—	0	—
6. Peptic ulcer	158	121	0	—
7. Peptic ulcer	177	30	0	—
8. Achlorhydria. Gastric cancer	126	—	0	—

[1] LINDELL, WESTLING and ZEDERFELDT, unpublished.

Recently we have had the opportunity to examine histamine formation in *human gastric mucosa* which is known to be rich in histamine. The specimens were obtained from gastric resection for ulcer or cancer. The tissues were minced with scissors and suspended in 0.1 M phosphate buffer and incubated with 40 μg C^{14}-labelled L-histidine for 3 hours in an atmosphere of nitrogen. The amount of C^{14}-histamine formed was measured with SCHAYER's isotope dilution technique. 1 μg histamine formed from this histidine should give 5100 cpm above background under our standardized conditions of assay. The results are given in Table 1.

There was thus a considerable histamine formation in the mucosa irrespective of whether the subject had achlorhydria or not.

Table 2 shows the formation of histamine in tissues *from human foetuses* (obtained at abortions for psychiatric reasons). The incubations were carried out as mentioned above.

Table 2. *Formation of C^{14}-histamine by various tissues from human foetuses in vitro*[1]

The figures refer to amounts of C^{14}-histamine formed from C^{14}-L-histidine by 1 g of tissue during 3 hours and are expressed as cpm/g. 1 μg histamine formed from this histidine is calculated to give 5100 cpm under the standardized conditions of assay used.

(Foetuses were 20—24 weeks old. Pregnancy terminated for psychiatric reasons.)

Tissue	1.	2.	3.	4.
Abdominal skin	45	58	18	44
Lung	4	8	0	2
Spleen	181	207	—	169
Liver	46	13	26	22
Stomach	55	31	33	19
Small intestine	11	—	29	10
Kidney	8	6	0	—
Heart	18	7	3	7
Adrenals	—	—	23	—
Cerebral hemisphere	25	21	5	6
Cerebellum	—	8	44	—
Brain stem	—	19	—	7
Hypothalamus	92	—	51	76
Spinal cord	—	—	14	—

[1] LINDBERG, LINDELL and WESTLING 1963.

The comparatively high activity found in the hypothalamus agrees with the observations in animals made by WHITE (1960). A great amount of histidine decarboxylase has been found in the rat foetus by KAHLSON et al. (1958) and notably in the liver (KAHLSON et al., 1959), and it is interesting to note that in comparison with other human foetal tissues the liver has a considerable activity, which, however, is low compared with the activity in the foetal liver of rats. So far very few data for histidine decarboxylase activity in normal adult tissues are available. The activity found in foetal skin may, however, be compared with the absence of activity in normal skin from healthy adults studied under identical conditions (LINDELL and WESTLING, unpublished). The higher histidine decarboxylase activity in foetal skin may be related to the rapid growth as discussed by KAHLSON (1960).

With the aid of SCHAYER's refined techniques it has thus been possible to demonstrate in vitro histamine formation from L-histidine in foetal tissues and also in some adult tissues.

C. Histamine formation in intact man

Histamine formation in intact man has yet to be demonstrated. Considerable difficulties may be expected in such a study. Only a very small part of histidine (less than 0.1%) given to animals is converted to histamine (SCHAYER, see Chapter 4, Section D). Of this newly formed histamine only a very small part may be expected to reach the urine in unchanged form. The time required for the newly formed histamine to leave its site and reach the blood and then the urine is not known. With the technique used now for the demonstration of formation of histamine from C^{14}-labelled histidine one will probably have to inject 1000 μC of C^{14}-histidine (free of C^{14}-histamine) to be able to get measurable quantities of C^{14}-histamine in the urine. To be conclusive the study will have to be performed in subjects with sterilized intestinal content and with precautions taken to prevent histamine formation by bacteria in the urine. Finally it should be mentioned that the possibility has not been excluded that histamine is synthesized directly, i.e. without passing through the state of histidine. There is, however, no evidence that such a histamine formation occurs in animal experiments (SCHAYER, 1952).

II. Catabolism of histamine in man

When investigating the cause of the transiency of the effects of injected histamine, BEST and MCHENRY (1930) discovered an enzyme that inactivated histamine. This enzyme which was abundantly present in the kidney and in the intestinal mucosa of the dog was called histaminase. ZELLER (1938) found that the same enzyme oxidized several diamines and for this reason suggested that it should be called diamine oxidase.

A. Histaminase or diamine oxidase

(See also Chapter 4, Sections A and B)

Histaminase or diamine oxidase inactivates histamine through oxidative deamination of the side chain. In this process oxygen is consumed and ammonia formed. The first product is imidazoleacetaldehyde which is usually but not always further oxidized to imidazoleacetic acid (LINDAHL et al., 1958; LINDAHL, 1960). The occurrence of diamine oxidase in a tissue can be demonstrated by incubation with histamine and measurement of the loss of biological activity or by manometric measurement of ammonia formation or oxygen consumption. If C^{14}-labelled histamine is used in the incubation the appearance of C^{14}-imidazoleacetic acid can be followed by SCHAYER's isotope dilution technique. To ensure the identity of the enzyme it is necessary to use specific and competitive inhibitors.

Table 3. *Diamine oxidase (histaminase) activity of various human tissues*

Tissue	Enzyme activity	Technique and comments	Author
Adult		Manometric measurement of oxygen consumption. Values are given in DoE, i.e. enzyme activity giving a consumption of 11.2 mm³ O_2 or formation of 17 μg ammonia per hour, per gram tissue	ZELLER, BIRKHÄUSER, MISLIN and WENK, 1939
Renal cortex	1.4		
Renal medulla	1.8		
Liver	1.3		
Adrenal	1.7		
Pancreas	0.6		
Placenta	>0.5		
Brain gray matter	0.1		
Brain white matter	0.2		
Brain stem	0.2		
Lung	+		
Newborn renal cortex	0.1		
Newborn renal medulla	1.6		
Liver	>0.2		
Adrenal	>0.3		
Brain	0		
Skin	17—25	μg histamine inactivated in 24 hours by 1 g at 37° C. Code's method	GRANROTH and NILZÉN, 1949
Skin	10	μg histamine inactivated by 1 g in 12 hours as determined by bioassay	STÜTTGEN, 1955
Skin	0	Bioassay and Kapeller-Adler's method	LEVI, MENEGHINI and RANTUCCIO, 1959
Uterus	0—2	μg histamine inactivated by 1 g in 1.5 hours at 37° C as determined by bioassay	EFFKEMANN and WERLE, 1940
Placenta	30—100		
Uterine mucosa	1—6		
Placenta	56—102	μg histamine base inactivated/g/hour. Code's method of assay	AHLMARK, 1944
Placenta normal	42—220	Simplification of Ahlmark's method. μg histamine inactivated/g/hour	WICKSELL, 1949a
Placenta normal	see Fig. 7	μg histaminedihydrochloride inactivated/g/hour. Ahlmark's method	SWANBERG, 1950 (Fig. 8, page 30)
Placenta normal	49800±10700	Permanganate units per placenta. Kapeller-Adler's method. Mean values and standard deviation	KAPELLER-ADLER, 1953
Placenta toxemia	38640±6100		
Pronounced toxemia	22520±7840		
Pronounced duplex	98040±12042		
Adult kidney	0.8—2.5	μg C^{14}-histamine converted to imidazoleacetic acid by 1g tissue in 3 hours at 37° C	LINDELL, 1958
Adult lung	0.1	As above	LILJA, LINDELL and SALDEEN, 1960
Placenta	50—180	μg histaminedihydrochloride metabolized/g/hour	LINDAHL, 1960

Table 4. *Histamine catabolism in human blood*

Diagnosis	Enzyme activity	Technique and comments	Author
	Inactivation of histamine in μg		
Healthy female	1.0—1.6	3 ml of defibrinated blood incubated with 3—50 μg histamine for 1.5 hours at 37° C. Assay of remaining histamine on isolated guinea pig ileum without chemical purification	Werle and Effkemann, 1940a
	0.0 (serum)		
Tuberculosis	0.3		
Cancer	1.0—1.8		
Pregnancy	5.0—47		
	17 (serum)		
Foetal	0.3—1.6	Blood from umbilical cord	
	0.0	Serum from umbilical cord	
	Inactivation of histamine in μg base per ml plasma per hour	Heparinized plasma incubated with histamine (0.6—1.5 μg/ml) for 10 minutes to 22 hours	Ahlmark, 1944
Healthy males	0.006±0.001	Code's method for extraction and bioassay	
Healthy non-pregnant females	0.005±0.0006		
Healthy pregnant females	0.005—5.0	See Fig. 6 (Ahlmark, 1944; p. 65 Fig. 12)	
Healthy non-pregnant females	0.007±0.001	Same as above but all values refer to histamine dihydrochloride	Swanberg, 1950
Foetus	0.012±0.002	Umbilical vein	
	0.014±0.003	Umbilical artery	
Pregnant	0.01 —3.5	Simplification of Ahlmark's method	Wicksell, 1949a
Foetal	0.007—0.023		Wicksell, 1949b
	Oxygen consumption in mm^3/3 ml serum/hour	Incubation with cadaverine for 6—20 hours. Serum dialysed	Zeller and Birkhäuser, 1940
Non-pregnant	0—6		
Pregnant	24—122		
	Permanganate units per ml serum	Kapeller-Adler's method. Incubation for 24 hours at 37° C	Kapeller-Adler, 1953
Pregnant	4.5—22		
Toxemia	1.5—12.2		
Foetal	0		Kapeller-Adler, 1952
Untreated cancer	0—4.5	Kapeller-Adler's method incubation with histamine for 24 hours	Benda and Miravet, 1960
Treated cancer	0—7		
Tuberculosis	0		

Systematic studies on the occurrence of diamine oxidase (histaminase) in human tissues have not been carried out. Available data are summarized in Table 3. A direct comparison of the data from different investigators is difficult or impossible because of variations in the techniques used. The identity of the active enzyme has not always been firmly established. When the incubation has lasted more than some hours it is not possible to exclude the action of bacterial enzymes unless the incubate is shown to be sterile.

The results of studies on the metabolism of histamine in human blood are given in Table 4.

The same reservations apply to these data as to those of Table 3. The measurement of histamine metabolism in blood is thoroughly discussed by AHLMARK (1944). The inactivation of histamine in blood from healthy non-pregnant subjects is so

Table 5. *The catabolism of C^{14}-histamine by human foetal tissues*[1]

Foetal tissues were obtained from abortions on psychiatric indication. 0.7—1.0 g minced tissue suspended in 2 ml 0.1 M phosphate buffer (pH 7.4) with 2 mg glucose per ml was incubated with C^{14}-histamine in an initial concentration of about 1.2 μg/ml. After 3 hours at 37° C in air the amount of C^{14}-histamine and its known metabolites in the samples was determined with Schayer's isotope dilution technique. Values are given in per cent of C^{14}-radioactivity added initially. The added histamine gave 13,000 cpm under our standardized conditions of assay.

Tissue	Case No.	Histamine	1,4-methyl-histamine	1,4-methylimidazoleacetic acid	Imidazole-acetic acid	sum of metabolites
Skin	1	48	58	0	0	106
	5	23	56	—	—	—
	6	38	—	—	—	—
	6	50[2]	—	—	—	—
Lung	1	3	108	14	0	125
	3	2	100	—	—	—
	5	2	92	—	—	—
	5	3[2]	92[2]	—	—	—
Liver	3	2	85	—	—	—
	5	1	77	—	—	—
	5	0[2]	85[2]	—	—	—
Kidney	1	0	9	19	66	94
	5	5	21	15	25	66
	5	27[2]	52[2]	12[2]	1[2]	92[2]
	6	8	33	31	36	108
	6	31[2]	86[2]	3[2]	0[2]	120[2]
Heart	1	37	68	1	0	106
	6	42	58	2	1	103
	6	51[2]	68[2]	2[2]	1[2]	122[2]
Small intestine	1	9	38	20	31	98
	3	3	24	—	—	—
	5	6	18	—	22	—
	5	28[2]	50[2]	1[2]	0[2]	79[2]
Brain hemisphere	1	58	46	0	0	104
	3	50	55	—	—	—
	4	18	52	—	—	—
	5	37	38	—	—	—
	6	43	62	1	1	107
	6	58[2]	44[2]	0[2]	0[2]	102[2]
Stomach	6	45	57	3	4	109
Brain stem	4	20	51	—	—	—
Cerebellum	5	42	36	—	—	—
	6	48	54	0	1	103
Hypothalamus	6	59	45	1	1	106

[1] LINDBERG, LINDELL and WESTLING, 1963.
[2] Aminoguanidine added to a concentration of 10^{-4} M.

small that it must be very difficult to demonstrate a decrease below normal. The phenomenon of "histaminopexy" will be discussed by PARROT (see Chapter 2, Section B).

The changes in histamine metabolism during pregnancy are discussed in part VIIb of this Section.

Urine which has been dialyzed for 16 hours has been found to inactivate histamine in amounts corresponding to roughly 1 μg histamine dihydrochloride per 3 ml urine per hour (WERLE, 1942). Dialyzed *sperm* incubated with cadaverine was found to consume oxygen at a rate of 2–3 mm^3 per ml sperm per hour (ZELLER, 1941).

The results of a study on the metabolism of C^{14}-histamine in human foetal tissues are given in Table 5. Since the experimental conditions were uniform the results with different tissues may be compared with each other.

It may be seen in the table that all tissues studied methylated histamine. Aminoguanidine in a concentration of 10^{-4} M did not inhibit the metabolism of histamine in lung or liver tissue where almost all the added histamine was methylated. There was thus no evidence for the presence of diamine oxidase in these tissues. In the kidney and in the wall of the intestine the metabolism of histamine was inhibited by aminoguanidine. This effect which was associated with a decrease in the amount of imidazoleacetic acid formed is very likely to be due to an inhibition of diamine oxidase.

B. Histamine-methylating enzyme (imidazole N-methyl transferase)

Published studies in vitro on the occurrence in human adult tissues of the histamine methylating enzyme discovered by SCHAYER are limited to observations on surgically obtained specimens of kidney and lung. LINDELL (1958) found that macroscopically normal renal tissue could form 1,4-methylimidazoleacetic acid from C^{14}-histamine. Human lung tissue can also form considerable quantities of 1,4-methylimidazoleacetic acid from C^{14}-histamine (LILJA et al., 1960).

LINDAHL (1960a, b) showed that methylation of histamine took place also in extracts of human placenta. She suggested that methylation may be the predominating reaction in vivo in the placenta. Blood from pregnant women does not methylate histamine (LINDAHL et al., 1958).

Acetylation of histamine by human tissues has not been demonstrated in vitro.

C. Histamine catabolism in vivo

Studies in intact man injected with non-radioactive histamine have shown that 1–4% of the injected histamine is excreted unchanged in the urine (ADAM et al., 1954; MITCHELL, 1956a; DUNÉR et al., 1961). Such studies do not allow any conclusions about the fate of the 96–99% which do not appear in the urine. Aminoguanidine which has been found to inhibit diamine oxidase in animals (SCHAYER, see Chapter 4, Section B) approximately doubled the part of the injected histamine which could be recovered in unchanged form in the urine (MITCHELL, 1956b). Thus 95% or more of the injected histamine could not be accounted for even though diamine oxidase probably was inhibited. An efficient inhibitor of the histamine methylating enzyme suitable for use in man is not known.

An advancement of our knowledge of histamine metabolism in intact man therefore required the application of SCHAYER's technique to man. SCHAYER and COOPER (1956) injected histamine labelled with C^{14} in the imidazole ring intradermally in 3 healthy men in a dose of 1 μg per kg body weight. Whithin 48 hours all the injected radioactivity was excreted in the urine. The urine was assayed for the known metabolites of histamine with SCHAYER's isotope dilution technique. 2–3% of the radioactivity of the urine was in the form of unchanged histamine. 4–8% was 1,4-methylhistamine, 42–47% was 1,4-methylimidazoleacetic acid. 9–11% was free imidazoleacetic acid, 16–23% was imidazoleacetic acid conjugated with ribose, and less than 1% was in the form of acetylhistamine.

SCHAYER (1956) gave 100 μg C^{14}-labelled histamine orally to a man. 66% of the radioactivity was excreted in the urine within 48 hours. There was no measurable amount of C^{14}-histamine in the urine and 1,4-methylimidazoleacetic acid accounted for 64% of the radioactivity in the urine.

Using the same method of analysis NILSSON et al. (1959) found that three human females metabolized C^{14}-histamine injected subcutaneously or intravenously in the same way as did SCHAYER's and COOPER's male subjects who had received about 10 times more C^{14}-histamine intradermally. Also in the female subjects there was little or no C^{14}-acetylhistamine in the urine.

These investigations showed clearly that in the subjects studied methylation was quantitatively the most important route of histamine metabolism.

BEALL and VAN ARSDEL (1960) found imidazoleacetic acid to be the most important metabolite of C^{14}-histamine in man. They did not use the isotope dilution technique with recrystallization to constant radioactivity as a means of separating the labelled metabolites from each other, but instead they used chromatography. It seems more likely that the divergency between their results and those of previous workers are due to this different technique than to individual differences in histamine metabolism. The small effect of aminoguanidine on the urinary excretion of free histamine after injection of histamine (MITCHELL, 1956b; ADAM and MITCHELL, 1957) does not support the idea that diamine oxidase is quantitatively important in the human metabolism of histamine.

The effects of some enzyme inhibitors on the metabolism of C^{14}-histamine in man have been studied by LINDELL et al. (1960). It was found that aminoguanidine in a dose of 0.1 mg per kg almost completely inhibited the formation of C^{14}-labelled imidazoleacetic acid. Aminoguanidine does not inhibit monoamine oxidase, and therefore these results do not support the hypothesis that monoamine oxidase is of importance for the oxidative deamination of histamine (ZELLER et al., 1956). Iproniazid inhibited both formation of 1,4-methylimidazoleacetic acid and imidazoleacetic acid. After iproniazid in a dose of 150 mg per day 40–50% of the injected C^{14} appeared in the urine as 1,4-methylhistamine. It is therefore evident that the methylating enzyme is capable of metabolizing the doses of histamine used here even when the oxidation of histamine and 1,4-methylhistamine are inhibited. In so far as it has been studied the methylation of histamine means that it becomes biologically inactive (LEE and JONES, 1949; WESTLING, 1957).

Chlorpromazine has been shown to inhibit the methylation of histamine in vitro (BROWN et al., 1959). However, in very large doses chlorpromazine did not inhibit the methylation of intravenously injected C^{14}-labelled histamine in man (JOHANSSON et al., 1961).

In the published studies of the metabolism of C^{14}-histamine in man the known metabolites, i.e. 1,4-methylhistamine, 1,4-methylimidazoleacetic acid, (free and conjugated) and acetylhistamine have accounted for 50–110% of the radioactivity excreted in the urine in 12–48 hours after injection of C^{14}-histamine. The unknown metabolite may be imidazoleacetaldehyde or 1,4-methylimidazoleacetaldehyde as discussed by NILSSON et al. (1959) and SCHAYER (1959). It is also possible that histamine may be methylated in the side chain (KAPELLER-ADLER and IGGO, 1957). Acetylation has not been found to be an important pathway in the metabolism of injected C^{14}-histamine in man. It is possible that acetylhistamine is formed when C^{14}-histamine is given orally to man or it may be that acetylation comes into play only when large doses of histamine are given.

Tables 6 and 7 summarize the results of studies of the metabolism of C^{14}-labelled histamine in man with the use of Schayer's technique. In addition to the

Table 6. *Catabolism of C^{14}-histamine in man.* Mean values for urinary excretion of total radioactivity, unchanged C^{14}-histamine and its main metabolites during 0—6 hours after an intradermal injection of 1 μg C^{14}-histamine per kg body weight

	No. of subjects	Excreted radioactivity in per cent of injected	Per cent of excreted radioactivity appearing as			
			Histamine	1,4-methylhistamine	1,4-methylimidazoleacetic acid	Total imidazoleacetic acid
Healthy males[1]	3	69	3	6	45	29
Healthy males[2]	7	55	4	6	59	28
Schizophrenics[2]	12	52	5	7	51	31

[1] SCHAYER and COOPER (1956).
[2] KOBAYASHI and FREEMAN (1961).

Table 7. *Catabolism of C^{14}-histamine in man.* Mean values for urinary excretion of "total" radioactivity, unchanged C^{14}-histamine and its main metabolites during 0—12 hours after a subcutaneous injection of about 10 μg C^{14}-histamine

Diagnosis	No. of subjects	Excreted radioactivity in per cent of injected	Per cent of excreted radioactivity appearing as				
			Histamine	Methylhistamine	Methylimidazoleacetic acid	Total imidazoleacetic acid	Sum of metabolites
Healthy[1 2]	4	82	1	8	60	25	93
Status asthmaticus[2]	3	64	2	7	63	33	103
Bronchial asthma, no symptoms[2] .	2	53	2	7	55	24	88
Bronchial asthma, steroid treatment[2]	2	50	1	7	60	28	96
Urticaria[2]	3	71	1	5	46	36	88
Pregnancy, 5th—6th month[1]	4	78	2	2	37	29	70
Psychiatric disease[3]	3	68	2	8	63	25	98

[1] NILSSON, LINDELL, SCHAYER and WESTLING, 1959.
[2] HELANDER, LINDELL, NILSSON and WESTLING, 1962.
[3] LINDELL, NILSSON, ROOS and WESTLING, 1960.

result of studies on normal male and female subjects mentioned above the table contains observations on 7 nonpsychotic male and 12 male schizophrenics studied by KOBAYASHI and FREEMAN (1961), 4 somatically healthy pregnant women studied by NILSSON et al. (1959), 10 allergic subjects from a study by HELANDER et al. (1962) and 3 subjects with psychiatric disease investigated by LINDELL et al. (1960). These studies will be discussed in the sections on pregnancy, allergy and mental disease. Suffice it to say here that the pattern of metabolism of injected C^{14}-histamine in all these subjects was remarkably uniform in spite of the fact that the dose of histamine varied between 10 and 100 μg.

D. Rate of elimination of C^{14} in the urine after injection of C^{14}-histamine

The rate of elimination into the urine of C^{14} after intravenous injection of C^{14}-labelled histamine has been studied by BEALL and VAN ARSDEL (1960). The recovery of the injected C^{14} is shown in Fig. 1 and 2. A subject with uremia differs markedly in the rate of elimination of C^{14}. Three patients of five with liver disease and one with bronchial asthma (of two studied) have a somewhat slower excretion of the injected C^{14} than the control subjects.

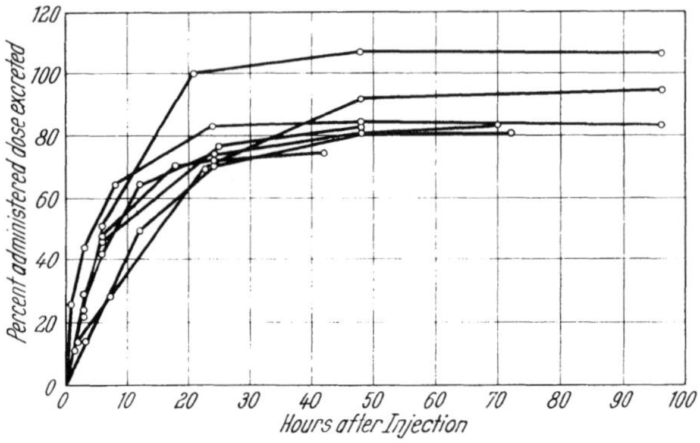

Fig. 1. Cumulative recovery of administered radioactivity from urine of seven control subjects

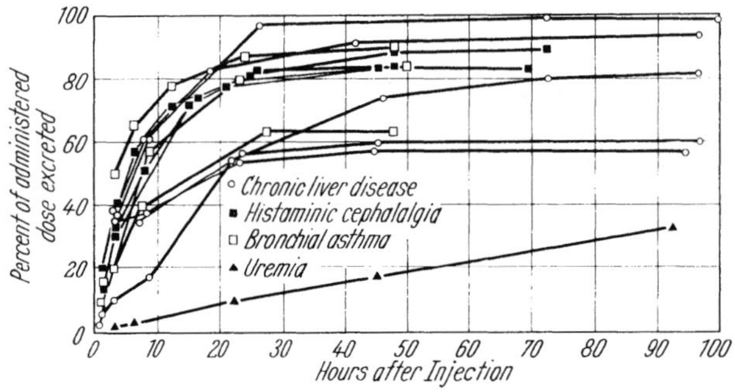

Fig. 2. Cumulative recovery of administered radioactivity from urine of subjects with various diseases

HELANDER et al. (1962) studied the rate of elimination of C^{14} after intravenous injection of C^{14}-histamine in allergic subjects. Attacks of severe asthma or urticaria were not associated with decrease in the elimination of C^{14}.

E. Rate of elimination of C^{14}-histamine from the blood

BEALL and VAN ARSDEL also measured the rate of elimination of the injected C^{14} from the blood. They did not find any significant differences between their patients with allergic, hepatic or renal disease and their control subjects. An attempt was also made to separate C^{14}-histamine from its metabolites. No experiment is however quoted to show how accurate the technique used was in separating C^{14}-histamine from its metabolites or to show the recovery of C^{14}-histamine added to blood.

When C^{14}-histamine was incubated with human blood (non-pregnant subject) 80–100% of the added histamine could be recovered in unchanged form with SCHAYER's isotope dilution technique (LINDELL and VISKE, 1961). A very small inactivation of histamine in blood from non-pregnant subjects has previously been observed by AHLMARK (1944). When C^{14}-histamine was given by vein at a constant rate a fairly steady concentration in arterial blood was reached after 20–30 min. The greater part of the labelled histamine was in the plasma fraction of the blood but some was in the red cell fraction (LINDELL and WESTLING, unpublished). See Fig. 3. When the infusion was interrupted the concentration of C^{14}-histamine in plasma fell within 3 min to a level which was not measurable. The disappearance of C^{14}-histamine from the cell fraction was much slower.

It should be mentioned that the amount of histamine given in the experiment illustrated here was enough to give tachycardia, flushing and a fall in blood pressure and yet the concentration of injected histamine in blood was only 1–2 μg per liter, that is less than can be measured with conventional bioassay.

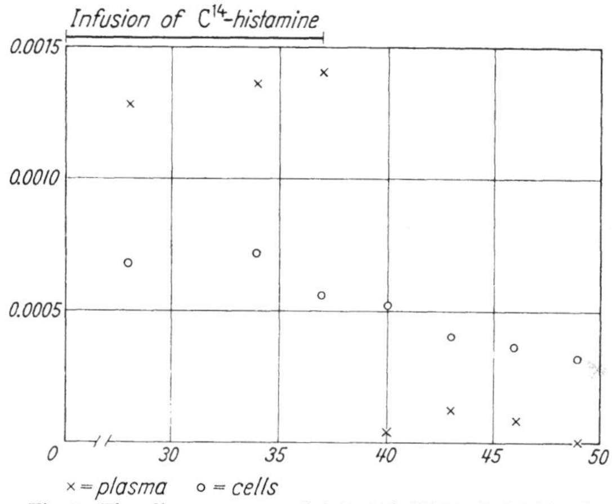

Fig. 3. The disappearance of injected C^{14}-labelled histamine from the blood in man. C^{14}-histamine was given in a steady intravenous infusion at a rate of 0.2 microgram histamine base per kg bodyweight per min. Ordinate: concentration of C^{14}-histamine in plasma or cell fraction (microgram/ml). Abscissa: time in min

If in an experiment similar to that illustrated in Fig. 3 blood samples are drawn from a renal vein or a hepatic vein at the same time as an arterial blood sample is taken it is found that 70–80% of the injected C^{14}-histamine is extracted from the blood during its passage through the renal or the splanchnic circulation. Some results of such experiments (ARNOLDSSON et al., 1962a) are shown in Table 8. It is evident from these studies that free histamine reaching the bloodstream is very rapidly removed from the circulation and that a great part of this removal takes place in the renal and splanchnic blood vessels.

Table 8. *Extraction of C^{14}-histamine from the blood in various human tissues. The concentration of C^{14}-histamine is expressed in per cent of the concentration in arterial blood taken at the same time*

	Concentration of C^{14}-histamine in blood from			
Clinical diagnosis	Renal vein	Hepatic vein	Cubital vein	Uterine vein
Healthy[1]	22	19	—	—
Non-pregnant[2]	—	—	89	64
Pregnant[2]	—	—	90	51
	Pulmonary artery	Internal jugular vein	Iliac vein	
Funnel chest or mitral disease[1]	99	—	—	
Mental disease[1]	—	105	75	

[1] From ARNOLDSSON et al. (1962).
[2] LINDBERG 1963.

III. The occurrence of histamine in human tissues

The actual concentration of histamine in a tissue depends on the capacity of the tissue to synthesize, store, release and catabolize histamine. As pointed out above there is evidence that the tissues do not take up histamine as such and store it for any longer period of time. Instead it would seem that histamine present in a tissue must be formed locally (probably from L-histidine). The mechanism of storage of histamine in human tissues has not been studied. It would seem that

Table 9. *Histamine content of human kidney, liver, lung, spleen and small intestine*

Diagnosis	Lung	Small intestine	Liver	Spleen	Kidney	Comments	Author
Healthy	33±10	14±0.9	2.2±0.76	3.4±0.97	2.5±1.2	2,4-dinitrofluorobenzene method. Autopsy material. Mean values and standard error	STONE, MERRILL and MENEELY (1955)
	6—21		1—2	2—4	1—4	Code's method. Histamine base. Range observed	DUNÉR and PERNOW (1960)
Urticaria pigmentosa			1250—1896			2,4-dinitrofluorobenzene method	GARDNER and TICE (1958)
Healthy.			5—12				

Table 10. *Histamine content of human bone marrow, pancreas, testis, thyroid, skeletal and uterine muscle*

Diagnosis	Pancreas	Testis	Thyroid	Bone marrow	Sceletal muscle	Uterine muscle	Comments	Author
Healthy . . .	4.8±1.5	4.6±0.98	1.0±0.13	3.3±1.5	0.97±0.13		2,4-dinitrofluorobenzene method. Autopsy material. Mean values and standard error	STONE, MERRILL and MENEELY (1955)
				2—6			Code's method. Histamine base. Range observed	DUNÉR and PERNOW (1960)
Non-pregnant .						8.58±1.60	Bioassay	GUNTHER and PATON (1960)
Pregnant . . .						0.93±0.22		

Table 11. *Histamine content of aorta, heart and nervous tissue*

Diagnosis	Heart	Aorta	Spinal roots	Peripheral nerves	Spinal cord	Comments	Author
Healthy. . .	1.6±0.07	4.2±2.4				2,4-dinitrofluorobenzene method. Autopsy material. Mean values and standard error	STONE, MERRILL and MENEELY (1955)
			0.4—0.5	3—10	0.05	Autopsy material. Range of mean values; Histamine dihydrochloride	WERLE (1956)

Table 12. *Histamine content of nasal mucosa membrane, nasal secretion, lymph, saliva and sweat*

Diagnosis	Nasal mucous membrane	Nasal secretion	Sweat	Saliva	Lymph	Comments	Author
Healthy							
♂ (2—12 year) . .	21 (5—54)					Bioassay	BAXTER and ROSE (1953)
♀ (3—12 year) . .	19 (6.0—48)					Histamine base	
♂ (18—43 year) . .	13 (4—30)						
♀ (15—39 year) . .	19 (6—39)						
(50—59 year) . .	28 (1—56)						
Nasal allergy . . .	14 (3—49)						
Rhinitis vasomotorica . . .		0.2				Bioassay μg/ml	HÄUSLER (1957)
			0.88 (0.4—1.4)			Bioassay μg/ml	DUNÉR and PERNOW (1960)
Healthy				146 (107—181)		2,4-dinitrofluorobenzene method.	SANDERS (1955)
24 hs after surgery .				669		μg/l	
					<0.1		DUNÉR and PERNOW (1960)

Table 13. *Histamine content of human oral and gastric tissues in μg/g and gastric juice in μ/g liter*

Diagnosis	Stomach	Fundus	Pylorus	Antrum	Ulcer	Gastric juice	Gingiva	Comments	Author
Healthy. . . .	14±4.0							2,4-dinitrofluorobenzene method. Autopsy material. Mean values and standard error	STONE, MERRILL and MENEELY (1955)
Duodenal ulcer		35.1±5.1	21.2±2.4					Bioassay. Mean values and standard error. See also Fig. 1 and 2 in SMITH (1959)	SMITH (1959)
Gastric carcinoma . .		33.7±4.5	20.1±2.1						
Ulcer		4—18	3—11	5—8	6—9			Code's method. Range	FAREDIN, BORBOLA and BIKICH (1954)
Cancer		15	10						
Healthy. . . .						13 (0—38)		Code's method. Mean values and range of concentration	FAREDIN, BIKICH and BORBOLA (1953)
Pern. anaemia .						44 (8—125)			
Duodenal ulcer.						15 (0—55)			
Duodenal ulcer									
"active" . . .						0—25		Code's method. Range of concentration	BIKICH, BORBOLA and HETÉNYI (1954)
"inactive". . .						0—700			
Gastric ulcer									
"active" . . .						0—20			
"inactive". . .						0—100			
Healthy. . . .							6.6 (5—8)	2,4-dinitrofluorobenzene method. Operation specimen	SANDERS (1955)

histamine is present in all tissue studied but in what form is not known. It seems likely, though, that in human tissues a great part of the histamine is in the mast cells as is the case in animal tissues. The greater part of the blood histamine seems to be located in the basophils. (See Part IV: Histamine in blood). The mechanism of release of histamine from the human tissues has not been studied extensively.

Allergens have been shown to release histamine from human skin in vivo (KATZ, 1942) and from human lung tissue in vitro (SCHILD, HAWKINS, MONGAR and HERXHEIMER, 1951; BROCKLEHURST, 1958). The mechanism of release of histamine in human blood by allergens has been studied by VAN ARSDEL, MIDDLETON, SHERMAN and BUCHWALD (1958) and MIDDLETON and SHERMAN (1961).

These studies indicate that the mechanism of histamine release in the allergic reaction is the same as in the anaphylactic reaction.

In many tissues histamine is present together with enzymes capable of inactivating histamine. This suggests that histamine in the tissues is bound in such a way that it is not available for the metabolizing enzymes. Thus, the tissue content of histamine does not simply reflect the net balance between the rate of formation and elimination. When examining the histamine content of a tissue care must be taken to prevent these enzymes from destroying the histamine during the preparation and extraction of the tissue. This may be checked by addition of known amounts of histamine. When interpreting measurements of histamine content in tissues it must be borne in mind that such measurements do not allow any conclusions about the rate of formation or destruction of histamine in the tissue.

Table 14. *Histamine content of human skin in µg/g*

Diagnosis	Skin	Comments	Author
Healthy	6.6 ± 0.6	2,4-dinitrofluorobenzene method. Autopsy material. Mean values and standard error	STONE, MERRILL and MENEELY (1955)
Outer zone	10	Bioassay. Mammary skin.	RILEY and WEST (1956)
Inner zone	3		
Healthy	18.1 (6.6—30.4)	2,4-dinitrofluorobenzene method. Autopsy material	JOHNSON (1957)
Healthy	9.2 (4.2—14.3)	2,4-dinitrofluorobenzene method. Mean values and range of concentration in antecubital skin.	JOHNSON, DE OREO, LASCHEID and MITCHELL (1960)
Eczematous	16.0 (9.7—24.8)		
Healthy	0.6—1.5	Code's method and chromatography	LEVI, MENEGHINI and RANTUCCIO (1959)
Urticatia pigmentosa	4—30		
Prurigo	3.1—11.4		
Eczema	4.9—10		
Urticaria	4.7—16.0		
Healthy	41 (19—68)	Code's method. Histamine base in µg/g *dried* tissue. Mean values and range	NILZÉN (1947)
10 min after mechanical stimulation	25 (10—53)		
Dermographism	52 (30—109)		
After mechanical stimulation	36 (17—76)		
Urticaria wheal	24 (22—31)		
Normal skin	47 (28—74)		
Various diseases	8.8 (2—27)	Bioassay. Histamine base. Specimens from surgery	FELDBERG and LOESER (1954)
Hypothyroidism	5.1 (3—8)		
Hyperthyroidism	13.3 (11—18)		
Various diseases		Bioassay. Histamine dihydrochloride in µg/g tissue. Autopsy material	HUKOVIĆ, SPUZIĆ and STERN (1957)
Skin from the neck	10.4		
Skin from the abdomen	3.7		
Skin from the thumb	2.6		

A tissue may have high rate of turnover of histamine and yet the actual histamine content may be low. This is probably the case of tissues in which histamine has recently been released (SCHAYER, 1961 b).

Tables 9–14 show the result of studies on the histamine content of various human tissues. The principle of assay is described briefly, and, if stated in the original publication, the means of obtaining the tissue, the diagnosis, and the way of expressing the histamine content in base or dihydrochloride.

A survey of the distribution of histamine in man conveys the impression that the concentration of histamine is greatest in tissues which have contact with the outside world, i. e. the nasal mucosa membrane, the lungs, the gastric and intestinal mucosa and the skin.

It is very interesting to find that the histamine content of gastric mucosa from subjects with gastric cancer is as high as that of gastric mucosa from healthy subjects or subjects with ulcer. These observations will be discussed in section VII f.

The low concentration of histamine in the skin of hypothyroid subjects and the comparatively high concentration of histamine in the skin of hyperthyroid subjects (FELDBERG and LOESER, 1954) suggest a relationship between histamine metabolism and thyroid activity. This is further discussed in section VII e.

IV. Histamine in the blood in man

Determinations of the amounts of histamine in the blood as well as the distribution of histamine in the various blood cells and in the plasma have been performed in man by a large number of workers. It is probably not wrong to say that the confusion about blood histamine is larger than that in any other area of histamine research.

The present section will contain some remarks about blood and plasma histamine in general; mention will also be made about the methods currently used for histamine determinations in man. Then a survey will follow of the variations in blood histamine under normal and pathological conditions in humans.

A. General remarks

For simplicity we can divide the blood histamine in cellular and non-cellular histamine. The former constitutes by far the largest fraction of the blood histamine (Table 15), and there is strong evidence that almost all of this histamine is contained in the white blood cells (e.g. CODE, 1952). There has been, in the past, much work which was taken to indicate that the eosinophil cell was the main carrier of blood histamine, but the painstaking work of, among others, CODE and ROSE and their co-workers has shown that this is not always so. During the last years the basophil leukocyte has attracted much interest by several groups and it is now certain that this cell type is, like its basophil fellow the tissue mast cell, an important storage place for histamine. Thus GRAHAM et al. (1955) find that the basophil leukocytes, in spite of their comparative rarity, contain more than half of the blood histamine, whereas the major part of the remaining histamine is present in the other leukocytes, notably the eosinophils (see Table 15). Simultaneous studies by CODE and MITCHELL (1957) and VALENTINE et al. (1955) also revealed a strong correlation between the total blood histamine and the number of basophil cells in normal conditions as well as in cases of myelogenous leukemia.

The riddle of the eosinophil leukocyte and histamine is still unsolved; the balance of the evidence suggests that this blood cell may sometimes contain histamine but certainly not regularly. The appearance of eosinophil leukocytes in conditions in which histamine is implicated, directly or indirectly, has caused a general feeling that the eosinophil still has something important to do with blood (and tissue) histamine, but its role is enigmatic.

There is some fresh evidence that the basophil leukocytes in man can synthesize histamine (HARTMAN et al., 1961; LINDELL et al., 1961 b) just like the tissue mast cells (see part I of this article), but it is not known whether the basophil leukocytes, or other white blood cells, can take up histamine from the outside by other means than passive diffusion, and thus be specially designed for the inactivation and/or transport of histamine from one tissue to another. The predominant

Table 15. *Distribution of histamine in blood according to* GRAHAM, LOWRY, WHEELWRIGHT, LENZ and PARISH (1955). Histamine values determined by the "microchemical" dinitrofluorobenzene method and expressed as the base

Cell type	Histamine content		
	μg/liter	μg/10⁹ cells	per cent of total blood histamine
Leukocytes, neutrophil	(7000)	3.3	14
Leukocytes, basophil	2400000	1080	51
Leukocytes, eosinophil	360000	160	29
Lymphocytes	?	0.6	1
Monocytes	(2600) ?	(1.2)	0.5
Platelets	1280	0.009	3
Plasma	2.6	—	1.5

localization of histamine to the leukocytes, notably the basophils, makes it clear that measurement of blood histamine in various conditions will, generally speaking, give information pertaining mainly to the number of these cells in the blood. Changes, or absence of changes in blood histamine under various conditions will give comparatively little positive evidence for or against the involvement of histamine itself. As an extreme example we may consider the blood histamine level in chronic myelogenous leukemia. Patients with this disease may have blood histamine values as high as 27 μg per ml. (SHIMKIN et al., 1951), that is more than 500 times the normal value. Such a patient has more than 100 mg of histamine (i.e. many lethal doses) circulating in his vessels, yet he has no symptoms which could be due to biological effects of this histamine and there is nothing to suggest that the large amounts of histamine in the blood are there for any other reason than as a regular constituent of the leukocytes, notably the basophils. In keeping with this are isolated findings that cases with chronic myelogenous leukemia have a normal plasma histamine (THIERSCH, 1947 b) and an essentially normal urinary excretion of free histamine (HELANDER and WESTLING, unpublished observations). The same argument as for leukemia is valid for the interpretation of changes of the blood histamine on a smaller scale, e.g. in certain allergic conditions. The poor relationship between the blood histamine level and biological actions of histamine in man was emphasized by ROSE (1940), who found that an injection of histamine could give biological effects in spite of unchanged or even lowered blood histamine levels. Animal experiments have substantiated this amply (EMMELIN et al., 1941).

It was mentioned in part II, E of this section that an infusion of C^{14}-histamine gave biological effects with a plasma concentration of 1–2 μg per liter. Such a small increase in histamine concentration cannot be established by conventional techniques for measuring whole blood histamine. The small amounts of injected (or liberated histamine) could not be distinguished from the comparatively large amounts of histamine ordinarily present in the blood.

In an effort to trace, in the blood, histamine liberated from a tissue, interest was therefore focused on the plasma. In spite of the fact that exogenous histamine is extremely rapidly eliminated from the blood (see part II, E) it should be possible to detect at least a temporary increase in the level of histamine in the plasma as a whole, or in the plasma emerging from an organ in which histamine was liberated. This promising approach has yielded surprisingly little information in man, as well as in laboratory animals. The reason for this may well be the methodological difficulties involved. These will be commented upon below (part IV, C).

B. Methodological considerations

1. Biological determination of blood histamine

(See Chapter 1, Section D)

In 1935 Barsoum and Gaddum introduced the first practicable method for the determination of *the histamine content of whole blood.* Code (1937) simplified and modified the extraction somewhat and his procedure has been used in most of the studies in man. Briefly, the method consists of precipitation of the proteins with trichloroacetic acid, which also extracts the histamine from the cells. The trichloroacetic acid filtrate is treated with strong hydrochloric acid and thereafter evaporated to dryness. The residue is then taken up in ethanol, and again evaporated to near dryness. Ethanol "washings" are performed three times and the residue is then taken up in some solution suitable for the biological estimation of the histamine content on the isolated ileum of the guinea-pig. The method as such should not present any difficulties for the worker with moderate experience in bioassay. It is sometimes forgotten that the method measures "histamine-like activity" and not histamine, specifically. This must be remembered above all in various pathological conditions in man, where it cannot be taken for granted that unknown compounds with biological activity may not appear. The usual tests (see part V, a, 2 of this article) for identity of the gut-contracting agent with histamine must be performed, i.e. graded antagonism with a specific antihistaminic agent and attempts to inactivate the unknown agent with a histaminase preparation.

For studies on whole blood histamine it is probably best to avoid the use of anticoagulants when taking the samples and add trichloroacetic acid quickly.

Adam and his co-workers have continued their painstaking methodological studies and have introduced ion-exchange resins in the preparation of blood samples for histamine determinations (Adam, Hardwick and Spencer, 1957).

Dunér and Pernow (1958a) introduced another technique for the primary extraction of histamine from the blood, namely by extraction with acetone and subsequent adsorption of histamine to an ion-exchange resin. This method should be less tedious to perform than the classical method of Code (1937).

The *plasma histamine level* appears to be exceedingly difficult to determine accurately. It appears, to the present authors, at least rather clear that this is dependent upon methodological difficulties. The work of Adam (Adam, Hardwick and Spencer, 1957) shows quite convincingly that the plasma level of normal humans is less than 0.001 μg/ml. Such a low value was obtained when the blood specimens were removed and treated very carefully (collection in chilled polythene tubes). The anticoagulant used was heparin. Each batch of heparin must be tested for its own content of histamine before use. Boiling with strong hydrochloric acid can apparently make accessible some histamine otherwise "bound" to the heparin (Adam et al., 1957). Code (1937) and Lowry et al. (1954), (see also Table 15) had found earlier that the plasma histamine level was less than 20 and 3 μg/l, respectively. Their methods for histamine assay and techniques for blood collection were not as sensitive and elaborate as that of ADAM et al. (1957).

2. Chemical estimations of blood histamine

(See also Chapter 1, Section C)

The chemical methods for histamine determination have been used most successfully in studies on blood. The present authors have practically no personal experience with these methods, but they appear to be useful and reliable under the conditions in which they have been tested. It would seem possible that their uncritical use in pathological conditions in man might lead to mistakes, and checks for accuracy and specificity must be made, just as with the biological methods.

The two methods currently in use are the spectrophotometrical dinitrofluorobenzene (DNFB) method devised by McINTIRE et al. (1950) and modified by LOWRY et al. (1954) and the fluorometrical o-phtalaldehyde (OPT) method of SHORE et al. (1959).

In the DNFB method histamine is coupled to DNFB after extraction with trichloroacetic acid and adsorption on an ion-exchange resin (Decalso). The coloured histamine-DNFB derivative is selectively extracted into methyl-n-hexyl ketone and the extinction measured spectrophotometrically. In the OPT method histamine is coupled to OPT after treatment with perchloric acid and extraction into butanol. The histamine-OPT derivative is fluorescent and can be measured in very small quantities on a spectrophotofluorometer or a spectrophotometer with suitable filters. It would seem that the OPT method has greater potential sensitivity and specificity than the DNFB method. Both methods have given values for blood histamine which are comparable to those obtained by bioassay.

The most specific of all methods, including current biochemical and biological techniques, is the one devised by SCHAYER, KOBAYASHI and SMILEY (1955). In this method histamine is coupled with p-iodophenylsulphonyl (pipsyl) chloride, in which the iodine is labelled with I^{131}. The radioactive pipsylhistamine is then "diluted" with a known, large amount of non-isotopic pipsylhistamine, which is recrystallized to constant radioactivity. The specificity is probably absolute for this method and its sensitivity is determined by the specific activity of the I^{131}, which can be made very high.

C. Histamine content of whole blood under various conditions

a) Normal values (Table 16)

There is a fairly large number of normal values for blood histamine reported in the literature and the values show a wide scatter ranging from 10–140 μg histamine base per liter. There are also conspicuous differences between the mean values obtained by various methods. However, the variations between mean values obtained by the same method (e.g. biological estimation of histamine) appear to be equally large as the differences between results obtained by radically different methods (e.g. biological and chemical). The reason for the individual variations in blood histamine is not known. There is apparently no sex difference. Fasting subjects have a slightly lower blood histamine content than non-fasting. Smoking habits may also influence the "normal" values (WERLE and EFFKEMANN, 1940b).

It is known that adrenocortical steroids and "stress" may lower the blood histamine (see later in this part). Samples from normal individuals obtained during heart catheterization had a lower histamine content than expected (ROSE,

RUSTED and FOWNES, 1950, and personal experience). This may be due to the emotional stress involved. This may well explain some other variations in normal values. For practical purposes histamine values below 20 and above 100 μg/liter may be regarded as probably abnormal.

Table 16. *Histamine levels in whole blood in normal cases*

Values refer to μg histamine base per liter blood. B & G = Method of Barsoum and Gaddum (1935). Code = Method of Code (1937). DNFB = Method of Lowry et al. (1954). D & P = Method of Dunér and Pernow (1958a). Lubschez = Chemical method of Lubschez (1950).

Cathegory	No. of cases	Range	Mean	Remark	Method	Reference
Normal adults	5	27—50	35		B & G	BARSOUM and GADDUM (1936)
Normal adults	8	50—110	80		B & G	BARSOUM and SMIRK (1936)
Normal adults	103	18—78	40		B & G	HAWORTH and MACDONALD (1937)
Normal adults	50	20—75	40		Code	ROSE and BROWNE (1940)
Normal adults	20	19—71	45		Code	RANDOLPH and RACKEMANN (1941)
Normal men } non-smokers	10	10—60	42	} values as histamine dihydrochloride	Code	WERLE and EFFKEMANN (1940b)
Normal women } non-smokers	11	18—60	44		Code	WERLE and EFFKEMANN (1940b)
Normal men } heavy smokers	18	65—200	99		Code	WERLE and EFFKEMANN (1940b)
Normal women } heavy smokers	11	50—200	81		Code	WERLE and EFFKEMANN (1940b)
Normal adults	30	45—84	60		Code	NILZÉN (1947)
Normal adults	39	38—80	59		Code	SERAFINI (1948)
Normal women	8	20—40	33		Code	KAPELLER-ADLER (1949)
Normal pulmonary artery	5	10—28	19	} during heart catheterization	Code	ROSE, RUSTED and FOWNES, (1950)
Normal femoral artery	5	12—28	19		Code	ROSE, RUSTED and FOWNES (1950)
Normal fasting	17	30—110	75		Code	VALENTINE et al. (1950)
Normal non-fasting	16	57—140	86		Code	VALENTINE et al. (1950)
Normal adults	47	—	82		DNFB	LOWRY et al. (1954)
Normal adults	12	12—67	40		Code	MITCHELL et al. (1954b)
Normal adults	17	—	60		Code	JIMENEZ-DIAZ et al. (1955)
Normal adults	12	—	89		DNFB	LOWETT DOUST et al. (1956)
Normal men	16	22—106	56		Code	GOOSZEN and DONKER (1956)
Normal women	38	22—114	58		Code	GOOSZEN and DONKER (1956)
Normal adults	25	15—88	45		D & P	DUNÉR and PERNOW (1958a)
Normal adults	19	10—110	58		Code	RORSMAN and ROSENGREN (1958)
Normal adults	18	<20—73	36		Lubschez	DEGARA (1951)
Normal children	15	20—80	49		Code	MITCHELL and CASS (1959)
Normal children	51	22—108	50		Code	MAAS et al. (1956)
Normal adults (indians)	12	20—130	57		Code	JHA and SINHA (1960)

The histamine content of the blood is apparently rather stable in one and the same individual when studied repeatedly (ROSE and BROWNE, 1940). This stability is not seen in pathological conditions, e.g. allergy (ROSE, 1941; MAAS et al., 1956) and schizophrenia (GOOSZEN and DONKER, 1956).

b) Blood histamine in conditions with abnormal cell content of the blood (Table 17)

It was not long after the introduction of practicable methods for the estimation of blood histamine (BARSOUM and GADDUM, 1935; CODE, 1937) that the discovery was made of a very high histamine concentration in blood from patients with chronic myelogenous leukemia (CODE and MCDONALD, 1937; MARCOU, GINGOLD and PARHON, 1937). The histamine content of the blood in chronic myelogenous leukemia has been raised to the amazing figure of 27,000 μg/l! (Normal values less than 100 μg/l). There is a clear tendency for blood histamine to be lower in more acute forms of myelogenous leukemia than in chronic cases. Histamine values are thus generally high in cases with a long survival time, but the variations are so large that histamine determinations are probably useless for prognostic assessments in individual cases.

Normal histamine values have been found in lymphatic and monocytic leukemias, as well as in leukemoid reactions and cases with leukocytosis. The high

Table 17. *Blood histamine in various haematological diseases.* Values are given in μg histamine base per lite of whole blood, if not otherwise indicated. The method of Code (1937) has been used

Diagnosis	No. of cases	Range of values	Mean	Reference	Remarks
Leukemia, myelogenous, chronic	5	1600—17500	8040	CODE and MCDONALD (1937)	
Leukemia, myelogenous, chronic	14	170—18300	4140	VALENTINE et al. (1950, 1955)	
Leukemia, myelogenous, chronic	16	80—6000	1230	THIERSCH (1947b)	
Leukemia, myelogenous, chronic	18	40—27000	5980	SHIMKIN et al. (1951)	High histamine cor tent of lei cocytes associated with bett prognosis
Leukemia, myelogenous, chronic with acute exacerbation	6	20—530	175	SHIMKIN et al. (1951)	
Leukemia, myelogenous, acute or subacute	6	30—5750	1510	SHIMKIN et al. (1951)	
Leukemia, acute	10	20—260	74	VALENTINE et al. (1950)	
Leukemia, monocytic	3	25—60	42	SHIMKIN et al. (1948—49)	
Leukemia, monocytic	4	30—100	58	THIERSCH (1947a)	
Leukemia, lymphatic	6	21—230	58	CODE and MCDONALD (1937)	
Leukemia, lymphatic	3	40—70[1]	—	WENT and REX-KISS (1941)	
Leukemia, lymphatic	9	20—180	70	SHIMKIN et al. (1948—49)	
Leukemia, lymphatic	5	20—200	85	THIERSCH (1947a)	
Leukocytosis or leukemoid reaction	35	5—290	63	VALENTINE et al. (1950)	
Polycythemia vera	17	110—750	350	VALENTINE et al. (1950, 1952)	
Polycythemia vera	18	23—500	119	SHIMKIN et al. (1948—49)	
Eosinophilia	5	40—1000	370	CODE and MCDONALD (1937)	
Eosinophilia	8	19—121	62	RANDOLPH and RACKEMANN (1941)	
Eosinophilia	4	70—100[1]	85[1]	WENT and REX-KISS (1941)	
Pernicious anemia	4	20—60[1]	—	WENT and REX-KISS (1941)	

[1] Values refer to histamine dihydrochloride.

blood histamine in myelogenous leukemia is therefore not due to the white cell mass as such or the presence in the blood of immature, rapidly growing cell forms. The available evidence suggests that the number of basophil cells is largely determining the blood histamine also in leukemia. There is apparently not much histamine in the plasma in myelogenous leukemia (THIERSCH, 1947b).

In patients with eosinophilia normal or high values may be found.

It appears certain that most patients with polycythemia have pathologically high blood histamine values. This is not dependent upon the red cells but due to associated abnormalities in the leukocytes, probably the basophils.

The blood histamine has been essentially normal in cases with anemia (e.g. MARCOU et al., 1937; WENT and REX-KISS, 1941).

c) *Blood histamine in bronchial asthma, urticaria and other allergic conditions*

Some observations on the blood histamine level in asthmatics are listed in Table 18. It will be seen that the blood histamine values are normal in asthmatic

Table 18. *Blood histamine levels in bronchial asthma.* For explanations: See Table 16

Condition	No. of cases	Range of values	Mean value	Method	Reference	Remark
Bronchial asthma, during attack	8	110—200	182	B & G	CERQUA (1936)	Several observations on each case; distinct rise of blood histamine *during* asthmatic attack
Bronchial asthma, towards end of attack	8	190—300	261	B & G	CERQUA (1936)	
Bronchial asthma, 10 hours after attack	8	80—140	101	B & G	CERQUA (1936)	
Bronchial asthma, further improvement	8	70—100	89	B & G	CERQUA (1936)	
Bronchial asthma, no symptoms	9	—	54	Code	RANDOLPH and RACKEMANN (1941)	Clear increase *during* attack
Bronchial asthma, during symptoms	9	—	88	Code	RANDOLPH and RACKEMANN (1941)	
Bronchial asthma, older pat., no symptoms	13	20—80	40	Code	ROSE (1941)	
Bronchial asthma, older pat., moderate sympt.	7	10—50	30	Code	ROSE (1941)	
Bronchial asthma, older pat., severe symptoms	6	10—90	41	Code	ROSE (1941)	
Bronchial asthma, young pat., no symptoms	6	30—120	69	Code	ROSE (1941)	Patients younger than 16 years have higher values than older patients
Bronchial asthma, young pat., moderate sympt.	4	15—190	81	Code	ROSE (1941)	
Bronchial asthma, young pat., severe symptoms	3	30—130	81	Code	ROSE (1941)	
Bronchial asthma, acute	5	27—416	149	Lubschez	DE GARA (1951)	
Bronchial asthma, no symptoms	20	—	53[1]	Code	JIMENEZ-DIAZ et al. (1955)	
Bronchial asthma, during attack	31	—	89[1]	Code	JIMENEZ-DIAZ et al. (1955)	
Asthmatic patients, no symptoms; pulmonary artery	12	4—120	37	Code	ROSE et al. (1950)	Samples taken during heart catheterization; higher values than in normal cases
Asthmatic patients, no symptoms; femoral artery	12	12—110	42	Code	ROSE et al. (1950)	
Allergic children (symptoms ?)	17	33—125	66	Code	MAAS et al. (1956)	No difference from control material

[1] Values refer to histamine dihydrochloride.

patients in a symptom-free period. During asthmatic attacks moderately elevated values were noted.

It will be apparent from the introduction to this section that this elevation of blood histamine does not permit the conclusion that histamine is released during the asthmatic attack. Anyhow, the finding suggests a connexion between histamine and asthma. This will be discussed later on (see part VII, d, of this section).

It is mentioned later on (part IV, c, d) that a reduction in blood histamine is seen in "stressful" conditions, probably as a result of increased adrenocortical secretion. It seems rather peculiar, then, that patients with severe asthmatic dyspnoea have a high blood histamine. It would be interesting to follow carefully the blood histamine level and the number of circulating basophil leukocytes during an asthmatic attack and its termination with adrenocortical steroids or hypophyseal adrenocorticotrophic hormone.

In urticaria two patterns of behaviour of the blood histamine may be distinguished (Table 19). First, it seems well established that an acute outbreak of urticaria is associated with a lowering of blood histamine (e.g. NILZÉN, 1947). RORSMAN and ROSENGREN (1958) could demonstrate that the fall in blood histamine in urticaria was associated with a corresponding diminution of the number of basophil leukocytes in the blood.

On the other hand the careful study of NILZÉN (1947) shows convincingly that patients with a more chronic type of urticaria generally have high blood histamine values during periods with symptoms, with decreases to below normal during the eruption of wheals.

The divergences in some other studies of the blood histamine in urticaria can perhaps be understood in the light of Nilzén's findings. It appears clear that the time of taking the blood sample must be rigidly defined in relation to the urticarial attack and the process of whealing. Moreover, it appears that the diagnosis of "urticaria" can cover diseases of different nature and this may also be an explanation of the varying results.

In patients with angioneurotic edema and during anaphylactic serum reactions low blood histamine values have been found (ROSE, 1941; CERQUA, 1936).

The reason why blood histamine (and the circulating basophil leukocytes) is diminished in urticaria, angioneurotic edema and anaphylactic serum reactions is entirely unkown. RORSMAN (1962) suggests that the low values in urticaria are not due to adrenocortical hyperactivity but to rather a more specific process. It could be that the basophil leukocytes are disrupted during antigen-antibody reactions, just as the tissue mast cells. It is also fully possible that the basophil cells leave the blood stream to reach the tissues and eventually release its histamine there. The latter possibility should be explored and it may well be that careful studies of the basophil leukocyte, the wandering mast cell, can contribute much to the understanding of the role of the mast cell and histamine in various normal and abnormal conditions in man.

d) Blood histamine level in various conditions

Changes in blood histamine have also been encountered in other conditions than allergic diseases. Table 20 gives references to some studies and it will be seen that some clinically important conditions are accompanied by pronounced changes in the blood histamine.

A pattern of decreased blood histamine during some stressful conditions can readily be seen. There is thus a decrease in blood histamine in pace with the development of surgical and posttraumatic shock, and in moribund patients the blood histamine values are excessively low (Rose and Browne, 1940). It seems rather clear, although not directly proven, that this effect of shock on the blood histamine is due to a decreased number of circulating basophil leukocytes in response to an increased secretion of adrenocortical hormones. It has been shown by several workers, e.g. Mitchell and Cass (1959) that the administration of cortisone will lower blood histamine and basophil cells in a parallel manner. The low blood histamine during a bout of fever in malaria may be explained in the same way, as can the relatively low blood histamine values encountered 1–4 days after a burn injury (Birke et al., 1957).

More intriguing, and perhaps worthy of further study, is the occurrence of rather high blood histamine values during congestive heart failure. These values were obtained by the original method of Barsoum and Gaddum, and may thus be subject to some criticism. However, the finding of Cerqua (1936), that the blood histamine is on the average 3 times the mean normal value, is so striking and regular that it would appear of interest even if it should prove to be caused by methodological errors.

Table 19. *Blood histamine levels in urticaria and some other allergic conditions.* For explanations: See Table 16

Diagnosis	No. of cases	Range of values	Mean value	Method	Reference	Remark
Urticaria, during attack	6	180—300	209	B & G	Cerqua (1936)	*High* values *during* symptoms
Urticaria, symptom-free, same cases	6	70—100	85	B & G	Cerqua (1936)	
Urticaria, uncomplicated, no symptoms	13	17—70	48	Code	Rose (1941)	Possibly slightly lower values during symptoms
Urticaria, uncomplicated, moderate symptoms	12	15—80	44	Code	Rose (1941)	
Urticaria, uncomplicated, severe symptoms	8	20—110	49	Code	Rose (1941)	
Urticaria, no wheals	4	24—156	90	Code	Nilzén (1947)	Clear *reduction* of blood histamine during *wheal* formation; each case carefully followed for a long time
Urticaria, wheals +	5	24—120	80	Code	Nilzén (1947)	
Urticaria, wheals ++	4	24—66	54	Code	Nilzén (1947)	
Urticatia, wheals +++	5	7—60	36	Code	Nilzén (1947)	
Urticaria, wheals ++++	2	7—23	21	Code	Nilzén (1947)	
Urticatia, no symptoms	8	—	100	Code	Jimenez-Diaz et al. (1955)	*Higher* values *during* attack
Urticaria, during attack	8	—	310	Code	Jimenez-Diaz et al. (1955)	
Urticaria, during attack	21	>5—160	21	Code	Rorsman and Rosengren (1958)	Values significantly *lower* than in control material
Angioneurotic oedema, no symptoms	3	30—50	43	Code	Rose (1941)	Very *low* values *during* severe symptoms
Angioneurotic oedema, moderate symptoms	3	10—30	19	Code	Rose (1941)	
Angioneurotic oedema, severe symptoms	6	5—10	6	Code	Rose (1941)	
Anaphylactic serum reaction, before	7	50—80	67	B & G	Cerqua (1936)	Clear reduction during the anaphylactic reaction
Anaphylactic serum reaction, during	8	10—30	15	B & G	Cerqua (1936)	
Anaphylactic serum reaction, after	8	60—80	66	B & G	Cerqua (1936)	
Eczema, moderate severity	6	50—140	73	Code	Rose (1941)	
Eczema, severe	4	60—280	123	Code	Rose (1941)	

Table 20. *Blood histamine in various conditions.* For explanations: See Table 16

Diagnosis	No. of cases	Range	Mean	Method	Reference	Remark
Normal persons, before muscular exercise	10	—	42	D & P	DUNÉR and PERNOW (1958c)	Increase also in serum: Parallel increase in white cell count
Normal persons, during muscular exercise	10	—	67	D & P	DUNÉR and PERNOW (1958c)	
Congestive heart failure, during symptoms	10	200—400	328	B & G	CERQUA (1936)	
Congestive heart failure, after treatment	9	50—110	97	B & G	CERQUA (1936)	
Congestive heart failure, during symptoms	8	80—300	250	B & G	BARSOUM and SMIRK (1936)	
Postoperative shock, slight or moderate	6	10—60	31	Code	ROSE and BROWNE (1940)	
Postoperative shock, slight or severe	5	10—20	13	Code	ROSE and BROWNE (1940)	
Postoperative shock, same patients, no shock	9	35—80	58	Code	ROSE and BROWNE (1940)	
Agonal states	6	1—15	8	Code	ROSE and BROWNE (1940)	
Malaria, no fever	6	60—90	73	B & G	CERQUA (1936)	
Malaria, 40—41° body temperature	6	10—20	15	B & G	CERQUA (1936)	
Malaria, attack over	6	50—80	63	B & G	CERQUA (1936)	
Burn injuries 1—3 hours after	7	60—230	135	D & P	BIRKE et al. (1957)	Increased blood histamine immediately after burn; parallel increase in urinary histamine
Burn injuries about 24 hours after	5	7—66	32	D & P	BIRKE et al. (1957)	
Burn injuries about 2 days after	3	13—34	23	D & P	BIRKE et al. (1957)	
Burn injuries about 3—4 days after	3	15—40	27	D & P	BIRKE et al. (1957)	
Burn injuries	1	—	—	Code	CODE and MACDONALD (1937)	Peak value of 140 at 12th day
Burn injuries	4	—	—	B & G	BARSOUM and GADDUM (1936)	Peak value at about the 7th day
Migraine, during attack	4	—	230	Code	JIMENEZ-DIAZ et al. (1955)	
Deep X-ray therapy	21	102—122	—	Code	LASSER and STENSTRÖM (1954)	
Cirrhosis of the liver	7	37—121	67	Code	MITCHELL et al. (1954a)	
Obstructive jaundice, mild pruritus	9	30—100	52	Code	MITCHELL et al. (1954a)	
Obstructive jaundice, severe pruritus	8	53—130	78	Code	MITCHELL et al. (1954a)	Slightly elevated values

The comprehensive study by BIRKE et al. (1957) shows quite clearly that the blood histamine level is elevated during the first few hours after a cutaneous burn. This is in all probability a result of the liberation of histamine from the large areas of skin involved, since a parallel increase occurs also in the urinary excretion of free histamine. The blood histamine drops to about half the normal value at 2–4 days after a burn. The reason why CODE and MCDONALD (1937) and BARSOUM and GADDUM (1936) find high blood histamine levels only about a week after the burn is not known. It may be that the severity of the burn and the methods for treatment can fully explain the slight discrepancy between the older results and those of BIRKE et al. (1957).

The elevated blood histamine levels in some mental abnormalities, particularly schizophrenia, (Table 21) have not yet received an explanation. Studies on the number of basophil leukocytes have apparently not been carried out. The observations in Table 21 will be commented upon in part VII, g, of this section.

Table 21. *Blood histamine levels in mental disease.* For explanations: See Table 16

Diagnosis	No. of cases	Range	Mean	Method	Reference	Remark
Schizophrenia, men . .	50	40—195	94	Code	GOOSZEN and DONKER (1956)	—
Schizophrenia, women	51	10—198	72	Code	GOOSZEN and DONKER (1956)	—
Schizophrenia	29	—	106	DNFB	LOWETT DOUST et al. (1956)	—
Schizophrenia, men . .	26	0—350	98	Code	STERN et al. (1957)	Higher values in early period of disease
Schizophrenia, women	14	0—135	43	Code	STERN et al. (1957)	
Various psychoses, men	26	15—110	57	Code	GOOSZEN and DONKER (1956)	—
Various psychoses, women.	16	25—107	59	Code	GOOSZEN and DONKER (1956)	—
Oligophrenia.	7	15—150	59	Code	STERN et al. (1957)	—
Postencephalitic syndromes, men	6	81—135	95	Code	GOOSZEN and DONKER (1956)	—
Epilepsy	5	—	139	DNFB	LOWETT DOUST et al. (1956)	—
"Progressive paralysis"	10	12—44	29	Code	STERN et al. (1957)	—

e) Blood histamine in human pregnancy (mother and new-born child)

Table 22 shows the results of some studies on the blood histamine level in pregnancy. It will be apparent from a comparison of Table 22 and Table 26 that the pregnant mothers have an essentially normal or slightly lowered blood histamine level, when studied not too close to delivery. At delivery low values for whole blood histamine have been recorded (MARCOU and ATHANASIU-VERGU, 1937; BJURÖ et al., 1961a). The reason for this lowering of the blood histamine at delivery is not known, but it is conceivably a phenomenon similar to the decrease in blood histamine during surgical shock and after the administration of adrenocortical steroids (see Section D, above).

The oxytocic action of histamine made it tempting to speculate about an eventual role of histamine during parturition also in the human female. However, measurement of both the plasma histamine level (WICKSELL, 1949b) and the urinary excretion of free histamine (WICKSELL, 1949b; BJURÖ et al., 1961a) have failed to support this view. Still, it would seem unjustified to disregard completely the possibility of histamine being instrumental in parturition.

In toxemic pregnancy the histamine values in whole blood are essentially unchanged (BJURÖ et al., 1961a) or slightly raised (KAPELLER-ADLER, 1949). KAPELLER-ADLER (1949) finds a larger proportion of the blood histamine in the plasma in toxemic pregnancy. The histamine in the blood cells was correspondingly lowered. If confirmed, this finding is of great interest for the interpretation of the

Table 22. *Histamine content in whole blood in pregnant mothers and new-born children (taken from umbilical vessels at delivery).* For explanations: See Table 16

Diagnosis	No. of cases	Range of values	Average	Method	Reference	Remark
Maternal blood; 2—4 days before delivery	8	—	about 140[1]	B & G	Marcou and Athanasiu-Vergu (1937)	Values taken from diagram
Maternal blood; delivery ± 2 hours	26	—	about 30[1]	B & G		
Maternal blood; 3—10 days after delivery	17	—	about 120[1]	B & G		
Maternal blood; pregnancy month VII—VIII	3	30—45	37	Code	Effkemann and Werle (1940)	
Maternal blood, normal pregnancy	8	—	31	Code	Bjurö et al. (1961 a)	Clear reduction at delivery and during pains
Maternal blood; toxemia	13	—	34	Code	Bjurö et al. (1961 a)	
Maternal blood; at delivery	10	6—18	13	Code	Bjurö et al. (1961 a)	
Maternal blood; hyperemesis	15	20—210	66	Code	Uuspää and Järvinen (1955)	
Maternal blood; hyperemesis after treatment	15	15—120	43	Code	Uuspää and Järvinen (1955)	
Foetal blood (umbilical artery)	6	130—277	248[1]	B & G	Marcou and Athanasiu-Vergu (1937)	
Maternal blood (at delivery)	7	9—75	40[1]	B & G		
Foetal blood (umbilical artery)	—	—	277[1]	B & G	Marcou et al. (1938)	25% reduction in blood histamine in placental passage
Foetal blood (umbilical vein)	—	—	208[1]	B & G	Marcou et al. (1938)	
Foetal blood (at birth)	5	40—130	71	Code	Effkemann and Werle (1940)	
Foetal blood (at birth)	4	85—400	181	Code	Wicksell (1949 b)	No difference in plasma histamine between mother and child
Maternal blood (at delivery)	4	50—92	74	Code	Wicksell (1949 b)	
Foetal blood (umbilical vein)	11	25—130	63	Code	Mitchell and Cass (1959)	
Foetal blood (umbilical artery)	9	40—135	87	Code	Bjurö et al. (1961 a)	15% lower values in umbilical vein
Foetal blood (umbilical vein)	13	33—125	69	Code	Bjurö et al. (1961 a)	

[1] Values probably not referring to histamine as the base.

role of histamine in toxemia. However, the difficulty of excluding increased fragility of the blood cells as a cause of the appearance of histamine in the plasma makes it desirable to repeat the studies of KAPELLER-ADLER (1949) with techniques for sampling and treatment of blood which are similar to those used by ADAM et al. (1957). There is also some uncertainty about the histamine content and behaviour of the white blood cells in Kapeller-Adler's experiments.

There is rather good agreement between different investigators as regards the whole blood histamine level in the new-born child, which has 2–5 times the histamine concentration of the mother. The possible implications of this will be discussed in part VII b.

f) Plasma histamine levels in man

Generally speaking, the figures for plasma histamine in man have become lower and lower as experience has accumulated about the many factors that may release histamine from the formed elements of the blood. The subject has been well treated by CODE (1952), who discusses several points that must be observed when obtaining the blood sample and separating the plasma. When taking the blood samples so as to prevent trauma to the cells (e.g. by shaking, bubble formation, contact with dry, "wetting" surfaces, clotting) and separating the plasma quickly, several workers (CODE, 1937; LOWRY et al., 1954, and ADAM et al., 1954) obtained values for plasma histamine that were below the limits of their methods for histamine assay.

ADAM, HARDWICK and SPENCER (1957) carried their methodological studies further and found after refinement of the blood sampling technique (collection in chilled polythene tubes, separation of plasma from white cells by two-stage centrifugation in the cold and total avoidance of glass contact) and increasing the sensitivity of the assay (by using the superfused guinea-pig ileum) that the plasma histamine level in man was less than 0.001 μg/ml (1 μg/liter). Small amounts of histamine added to the plasma could be adequately recovered. Similarly low values for plasma histamine were obtained in the cat. During infusion of relatively small amounts of histamine by vein to the cat measurable plasma levels of histamine were observed, which indicated that the method used was adequate for detecting histamine released or injected into the blood stream.

In the opinion of the present authors, the experiments cited give firm support to the belief that there is normally no free histamine in the plasma in man. The histamine in the blood must be considered physiologically inactive.

There is surprisingly little information about the plasma histamine in various conditions in man, estimated by methods similar to those just described. It is difficult to find a single study in the literature in which a measured increase of plasma histamine has been obtained with the precautions for blood sampling and separation of plasma suggested by ADAM, HARDWICK and SPENCER (1957). Indeed, if an increase in plasma histamine could be demonstrated by suitable methods in some physiological or pathological condition, one would immediately have to consider the possibility that the appearance of histamine in the plasma was due to increased fragility of the blood cells.

V. Urinary histamine in man

A. Urinary excretion of free histamine

1. General considerations

The frequent failure to obtain information about the release or formation of histamine from analysis of its concentration in whole blood or in plasma made it desirable to study the urinary excretion of histamine. Thanks mainly to ADAM (1949) and his subsequent co-workers it is now known that the urinary excretion is a more sensitive indicator of histamine release than the plasma or blood concentration.

ADAM et al. (1954) infused various amounts of histamine by vein to normal humans. Even during the infusion of high doses of histamine, causign headache, flush and copious gastric secretion, there was no measurable increase in the plasma histamine level as determined by conventional methods. On the other hand the urinary excretion of free histamine increased in proportion to the amount of histamine infused, about 1% of the amount being excreted (See Fig. 4.).

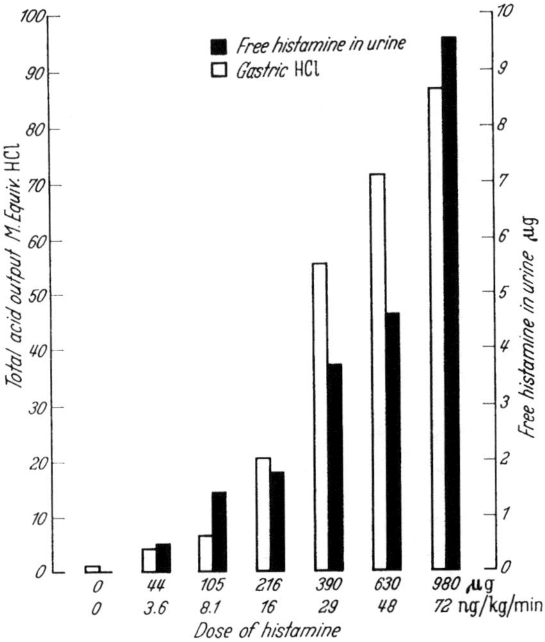

Fig. 4. Subject J.A.S. Effect of intravenous infusions of histamine on acid gastric secretion and on urinary excretion of free histamine. The duration of each infusion was about 180 min. The dose is shown as the total amount infused (µg) and as the rate of infusion (ng/kg/min)

ADAM et al. (1954) could also show that detectable amounts of histamine in the urine appeared at dose levels of histamine which just caused a barely detectable increase in the rate of hydrochloric acid secretion from the stomach. The urinary excretion of histamine is therefore as sensitive an indicator as measurements of its biological actions for detecting the release of histamine into the blood stream. The superiority of "biological indicators" over estimations of plasma histamine in detecting histamine release in animals was pointed out already by EMMELIN et al. (1941).

Unfortunately, several disturbing factors exist, which make the urinary histamine in man much less useful than was originally expected. Even if some of these factors may be eliminated with proper precautions and experimental conditions, their possible interference must constantly be borne in mind, and due caution exerted when drawing conclusions about the release and formation of histamine in the body from analyses of the urinary histamine.

The following factors must thus be considered.

a) The highly efficient catabolism of histamine

As pointed out already by ADAM (1949) and ADAM et al. (1954) and discussed in part II the histamine-catabolizing enzymes are so efficient that only about 1% of intravenously infused histamine reaches the urine unchanged and measurable by current methods, i.e. as "free histamine." It seems likely that also endogenous histamine reaching the blood stream will be metabolized in a similar manner or possibly even more efficiently. The fact that only a minute fraction of released histamine is detectable in the urine need not by itself invalidate the use of urinary histamine, but the efficiency of the histamine-catabolizing enzymes (histamine-N-methyl transferase and diamine oxidase) may well vary under different physiological and pathological conditions. Thus a ten-fold increase of the urinary histamine, say from 10–100 μg/day, could be explained by a decrease in histamine inactivation from 99–90%, and need not be due to ten-fold increase in histamine formation or release. This makes it necessary to analyse the catabolic pathways for histamine in conditions which are accompanied by increase *or* decrease in the urinary excretion of free histamine (see part II).

Since the normal urinary excretion of free histamine may vary with 5–10 μg from day to day, a barely demonstrable increase in the urinary histamine would have to involve the liberation or formation of 0.5–1 mg per 24 hrs. Urinary excretion of histamine will therefore give information mainly in conditions involving relatively large and preferably rapid mobilizations of tissue histamine.

b) Urinary histamine may come from the intestinal lumen

where it has been formed by bacteria or it may have been present in the food (e.g. IRVINE et al., 1959b).

c) Urinary histamine may have been formed in the kidney

Such histamine may, although small in absolute amounts, be a relatively important part of the urinary histamine, since it might reach the urine without having been exposed to the histamine-metabolizing enzymes in the kidney (SCHAYER et al., 1954; LINDELL and SCHAYER, 1958). It is not yet known if some of the free urinary histamine in man is derived from the kidney.

d) Technical difficulties are present

Histamine may be formed or inactivated by bacteria. These processes may occur not only in the urine bottle, where they can be prevented, but also in the urinary bladder. Checks for urinary infection must therefore be carried out, especially in clinical studies.

2. Methodological considerations

Two useful methods exist for the estimation of the urinary excretion of free histamine. Both methods involve a concentration of the histamine by absorption to a cation exchanger and subsequent biological assay of the histamine content of the eluate on the isolated ileum of the guinea-pig.

ADAM (1949) initially used a modification of the method described by ANREP et al. (1944), in which histamine was concentrated by adsorption to charcoal. Then ROBERTS and ADAM (1950) succeeded in developing a more sensitive and reliable method for urinary histamine, namely:

a) By the absorption of histamine to the cation exchanger Decalso

Urine, with pH adjusted, is run through a column of Decalso F. Histamine is eluted from the column by concentrated ammonium hydroxide and chloroform, saturated with ammonia gas. After evaporation of the eluent the extract is taken up in a saline solution, the histamine content of which is estimated on the guinea-pig ileum.

The method has given reliable results and its main advantage appears to be that inorganic ions are present only in negligible amounts in the final extract.

The mean recovery of added histamine, 67%, appears to be constant, and may be corrected for.

b) The absorption of histamine to the cation exchanger Amberlite IRC-50

Bergström and Hansson (1951) showed that the weak carboxylic acid cation exchanger Amberlite IRC-50 absorbed histamine quantitatively, and that the histamine could be easily eluted by weak acids. This principle was adopted by Dunér and Pernow (1956a) who used it for determination of urinary histamine in man. The method is technically much simpler than that of Roberts and Adam (1950), because there is no need for evaporation. On the other hand, large amounts of urinary salts may appear in the final extract and disturb the assay on the guinea-pig ileum. This complication may be overcome by precipitation of most of the salts with an alcohol-acetone mixture in the cold. The recovery of added histamine from urine is similar to that with the Decalso method, about 70%.

With both methods a and b there is the possibility of other agents interfering with the bioassay of histamine. *These agents might cause contraction of the gut by themselves* (e.g. 5-hydroxytryptamine, potassium and slow-contracting substances). It is possible, however, to ascertain that a gut contraction caused by a urine specimen is due to histamine specifically, by adding antihistaminic agents in threshold doses and by using other antagonists, e.g. to 5-hydroxytryptamine (Cf. Dunér and Pernow, 1958a). Another possibility is to assay the urine for its histamine-like activity also on the cat's blood pressure. The result should be the same as on the guinea-pig ileum. Further biochemical confirmation may be derived from paper chromatography or incubation of the urinary extract with a purified preparation of diamine oxidase, which should destroy the histamine-like activity.

It appears certain that the agent called histamine in extracts prepared according to the methods of Roberts and Adam (1950) or Dunér and Pernow (1956a) and assayed with proper precautions is really identical with histamine. However, some doubt about this originates from the study of Kapeller-Adler and Iggo (1957) who found derivatives of histamine methylated on the side chain nitrogen in human urine. N-methylation on the side chain will not deprive histamine of its biological effects, like the ring-N-methylation does. Most workers have actually not excluded that part of the histamine-like activity in their urine samples was due to the presence of chain-N-methylated histamine. However, such an admixture would make little difference from the biological point of view.

More difficult to handle are urinary extracts in which *substances are present that inhibit the contraction of the guinea-pig ileum* in response to histamine. A drastic example is provided by a urine sample from a patient that has received treatment with antihistaminic agents. Extract from such a urine may depress the response of the intestine to histamine for a long time, and the histamine eventually present in the extract can therefore not be estimated. In practice it seems preferable to withhold antihistaminics while histamine studies are being carried out. However, Dunér and Pernow (1958a) succeeded in extracting promethazine from urine samples while not destroying the histamine. They were thus able to follow the urinary histamine in cases under treatment with promethazine (Birke et al., 1958).

Treatment with antihistaminic agents should be easy to recognize and prevent, but other substances, administered by the physician or formed in the body, may also interfere. Particularly striking is the finding of an endogenous "antihistaminic agent" in the urine during asthmatic symptoms (Dunér and Pernow, 1958d). While a long lasting inhibition of the histamine sensitivity of the ileum is easily recognized, it should be borne in mind that it may be difficult or impossible to assay the histamine content of a urine extract, which contains substances that inhibit the response of the gut for a brief period only, possibly only while the extract is kept in the bath. Such a depression of gut contractility can occur with salt-rich urine extracts and may easily pass unnoticed. Comparison of the gut-contracting activity of the sample without and with the addition of a small amount of histamine (as "internal standard") should reveal whether the expected increase in contraction height does occur or not. The presence of interfering agents in a urinary extract may sometimes also be revealed by different dose-response curves for the extract and the histamine standard, or by a conspicuous difference in "histamine activity" on different pieces of guinea-pig ileum.

After the preceding remarks, it is perhaps unnecessary to emphasize that the estimation of free histamine in human urine by bioassay may be a tricky business, requiring some experience. It may be risky to regard it as a routine technique, to be performed by a laboratory assistant. The problems of interfering agents, causing contractions or inhibitions of the gut, must be solved individually and no standard procedure can be recommended.

3. The urinary excretion of free histamine under various conditions

(Tables 23–28)

The urinary excretion of free histamine in normal adults appears to vary only little in different materials. Thus the mean values range from 8.6–21.6 μg/24 hours (Table 23). The composition of the food has not been specified in some of the reports, but it has presumably been "mixed." It would probably be possible to reduce variations in urinary, free histamine by keeping a rigidly fixed diet during the experimental periods. This is emphasized by the findings of MITCHELL and CODE (1954a) who showed that fasting lowered, and a meat diet increased the urinary histamine. These observations have been confirmed and extended by IRVINE et al. (1959b) who found that the urinary excretion of free histamine increased if a meal of meat was given. A similar increase was seen after the administration of 4.5 g of L-histidine by mouth. Because the urinary histamine peak after meat or L-histidine disappeared after treatment with succinylsulphathiazole, IRVINE et al. (1959b) concluded that intestinal bacteria can contribute to the urinary histamine by decarboxylating histidine in the food. The variability of the dietary intake of meat and other food with a high content of histamine and histidine may well obscure interesting variations in the excretion of endogenous histamine. There is apparently no sex difference in histamine excretion in man (DUNÉR and PERNOW, 1956a). The urinary excretion of free histamine is lower at night than during daytime (ROBERTS and ADAM, 1950; DUNÉR and PERNOW, 1956a).

The upper limit of normal values is of interest for the clinical use of histamine determinations in urine. This limit has not been rigidly defined. It would appear probable that an individual which excretes more than 30 μg of free histamine per 24 hours in two or three samples has a pathologically high urinary histamine, but possible abnormalities in the diet and in the intestinal bacterial population will have to be considered in each case. In children urinary histamine is proportional to the body weight (Table 24), the daily excretion being 0.30–0.40 μg/kg body weight over a weight range of 5–30 kg. On a weight basis children thus have a larger amount of free histamine in the urine than adults, which excrete about 0.2 μg/kg.

An increased excretion of urinary histamine has been found in cases of acute urticaria, eosinophilic lung infiltrations, pregnancy, urticaria pigmentosa, carcinoid tumour and after large burns of the skin. The significance of the increased urinary histamine in some of these conditions will be considered in part VII.

Table 23. *Observations on urinary excretion of free histamine in normal adults. For simplicity and to facilitate comparisons the range of values and the mean values are given. These mean values may sometimes be misleading due to the wide variations between individuals, notably in pathological conditions.*

Experimental conditions	No. of cases	Range	Mean value	S.E.M.	Method	Reference	Remark
Normal men	5	12.1—41.4	21.6	—	I	Roberts and Adam (1950)	—
Normal adults	10	traces—27.0	8.6	2.3	I	Adam et al. (1951-52)	—
Normal adults	—	8.0—26.9	17.7	1.2	I	Mitchell et al. (1954)	—
Normal adults	17	6.1—19.0	11.9	0.8	II	Dunér & Pernow (1956 a)	Urinary histamine lower at night.
Normal men	5	10.8—20.5	17.9	—	I	Mitchell & Code (1954 a)	—
Normal women	12	3.8—23.0	12.5	2.0	II	Bjurö et al. (1961 a)	—
Normal adults mixed diet	5	7.9—18.0	15.0	—	I	Mitchell and Code (1954 a)	Same subjects on 3 different diets and fasting
Normal adults fasting	5	7.1—14.5	10.8	—	I	Mitchell and Code (1954 a)	
Normal adults bread and milk	5	6.7—17.1	12.8	—	I	Mitchell and Code (1954 a)	
Normal adults meat	5	9.1—40.0	25.4	—	I	Mitchell and Code (1954 a)	

Unless otherwise stated the values denote free histamine in μg base/24 hrs (± S.E.M.). Method I = Decalso method of Roberts and Adam (1950). Method II = Amberlite method of Dunér and Pernow (1956 a).

Table 24. *Urinary excretion of free histamine in healthy children*

Experimental conditions	No. of cases	Mean age (years)	μg/24 hours		μg/kg/24 hours		Method	Reference	Remark
			range	mean	range	mean			
Healthy children	10	<1	0.3—2.8	1.7	0.13—0.48	0.30	I	Adam and Mitchell (1953)	Excretion related to body weight
Healthy children	10	2—5	2.5—8.1	5.1	0.16—0.55	0.33	I	Adam and Mitchell (1953)	
Healthy children	10	6—9	6.1—12.3	9.4	0.28—0.61	0.42	I	Adam and Mitchell (1953)	
Healthy children	10	10—12	7.2—18.5	12.7	0.25—0.63	0.42	I	Adam and Mitchell (1953)	
Healthy children	14	<1	—	—	0.10—0.46	0.28	I	Dieckhoff (1957 a)	
Healthy children	10	1—4	—	—	0.14—0.52	0.36	I	Dieckhoff (1957 a)	
Healthy children	12	4—8	—	—	0.12—0.64	0.40	I	Dieckhoff (1957 a)	
Healthy children	10	8—14	—	—	0.21—0.62	0.42	I	Dieckhoff (1957 a)	
Healthy children	4	—	—	—	0.21—0.40	—	II	Bloom et al. (1958)	

Values are given in μg histamine base per 24 hours and as μg/kg body weight per 24 hours. Method I: Roberts and Adam (1950). Method II: Dunér and Pernow (1956 a).

There are a few cases recorded in which the urinary histamine has been raised to very high values (Tables 27 and 28). Such an excretion has been found in pregnant women with preeclamptic toxemia, and in cases of urticaria pigmentosa or carcinoid tumours. Urinary free histamine in such cases has reached values from several hundred μg up to several thousand μg per day. In striking contrast to these enormous figures are the observations in wide-spread acute urticaria and large cutaneous burns, in which the urinary histamine has been in the order of 100 μg per day, in spite of the fact that a large part of the skin histamine probably was mobilized under these conditions. In some cases of urticaria pigmentosa with a high urinary histamine there have been signs indicative of biological effects of histamine, and even shock-like states (Bloom et al., 1958). In these cases, one is reasonably certain that the urinary histamine reflects the rate of release of endogenous histamine from the mast cells. In the cases of carcinoid tumour having a high urinary histamine there has been a more red and warm flushing of the skin than in other cases and this may conceivably reflect an increased synthesis and liberation of histamine.

However, it is well known that histamine infused by vein will produce drastic circulatory changes and a copious gastric secretion at a dose level of about 0.3 μg/kg/min. A tentative 24 hour infusion of histamine giving biological effects would thus deliver some 30 mg to a patient. Assuming that histamine catabolism is unchanged, one would expect about 1% of 30 mg to reach the urine, i.e. 300 μg per 24 hours. The histamine values in urticaria pigmentosa and burns are of this order of magnitude, but it seems very difficult to explain why patients that excrete 1000–7000 μg histamine daily (pregnancy, carcinoid tumour) do not have severe symptoms of histamine shock. Adaptation to the actions of histamine might occur, but the question must be asked, whether this urinary histamine really comes from the plasma. It may have been formed in the kidney and excreted directly. Urinary infection has been excluded in some cases, but not in all. The high urinary histamine in carcinoid disease and in pregnancy may also be due to a diminished rate of catabolism. This point could be settled in carcinoid tumours at least by the use of C^{14}-histamine, but in pregnant women, who are going to bear a live child, the administration of C^{14}-histamine might be inappropriate.

Comment must also be made upon some observations of *an abnormally low histamine excretion*. The lower normal limit for the excretion of free histamine has not been well defined, and estimations of urinary histamine by bioassay appear to be more difficult at low excretion rates. It appears certain, however, that a low histamine excretion is sometimes found during symptoms of bronchial asthma (Tables 25 and 26) and food allergy (Table 25) and during severe preeclamptic toxemia or eclampsia in pregnant women (Table 27). It is tempting to assume that the lowered urinary histamine might be an important pathophysiological mechanism in these conditions, and one could imagine a retention of histamine in the blood or in certain tissues. Studies with C^{14}-histamine (see part II) have shown that the kidney is able to excrete injected histamine during asthmatic symptoms. Another alternative is that urinary histamine normally is formed by renal histidine decarboxylase (Section V, A, 1, c) and that this formation is depressed under certain conditions.

It seems that an abnormally low urinary histamine might be an equally interesting phenomenon as an increased excretion, and merits further research.

To test the validity of the "free" urinary histamine as an indicator of endogenous formation and/or liberation of histamine in the body, Dunér and Pernow (1958b) studied blood and urinary histamine levels simultaneously in healthy persons and in some pathological conditions (i.e. leukemia, carcinoid tumor, burns). They

Table 25. *Urinary excretion of free histamine in some allergic conditions.* Explanations: See Table 23

Experimental conditions	No. of cases	Range	Mean	Method	Reference	Remark
Urticaria, acute, adults	2	46; 104	75	I	Adam et al. (1951—52)	
Urticaria, chronic, adults	7	traces—67	23	I	Adam et al. (1951—52)	
"Various diseases"	10	traces—54	15	I	Adam et al. (1951—52)	Convalescents used as control material
Bronchial asthma, adults during symptoms	10	0 or traces	<1.0	II	Dunér and Pernow (1958d)	Endogenous "antihistaminic" present in 3 cases during symptoms
Bronchial asthma, adults symptom-free	10	4.2—32	9.8	II	Dunér and Pernow (1958d)	
Eosinophilic pulmonary infiltrations (Loeffler's syndrome)	1	—	120	II	Dunér and Pernow (1956b)	Normalized excretion after treatment
Food allergy	1	very low during symptoms		II	Dunér and Pernow (1960)	
Hereditary, periodic edema	2	low excretion during symptoms; high excretion on other occasions		II	Arnoldsson et al. (1962b)	

Table 26. *Urinary excretion of free histamine in children with allergic or other diseases.* For explanations: See Table 24

Experimental conditions	No. of cases	μg/24 hours range	μg/24 hours mean	μg/kg/24 hours range	μg/kg/24 hours mean	Method	Reference	Remark
Allergic children, no symptoms	14	6.7—17.8	11.5	0.21—0.57	0.38	I	Mitchell et al. (1954b)	Not different from normal values
Allergic children, *during asthma*	5	3.7—19.7	10.3	0.17—0.52	0.32	I	Mitchell et al. (1954b)	Lower excretion per kg body weight than in normal cases (cf Table 24)
Allergic children, during pollinosis	5	5.4—16.4	12.7	0.16—0.43	0.30	I	Mitchell et al. (1954b)	
Asthmatic children, no symptoms	5	—	—	0.19—0.58	0.33	I	Dieckhoff (1957a)	Normal excretion
Asthmatic children, *during attack*	5	—	—	0.14—0.29	0.21	I	Dieckhoff (1957a)	Lower excretion during asthmatic attack
Children with eczema	5	—	—	0.21—0.41	0.32	I	Dieckhoff (1957a)	Normal excretion
Gastroenteritis, acute	10	0.5—2.8	1.1	—	—	I	Adam and Mitchell (1953)	Values about the same during symptoms as in convalescence
Gastroenteritis, in convalescence	10	0.6—3.3	1.6	—	—	I	Adam and Mitchell (1953)	
Acute "dyspepsia"	12	—	—	0.31—0.49	0.38	I	Dieckhoff (1957a)	Normal excretion
Dyspeptic "intoxication"	5	—	—	0.47—1.24	0.78	I	Dieckhoff (1957a)	High excretion; children in shock stage
Acute nephritis	8	—	—	0.41—1.75	0.92	I	Dieckhoff (1957a)	High excretion; children in shock stage
Chronic nephritis	5	—	—	0.25—0.68	0.46	I	Dieckhoff (1957a)	
Child with urticaria pigmentosa	1	—	—	0.8; 1.6	1.2	II	Bloom et al. (1958)	Child showing sings of "histamine shock"

Table 27. *Urinary excretion of free histamine in human pregnancy.* Explanations: See Table 23

Experimental conditions	No. of cases	Range	Mean value	Method	Reference	Remark
Normal pregnancy	19	traces[1]	—	X	Kapeller-Adler and Adler (1943)	
Pregnancy with heart disease, hypertension, anemia or pyelitis	11	traces[1]	—	X	Kapeller-Adler and Adler (1943)	
Hyperemesis gravidarum	3	traces[1]	—	X	Kapeller-Adler and Adler (1943)	
Hyperemesis gravidarum	8	16—63[1]	—	X	Kapeller-Adler and Adler (1943)	
Preeclamptic toxaemia, mild	4	traces[1]	—	X	Kapeller-Adler and Adler (1943)	
Preeclamptic toxaemia, mild	12	0.9—181[1]	—	X	Kapeller-Adler and Adler (1943)	
Preeclamptic toxaemia, severe	8	0-trace[1]	—	X	Kapeller-Adler and Adler (1943)	
Eclampsia	2	0	—	X	Kapeller-Adler and Adler (1943)	
After birth	5	0-trace[1]	—	X	Kapeller-Adler and Adler (1943)	
Normal pregnancy (>30 weeks)	10	18.0—24.0	20.4	I	Rockenschaub (1953)	
Preeclamptic toxemia, mild	10	10.8—40.0	20.2	I	Rockenschaub (1953)	
Preeclamptic toxemia, severe	10	1.4—11.0	6.3	I	Rockenschaub (1953)	
Normal pregnancy (near birth)	14	3.0—82.0	29.5	II	Bjurö et al. (1961a)	Reduction after delivery in 9 cases
Prolonged pregnancy	3	180—300	253	II	Bjurö et al. (1961a)	Reduction after delivery in 3 cases
Preeclamptic toxemia, mild	7	7.5—132	52.6	II	Bjurö et al. (1961a)	Reduction after delivery in 6 cases
Preeclamptic toxemia, moderate to severe	8	7—1200[2]	42.5	II	Bjurö et al. (1961a)	Reduction after delivery in 5 cases
Eclampsia	2	2—3	2.5	II	Bjurö et al. (1961a)	
After birth (normal cases)	10	—	—	II	Lindberg and Westling (1961)	Short-lasting elevation of urinary histamine at days 4—7 after birth

[1] Histamine values refer to mg histamine diflavianate crystallized from 3 l urine (Method X).
[2] Highest value, 1200 μg/24 hrs, not included in the average.

Table 28. *Observations on free urinary histamine in some other conditions where changes might be expected.* Explanations: See Table 23

Experimental conditions	No. of cases	Range	Mean value (approximate)	S.E.M.	Method	Reference	Remark
Urticaria pigmentosa adults	7	42—555	170	—	II	Brogren et al. (1959)	High excretion also in children
Urticaria pigmentosa adults	5	60—850	290	—	II	Demis et al. (1961)	
Urticaria pigmentosa adults	2	100; 260	180	—	II	Demis and Brown (1961)	—
Carcinoid tumor adults	9	15—6800	—	—	II	Pernow and Waldenström (1957)	Cases showing bright, red flush
Carcinoid tumor adults	1	480—940	—	—	I	Sandler and Snow (1958)	
Burns, large adults first 24 hours	8	2.0—6.1 µg/hr	4.0 µg/hr	—	II	Birke et al. (1958)	High urinary histamine immediately after burn
Burns, large adults later on	6	0.2—1.0 µg/hr	0.50 µg/hr	—	II	Birke et al. (1958)	
Cirrhosis of the liver	7	8.5—20.9	14.9	2.3	I	Mitchell et al. (1954a)	—
Obstructive jaundice; mild pruritus	9	6.1—25.5	13.5	2.6	I	Mitchell et al. (1954a)	—
Obstructive jaundice; severe pruritus	8	6.9—31.1	15.7	3.7	I	Mitchell et al. (1954a)	—

found a good correlation between blood and urinary histamine (correlation coefficient = 0.88 for 19 cases).

It should be emphasized that such a correlation is not found in many conditions involving changes of blood and urinary histamine in either direction. A correlation may exist in conditions which are characterized by a rapid flooding of the blood stream with histamine and subsequent increase in urinary histamine (e.g. the cases of burn injuries mentioned by Dunér and Pernow, 1958b). The lack of such a correlation in bronchial asthma was pointed out by Dunér and Pernow (1958d). In bronchial asthma the urinary histamine may be low (Dunér and Pernow, 1958d) but the blood level of histamine is unchanged or even raised (Serafini, 1948, and Rose, Rusted and Fownes, 1950). Another striking example is found during the administration of cortisone or related steroids, which decrease blood histamine in normal and pathological conditions (Code and Mitchell, 1957; Noah and Brand, 1957), but increase the urinary excretion of free histamine (Mitchell and Code, 1954b, and Mitchell et al., 1954b). Cases of acute urticaria may have a high excretion of urinary histamine (Adam, Hunter and Kinnear, 1951), but the blood histamine is lowered during attacks (e.g. Rorsman and Rosengren, 1958). In some pregnant women the urinary excretion of free histamine may be high but the blood histamine is not appreciably changed (Bjurö et al., 1961a).

Most of the blood histamine is bound to the white cells, notably the basophils (see part IV) and there is thus reason to believe that the histamine in the blood is of a different physiological nature than the urinary histamine, which probably comes from the plasma or is newly formed in the kidney. A lack of correlation between blood and urinary histamine under various conditions is therefore not surprising. It may in fact be said, that changes in blood histamine largely reflect changes in the blood content of basophils.

It was mentioned above, and in part IV, C, c, that cortisone could produce changes in the blood histamine level and in the urinary histamine. These actions of cortisone appear to be related and may well throw light upon the mechanism of action of adrenocortical steroids in conditions of allergic nature. MITCHELL and CODE (1954b) and DIECKHOFF (1957a) found that cortisone caused only a scarcely detectable increase in the free urinary histamine in normal persons. The number of experimental subjects was small, but the available observations are probably sufficient to delineate the "normal" effect of cortisone from that observed in certain allergic states. In 2 cases out of 6 examined, with allergic diseases, MITCHELL et al. (1954b) found a substantial increase in the urinary histamine after cortisone. This "abnormal" effect of cortisone appears to have been studied further only by DIECKHOFF (1957a, b). DIECKHOFF (1957a) found a regular and relatively pronounced increase in the urinary histamine upon the administration of cortisone to children with asthma and eczema. The healthy child did not exhibit any clearcut

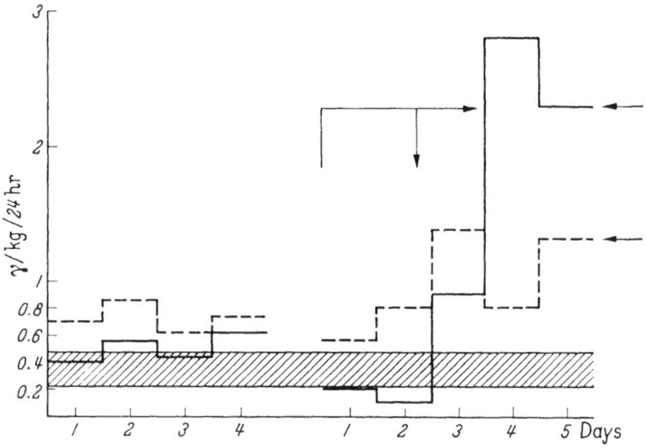

Fig. 5. Urinary excretion of free (whole-drawn line) and conjugated (interrupted line) histamine in a child with bronchial asthma. Values are first given for 4 days in a symptom-free interval. Then values are given during a period of asthma, which was interrupted by cortisone (2 × 50 mg daily) on the 2nd day. Hatched area = normal range

changes in the urinary histamine during treatment with cortisone (DIECKHOFF, 1957b). Particularly striking is the nice observation by DIECKHOFF (1957b) that cortisone, given to a child with asthmatic symptoms, could reverse the urinary excretion of histamine from the low level characteristic of the asthmatic attack to a pathologically high level (Fig. 5 from DIECKHOFF, 1957b). These results appear to provide new evidence both for the participation of histamine in asthma and for the view that adrenocortical steroids may affect the metabolism of histamine, at least in abnormal conditions.

a) Urinary excretion of "conjugated" histamine

ANREP et al. (1944) observed that the urine of man and some animals contained a histamine derivative that became physiologically active after acid hydrolysis. Subsequent work (URBACH, 1949; TABOR and MOSETTIG, 1949) showed that this "conjugated histamine" was identical with N-acetylhistamine, the acetate being bound to the side chain nitrogen.

Conjugated histamine may be estimated by the same methods as used for free histamine; the only requirement being that the sample is subjected to a thorough hydrolysis with hydrochloric acid before extraction (e.g. ROBERTS and ADAM, 1950). Conjugated histamine is present in highly varying amounts in human urine. Most workers have not rigidly identified the "conjugate" with N-acetylhistamine. It is well established (ANREP et al., 1944; ADAM et al., 1951–1952)

Table 29. *Occurrence of histamine in human faeces*

Cathegory	No. of cases	Range of values or average	Method	Reference	Remark
Normal men	13	0—4 μg/ml	Code	Myhrman and Tomenius (1939)	
"Various diseases"	8	0—5 μg/ml	Code	Myhrman and Tomenius (1939)	
Various gastrointestinal diseases	10	0—14 μg/ml	Code	Myhrman and Tomenius (1939)	Including dyspepsia and enteritis
Ulcerous colitis	8	0.25—20 μg/ml	Code	Myhrman and Tomenius (1939)	High values in 2 of 8 cases
Bronchial asthma	10	0.5 —256 μg/ml	Code	Myhrman and Tomenius (1939)	High values in 5 of 10 cases
Normal subjects, males	—	average 0.03 μg/ml	Code	Jimenez Diaz et al. (1955)	Faeces from asthmatics form more histamine and/or destroy less histamine. Presumably entirely dependent upon bacterial population in gut
Normal subjects, females	—	avergae 0.44 μg/ml	Code	Jimenez Diaz et al. (1955)	
Asthmatics, males	—	average 29.0 μg/ml	Code	Jimenez Diaz et al. (1955)	
Asthmatics, females	—	average 116.0 μg/ml	Code	Jimenez Diaz et al. (1955)	

that the excretion of conjugated histamine is increased much more after giving histamine by the mouth than after intravenous injection, the latter causing a preferential increase in the urinary excretion of free histamine. There is also evidence that the excretion of conjugated histamine varies much with the type of food eaten by the subject (Mitchell and Code, 1954a). A diet rich in meat thus causes large amounts of conjugated histamine to appear in the urine, presumably because the meat contained histamine or because intestinal bacteria formed histamine from histidine in the meat. There is some evidence that acetylation of histamine may occur in the tissues of the body (for discussion see Gaddum, 1956; Dunér and Pernow, 1960). On the other hand, studies with C^{14}-histamine (see Schayer, 1959) show that only a small fraction of injected histamine is acetylated, and it seems probable that this holds also for endogenous histamine.

In our opinion analysis of the urinary content of conjugated histamine does not materially increase the validity of urinary histamine measurements, except if the excretion of conjugated histamine is elevated out of proportion to that of free histamine. This will direct attention to the food or the intestinal bacteria as important sources of histamine. In the present review data for the excretion of conjugated histamine are therefore given comparatively little attention.

VI. Occurrence of histamine in human faeces

Table 29 shows some observations on the histamine content of human faeces. One is inclined to believe that the content of histamine in the faeces is dependent upon the balance between the activity of histamine-forming and histamine-inactivating bacteria, and upon the passage time through the colon. The presence of large amounts of histamine in the faeces of some asthmatic patients is nevertheless of some interest. The resorption rate of histamine from the colon is not specifically known; histamine in the colon may reach the blood in larger amounts than histamine given by the mouth. 133 mg histamine have been given orally without any significant increase in urinary free histamine (Adam, 1949).

VII. Remarks about the possible involvement of histamine in some physiological and pathological conditions in man

a) General remarks

The preceding sections concerning histamine metabolism will have made it apparent that nothing is known about the physiology of histamine in man. Moreover, the role of histamine in most of the pathological conditions in which it has been studied, remains entirely unclear. However, much work is still being carried out in the belief that histamine is of importance both in health and disease. This is not only a matter of stubborn belief but a reflection of the many suggestive hints that exist.

In recent years histaminologists have become stronger in their conviction as a result of fundamental work in animals. SCHAYER has thus not only enriched physiologists with useful isotopic methods for histamine work but has also cleared up the catabolism and formation of histamine (see Chapter 4, Sections B and D of this book). In addition to this he has provided a new theory for the function of histamine in normal conditions as well as in various abnormal conditions in laboratory animals. SCHAYER suggests that the function of histamine is to secure an adequate circulation to the tissues. To this end, the histamine-forming enzyme histidine decarboxylase, is activated (maybe in the very endothelium of the small vessels). The histamine thus formed dilates the small vessels and is then removed rapidly, escaping detection by conventional methods for measuring tissue histamine content. Such a histamine formation can be induced in every tissue examined, and in several species.

At about the same time, KAHLSON (for a review see: KAHLSON, 1960) demonstrated an extremely rapid formation of histamine during pregnancy in the rat. It could also be shown that the foetuses of the rat contained an extremely active histidine decarboxylase. This lead to the hypothesis that the process of histamine formation was in some way connected with the intra-uterine growth of the rat foetus. Further experiments by KAHLSON's group showed that histamine was formed in regenerative and reparative growth as well as in certain tumours in the rat. The histamine which has been related to growth processes by KAHLSON is not bound in the tissues in the conventional way. In growing tissues where histamine formation is rapid, the actual content is generally quite low. The status of the "nascent histamine" of KAHLSON in growing tissues is thus similar to that of Schayer's "inducible histamine," both being formed in the tissue but not staying there for a long time. The physiological effects of this "sustained histamine action" may well be radically different from those of exogenous or suddenly liberated histamine, and it is not certain whether antihistaminics counteract the effects of nascent or induced histamine.

Thus, about 50 years after its isolation, histamine has been firmly linked with two fundamental biological processes, namely circulatory control, pregnancy and growth in general. It would seem appropriate to discuss here the possibility of histamine being associated with circulatory control, pregnancy and growth processes also in man. In doing so, we are aware that the evidence, for or against, is presently scarce.

In addition we shall attempt to discuss briefly the possible role of histamine for allergic diseases as well as the relationship of histamine to the endocrine glands. Histamine as a possible factor in gastric secretion and mental diseases will also be discussed.

b) *Histamine and pregnancy*

Several observations point to a connexion between histamine and pregnancy. Thus histamine contracts the uterine smooth muscle in several species (DALE and LAIDLAW, 1910). There is, however, no conclusive evidence that histamine is connected with the process of parturition.

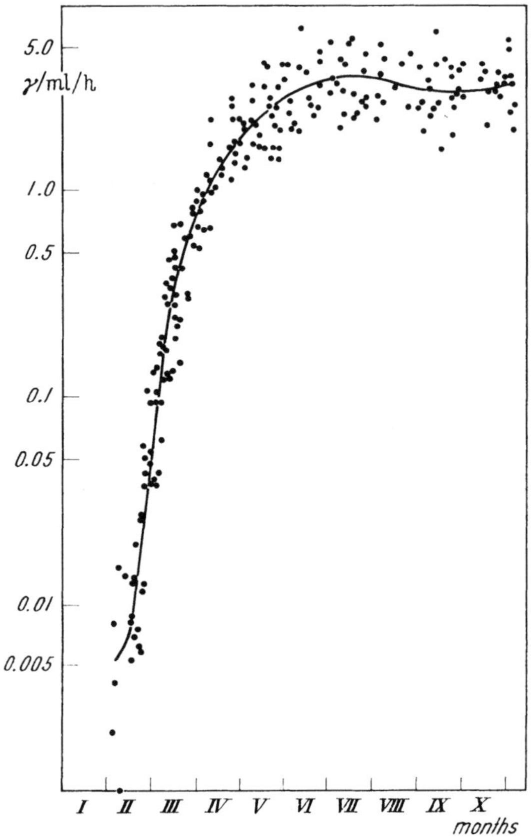

Fig. 6. Histaminolytic power of plasma from ca. 45 healthy pregnant women. Abscissa: months of pregnancy calculated from first day of last menstruation. Ordinate: histaminolytic power expressed in γ inactivated histamine per ml plasma per hour

The strongest link between histamine and pregnancy was for a long time an indirect one, namely the high histaminolytic activity of placental extracts and, in man, of the pregnant mother's plasma.

It was first shown by MARCOU, ATHANASIU-VERGU, CHIRICEANU, COSMA, GINGOLD and PARHON (1938) that blood from pregnant women contains increased amounts of a histaminolytic agent. This histaminolysis has been shown to be due to oxidative deamination catalyzed by an enzyme. Whether this histaminase is identical with diamine oxidase has been debated by KAPELLER-ADLER (1953). The histaminolytic activity in plasma increases in a regular fashion during normal pregnancy.

Fig. 6 shows the range of activity observed by AHLMARK (1944). The increased plasma histaminase has been used to determine the duration of a pregnancy in forensic medicine. Measurements of the histaminolytic activity in plasma have been used to judge the prognosis in cases of threatening abortion. A histaminolysis within the normal range in a case of uterine bleeding indicates a good prognosis for the pregnancy. In the experience of BORGLIN and WILLERT (1957) this is so reliable that if an abortion occurs in spite of a normal histaminase activity in plasma there is reason to suspect a criminal induction.

As first demonstrated by DANFORTH (1939), the human placenta contains a histaminolytic agent. According to ZELLER and BIRKHÄUSER (1940) this histaminase is indistinguishable from diamine oxidase. The distribution of the enzymatic activity in placenta is shown in Fig. 7.

SWANBERG (1950) found that the concentration of the enzyme usually was a little higher in blood from the uterine vein than in arterial blood or blood from a peripheral vein. This was taken to indicate that the histaminolytic activity in plasma comes from the placenta.

LINDAHL (1960a, b) showed that placenta also contains a histamine-methylating enzyme. However, blood from pregnant women did not methylate histamine (LINDAHL et al., 1958).

The significance of the histaminolytic activity in placenta and plasma is not known. The possibility has been discussed that the enzymes protect the uterine muscle which is sensitive to histamine during pregnancy (EFFKEMANN and WERLE, 1940; GUNTHER and PATON, 1960). Another possibility is that the foetus needs protection for histamine and/or other diamines possibly produced in the maternal body, e.g. in the intestines.

Several workers have found that the sensitivity of the mother towards exogenous histamine is not different from that in non-pregnant women. This has been found for several actions of histamine, e.g. metallic taste, dizziness and headache (JANOWITZ and GROSSMAN, 1949) the size of the flare of the triple response (WICKSELL, 1949b), eosinopenia (KULLANDER, 1952) and gastric secretion (CLARK and TANKEL, 1954). These observations could indicate that the plasma histaminase was not active *in vivo*. Another explanation is that the addition of histaminolytic activity provided by the plasma and placenta in pregnancy is comparatively small in relation to the eliminating mechanisms normally present in various tissues, e. g. the liver and the kidneys (Cf. NILSSON, LINDELL, SCHAYER and WESTLING, 1959).

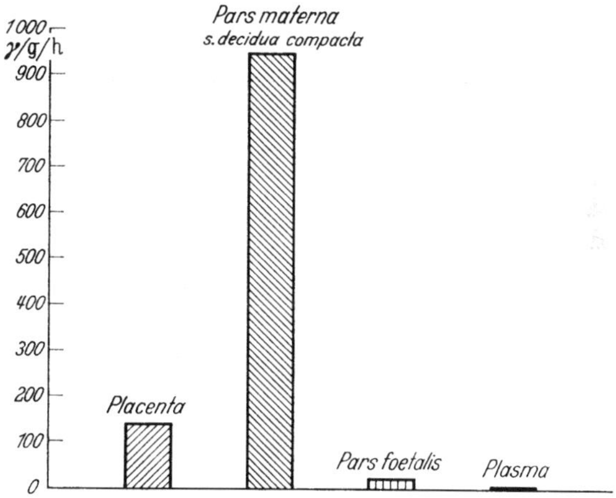

Fig. 7. Histaminolytic activity of the placenta as a whole, its two components and the maternal plasma

It may be mentioned here that the histaminase inhibitor aminoguanidine in a dose of 50 mg three times daily did not cause a particularly large increase in the urinary excretion of free histamine in pregnant women (20–24 weeks). Nor did it cause abortion or any other harmful effects (BJURÖ, LINDBERG and WESTLING, unpublished).

The connexion between histamine and pregnancy became stronger when it was found that the pregnant rat excreted large amounts of histamine in the urine (KAHLSON, ROSENGREN and WESTLING, 1958). Evidence was also obtained that the excess urinary histamine was produced by the foetuses which contained a very active histidine decarboxylase (KAHLSON, ROSENGREN, WESTLING and WHITE, 1958).

There are some observations which support the belief that also the human foetus can produce histamine. Some observations on the urinary excretion of free histamine were recorded in part V, Table 27. It can be seen from this table that a high urinary histamine is sometimes seen during normal pregnancy and in such cases a prompt reduction occurs at delivery (BJURÖ et al., 1961a). It has been pointed out (part V), that conclusions about the significance of changes in the urinary histamine must be made with caution. The analogous findings in the pregnant rat, however, strengthen the belief that the increase in urinary histamine sometimes seen in human pregnancy is the result of increased histamine formation in the mother and/or the foetus. There is also some evidence, apart from that provided by analogy with the rat, that the human foetus may be a source of histamine. First, the urinary excretion of histamine is promptly reduced at delivery. Second, there is evidence that the foetal blood, and possibly also the plasma, contains more histamine than the mother's blood (Table 22, part IV).

Most workers agree that the whole blood of the new-born human child is richer in histamine than blood from adults. The child's blood contains roughly 2–3 times more histamine than the adult, but the difference is more striking if the comparison is made with the mother's blood obtained simultaneously at parturition. The maternal blood histamine is then lowered (see part IV), and the foetal level is 5–7 times that of the mother. MITCHELL and CASS (1959) concluded that the tendency to higher blood histamine levels in the umbilical vein simply reflected differences in the numbers of circulating basophils and eosinophils. MARCOU et al. (1938) and BJURÖ et al. (1961a) found that whole blood from the umbilical vein often contained less histamine than blood from the umbilical artery. This difference suggests removal of histamine from the foetal blood during the placental passage, and could be explained either by the presence of some diffusible histamine in the plasma, by liberation of histamine from blood cells or by the disappearance of cells from the foetal blood.

WICKSELL (1949b) investigated the concentration of histamine in plasma from the umbilical vessels at birth. Using Code's method or ultrafiltration of plasma he found no difference between the plasma level of histamine in the umbilical artery, umbilical vein and venous blood from the mother. On the other hand, PETTAY (1950) found quite high plasma histamine levels in "umbilical cord blood," levels that were higher than those in adults. The findings of PETTAY were criticized by MITCHELL and CASS (1959) who found that the plasma histamine level in the umbilical vein at birth was so low that it could not be measured, just as it is in adults (ADAM, HARDWICK and SPENCER, 1957). MITCHELL and CASS did not examine blood from the umbilical artery. The findings of PETTAY (1950) were confirmed by KAHLSON, ROSENGREN and WHITE (1959), who found that plasma from foetal arterial blood mostly contained histamine in measurable amounts, while the plasma histamine in the mother was not detectable. Further, they found that the umbilical vein plasma contained less histamine than that in the artery, which again suggests removal of histamine by the placenta.

Although somewhat divergent, the studies on blood and plasma histamine in the umbilical vessels may be said to support the view that histamine formation can take place also in the human foetus.

As mentioned in part I there is a measurable formation of histamine in most tissues from human foetuses. The rate of formation appears to be higher than in some adult tissues examined but is still very much lower than in rat foetuses (KAHLSON, ROSENGREN, WESTLING and WHITE, 1958).

Summarizing, it can perhaps be said that in man pregnancy is the only normal condition so far examined in which histamine seems to be implicated. The evidence is, however, not yet fully conclusive, but it suggests that histamine may be produced by the foetus. The powerful histamine-inactivating enzymes in the maternal placenta (and plasma) then become biologically more meaningful.

c) Histamine and circulatory control

There is no evidence available that gives information whether SCHAYER's conception of histamine as a circulatory regulator can be applied to man. So far SCHAYER (see Chapter 4, Section D) has demonstrated the appearance of inducible histidine decarboxylase in all species examined. The methods presently applicable to human experimentation are insufficient and further extension of the theory to man will have to await newer techniques.

Anyhow, it may be pointed out that blood histamine levels vary in a few conditions involving circulatory adjustments. The elevation of whole blood histamine during muscular exercise, reactive hyperemia and congestive heart failure is in all probability connected with an increased number of circulating basophil leukocytes, and these observations do not therefore directly implicate histamine in itself. On the other hand, it may well be imagined that the basophil leukocyte (and its load of i. c. histamine) may be of importance for the maintenance of blood flow in the small vessels. The role of histamine as an endogenously liberated vasodilatator in man was thoroughly discussed by WHELAN (1956) who concluded that histamine was not the cause of the vasodilatation after adrenaline infusion, short periods of muscular work or circulatory arrest or exposition to cold. Whelan obtained some reduction by antihistaminics of the reactive hyperemia following long periods (10–25 min) of circulatory arrest, indicating that histamine was a contributory factor.

d) Histamine in allergy

The fact that histamine can mimic many of the symptoms of the allergic reaction is well known and many investigators have studied the role of histamine in allergy. If, as seems reasonable, we assume that histamine in fact is responsible for some of the allergic manifestations, we must consider the following possible mechanisms behind these reactions.

A. The concentration of histamine at the site of the reaction is increased. This may be caused by:

1. A release of preformed histamine (probably mainly from the mast cells) elicited by allergen-antibody reaction or by a histamine releaser.

2. An increased formation of histamine through an increased activity of histidine decarboxylase (Schayer's inducible histamine).

3. A decreased catabolism of histamine, which might explain the well known supersensitivity to exogenous histamine in many allergic subjects.

B. An increased sensitivity to histamine brought about by other means than a defect in the catabolism.

Ad A: 1. That histamine is actually released in sensitized human tissues on addition of the specific allergen has been demonstrated by KATZ (1942) who studied skin and by SCHILD et al. (1951) who studied lung tissue. It has also been found that allergens added to blood from an allergic subject may release histamine from the blood cells (VAN ARSDEL et al., 1958; MIDDLETON and SHERMAN, 1961). The mechanism of this release seems to be the same as the mechanism of histamine release in the anaphylactic reaction (SCHILD, 1958; BROCKLEHURST, 1958; HÖGBERG and UVNÄS, 1960). It seems likely that the released histamine comes mainly from the mast cells (BORÉUS and CHAKRAVARTY, 1959) or the basophil leukocytes.

Ad A: 2. The histidine decarboxylase activity at the site of the allergic reaction has not been studied in man. An increased histamine formation has however been demonstrated at the site of the tuberculin reaction in guinea-pigs (SCHAYER and GANLEY, 1959). It has also been found that histidine decarboxylase activity increases following release of histamine by compounds 48/80 and polymyxin B (SCHAYER, ROTHSCHILD and BIZONY, 1959; SCHAYER and GANLEY, 1959). Thus it is conceivable that in man, too, a histamine release may be followed by an increased formation of histamine.

Ad A: 3. The possibility that a decreased capacity to catabolize and excrete histamine contributes to the allergic reaction has been discussed several times. MITCHELL (1959) gave histamine to asthmatic children and found that the fraction of the injected histamine which appeared in the urine was the same as in healthy children. HELANDER et al. (1962) studied the catabolism of injected C^{14}-histamine in allergic subjects, symptom-free as well as during allergic reactions. The catabolism of subcutaneously or intravenously injected C^{14}-histamine was the same irrespective of whether the subjects had symptoms or not and the pattern and rate of metabolism did not differ significantly from that in healthy subjects. There is thus *no* experimental support for the belief that a reduction of the capacity to destroy or excrete histamine is a cause of the allergic reaction. On the contrary it would seem that the human organism is very well equipped to eliminate histamine reaching the circulating blood (Fig. 7 and ARNOLDSSON et al., 1962a). The possibility that the inactivation of histamine is reduced at the site of the allergic reaction has not been studied.

Ad B. It is well known that asthmatic subjects are very sensitive to inhaled histamine. BOUHUYS et al. (1960) found that this supersensitivity could be reduced by a ganglion blocking agent (hexamethonium). This suggests that nervous mechanisms may be responsible for the increased reactivity of the bronchial muscle in asthmatic subjects. Another explanation for the supersensitivity to histamine in allergic subjects has been suggested by SCHAYER (1961a). According to him a continuous increased formation of histamine in the allergic tissue might explain the pronounced sensitivity to exogenous histamine.

It is the opinion of the present authors that we must accept as a fact that the allergen-antibody reaction leads to liberation of histamine (and other substances) in man. What chance is there that histamine released or newly formed at the site of the allergic reaction will appear in the blood or in the urine? The local concentration of histamine may be sufficient to cause a local reaction and yet the actual amount of free histamine may be very small. Most human tissues can metabolize histamine (see Table 3).

Human lung tissue can methylate considerable quantities of histamine (LILJA et al., 1960). For this reason it is possible that a great part of the histamine liberated in the allergic reaction is metabolized locally, before reaching the circulating blood. If some of it ever escapes into the blood it will be very efficiently taken up and metabolized in other organs (ARNOLDSSON et al., 1962b). Here one must remember that histamine may be injected intravenously in doses which have general circulatory effects and yet the presence of the injected histamine in the blood cannot be demonstrated by conventional methods of assay (part IV). Measurements of blood histamine are therefore not likely to give any information about release of histamine. It is possible that measurement of plasma histamine with the technique developed by ADAM et al. (1957) may be more helpful, but even so the amount of histamine released into the blood must be great enough to give circulatory effects. Unless this is the case it is probably useless to search for the liberated histamine in the blood.

An increased urinary excretion of histamine has been observed during attacks of urticaria (ADAM et al., 1951–1952).

Other investigators have actually found a decrease in the urinary excretion of free histamine during allergic manifestations. In interpreting these results it must be borne in mind that only 1–2 (4) % of injected histamine is excreted in unchanged form in the urine.

A positive finding of increased excretion of histamine during an allergic attack indicates but does not prove the participation of histamine in the reaction. The absence of such an increase can however not be used to prove that histamine was not liberated at the site of the reaction. Similar arguments may be applied in the interpretation of changes in blood histamine. It must also be borne in mind that changes in the histamine content of whole blood are likely to be due to changes in the number of white blood cells.

Cold urticaria is regarded by some workers as a "supersensitiveness to cold" and some studies provide fairly strong evidence that histamine may be involved in this condition. HORTON, BROWN and ROTH (1936) and ROTH and HORTON (1940) found that exposure to cold of a sensitive subject led to an increase in the gastric secretion of hydrochloric acid and other symptoms similar to histamine intoxication. ROSE (1941) found an increase in the histamine content in venous blood from the extremity exposed to cold in 3 subjects, while no increase was seen in a control subject. An increase in whole blood (and plasma) histamine after exposure to cold was also reported by ROSE (1954). At the same time the blood pressure decreased and the heart rate was increased, both effects compatible with systemic effects of liberated histamine. A comprehensive study on a subject with thermal intolerance was performed by HENDERSON, CODE and ROTH (1958). Their patient developed intense local symptoms in the hand after exposure to 10° C. A blood pressure cuff first prevented blood from the hand to reach the general circulation, but after deflation of the cuff a systemic reaction occurred, consisting of flushing of the skin, asthmatic symptoms, rhinitis, injection of conjunctivae, nasal congestion and faintness. These symptoms suggest histamine as a causative factor, and this belief is substantiated by the finding of an enormous increase in the histamine (10 to 26 times) in the venous blood from the chilled hand. The number of basophil and eosinophil leukocytes was not increased. The histamine was apparently present in the plasma and an increase in the urinary histamine could also be demonstrated. The study of HENDERSON, CODE and ROTH (1958) presents the most convincing example of histamine liberation in a pathological condition in man.

The role of histamine for cold urticaria was questioned by DUNÉR, PERNOW and STERKY (1960)[1], who found increased histamine levels in the venous blood from arms exposed to cold. However, the increase in blood histamine was the same in normal subjects as in patients with cold urticaria. The total number of leukocytes did not change after exposure to cold. If the increased blood levels of histamine in these experiments are the result of histamine liberation by cold, one would have to assume that the histamine-like symptoms in the patients with cold urticaria were caused by a supersensitiveness to the histamine normally released during exposure to cold.

e) Endocrine control of histamine metabolism in man

Animal experiments indicate that the rate of formation, the tissue content, the inactivation, the urinary excretion and the biological effects of histamine are influenced by some endocrine glands, notably the anterior lobe of the pituitary, the adrenals and the thyroid (DALE, 1920; ROSE and BROWNE, 1941; CARLSTEN, 1950; HAEGER and KAHLSON, 1952; HAEGER, JACOBSOHN and KAHLSON, 1952; SCHAYER et al., 1955a; TELFORD and WEST, 1960, 1961; ANGERVALL et al., 1961; GOTZL and DRAGSTEDT, 1940; PARRATT and WEST, 1960; BJURÖ et al., 1961b).

Some fragmentary evidence suggests that also in man the metabolism of histamine may be similarly influenced by adrenocortical hormones and the thyroid gland. The decrease in blood histamine (part IV) and the concomitant increase in the urinary histamine (part V) occurring after the administration of cortisone shows that at least from the pharmacological point of view the adrenocortical hormones can cause changes in the histamine metabolism in man. The accentuated effect of cortisone on the urinary histamine in certain allergic diseases (part V) seems to be worthy of further study as a possible mechanism of the therapeutic action of cortisone. It may be pointed out here that a similar "outflow" of histamine into the urine after cortisone has been observed in rats, especially after adrenalectomy (BJURÖ and WESTLING, 1960).

[1] The histamine values given in the paper of DUNÉR et al. (1960) refer to histamine diphosphate (DUNÉR, personal communication).

The high content of histamine in the skin in thyreotoxicosis, and the reduced values in myxoedema (part III), also point to an effect of the thyroid hormones on histamine metabolism. Corresponding changes have been found in the skin of rats (Gotzl and Dragstedt, 1940).

f) Histamine and gastric secretion in man

The role of histamine in gastric secretion will be discussed by Ivy (Chapter 2, Section G, and Chapter 5, Section B). It has been shown that the histamine content of gastric mucosa is the same in subjects with duodenal ulcer and in subjects with gastric cancer (Table 13). The histamine content of gastric juice was, if anything, higher in cases of achlorhydria (pernicious anemia) than in cases of duodenal ulcer. Finally the rate of histamine formation in gastric mucosa was the same whether the tissue came from subjects with duodenal ulcer or subjects with achlorhydria (Table 1).

These observations do not support the idea that histamine in the gastric mucosa is there only to serve in the process of secretion of hydrochloric acid.

The distribution of histamine in the wall of the stomach has thoroughly been studied by Smith (1959).

g) Histamine and mental disease

The ability of the brain, particularly the hypothalamus, to form and inactivate histamine is probably common to man (part I) and other species (see White, Chapter 4, Section G in this book). The distribution of histamine, as well as of the enzymes relevant for its metabolism, is rather similar to that of 5-hydroxytryptamine and some catechol amines. The biochemical similarities in the metabolism of histamine and the other amines mentioned make histamine another potential candidate for a role in the normal physiology of the central nervous system. Positive evidence for a function of histamine in the normal brain is lacking, but it has nevertheless been suggested that histamine might have something to do with mental disease, notably schizophrenia. The main observation that has led to this hypothesis is that schizophrenic patients are much less sensitive to histamine (e.g. Lucy, 1954) than others. Unfortunately this high resistance is not confined to histamine, and it is not even specific for schizophrenic patients since also patients with other types of chronic mental disease may be resistant to histamine.

Schizophrenic patients have about 50% higher blood histamine levels than normal cases (part IV C, d, Table 21). This is again not specific for schizophrenia since high blood histamine values are also found in epilepsy and in postencephalitic disturbances. The urinary excretion of free histamine is not abnormal in schizophrenia (Adam and Mitchell, 1957). These workers also found that a normal percentage of injected histamine was excreted into the urine. Lindell et al. (1960) found a normal catabolism of injected C^{14}-histamine in three patients with mental disease, two of which had a schizophrenia-like condition.

Kobayashi and Freeman (1961) studied the metabolism of intradermally injected C^{14}-histamine in 12 patients with the diagnosis of chronic schizophrenia and in 7 non-psychotic subjects. It was found that the schizophrenics excreted less C^{14}-labelled 1,4-methylimidazoleacetic acid and more conjugated imidazoleacetic acid. The difference, although statistically significant, was not "a parameter which can be used as an individual test for schizophrenia."

It may be mentioned that iproniazid in a dose which was clinically effective in the treatment of depression inhibited the oxidation of both histamine and 1,4-

methylhistamine, but had no effect on the methylation of histamine (LINDELL et al., 1960). Chlorpromazine which inhibits the methylation of histamine in vitro had no significant effect on the metabolism of C^{14}-labelled histamine injected intravenously (JOHANSSON et al., 1961). This does, of course, not exclude the possibility that the methylation of histamine in the brain was inhibited although this seems less likely.

To sum up, there is as yet no direct evidence that histamine is of importance in mental disease. The increased tolerance to histamine, and the high blood histamine values sometimes found in schizophrenia are probably unspecific and secondary phenomena. The eventual function of histamine in the human brain is as obscure as in other species.

h) Future approaches to the study of histamine in man

The very limited possibilities of drawing any conclusion with regard to the liberation, formation or catabolism of histamine from measurements of whole blood histamine have already been pointed out. With the technique developed by ADAM and his co-workers (1957) it has been found that the amount of free histamine in plasma is less than 1 μg per liter. This finding is indirectly supported by studies made with injected C^{14}-labelled histamine (ARNOLDSSON et al., 1962a). It is possible that the applications of the method of ADAM et al. (1957) may yield useful informations about the release of histamine into the circulating blood under various pathological conditions. However, even with this very sensitive method one would expect to have clinical signs of histamine effects on the circulation when a definite increase in the concentration of free histamine in plasma is found.

Measurements of the urinary excretion of free histamine are more likely to give information about changes in histamine metabolism than studies of blood histamine (ADAM et al., 1954). However, it must always be kept in mind that only a very small part of the histamine which enters the circulation is excreted in unchanged form in the urine. If changes in the urinary output of free histamine occur it is usually impossible to say whether this reflects a change in the production and release or in the catabolism and excretion of histamine. To facilitate the interpretation one can inject C^{14}-labelled histamine in trace amounts and see if catabolism and excretion are changed.

The study of the metabolism of 5-hydroxytryptamine was greatly aided when it was discovered that its major metabolite, 5-hydroxyindoleacetic acid, could be easily measured. The major metabolite of histamine is 1,4-methylimidazoleacetic acid. Unfortunately there is yet no known method of measuring this compound in tissues or body fluids. The development of such a method is of utmost importance for further studies of histamine and its significance in health and disease.

The other metabolite of quantitative importance is imidazoleacetic acid. This compound may however be formed directly from histidine and changes in its excretion in urine cannot be taken to reflect changes in histamine metabolism (BALDRIDGE and TOURTELLOTTE, 1958; LINDELL and SCHAYER, 1958, and DUNÉR et al., 1961).

As pointed out in the part on histamine in allergy (this part, d), it is likely that the histamine which takes part in the allergic manifestation is both formed and liberated locally in the reacting tissue. It is also likely that a great part of this histamine is inactivated locally without ever reaching the circulating blood. It would seem that many of the problems connected with the liberation of histamine, the induction of increased histamine formation and the local catabolism of histamine could with advantage be studied in vitro with biopsy specimens of various tissues.

References

ADAM, H. M.: Excretion of histamine in human urine. Quart. J. exp. Physiol. **35**, 281 (1949).

— W. I. CARD, M. J. RIDDELL, M. ROBERTS, and J. A. STRONG: The effect of intravenous infusions of histamine on the urinary histamine and on gastric secretion in man. Brit. J. Pharmacol. **9**, 62 (1954).

— D. C. HARDWICK, and K. E. V. SPENCER: A method of estimating histamine in plasma. Brit. J. Pharmacol. **12**, 397 (1957).

— R. B. HUNTER, and T. W. G. KINNEAR: Observations on the urinary excretion of histamine in urticaria. Quart. J. exp. Physiol. **36—37**, 49 (1951—1952).

—, and R. G. MITCHELL: The urinary excretion of histamine in children. Arch. Dis. Child. **28**, 61 (1953).

ADAM, J., and R. G. MITCHELL: The urinary excretion of histamine in schizophrenia. J. Neurol. Neurosurg. Psychiat. **20**, 114 (1957).

AHLMARK, A.: Studies on the histaminolytic power of plasma with special reference to pregnancy. Acta physiol. scand. **9**, suppl. XXVIII (1944).

ANGERVALL, L., T. BJURÖ, and H. WESTLING: The effect of adrenalectomy on the urinary excretion of histamine in the rat. Acta endocr. (Kbh.) **36**, 467 (1961).

ANREP, G. V., M. S. AGADI, G. S. BARSOUM, J. R. SMITH, and M. M. TALAAT: The excretion of histamine in urine. J. Physiol. (Lond.) **103**, 155 (1944).

ARNOLDSSON, H., C.-G. HELANDER, E. HELANDER, S.-E. LINDELL, B. LINDHOLM, O. OLSSON, B.-E. ROOS, A. SVANBORG, B. SÖDERHOLM, and H. WESTLING: Elimination of C^{14}-histamine from the blood in man. Scand. J. clin. Lab. Invest. **14**, 241 (1962a).

— L. BELIN, L. HALLBERG, B. LINDHOLM, S.-E. LINDELL, and H. WESTLING: Unpublished observation (1962b).

ARSDEL, P. P. VAN, and G. N. BEALL: The metabolism and functions of histamine. Arch. intern. Med. **5**, 714 (1960).

— E. MIDDLETON, W. B. SHERMAN, and H. BUCHWALD: A quantitative study on thein vitro release of histamine from leukocytes of atopic persons. J. Allergy **29**, 429 (1958)

BALDRIDGE, R. C., and C. D. TOURTELOTTE: The metabolism of histidine. J. biol. Ch.em. **233**, 125 (1958).

BARSOUM, G. S., and J. H. GADDUM: The pharmacological estimation of adenosine and histamine in blood. J. Physiol. (Lond.) **85**, 1 (1935).

— — The effect of cutaneous burns on the blood-histamine. Clin. Sci. **2**, 357 (1936).

—, and F. H. SMIRK: Observation on the histamine yielding substance in the plasma and red cells of normal human subjects and of patients with congestive heart failure. Clin. Sci. **2**, 337 (1936).

BAXTER, J. D., and B. ROSE: The histamine content of allergic and nonallergic human nasal membrane with simultaneous observations on the eosinophils. J. Allergy **24**, 18 (1953).

BEALL, G. N., and P. P. VAN ARSDEL: Histamine metabolism in human disease. J. clin. Invest. **39**, 676 (1960).

BENDA, R., et L.-F. MIRAVET: Histaminase sérique et cancer. Bull. Soc. med. Hôp. Paris **76**, 184 (1960).

BERGSTRÖM, S., and G. HANSSON: The use of Amberlite IRC-50 for purification of adrenaline and histamine. Acta physiol. scand. **22**, 87 (1951).

BEST, C. H., and E. W. MCHENRY: The inactivation of histamine. J. Physiol. (Lond.) **70**, 349 (1930).

BIKICH, G. Y., J. BORBOLA, and G. HETÉNYI: Experimental approach to the role of histamine in peptic ulcer formation. Acta med. Acad. Sci. hung. VI, 207 (1954).

BIRKE, G., H. DUNÉR, S.-O. LILJEDAHL, B. PERNOW, and L. O. PLANTIN: The effect of antihistamine treatment in severe burns. Acta chir. scand. **115**, 401 (1958).

— — — — —, and L. TROELL: Histamine, catechol amines and adrenocortical steroids in burns. Acta chir. scand. **114**, 87 (1957).

BJURÖ, T., and H. WESTLING: Observations on the urinary excretion of histamine in adrenalectomized rats. Acta physiol. scand. **50**, suppl. **175**, 25 (1960).

— S. LINDBERG, and H. WESTLING: Observations on histamine in pregnancy and the puerperium. Acta obstet. gynec. scand. **40**, 152 (1961a).

— H. WESTLING, and H. WETTERQVIST: The effect of thyroid hormones on histamine formation in the rat. Brit. J. Pharmacol. **17**, 479 (1961b).

BLASCHKO, H., P. J. FRIEDMAN, ROSEMARY HAWES, and KAREN NILSSON: The amine oxidase of mammalian plasma. J. Physiol. (Lond.) **145**, 384 (1959).

BLOOM, C., H. DUNÉR, B. PERNOW, J. WINBERG, and R. ZETTERSTRÖM: Spontaneous histamine shocks in urticaria pigmentosa. Acta paediat. (Uppsala) **47**, 152 (1958).

BORÉUS, L.O., and N. CHAKRAVARTY: Tissue mast cells, histamine and "slow reacting substance" in anaphylactic reaction in guinea-pig. Acta physiol. scand. **48**, 1 (1959).

BORGLIN, N. E., and B. WILLERT: The prognostic value of histaminase and pregnandiol determination in threatening abortion. Acta obstet. gynec. scand. **36**, 382 (1957).

BOUHUYS, A., R. JÖNSSON, S. LICHTNECKERT, S.-E. LINDELL, C. LUNDGREN, G. LUNDIN, and T. R. RINGQUIST: Effects of histamine on pulmonary ventilation in man. Clin. Sci. **19**, 79 (1960).

BROCKLEHURST, W. E.: Histamine and other mediators in hypersensitivity reactions. IIIe congrès international d'allergologie 361. Paris: Editions Médicales Flammarion 1958.

BROGREN, N., H. DUNÉR, B. HAMRIN, B. PERNOW, G. THEANDER, and J. WALDENSTRÖM: Urticaria pigmentosa (Mastocytosis). A study of nine cases with special reference to the excretion of histamine in urine. Acta med. scand. **163**, 223 (1959).

BROWN, D. D., R. TOMCHICK, and J. AXELROD: The distribution and properties of a histamine-methylating enzyme. J. biol. Chem. **234**, 2948 (1959).

CARLSTEN, A.: Effect of adrenalectomy on lymph and plasma histaminase. Acta physiol. scand. **20**, Suppl. 70, 33 (1950).

CERQUA, S.: L'equivalente istaminico nel sangue in diverse condizioni patologiche. Minerva med. **27**, 542 (1936).

CLARK, D. H., and H. I. TANKEL: Gastric acid and plasma histaminase during pregnancy. Lancet **1954**, 886.

CODE, C. F.: The quantitative estimation of histamine in the blood. J. Physiol. (Lond.) **89**, 257 (1937).

— Histamine in blood. Physiol. Rev. **32**, 47 (1952).

—, and A. D. McDONALD: The histamine-like activity of blood. Lancet **233**, 730 (1937).

—, and R. G. MITCHELL: Histamine, eosinophils and basophils in the blood. J. Physiol. (Lond.) **136**, 449 (1957).

DALE, H. H.: Conditions which are conducive to the production of shock by histamine. Brit. J. exp. Path. **1**, 103 (1920).

—, and P. P. LAIDLAW: The physiological action of β-iminazolylethylamine. J. Physiol. (Lond.) **41**, 318 (1910).

DANFORTH, D. N.: Concentration and possible significance of histaminase in the human placenta. Proc. Soc. exp. Biol. (N. Y.) **40**, 319 (1939).

DEMIS, J. D., and D. D. BROWN: Histidine metabolism in urticaria pigmentosa. J. invest. Derm. **36**, 253 (1961).

— M. D. WALTON, and R. HIGDON: Histaminuria in urticaria pigmentosa. Arch. Derm. **83**, 181 (1961).

DIECKHOFF, J.: Histaminstoffwechseluntersuchungen bei toxischen und allergischen Symptomen im Kindesalter. Allergie u. Asthma **3**, 274 (1957a).

— Die patho-physiologische Bedeutung des Histamins bei toxischen und allergischen Krankheitszuständen im Kindesalter. Kinderärztl. Prax. **25**, 189 (1957b).

DUNÉR, H., B. HAMRIN, B. PERNOW, and J. WALDENSTRÖM: Histamine and urticaria pigmentosa. Nord. Med. **61**, 80 (1959).

— S. O. LILJEDAHL, and B. PERNOW: Does the urinary excretion of imidazoleacetic acid reflect the endogenous histamine metabolism in man? Acta physiol. scand. **51**, 41 (1961).

—, and B. PERNOW: Urinary excretion of histamine in healthy human subjects. Scand. J. clin. Lab. Invest. **8**, 296 (1956a).

— — The urinary excretion of histamine in a case of Loeffler's syndrome. Acta med. scand. **156**, 313 (1956b).

— — The correlation between the occurrence of histamine in blood and urine. Scand. J. clin. Lab. Invest. **10**, 390 (1958b).

— — Determination of histamine in blood and urine by absorption on Amberlite IRC-50. Scand. J. clin. Lab. Invest. **10**, 233 (1958a).

— — Histamine and leukocytes in blood during muscular work in man. Scand. J. clin. Lab. Invest. **10**, 394 (1958c).

— — Urinary excretion of histamine in bronchial asthma. Acta med. scand. **161**, 361 (1958d).

— — Histamine in man under physiological and pathological conditions. Acta med. scand. **168**, 307 (1960).

— —, and G. STERKY: The histamine concentration of the blood on exposure to cold and heat. Acta allerg. (Kbh.) **15**, 417 (1960).

EFFKEMANN, G., and E. WERLE: Die Bedeutung des Histamin-Stoffwechsels im weiblichen schwangeren und nichtschwangeren Organismus. Arch. Gynäk. **170**, 173 (1940).

EGGERTH, A. H.: The production of histamine in bacterial cultures. J. Bact. **37**, 205 (1939).

EMMELIN, N., G. KAHLSON, and F. WICKSELL: Histamine in plasma and methods of its estimation. Acta physiol. scand. **2**, 123 (1941).

FAREDIN, I., G. Y. BIKICH, and J. BORBOLA: Determination of histamine in human gastric juice. Gastroenterologia (Basel) **79**, 185 (1953).

FAREDIN, I., J. BORBOLA, and G. Y. BIKICH: Studies on gastric mucosa histamine. Acta med. Acad. Sci. hung. **6**, 195 (1954).
FELDBERG, W., and A. A. LOESER: Histamine content of human skin in different clinical disorders. J. Physiol. (Lond.) **126**, 286 (1954).
GADDUM, J. H.: The origin of histamine in the body. Ciba Foundation Symposium on histamine 285. London: J. & A. Churchill Ltd. 1956.
DE GARA, P. F.: Chemical determination of histamine in blood in health and disease. J. Allergy **22**, 429 (1951).
GARDNER, L. J., and A. A. TICE: Histamine and related compounds in urticaria pigmentosa: Analyses of tissues having mast-cell infiltration. Pediatrics **21**, 805 (1958).
GOOSZEN, J. A. H., and JACOBA DONKER: A study of histamine metabolism in schizophrenic patients. Acta allerg. (Kbh.) **10**, 149 (1956).
GOTZL, F. R., and C. A. DRAGSTEDT: Effect of thyroidectomy and of experimental hyperthyroidism upon histamine content of rat tissue. Proc. Soc. exp. Biol. (N. Y.) **45**, 688 (1940).
GRAHAM, H. T., O. H. LOWRY, F. WHEELWRIGHT, M. A. LENZ, and H. H. PARISH: Distribution of histamine among leukocytes and platelets. Blood **10**, 467 (1955).
GRANROTH, T., and Å. NILZÉN: On the histaminolytic activity of skin extracts. Acta physiol. scand. **15**, 188 (1948).
GUNTHER, M., and W. D. M. PATON: The histamine content of human uterus. J. Physiol. (Lond.) **154**, 417 (1960).
HAEGER, K., DORA JACOBSOHN, and G. KAHLSON: The levels of histaminase and histamine in gastro-intestinal mucosa and kidney of the cat deprived of the hypophysis or the adrenal glands. Acta physiol. scand. **25**, 243 (1952).
—, and G. KAHLSON: Disappearance of histaminase from the whole body following adrenalectomy in cats. Acta physiol. scand. **25**, 255 (1952).
HARTMAN, W. J., W. G. CLARK, and SHIRLEY D. CYR: Histidine decarboxylase activity of basophils from chronic myelogenous leukemia patients. Origin of blood histamine. Proc. Soc. exp. Biol. (N. Y.) **107**, 123 (1961).
HÄUSLER, H. F.: Differentialdiagnose durch Histamin-Nachweis im Nasensekret bei „Rhinitis vasomotorica". Wien. klin. Wschr. **69**, 440 (1957).
HAWORTH, E., and A. D. MACDONALD: On histamine in cotton dust, and in the blood of cotton workers. J. Hyg. (Lond.) **37**, 234 (1937).
HELANDER, E., S.-E. LINDELL, KAREN NILSSON, and H. WESTLING: Catabolism of C^{14}-labelled histamine in patients with allergic disease. Acta allerg. (Kbh.) **17**, 86 (1962).
HENDERSON, L. L., C. F. CODE, and G. M. ROTH: Increased blood histamine in thermal intolerance. J. Allergy **29**, 122 (1958).
HÖGBERG, B., and B. UVNÄS: Further observations on the disruption of rat mesentery mast cells caused by compound 48/80, antigen-antibody reaction, lecithinase A and decylamine. Acta physiol. scand. **48**, 133 (1960).
HORTON, B. T., G. E. BROWN, and G. M. ROTH: Hypersensitiviness to cold with local and systemic manifestations of a histamine-like character: Its amenability to treatment. J. Amer. med. Ass. **107**, 1263 (1936).
HUKOVIĆ, S., I. SPUZIĆ, u. P. STERN: Über die Übertragung des Schmerzempfindens in der Haut des Menschen. Arch. int. Pharmacodyn. **109**, 285 (1957).
MCINTIRE, F. C., F. B. WHITE, and MURIEL SPROULL: The determination of histamine with 2,4-dinitrofluorobenzene. Arch. Biochem. **28**, 376 (1950).
IRVINE, W. T., H. L. DUTHIE, and N. G. WATON: Urinary output of free histamine after a meat meal. Lancet **1959**, 1061.
JANOWITZ, H., and M. I. GROSSMAN: Minimal effective dose of intravenously administered histamine in pregnant and non-pregnant human beings. Amer. J. Physiol. **157**, 94 (1949).
JHA, C. D., and Y. K. SINHA: Histamine content of blood and skin sensitivity to histamine. Indian J. med. Res. **48**, 41 (1960).
JIMENEZ-DIAZ, C., E. ARJONA, and J. PERIANES: Studies on histamine in allergic patients. Int. Arch. Allergy **6**, 243 (1955).
JOHANSSON MAJ-BRITT, S.-E. LINDELL, B. E. ROOS, and H. WESTLING: Histamine catabolism during treatment with chlorpromazine. Med. Exp. **4**, 239 (1961).
JOHNSON, H. H.: Histamine levels in human skin. Arch. Derm. **76**, 726 (1957).
— G. A. DE OREO, W. P. LASCHEID, and F. MITCHELL: Skin histamine levels in chronic atopic dermatitis. J. invest. Derm. **34**, 237 (1960).
KAHLSON, G.: A place for histamine in normal physiology. Lancet **1960 I**, 67
— ELSA ROSENGREN, and H. WESTLING: Increased formation of histamine in the pregnant rat. J. Physiol. (Lond.) **143**, 91 (1958).
— — —, and T. WHITE: The site of increased formation of histamine in the pregnant rat. J. Physiol. (Lond.) **144**, 337 (1958).
— —, and T. WHITE: Formation of histamine by the foetus in the rat and man. J. Physiol. (Lond.) **145**, 30 (1959).

KAPELLER-ADLER, REGINE: Histamine metabolism in pregnancy. Lancet **1949 II**, 745.
— Histamine metabolism in the human placenta and in the umbilical cord blood. Biochem. J. **51**, 610 (1952).
— Zur Kenntnis der Histaminase. Naunyn-Schmiedebergs Arch. exp. Path. Pharmak. **219**, 491 (1953).
—, and E. ADLER: Further investigations on the histidine and the histamine metabolism in normal and pathological pregnancy. J. Obstet. Gynaec. **50**, 177 (1943).
—, and B. IGGO: Histamine and its derivatives in human urine. Biochem. biophys. Acta **25**, 394 (1957).
KATZ, G.: Histamine release in the allergic skin reaction. Proc. Soc. exp. Biol. (N.Y.) **49**, 272 (1942).
KOBAYASHI, Y., and H. FREEMAN: Histamine metabolism by schizophrenic and normal subjects. J. Neuropsychiat. **3**, 112 (1961).
KULLANDER, S.: Studies on eosinophil leukocytes in pregnancy. Acta endocr. (Kbh.) **10**, 135 (1952).
LASSER, E. C., and K. W. STENSTRÖM: Elevation of circulating blood histamine in patients undergoing deep roentgen therapy. Amer. J. Roentgenol. **72**, 985 (1954).
LEE, H. M., and R. G. JONES: The histamine activity of some β-aminoethyl heterocyclic nitrogen compounds. J. Pharmacol. exp. Ther. **95**, 71 (1949).
LEVI, L., C. L. MENEGHINI, et F. RANTUCCIO: Activité cholinestérasique: Pouvoir histaminolytique et dosage de l'histamine dans la peau de sujets sains et atteint de certaines dermatoses allergiques. Rapport Histamine-Mastocytes. Acta allerg. (Kbh.) **13**, 332 (1959).
LILJA, B., S.-E. LINDELL, and T. SALDEEN: Formation and destruction of C^{14}-histamine in human lung tissue in vitro. J. Allergy **31**, 492 (1960).
LINDAHL, KERSTIN M.: In vitro studies on histamine metabolism in placenta. Arkiv kemi **16**, 1 (1960a).
— Paperchromatographic indication of imidazole-4(5)-acetic acid and 1-methylimidazole-4-acetic acid as histamine metabolites in human placental tissue. Arkiv kemi **16**, 15 (1960b).
— S.-E. LINDELL, KAREN NILSSON, R. W. SCHAYER, and H. WESTLING: Studies on the metabolism of C^{14}-labelled histamine in human plasma during pregnancy. Arkiv kemi **13**, 379 (1958).
LINDBERG, S.: ^{14}C-Histamine elimination from the blood of pregnant and non-pregnant women with special reference to the uterus. Acta Obst. et Gynec. Scandinav. **42**, suppl. 1, 3 (1963).
— S.-E. LINDELL, and H. WESTLING: Formation and inactivation of histamine by human foetal tissues in vitro. Acta Obst. et Gynec. Scandinav. **42**, suppl. **1**, 49 (1963).
—, and H. WESTLING: The urinary excretion of histamine in the puerperium. Med. Exp. **5**, 423 (1961).
LINDELL, S.-E.: Observations on the inactivation of C^{14}-histamine by human renal tissue in vitro. Kungl. fysiogr. Sällsk. Lund Förh. **28**, 15 (1958).
— KAREN NILSSON, B.-E. ROOS, and H. WESTLING: The effect of enzyme inhibitors on histamine catabolism in man. Brit. J. Pharmacol. **15**, 351 (1960).
—, and R. W. SCHAYER: Formation of histamine in the kidney of the dog. Brit. J. Pharmacol. **13**, 89 (1958).
— H. RORSMAN, and H. WESTLING: Histamine formation in urticaria pigmentosa. Acta derm.-venereol. (Stockh.) **41**, 277 (1961a).
— — — Histamine formation in human blood. Acta allerg. (Kbh.) **16**, 216 (1961b).
—, and K. VISKE: A note on the distribution of C^{14}-histamine added to blood. Brit. J. Pharmacol. **17**, 131 (1961).
LOWETT DOUST, J. W., H. HUSDAN, and M. E. SALNA: Blood-histamine and tissue cell anoxia in mental disease. Nature (Lond.) **178**, 492 (1956).
LOWRY, O. H., HELEN T. GRAHAM, F. B. HARRIS, M. K. PRIEBAT, A. R. MARKS, and R. U. BERGMAN: The chemical measurement of histamine in blood plasma and cells. J. Pharmacol. exp. Ther. **112**, 116 (1954).
LUBSCHEZ, R.: Chemical determination of histamine in human blood. J. biol. Chem. **183**, 731 (1950).
LUCY, J. D.: Histamine tolerance in schizophrenia. Arch. Neurol. Psychiat. (Chic.) **71**, 629 (1954).
MAAS, J. W., G. A. FEHMERS, and T. STRENGERS: Some aspects of blood histamine in normal allergic and tuberculous children. Acta allerg. (Kbh.) **10**, 170 (1956).
MCINTIRE, F. C., F. B. WHITE and M. SPROULL: The determination of histamine with 2,4-dinitrofluorobenzene. Arch. Biochem. **29**, 376 (1950).
MARCOU, I., et E. ATHANASIU-VERGU: L'histamine dans le sang des parturientes. Bull. Acad. Méd. Roum. **3—4**, 359 (1937).
— N. GINGOLD et C. C. PARHON: L'histamine dans les maladies du sang. Bull. Acad. Méd. Roum. **3**, 366 (1937).
— E. ATHANASIU-VERGU, D. CHIRICEANU, G. COSMA, N. GINGOLD et C.-C. PARHON: Sur le rôle physiologique de l'histamine. Presse méd. **46**, 371 (1938).

MIDDLETON, E., and W. B. SHERMAN: Studies of histamine release from leukocytes of subjects with atopic hypersensitivity. IV Int. Congr. of Allerg., Excerpta Medica Int. Congr. Series **42**, 3 (1961).
MITCHELL, R. G.: The urinary excretion of subcutaneously injected histamine. Brit. J. Pharmacol. **11**, 462 (1956a).
— The effect of enzyme inhibitors on the excretion of free histamine in human urine. Brit. J. Pharmacol. **11**, 467 (1956b).
— Excretion of injected histamine by asthmatic children. J. Allergy **30**, 506 (1959).
— H. R. BUTT, and C. F. CODE: Histamine metabolism in diseases of the liver. J. clin. Invest. **33**, 1199 (1954).
—, and ROSEMARY CASS: Histamine and 5-hydroxytryptamine in the blood of infants and children. J. clin. Invest. **38**, 595 (1959).
—, and C. F. CODE: Effect of diet on urinary excretion of histamine. J. appl. Physiol. **6**, 387 (1954a).
— — Urinary excretion of histamine after administration of cortisone. J. clin. Endocr. **14**, 707 (1954b).
— G. B. LOGAN, G. A. PETERS, and L. L. HENDERSON: Urinary excretion of histamine in patients having asthma hay fever: Observations on changes produced by administration of cortisone. J. Allergy **25**, 504 (1954).
MYHRMAN, G., u. J. TOMENIUS: Über das Vorkommen von Histamin in menschlichen Faeces. Naunyn-Schmiedebergs Arch. exp. Path. Pharmak. **193**, 14 (1939).
NILSSON, KAREN, S.-E. LINDELL, R. W. SCHAYER, and H. WESTLING: Metabolism of C^{14}-labelled histamine in pregnant and non-pregnant women. Clin. Sci. **18**, 313 (1959).
NILZÉN, Å.: Studies in histamine (H-substance) with special reference to the conditions obtaining in urticaria and related skin-changes. Acta derm.-venereol. (Stockh.) **27**, suppl. 17 (1947).
NOAH, J. W., and A. BRAND: The effect of corticosteroid administration upon blood histamine content. J. Allergy **28**, 405 (1957).
PARRATT, J. R., and G. B. WEST: Hypersensitivity and the thyroid gland. Int. Arch. Allergy **16**, 288 (1960).
PERNOW, B., and J. WALDENSTRÖM: Determination of 5-hydroxytryptamine, 5-hydroxindoleacetic acid and histamine in thirty-three cases of carcinoid tumour (Argentaffinoma). Amer. J. Med. **23**, 16 (1957).
PETTAY, O.: Investigations into the histamine content of umbilical blood. Acta paediat. (Uppsala) **39**, 283 (1950).
RANDOLPH, T. G., and F. M. RACKEMANN: The blood histamine level in asthma and eosinophila. J. Allergy **12**, 450 (1940—1941).
RILEY, J. F., and G. B. WEST: Skin histamine. Its location in the tissue mast cells. Arch. Derm. **74**, 471 (1956).
ROBERTS, M., and H. M. ADAM: New methods for the quantitative estimation of free and conjugated histamine in body fluids. Brit. J. Pharmacol. **5**, 526 (1950).
ROCKENSCHAUB, A.: The urinary excretion of histamine in pregnancy and in preeclampsia. J. Obstet. Gynaec. **60**, 398 (1953).
RORSMAN, H.: Personal communication (1962).
—, and ELSA ROSENGREN: Basophil leukocytes and blood histamine in urticaria. Acta derm.-venereol. (Stockh.) **38**, 377 (1958).
ROSE, B.: Production of symptoms by subcutaneous injection of histamine without increase of the blood histamine. Science **92**, 454 (1940).
— Studies on blood histamine in cases of allergy. I. Blood histamine during wheal formation. J. Allergy **12**, 327 (1941).
— Histamine, hormones and hypersensitivity. J. Allergy **25**, 168 (1954).
—, and J. S. L. BROWNE: Alterations in the blood histamine in shock. Proc. Soc. exp. Biol. (N. Y.) **44**, 182 (1940).
— — The effect of adrenalectomy on the histamine content of the tissues of the rat. Amer. J. Physiol. **131**, 589 (1941).
— I. RUSTED, and A. J. FOWNES: Intravascular catheterization studies of bronchial asthma. I. Histamine levels in arterial and mixed venous blood of asthmatic patients before and during induced attacks. J. clin. Invest. **29**, 113 (1950).
ROTH, G. M., and B. T. HORTON: Histaminase: physiological effects on man and its therapeutic value in medicine. Bull. N. Y. Acad. Med. **16**, 570 (1940).
SANDERS, S. G.: Chemical determination of histamine content of oral tissues and saliva. J. oral Surg. **13**, 193 (1955).
SANDLER, M., and P. J. D. SNOW: An atypical tumour secreting 5-hydroxytryptamine. Lancet **1958I**, 137.

SCHAYER, R. W.: Biogenesis of histamine. J. biol. Chem. **199**, 245 (1952).
— The metabolism of histamine in various species. Brit. J. Pharmacol. **11**, 472 (1956).
— Catabolism of physiological quantities of histamine in vivo. Physiol. Rev. **39**, 116 (1959).
— Role of histamine in allergy. Report of the thirty-eighth Ross conference on pediatric research, p. 52 (1961a).
— Significance of induced synthesis of histamine in physiology and pathology. Chemotherapia **3**, 128 (1961b).
—, and J. A. D. COOPER: Metabolism of C^{14}-histamine in man. J. appl. Physiol. **9**, 481 (1956).
— K. J. DAVIS, and ROSA L. SMILEY: Binding of histamine in vitro and its inhibition by cortisone. Amer. J. Physiol. **182**, 54 (1955a).
—, and O. H. GANLEY: Adaptative increase in mammalian histidine decarboxylase activity in response to nonspecific stress. Amer. J. Physiol. **197**, 721 (1959).
— Y. KOBAYASHI, and ROSA L. SMILEY: Determination of histamine as an isotopic derivative. J. biol. Chem. **212**, 593 (1955b).
— ZULEIKA ROTHSCHILD, and PIROSKA BIZONY: Increase in histidine decarboxylase activity of rat skin following treatment with compound 48/80. Amer. J. Physiol. **196**, 295 (1959).
— K. Y. T. WU, and ROSA L. SMILEY: Sources of urinary histamine in the rat. Amer. J. Physiol. **179**, 481 (1954).
SCHILD, H. O.: Mechanism of anaphylaxis. IIIe congrès international d'allergologie, p. 351. Paris: Editions Médicales. Flammarion 1958.
— D. F. HAWKINS, J. MONGAR, and H. HERXHEIMER: Reactions of isolated human asthmatic lung and bronchial tissue to a specific antigen. Lancet **1951 II**, 376.
SERAFINI, U.: Studies on histamine and histamine antagonists. J. Allergy **19**, 256 (1948).
SHIMKIN, M. B., H. R. BIERMAN, B. V. A. LOW-BEER, P. M. WHEELER, and F. R. GOTZL: Blood histamine in myelogenous leukemia. Cancer **4**, 570 (1951).
— L. SAPIRSTEIN, F. R. GOTZL, P. M. WHEELER, and N. I. BERLIN: Blood histamine in leukemia and erythremia. J. nat. Cancer Inst. **9**, 379 (1948—1949).
SHORE, P. A., A. PARKHURST, A. BURKHALTER, and V. H. COHN: A method for the fluorometric assay of histamine in tissues. J. Pharmacol. exp. Ther. **127**, 182 (1959).
SMITH, A. N.: The distribution and release of histamine in gastric tissues. Clin. Sci. **18**, 533 (1959).
STERN, P., S. HUKOVIĆ, Z. MADJEREK, u. S. KARABIC: Histamingehalt im Blut von Schizophrenikern. Arch. int. Pharmacodyn. **109**, 294 (1957).
STONE, JANET, J. M. MERRILL, and G. R. MENEELY: Distribution of histamine in human tissue. Fed. Proc. **14**, 147 (1955).
STÜTTGEN, G.: Der fermentative Abbau von Tyramin, Histamin und Acetylcholin in den Schichten der menschlichen Haut. Arch. klin. exp. Derm. **201**, 564 (1955).
SWANBERG, H.: Histaminase in pregnancy with special reference to its origin and formation. Acta physiol. scand. **23**, Suppl. 79 (1950).
TABOR, H., and E. MOSETTIG: Isolation of acetylhistamine from urine following oral administration of histamine. J. biol. Chem. **180**, 703 (1949).
TELFORD, J. M., and G. B. WEST: The effects of corticosteroids and related compounds on the histamine and 5-hydroxytryptamine content of rat tissues. Brit. J. Pharmacol. **15**, 532 (1960).
— — Some effects of corticosteroids on the metabolism of histamine and 5-hydroxytryptamine in the rat. Brit. J. Pharmacol. **16**, 360 (1961).
THIERSCH, J. B.: Histamine and histaminase in the blood of cases of lymphoid and monocytic leukemia. Aust. J. exp. Biol. med. Sci. **25**, 73 (1947a).
— Histamine and histaminase in chronic myeloid leukemia of man. Aust. J. exp. Biol. med. Sci. **25**, 79 (1947b).
URBACH, K. F.: Nature and probable origin of conjugated histamine excreted after ingestion of histamine. Proc. Soc. exp. Biol. (N. Y.) **70**, 146 (1949).
UUSPÄÄ, V. J., and P. A. JÄRVINEN: The blood histamine content in hyperemesis gravidarum. Ann. Med. exp. Fenn. **33**, 89 (1955).
VALENTINE, W. N., W. S. BECK, J. H. FOLLETTE, H. MILLS, and J. S. LAWRENCE: Biochemical studies in chronic myelocytic leukemia, polycythemia vera and other idiopathic myeloproliferative disorders. Blood **7**, 959 (1952).
— J. S. LAWRENCE, M. L. PEARCE, and W. S. BECK: The relationship of the basophil to blood histamine in man. Blood **10**, 154 (1955).
— M. L. PEARCE, and J. S. LAWRENCE: Studies on the histamine content of blood, with special reference to leukemia, leukemoid reactions and leukocytoses. Blood **5**, 623 (1950).
WATON, N. G.: Studies on mammalian histidine decarboxylase. Brit. J. Pharmacol. **11**, 119 (1956).
WENT, FR., u. B. REX-KISS: Über den Histamingehalt des Blutes bei pathologischen Änderungen des Blutbildes und Blutdruckes. Z. klin. Med. **139**, 157 (1941).

WERLE, E.: Über das Vorkommen von Diaminoxydase und Histidin-Decarboxylase in Mikroorganismen. Biochem. Z. **309**, 61 (1941).
— Vorkommen der Diaminoxydase im Urin des Menschen. Biochem. Z. **311**, 329 (1942).
— Histamine in nerves. Ciba Foundation Symposium on histamine, p. 264. London: J. & A. Churchill Ltd. 1956.
—, u. G. EFFKEMANN: Über die histaminzerstörende Fähigkeit des Schwangerenblutes. Arch. Gynäk. **170**, 82 (1940a).
— — Der Histamingehalt des Blutes von Rauchern. Klin. Wschr. **19**, 1160 (1940b).
WESTLING, H.: Observations on the action of histamine and related substances on the bronchial resistance in the guinea-pig. Acta physiol. scand. **40**, 75 (1957).
WHELAN, R. F.: Histamine and vasodilatation. Ciba Foundation Symposium on histamine, p. 220. London: J. & A. Churchill Ltd. 1956.
WHITE, T.: Formation and catabolism of histamine in brain tissue in vitro. J. Physiol. (Lond.) **149**, 34 (1960).
WICKSELL, F.: A simplified method for estimating the histaminolytic activity of plasma in pregnancy. Acta physiol. scand. **17**, 359 (1949a).
— Observations on histamine and histaminolysis in pregnancy. Acta physiol. scand. **17**, 395 (1949b).
ZELLER, E. A.: Über den enzymatischen Abbau von Histamin und Diaminen. Helv. chim. Acta **21**, 880 (1938).
— Über das Vorkommen der Diamin-Oxydase im menschlichen Sperma. Helv. chim. Acta **24**, 117 (1941).
—, u. H. BIRKHÄUSER: Über eine in vitro Schwangerschaftsreaktion. Schweiz. med. Wschr. **21**, 975 (1940).
— — H. MISLIN, u. MARIANNE WENK: Über das Vorkommen der Diamin-Oxydase bei Mensch, Säugetier und Vogel. Mit einem Anhang über das Vorkommen der Cholin-Esterase beim Vogel. Helv. chim. Acta **22**, 1381 (1939).
— P. STERN, and L. A. BLANKSMA: Degradation of histamine by monoamine oxidase. Naturwissenschaften **43**, 157 (1956).

Section G

Histamine in the Brain

By

T. White

During the last few years much interest has been focused on the biologically active amines in the brain, but much less attention has been paid to histamine than to 5-hydroxytryptamine (serotonin) and the catecholamines. Although there is still much uncertainty about the physiological significance of 5-hydroxytryptamine and the catecholamines in the brain, these substances are included in modern concepts of "psychopharmacology". Our knowledge of brain histamine is even more incomplete, but the available evidence tends to show that there are several similarities between all these substances as regards their distribution and general pattern of metabolism in the brain. The present account is an attempt to summarize observations on the pharmacological effects of histamine on the brain, after giving a survey of the general pattern of the distribution and metabolism of histamine in the brain. Finally, some physiological implications of the facts and speculations about brain histamine will be discussed.

I. Occurrence of histamine in the brain

Kwiatkowski (1943) claimed that the cerebellum of dogs and cats contained 1.5–2.0 μg histamine equivalent/g tissue, whereas other parts of the brain contained less or none. Subsequent work (Table 1) has confirmed that histamine is present in the brain tissue of various species. In contrast to Kwiatkowski (1943), Harris et al. (1952) and Crossland (1961) could not detect histamine in the cerebellum, whereas Shore et al. (1959) found a relatively uniform distribution in all parts of the dog and rabbit brain examined, including the cerebellum. The recent investigation by Adam (1961) on histamine in canine brain is the most detailed study so far on the distribution of histamine in the brain, and it largely confirms the findings by Harris et al. (1952). As a rule higher concentrations of histamine have been found in peripheral nerves, particularly autonomic nerves, than in the brain (von Euler, 1949; Werle and Weicken, 1949; West, 1957). Although rather low concentrations of histamine have been found in whole brain, histamine seems to be concentrated in some regions of the brain stem, such as the hypothalamus and the median eminence (Harris et al., 1952; Crossland, 1960; Adam, 1961). It would thus seem that histamine is one among several biologically active amines that are concentrated in the hypothalamus and other parts of the brain stem (Amin, Crawford and Gaddum, 1954; Vogt, 1954; von Euler, 1946). It is well known that the administration of drugs such as monoamine oxidase inhibitors, reserpine, and others, to various species of laboratory animals can change the concentrations of 5-hydroxytryptamine and of noradrenaline in the brain (Vogt, 1954; Holzbauer and Vogt, 1956; Paasonen and Vogt, 1956; Wolley, 1959).

Table 1. *Distribution of histamine (μg/g) in brain*

	Total brain	Cerebrum	Cerebellum	Hypothalamus	Median eminence Hypophysial stalk	Pituitary gland	Nucleus caudatus	Brain stem
Rat . .	4.3±1.0 S.D. (3)	1.0±0.1 (10)		4.3±0.3 (10)				
		0.05—0.09† (11)	<0.05 (11)			2.3—15.2 ant (11)		
Dog . .	9.8—17.3 (2)	0.2—0.4 (5)	<0.2 (6)	0.24—1.6 (11)	8.0—27.0 (11)	2.0—23.0 post (11)		
		0.1—0.16† (1)	0.2—0.4 (5)	<0.2—6.2 (6)	5.7—30.0 (6)	1.0—19.0 ant (6)	<0.2 (6)	0.2—0.4 (5)
			1.5 (1)			<0.4—26.5 post (6)		
Pig . .			<0.02 (6)	0.12—0.75 (6)	2.3—11.0 (6)	0.1—1.0 ant (6)	<0.06 (6)	
						1.2—7.0 post (6)		
Cat. . .	0.2 (9)	0—0.12† (1)	<0.5 (6)	0.7—8.3 (6)	3.6—25.5 (6)	0.26—43.0 ant (6)	<0.6 (6)	
	<0.06 (6)		1.5 —2.0 (1)			1.0—76.0 post (6)		
Guinea pig	0.2 —0.4* (8)	0.05† (1)						
	<0.1 (6)							
Cattle .	0.1—0.7* (4)	1—1.5* (7)	2—3* (7)			9—11* (7)	<0.02 (6)	1* (4)
Rabbit .	0.06 (9)	0.20—0.25† (5)	0.19 —0.24 (5)					
	0.20—0.40 (5)	0.044—0.05† (1)						0.30—0.35 (5)
Man . .						5—6.5* (7)	1* (7)	

* Figures given in terms of histamine dihydrochloride; † Cortex; ant Anterior lobe; post Posterior lobe. (1) Kwiatkowski, 1943; (2) Cicardo and Stoppani, 1949; (3) Clouet, Gaitonde and Richter, 1957; (4) von Euler, 1949; (5) Shore, Burkhalter and Cohn, 1959; (6) Harris, Jacobsohn and Kahlson, 1952; (7) Werle and Weicken, 1949; (8) Strengers and Maas, 1956; (9) West, 1957; (10) Szeberényi and Kovács, 1959; (11) Adam, 1961.

It is not known if the histamine content of the mammalian brain can be influenced in a similar manner. However, it has been reported that the histamine content of the hypothalamus of the rat decreases after hypophysectomy (Szeberényi and Kovács, 1959). The pituitary gland itself contains high amounts of histamine (Abel and Kubota, 1919; Harris et al., 1952). Adam (1961) suggested that in the hypophysis the histamine content is related to the mast cell content, although it has not been shown that all the histamine of the gland is in mast cells.

Various authors have reported low concentrations of histamine, usually less than 0.1 μg/ml, in the cerebrospinal fluid (for references, see Schain, 1960). When perfusing the ventricular system of cats histamine could not be detected in the effluent, either before or after strong electrical stimulation of the hypothalamus (Hilton and Schain, 1961).

II. Formation of histamine in the brain

The formation of histamine by decarboxylation of histidine is catalyzed by the enzyme histidine decarboxylase which is present in several tissues of various species (for references, see Waton, 1956). Formation of histamine from histidine by brain tissue has been demonstrated *in vitro* in cattle (Holtz and Westermann, 1956), rat (Schayer, 1956a), cat, pig, and dog (White, 1959). Injected histamine is said to penetrate slowly, or not at all, from the blood into the brain

(HALPERN, NEVEU and WILSON, 1959). This would imply that the histamine present in the brain is formed there. Formation of radioactive histamine in the brain has also been demonstrated *in vivo* in cats after intraventricular administration of radioactive histidine (WHITE, 1960). In the rat, where comparative studies on different organs have been made with a sensitive method, the histamine forming capacity of the whole brain is not great as compared to the singularly high activities in the embryonic tissues (KAHLSON, ROSENGREN, WESTLING and WHITE, 1958), but it is higher than in most adult tissues, stomach and lung excepted (SCHAYER, 1956a). In cat, pig, and dog the histamine forming capacity is much higher in the hypothalamus than in other parts of the brain (WHITE, 1959). As already mentioned, the hypothalamus and adjacent structures also contain high concentrations of histamine (HARRIS et al., 1952; ADAM, 1961). Thus it would seem that the hypothalamus both contains and can form more histamine than other parts of the brain, and further that the hypothalamus is among the most active tissues of adult animals in forming histamine. It is not known what component of the brain tissue is responsible for the formation of histamine. Mast cells are very effective in forming histamine (SCHAYER, 1956b) but seem to be absent from brain tissue (for references, see RILEY, 1959 and Chapter 1, Section E of this book.)

III. Catabolism of histamine in the brain

Monoamine oxidase is thought to play an important role in the inactivation of 5-hydroxytryptamine and noradrenaline in the brain (for references, see DAVISON, 1958; WOLLEY, 1959). Although there is some evidence that monoamine oxidase can catalyze the oxidation of histamine (SCHAYER, 1959), this reaction does not seem to be an important pathway for the catabolism of histamine in the brain. In fact, brain tissue *in vitro* transforms histamine into ring-N-methyl derivatives (i.e. methylhistamine: 1-methyl-4(β-aminoethyl)-imidazole, and methylimidazoleacetic acid: 1-methyl-imidazole-4-acetic acid), whereas the oxidation of histamine to imidazoleacetic acid is insignificant (WHITE, 1959). Also *in vivo*, on intraventricular administration in the cat, histamine is methylated, and again practically no imidazoleacetic acid is formed (WHITE, 1960). These findings are in agreement with observations by BROWN, TOMCHICK and AXELROD (1959), who found that brain tissue is particularly rich in the enzyme imidazole-N-methyl transferase. The highest activities of this enzyme are present in the hypophysis and the lowest in the cerebellum (AXELROD, MACLEAN, ALBERS and WEISSBACH, 1961). The question then arises why brain contains histamine at all. It might simply be that the rate of formation exceeds that of destruction. It seems more probable, however, that the newly formed histamine and the methylating enzyme are present in distinct structures, e.g. different cells, or intracellular compartments, so that enzyme action on the substrate is prevented. The histamine methylating enzyme is present in brain tissue exclusively in the soluble supernatant fraction (BROWN et al., 1959). Therefore, it seems possible that histamine administered to the brain might be treated differently (e.g. catabolized more rapidly) from histamine formed in the brain. Yet, even newly formed histamine is methylated to some extent (WHITE, 1959, 1960). Anyhow, the physiological meaning of the histamine methylating enzyme in the brain is not likely to be a protective device against excessive amounts of histamine from the blood, as histamine does not seem to penetrate the so called "blood-brain barrier" (HALPERN, NEVEU and WILSON, 1959).

Although there is, on the whole, little information on the inhibition of the methylation of histamine *in vivo*, it has been found that chlorpromazine and cupric ions inhibit the methylation of histamine administered intraventricularly in anaesthetized cats (White, 1961a). There is no precise evidence as to the mechanism responsible for this effect of chlorpromazine and of copper. It is possibly due to inhibition of the histamine methylating enzyme in the brain (Brown et al., 1959).

Noradrenaline, 5-hydroxytryptamine, and histamine are all formed and are present in distinct areas of the brain, whereas the capacity of inactivation by monoamine oxidase, catechol-N-methyl transferase, and imidazole-N-methyl transferase is present in most parts of the brain (Bogdanski, Weissbach and Udenfriend, 1957; Udenfriend and Creveling, 1959; Axelrod, Albers and Clemente, 1959; Brown et al., 1959; Axelrod et al., 1961).

IV. Pharmacological effects of histamine on the brain

The pronounced effects of histamine on the circulation and respiration make the effects on separate organs difficult to interpret, especially when histamine is administered intravenously, or by other routes of administration leading to the appearance of considerable quantities of histamine in the blood. This is particularly true for the brain. For instance, an injection of histamine into an experimental animal causing acute hypotension and/or hypoxemia could conceivably influence brain function by these effects *per se*, and it would be difficult to demonstrate direct actions of histamine on the brain (for references, see Sokoloff, 1959; Virno, Gertner and Bovet, 1956). These considerations make it difficult to evaluate some experiments on the effects of histamine, at least in terms of *direct* effects. Thus histamine has been reported to change the EEG pattern in rats (Brandon, 1955; Bovet, Kohn, Marotta and Silvestrini, 1958), and to stimulate the vasomotor centre in cats and dogs (Feldberg and Kwiatkowski, 1933; Pilcher and Sollman, 1914—15). Of greater interest are the effects of small amounts of histamine injected into the carotid artery. Histamine has been reported to inhibit transcallosally evoked potentials in the cat after intraarterial injection (Gilfoil, Hart and Marrazzi, 1960). Intracarotid injection of histamine, in the rabbit, is reported to increase the electrical activity of the cerebellar cortex (Crossland and Mitchell, 1956). In guinea-pigs characteristic posture and movements have been observed after intra-carotid injections of histamine in doses lower than those producing bronchoconstriction (Schmidt and Stähelin, 1929).

Histamine injected into the ventricular system of cats penetrates to some extent into the brain tissue and only a small portion enters the blood stream (Bhawe, 1958; Draškoci, Feldberg, Fleischhauer and Haranath, 1960; White, 1960). Feldberg and Sherwood (1954) showed that intraventricular injections of histamine into conscious cats caused marked changes in the behaviour of the animals, including salivation, tachypnoe, sedation, and muscular weakness. Similar effects have been obtained in mice (Haley, 1957), where large doses produce convulsions (Kohn and Millichap, 1958). Intraventricular injections of the histamine liberator 48/80 in mice produce exitation (delirium ambulatorium) which is not prevented by pretreatment with mepyramine (Rocha e Silva, 1959). Intraventricular injections of histamine into anaesthetized cats cause a rise in blood pressure of central origin which can be prevented by intraventricular mepyramine (Trendelenburg, 1957a). This pressor effect is not produced in dogs (Bhargava and Tangri, 1959), but histamine intraventricularly antagonizes the circulatory effects of intraventricular injections of 5-hydroxytryptamine and of noradrenaline (Kaneko, McCubbin and Page, 1960). Trendelenburg (1957a) suggested that intraventricular histamine stimulated sympathetic ganglion cells in the brain. This view would be in accordance with the findings, also in cats, that histamine stimulates peripheral sympathetic ganglion cells, and, in smaller doses, potentiates ganglionic transmission (TRENDELENBURG, 1954; 1957b; 1959).

The major product of histamine catabolism in the brain, methylhistamine, lacks the pharmacological effects of intraventricular histamine (WHITE, 1961b). If the pharmacological effects of intraventricular histamine are related to the physiological actions of histamine in the brain, if any, then the methylation of histamine in the brain can be regarded as a process of physiological significance.

Various authors (e.g. BELOUS, 1955; BLACKMORE and CHERRY, 1955; FUCHE and KAHLSON, 1957; GRAY and MUNSON, 1951; SAWYER, 1955) have described a stimulating action of histamine on the pituitary gland, on the adenohypophysis or the neurohypophysis. However, it has not been definitely established whether these effects are direct, or mediated through the hypothalamus.

V. The physiological significance of histamine in the brain

"The uneven distribution of a pharmacologically active substance in the brain strongly suggests that the agent has a role to play in the specialized function of those regions where its concentration is high" (VOGT, 1959). This general statement, quoted from a discussion of the catecholamines in the brain, may equally well be applied to the histamine in the brain. A role for histamine is further indicated by the similarly uneven distribution of the capacity to form histamine (WHITE, 1959). Further still, the brain possesses a powerful mechanism for the inactivation of histamine by means of ring-N-methylation (BROWN et al., 1959; WHITE, 1959; 1960; AXELROD et al., 1961). At present one can only speculate as to what sort of function in the brain, if any, is effected by histamine. The pharmacological actions may give some clue but it is difficult to see a common denominator for all the different actions of histamine on the brain. Some of the most interesting experiments, so far, have involved intraventricular administration of histamine. It must be emphasized that in these experiments huge doses been used, about 100–1000 times those required for a depressor response in the cat after intravenous injection. These large amounts exceed those which are normally present in the brain and would thus seem to be of little interest from the physiological standpoint. On the other hand, it should be realized that in these experiments histamine in all probability does not act by its presence in the ventricular fluid, but by its presence in the brain tissue, where much lower concentrations are produced (DRAŠKOCI et al., 1960; WHITE, 1960). DRAŠKOCI et al. (1960) also demonstrated that histamine does not infiltrate the brain tissue diffusely; more being taken up by the grey than by the white matter.

The findings of HARRIS et al. (1952) "might be taken to indicate the possibility that in the median eminence histamine may be related to nerve terminals from where histamine, dependent on the state of activity, is carried to the anterior lobe in quantities anywhere between minimal and maximal." Hyperhistaminemia has been discussed as a possible "symptom of a disturbance in the middle brain" (GOOSZEN and DONKER, 1956). "Histamine is present in nervous tissue to perform some physiological function, though it is unlikely that it is concerned with nerve conduction" (WEST, 1957). SHORE et al. (1959) suggested that "brain histamine may be associated with non-nervous, perhaps vascular tissue." Histamine (and adrenaline) "through their local action may play a role in the physiologic and pathologic regulation of the cerebral circulation in man" (WEISS, LENNOX and ROBB, 1929). "A new cerebral synaptic neurohumoral inhibitor is suggested"

(GILFOIL, HART and MARRAZZI, 1960). Histamine "still warrants consideration in any discussion of chemical transmission" (CROSSLAND, 1960). "Histamine in the CNS has been ignored for a long time by several investigators as a second-class amine. But this amine, however annoying the fact may be, has the same citizenship rights in the CNS as catecholamines and 5-HT, whose function in the CNS is approximately as obscure as that of histamine" (ERSPAMER, 1961).

These quotations from the literature reflect the wide diversity in speculation as to the function of histamine in the brain. It is not even known to what tissues, vascular, neural or others, the occurrence and function of the brain histamine is primarily related. In the light of current work in this laboratory even the possibility of a role for histamine in the intracellular metabolism of brain tissues should be mentioned (KAHLSON, 1960). Histamine should now be included among the biologically active amines in the brain, such as the catecholamines and 5-hydroxytryptamine, which are formed, stored and inactivated in the brain. Despite intense research it has so far been impossible to ascribe a definite function in the brain to any of them. It seems probable that future work on the elaboration of suitable means of increasing and decreasing the formation and content of histamine in the brain, and a closer analysis of the effects of histamine on brain function, will shed more light on the functional significance of the histamine in the brain.

References

ABEL, J. J., and S. KUBOTA: On the presence of histamine (β-iminazolyl-ethylamine) in the hypophysis cerebri and other tissues of the body and its occurrence among the hydrolytic decomposition products of proteins. J. Pharmacol. exp. Ther. **13**, 243 (1919).

ADAM, H. M.: Histamine in the central nervous system and hypophysis of the dog. In: Regional Neurochemistry, ed. KETY, S. S. and ELKES, J. Oxford, London, New York, Paris: Pergamon Press 1961.

AMIN, A. H., T. B. B. CRAWFORD, and J. H. GADDUM: The distribution of substance P and 5-hydroxytryptamine in the central nervous system of the dog. J. Physiol. (Lond.) **126**, 596 (1954).

AXELROD, J., W. ALBERS, and C. D. CLEMENTE: Distribution of catechol-0-methyl transferase in the nervous system and other tissues. J. Neurochem. **5**, 68 (1959).

— P. D. MACLEAN, R. W. ALBERS, and H. WEISSBACH: Regional distribution of methyl transferase enzymes in the nervous system and glandular tissues. In: Regional Neurochemistry, ed. KETY, S. S. and ELKES, J. Oxford, London, New York, Paris: Pergamon Press 1961

BELOUS, A. A.: Influence of histamine on the secretion of the neurohypophysis. Fiziol. Zh. S.S.S.R. **41**, 666 (1955). Cited in: Int. Abstr. biol. Sci. **7**, 190 (1957).

BHARGAVA, K. P., and K. K. TANGRI: The central vasomotor effects of 5-hydroxytryptamine. Brit. J. Pharmacol. **14**, 411 (1959).

BHAWE, W. B.: Experiments on the fate of histamine and acetylcholine after their injection into the cerebral ventricles. J. Physiol. (Lond.) **140**, 169 (1958).

BLACKMORE, W. P., and G. R. CHERRY: Antidiuretic action of histamine in the dog. Amer. J. Physiol. **180**, 596 (1955).

BOGDANSKI, D. F., H. WEISSBACH, and S. UDENFRIED: The distribution of serotonin, 5-hydroxytryptophan decarboxylase, and monoamine oxidase in brain. J. Neurochem. **1**, 272 (1957).

BOVET, D., R. KOHN, M. MAROTTA, and B. SILVESTRINI: Some effects of histamine in the normal and Haemophilus pertussis vaccinated rat. Brit. J. Pharmacol. **13**, 74 (1958).

BRANDON, A.: Étude électrocorticographique et électromyélographique de l'action de l'histamine. Arch. int. Physiol. **63**, 62 (1955).

BROWN, D. D., R. TOMCHICK, and J. AXELROD: The distribution and properties of a histamine-methylating enzyme. J. biol. Chem. **234**, 2948 (1959).

CICARDO, V. H., and A. O. M. STOPPANI: Presence of histamine in central nervous system extracts. Nature (Lond.) **163**, 365 (1949).

CLOUET, D. H., M. K. GAITONDE, and D. RICHTER: The free histidine, histamine, and arginine content of the rat brain. J. Neurochem. **1**, 228 (1957).

CROSSLAND, J.: Chemical transmission in the central nervous system. J. Pharm. Pharmacol. **12**, 1 (1960).

Crossland, J.: Biologic estimation of histamine. In: Methods med. Res., ed. Quastel, J. H. Chicago: Year Book Medical Publishers, Inc. 1961.
—, and J. F. Mitchell: The effect on the electrical activity of the cerebellum of a substance present in cerebellar extracts. J. Physiol. (Lond.) **132**, 391 (1956).
Davison, A. N.: Physiological role of monoamine oxidase. Physiol. Rev. **38**, 729 (1958).
Draškoci, M., W. Feldberg, K. Fleischhauer, and P. S. R. K. Haranath: Absorption of histamine into the blood stream on perfusion of the cerebral ventricles, and its uptake by brain tissue. J. Physiol. (Lond.) **150**, 50 (1960).
Erspamer, V.: Pharmacologically active substances of mammalian origin. In: Ann. Rev. Pharmacol., ed. Cutting, W. C. Palo Alto: Annual Reviews, Inc. 1961.
Euler, U. S. von: A specific sympathomimetic ergone in adrenergic nerve fibres (sympathin) and its relations to adrenaline and nor-adrenaline. Acta physiol. scand. **12**, 73 (1946).
— Histamine as a specific constituent of certain autonomic nerve fibres. Acta physiol. scand. **19**, 85 (1949).
Feldberg, W., and H. Kwiatkowski: Untersuchungen über primären und sekundären Histaminschock am arteriellen Blutdruck. Naunyn-Schmiedebergs Arch. exp. Path. Pharmak. **170**, 551 (1933).
—, and S. L. Sherwood: Injections of drugs into the lateral ventricle of the cat. J. Physiol. (Lond.) **123**, 148 (1954).
Fuche, J., and G. Kahlson: Histamine as a stimulant to the anterior pituitary gland as judged by the lymphopenic response in normal and hypophysectomized rabbits. Acta physiol. scand. **39**, 327 (1957).
Gilfoil, T. M., E. R. Hart, and A. S. Marrazzi: Cerebral synaptic inhibition by histamine. Fed. Proc. **19**, 262 (1960).
Gooszen, J. A. H., and J. Donker: Studies on histamine. VI. A study of histamine-metabolism in schizophrenic patients. Acta allerg. (Kbh.) **10**, 149 (1956).
Gray, W. D., and P. L. Munson: The rapidity of the adrenocorticotropic response of the pituitary to the intravenous administration of histamine. Endocrinology **48**, 471 (1951).
Haley, T. J.: Pharmacological effects produced by intracerebral administration of drugs of unrelated structure to conscious mice. Arch. int. Pharmacodyn. **110**, 239 (1957).
Halpern, B. N., Th. Neveu, and C. W. M. Wilson: The distribution and fate of radioactive histamine in the rat. J. Physiol. (Lond.) **147**, 437 (1959).
Harris, G. W., D. Jacobsohn, and G. Kahlson: The occurrence of histamine in cerebral regions related to the hypophysis. Ciba Found. Colloq. Endocr. **4**, 186 (1952).
Hilton, S. M., and R. J. Schain: A search for pharmacologically active substances in fluid from the cerebral ventricles. J. Physiol. (Lond.) **157**, 46P (1961).
Holtz, P., u. E. Westermann: Über die Dopadecarboxylase und Histidindecarboxylase des Nervengewebes. Naunyn-Schmiedebergs Arch. exp. Path. Pharmak. **227**, 538 (1956).
Holzbauer, M., and M. Vogt: Depression by reserpine of the noradrenaline concentration in the hypothalamus of the cat. J. Neurochem. **1**, 8 (1956).
Kahlson, G.: A place for histamine in normal physiology. Lancet **1960 I**, 67
— E. Rosengren, H. Westling, and T. White: The site of increased formation of histamine in the pregnant rat. J. Physiol. (Lond.) **144**, 337 (1958).
Kaneko, Y., J. W. McCubbin, and I. H. Page: Mechanism by which serotonin, norepinephrine and reserpine cause central vasomotor inhibition. Circulat. Res. **8**, 1228 (1960).
Kohn, R., and J. G. Millichap: Properties of seizures induced by histamine. Proc. Soc. exp. Biol. (N. Y.) **99**, 623 (1958).
Kwiatkowski, H.: Histamine in nervous tissue. J. Physiol. (Lond.) **102**, 32 (1943).
Paasonen, M. K., and M. Vogt: The effect of drugs on the amounts of substance P and 5-hydroxytryptamine in mammalian brain. J. Physiol. (Lond.) **131**, 617 (1956).
Pilcher, J. D., and T. Sollmann: Studies in the vasomotor centre. XII. The action of ergot and its constituents, ergotoxin, and histamine. J. Pharmacol. exp. Ther. **6**, 385 (1914—1915).
Riley, J. F.: The mast cells, p. 13. Edinburgh and London: E. & S. Livingstone Ltd. 1959.
Rocha e Silva, M.: Central effects produced by injection of 48/80 into the cerebral ventricles of mice. Brit. J. Pharmacol. **14**, 243 (1959).
Sawyer, C. H.: Rhinencephalic involvement in pituitary activation by intraventricular histamine in the rabbit under nembutal anesthesia. Amer. J. Physiol. **180**, 37 (1955).
Schain, R. J.: Neurohumors and other pharmacologically active substances in cerebrospinal fluid: A review of the literature. Yale J. Biol. Med. **33**, 15 (1960).
Schayer, R. W.: Formation and binding of histamine by rat tissues *in vitro*. Amer. J. Physiol. **187**, 63 (1956a).
— Formation and binding of histamine by free mast cells of rat peritoneal fluid. Amer. J. Physiol. **186**, 199 (1956b).
— Catabolism of physiological quantities of histamine in vivo. Physiol. Rev. **39**, 116 (1959).

SCHMIDT, G. W., u. A. STÄHELIN: Histaminempfindlichkeit und anaphylaktische Reaktionen. Z. Immun.-Forsch. **60**, 222 (1929).
SHORE, P. A., A. BURKHALTER, and V. H. COHN JR.: A method for the fluorometric assay of histamine in tissues. J. Pharmacol. exp. Ther. **127**, 182 (1959).
SOKOLOFF, L.: The action of drugs on the cerebral circulation. Pharmacol. Rev. **11**, 1 (1959).
STRENGERS, TH., and J. W. MAAS: Studies on histamine. IV. On free and bound histamine. Acta allerg. (Kbh.) **10**, 130 (1956).
SZEBERÉNYI, SZ., u. K. KOVÁCS: Über den Einfluß endokriner Faktoren auf den Histamingehalt des Hypothalamus der Ratte. Naturwissenschaften **46**, 581 (1959).
TRENDELENBURG, U.: The action of histamine and pilocarpine on the superior cervical ganglion and the adrenal glands of the cat. Brit. J. Pharmacol. **9**, 481 (1954).
— Stimulation of sympathetic centers by histamine. Circulat. Res. **5**, 105 (1957a).
— The action of histamine, pilocarpine, and 5-hydroxytryptamine on transmission through the superior cervical ganglion. J. Physiol. (Lond.) **135**, 66 (1957b).
— Non-nicotinic ganglion-stimulating substances. Fed. Proc. **18**, 1001 (1959).
UDENFRIEND, S., and C. R. CREVELING: Localization of dopamine-β-oxidase in brain. J. Neurochem. **4**, 350 (1959).
VIRNO, M., S. B. GERTNER, and D. BOVET: Action of histamine on the jugular venous pressure and cerebral circulation of the dog. Effects of antihistaminic drugs (pyrilamine and chlorpheniramine) and a histamine liberating agent (48/80 B. W.). J. Pharmacol. exp. Ther. **118**, 63 (1956).
VOGT, M.: The concentration of symphatin in different parts of the central nervous system under normal conditions and after the administration of drugs. J. Physiol. (Lond.) **123**, 451 (1954).
— Catecholamines in brain. Pharmacol. Rev. **11**, 483 (1959).
WATON, N. G.: Studies on mammalian histidine decarboxylase. Brit. J. Pharmacol. **11**, 119 (1956).
WEISS, S., W. G. LENNOX, and G. P. ROBB: The dilator effect of histamine on the cerebral vessels in man. Proc. Soc. exp. Biol. (N. Y.) **26**, 706 (1929).
WERLE, E., u. G. WEICKEN: Über das Vorkommen von Histamin in Nerven. Biochem. Z. **319**, 457 (1949).
WEST, G. B.: Histamine in nervous tissue. In: Metabolism of the nervous system, ed. RICHTER, D. London, New York, Paris, Los Angeles: Pergamon Press 1957.
WHITE, T.: Formation and catabolism of histamine in brain tissue *in vitro*. J. Physiol. (Lond.) **149**, 34 (1959).
— Formation and catabolism of histamine in cat brain *in vivo*. J. Physiol. (Lond.) **152**, 299 (1960).
— Inhibition of the methylation of histamine in cat brain. J. Physiol. (Lond.) **159**, 191 (1961a).
— Some effects of histamine and two histamine metabolites on the cat's brain. J. Physiol. (Lond.) **159**, 198 (1961b).
WOOLLEY, D. W.: (chairman). Amine oxidase inhibitors. Ann. N. Y. Acad. Sci. **80**, 551 (1959).

Chapter 5

Physiological Significance of Histamine

Section A

Rôle de l'histamine dans la vasodilatation d'origine postéro-radiculaire

Par

JEAN-LOUIS PARROT et BERNARD VASSEUR

Avec 8 figures

La stimulation du bout distal de certaines racines postérieures de la moelle, ou du bout périphérique d'un nerf qui contient des fibres postéro-radiculaires provoque chez l'animal une vasodilatation dans le territoire cutané correspondant.

D'autre part, diverses agressions de la peau, qu'elles soient d'ordre physique ou chimique, déterminent chez l'Homme une triple réponse vasculaire et l'un des éléments de celle-ci relève d'un phénomène axonique qui intéresse certaines fibres postéro-radiculaires.

Tels sont les deux cas de vasodilatation cutanée d'origine nerveuse où le rôle de l'histamine a pu être discuté.

I. Effets de la stimulation de fibres postéro-radiculaires

L'existence de fibres vasodilatatrices dans les racines postérieures est mise en évidence pour la première fois par STRICKER (1876). Cet auteur stimule électriquement ou mécaniquement les 6e et 7e racines postérieures lombaires chez le Chien. Il enregistre toutes les minutes les variations d'un thermomètre placé entre les orteils de la patte du même côté. Une augmentation de la température témoigne de la vasodilatation consécutive à la stimulation nerveuse.

GÄRTNER (1889) et WERZILOFF (1896) ont confirmé ce phénomène en utilisant la même technique.

MORAT (1892), qui préférait apprécier «à l'oeil nu» les variations de couleur de la peau, voit apparaître une «belle rougeur» après avoir stimulé les dernières racines postérieures lombaires chez le Chien et le Chat.

L'enregistrement continu et objectif des réactions vasomotrices provoquées par la stimulation des racines postérieures fut réalisé par BAYLISS (1900–1901) grâce à la technique pléthysmographique. Cette amélioration technique lui permit de décrire avec précision les caractères de la vasodilatation. Cette dernière débute après un temps de latence prolongé, de l'ordre de plusieurs secondes. Elle se développe progressivement et se maintient longtemps.

LEWIS et MARVIN (1927) ont clairement dégagé trois faits qui suggèrent la libération d'une substance vasodilatatrice dans ce phénomène:

a) Une stimulation relativement brève des fibres nerveuses vasodilatatrices détermine une réponse remarquablement prolongée. Le fait devait être maintes fois confirmé; ainsi HOLTON et PERRY (1951) montreront que la stimulation du nerf grand auriculaire chez le Lapin, par un choc unique, déclenche une vasodilatation qui atteint son maximum au bout d'une minute et disparaît après trois à quatre minutes.

b) La réaction vasculaire atteint son maximum après la fin de la stimulation.

c) La durée de la réponse est, dans une large mesure, fonction de la durée de la stimulation. Ainsi la stimulation du bout périphérique de fibres postéro-

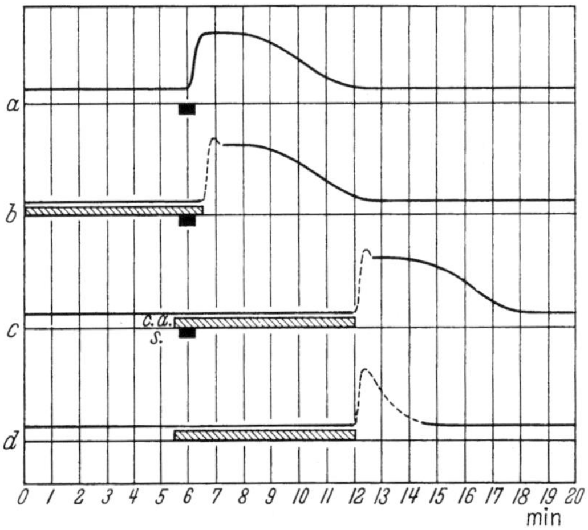

Fig. 1

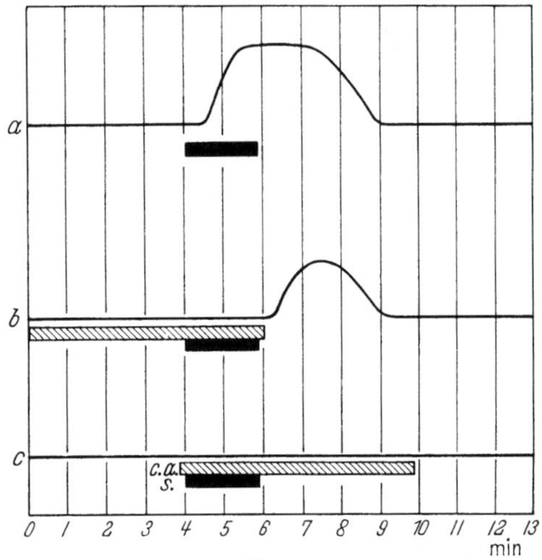

Fig. 2

Fig. 1. Schéma destiné à montrer la vaso-dilatation qui survient dans la patte du Chat à la suite d'une stimulation centrifuge des racines postérieures (*a*) et à la suite d'un simple arrêt circulatoire (*d*). En *b* et *c*, la stimulation nerveuse a lieu pendant l'arrèt circulatoire; on voit en *c* que l'arrêt circulatoire a retardé l'effet de la stimulation nerveuse: *s*, période de stimulation; *c*, *a*, période d'arrêt circulatoire (LEWIS et MARVIN, 1927)

Fig. 2. Schéma destiné à montrer, par comparaison avec la fig. 1, l'effet de l'arrêt circulatoire (*c.a.*) sur l'action vaso-dilatatrice du parasympathique; en *s*, stimulation du nerf érecteur (LEWIS et MARVIN, 1927)

radiculaires pendant 10, 20 et 40 secondes provoquent des réponses de 3–3,5 et 7,5 minutes (LEWIS et MARVIN, 1927).

Ajoutons un autre caractère qui évoque l'intervention d'un médiateur: l'effet des stimulations s'épuise lorsqu'elles sont répétées (WYBAUW, 1938; CAPON, 1957).

En outre, l'activité vasodilatatrice des fibres postéro-radiculaires est différée par un arrêt circulatoire. LEWIS et MARVIN stimulent chez le Chat des filets nerveux cutanés de l'extrémité d'une patte, alors que la circulation est interrompue dans celle-ci. La réponse vasculaire est suspendue jusqu'à la reprise de la circulation, plusieurs minutes après la fin de la stimulation nerveuse (fig. 1).

Or la vasodilatation provoquée par la stimulation des fibres cholinergiques est toute différente. Ces mêmes auteurs, en effet, étudient la vasodilatation pénienne provoquée chez le Chat par stimulation des nerfs érecteurs. Le temps de latence est beaucoup plus court. La vasodilatation décroît dès la fin de la stimulation. Enfin, il n'y a aucune réponse ni immédiate, ni différée, lorsque la stimulation du nerf a lieu pendant l'arrêt circulatoire obtenu par clampage de l'aorte (fig. 2).

Ainsi apparaît-il que le médiateur libéré par la stimulation des fibres postéro-radiculaires est plus stable que l'acétylcholine

II. Analogies pharmacologiques entre le médiateur et l'histamine

Le rôle de l'histamine fut envisagé par LEWIS et MARVIN (1927) qui rapprochèrent cette vasodilatation d'un autre phénomène vasculaire cutané; il s'agit de la triple réaction cutanée que LEWIS et GRANT (1924) avaient précédemment étudiée chez l'Homme.

La stimulation mécanique de la peau (friction avec une pointe mousse) détermine des réactions vasculaires que LEWIS et GRANT analysent ainsi:

D'une part:

a) Dilatation locale des petits vaisseaux.

b) Augmentation de la perméabilité des capillaires qui provoque l'apparition d'une boule d'oedème ou papule.

D'autre part:

c) Dilatation des artérioles voisines qui détermine un érythème environnant.

Cette réponse complexe est particulièrement bien marquée chez les sujets atteints de dermographisme. Elle apparaît également après d'autres stimulations cutanées: ainsi le chaud ou le froid, appliqués localement, provoquent une réponse qui paraît très analogue à l'érythème environnant de LEWIS.

L'histamine elle-même détermine une triade caractéristique. Et ce test cutané permet à LEWIS d'établir qu'il existe des analogies pharmacologiques entre l'intermédiaire chimique responsable de la réaction et l'histamine.

a) Ainsi l'érythème environnant ne se manifeste jamais lorsque les fibres postéro-radiculaires ont dégénéré après section.

Expérimentalement LEWIS et GRANT (1924) établissent que l'anesthésie des extrémités nerveuses par infiltration de novocaïne dans la peau supprime l'érythème environnant. Par contre il persiste à l'avant-bras après anesthésie du nerf musculo-cutané qui réalise une section physiologique et temporaire du tronc nerveux. Ainsi la substance libérée par friction de la peau détermine l'érythème environnant en mettant en jeu un phénomène axonique. Des expériences semblables établissent que l'histamine agit aussi par l'intermédiaire de ce mécanisme.

b) D'autre part l'érythème environnant consécutif à l'agression de la peau est différé par arrêt temporaire de la circulation. La stimulation mécanique de la peau libère donc une substance vasodilatatrice qui est relativement stable. L'érythème environnant provoqué par l'histamine est semblablement différé.

c) Le liquide d'une papule provoquée par l'agression cutanée contient une substance douée de propriétés pharmacologiques analogues à celles de l'histamine.

Ce liquide injecté dans la peau d'un sujet normal détermine une nouvelle triade. LEWIS et GRANT évaluent l'équivalent histaminique de ce liquide à 10^{-6} d'histamine base.

D'autre part, ce liquide stimule l'utérus isolé de Cobaye; il détermine une contraction analogue à celle que donne l'histamine à la concentration de 7×10^{-7} (histamine base).

d) Enfin LEWIS et HARMER (1927) ont mis en évidence la libération d'une substance «histaminique» chez 4 sujets prédisposés au dermographisme. La friction d'une large surface cutanée détermine, dans les minutes qui suivent, une élévation de la température cutanée et un érythème de la face. Une injection sous-cutanée d'histamine, à la dose de 0,03 mg (histamine base), provoque une réaction tout à fait semblable.

En conclusion, les réactions cutanées de l'animal consécutives à la stimulation de fibres postéro-radiculaires sont étroitement comparables aux réactions qui surviennent dans la peau humaine quand elle répond à une friction vigoureuse ou à d'autres formes d'agression. Ces réponses sont attribuées à la libération de substances histaminiques dans la peau et à partir de cellules de la peau (LEWIS et MARVIN, 1927).

III. Nouvelles analogies pharmacologiques entre le médiateur postéro-radiculaire et l'histamine

UNGAR (1935) eut l'idée de caractériser l'éventuelle libération d'histamine consécutive à la stimulation des fibres vasodilatatrices postéro-radiculaires en observant la sécrétion gastrique du chien en expérience. Les cellules sécrétrices gastriques sont en effet parmi les plus sensibles de l'organisme à l'histamine; POPIELSKI (1920) rapporte que 0,0033 mg/kg suffisent à stimuler la sécrétion gastrique chez le Chien.

UNGAR constate ainsi que la stimulation du bout périphérique du nerf saphène interne déclenche chez le Chien choralosé et atropinisé une augmentation considérable de la sécrétion gastrique. Après un temps de latence important de 8 à 10 minutes (qui exclut la possibilité d'une réponse directe ou réflexe à la stimulation nerveuse), le volume de la sécrétion s'accroît considérablement pendant une quinzaine de minutes (fig. 3).

L'arrêt de la circulation veineuse fémorale abolit cette réponse gastrique, ce qui confirme bien la nature humorale de son mécanisme. De plus, au cours d'expériences de circulation croisée entre deux chiens réunis par une anastomose carotido-jugulaire, UNGAR établit que la stimulation du bout périphérique du nerf saphène interne de l'un active la sécrétion gastrique de l'autre.

Occasionnellement, un autre test sert à identifier la substance: UNGAR (1936) observe, en effet, que des contractions des cornes utérines *in situ* chez la Chienne se développent parallèlement à la réaction gastrique.

Enfin, TINEL et UNGAR (1935), rapportent qu'une substance semblable est libérée lors des réactions vasodilatatrices à la chaleur. En effet, l'immersion de la patte d'un chien chloralosé et atropinisé dans l'eau à 50° active la sécrétion gastrique.

UNGAR retient de ces faits que, parmi les substances alors connues, seule l'histamine est capable chez un chien atropinisé d'agir sur la sécrétion gastrique aux doses qui peuvent être libérées au cours de telles expériences. C'est là le principal argument en faveur de la nature histaminique de la substance vasodilatatrice. D'ailleurs, par sa nature, le suc gastrique recueilli dans ces circonstances est comparable à la sécrétion déclenchée par l'injection d'histamine (UNGAR et coll., 1935). Enfin, l'histamine seule est capable de reproduire à la fois les trois phénomènes vasculaire, gastrique et musculaire, déclenchés par la stimulation des racines postérieures.

Par la suite, d'autres expériences permirent d'étendre ces constatations à d'autres contingents de fibres postéro-radiculaires. Ainsi, la stimulation du bout périphérique du splanchnique d'un chien perfuseur détermine une augmentation de la sécrétion gastrique chez le chien perfusé (UNGAR, CONTIADÈS et GROSSIORD, 1935). De même la stimulation du bout distal des racines postérieures de C_3 à C_7, ou du nerf phrénique dans sa partie cervicale, provoque une vasodilatation de la petite circulation objectivée par une baisse de pression dans l'artère pulmonaire (UNGAR et coll. 1936). Ces fibres libèrent donc une substance dont les propriétés pharmacologiques sont analogues à celles de l'histamine. UNGAR (1936) crée le terme d'«histaminergie» directement inspiré de la terminologie inaugurée par DALE (cholinergie et adrénergie).

Divers résultats expérimentaux devaient confirmer l'analogie pharmacologique qui existe entre l'histamine et le médiateur postéro-radiculaire.

1. KWIATKOWSKI (1943) étudie l'action du sang veineux fémoral du Chat sur l'iléon isolé de Cobaye. Les échantillons de sang total, recueilli une à quatre minutes après la stimulation des racines postérieures correspondant à la patte, possèdent une activité nettement supérieure à celle du sang recueilli avant ou pendant la

stimulation (fig. 4). Le principe actif de ces extraits provoque également une hypotension artérielle chez le Chat. Or ce principe actif peut être extrait suivant la technique que Barsoum et Gaddum ont décrite pour extraire l'histamine. Les équivalents d'histamine ainsi évalués par Kwiatkowski dans le sang *total* de la veine fémorale varient de 0,03 à 0,18 μg/ml. Ils sont nettement supérieurs à ceux du sang témoin (0,01 μg/ml).

Ibrahim et coll. (1951) rapportent des résultats semblables chez le Chien chloralosé: l'histaminémie du sang veineux total (0,021 μg/ml) s'élève après stimulation des racines postérieures pendant 10 minutes à 0,077 μg/ml (moyenne de deux expériences).

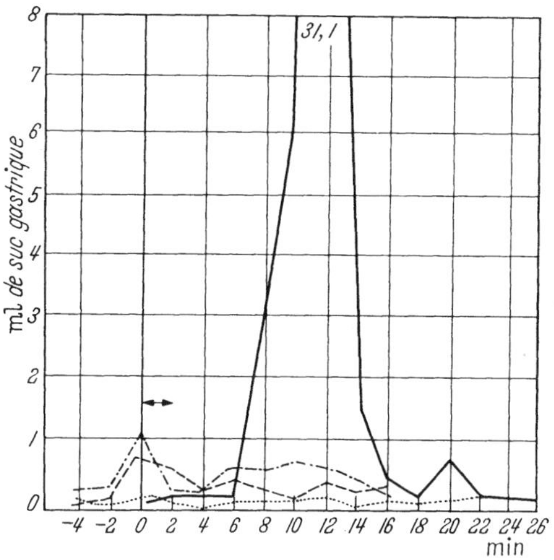

Fig. 3

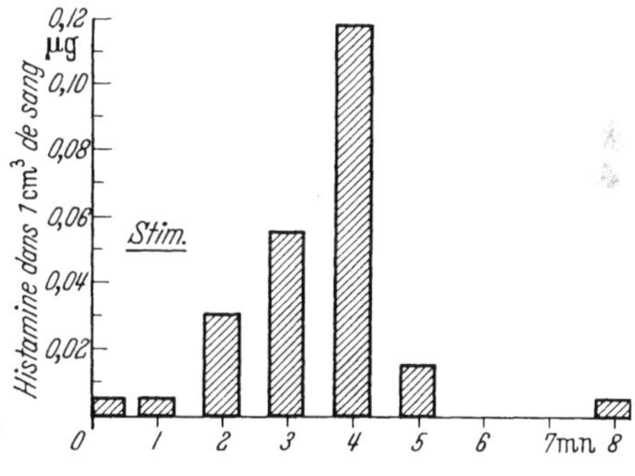

Fig. 4

Fig. 3. Modifications de la sécrétion gastrique par excitation des nerfs de la patte. En traits pleins, excitation du bout periphérique du nerf saphène interne; — — —, bout central du crural; — · — · —, bout périphérique de le branche motrice du crural; · · · · · bout périphérique du saphène interne, la veine fémorale étant comprimée pendant 10 minutes depuis le début de l'excitation (Ungar, 1936)

Fig. 4. Chat (2,3 kg) sous anesthésie au chloralose. Stimulation du bout périphérique sectionné des racines postérieures lombaires (5—7) pendant 1 mn. Les colonnes représentent l'équivalent histaminique du sang veineux évalué de minute en minute (Kwiatkowski, 1943)

Cependant la signification de tels résultats se prête à discussion: c'est dans le plasma qu'il faut rechercher, et que l'on trouve, en effet, le médiateur. De fait, la concentration de l'histamine *plasmatique* évaluée simultanément en deux occasions par Kwiatkowski est certes plus élevée que dans le sang témoin: 0,03 et 0,025 μg/ml dans le plasma de stimulation pour moins de 0,01 μg/ml dans le plasma témoin. Mais ces valeurs de l'histaminémie plasmatique ne rendent pas compte de l'hyperhistaminémie totale. C'est donc la fraction de l'histamine présente dans les éléments figurés qui assure la majeure partie de l'augmentation de l'histaminémie observée. Il est possible que la vasodilatation entraîne dans le sang veineux certains éléments particulièrement riches en histamine qui rendraient compte de l'hyperhistaminémie observée dans le sang total. Quant à la discrète élévation de l'histaminémie plasmatique, elle pourrait s'interpréter par la diffusion de l'histamine des éléments figurés dans le plasma. Telle est l'explication que proposent Parrot et Reuse (1954).

2. D'autre part, Kwiatkowski (1943) montre que la partie périphérique des nerfs sensitifs de la peau est particulièrement riche en une substance qui agit comme l'histamine: en effet des extraits de tissu nerveux, provenant de diverses espèces animales, font contracter l'iléon isolé de Cobaye et abaissent la pression artérielle chez le Chat chloralosé, en dépit de la présence d'atropine. En revanche,

les racines postérieures et le ganglion rachidien, les racines antérieures, les fibres motrices en contiennent peu.

Ainsi les fibres nerveuses auxquelles on attribue une action vasodilatatrice semblent caractérisées par leur richesse en une substance dont les propriétés pharmacologiques sont analogues à celles de l'histamine.

Une répartition préférentielle de l'histamine dans les nerfs périphériques fut également montrée par von Euler (1949) (fig. 5); mais selon cet auteur la distribution de l'histamine serait anatomiquement associée au système sympathique, comme la noradrénaline elle-même.

En résumé, la stimulation de fibres nerveuses postéro-radiculaires, soit directement par stimulation des racines postérieures, soit par agression cutanée détermine une vasodilatation qui a semblé analogue à celle qu'on observe après injection d'histamine.

Cette même stimulation déclenche des réactions à distance, notamment gastriques, que, seule parmi les substances étudiées, l'histamine paraissait capable de reproduire. A ce moment d'ailleurs le sang veineux s'est enrichi en une substance pharmacologiquement analogue à l'histamine.

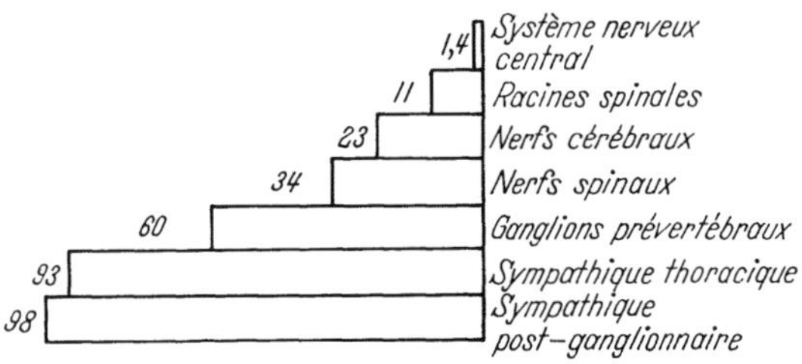

Fig. 5

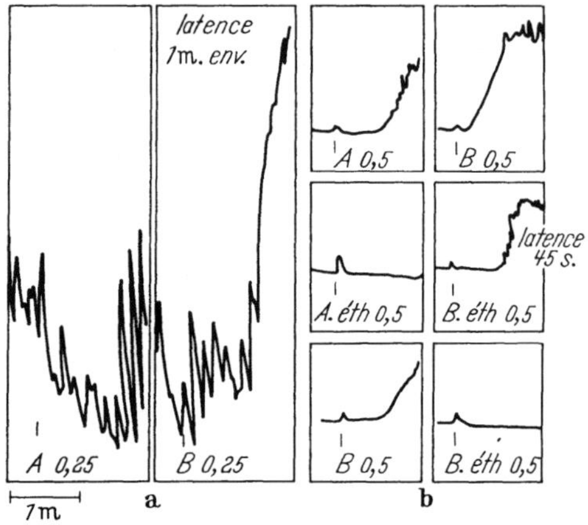

Fig. 6

Fig. 5. Répartition de l'histamine dans divers tissus nerveux (μg de dichlorhydrate d'histamine par g de tissu) (U. S. v. Euler, 1949)

Fig. 6. *a*) Contractions de l'intestin isolé du Chien sous l'influence de 0,25 cm³ de plasma du sang de la veine fémorale recueilli avant (A) et pendant (B) la stimulation faradique de la dernière racine postérieure lombaire chez le Chien. *b*) Contractions de l'intestin isolé du Cobaye: en haut sous l'influence de 0,5 cm³ de plasma du sang veineux fémoral recueilli avant (A) et pendant (B) la stimulation faradique de la dernière racine postérieure lombaire chez le Chien; au milieu, action des extraits éthérés correspondants; en bas, action du plasma de stimulation (B) et de son extrait éthéré (B. éth.) lorsque l'intestin est soumis à l'action du sulfate d'atropine (5×10^{-7}). (Ungar et Parrot, 1938)

IV. Différence entre le médiateur et l'histamine

a) On peut déjà remarquer que l'histamine ne reproduit pas tous les caractères de l'action vasculaire des fibres postéro-radiculaires: dans cette action nerveuse les artérioles augmentent de diamètre; or l'histamine fait contracter les artérioles par son action directe.

D'autre part, Holton et Perry (1951) devaient remarquer que la vasodilatation observée sur l'oreille du Lapin, après stimulation du nerf grand auriculaire, dure toujours beaucoup plus longtemps que la vasodilatation provoquée par l'injection intra-artérielle locale d'histamine. La même observation est formulée par Celander et Folkow (1953), à propos de la vasodilatation déclenchée sur la patte du Chat par stimulation des racines postérieures L 6, L 7 et S 1.

b) Une étude des propriétés pharmacologiques, physiques et chimiques du médiateur postéro-radiculaire ne permet pas d'identifier ce corps à l'histamine, comme le montrèrent Ungar et Parrot (1938, 1939) (fig. 6). Ces auteurs étudient la substance vasodilatatrice qui apparaît dans le sang veineux fémoral, chez le Chien chloralosé, après stimulation de la dernière racine postérieure lombaire et constatent les faits suivants. L'atropine (5×10^{-7}) s'oppose à l'action du médiateur sur l'intestin isolé de Cobaye, alors qu'elle n'empêche pas celle de l'histamine. D'autre part une dose d'histamine équivalente au médiateur sur l'iléon isolé de Cobaye se montre moins active que lui sur l'intestin de Chien. Le médiateur agit sur les organes isolés après un temps de latence prolongé, qui peut atteindre plusieurs dizaines de secondes, alors que l'action de l'histamine se manifeste presque immédiatement après son introduction dans le bain. Enfin, l'adsorption du médiateur sur la permutite, son passage dans l'éther et sa destruction par ébullition acide sont autant de propriétés qui le distinguent de l'histamine.

c) Les antagonistes de l'histamine permirent d'éprouver la nature de la substance vasodilatatrice libérée par les fibres postéro-radiculaires.

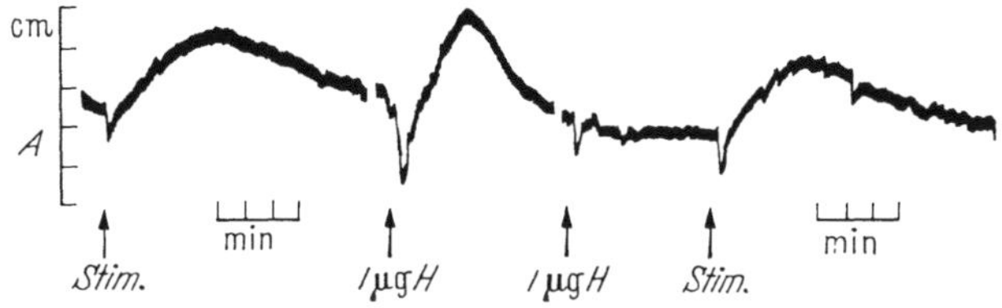

Fig. 7. Vaso-dilatation de l'oreille du Lapin. Enregistrement photoélectrique. Stim., stimulation centrifuge du grand nerf auriculaire (5 stimuli, 30 V, 1 msec à 1/sec). 1 μg H, injection intra-artérielle de 1 μg d'histamine. Entre les deux injections d'histamine, injection intraveineuse de néoantergan (2 mg/kg). On voit que l'antihistaminique supprime complètement l'action vaso-dilatatrice de l'histamine, sans modifier l'action nerveuse. (D'après Holton et Perry, 1951)

Parrot et Lefebvre (1943), essayèrent pour la première fois l'action d'un antihistaminique sur la vasodilatation d'origine nerveuse. Ils injectent par voie intra-veineuse chez le Chien chloralosé, du chlorhydrate de N-diméthyl-amino-éthyl-N-benzylaniline (Antergan) ou 2339 RP à la dose de 10 mg/kg et stimulent le bout périphérique de la première racine sacrée postérieure. Ils enregistrent toujours une vasodilatation de la patte cependant qu'une dose d'histamine, capable de produire une réaction vasculaire de même importance, devient inefficace.

Holton et Perry (1951) injectent par voie intra-veineuse chez le Lapin du N-diméthyl-amino-éthyl-N-p-méthoxybenzyl-α-amino-pyridine (Néoantergan) ou 2768 RP à la dose de 2 mg/kg. La vasodilatation de l'oreille provoquée avant le traitement par l'injection intra-artérielle locale d'histamine (0,1 mg) est abolie alors que la réponse à la stimulation du nerf grand auriculaire persiste (fig. 7).

Chez le Chien, Frumin, Ngai et Wang (1953) constatent que le débit artériel fémoral, mesuré par rotamètre, augmente en réponse à la stimulation centrifuge des racines postérieures même après l'injection intra-veineuse de N-benzyl-N-diméthyl-aminoéthyl-α-aminopyridine (Pyribenzamine) à la dose de 5 mg/kg.

Seuls, Ibrahim, Stella et Talaat (1951) ont observé une inhibition de la vasodilatation postéro-radiculaire par un antihistaminique. Ils mesurent le débit de la veine saphène, chez le Chien chloralosé, avant et après stimulation centrifuge des racines postérieures. L'accroissement de ce débit est moins important et moins prolongé sous l'influence d'un antihistaminique (antistine, néoantergan ou pyribenzamine) injecté par voie intraveneuse à la dose de 5 mg/kg. On remarquera cependant que le médiateur vasodilatateur est plus résistant à l'action des antihistaminiques qu'une forte dose d'histamine. En effet, dans la même expérience, l'effet vasodilatateur de 100 μg d'histamine, injecté à contre-courant dans une artère collatérale se trouve complètement supprimé.

D'une façon générale, il semble que les antihistaminiques, aux doses qui agissent sur l'action vasculaire de l'histamine, ne modifient pas la vasodilatation cutanée évoquée par la stimulation des racines postérieures, ou la modifient peu.

En conclusion, on peut affirmer que la substance vasodilatatrice libérée par la stimulation de certaines fibres nerveuses postéro-radiculaires n'est pas l'histamine, ou du moins qu'il ne s'agit pas de l'histamine seule.

V. Hypothèses sur la nature du médiateur postéro-radiculaire

A. UNGAR et PARROT (1939), ont constaté que l'adrénaline, mise *in vitro* en présence de certains tissus animaux, suscite une nouvelle activité qui se manifeste par une hypotension chez le Chat et le Chien, et par une contraction de l'intestin isolé de Cobaye. Or cette nouvelle activité, qui reproduit l'action «inverse» de l'adrénaline se montre pharmacologiquement semblable à l'activité de la substance libérée par stimulation des racines postérieures.

B. D'autre part, UNGAR, PARROT et GROSSIORD (1936) ont constaté que la stimulation de la corde du tympan ou du nerf lingual chez le Chien libère dans la salive sous-maxillaire une substance hypotensive qui stimule la sécrétion gastrique.

Ces auteurs ont envisagé que cette substance pourrait intervenir dans le mécanisme de la vasodilatation des glandes salivaires dont la nature cholinergique est contestable. Comme la vasodilatation postéro-radiculaire, l'hyperémie qui accompagne l'activité des glandes salivaires résiste en effet à l'atropine.

UNGAR et PARROT (1936) ont identifié cette substance à une enzyme protéolytique, la callicréine.

C. Qu'une enzyme protéolytique intervienne dans divers phénomènes de vasodilatation est une notion qui a reçu une extension considérable. En effet HILTON et LEWIS (1955a, b) ont établi que la vasodilatation fonctionnelle de la glande sous-maxillaire du Chat est due à un polypeptide vasodilatateur, la bradykinine. Ce polypeptide est formé sur place par un système enzymatique, libéré en quantités importantes par l'activité des glandes salivaires.

L'existence d'un système enzymatique analogue, aboutissant à la formation de polypeptides vasodilatateurs a été confirmée dans la peau (FOX et HILTON, 1958). C'est l'activité des glandes sudoripares qui conditionne la formation de ces substances vasodilatatrices. La bradykinine est probablement le polypeptide responsable de la vasodilatation secondaire à la sudation.

Qu'une série de réactions chimiques, aboutissant à la formation d'un polypeptide, explique la vasodilatation postéro-radiculaire, est une hypothèse qui a été formulée (HILTON, 1962). CHAPMAN et coll. (1961) ont mis en évidence l'apparition d'un polypeptide consécutive à une agression cutanée ou à la stimulation de racines postérieures chez l'Homme. Ce polypeptide serait spécifique et distinct pharmacologiquement des autres polypeptides connus (bradykinine, kallidine, ocytocine).

HELLAUER et UMRATH (1947) ont constaté l'existence dans des extraits de racines postérieures d'une substance analogue à la substance P. La concentration de ce polypeptide vasodilatateur dans les nerfs afférents diminue parallèlement avec leur dégénérescence après section, de même que l'acétylcholine disparaît des fibres cholinergiques au cours de leur dégénérescence.

D. D'autres substances vasodilatatrices ont été proposées. Si le rôle de l'acétylcholine, soutenu par DALE et GADDUM (1930) puis par WYBAUW (1938), paraît difficile à défendre, le rôle de l'ATP a été envisagé par HOLTON et HOLTON (1953). L'ATP est en effet présent dans les extraits de racines postérieures et de nerfs périphériques. HOLTON (1959) a montré que la concentration de cette substance augmente dans le perfusat d'une oreille de Lapin après stimulation du nerf grand auriculaire. Cependant l'ATP ne semble pas avoir la stabilité que l'on a reconnue au médiateur postéro-radiculaire qui, libéré dans un territoire périphérique, peut atteindre l'estomac et stimuler sa sécrétion. D'autre part, il paraît difficile d'admettre qu'un métabolite aussi banal et aussi répandu que l'ATP puisse jouer un rôle physiologique spécifique.

En somme, la nature du médiateur n'est pas établie, et, dans l'incertitude où nous sommes à son sujet, il n'est pas absolument exclu qu'il s'agisse d'une médiation mixte, par exemple histamine et acétylcholine, ou histamine et bradykinine.

VI. L'histamine comme stimulant nerveux

Il n'est pas établi que l'histamine soit la substance libérée par les fibres vasodilatatrices des racines postérieures. Cependant les anti-histaminiques abolissent la vasodilatation cutanée que déclenche une agression locale par phénomène axonique.

Parrot (1942) constate chez l'Homme que l'ingestion d'un antihistaminique (2339 RP) abolit l'érythème environnant provoqué par l'injection intracutanée d'une solution diluée de venin de Vipère. De même est supprimée pour quelques heures la vasodilatation périphérique provoquée par le frottement cutané chez les sujets prédisposés au dermographisme. Cette observation fut depuis lors maintes fois confirmée dans des conditions diverses: avec la pyribenzamine par Arbesman, Koepf et Miller (1946) dans le cas de la réaction anaphylactique locale de la peau, par Baer et Sulzberger (1946) sur l'urticaire factice, par Claman (1947) sur la rubéfaction provoquée par la Jacobée, avec la pyribenzamine et le bénadryl par Grob, Lilienthal et Harvey (1947) sur les réactions cutanées que déterminent le curare et la D-tubocurarine, avec le thénylène par Feinberg et Bernstein (1947) dans 7 cas de dermographisme sur 9, etc. Cependant l'injection intra-artérielle de maléate de mépyramine (2,5 mg/min pendant 8 min) n'a pas permis de modifier la vasodilatation du doigt consécutive à un refroidissement local (Whelan, 1956).

Chez le Chien, Cier et Froment (1954) constatent que divers antihistaminiques (antergan, néoantergan, phénergan) ralentissent la réaction vasodilatatrice consécutive au refroidissement de la patte: son réchauffement dure alors deux à trois fois plus longtemps que chez l'animal normal.

Or pour interpréter de tels résultats expérimentaux observés chez l'Homme ou chez le Chien, il faut se rappeler que dans l'une et l'autre espèce, les mêmes antihistaminiques paraissent incapables de diminuer la vasodilatation provoquée par la stimulation électrique des nerfs. Nous avons vu (voir IV c) que ce fait plaide contre le rôle de médiateur que l'on a voulu attribuer à l'histamine.

Une seule interprétation reste donc ici possible, c'est que l'histamine intervienne à l'origine même du phénomène axonique et qu'elle stimule les origines nerveuses (fig. 8).

Ainsi est-on ramené à la conception originelle de Lewis (1927) qui attribuait à l'histamine le rôle de stimulant des terminaisons nerveuses. Dans cette conception, réaffirmée par Parrot et Lefebvre (1943), l'histamine est non pas le médiateur des fibres vasodilatatrices des racines postérieures, mais bien l'agent stimulant qui est à l'origine du phénomène axonique.

Libérée par les tissus lors d'une agression cutanée, l'histamine agit localement de deux façons:

a) Par une action vasculaire directe: elle modifie le diamètre et la perméabilité des capillaires.

b) Par une action nerveuse: elle met en jeu un mécanisme axonique et détermine alentour une vasodilatation artériolaire.

En somme, cette conception suppose:

a) la libération d'histamine dans la peau lors d'une agression;

b) l'action de l'histamine sur certains nerfs de la peau.

a) Le premier terme est très généralement admis: rappelons, par exemple, que dès 1939 Rosenthal et Minard avaient prouvé la libération d'histamine par stimulation de la peau. Ces auteurs découpent des lambeaux lamellaires de peau humaine ou de différentes espèces animales. Ces fragments cutanés sont adaptés à l'extrémité d'un tube de façon que leur face profonde est baignée par la solution physiologique présente dans le tube. La face externe de la peau est stimulée par un courant électrique.

Il apparaît alors par diffusion dans la solution physiologique une substance qui possède les propriétés de l'histamine. Fait significatif, cette libération d'histamine a lieu même après des stimulations faibles qui ne provoquent pas de lésions cellulaires.

Cependant d'autres substances que l'histamine sont libérées par la peau lors d'une agression.

b) D'autre part, il semble que l'histamine est capable de stimuler certaines fibres nerveuses. Cela est suggéré par les sensations prurigineuses ou douloureuses évoquées par l'histamine.

Habgood (1950), isole deux lambeaux cutanés de Grenouille ayant conservé chacun leur innervation, et les dispose de façon que leurs surfaces internes soient contiguës; ou bien encore il isole un seul lambeau de peau innervé par plusieurs fibres nerveuses voisines. Cet auteur constate que la stimulation de l'un des nerfs favorise la mise en activité des fibres nerveuses voisines. Tantôt le seuil d'excitation du nerf non stimulé est abaissé, tantôt les nerfs non stimulés déchargent spontanément. Habgood attribue cette facilitation à la libération d'une substance par la stimulation électrique des filets nerveux, substance qui pourrait être l'histamine.

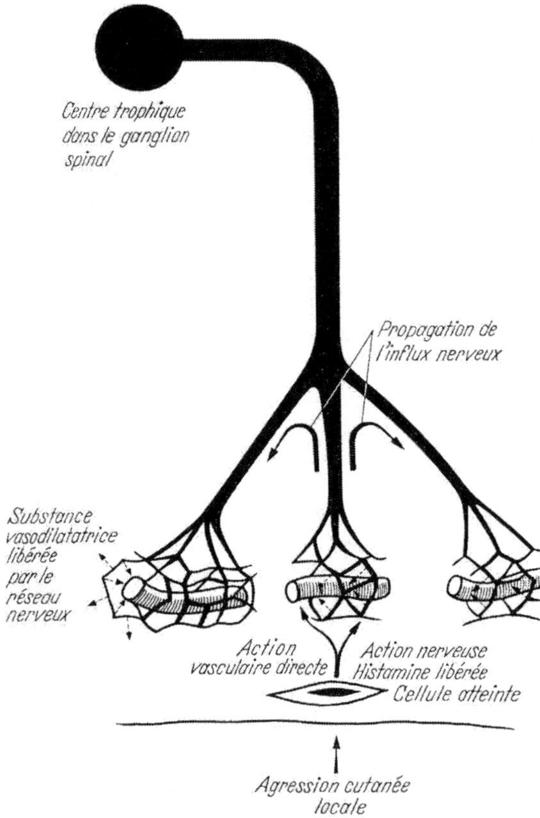

Fig. 8. Schéma du réflexe d'axone vaso-dilatateur. L'agression libère l'histamine d'une cellule cutanée. La substance exerce localement: *a*) une action vasculaire, *b*) une action nerveuse. Cette dernière action déclenche un réflexe d'axone. Les flèches en pointillé representent le médiateur libéré. Dans ce schéma, la fibre intéressée est considérée comme centrifuge et toutes ses extrémités sont équivalentes. (D'après Parrot, 1942)

Pour intégrer cette très intéressante constatation dans le cadre général des conceptions de Lewis que, dans l'ensemble, nous avons adoptées dans cet exposé, il faudrait admettre que l'histamine ne joue pas, au sens propre, le rôle de médiateur nerveux dans cette expérience, mais qu'elle est libérée des tissus à la suite de l'influx nerveux centrifuge.

FJÄLLBRANT et IGGO (1961) d'autre part, montrent que l'histamine, l'acétylcholine, la sérotonine, sont capables de déclencher des influx centripètes, dans les nerfs périphériques chez le Chat. Ils enregistrent l'activité électrique de fibres afférentes cutanèes en réponse à l'injection de ces substances dans le courant sanguin artériel. L'histamine, de même d'ailleurs que l'acétylcholine et la 5-hydroxytryptamine, augmente la fréquence de décharges de certaines fibres nerveuses, ou abaisse le seuil de sensibilité de certains récepteurs.

En réalité ce sont des récepteurs à adaptation lente, des mécanorécepteurs et des thermorécepteurs qui sont stimulés par l'injection intra-artérielle d'histamine; et dans ces mêmes conditions expérimentales, la mise en jeu de fibres lentes telles que les fibres postéro-radiculaires vasodilatatrices n'a pas été observée.

Conclusion

1. La stimulation centrifuge de certaines racines postérieures de la moelle chez l'animal donne lieu à une vasodilatation cutanée qui s'exerce grâce à un intermédiaire chimique relativement stable.

2. Des progrès importants dans la connaissance de ce corps ont pu être accomplis grâce à sa comparaison avec les propriétés pharmacologiques de l'histamine. Le médiateur donne lieu, comme l'histamine à deux réactions caractéristiques: la triple réaction cutanée (LEWIS) chez l'Homme, et la stimulation de la sécrétion gastrique chez le Chien atropinisé (UNGAR).

3. Cependant ses propriétés chimiques et physiques ne permettent pas d'identifier ce médiateur à l'histamine elle-même. Si l'intervention de l'histamine n'est peut-être pas définitivement exclue, on peut affirmer du moins qu'une autre substance à côté d'elle joue un rôle important. Diverses recherches ont attiré l'attention soit sur l'acétylcholine, soit sur une substance qui serait en relation chimique ou fonctionnelle avec l'adrénaline, soit sur un polypeptide vasodilatateur, soit sur la substance P, soit sur l'ATP. En dépit de ces divers travaux la nature du médiateur reste inconnue.

4. L'histamine intervient dans la vasodilatation postéro-radiculaire d'une tout autre manière: il semble bien que, libérée par l'agression cutanée, elle soit capable de stimuler les terminaisons nerveuses et de mettre ainsi en jeu le phénomène axonique vasodilatateur. C'est l'emploi des antihistaminiques chez l'Homme et chez le Chien qui permet de remettre en honneur cette conception, conforme d'ailleurs à celle de LEWIS. L'électrophysiologie montre que l'histamine peut, en agissant à la périphérie, activer certaines fibres nerveuses; cette méthode n'a pas permis cependant jusqu'ici de reconnaître l'activation des fibres postéro-radiculaires vasodilatatrices dont les potentiels d'action doivent être faibles et lents.

Bibliographie

ARBESMAN, C. E., G. F. KOEPF, and G. E. MILLER: Some antianaphylactic and antihistaminic properties of N'-pyridyl-N'-benzyl-dimethylethylene-diamine monohydrochloride (pyribenzamine). J. Allergy **17**, 203—209 (1946).

BAER, R. L., and M. B. SULZBERGER (1946): Cité d'après HALEY (1948).

BAYLISS, W. M.: On the origin from the spinal cord of the vasodilator fibres of the hind-limb, and on the nature of these fibres. J. Physiol. (Lond.) **27**, 173—209 (1900—1901).

CAPON, A.: Analyse des réactions vasodilatatrices de l'oreille du Lapin. Arch. int. Physiol. **65**, 515—546 (1957).

CELANDER, O., and B. FOLKOW: The correlation between the stimulation frequency and the dilator response evoked by "antidromic" excitation of the thin afferent fibres in the dorsal roots. Acta physiol. scand. **29**, 371—376 (1953).

CHAPMAN, L. F., A. O. RAMOS, H. GOODELL, and H. G. WOLFF: Neuro-humoral features of afferent fibres in man. Arch. Neurol. (Chic.) **4**, 617—650 (1961).

CIER, J. F., et O. FROMENT: Arguments pharmacodynamiques en faveur de la nature histaminergique de la réaction vasodilatatrice de réchauffement de la patte chez le Chien. J. Physiol. (Paris) **46**, 300—302 (1954).
CLAMAN, (1947): Cité d'après HALEY (1948).
DALE, H. H., and J. H. GADDUM: Reactions of denervated voluntary muscle, and their bearing on the mode of action on parasympathetic and related nerves. J. Physiol. (Lond.) **70**, 109—144 (1930).
VON EULER, U. S.: Histamine as a specific constituent of certain autonomic nerve fibres. Acta physiol. scand. **19**, 85—93 (1949).
FEINBERG, S. M., et T. B. BERSTEIN (1947): Cité d'après HALEY (1948).
FJÄLLBRANT, N., and A. IGGO: The effect of histamine, 5-hydroxytryptamine and acetylcholine on cutaneous afferent fibres. J. Physiol. (Lond.) **156**, 578—590 (1961).
FOX, R. H., and S. M. HILTON: Bradykinin formation in human skin as a factor in heat vasodilatation. J. Physiol. (Lond.) **142**, 219—232 (1958).
FRUMIN, M. J., S. H. NGAI, and S. C. WANG: Evaluation of vasodilator mechanisms in the canin hind leg; question of dorsal root participation. Amer. J. Physiol. **173**, 428—436 (1953).
GÄRTNER, G.: Über den Verlauf der Vasodilatatoren. Wien. klin. Wschr. **1889**, 908.
GROB, D., J. L. LILIENTHAL, and A. M. HARVEY: On certain vascular effects of curare in man; "histamine" reaction. Bull. Johns Hopk. Hosp. **80**, 299—322 (1947).
HABGOOD, J. S.: Sensitization of sensory receptors in the frog's skin. J. Physiol. (Lond.) **111**, 195 (1950).
HALEY, T. J.: The antihistaminic drugs, a review of the literature. J. Amer. Pharm. Ass. **37**, 383—408 (1948).
HELLAUER, H., and K. UMRATH: The transmitter substance of sensory nerve fibres. J. Physiol. (Lond.) **106**, 20P (1947).
HILTON, S. M.: Local mechanisms regulating peripheral blood flow. Physiol. Rev. **42**, Suppl. N° 5, 265—275 (1962).
—, and G. P. LEWIS: Mechanism of the functional hyperemia in the submandibular salivary gland. J. Physiol. (Lond.) **129**, 253—271 (1955a).
— — Cause of the vasodilatation accompanying activity in the submandibular salivary gland. J. Physiol. (Lond.) **128**, 235—248 (1955b).
HOLTON, F. A., and P. HOLTON: The possibility that ATP is a transmitter at sensory nerve endings. J. Physiol. (Lond.) **119**, 50P (1953).
HOLTON, P.: The liberation of adenosine triphosphate on antidromic stimulation of sensory nerves. J. Physiol. (Lond.) **145**, 494—504 (1959).
—, and W. L. M. PERRY: On the transmitter responsible for antidromic vasodilatation in the rabbit's ear. J. Physiol. (Lond.) **114**, 240—251 (1951).
IBRAHIM, F. D., G. STELLA, and M. TALAAT: The mechanism of antidromic vasodilatation. Quart. J. exp. Physiol. **36**, 189—198 (1951).
KWIATKOWSKI, H.: Histamine in nervous tissue. J. Physiol. (Lond.) **102**, 32—41 (1943).
LEWIS, TH: The blood vessels of the human skin and their responses. London: Show & Sons 1927.
—, and R. T. GRANT: Vascular reactions of the skin to injury. Part. II. The liberation of a histamine-like substance in injured skin: the underlying cause of factitious urticaria and of wheals produced by burning, and observations upon the nervous control of certain skin reactions. Heart **11**, 209—265 (1924).
—, and I. M. HARMER: Vascular reactions of the skin to injury. Part. IX. Further evidence of the release of a histamine-like substance from the injured skin. Heart **14**, 19—26 (1927).
—, and H. M. MARVIN: Observations relating to vasodilatation arising from antidromic impulses, to herpes zoster and trophic effects. Heart **14**, 27—47 (1927).
MORAT, J. P.: Les fonctions vasodilatatrices des racines postérieures. Arch. Physiol. **4**, 688 à 698 (1892).
PARROT, J.-L.: Les modifications apportées par un antagoniste de l'histamine (2339 R.P.) à la réaction vasculaire locale de la peau. C. R. Soc. Biol. (Paris) **136**, 715 (1942).
—, et J. LEFEBVRE: Analyse de la triple réaction cutanée au moyen d'un antagoniste de l'histamine. C. R. Soc. Biol. (Paris) **137**, 316 (1943).
—, et J. REUSE: Rôle physiologique et physiopathologique de l'histamine. J. Physiol. (Paris) **46**, 99—221 (1954).
POPIELSKI, L.: β-Imidazoläthylamin und Organextrakte. Imidazolyläthylamin als mächtigen Erreger der Magendrüsen. Pflügers Arch. ges. Physiol. **178**, 214—236 (1920).
ROSENTHAL, S. R., and D. MINARD: Experiments on histamine as the chemical mediator for cutaneous pain. J. exp. Med. **70**, 415—425 (1939).
STRICKER, S.: Untersuchungen über die Gefäßnervenwurzeln des Ischiadicus. S.-B. Akad. Wiss. Wien **74** (6), 173 (1876).

TINEL, J., et G. UNGAR: Vasodilatation et libération locale de substances histaminiques. C. R. Soc. Biol. (Paris) **118**, 1148 (1935).

UNGAR, G.: Effet de l'excitation du bout périphérique des nerfs sensitifs sur la sécrétion gastrique. Transmission neuro-humorale histaminique. C. R. Soc. Biol. (Paris) **118**, 620 (1935).

— Démonstration de la mise en liberté de substances histaminiques. Transmission neuro-humorale histaminergique. J. Physiol. Path. gén. **34**, 77—91 (1936).

— X. J. CONTIADÈS et A. GROSSIORD: Libération de substances histaminiques, par excitation du bout périphérique du nerf splanchnique. Lésions hémorragiques de l'intestin par injection intra-artérielle d'histamine. C. R. Soc. Biol. (Paris) **120**, 328 (1935).

— A. GROSSIORD, J. BRINCOURT et J-L. PARROT: Sur l'origine, le trajet et la nature des fibres vasomotrices pulmonaires contenues dans la portion cervicale du nerf phrénique. C. R. Soc. Biol. (Paris) **121**, 115 (1936).

—, et J.-L. PARROT: Sur la présence de callicréine dans la salive et la possibilité de son intervention dans la transmission chimique de l'influx nerveux. C. R. Soc. Biol. (Paris) **122**, 1052 (1936).

— — Sur la nature de la substance libérée au cours de la vasodilatation dite antidromique. C. R. Soc. Biol. (Paris) **129**, 753 (1938).

— — Sur les rapports entre la substance libérée au cours de la vasodilatation antidromique et le corps hypotenseur produit par la transformation enzymatique de l'adrénaline. C. R. Soc. Biol. (Paris) **131**, 1165 (1939).

— — et A. GROSSIORD: Stimulation de la sécrétion gastrique par excitation du bout périphérique du nerf lingual. Passage d'une substance active dans la salive. C. R. Soc. Biol. (Paris) **121**, 1077 (1936).

— M. R. ZERLING et A. POCOULÉ: Sur la nature histaminique de la substance libérée par l'excitation antidromique des nerfs sensitifs. C. R. Soc. Biol. (Paris) **118**, 778 (1935).

WERZILOFF, N. M.: Zur Frage über die vasomotorische Funktion der hinteren Wurzeln. Zbl. Physiol. **10**, 194—198 (1896).

WHELAN, R. F.: Histamine and vasodilatation. In: Ciba Foundation Symposium on Histamine, p. 229. London: Churchill Ltd. 1956.

WYBAUW, L.: Contribution à l'étude du rôle vaso-moteur et trophique des nerfs sensitifs. Arch. int. Physiol. **46**, 293—344 (1938).

Section B

Physiological Significance of the Effect of Histamine on Gastric Secretion

By

A. C. Ivy and W. H. Bachrach

With 8 Figures

I. Introduction

Histamine stimulates the gastric secretion of acid and in blood concentrations below the threshold for other physiological responses. Furthermore, histamine is especially concentrated in the gastric and intestinal mucosa. The gastric mucosa of man and carnivora is devoid of the enzyme, histaminase, which inactivates histamine. The gastric juice contains histamine, the amount apparently being proportional to the output of HCl. These four observations, generally considered to be well-established, render it logical to investigate the theory that the release of histamine by the gastric mucosa might be the or a physiological, circulating or local hormone involved in the gastric secretion of HCl.

A historical survey of the subject will first be presented because it will provide a general orientation to facilitate a more rapid comprehension of the meaning of the various experiments performed to elucidate this intriguing but complicated subject.

In 1920 Popielski published the observation that histamine stimulates gastric secretion. At the same time Keeton, Luckhardt and Koch (1920) had made the same discovery. As the result of an extensive series of experiments, the latter investigators suggested that histamine may be the final mediator concerned in the stimulation of acid secretion, regardless of the nature of the initial excitatory stimulus (nervous, mechanical, or chemical).

In 1925, Ivy and Farrell transplanted a pouch of the corporic or acid secreting mucosa subcutaneously in dogs and it was found that the transplanted pouch secreted after a meal was ingested. This proved unequivocally that on feeding some agent passed into the blood and stimulated gastric secretion. The nature of the agent remained to be determined. In 1930 Best and McHenry discovered an enzyme, histaminase, with the property of destroying histamine. This enzyme, however, was not in the gastric mucosa. In the same year, Sacks, Ivy, Burgess and Vandolah (1932 a, b; see Ivy, 1930) isolated histamine in crystalline form from the pyloric mucosa of hogs. They found that the ratio of vasodepressor to gastric secretory units remained approximately the same in all fractions up to and including the final step of crystallization. Furthermore, the active principle was destroyed by histaminase. This was confirmed by Gavin, McHenry and Wilson (1933). Sacks et al. (1932 b) concluded that histamine was the only active secretory agent in the acid extracts made by them and others at that period, and that "histamine may be the gastric hormone." They did not conclude that it was the hormone because the evidence did not permit such a conclusion. They also indicated that perhaps "the gastric hormone has never been extracted from pyloric mucosa." MacIntosh (1938), using the method of Code (1937) for extracting histamine from tissues, found histamine in gastric juice. In 1944 and again in 1950, Babkin summarized the evidence in support of the view (Keeton et al., 1920) that, although it could not be concluded at that time that histamine is a gastric hormone, it is very likely that histamine is the agent which serves as the common stimulator of the parietal cell, regardless of the source of the initial stimulus. In 1956, Code interpreted the evidence then available as establishing that histamine is the final common stimulator of the parietal cells.

In 1938 Komarov made an extract of the pyloric mucosa and found that it contained a gastric secretory excitant in what is usually called the polypeptide fraction of tissue extracts. This new agent will be referred to as "non-histamine gastrin" or Komarov's "gastrin". Komarov injected the extract slowly intravenously, as is done in the case of secretin and cholecystokinin and the other gastrointestinal hormones. The extract had no, or only a little, effect on blood pressure. This observation was confirmed by Uvnäs (1942a, 1944). Bauer and Uvnäs (1944) reported that *histaminase did not destroy the gastric secretory excitant* in their extract made from the pyloric mucosa; that is a very interesting and important observation. In 1950, Roberts and Adam developed a chemical method for separating acetyl or conjugated histamine from "free" histamine in the urine. This rendered it possible to study the excretion of "free" and conjugated histamine in the urine. Unfortunately the method yielded only a recovery of 67% of added histamine. It yielded consistent comparative data, however. In 1957, Adam et al. published a method for the extraction of histamine from blood plasma. Though it yields consistent data, it may not be sensitive enough to detect in blood plasma the very small concentrations of histamine and some of its analogues which stimulate the parietal cells to secrete HCl.

In 1956, Lin et al. and Ivy et al. found that antihistaminase compounds, such as aminoguanidine, augment and stimulate gastric secretion under basal conditions, or after stimulation by a submaximal dose of histamine or a submaximal meal containing *no* histamine. Schayer and Ivy (1957, 1958) and Ivy (1958b, c) by using C^{14}-L-histidine in rats and one dog, found that C^{14}-histamine excretion in the urine increased after a meal, and that the C^{14}-histamine in the gastric and intestinal mucosa diminished approximately to the same extent. This circumstantially proved, in the rat and one dog, that histamine or a very closely related substance is or can serve as a gastric secretory hormone.

So, in the following discussion it must be kept in mind either (a) that histamine may be a gastric hormone in the sense that it is released by the gastric and/or intestinal mucosa into the blood which carries it to the parietal cells, or (b) that it is only a local tissue hormone and is released only in close proximity to or inside the parietal cells in the acid secreting mucosa. Its release locally as a stimulator, may occur either at the end of post-ganglionic nerve endings of the vagus or of the Meissner's plexus, or as the result of the release of a "hormone" or a substance by the pyloric or gastric mucosa into the blood, to act in turn by releasing histamine from cells located in proximity to or inside of the parietal cells. These concepts must be distinguished from Komarov's "gastrin" – *a non-histamine or histamine-like hormone* – one not destroyed by histaminase – which is produced and presumed to be released by the pyloric mucosa into the blood, to act directly on the parietal cells or perhaps to release histamine inside of or in the region of the parietal cells.

Table 1

I	IIA	IIB	IIIA	IIIB
Histamine is the hormone gastrin	Histamine is the final stimulator of parietal cell released only in or in region of parietal cell		Non-histamine "gastrin" is the hormone gastrin	
Histamine released by pyloric mucosa on appropriate stimulation	Histamine released by post-gang. nerve endings instead of acetylcholine, or nerve endings of Meissner's plexus	Post-gang. cholinergic nerve endings release ACh which acts on histamine containing cells located near parietal cells to release histamine	Non-histamine "gastrin" released by pyloric mucosa on appropriate stimulation	Non-histamine "gastrin" released by pyloric mucosa on appropriate stimulation
In blood	Enters blood when produced in excess Enters juice when cell secretes		In blood	In blood
		ACh enters parietal cell to release histamine which stimulates secretion and enters juice	Acts on histamine containing cells located near parietal cells which release histamine	Acts on parietal cell to release histamine which stimulates secretion and enters juice
Histamine acts on parietal cells	Histamine acts on parietal cells	Histamine acts on parietal cells	Histamine acts on parietal cells	
Histamine is inactivated by histaminase				Not inactivated by histaminase
Anti-histaminase compounds would augment response to stimuli or would stimulate basal secretion, if histamine is being produced slowly in the gastric mucosa or elsewhere during digestion or fasting. The action would be additive — histamine plus histamine —; it would not be synergistic or potentiating in type				Anti-histaminase compounds would augment secretion due to a synergistic or additive action due to histamine accumulation
Anti-histaminase compounds, such as aminoguanidine, which have been studied most, augment the response to a meal in the dog. The only statistically reliable evidence shows that the response is additive in type; it is not synergistic or potentiating in type				
Since we are dealing with three substances, namely, histamine, acetylcholine, and Komarov's "gastrin", the possibility that all three mechanisms are involved in the secretory response to a meal has to be considered.				

The outline in Table 1 and Figure 1 has been prepared as a guide for the reader who is not already familiar with the complicated literature on this subject.

The literature has been reviewed at different stages by IVY (1930), BABKIN (1950), GROSSMAN (1950), FELDBERG (1954), PARROTT and REUSE (1954), CODE (1956), and IVY (1958c).

"Gastrin" historically refers to the gastric secretory excitatory substance in acid extracts of the pyloric mucosa, which is assumed to be released into the blood on appropriate stimulation and carried to the parietal cells causing them to secrete HCl. *Gastrin* when not in quotes will be used to refer to the physiological hormone postulated by EDKINS in 1905 and unequivocally demonstrated to exist by the secretion of a transplanted pouch in 1925 by IVY and FARRELL and by the secretion of a transplanted pouch when a pyloric pouch was distended with a balloon in 1948 by GROSSMAN, ROBERTSON and IVY, without any reference to what its chemistry may be. "*Gastrin*" used in quotes will refer to any agent derived from tissue extracts which stimulates the secretion of HCl by the stomach, when given parenterally.

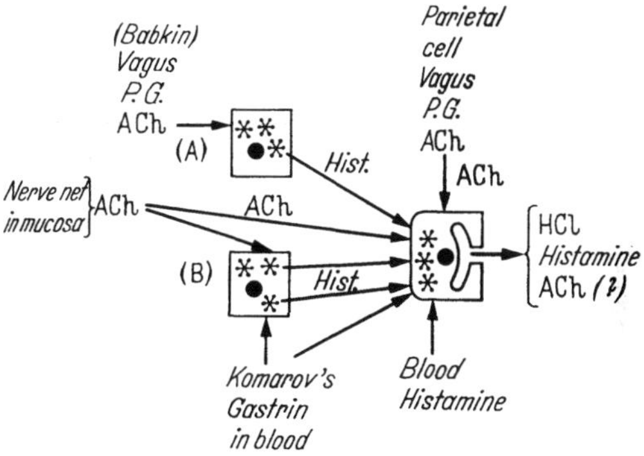

Fig. 1. Possible modes of action of a circulating or a local hormone in the acid secreting corporic mucosa. * Histamine; P.G., postganglionic fiber of vagus; ACh, acetylcholine. (A) and (B), cells which release histamine in response to ACh or KOMAROV's "gastrin". The possibility that the postganglionic nerve endings of the vagus release histamine has no evidence in its support, and is not illustrated. See also KAHLSON: Brit. med. J. **1948 II**, 1091; HEINZ and ÖBRINK Physiol. Rev. **34**, 643 (1954); HAKKINEN: Acta physiol. scand. **51**, Suppl. 177 (1960)

The acid secreting mucosa will be referred to as the corporic or fundic mucosa. The slightly alkaline secreting mucosa will be referred to as the pyloric mucosa, or pyloric portion of the stomach in contradistinction to the corporic part. The corporic glandular area could be referred to as the CGA and the pyloric as the PGA. In the rat, the secretory mucosa is referred to as the glandular stomach which includes CGA and PGA, but not the squamous stomach or rumen.

II. Historical background

Prior to the discovery of the hormone secretin by BAYLISS and STARLING, in 1902, it was believed that the secretion of acid by the gastric glands was stimulated via long reflexes through the cerebro-spinal nervous system, excited by conditioned reflexes or by the chemical action of secretagogues on the stomach or intestinal mucosa. When it was found that these nervous pathways could be dispensed with by the section of all extrinsic nerves, it was suggested that the application of meat extract to the gastric or pyloric mucosa stimulated secretion through a local reflex mechanism. This latter view was emphasized by POPIELSKI, in 1902, when he found that the application of a meat extract to the stomach would stimulate acid secretion, whereas its intravenous injection would not.

In 1905, the effect of the discovery of the hormone *secretin* by BAYLISS and STARLING on the subject of gastric secretion became apparent. EDKINS (1905, 1906) made extracts of the cardiac and pyloric mucosa of hogs, using aqueous solutions of dextrin, dextrose, peptone and 0.4% HCl. The extracts were administered intravenously to an anesthetized cat. He observed that extracts made from the pyloric and cardiac mucosa stimulated the secretion of acid, whereas an extract of the corporic or acid secreting mucosa did not. He called the active principle of these extracts "gastric secretin", or "*gastrin*".

During the same year of EDKIN's report, 1906, GROSS in PAVLOV's laboratory using a multiple pouch dog obtained results which suggested that a hormone was released into the blood when meat extract was applied to the pyloric mucosa. In 1909, EDKINS and TWEEDY performed a physiological experiment on cats similar to that of GROSS and obtained the same results as GROSS. However, ORBELI (1906) in PAVLOV's laboratory performed experiments which caused him to conclude that part of the pyloric secretagogue effect of meat extract was due to local nervous connections. POPIELSKI (1909–1913), then found that tissue extracts from widely varying sources contained a blood pressure reducing substance (or substances) which would stimulate gastric secretion on parenteral administration. This caused him and others (IVY, 1930) to conclude that the secretory activity in the extracts made by EDKINS was due to the presence in them of a vasodilatin and not of a specific hormone. He, for example, suggested that the reason for EDKIN's failure to obtain a stimulation of gastric secretion with his extract of fundic or acid secreting mucosa was probably due to a marked reduction of blood pressure from a too large dose of the extract, since the stomach would not secrete if the blood pressure is too low.

KOCH et al. (1920) in the last of a series of five important publications pointed out that on the basis of physiological studies and the use of tissue extracts the investigators at that period were divided into two schools. "One school considers pancreatic secretin on the one hand and 'gastrin' on the other to be different chemical substances and to act as distinctly specific hormones. The other school considers the substances to be identical, that they are widely distributed 'vasodilatins', and that they do not act as specific secretagogues or hormones".

These two schools persisted until 1925 when it was shown by IVY and FARRELL (1925) that an autotransplanted pouch of the stomach and an autotransplanted tail of the pancreas would respond to the ingestion of a meal (FARRELL and IVY, 1926). This physiologically proved the existence of a humoral mechanism for gastric and pancreatic secretion, but did not disclose the chemical nature of the humoral agents.

The view that secretin was histamine or some form of a generally distributed vasodilatin, was disproven first by PARSONS (1925) who showed by chemical analysis that histamine was not the vasodilator agent in the secretin preparation she studied, and by VOLBORTH (1925), by MELLANBY (1926), and by WEAVER, et al. (1926), all of whom made vasodilatin free or almost free preparations of secretin.

The views that the circulating humoral agent may be histamine, or that, "gastrin" and histamine may be identical, or that histamine can be released by the pyloric mucosa and serve as a hormone, or that histamine is a local hormone located in the corporic mucosa or acid secreting mucosa and is released by ACh from nerve endings or cells which contain histamine, have been supported by an accumulation of strongly presumptive but not categorical evidence.

III. Histamine as a possible gastric hormone

If histamine is the chemical agent for gastric secretion, it is appropriate to investigate the status of histamine in the gastric mucosa, the blood, the gastric juice, and the urine in relation to gastric secretory activity.

A. Histamine is present in the gastric mucosa

1. The proof of its presence there

BARGER and DALE, in 1911, isolated histamine in crystalline form from an extract of the intestinal mucosa containing *secretin*. They suggested that *secretin* and histamine were identical. This view, at the time, was plausible especially since histamine was known to stimulate pancreatic secretion, but we now know it is not a very potent stimulant of pancreatic secretion. DALE and LAIDLAW (1910–11) compared the "tissue vasodilatins" of POPIELSKI with histamine and concluded that they were identical. In 1912 POPIELSKI started a study of histamine and reported that, when given intravenously in a relatively large dose, a stimulation of acid secretion did not result. (See G. MODRAKOWSKI 1912). In 1915, KEETON and KOCH made acid extracts of many tissues and of the various portions of the gastric mucosa. The potency of these extracts, when given subcutaneously to gastric pouch dogs, varied considerably. They found that "gastrin" was present in acid extracts of the different parts of the gastric mucosa, there being more there than in the duodenal mucosa, and perhaps more in the fundic than the pyloric mucosa. They suggested that "gastrin", the active secretory principle in the gastric mucosa, was a specific substance and did not act as the result of an ordinary vasodepressor or vasodilatin. Their extracts caused vasodilation when given intravenously at a relatively rapid rate, but not when given subcutaneously after which the secretion of acid was started in ten minutes and continued for an hour or more. Later they found that histamine acted similarly. In 1919, ABEL and KUBOTA obtained crystalline histamine in a large yield from the combined gastric and intestinal mucosa of a dog. In 1920, KEETON *et al.* (1920a,b) found that histamine given subcutaneously stimulated gastric secretion in a large variety of laboratory animals (dog, cat, rabbit, guinea pig, duck, frog). In 1920, POPIELSKI had likewise found that histamine stimulates acid production in the vagotomized dog, which KEETON et al. (1920a,b) had found. He reported that it stimulated acid production in a human subject, namely, his assistant Dr. W. KOSKOWSKI. In the same year ROTHLIN and GUNDLACH (1921) as a result of their study of the effect of histamine on gastric secretion concluded that histamine and "gastrin" were identical. In 1922, CARNOT et al. found that histamine was an excellent stimulus of gastric acid production in man. This was followed by a more extensive study on man by MATHESON and AMMON (1923).

In 1920, KEETON et al. (1920b) after finding that only large, toxic doses of atropine would block the secretory response to "gastrin" or histamine, *suggested that if either of the two is physiologically important, it would appear to be liberated by secretory nerves and then become the exciting agent of the cell to acid secretion.* These investigators, (KEETON at al., 1920a, b; KOCH et al., 1920–1921) in the same year reported a series of physiological and chemical studies in which they compared some of the chemical properties of "gastrin" (gastric secretory excitant in acid extracts of gastric mucosa) with those of histamine. They found a striking similarity between histamine and "gastrin", both being basic imidazole derivatives extractable by amyl alcohol from aqueous solutions containing the free base. The only difference found between them was that the "gastrin" solution obtained from amyl alcohol extraction did not yield a physiologically active picrolonate or picrate, as it did when some histamine was added to it. They found that "gastrin" was inactivated when a dry alkaline mixture of crude "gastrin" was extracted continuously with amyl alcohol by the Soxhlet method. They wrote, however, that histamine and gastrin "may later be found to be identical or closely related."

In 1932, Sacks, Ivy, Burgess and Vandolah confirmed the chemical observations of Koch et al. However, they found that chloroform will not extract "gastrin" from aqueous solutions like amyl alcohol, but will do so when the concentrated aqueous "gastrin" solution is mixed with anhydrous sodium carbonate and the dry powder extracted in a Soxhlet apparatus with chloroform for 24 to 48 hours (chloroform boils at 61° C and amyl alcohol at 135° C). As the result of this procedure they, for the first time, obtained histamine from the pyloric mucosa of hogs in pure crystalline form. Furthermore, they found that the ratio of the vasodepressor and the intensity of the Pauly reaction for histamine to the gastric secretory units in the fractions of the extraction process remained essentially the same. Also, histaminase destroyed the secretory activity. They concluded that "histamine is the sole gastric secretory excitant in dilute acid extracts of pyloric mucosa (as usually prepared), and that histamine may be the gastric hormone. It has not been proved that histamine is the gastric hormone, ..." They also indicated that if histamine is not the active humoral or hormonal secretory principle in gastric mucosa, then the true "gastric hormone" had never been extracted from gastric mucosa because of the current practice of starting the extraction process with dilute aqueous HCl solution[1]. The observations of Sacks et al. (1932) were confirmed by Gavin et al. (1933). They used the methods of Best and McHenry for making their extracts, and a gastric fistula dog for their secretory assay. Incubation of the active extracts with histaminase destroyed the depressor and secretory activity of their extract.

2. The concentration of histamine in the gastric mucosa

It is of theoretical interest to consider the question of the quantity of histamine or "gastrin" in the gastric mucosa. Keeton and Koch (1915) found one secretory dose in 4 or 5 grams of pyloric mucosa of the hog in their crude preparation. One of us (A.C.I.) using their method obtained the same yield. The yield of Sacks et al. (1932) for their crude extract (the eluate of the hydrous aluminium silicate) was a secretory dose in 4 or 5 gm of hog's pyloric mucosa, which was roughly equivalent to 0.4 or 0.5 mg of histamine dihydrochloride or 0.25 to 0.3 mg of the base in dogs weighing 10 to 15 kg. The average yield of histamine obtained from the pyloric mucosa of the dog by several groups of investigators, shown in Table 2, was 61 μg per gram of wet tissue. This would amount to 0.244 mg of the base in 4 grams of mucosa, which is not a bad check for the two methods of approach. (See Appendix for methods of extraction of gastric mucosa for "gastrin".) Trach et al. (1944) found enough histamine by biological assay in 5 gms of *human* gastric mucosa, to stimulate acid production in a Heidenhain pouch dog. They concluded that enough "histamine activity to allow local and humoral stimulation of gastric secretion" was present in human gastric mucosa. Table 2.

3. The concentration of histamine in different anatomical parts of the gastric mucosa

Using the gastric secretory test for determining the concentration of histamine or "gastrin" in the gastric mucosa, Keeton and Koch (1915) found slightly more in the fundic or acid secreting mucosa, than in the mucosa of the pyloric portion which in turn contained slightly more than the cardiac portion. Later the same group (Luckhardt et al., 1919—1920) found about the same amount of "gastrin"

[1] Unless the pepsin in the mucosa, for example, had been inactivated by heat before the mucosa was placed in 0.4% HCl solution, the pepsin might have destroyed the true "gastric" hormone".

in the different parts of the gastric mucosa and about the same in duodenal mucosa.

In Table 2 it will be observed that, on the average, the acid secreting mucosa contains about 40 % more histamine than the pyloric. The data (DOUGLAS et al.,

Table 2. *Histamine in gastric mucosa (fresh or wet tissue); estimation by biological methods*

Animal	Average Micrograms of base/gm of mucosa of fundus	pylorus	Author	Year
Dog (fasting)	69	39	GAVIN et al.	1933
Dog (fed)	92	63	GAVIN et al.	1933
Dog (fasting)	84	40	EMMELIN and KAHLSON	1944
Dog (fasting)	87 (*1*)	51 (*1*)	DOUGLAS et al.	1951
Dog (fasting)	90	46	FELDBERG and HARRIS	1953
Dog (fasting)	115	126	YOUNG	1948/49
Average.	89	61		
(2) Cat	29	23	SMITH	1953b
Cat	19	23	EMMELIN and KAHLSON	1944
Cat (mucosa whole st.) . .	21.5 (Intestine-17.7)		HAEGER and KAHLSON	1952a
(1) Rat (glandular st.) . . .	13.0		FELDBERG and TALESNIK	1953
Guinea pig	6.7[3]	3.4[3]	PARROT and VASSEUR	1960
Lizzard (whole st.)	75		WRIGHT and TRETHEWIE	1956
Man[1] (mucosa)	10	6	TRACH et al.	1944
Man[1] (mucosa)	38.8±6.1	24.0±3.8	SMITH	1959
Man[1] (Full thickness)	35±5.1	21 ±2.4	SMITH	1959
Man[2]	10.5	12.6	BLOOMER	1942

The "gastrin" yield from 4 g of pyloric mucosa by the use of the methods of KEETON and KOCH (1915) and of SACKS et al. (1932), when tested on gastric secretion is roughly equivalent to 0.25 to 0.3 mg of histamine base. Multiplying 61 μg (ave., Table 2) by 4 g of mucosa, a figure of 0.244 mg of histamine base is obtained. This "gastrin" yield is from hog's pyloric mucosa. The amount of histamine found in the intestinal mucosa of the dog was 35 μg/g of fresh tissue (GADDUM, 1936).

(*1*) Mucosa without submucosa.

(1) See FELDBERG and TALESNICK (1953), glandular stomach 14 and duodenum 14 μg.

(2) See SMITH (1953b), duodenal whole wall value was 40 μg/g of fresh tissue.

[1] Surgical specimens from patients; values may be too low.

[2] Post mortem specimens.

[3] Converted from diHCl to base.

1951) in Table 3 show that the alkaline secreting *duodenal mucosa* contains about the same amount of "gastrin" or histamine as the acid secreting mucosa of the stomach and twice that of the alkaline secreting mucosa of the pylorus.

4. Deficiencies in the methods used is the most probable cause of the discrepancies in the old and more recent literature

The older literature on this subject is replete with discrepancies. For example, EDKINS and TWEEDY (1909), EMSMANN (1911–1912), EHRMANN (1911–1192), TOMASZEWSKI (1913, 1918), MAYDELL (1913, 1917–1918), KEETON and KOCH (1915), KOCH et al. (1920–1921), ROGERS et al. (1915), FAWCETT et al. (1915) found their acid extracts of the pyloric mucosa to stimulate acid production. On the other hand EDKINS and TWEEDY (1909) and MAYDELL (1913, 1917–1918) found their extracts of the fundic or acid secreting gastric mucosa to be inactive, but KEETON and KOCH (1915), KEETON et al. (1920), TOMASZEWSKI (1913, 1918), EHRMANN (1911–1912) and GAVIN et al. (1933) found theirs to be active. EMSMANN (1911–1912) and EHRMANN (1911-1912) like KEETON and KOCH (1915) found their acid extracts of the duodenal mucosa to be active. The latter group found the duodenal mucosa less active than the stomach (KEETON and KOCH, 1915), but later found it to be about the same as gastric mucosa (LUCKHARDT et al., 1919–1920).

Reference to the average data in the more recent literature in Table 2, and especially to the data in the original articles, will show that wide variations in the results obtained with the extract of various specimens occur. However, the yield

Table 3. *Histamine (biological assay) in alimentary tract of dog, in micrograms of the base/g of wet tissue*

Averages are from the data of DOUGLAS et al. (1951)

Average values																		
Tissue site	Esoph.		Stomach			Tissue site	Small intestine									Colon	
	U 1	L 2	F 3	C 4	P 5		D 6	D 7	8	9	10	11	12	13	14	P 15	D 16
M[1]			126	87	51	GM[2]											
M[1]			126	87	51	GM[2]	84	91	94	77	83	65	38	42	34	9	7
M + SM	29	27				MM	129	127	143	93	117	125	103	130	111	143	130
SM			58	97	48	SM	79	70	54	55	50	43	28	31	32	29	31
ME	7	4	32	30	14	ME	40	39	26	22	27	20	18	24	21	7	14
WW	19	14	69	66	28	WW	94	86	81	66	71	68	57	59	50	44	42

[1] M mucosa; SM submucosa; ME muscularis externa. Esophagus; U upper; L lower. Stomach; F fundus or proximal; C corpus or middle; P pyloric or distal. Small intestine; D duodenum proximal and distal; 8 jejunum; 14 distal ileum. Colon: proximal and distal.

[2] GM glandularis mucosae; MM muscularis mucosae; WW whole wall.

per gram of mucosa of KEETON and KOCH (1915) and SACKS et al. (1932) is the same as the average for the dog in Table 2. It should be noted, however, that the standard deviations of the results of SMITH (1959) are not large.

According to one of us (A.C.I.) who has had much first hand experience with the chemical extraction methods, as well as all of the assay methods, the blood pressure and intestinal strip method (when properly used) yield the most quantitative, easily obtained values. The biological assays yield more consistent values than the chemical extraction methods, especially when applied to different small portions of the same large specimen of mucosa. This is an impression since no data can be submitted in support of it; but no data have been found in the literature contrary to it. The best extraction methods for urine and plasma yield a recovery of added histamine of from 50 to 80 %. In fact, there is a paucity of data in the literature showing the consistency of the results on the assay of adjacent pieces of mucosa although there is much data on the consistency of the assay of "an extract" on a "strip" or on the blood pressure in relation to the "histamine" control. But, there are no reports showing the consistency of the histamine or "gastrin" yield from 10 batches of 400 grams each of pyloric mucosa. Those data in Table 2 showing a standard deviation or error represent a "step in the right direction".

There are difficulties inherent to the "anesthetized cat or dog" method for the assay of secretory potency. Histamine can be used for a "control response" but when this is done it will be found that the variation even in the same animal is sometimes quite marked, especially as the anesthesia is prolonged. And, after the unknown "gastrin" has been assayed another histamine control response should be determined. *If the results are to be considered to be quantitative or comparative rather than qualitative, then statistical methods must be applied to the design and results of the experiment.* If chronic gastric preparations are used, it must be realized that pitfalls exist. The gastric fistula dog with vagi intact is the most sensitive, but such an animal is subject to psychic influences as well as conditioning. The same holds for the PAVLOV type of pouch, which can become a HEIDENHAIN pouch in time due to the contraction of scar tissue. No gastric pouch should be called a PAVLOV pouch unless it has been shown to respond well to psychic stimulation, sham feeding or hypoglycemia. The pouch of the entire stomach with vagi cut is ideal, except some such dogs have to be specially fed. They are more refractory than the gastric fistula dog. The denervated or transplanted pouch is used for studies on blood borne agents (GREGORY, 1950,58; LIM et al., 1925). When quantitative or comparative conclusions are desired then the experiments must be designed and the results analyzed statistically. With few exceptions, the studies in the literature in this field are qualitative rather than quantitative. This obviously breeds discrepancies.

Because of the lack of quantitatively established reliable extraction and assay procedures, it cannot be concluded whether the discrepancies represent errors in, or lack of reliability of methods, or true variations, in the concentration of histamine per gram of mucosa.

A chemical method of extraction and assay which will yield statistically significant values on small samples of mucosa and will also yield at least a 90% recovery of added histamine is sorely needed.

5. "Histamine profile" of the gastric and intestinal mucosa, or the concentration of histamine in the different histological layers

The concentration of histamine in the different anatomic layers of the mucosa was first studied by DOUGLAS et al (1951). The averages of their results are summarized in Table 3. A more extensive study of this problem was made by FELDBERG and HARRIS in 1953. They excised small pieces of the gastric wall, flattened and then froze them on the freezing microtome. Serial sections were made in a horizontal plane of two adjacent blocks of mucosa. The sections from one block were stained for histological study and identification, and those from the other block were used to assay for histamine concentrations. In this way the results could be put together to form a "histamine profile" of the gastric or intestinal mucosa. Two peaks of histamine concentration were found. One was located at and just below the neck of the glands, where the parietal or acid forming cells are especially concentrated, and the other was located in the region of the muscularis mucosae. In the pyloric mucosa only one peak located at the level of the pyloric glands was found (Fig. 2).

SMITH (1959) made a "histamine profile" from the acid secreting portion of the stomach and the pyloric portion of the stomach of man. The "histamine profiles" of human mucosa closely resembled those obtained by FELDBERG and HARRIS (1953) on canine mucosa.

These findings suggest that histamine plays a definite physiological role. If not, why is histamine in or adjacent to the cells it stimulates to secrete? The histamine may serve to act directly on the parietal and intestinal glands to stimulate secretion, or it may serve to augment blood flow in relation to secretion caused by stimuli other than histamine. Or, it may do both in certain instances.

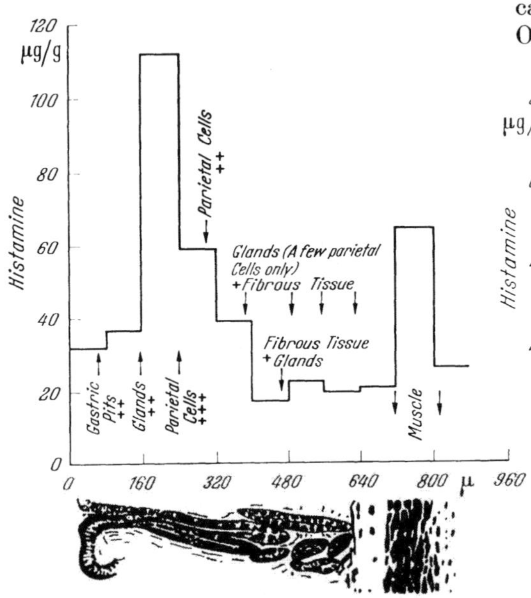

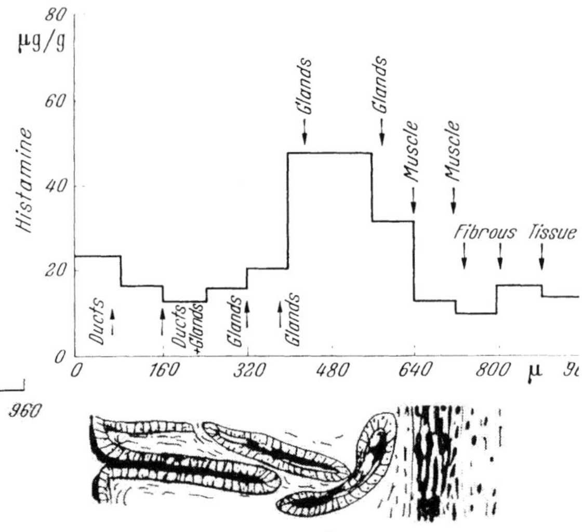

a b

Fig. 2 a/b. The histamine profile of the layers of the acid secreting or corporic region of the stomach of man. The muscularis externa is not included. The horizontal axis indicates the depth of the layer in micra. The vertical axis indicates the concentration of histamine in micrograms per gram of tissue

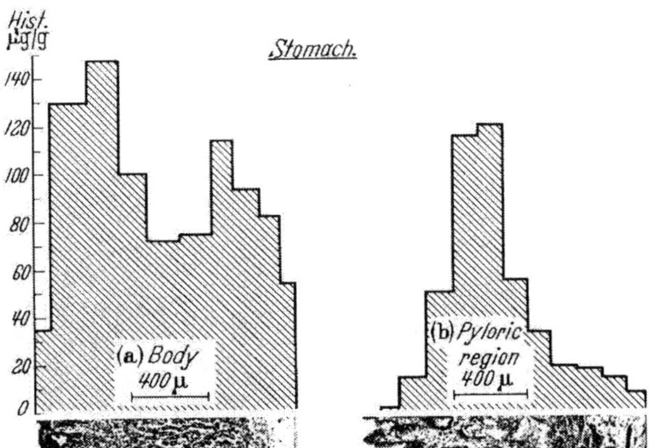

c d

Fig. 2 c/d. The histamine profile of the pyloric region of the stomach of man. See Smith (1959). The use of these illustrations has the permission of the author and publisher

6. The relation of the location of histamine to mast cells in the gastric mucosa. Non-mast cell histamine in the gastrointestinal mucosa

It is well-known that histamine is located in mast cells from which it is released following the action of certain histamine releasers (Riley, 1959). Riley and West (1953) found a strong correlation between the histamine content and mast cell population in different tissues. However, FELDBERG and TALESNIK (1953) found that the repeated intraperitoneal injection of 48/80, a potent histamine releaser, markedly reduced the histamine content of various tissues with the exception of the liver, stomach and duodenum. MOTA, et al (1956) found only a few mast cells in the gastric and intestinal mucosa. They found in the esophagus, cardia, fundus, duodenum, ileum, rectum and liver the following amounts of histamine/gm of wet tissue 4.5, 3.0, 15.1, 14.8, 5.5, 2.5, 0.5 μg, respectively. When 48/80 was injected intraperitoneally repeatedly, the histamine content of the glandular stomach, duodenum and small intestine and distal colon decreased as it did in the skin and tongue. MOTA et al. (1956) found more mast cells in the mucosa of the corpus or acid secreting mucosa than any place else in the alimentary tract. RILEY (1959) found also that the mucosa of the stomach, except for the corpus, was almost devoid of mast cells but some were present in the submucosa, throughout. They found 25, 18, 10, 9 μg of histamine/gm of fresh tissue in the pylorus, duodenum, ileum, and cecum, respectively. After 5 days of injection of 48/80, they found 15, 12, 14, 9 μg, respectively. On the eleventh day, 6 days after the last 48/80, the values were 55, 12, 16, 16, respectively. No explanation was available for this "rebound effect" in the pyloric mucosa. It appeared to involve the mucosa chiefly. When they separated the mucosa from the muscularis and assayed for histamine, they found 63 μg/gm in the mucosa and 18 in the muscularis propria. MONGAR and SCHILD (1952) found that the mucosa of the gastrointestinal tract of guinea pigs was resistant to histamine liberators. In cats, SMITH (1953 b) found that a very small amount of histamine was released by 48/80 from the gastric mucosa of the corpus but not from the remainder of the gastrointestinal tract. Cats pretreated with 48/80 showed a decreased gastric secretory response to histamine, "gastrin" and vagal stimulation. RILEY (1959) in the hog found mast cells in the submucosa in relation to blood vessels. A few smaller mast cells were in the mucosa located in relation to the glands. A mast cell and histamine profile of the hog's pyloric mucosa, was made. It was found that the high histamine content of the submucosa could be accounted for by the high mast cell count. This was not true for the mucosa, which shows that cells other than mast cells in the parietal cell region contain histamine; perhaps the histamine is in the oxyntic granules of the parietal cells. It is possible that mucus in the goblet cells in the lower two-thirds of the pyloric glands binds histamine, since there is evidence that gastric mucus binds histamine (NEUGEBAUER and SCHMID, 1949). This mucus stains metachromatically with toluidine blue, but there is no stain to show that the granules are histamine.

The larger concentration of mast cells in the fundic mucosa (SMITH, 1953 b) might account for the higher histamine content of the acid secreting mucosa. The remaining portion, which is about equal to the non-mast cell histamine in the pyloric mucosa (Table 2), could be bound with mucus in the pyloric glands or the mucin in the cells of the neck of the acid secreting glands in the corpus and fundus. *It is evident that more than half of the histamine in the gastrointestinal tract is non-mast cell histamine.* This morphological observation must have significance, since histamine stimulates to a variable extent all the digestive secretory processes.

7. Comparison of histamine concentration in gastric mucosa and mast cell tumors

Regardless of the variations or discrepancies just emphasized, it is interesting to indicate that RILEY and WEST (1953) found a concentration of 103 to 295 micrograms of histamine per gram of tissue in mast cell tumors. The lower value approximates that found in the duodenal and gastric mucosa in some cases

(Table 2). In solitary mast cell tumors of the human skin, the histamine concentration may be as high as 950 micrograms/gm of fresh tissue. In mast cell tumors of the dog it may be as high as 1290 micrograms/gm.

Thus in the gastric mucosa, *mast-cell histamine* exists in the submucosa along the blood vessels and to some extent along the blood vessels in the stroma of the acid secreting mucosa especially and in the pyloric mucosa about the base of the glands. *Non-mast cell histamine* is located in the base of the pyloric glands and seems to be found with mucin granules and either in the region of or inside the parietal cells in the acid secreting (corpus or fundus) mucosa.

8. Relation of histamine to eosinophiles in the gastric mucosa

Eosinophilic granular cells have often been described in the stroma of the gastric mucosa. More recently GRANT (1961), studying the rat in the senior author's laboratory, observed a statistically significant increase in the gastric mucosa after feeding, especially in the acid secreting mucosa. In the pyloric portion or mucus secreting mucosa, higher counts were found outside the glands in the stroma than inside the gland area, in both the fed and fasting groups.

The work was done because the eosinophile is no longer considered to be a carrier of histamine or involved in its production. Instead these cells are believed to be concerned with the disposal and "detoxification" of tissue histamine (RILEY, 1959). RILEY (1959) writes that eosinophiles are frequently seen in tissues in which histamine is being released from mast cells. In GRANT's observations the increase in eosinophile count occurred in tissues where there is a relative paucity of mast cells, but nevertheless in tissues where non-mast-cell histamine is produced and is acting in relation to gastric secretion.

In other words, the increase in eosinophiles in the gastric mucosa during digestion in the rat suggests that histamine is in some way involved.

9. Changes in histamine content of the gastric mucosa under various conditions

Several studies have been made to determine whether the histamine content of the gastric mucosa changes under various conditions. GAVIN et al. (1933) found an average of 39 and 69 mg of "histamine" per kilogram in the pyloric and fundic mucosa, respectively, of 24-hour fasting dogs, and 63 and 92 mg per kilogram in the pyloric and fundic mucosa of dogs which had been fed from 1 to 2 hours previously. HAEGER and KAHLSON (1952 a) found that starvation for one week did not have an effect on the concentration of histamine in the gastric mucosa of cats, the concentration being the same in fasted and fed cats. HILL and CODE (1959) obtained the same result in dogs, and even when they injected 0.2 mg of histamine subcutaneously every 10 min after the meal. It is interesting that hypoglycemia *significantly* increased the histamine in the mucosa of the corpus from a control of 80 $\pm$ 5.4 μg/gm of mucosa to 105 $\pm$ 6 and of the mucosa of the pars pylorica from 57 $\pm$ 5.0 to 83 $\pm$ 7.6 μg/gm of mucosa. A meal, or a meal plus histamine, or cortisone had no effect.

In the light of what is now known regarding the production of histamine in the gastric mucosa, namely, by the decarboxylation of L-histidine, there is no reason why the histamine content of the mucosa should not be held in a homeostatic balance. It may be produced as fast as it is released into the gastric juice and blood. This should be rather readily accomplished because of the small amounts of histamine released in the gastric juice and the very small amount that would have to be released into the blood to stimulate gastric secretion.

The increase in histamine in the mucosa during hypoglycemia, as HILL and CODE suggest, may be due to a local disturbance of the histamine metabolism. For example, hypoglycemia may speed decarboxylation of L-histidine or the accumulation may occur because hypoglycemia releases acetylcholine instead of histamine and acetylcholine increases the rate of decarboxylation in the parietal cell, or other cells in the region of the parietal cells. *This suggestion is supported by the observation of* BIKICH *et al. (1954) who found an increase in histamine in the gastric mucosa after vagal stimulation and acetylcholine.*

YOUNG (1948-1949) used the method of GILMAN and LINDSKOG (1942) for the extraction of the gastric mucosa in a study on the effect of injections of histamine in beeswax on the concentration of histamine in the gastric mucosa. Specimens of the gastric mucosa were removed at laparotomy in dogs. The histamine-beeswax intramuscular injections were made for 2 or 3 weeks, then the mucosa was assayed again. No difference was found between the pyloric and corporic mucosa after the continuous exposure to histamine. (The same was true of the lung.) SMITH (1953 b), when he administered histamine in beeswax to cats, found the histamine content of the pyloric mucosa increased 30 %, especially in the submucosa (100 %). In the corporic mucosa the histamine concentration was either the same or reduced.

10. Changes in histamine in gastric mucosa after exposure to the histamine releaser 48/80

FELDBERG and TALESNIK (1953) in rats did not detect a reduction in the histamine content of the gastric mucosa after the subcutaneous administration of 48/80. The same was true for the liver. SMITH (1959) found a slight reduction in cats when the 48/80 was injected into the coeliac artery. On repeated injections of 48/80 the histamine content of the mucosa was only slightly decreased, but the HCl output which normally occurs in response to the injections of 48/80 was decidedly decreased. The control dose of 20 μg/kg of 48/80 caused a decided stimulation of acid output before repeated treatment with 48/80, but after repeated treatment a dose of 50 to even 2000 μg of 48/80 did not cause as much output of HCl as the control dose did before repeated treatment. These results were due primarily to the depletion of histamine from the skin. However, a decrease in the sensitivity of the parietal cells to UVNÄS "gastrin" and vagal stimulation occurred. This may have been due to the presence of inflammation and multiple ulcers, or an intoxication.

The resistance of the gastric mucosa to the release of histamine in response to 48/80, which otherwise is a powerful releaser, suggests that the release of histamine by the gastric mucosa occurs only in response to specific agents, if it occurs at all, and represents a specialized physiological adaptation. SMITH (1953 a, b) in a previous paper suggested that, since the HCl output is greater when 48/80 is injected into the coeliac artery than when the same dose is injected into the portal vein, only a small fraction of the gastric-mucosal histamine is or could be released to participate in the secretory response. In a preliminary study on two total gastric pouch dogs, one of the reviewers (A.C.I.) found no increase in HCl production when 48/80 in a 1 % solution in saline (50 ml) was applied to the mucosa of the pouch for one hour.

SMITH (1959) found no difference in the histamine content of patients with gastric cancer or duodenal ulcer. But when he made sections 10 microns thick of the mucosa and submucosa in order to make a "histamine profile", and applied 48/80 to the sections to obtain a release of histamine, he found that more histamine was released from the duodenal ulcer specimens than from the cancer specimens. He also found a greater release from the sections of the corporic than the pyloric mucosa. The submucosa of the corporic sections released a higher percentage of its histamine content than the mucosa. These results show that 48/80 does release histamine from the corporic mucosa, but in small amounts.

Tsukamoto (1961) using an acutely semi-exteriorized stomach of the rat with the mucosa exposed found that the submucosal injection of 10^{-5} dilution of histamine base would stimulate acid secretion, and that the submucosal injection of 48/80 did not cause acid secretion. The difference between the rat and cat, according to the observations of Smith (1959), may be due to the much greater susceptibility of the cat's stomach to histamine than that of the rat.

Parrot and Vasseur (1960) could find no histidine-decarboxylase in the gastric mucosa of guinea pigs. Since then Schayer (1956 a,b) and Schayer et al. (1955) found that gastric mucosal histidine decarboxylase cannot be detected in the gastric mucosa by the assay method for renal histidine decarboxylase which they used. When Schayer used his method, histidine decarboxylase was found. The rat's glandular stomach is very rich in this enzyme.

B. Histamine diamine oxidase (HDO) in the gastric mucosa

1. Species distribution

It has been known since its discovery by Best and McHenry in 1930 that a diamine oxidase, histaminase (HDO), which deaminates histamine, is present in numerous tissues including that of the intestine of all species studied (Zeller, 1942,) but is absent from the gastric mucosa of the dog (Best and McHenry, 1930; Dworetzky and Code, 1951) and cat (Haeger and Kahlson, 1952 a, b; Haeger et al., 1952). Oddly, it is absent from the kidney of the rat (Zeller, 1942; McHenry and Gavin, 1932; Rose et al., 1940), guinea pig (Zeller, 1942; McHenry and Gavin, 1932; Rose et al., 1940) and chicken (Zeller, 1942; McHenry and Gavin, 1932), but is present in the glandular stomach of the rat (Kobayashi and Ivy, 1958) and guinea pig (Dworetzky and Code, 1951). The chicken has not been studied.

2. Use of C^{14}-histamine for study of presence or absence of HDO

Kobayashi and Ivy (1959) used C^{14} histamine for the determination of the HDO in the mucosa of the fundic and pyloric glandular areas of the dog. It was thought that traces might be found. None or only a trace was found in the pyloric or fundic mucosa in contrast to the intestinal mucosa where much was found. However, a small amount of histamine destruction occurred which was not due to HDO but to some other type of enzyme action. On studying the mucosa of the glandular stomach and intestine of the rat with the same method, Kobayashi and Ivy (1958) found that the intestinal mucosa oxidized 92 % of the C^{14}-histamine, the glandular stomach (pyloric and fundic) 40 % and the squamous stomach 70 %. When the HDO was inactivated another agency destroyed about 12 %. The nature of the non-HDO destruction requires further study. It was probably due to a methylating enzyme.

The gastric mucosa of the bull frog (Buffo) contains only a slight amount of HDO, slightly more than found in the dog, and is completely inhibited by aminoguanidine. The intestine of the frog possesses two very active histamine destroying enzyme systems, one (HDO) inhibited by aminoguanidine and the other not (Kobayashi and Ivy, in press). Since the gastric mucosa of the bull frog will secrete HCl *in vitro* some very interesting basic and perhaps important observations may be made on the relation of histamine, aminoguanidine and histaminase.

3. Physiological significance of HDO

The physiological significance of histaminase has been studied and because of its absence in the gastric mucosa of some animals, it has to be considered in relation to the mechanism of gastric secretion. ROSE et al. (1940), ROSE and BROWNE (1938,1940-1941) and ROSE and KARADY (1939) found that adrenalectomy decreased the HDO in the lung of the rat, increased the susceptibility of the rat to histamine, and increased the histamine content of the stomach and lung. The sensitivity of the adrenalectomized rat and the accumulation of histamine in the tissues was corrected by ACTH and corticoids. KAHLSON and his colleagues made an extensive study of the significance of histaminase on the basis of the lead provided by ROSE et al. HAEGER and KAHLSON (1952 a) made an extensive study of the histaminase and histamine concentration of tissues in the cat — the most extensive in the literature. It was found that fasting for 7 days did not alter the histamine concentration of the gastrointestinal mucosa. A strict correlation between histaminase and histamine concentration was not found. After removal of the adrenals or pituitary gland the histaminase in the intestinal mucosa and kidney are remarkably decreased. This starts within 2 to 4 hours and an increase in the histaminase in the chyle is found. The histaminase content of the whole body decreases 75 %, due to the decrease in the viscera. However, the histamine content of the gastric and intestinal mucosa did not increase as was reported by ROSE et al. for the rat. This observation is in apparent conflict with the observation that histamine infused intravenously is more rapidly destroyed by those tissues with the highest concentration of histaminase (EMMELIN, 1951). It is not necessarily in conflict, however, if it is assumed that the function of histaminase is to deal with histamine which enters the circulation or is released so that histaminase may act on it. Until released, histamine is probably located inside cells in such a relation that it cannot be affected by histaminase.

4. Comment

Histamine may be inside the parietal cell to be released on appropriate stimulation. Histaminase may be partly intracellular and partly extracellular to deal with circulating or locally released histamine. Since there is no histaminase in the acid secreting mucosa of the dog and cat and probably man, the parietal cells of these species, being permeable to histamine, have a low threshold for circulating histamine; whereas the rat (LANE et al. 1957) and probably the guinea pig, which have histaminase in the gastric glandular mucosa, have a high threshold.

5. Effect of intravenous histaminase on gastric secretion

Histaminase intravenously should at least partially block the formation of acid due to histamine, but not to KOMAROV's "gastrin," since it is not affected *in vitro* by histaminase (BAUER and UVNÄS 1944). ROTH and HORTON (1940) reported that intraduodenal or intramuscular histaminase prevented the acid response to subcutaneous histamine given 30 minutes later. ATKINSON and IVY (1934) and ATKINSON et al. (1941) used the best histaminase then available and gave it by various routes without obtaining an effect. GROSSMAN and ROBERTSON (1948) used the best concentrate of histaminase then available and found it to reduce greatly or abolish the secretory response to histamine. Though the depression of secretion observed was very marked and impressive, the authors pointed out that the result was theoretically equivocal due to the impurity of the product though no toxicity and fever was observed. *The results were such that it would appear that pure histaminase would completely block the response to parenteral histamine, cholinergic drugs and food.*

6. General summary

Histaminase or histamine diamine oxidase is absent from the gastric mucosa of the dog, cat and man, but is present in the rat. Since the parietal cells of the former have a decidedly lower threshold for stimulation with histamine than the rat it would appear that histaminase may be involved in determining the threshold level. There is a non-HDO enzyme in small amount in the gastric mucosa of the dog which destroys a small amount of histamine; it is probably a methylating enzyme.

After removal of the pituitary gland or adrenals, the histaminase content of the intestinal mucosa and entire body dramatically decreases in the cat, and an increase in the sensitivity of the rat to exogenous histamine occurs. It would appear from these latter studies that histaminase may function to deal only with circulating histamine after it is released locally or generally. It would be of interest to determine, in the rat, if hypophysectomy or adrenalectomy renders the gastric glands more sensitive to parenteral histamine. It is also important to make a more concentrated preparation of histaminase. Histaminase may be involved only under conditions of stress.

C. Plasma histamine during digestion

Histamine is probably present in blood plasma at all times (Best and McHenry, 1930; Code, 1952; Hartman et al., 1961; Barsoum and Gaddum, 1935; Koskowski and Kubikowski, 1929; Koskowski, 1933). The amount is very small and is too small to detect in small quantities of plasma. The approximate average value for dogs, rabbits and cats is 0.05 μg/ml and for guinea pigs and rats 0.1 to 0.3 μg/ml (Code, 1952), according to the literature prior to 1952.

Roberts and Adam (1950), Adam (1950) and Adam et al. (1954a, b) found less than 0.01 μg/ml in the plasma of man. They found 0.02 to 0.03 μg/ml of histamine in the plasma of a patient during an acute urticarial reaction (Adam et al., 1950-1951), during which reaction the gastric secretion of HCl is reported to be increased (Kalk, 1929; Horton et al., 1936; Baker, 1940; Ivy et al., 1948; Grossman and Robertson, 1948; Sangster et al., 1946). An improved method was reported by Adam et al. (1957). Less than 0.001 μg/ml of plasma was found. Unfortunately the method recovers only 85% of small amounts of histamine added to plasma. The authors wrote that the method might be as sensitive as that of the parietal cells for detecting histamine. When C^{14}-histamine is injected its catabolism starts immediately. The percentage of non-catabolized histamine excreted in the urine is small. But some has been found in the rat, cat and human subject (Schayer, 1959).

But, the pertinent question under this topic is, whether histamine is released from the gastric and intestinal mucosa into the blood plasma during digestion in amounts which stimulate the parietal cells minimally and/or maximally, and in such amounts which can or cannot be detected by any method used to date for the detection of histamine.

After the unequivocal demonstration (Ivy and Farrell, 1925; Grossman et al., 1948) that a blood borne hormone or agent is concerned in part with the gastric secretory response to a meal, several groups of investigators have tried to detect and to ascertain the nature of the humoral agent by studying the blood. Several methods have been used.

1. Cross-circulation of anesthetized and unanesthetized gastric pouch dogs

Ivy et al. (1925) performed a "carotid-to-carotid cross circulation" in cross-matched Pavlov pouch dogs. When one of the pair was fed after full recovery from anesthesia, suggestive but unconvincing increases in acid output occurred in the unfed dog of the pair. When an ordinary dose of histamine was injected into one of the pair, the other of the pair secreted only slightly or not at all. In acute experiments it was estimated that not more than one-sixth to one-eighth of the cardiac output passed through the carotid artery per unit of time.

This indicated that vividialysis should be tried on the portal and arterial blood, so as to avoid the dilution inherent in the cross circulation method.

2. Dialysis

Necheles and Lim (1928) vividialyzed the portal blood of dogs and obtained a dialysate which stimulated gastric secretion on subcutaneous injection. It gave a positive Pauly reaction but its vasodepressor property was variable. Sacks et al. (1932 b) and Vandolah and Ivy (1928-1929) made dialysates of the total blood of three groups of large "fed" and "unfed" dogs (10 dogs in each group), bacterial action being prevented. They obtained an organic substance which was soluble in 90% alcohol containing N/10 HCl. In two groups of the "fed" dogs one dose of "gastrin" equivalent to 0.2 mg histamine base was obtained. All other results were negative. The experiment was not continued because it was suspected that histamine might come from blood cells. Emmelin (1951) ultra-filtered plasma *in vitro* in guinea pigs, rats, cats, dogs and rabbits and also made an extract of the same plasma by Code's method. He found approximately the same amount of histamine-like material present in both extracts. The aqueous humor caused a contraction of g.p. ileum when applied directly to it. He also performed ultrafiltration *in vivo* in rabbits and found a histamine-like material. He performed an ingenious type of cross-circulation in guinea pigs in which bronchoconstriction was the target reaction to the histamine-like material. The tests showed that a histamine-like material is in the blood plasma. But, no tests involved the effect of feeding on the plasma level. Emmelin's results showed the existence of a circulating diffusible histamine in the blood. Sacks et al. (1932 b) and Vandolah and Ivy (1928, 1929) vividialyzed the blood of fed and unfed dogs using a modified Abel apparatus. They also dialyzed the plasma of five dogs which had been fed and ultrafiltered (Viscose sausage casing diaphragms). The dialysates and filtrates were concentrated at 40°C under vacuum. A product soluble in 95% alcohol and giving a positive Pauly reaction was obtained. It depressed the blood pressure if given rapidly intravenously, but the secretory response was too slight and variable to permit a definite conclusion. They also collected thoracic duct lymph (Sacks et al. 1932 b) in dogs after a meal and found in it a substance which gave a Pauly reaction but had no effect on blood pressure or gastric secretion (Vandolah and Ivy, 1928-1929). The difference between the results of these investigators may have been due to a difference in the membrane used for dialysis and the chemical methods used for the concentration and extraction of the dialysate.

3. Direct assay of the blood for gastric secretory excitants

Vandolah and Ivy (1928) extracted the "total plasma" of 10 unfed and of 10 fed dogs by an adaptation of the Keeton and Koch method (1915) for "gastrin." The dogs were bled two hours after feeding. The plasma amounted to about 5 liters in each group. The total extract of the "non-fed plasma" when given subcutaneously to a gastric pouch dog did not stimulate; that from the "fed plasma" did in a histamine dose equivalent of 0.1 mg of the base. This experiment was not repeated because it was indicated that with the chemical extraction method used, there was not enough gastric secretory excitant in the total plasma of 10 fed dogs at one time to provide more than one mild stimulating dose of "gastrin" or "histamine". Just how efficient the extraction method was, is unknown. If dog's plasma should contain 0.005 μg/ml, then 5 liters should contain 25 μg of histamine base, which is too little to stimulate a PAVLOV pouch dog when given subcutaneously. It is now known that most of the total blood histamine is in the leucocytes and platelets (CODE, 1952; HARTMAN et al. 1961). These could be fractured during the preparation of the plasma, yielding histamine and an equivocal result. This experimental approach was abandoned by VANDOLAH and IVY because of the equivocal nature of any positive results which might be obtained. BEST and MCHENRY (1930) found 0.4 mg of histamine base in one kilogram of dog's whole blood. This would be a good gastric stimulating dose, but again the result would be obviously equivocal.

KOSKOWSKI and KUBIKOWSKI (1929) and KOSKOWSKI (1933) observed that defibrinated blood when applied directly to the virgin uterus of a guinea pig caused contraction. In addition to histamine we now know that other agents may have been involved in the genesis of such a result.

MCINTOSH (1938) used a slight modification of the CODE (1937) method for extracting histamine from the blood and the ileal strip for assay. The CODE method is a modification of the method of BARSOUM and GADDUM (1935). His extraction method would remove 85 to 95% of 0.2 micrograms of histamine added to 10 ml of blood, which approximates the limits of biological assay. He used venous blood in which the histamine content was undoubtedly reduced as compared to arterial blood as a result of loss in the tissues. He failed to find an increase in the histamine equivalent of the systemic venous blood after feeding, and of the gastric venous blood after stimulation of the peripheral vagi. Furthermore, he could not detect an increase in blood histamine after giving subcutaneously 1 mg of histamine dihydrochloride (0.6 mg of base) which decidedly stimulated gastric secretion. When he gave a dose of 2.0 mg of the dihydrochloride (1.2 mg of base), a definite increase in blood histamine was believed to have been found. In other words about twice the usual dose of histamine, a dose which produces a marked stimulation of gastric secretion, had to be given before a result indicating an increase in histamine in the blood could be detected by the method then available. In 1941, EMMELIN et al. gave histamine slowly intravenously to cats and dogs, and found that gastric secretion was stimulated before an increase in blood histamine could be detected by the CODE 1937-method. Similar observations have been made by ÖBRINK (1946, 1948) who in addition found that, when intravenous infusions of histamine are given, a detectable rise in blood histamine does not occur in some experiments until a dose greater than that required for maximal secretion is given. BIKICH et al. (1954) obtained results similar to those of MCINTOSH. GREGORY (1950 b) found no increase in histamine in portal or gastric venous blood after a meal. IRVINE et al. (1961) found no increase in portal blood after alcohol and insulin stimulation of gastric secretion.

4. Gastric secretory threshold for histamine and the difficulty of its detection in the blood plasma

The gastric secretory threshold dose for histamine is very small. HANSON et al. (1948) found it to be an average of 0.04 micrograms of histamine per kilogram per minute for the dog and 0.004 for man. ÖBRINK (1946, 1948) in a HEIDENHAIN pouch dog found a minimal dose to be 0.05 μg/kg/min. He extrapolated the dose-response curve and came to the conclusion that there is no threshold dose for histamine. EMMELIN and KAHLSON (1944) found the minimal rate of histamine

Table 4. *Threshold dose of histamine given by intravenous infusion for stimulation of gastric secretion*

Source	Reference No. (Year)	Animal	μg/kg/min
IVY-JAVOIS . . .	(1924/25)	Dog (pouch)	1 μg[1]
EMMELIN et al. . .	(1941)	Dog (pouch)	0.5—6.0 μg
ÖBRINK	(1948)	Dog (pouch)	0.05 (no thresh.)
HANSON et al. . .	(1948)	Dog (pouch)	0.04
IRVINE-CODE . . .	(1958)	Dog (pouch)	0.08
EMMELIN et al. . .	(1941)	Cat (decer.)	0.5—1.5
EMMELIN-FROST .	(1947)	Cat (anest.)	2—3[1]
WOOD	(1948)	Cat (anest.)	2—3[1]
IVY and LIN . . .	(1958)	Cat (anest.)	0.01—0.005 (ave. 0.015)
MCELIN-HORTON .	(1946)	Man	Less than 0.030
HANSON et al. . .	(1948)	Man	Ave. 0.004 (0.002—0.016)
ADAM et al. . . .	(1954)	Man	Ave. 0.010 (0.0036—0.013

[1] The objective was not to obtain a true measure of a threshold dose. See also: KALK (1929); WEISS et al. (1932); UNGAR (1935); FELDBERG and HOLMES (1941); GROB et al. (1947).

administration to produce a detectible rise in plasma histamine, is from 2 to 5 μg/kg/min in the dog by their method of extraction and assay; that is a supermaximal dose for gastric secretion (Table 4).

Everyone agrees that the dose or concentration of histamine in the blood required to stimulate gastric secretion is well below that which can be detected by the methods used in the past (ADAM et al., 1957). This confirms the initial findings of ROSE (1940, 1941), and the more recent findings of ADAM (1950) and of ADAM et al. (1954 a,b). In human subjects headache occurred with large doses of histamine before an increase was detectible in the blood. The plasma level of histamine infusion required to produce it was more than 0.03 μg/ml (Figure 3).

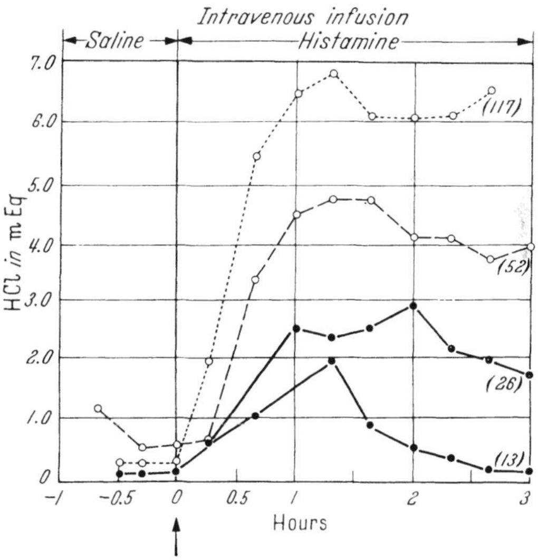

Fig. 3. An intravenous infusion of histamine was started at zero hours in a human subject. The dose of histamine in ng/kg/min is shown in brackets. The total HCl output for 20-min intervals in mEq is shown on the ordinate. The curves show an accumulative effect followed by a fall, indicating an adaptation, or a depression of the sensitivity of the "parietal cells" by histamine as indicated by IVY and JAVOIS (1924/1925) and others. Figure from ADAM et al. (1954) (Fig. 1)

These findings on the plasma are obviously compatible with the view that, "histamine" is a local hormone in the acid secreting mucosa serving as the final stimulator of the parietal cell, regardless of the nature of the original stimulus. All agree that the findings do not rule out the possibility that histamine may be gastrin or "the true hormone" or "a hormone" released into the plasma during digestion. Too large or maximal doses cause flushing and headache, especially if the dose is quickly increased. Because of this ADAM et al. (1954, b) suggested that their findings were compatible with the view that histamine in the systemic circulation could contribute to the maintenance of a basal secretion of acid. But they found that 0.026 μg/kg/min would cause a good gastric secretory response without symptoms. See Figure 3.

MALLIK and BHATTACHARYA (1958) could not find a correlation between fasting acidity and blood histamine in patients with chronic peptic ulcer, but their data do not make it clear whether they were measuring "basal secretion" or the "fasting residuum" of the stomach.

EMMELIN (1945) has suggested, as the result of his studies, that a small amount of histamine is normally present in the plasma and that responsive cells become adapted to a constant level, and a response occurs only with an increment. The phenomenon of the inhibitory effect or adaptation to histamine, when given particularly in large doses, was pointed out by IVY and JAVOIS (1924-1925) and also ADAM et al. (1954 b). See Figure 3.

5. Assays on portal blood plasma for histamine

GREGORY (1950 b) used the method of CODE (1937) for extracting portal blood and the 4-point biological assay method of SCHILD. The portal blood samples were obtained by a plastic tube installed into the portal vein at an asceptic operation. Samples of blood before and after a meal of meat were removed for assay. In 12 experiments on 3 dogs, after feeding, a significant increase in plasma histamine did not occur. The author realized that his method may not have been sensitive enough to detect an increase in histamine which if present for an hour would stimulate gastric secretion.

More recently, IRVINE et al. (1961) in a study of the mechanism by which alcohol stimulates gastric acid secretion failed to find a detectible increase of histamine in gastric venous blood after the intravenous infusion of 300 ml of 10 % ethyl alcohol into the splenic artery through an indwelling plastic cannula in anesthetized dogs. Conscious dogs received 200 ml of 7 % ethyl alcohol over a period of 30 min. in both instances. The gastric juice was collected from the intact stomach. For the determination of plasma and urinary free histamine, they used the method of ADAM et al. (1957). The method yielded a mean recovery of 82.5 % ± 2 (S. E.) of added histamine in a range of from 25 to 100 nanograms. The method was sensitive enough to detect changes in the plasma of a cat when 0.33 μg/kg/min of histamine was injected over a period of 20 min (total 20 μg in 20 min injected). In one experiment the plasma histamine increased from 0.0016 μg/ml to 0.0056 μg/ml. The alcohol yielded a good secretion of HCl, but no histamine was found in the gastric venous effluent. The authors realized that their method may not have been sensitive enough to detect a physiological increase in histamine. When they infused histamine into the splenic artery of their dogs at a rate of 1.0 μg/kg/min, there was a definite increase in acid output and the concentration of histamine in gastric and femoral vein plasma. But when 0.2 μg/kg/min of histamine was given, the gastric venous plasma increased to 0.0024 μg but the femoral venous blood did not change. 0.2 μg/kg/min is more than a mean threshold dose for a dog, which is 0.04 μg/kg/min. But when injected into the portal vein, the dose of 0.04 μg would be reduced to 0.02 μg/kg/min due to the removal of about 50 % of the histamine by the liver. The method would not detect such a small change.

IRVINE et al. (1961) also gave 2 units/kg of insulin into the splenic artery, the gastric glands were stimulated decidedly but there was no increase in the histamine concentration of portal or femoral venous plasma. This is interesting because

IRVINE and CODE (1958) in another group of dogs obtained a good acid secretion in response to hypoglycemia, but the urinary concentration of free histamine did not increase. It should be pointed out that perhaps histamine is not released on vagal excitation as occurs in hypoglycemia; instead acetylcholine may be released, as in the case of other post-ganglionic parasympathetic nerve endings, and stimulate the parietal cells directly. The results of experiments by HIRSCHOWITZ et al. (1956) indicate that alcohol stimulates acid output by acting on the center of the vagus nerve in the medulla *(vide infra)*.

6. The histamine plasma level and threshold stimulation of gastric secretion

Most studies made on the blood histamine levels have been made on whole blood and it is well known that most of the blood histamine is in the cellular elements and less than 0.01 μg/ml is in blood plasma. It would seem most logical then to look in the plasma for histamine released from cells or tissues.

Some students of the "gastrin problem" would insist that to prove the existence of histamine, or KOMAROV's "gastrin", as a true hormone, an increase in plasma level of either one or both after feeding must be established. We agree with this view in so far as categorical proof is concerned, with one important exception. But, let us examine this problem on the basis of the existing facts to ascertain the nature of the problem. *Basically it is the problem of the regulation of the blood plasma histamine level and of a method sensitive and accurate enough to detect a very small physiologically significant plasma increment, in so far as gastric secretion is concerned.*

The problem of regulation and method is set forth by the results of an experiment of ADAM et al. (1954a). They gave a human subject an intravenous infusion of histamine for 180 min at a rate of 0.008 μg/kg/min. The effect on gastric secretion was slight but definite, the average threshold dose for man being 0.004 μg/kg/min (HANSON et al., 1948), but the renal excretion of free histamine was doubled over the control period, and the change in plasma histamine level was less than 0.001 μg/ml, or smaller than they could detect by their method.

That the kidney would show an increase in excretion when the plasma change was not detectible is not surprising. BEST and MCHENRY (1930) found that the kidney of the dog removes histamine from blood faster than any other organ. STEGGERDA et al. (1935) found that the dog's kidney in a "heart-lung-kidney" preparation would remove 25 mg of histamine from the blood in 15 min, whereas the lung removed only traces. VALETTE *et al.* (1955) obtained similar results.

CODE (1956) has pointed out, that the recovery in the urine of a small amount of histamine given intravenously during a period of 180 minutes, amounts to from 0.7 to 1.9 % during a 6-hour period after the start of the injection, and that the recovery of heavy (deuterium) water in the urine by SCHOLER and him, when it was injected over a period of 2 to 5 hours, was 0.5 to 1.3 %. The similarity in these percentages indicates that a definite portion of each amount of histamine which enters the blood is removed and excreted by the kidney, as was true in the case of deuterium. This fact, as ADAM (1950) recognized, should render the output of free histamine in the urine an excellent indicator of changes in plasma histamine level, or in the total circulating histamine.

Only an average of 1 % of parenterally administered histamine is excreted in the urine without being catabolized (SCHAYER, 1959). The remaining 99 % is changed into methylimidazoleacetic acid or imidazoleacetic acid by special methylating and oxidizing enzymes (SCHAYER, 1959). Thus, a large increase in plasma histamine level, such as up to 0.02 to 0.03 μg/ml, or up to over 0.001 μg/ml with the most recent method, should *not* be expected, until the capacity of the tissues to destroy it and the kidney to eliminate it, is encroached on. This is why EMMELIN et al. (1941) with an "intensive method" did not detect a rise in plasma histamine until the rate of intravenous infusion of histamine in the dog reached a rate of 2 to 5 μg/kg/min. Such a dose, of course, causes symptoms and is a supermaximal dose for the gastric glands of the dog. Somewhere between the mean gastric secretory threshold dose for the dog of 0.04 μg/kg/min and the 2 to 5 μg/kg/min dose injected, the capacity of the kidney and tissues to regulate the plasma level was overtaxed. If, in order to obtain a rise in plasma histamine level and to overtax the histamine plasma level regulatory mechanism, it is necessary to give histamine at a rate which produces symptoms and represents a supermaximal gastric secretory dose, then we are looking for something abnormal.

This situation will continue to prevail unless it is fully realized how small the increment required to stimulate acid secretion is, and how sensitive the method to detect that increment in the plasma must be.

The evidence indicating the size of the increment will be briefly outlined. Assuming the average *fasting* plasma level of histamine in the dog to be 0.01 μg/ml, (CODE, 1952) and since 0.04 μg/kg/min of histamine must be intravenously infused to obtain a minimal stimulation of gastric secretion, then *either (a) a rise in the plasma histamine level above 0.01 μg/ml must have occurred, or (b) the minute volume delivery of histamine to the gastric glands must have increased the histamine concentration or the supply of histamine in the mucosa to the secretory threshold.* Since under analogous conditions in man the renal output of free histamine is doubled over the control output, there must have been an increase in the plasma histamine level or in the amount of histamine being delivered to the renal excretory mechanism per unit of time.

Intravenously infused histamine at a rate of 0.04 μg/kg/min for 30 min is the average infusion dose required to stimulate. This represents a total of 12 μg in a 10 kg dog. This amount would be diluted roughly in a minimum of 400 ml of plasma yielding an increment of 0.03 μg/ml, providing none were removed from the plasma and lymph. If the histamine were diluted in the 6000 ml of extracellular water, then the dilution would be 0.002 μg/ml (12 : 6000 = .002 μg/ml). The average dose to produce a maximal secretion of HCl in the dog is 1.8 μg/kg/min for 30 min. This represents a total of 54 μg in a 10 kg dog. It would be diluted roughly in a minimum of 400 ml of plasma and lymph yielding an increment of 0.13 μg/ml. If diluted in 6000 ml of fluid, the increment would be 0.009 μg/ml.

These increments are obviously excessive because during the 30-minute period a large portion of the injected histamine has been removed from the blood and another portion has been destroyed, so that it cannot be detected by ordinary chemical and biological methods. The recent method of ADAM et al. (1957) might solve this problem, but it is doubtful.

More recently LINDELL and SCHAYER (1958) have published some data bearing directly on this problem. They injected dogs with C^{14}-histamine by intravenous infusion and determined the C^{14}-histamine in renal arterial and venous blood and in the urine. The doses ranged from 0.4 μg/kg/min to 0.5 μg/kg/min, which is 10 times larger than the dose required to minimally stimulate the secretion of acid in the dog, and 5 times less than that required to maximally stimulate. After 30 min of such an infusion the renal arterial blood contained 0.00255 μg/ml of C^{14}-histamine. The renal venous blood contained 0.00055 μg/ml. If arterial blood is used, then 10 ml of plasma would contain a total increment of 0.0255 μg. This could be detected by an experienced and skilled assayist.

Venous blood has been used most frequently in attempts to detect an increment in the histamine plasma level. In the case of renal venous blood, 10 ml of plasma would contain only 0.0055 μg. Of course, renal venous blood is not a good choice because the kidney is so effective in removing histamine and its metabolic derivatives (SCHAYER, 1959).

The data of LINDELL and SCHAYER (1958) emphasize another important point. At the end of 30 min of the i. v. infusion of 0.4 μg/kg/min of histamine, the total blood of the 9 kilo dog could not have contained an increment of more than 1.836 μg which was chiefly in a total of about 360 ml of plasma, whereas 108 μg had been given. (720×0.00255 μg/ml $= 1.836$).

This forcibly indicates that an increment in the histamine concentration of the acid secreting mucosa could occur without a detectible increase in the concentration of histamine in the blood plasma. This possibility has to be considered especially because (a) of the great sensitivity of the parietal cells to histamine, (b) of the greater physiological tendency of the kidney, stomach and intestine to take up infused histamine (BEST and MCHENRY, 1930; EMMELIN, 1951; SCHAYER, 1959; STEGGERDA et al., 1935) and of the absence in the gastric mucosa of man, dog and cat of histaminase or any important means of destroying histamine.

Thus, *if there were an increase/min release of histamine into the circulating blood, and if at the same time the circulatory rate/min increased due to the effect of a concomitant physiological stimulus such as a meal, more blood and a proportional increment of histamine could be delivered to the acid secreting mucosa without any increment in the concentration of the arterial plasma.* Furthermore, the histamine delivered to the stomach would remain there longer and without being metabolized, whereas the concomitant increments delivered to the intestine, liver, and kidney would be metabolized. It is well established that the circulation rate, blood flow and cardiac output increases shortly after eating (SHEARD et al., 1934; BAZETT et al., 1936). The greater uptake and retention in the gastric mucosa without metabolic change is probably more true of the gastric mucosa than any other visceral and perhaps parenchymatous tissue, and is potentially a beautiful adaptation wherein a primitive histamine production and release mechanism has been developed into a specialized mechanism for secreting HCl. *At least, it should be clear that gastric secretion could be easily stimulated without an increment in the concentration in the arterial plasma, because an increase in the total histamine delivered to the gastric mucosa can occur without an increase in concentration.* The same would hold for the release of histamine or KOMAROV's "gastrin" from the pyloric and corporic mucosa. More study needs to be devoted to rates of blood flow in the gastric mucosa during digestion (LIM et al., 1925).

We need then to direct our attention toward ascertaining whether increases in histamine or KOMAROV's "gastrin" supply to, or concentration in the corporic mucosa and gastric juice, and urine, as well as the blood, occur during and after the digestion of a meal. For this complete extraction and very sensitive chemical methods seem to be required. Perhaps, as will be pointed out later, C^{14}-histidine and C^{14}-histamine techniques may provide the evidence required.

7. Stimulation of gastric secretion and histamine release from the skin in the urticarial reaction

There are a number of articles in the literature showing that gastric secretion is stimulated when an urticarial reaction is produced in dermatographia or whealing (KALK, 1929; HORTON et al., 1936; BAKER, 1940).

It was observed by IVY et al. (1948) that the intravenous injection of the detergent Tween 20 into dogs would produce urticaria. This provided an opportunity to determine whether gastric secretion was stimulated, and whether the humoral borne agent was histamine. GROSSMAN and ROBERTSON (1948b) made 18 tests in 8 dogs. The test consists of injecting 0.8 mg/kg of Tween 20 in a 1% aqueous solution intravenously. The gastric secretory response begins in 15 to 45 min following the injection, reaches its peak during the second half-hour period, and has returned to the basal level by the end of 2 hours. Urticaria begins to occur 3 to 5 min after the injection, reaches a maximum in 10 to 15 min, and has usually subsided completely within 30 min after injection. When Tween 20 was injected one-half hour after benadryl had been given, both urticaria and gastric secretion were either completely abolished or definitely diminished in 14 out of 18 tests on 7 of the dogs. In the remaining 4 tests on 3 dogs, urticaria was only questionably or moderately reduced and gastric secretion was the same or slightly greater than in the tests with Tween 20 alone. Statistical analysis reveals that the difference between the results, with and without benadryl, could be expected to occur by chance variation due to random sampling error in less than 4 out of 100 similar experiments. Since benadryl (10 mg/kg) intravenously does not inhibit histamine stimulated gastric secretion, the benadryl most probably acts in the skin to inhibit the release of histamine (SANGSTER et al. 1946). The only other possibility is that another substance is released instead of histamine, and benadryl blocks its action on the gastric glands.

D. Histamine in the gastric juice

1. Historical outline

LUCKHARDT et al. (1919—1920) failed to find a gastric secretory dose of "gastrin" in 11.5 ml of gastric juice. IVY and OYAMA (1921) extracted 100 ml of clear pyloric secretion by the KEETON-KOCH method for "gastrin" production. A gastric secretory dose was not found. IVY and OYAMA also collected two liters of dog's gastric juice having a pH below 2.0, filtered it while fresh and kept it in an ice box under toluol while it was accumulating. It was secreted in response to a meal. A gastric secretory dose, 0.1 mg of the base, was not found in one liter of such juice. The fasting gastric residuum of man and histamine stimulated juice contained from 0.0013 to 0.005 mg of base/100 ml when extracted and assayed by the BEST-MCHENRY method (1930). This is not enough to constitute a gastric secretory dose. KOMAROV (1936) found that the histidine fraction of the protein in gastric juice had a histamine-like effect. BLOCK and NECHELES (1938) did not find histamine in gastric juice but did find a substance resembling acetyl choline and another resembling "substance P" of GADDUM and EULER.

BROWN and SMITH (1935), using the method of BEST and MCHENRY, found in "fasting juice" from 13 μg/l to 535 μg/l. and in "histamine juice" from 23 μg/l to 411/l of histamine equivalent. These amounts are much larger than found by later investigators.

In 1938, MACINTOSH in dogs, and EMMELIN and KAHLSON (1944) in cats and dogs and CODE *et al.* (1947) in dogs, and ADAM *et al.* (1954a, b) have found histamine in gastric juice in small quantities and under diverse types of stimulation of gastric secretion.

2. Amounts found

Although histamine has not been isolated in crystalline form from gastric juice, as in the case of the gastric mucosa, either it or something very closely related to it is present in small amounts. When the flow of juice is copious, as induced by histamine in beeswax, the presence of histamine has not been detected even when the juice was twice concentrated (CODE et al., 1947), probably because the method was not sensitive enough. The highest concentration, except in some specimens of fasting secretion, has been found *when mecholyl was the stimulus* (CODE et al., 1947; BORBOLA et al., 1951).

MACINTOSH (1938) in sham-feeding juice obtained a histamine-equivalent of from 2 to 15 μg/l. Under vagal stimulation, the values ranged from 3 to 22 μg/l.; under histamine stimulation from 8 to 95 μg/l. The histamine equivalent of the canine gastric juice was higher than that of the plasma, a situation found by everyone who has made the comparison. So, histamine does not simply diffuse from the plasma into the gastric juice.

EMMELIN and KAHLSON (1944), using chiefly the CODE (1937) procedure for extraction, found in cats from 5 to 55 μg/l in "fasting juice", in dogs from 35 μg/l to 45 μg/l. in "sham feeding juice". On stimulation of the vagus in cats over a period of from 20 to 80 min they found from 6 to 150 μg/l of histamine, in dogs they obtained from 8 μg/l to 120 μg/l. When acetylcholine was placed in the cerebral ventricles, the juice contained from 25 to 45 μg/l. When aqueous meat extract was placed into the main stomach, the juice secreted by the PAVLOV pouch ranged from 30 to 80 μg/l. In the cat the juice after eserine contained from 30 to 35 μg/l; after injecting KOMAROV's "gastrin" made by UVNÄS (1942a, 1944), the histamine equivalent of the juice ranged from 20 to 55 μg/l. In cats which received UVNÄS "gastrin" and vagus stimulation simultaneously, the histamine ranged from 14 to 45 μg/l. In three cats which were given "Priscol", an imidazole which is used as a vasodilator, intravenously at a rate of 0.5—1.0 mg/kg/min for from 30 to 60 minutes, the juice contained from 30 to 65 μg/l. In cats stimulation of the vagi for 2 to 10 hours was not associated with a decrease in the concentration of histamine in the juice. They gave very large unphysiological doses of histamine by continuous intravenous infusion for from 5 to 115 min and found the juice to contain from 16 to 180 μg/l (Fig. 4). The low concentration of histamine found in some samples stimulated by various physiological procedures, they suggested might be due to the presence of an inhibitory substance for smooth muscle in the extract. They interpreted their results as showing no correlation between the rate of secretion and the histamine concentration of the juice, except when histamine was infused intravenously. They believed it reasonable to assume that the liberation of histamine in the fundic mucosa served as an integral link in the genesis of parietal cell secretion. They suggested that KOMAROV's "gastrin" might release histamine, histamine being the final stimulator of the parietal cell. (Figure 1.)

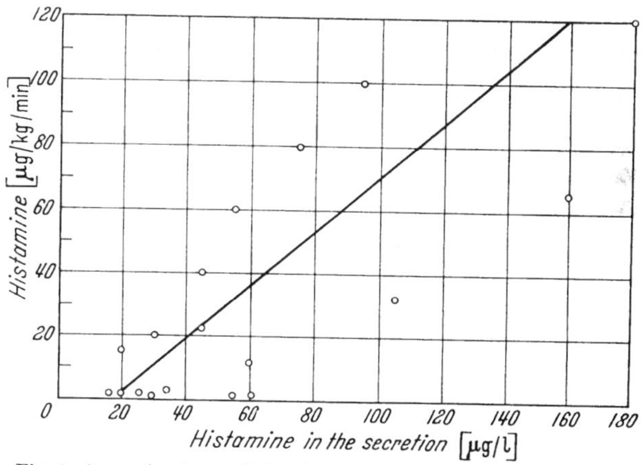

Fig. 4. Approximate correlation between rate of injection of histamine by intravenous infusion and the concentration of histamine in the *gastric juice* in 19 tests on 7 anesthetized cats. From EMMELIN and KAHLSON (1944)

CODE *et al.* (1947) extracted gastric juice of dogs by a modification of CODE's method consisting chiefly of an alcoholic extraction to reduce the potassium content of the extracts, since potassium can cause a contraction of an ileal strip. With their method, they were able to recover 79 to 81% of added histamine.

A concentration of 5 μg/l could be determined quantitatively. They gave 1.0 mg histamine (base) subcutaneously and histamine-in-beeswax intramuscularly. Combining the results of the two methods on 58 specimens of juice, in 5 specimens

Table 5. *Histamine in gastric juice and the percentage recovery of added histamine as a check in the method used*

Author	Ref.	Animal	μg per liter of juice*	Type of secretory stimulus	% Added hist. recov.	Extraction method
IVY-OYAMA	1921	Dog	Less than 100 in filtered juice	Food	70%	KEETON and KOCH "gastrin" method (1915)
BROWN-SMITH	1935	Man	13—535	Histamine sub-cut.	60%	BEST and MCHENRY (1930)
KOMAROV	1936	Dog	250	Sham feeding	?	Histidine fraction of juice
MACINTOSH	1938	Dog	Ave. 24 (8—95)	Histamine I.V.	90%	Own method
MACINTOSH	1938	Dog	Ave. 8 (3—22)	Vagal stim.	90%	Own method
MACINTOSH	1938	Dog	Ave. 7[1] (2—15)	Sham feeding	90%	Own method
EMMELIN-KAHLSON	1944	Cat	Ave. 25[1] (5—55)	Spontaneous	90—103%	CODE (1937) for blood
	1944	Cat	Ave. 37 (4—150)	Vagal stim.	90—103%	
	1944	Dog	Ave. 34 (25—40)	Vagal stim.	90—103%	
	1944	Dog	Ave. 40 (35—45)	Sham feeding	90—103%	
	1944	Dog	— (30—80)	Meat extract into stomach	90—103%	
	1944	Dog	More than 33; 610 cc juice extracted by CODE method and total injected I.V. into a cat.			
	1944	7 cats	Ave. 34 (20—55)	Uvnäs gastrin	90—103%	
	1944	3 cats	14, 25, and 45	Gastrin + vagal stim.	90—103%	
	1944	Cat	(30—35)	Eserine	90—103%	
	1944	Cat	Ave. 34 (25—40)	Acetyl. choline		
	1944	Cat	Ave. 47 (30—65)	"Priscol", 0.5—1.0 mg/kg/min for 30 to 60 min		
	1944	Cat	Ave. 40 (30—45)	Vagal stim. for 2 to 10 hr, no change in output		
	1944	7 cats	Constant output 16 to 180	Continuous histamine over a 5- to 115-min period		
CODE-HALLENBECK-GREGORY	1947	Dog	Ave. 14 (5—58)[2]	Meat meal	79—81%	CODE (1937)
	1947	Dog	Ave. 16[1] (8—40)	Hypoglycemia		
	1947	Dog	Ave. 16 (5—36)	Histamine sub. cut.		
	1947	3 dogs	Ave. 16 (8—40)	Mecholyl		
	1947	4 dogs	Ave. 44 (7—140)	Mecholyl		
ADAM et al.	1954	Man (3)	Ave. 14 (0.8—1.4)	Spontaneous secretion	67%	ROBERTS ADAMS
	1954	Man (2)	Increased in 8 of 10 Expt. 0.3—31	Histamine I.V. infusion	Increase had no close relation to amount	

[1] BLOCK and NECHELES found none.
[2] 59 of 124 specimes of juice yielded no histamine.

(8 %) histamine could not be detected, in 10 there was only a trace, and in 43 the amount of histamine ranged from 5 to 80 μg/l. The administration of mecholyl subcutaneously or by intravenous infusion produced a juice relatively high in histamine concentration. All the specimens of juice from this type of stimulus contained detectible amounts of histamine, the values ranging from 8 to 140 μg/l. They

could find no good correlation between the *concentration* of histamine and the rate of acid secretion which is in agreement with EMMELIN and KAHLSON. They produced insulin hypoglycemia, which simulates vagal stimulation, in four dogs with PAVLOV pouches. In 11 samples of juice no histamine was found in 3, a trace in 1, and from 6.3 to 25 μg/l in the remainder. No correlation was found between *concentration* of histamine and output of HCl. In 8 PAVLOV pouch dogs 124 specimens of juice, secreted in response to a meal, were assayed. No histamine was found in 31 (25%), a trace in 34 and from 5.0 to 58.8 μg/l in 59 (47%). In 17 experiments in which the histamine was measurable in sequential specimens of juice, it was observed that the *highest concentration* occurred during the first hour after the meal (up to 60 μg/l) and then it leveled off at about 10 μg/l. This suggested a "washing out" process. To check on this suggestion from 0.5 to 10 mg of histamine was given 45 to 90 minutes before feeding the meal. By 45 to 90 minutes the response to histamine was over and "washing out" was completed. When a meat meal was fed after the histamine injection, the initial rise still occurred. The acid output, of course, was highest during the second to third hours when the concentration of histamine in the juice was 5 to 10 μg/l. (One dog consistently secreted so little histamine that no correlation of any kind was possible.)

ADAM et al. (1954a, b), using their method for the extraction of histamine in a study on two human subjects, found histamine to be present in the overnight fasting secretion; the amounts "varied widely." In nine experiments an intravenous infusion of histamine was given. The doses varied from 0.0036 μg/kg/min to 0.1162 μg/kg/min. The concentration of histamine in the resting secretion ranged from 0.8 to 1.4 μg/l; and after intravenous infusion of histamine from 0.3 to 31 μg/l. The histamine excreted in the juice during the infusion increased in 7 of the 9 experiments. The authors state that the increase in excretion bore no close relation to the dose infused. The concentration of histamine in the juice rose slightly in 6 of the 9 experiments. *They point out that the concentration of histamine in "fasting juice" is more variable but in the same range as that in the urine*, which is interesting in that the parietal cells and renal cells both concentrate the substance. Histamine appears to be secreted by the tubular cells of the kidney (LINDELL and SCHAYER, 1958).

No correlation in man between the amount of histamine in the gastric content and the level of gastric secretion (BORBOLA et al., 1951) and no increase in histamine output in the gastric juice was found after a single injection of the histamine (GIBERTINI, 1942). These observations fall within the variations indicated above (Table 5).

3. Relation of histamine in the gastric juice to the output of gastric juice and HCl

MACINTOSH, EMMELIN and KAHLSON, ADAM et al., and CODE et al. in their original publications concluded that there appeared to be no good correlation between the *concentration* of histamine in the gastric juice and the *output* of juice or of the HCl. In 1956, CODE studied the literature regarding the question of the relation of histamine output in micrograms/unit of time (not the μg/l) to the volume and HCl output/unit of time. None of the prior investigators had done this. When he examined MACINTOSH's (1938) data a correlation of 0.86 ($P < .001$) was found between histamine output and the volume of gastric juice secreted by dogs during sham feeding, vagal stimulation and histamine injection. The data of EMMELIN and KAHLSON (1944) obtained on cats during stimulation of the vagus showed a correlation of 0.98 ($P < .001$). The data of ADAM et al. (1954a, b) could not be correlated because the volumes of juice were not published.

CODE et al. (1947) restudied their own data on the juice collected after a meal. *They found that the output of histamine in micrograms in the juice during 30-min periods correlated with the HCl and volume output, except in the first half hour after feeding.* In the first half-hour 0.089 μg of histamine/ml of juice was present; then during the subsequent half-hour periods 0.011 μg/ml was secreted, the correlation being 0.8 ($P<0.001$). Apparently more histamine was required to get the secretion started than to maintain it. After the glands were stimulated an average of 0.048 μg of histamine was excreted for each mEq. of HCl, the correlation coefficient being 0.9 ($P<0.001$). As indicated above, it was found in the original article that the high concentration of histamine during the first half hour was not necessarily due to a "washing out" process.

More recently, BUGAJSKI and KAULBERSZ (1960) found in gastric juice during the first 15 min. of sham feeding, a correlation between the histamine output and HCl output.

4. Comment

The observations made by CODE et al. (1947), and just referred to, suggests the existence of an inertia in the resting parietal cell or the cell that has come to rest after having been recently stimulated, so that more histamine than otherwise is required to enter the cell or to act on the membrane of the cell to start it operating. After it is operating, less histamine is required. Since the histamine entering the cell is greater initially, there will be more excreted in the initial juice per unit of time. Then as the mechanism in the cell operates smoothly on an "all or none" basis, a specific and constant quantity of HCl will be produced and excreted per unit of histamine entering the cell and being excreted. When the available histamine is increased, then more cells are recruited and the volume and HCl output/unit of time increases along with a proportional amount of histamine excreted with it. The recruitment of cells on an "all or none" response basis with an increase in the amount of histamine is best supported by the histological evidence (DAWSON and IVY, 1926). The alternative view is that all the parietal cells are stimulated equally but each one produces gastric juice not on an "all or none" basis but to the extent that histamine enters it and up to its capacity to form secretion. The amount of secretion formed after the cell has started working efficiently will bear a proportion to the histamine excreted.

Why is it physiologically significant to know whether histamine is or is not excreted in the gastric juice quantitatively?

It appears certain that the histamine in the acid secreting mucosa is located in the region of the parietal or acid secreting cells (Figure 2). Whether it is located inside the parietal cells or in adjacent cells is not known. *If, after the ingestion of a meal, histamine is not released into the gastric venous blood to be carried to the parietal cells, where it is excreted into the gastric juice, then the histamine must come from one of the two sources just mentioned. If histamine is not carried away in the blood and is not destroyed because of the lack of histaminase in the mucosa, then it must be secreted quantitatively into the gastric juice; otherwise it would accumulate in the gastric mucosa.*

However, it has not been established that an increment of histamine does *not* enter the gastric venous blood. If it did, a portion (50 %) could enter the systemic arterial blood; then a portion could reach the gastric glands and a portion could be removed by the kidney to prevent histamine in physiological amounts from accumulating in the blood to cause headache. In the latter case, histamine would not have to be excreted quantitatively in the gastric juice. Blood flow would prevent accumulation in the mucosa, and the liver and kidney would maintain a systemic physiological homeostasis of histamine concentration in the plasma.

Unfortunately the evidence presented above is not entirely conclusive. Some of the data show an excellent quantitative excretion of histamine into the juice in relation to the HCl or volume of juice secreted; other data do not. The lack of a better correlation might be expected in view of the inadequacies of the methods. However, the most disturbing feature of the observations of CODE et al. (1947) is the failure to find histamine in detectible amounts in 25 %, and to find only traces in an additional 28 % of specimens of gastric juice secreted after a meal. ADAM et al. (1954a, b) failed to find increments of histamine in the gastric juice in 3 of 9 instances when histamine was infused intravenously at a physiologically rapid rate. The absence of histamine or its presence in only traces may be ascribed to the methods used, and to the factor of dilution. The results may not be consistently reliable for some subtle physiological reason because in certain instances indicated above the correlation coefficients are excellent. Obviously better methods are needed for this type of work because the method used by CODE et al. recovers only about 80 % and that of ADAM et al. only about 66 % of added histamine.

If the methods used are consistently trustworthy, then it must be assumed that under certain types of stimulation, a quantitative relation exists and under others it does not. And, if all the histamine in the corporic mucosa resides in the parietal cells, the possibility that some is used up in the secretory process or is methylated, has to be considered. On the other hand if histamine acts by changing the permeability of the vascular side of the parietal cell membrane, so as to permit the entrance of chloride ions and water, then the extent of the presence of histamine in the juice could be dependent on differences in blood and lymph flow, variations in the permeability of the parietal cell and the rate of its destruction by the methylating enzyme probably present in small amounts in the gastric mucosa (KOBAYASHI and IVY, 1958, 1959; SCHAYER, 1959). Another possibility is that histamine is located in the parietal cells in relation to the oxyntic granules. If so, histamine, like pepsinogen, may move out of the parietal cell into the blood and into the secretion. Since cholinergic agents act synergistically with histamine on the parietal cells, the degree of vagal tone or activity may be involved in the genesis of the variations in the histamine output in the gastric juice.

5. Significance of the amount of histamine in the gastric secretion

This raises the question of the significance of the amount of histamine found in the gastric juice. CODE et al. (1947) found in the juice secreted after a meal 0.006 μg/ml of histamine, and 0.043 μg of histamine was present for each mEq of HCl.

EMMELIN and KAHLSON (1944) intravenously infused 5 anesthetized cats at rates varying from 1.2 μg to 3.0 μg/kg/min for from 10 to 115 minutes. They recovered an average of 0.0025 % in the gastric juice in an average concentration in the juice of 0.045 μg/ml. They pointed out that the concentration of histamine in this histamine stimulated secretion is in the same range as that in the juice obtained under a variety of stimuli, including that which is associated with a "spontaneous" or fasting secretion. ADAM et al. (1954a) in two human subjects intravenously infused histamine in total doses ranging from 44 μg up to 1650 μg over a period of from 162 to 217 min. In nine experiments the increment excreted in the gastric secretion averaged only 0.006 %. The concentrations were within the usual range. The average concentration of histamine in the secretion was 16.5 μg/l or 0.0165 μg/ml. (The CODE et al. and EMMELIN values may be increased by 20 % and the ADAM values by 33 % because of the percentage error of the methods.)

So, when histamine is infused intravenously into cats and human subjects, there may be no increase in histamine concentration in the juice. The same is apparently true of the dog (CODE et al., 1947). When large quantities are infused, the results of some tests suggest that an increase in concentration occurs. The concentration of histamine in the dog's "meal" juice was 0.006 μg/ml, and in the "histamine" juice of the cat 0.045 μg/ml and of man 0.0165 μg/ml.

If, when histamine is intravenously infused in physiological amounts, no increase in histamine output in the gastric secretion occurs, then either the *injected* or exogenous histamine does not enter the parietal cell, or if it does, it only replaces the intrinsic histamine of the cell which was excreted.

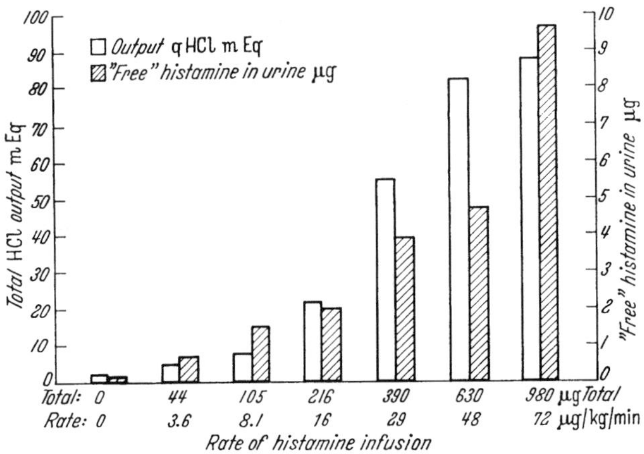

Fig. 5. Effect of intravenous infusion of histamine on gastric secretion and on urinary excretion of "free" histamine in man. Duration of each infusion about 180 min. The dose is shown as the total amount infused (μg) and as the rate (ng/kg/min). From ADAM et al. (1954a). The rough correlation is strong presumptive evidence that the urinary histamine does not come from the renal metabolism. On the basis of histamine infusion (i.v.) studies, only an average of about 1% of that infused is recovered in the urine

So, this discussion teaches that, until we know where the histamine in the juice comes from and more about the plasma-secretion exchange, we cannot with certainty appraise the significance of the presence of histamine in the juice. Data are not now available showing how much of intravenously infused histamine, at physiological rates in the dog of from 0.04 to 1.5 μg/kg/min, actually reaches the stomach. Data are not available for a rough estimate. Granted a guess, it is probably less than one-tenth of that infused.

This leaves us with the established situation that if histamine enters the blood, and if an increment occurs in the amount reaching the stomach and the increment is adequate, secretion will occur. KOMAROV's "gastrin" could act directly on the parietal cell to cause histamine to be released by the oxyntic granules. Mecholyl could act directly on the oxyntic granules. The relation of the action of atropine to the source of histamine in the secretion will be considered later.

When C^{14}-histamine is given by intravenous infusion, some enters the gastric juice unchanged and some in an inactive form with a CH_3 group in the ring. The distribution of the radioactivity is variable (GROSSMAN and KOBAYASHI, personal communication). Since unchanged histamine appears in the secretion, it is now known that exogenous histamine is excreted by the parietal cell. The methylated histamine could come from the methylating enzyme in the gastric mucosa or in the liver. The dog and man have methylating enzyme in the liver. Most of the methylated histamine would be removed by the kidney but some would reach the stomach. It may be excreted like histamine, but is inactive on gastric secretion (IVY and LIEPINS, 1958). This supports in a crucial way those data in the literature obtained by the chemical-extraction method, which show that after an infusion of histamine some of it is excreted or secreted into the gastric juice.

The variation in histamine output may be due to a variation in the methylating enzyme, and perhaps to ACh stimulated secretion, as stated before.

Reference to Figure 5 shows a good correlation between the excretion of "free" histamine in the urine and the HCl in the gastric juice with increasing doses of histamine infused intravenously in man.

E. Histamine in urine

1. Historical background

Although several attempts to find histamine in the urine were made prior to 1936, GADDUM in that year concluded that histamine was not normally excreted by the kidneys. However, in 1921, IVY and OYAMA, when they applied the KEETON-KOCH method for "gastrin" to the secretion of a pyloric pouch dog, also applied it to the 24-hour output of the urine of canine and human subjects on a mixed diet, finding in it a gastric secretory response equivalent from 0.2 to 0.3 mg of histamine dihydrochloride. The possible significance of the observation at the time was not appreciated. BEST and MCHENRY (1930) also using a method of acid hydrolysis, found 0.2 mg of histamine in one kilogram of dog's urine. ACKERMANN and FUCHS, in 1939, isolated 0.9 mg (0.18 mg of the base) of histamine dipicrate from a liter of normal urine. It was not chemically identified because of the small quantity.

This subject was greatly clarified in 1944 when ANREP et al. found very small amounts of "free" histamine and a relatively large amount of a conjugated histamine in dog's urine. They converted the relatively "inactive" conjugated histamine into "free" histamine by hydrolysis with HCl for biological assay of the quantity of histamine base present.

When a dog was fed a meat diet they found in a 72-hour specimen of urine 20 mg of histamine expressed as the phosphate. Sixty per cent of this amount was excreted in 24 hours after a meal of meat. When histamine was given orally to a dog, 5% of it was eliminated in the urine in the conjugated form. Parenterally administered histamine was eliminated in traces only in a "free" form. Carnivora excreted chiefly the conjugated form and Herbivora the free form. Both in varying proportions were present in rat's urine. The work of ANREP et al. (1944) was confirmed by ROSENTHAL and TABOR (1948). URBACH (1949), using paper chromatography, separated the free from the conjugated histamine in the urine and found that the conjugated histamine in urine was probably identical with N-acetyl histamine. The observations of TABOR and MOSETTIG (1949) demonstrated that the substance was N-acetyl histamine and that it was produced by the action of intestinal bacteria. The bacterial source of urinary conjugated histamine was clearly established by LIVINGSTONE and CODE (1955).

So, it is now evident that the failure to find a gastric secretory dose, or any other signs of histamine activity in the urine of canine and human subjects on a mixed diet, was apparently due to inadequate methods.

2. Methods for determination of histamine and acetyl histamine in urine

In 1950, ADAM reported a new method for the determination of "free" and conjugated histamine in the urine, which they considered to be an improvement over the method of ANREP et al. (1944). The ANREP method consists in determining the free histamine by charcoal adsorption since conjugated histamine was not adsorbed. The total histamine is determined on a second sample of urine after it is hydrolized. The difference between the free and total represents the conjugated histamine. The percentage recovery of added histamine by charcoal absorption ranged from 83 to 100 (mean, 90) and by hydrolysis from 90 to 110 (mean, 99). ROBERTS and ADAM (1950) found that acetyl histamine could be separated from histamine because the former was all absorbed at pH 8 and none of the latter until a pH of 9.5 was reached. They reported that their method recovered 67 ± 1.1 % (S.E.) of added histamine in a range of from 10 to 250 μg/liter. Added acetyl or conjugated histamine was recovered to the extent of 80 to 90 % in a range of from 0.5 to 20 μg/ml.

3. Observations in Man

Using their method, ADAM (1950), ROBERTS and ADAM (1950) and ADAM et al. (1950—1951, 1954a, b) found that when 133 mg of histamine base was given by mouth to fasting human subjects from 0.17 to 1.0 % of that given was obtained as the conjugate in the urine. The "free" histamine increased from 4 for the control to 17 μg in the first 6-hour period in one subject and from 5 to 16 μg in a second subject. In two other subjects 0.55 and 1.2 % of the oral dose of 133 mg was recovered in the urine, the free histamine output increasing from a trace to 7 μg/6-hour period in one and from a trace to 15 μg/6-hour period in another. The first 6-hour specimen after taking the histamine was the highest for "free" histamine and the 6- to 12-hour specimen was the highest for the conjugated. In a total of five subjects receiving 133 mg of histamine orally, the average increment of "free" and conjugated histamine in the first 12-hour specimen was 21 and 806 μg, respectively. This is a ratio of 1 μg of "free" to 36 μg of the conjugated. The increment in the "free" and conjugated histamine was 0.016 % and 0.66 % of the 133 mg of the histamine orally administered.

4. Observations in animals

In the dog, rabbit and guinea pig 10 to 20 % of the orally administered histamine is excreted in the urine in a conjugated form and only traces of an increment of "free" histamine are detected when relatively large amounts are given. In the mouse and rat, the excretion of both forms is relatively quite large. In two rats receiving 40 mg of histamine orally, 22 % and 11 % appeared in the urine in the "free" and conjugated forms, respectively. In 2 rats receiving 20 mg, 15 % and 8 % was excreted, respectively, in the "free" and conjugated form (MILLICAN et al., 1949). According to body weight the amounts of histamine given the animals was out of proportion to that given in the human tests (ANREP et al., 1944; URBACH 1949; MILLICAN et al., 1949).

5. Parenterally administered histamine

ADAM et al. (1950—1951, 1954a, b) confirmed ANREP et al. (1944) in finding that parenterally administered histamine increased the renal excretion of "free" but not conjugated histamine. When 5 mg of histamine was injected intravenously 1 % was recovered in the urine in the "free" form and none in the conjugated form. In six experiments, human subjects received 3.3 to 7.25 mg of histamine intravenously during a period of 180 min. The control 6-hour output of urinary "free" histamine averaged 8 μg and that for the first 6-hour output after the infusion 71 μg.

In five healthy men consuming their ordinary mixed diet, the 24-hour output of "free" histamine in the urine on six different days ranged from 12.1 to 41.4 μg daily. The values for the conjugated histamine ranged from 16 to 727 μg. The mean of 30 daily outputs was 21.6 μg for free and 125 μg for conjugated histamine. The range of the concentration of free histamine in the urine was 8 to 33 μg/liter. ADAM et al. (1950—1951) in 10 normal and convalescent subjects on a mixed hospital diet found a mean "free" histamine excretion of 8.6 ± 2.3 (S.E.) μg/24-hr and of 29.6 ± 3.4/24-hr for conjugated histamine. In 9 patients with urticaria the average free and conjugated histamine was 35.8 ± 8.4 (S.E.) and 44.1 ± 8.8, respectively. In 10 patients with other diseases the values for "free" and conjugated histamine were 15.4 ± 3.4 and 24.3 ± 7.4, respectively. The higher value for the urticarial patients was due to two patients with acute urticaria due to penicillin at the time the urine was collected. It should be mentioned that these values for free and conjugated histamine represent a recovery of only 67 % and 95 %, respectively.

So, it is now clear why so many early investigators failed to find histamine in the urine in detectible quantities. In the case of "free" histamine, only an average of 21 μg or 0.021 mg was present in the 24-hour output of urine, and if isolated completely, it would not be enough to stimulate gastric secretion in a dog when given subcutaneously. However, if a method which hydrolyzed the acetyl histamine were used, then an average output of 146μg (21 + 125 μg) or 0.146 mg would be obtained on the average, and at times as much as 0.5 mg on a meat diet (ANREP et al. 1944). This checks well with the yields obtained by IVY and OYAMA when they used the KEETON-KOCH "gastrin" method and by BEST and McHENRY (1930) when they used their method.

6. Infusion into the portal vein

LIVINGSTONE and CODE (1955) have reported that when histamine was injected by continuous infusion into the portal vein, the recovery of free histamine is about one-half of that recovered when a similar infusion is given into a systemic vein. IRVINE et al. (1959a) found that the rate of histamine infusion in the portal vein must be twice greater than in the femoral vein in order obtain about the same degree of HCl output by a gastric pouch and of urinary free histamine output.

7. Relation of histamine excretion in urine and gastric juice

ADAM et al. (1954a) studied the relation of the rate of the intravenous infusion of histamine to the HCl output in the gastric juice and the output of histamine in the urine in three human subjects. As indicated before, they found a good correlation between the rate of infusion and the HCl output, as others had found (Figure 5). More important, they observed that the threshold rate for an increase in the output of HCl and for an increase in "free" histamine output in the urine was the same, namely, from 0.0074 μg/kg/min to 0.013 μg/kg/min. They found that only 1 % of the histamine infused was recovered in the urine and this was independent of the rate of infusion or the amount infused. Headache and flushing did not occur until the dose exceeded 0.030 μg/kg/min. A dose of 0.026 μg/kg/min produced an average output of 2.5 mEq (91.2 mg) of HCl every 20 minutes without headache and flushing. If this secretion continued at the same rate for 24 hours, the output of HCl would be approximately equivalent to the 1800 ml of N/10 gastric juice.

8. Gastric secretory equivalent of free histamine values in the urine of man

At the rate of a "free" histamine excretion of 0.02 μg/kg/min ADAM et al. (1954a,b) calculated that a 70 kilo man would produce endogenously 2000 μg in 24 hours, which if infused slowly intravenously would maintain the basal acid secretion. It would be even more if the threshold of the gastric glands in a subject was 0.004 μg/kg/min of histamine, the mean threshold, rather than 0.010 μg/kg/min. Furthermore, their value of 0.02 μg/kg/min was the amount found which represented probably only 67 % of the free histamine found in the urine in the experiment on which they based their calculation.

The foregoing data on the free histamine found in the urine of human subjects under certain conditions, represents an amount which would stimulate HCl output. It would appear that if such an experiment were performed on a larger group of human subjects the gastric secretory equivalent of "free" histamine in the urine might be established.

MITCHELL and CODE (1954) employed the method of ADAM et al. for the assay of "free" and conjugated histamine in the urine in a study of the effect of diet. They obtained an average recovery of added histamine of 67 %, the same reported by ADAM et al. They gave orally to 3 human subjects 30 mg of histamine base after they had fasted for 24 hours. During the first 12-hour period, 1.7 % of the histamine was recovered from the urine in the conjugated form without obtaining a significant increase in the excretion of "free" histamine. Similarly, when ADAM (1950) and ADAM et al. (1950—1951) gave to human subjects a larger oral dose, namely, 67 mg of the base, no significant increase in the urinary excretion of free histamine was obtained. However, when ADAM (1950) and ADAM et al. (1950—1951) gave 133 mg of the base orally a small but definite increase in "free" histamine was observed in 4 of 5 subjects. This is significant because IVY and JAVOIS (1924—1925) found that, when 225 mg of histamine di-HCl or 150 mg of the base was given orally to human subjects, gastric secretion was stimulated. Sixty to 100 mg of the base orally stimulated gastric secretion in pouch dogs. *Thus it appears that when enough histamine is given orally to result in an increase in the urinary excretion of "free" histamine, a stimulation of gastric secretion occurs.* This observation supports the suggestion that a gastric secretory equivalent of orally administered histamine might be established on the basis of the "free" histamine in the urine and confirms the report (ADAM et al., 1954a) that the threshold dosage rate of histamine for an increase in HCl output and for an increase in "free" histamine in the urine is the same.

9. Effect of diet in man on the urinary excretion of histamine

MITCHELL and CODE (1954) used the method of ADAM et al. in a well designed experiment on 5 human subjects to ascertain the relation of the diet to the urinary excretion of free and conjugated histamine (Tables 6 and 7). The subjects after

Table 6. *Mean and range values for the 24-hr renal excretion of free and conjugated (acetyl) histamine by human subjects under various dietary conditions.* (Values not corrected for a 67 % recovery)

Author	Diet	No. Subj.	Urinary histamine μg/24 hr				Method for histamine
			Free		Conjugated		
			Mean	Range	Mean	Range	
ADAM et al.[3] (1954a, b)	mixed	10	8.6±2.3[1]	tr—27	29.6±3.4[1]	6— 48	ADAM et al.
ROBERTS-ADAM[4] (1950)	mixed	5	21.6[2]	12.1—41.4	125	16— 727	ADAM et al.
MITCHELL-Code (1954)	fasting	5	10.7	5.6—15.6	28	6— 60	ADAM et al.
MITCHELL-CODE (1954)	mixed	5	15.0	7.5—21.2	160	22— 900	ADAM et al.
MITCHELL-CODE (1954)	bread-milk	5	10.9	6.2—22.2	42	10— 235	ADAM et al.
MITCHELL-CODE (1954)	meat 700—800 g	5	25.4	7.6—48.5	340	17—2311	ADAM et al.

[1] S. E. [2] When corrected for 67 % recovery of added histamine, the 21.6 μg represents 32.4 μg.
[3] Convalescent patients and healthy subjects. [4] Healthy subjects.

consuming a mixed diet for three days, fasted for three days, then ingested a diet of bread and milk on the 7th and 8th days, and then 700 to 800 gm of meat daily on the 9th through the 11th day (Table 7). During fasting the excretion of "free" histamine ranged from 5.6 to 15.6 μg/24-hour, the mean being 10.7. On a mixed diet the subjects showed a mean excretion of 15 μg/24-hour, with a range of from 7.5 to 21.2 μg. As indicated above, the value of ADAM et al. for 10 subjects on a mixed diet was a mean of 8.6 ± 2.3 μg for free histamine, the range being from a trace to 27. These are good checks. When the diet of bread and milk was consumed, the mean for free histamine was 12.9 μg/24-hour, the range 6.2 to 22.2.

When the subjects consumed a diet of meat, the mean output for free histamine was 25.4 μg/24-hour and the conjugated was 340. Their observations on the

Table 7. *Output of free histamine in the urine of five human subjects on various diets.* Data from MITCHELL and CODE (1954)

Diet	Days of test	Ave. daily free histamine in urine, micrograms/24 hours										Total daily for group		Ave. daily for group		% Free H of total
		Subject														
		A		B		C		D		E						
		F	C	F	C	F	C	F	C	F	C	F	C	F	C	
mixed	1-3	7.8	22	17.5	531	14.4	38	17.9	80	13.8	128	71.4[1]	800	14.3[1]	160	8% of 174
fasting	4-6	7.1	12	14.5	52	9.6	21	12.9	39	9.6	14	53.7	178	10.7	36	23%
bread and	7-8	7.1	12	14.7	103	11.3	16	14.1	16	17.1	9	64.3	156	12.8	31	30%
meat	9-11	9.1	42	40	1200	18.0	322	40.3	82	29.7	42	127.1	1688	25.4	338	7% of 363

[1] 71.4 : 5 = 14.3. F = free histamine; C = conjugated histamine.

effect of a meat diet (700–800 gm daily) confirmed those of ANREP et al. (1944) on the rat, dog and man. ANREP et al. (1944) in the rat, in one experiment, found that free histamine excretion in the urine on feeding meat was increased from 8 to 18 μg/24-hour and that conjugated histamine was increased from 3 to 60 μg/24-hour. In dogs the conjugated histamine increased very markedly (10 mg/24-hour) and "free" histamine was not found. This may have been due to a difficulty in the method in view of the very large amount of conjugated histamine present. In one man on a meat diet they found free histamine in the urine, and a much larger quantity of conjugated histamine.

10. Source of the urinary histamine on a meat diet

Fasting: MITCHELL and CODE (1954) suggested that the basal or fasting output of free histamine (5.6 to 15.6, ave. 10.7 μg/day) represents a small portion, 1% or perhaps 2%, of the daily basal metabolic release or turn-over of the body and is independent of digestion (Table 6). A question arises then regarding whether the average 10.7 μg/24-hour output of "free" histamine is enough to account for the occasional appearance of acid in the fasting secretion of some persons. If the mean of 10.7 μg/24-hour represents 67% recovery of the free histamine in the urine by the method used, then 16 μg were actually present. If the 16 μg represents 1% of the fasting metabolic release, then 1600 μg were released into the blood in 24 hours. This would amount to 0.016 μg/kg/min in a 70 kg man. Histamine infused at this rate would stimulate the output of HCl in more than 50% of human subjects, since the average required is 0.004 μg/kg/min (HANSON et al., 1948). See Table 4.

Meat: In regard to the increase in "free" and conjugated histamine in the urine when a meal is ingested ANREP et al. (1944) and MITCHELL and CODE (1954) believed that they might come from the histamine in the meat. MITCHELL and CODE also suggested that some of the "free" histamine might come from the release of histamine as a result of the operation of digestive mechanisms set in motion by the meat meal. Both, of course, may be involved. This was reasonable for the conjugated histamine for the following reasons: ANREP et al. (1944) had found that 60 % of orally administered and 100 % of intravenously administered conjugated histamine was excreted in the urine, and that when histamine was given *parenterally* all of it was excreted in the "free" form in the urine.

Since skeletal muscle of cattle contains approximately 5 μg/gm of histamine (FELDBERG, 1956) and since 700 gm of cattle meat was ingested daily by the human subjects of MITCHELL and CODE, they consumed about 3500 μg or 3.5 mg of histamine daily. The subjects excreted in the urine an average of 340 μg or 10 % of the ingested histamine as conjugated histamine. This 340 μg represents the total absorption of conjugated histamine because, according to ANREP et al. (1944), all conjugated histamine which is given into the blood is excreted as such in the urine. *Thus, the excretion of the observed conjugated histamine excreted can easily be accounted for by the histamine in the meat.*

But, 3500 μg or 3.5 mg of histamine taken orally is far too small to stimulate gastric secretion. At least 133 to 150 mg of histamine base orally is required. Furthermore, with such doses ADAM (1950) and ADAM et al (1950-51) recovered in the urine only about 1 % of the oral dose of histamine, which in this case would be only 35 μg, instead of the 340 μg found. So, the meat contributed to the production of acetyl histamine to the extent of 35 μg. The remainder, 325 μg, must have come from the bacterial production of histamine and then acetyl histamine from histidine in the meat and also from substances such as *beta-alanylhistamine* which chemically react like acetyl histamine.

Regarding the increase in "free" histamine in the urine observed after a meat meal in man, it should be recalled that the increment in the output over the fasting output represents only 1 % of the total available in the circulation for the stimulation of gastric secretion. The observed increment over the fasting output amounted to about 15 μg (25.4 after the meal minus 10.7, mean fasting output = 14.7, or 15) (Table 6). It is very unlikely that any of this 15 μg came from histamine in the meat for two reasons. One is that when 133 mg of histamine base is given orally to man, the increment in the free histamine in the urine amounts to only 11 to 13 μg, and only 3.5 mg of histamine was in the meat. The other is that when C^{14}-histamine was given orally to a man (SCHAYER, 1956 c), it all appeared in the urine as methylimidazole acetic acid, not histamine. This might be expected in view of the large amount of histaminase in the intestinal mucosa, as well as of the methylating enzyme in the intestinal mucosa and the liver. So, the increment of 15 μg of free histamine or most probably 22 μg[1], represented a total of 2200 μg of free histamine released into the circulation by digestive mechanisms (Table 6).

11. The use of urinary "free" histamine in the study of various phases of gastric secretion in dogs

a) Meat meal

UPDIKE et al.(1958) collected the urine and gastric secretion in 6 dogs with gastric pouches (HEIDENHAIN type). For the determination of urinary free hista-

[1] 15 ÷ 67% recovery = 0.22 × 100 = 22 μg, or 100% recovery. 22 μg represents a 1% recovery in the urine of the total circulating histamine resulting from eating the meal. 2200 ÷ 1440 = 1.53 μg/min which would be 0.022 μg/kg/min in a 70 kg person. The threshold stimulus for an average man is 0.004 μg/kg/min. So, there is plenty of histamine released from some source to stimulate gastric secretion.

mine they used the method of ROBERTS and ADAM (1950), and with it recovered 65 % ± 4.4 (S.E.) of added histamine. After feeding a meal of 170 gm of horse meat, they found a remarkable correlation in most dogs between the hourly output of free HCl in the gastric juice and of free histamine in the urine. The correlation

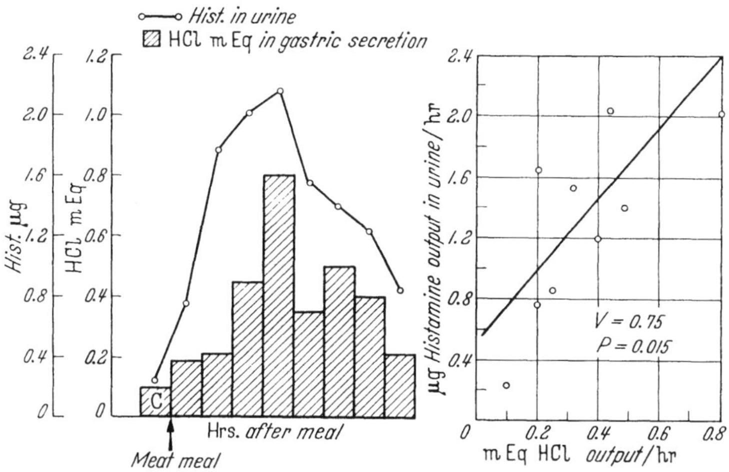

Fig. 6. Correlation between mean hourly outputs of free histamine in the urine and free HCl in the gastric juice from 4 Heidenhain pouch dogs after the ingestion of a meal of meat. The histamine in the urine on the basis of histamine infusion (i.v.) studies represents a mean recovery of only 1%. From IRVINE and CODE (1958)

was good in all dogs. In one dog 20 such experiments were performed. The HCl secreted in mEq was plotted against the μg output of free histamine in the urine. A correlation coefficient of 0.68 (P < 0.001) was found. IRVINE and CODE (1958) repeated the foregoing experiment in four gastric pouch dogs (HEIDENHAIN) and

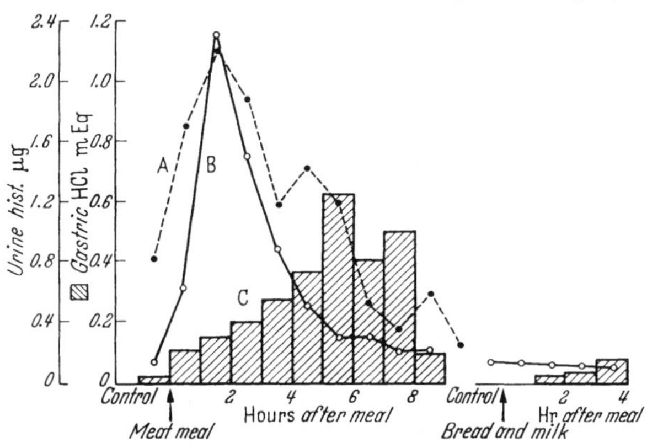

Fig. 7. Correlation between urinary histamine output in 3 total gastrectomized dogs and 3 Heidenhain pouch dogs with a gastric and jejunal fistula before and after a meal of 170 gm meat in 10 tests and bread and milk in 4 tests, the food being injected into the jejunum. Infusion (i.v.) studies on histamine show that the μg recovered in the urine by the method amounts to a mean of about 1% of that infused, and the value for the urine represents only about 66% of that actually present. From IRVINE and CODE (1958)
A = ● - - - ● Urinary output of "free" histamine in 3 gastrectomized dogs in 5 tests before and after meal of meat (Fig. 4, Ref.). B = ○—○ Urinary output of "free" histamine in 3 Heidenhain pouch dogs with gastric and jejunal fistula before and after a meal of meat in 10 tests and bread and milk in 4 tests on 4 dogs was injected into *jenunum*. C = Columns give mEq HCl output from pouch (Fig. 3, Ref.)

after a meal of 170 gm of horse meat found a good correlation between the hourly output of free histamine in the urine and the mEq of HCl output in the gastric secretion (Figures 6 and 7). In 10 tests on one dog the correlation coefficient between the two values was 0.75 (P = 0.015) (Figure 6).

b) Bread-milk meal

IRVINE and CODE (1958) fed their dogs a meal consisting of 150 gm of milk and 50 gm of bread. (It is well known that dogs in the U.S.A. do not secrete well in response to such a meal; also, they do not respond well to sham-feeding with such a meal. This is stated because exceptions are seen in the U.S.A., and the older literature is replete with examples of good secretory responses on "black bread" and milk or without milk in dogs.) In four tests on 4 dogs, very little secretion of HCl occurred and the free histamine in the urine remained the same (Figure 7).

c) Comment

On the basis of the data obtained in the experiments on the response to meat, one could hardly desire a better comparative method for the assay of "free" histamine in the urine; and, in view of the inherent difficulties in such experiments, could not expect better correlations than those obtained. This was also true of the observations of MITCHELL and CODE (1954) referred to above in their studies on fasting, oral histamine administration and diets of meat and bread and milk.

d) Control intravenous infusion of saline solution

Since in all experiments of IRVINE and CODE a catheter was in the urinary bladder and saline (0.45 %) was given intravenously to insure a good urinary volume output, a control test of the effect of such an infusion on the output of HCl in the gastric secretion and of "free" histamine in the urine was performed. The control infusion was given over a period of six hours to 2 dogs. Surprisingly the hourly "free" histamine output in the urine remained unchanged, testifying to the apparent validity of the method, but the HCl output increased the first hour from a control level of about 0.1 to 0.6 mEq and remained at an average level of 0.4 mEq for 6 hours. In a second dog the same type of data were obtained except the acid output was not so much.

e) Continuous intravenous infusion of histamine

Two dogs with HEIDENHAIN pouches were used. They received histamine at a rate of 2 μg/kg/hr or 0.033 μg/kg/min., and at a rate of 20 μg/kg/hr, or 0.33 μg/kg/min. The first is a threshold secretory rate for the dog and the second a decided stimulatory rate. With the low rate, one dog secreted 1.4 mEq of HCl in 4 hours and the other about 0.8 mEq, and the urinary "free" histamine was roughly increased correspondingly. With the larger rate the first dog secreted quite copiously, more than in response to the meat meal; the second dog secreted likewise. *The urinary "free" histamine in the first dog increased from an hourly control level of 0.1 μg/hr to a level of 2.4 μg/hr for four hours*, the second dog increased to an average output of 2.8 μg/hr for 4 hours. In these tests, as in most of the others, *the effect of the saline solution alone was controlled for one hour prior to the introduction of histamine;* in other tests two hours before introducing the stimulus. UPDIKE et al. (1958) gave intravenous infusions of histamine to 5 dogs with HEIDENHAIN pouches. The rate of infusion of 0.083 μg/kg/min. produced not quite as much HCl as the meat meal and a rate of infusion of 0.33 μg/kg/hr produced more HCl than the meat meal. The meat meal was associated with the secretion of twice as much free histamine in the urine/mEq of HCl secreted than when 0.083 μg/kg/min. of histamine was given by intravenous infusion.

f) Comment

A portion of the increase in HCl output may have been due to the infusion fluid, but not all; and none of the increase in urinary histamine output can be due to the saline infusion, because of the prior control. The data provide no explanation of why twice as much "free" histamine per mEq of HCl was found in the urine after a meat meal than after an intravenous histamine infusion. This would be of considerable interest if the difference had been shown to be statistically significant.

g) Hypoglycemia

Hypoglycemia was induced with insulin in 5 tests on two dogs. *The histamine output in the urine did not increase above that of the two hour control period* for a period of four hours. Gastric secretion increased decidedly and during four hours the average output of HCl was 1.4 mEq/hr (Irvine and Code, 1958).

This is a very provocative result. Its implications will be discussed now because, like the control intravenous saline solution, it is contrary to the results of other tests because urinary "free" histamine did not increase with the HCl output.

Since the output of urinary "free" histamine was approximately the same during each of the two hours of control, and during each of the four hours after the increased HCl output due to hypoglycemia occurred, it is difficult to suspect the method. Furthermore, the use of the method yielded consistent results in numerous other tests. So, the result strongly indicates that *in a type of vagal stimulation of the parietal cells enough histamine is not released into the blood to increase the output of free histamine in the urine.* On the contrary, the literature indicates that sham-feeding, hypoglycemia, electrical vagal stimulation, and acetylcholine and mecholyl increase the output of histamine in the gastric secretion. And, when histamine is infused, its output in the urine is increased. Why then did not the urinary histamine go up when the vagal center was excited by hypoglycemia? If the experimental data are accepted as they appear to be, they clearly teach either (a) that histamine is located in the parietal cell and that postganglion vagal nerve endings in contact with the parietal cell stimulate the parietal cell to release histamine and HCl, under which condition no histamine enters the blood to reach the urine, or (b) that the vagal nerve endings release acetylcholine which in turn stimulates the parietal cell to release histamine and HCl, under which condition no histamine enters the blood. If histamine were released by vagal nerve endings outside the cell, then some histamine would or could enter the blood and increase the "free" histamine output in the urine. This subject merits further study.

The remainder of the findings of Code and his collaborators in which an increase in the output of free histamine occurred in the urine along with an increase in acid output, are explicable on the basis either (a) that histamine was released into the blood by the gastric and intestinal mucosa, or (b) that Komarov's "gastrin" was released by the meat and in turn released histamine outside the parietal cell, so that it could pass into the blood and gastric juice.

Irvine and Code (1958) wrote that their results were perplexing and that the method they used was not very accurate in their hands. The method admittedly recovers only 67 % of added histamine. Nevertheless it yielded very consistent results, as evidenced by the curves published, except in two experiments.

Instead of being perplexing, the results of Irvine and Code may be considered to be very challenging because they place in jeopardy the theory that histamine is the final common stimulator of the parietal cell. Their results suggest a way to test, probably in a crucial manner, whether sham-feeding, hypoglycemia, vagal stimulation, and cholinergic drugs act on the parietal cells and cause them to release HCl and histamine into their secretion, without any histamine passing into the blood and then into the urine. *The use of C^{14}-L-histidine to label the histamine in the gastric mucosa and which should be released on vagal stimulation, according to the final common stimulator theory, may facilitate the task.*

h) *Intestinal phase*

Irvine and Code (1958) *assayed* the urine for "free" histamine in three totally gastrectomized dogs. Five tests were made. The urine was collected hourly before and for 10 hours after ingestion of a meal of meat, consisting of 170 gm of horse meat which is low in histamine (Feldberg, 1956). The urinary excretion of free histamine increased from a control of 0.41 to 1.7 μg in the first hour, 2.2 in the second, 1.8 in the third, and then decreased to the control level after 6.5 hours.

The rise and fall in the curve of the urinary "free" histamine output was almost the same as that of the average curves obtained with the meat meal in Heidenhain pouch dogs (Figure 7). This indicated, as pointed out above, that *perhaps no histamine is released into the blood to appear in the urine during the cephalic phase, only during the gastric and intestinal phases.*

i) *Gastric and intestinal phase*

Irvine and Code (1958) attempted to determine the effect of placing a meat meal into the stomach or into the intestine on the urinary excretion of "free" histamine. They first used three dogs with Heidenhain pouches and an upper jejunal fistula. When they introduced the meat meal into the jejunum, the urinary output of free histamine increased as though the animal had received the meal by mouth. The HCl output also increased to reach a peak during the third and fourth hour, as is usually the case with Heidenhain pouch dogs.

It was thought that the similarity in the HCl and urinary output curves might be due to the regurgitation of some of the food into the stomach. The experiments were repeated with gastric suction. The results were essentially the same. The peak output of histamine in the urine being reached 1 to 3 hours before the peak output of HCl. It requires a longer period of stimulation for a Heidenhain pouch to start secretion, because the vagus nerves to it have been cut, than a Pavlov pouch which still has some vagal innervation. It would be of interest to repeat the experiment in the presence of subthreshold mecholyl sensitization of the vagally denervated pouch.

To avoid the mechanical effects of the suction tubes in the stomach, and such effects are well known to exist, five dogs with a Heidenhain pouch were prepared with an operative occlusion of the pyloric orifice and an upper jejunal fistula. The meat meal was placed into the stomach for four hours and then removed and placed into the jejunum for four hours. The urinary histamine was not increased with the food in the stomach although the HCl output was increased. But, when the meat was placed into the intestine, the histamine output in the urine increased, and the HCl output increased but not as much as when the meal was in the stomach. The failure for the urinary output to increase when the meat was in the stomach was unexpected since histamine or Komarov's "gastrin" should have been released. However, when a control test was performed with the tube in the stomach and jejunum and an intravenous infusion of saline was given and no meat introduced, the urinary excretion of "free" histamine did not increase but the output of acid did, indicating cholinergic stimulation of the parietal cell.

As IRVINE and CODE (1958) indicate in their article, some of their results are unexpected and difficult to explain. A completely tenable explanation cannot be offered until further experiments are done.

However, the only two experiments in which IRVINE and CODE observed a rise in output of HCl without a rise in "free" histamine output in the urine, was (a) in the presence of hypoglycemia, which is associated with vagal excitation of the gastric glands, and (b) in the presence of tubes in the stomach and jejunum with an infusion of saline solution. Since the stomach was obstructed and filled with a 170 gm meal, the release of histamine or KOMAROV's "gastrin" may have been inhibited, (GROSSMAN et al., 1945) and the secretion of HCl observed may have been due to ACh or to the intravenous infusion of saline which is not consistent in its effect on secretion (HALE et al., 1950).

j) *Urinary histamine excretion before and after transplantation of the pyloric portion of the stomach to the colon*

This operation was done in three dogs by UPDIKE et al (1958). Before the transplantation the results of 17 tests on the three dogs showed a mean fasting 24-hour output of HCl of 0.11 mEq and a mean urinary "free" histamine output of 1.98 μg. In 9 tests after the operation the average 24-hour fasting output of HCl increased to 5.55 mEq and the urinary output of histamine to 2.25 μg. An increase in acid output occurred with an increase in "free" histamine excretion in the urine.

The cause of the hypersecretion which occurs after the transplantation of the pyloric portion of the stomach into the colon, is in a state of controversy at present. Some have failed to see it. Some believe the hypersecretion is due to a hypersecretion of KOMAROV's "gastrin" or of histamine, and others believe it is due to the absence of acid inhibition resulting from the production of an inhibitory hormone by the pyloric mucosa which inhibits HCl formation, or the absence of an inhibition of the release of "gastrin", or the absence of a reflex vagal inhibition of HCl formation (GROSSMAN, 1960; WOODWARD, 1960; IVY and MCILVAIN, 1923).

It would be of interest to transplant a portion of the colon into the colon by the same method used to transplant the pyloric portion of the stomach into the colon, and to study acid and "free" histamine outputs. Also, the dogs used in this work in many instances had not fully recovered from the trauma of the operation, and the post-operative dates of the tests have not been published. A post-operative period of 3 or 4 weeks is required for the secretion of pouches to become stabilized.

12. Effect of antibacterial agent on urinary free histamine excretion after a meal of meat

The stimulation of gastric secretion after the oral administration of histamine in the dog, was shown by observations of IVY and JAVOIS (1924-25), who also found that this would occur in the human subject without the appearance of systemic effects.

IRVINE et al. (1959 b) used the method of ROBERTS and ADAM (1950) to assay the urine for "free" histamine after a meal of meat (150 gm) with and without reducing the bacterial flora with succinylsulphathiazole. After a meat meal in four subjects, the control excretion of free histamine in the urine rose from a control output of 0.7 μg/hr to 3.6 μg/hr the third hour after which it returned to about 1 μg/hr. After the sulfa drug (12 gm daily) had been given for five days, the meat meal caused no rise in the "free" histamine in the urine. When 4.5 gm of L-histidine (the amount in the meat meal) was given orally without pretreatment with sulfa drug, the curve of increase in urinary "free" histamine output was like that obtained with 150 gm of meat. When the L-histidine was given after antibiotic treatment for 5 days, no increase in urinary "free" histamine occurred. A dog was given, orally, 10 mg of histamine with and without oral pretreatment with succinylsulphathiazole and the gastric HCl output and urinary output of "free" histamine was followed hourly. The gastric secretory response to the oral histamine (100 mg) and the urinary "free" histamine output was decidedly greater after the succinylsulphathiazole.

The dog weighed about 20 kg and when given the 100 mg dose of histamine orally without the sulfa drug, showed a slight but definite increase (0.3 mEq in 4 hours) in HCl output. The mean intravenous threshold rate for the stimulation of gastric secretion in the dog is 0.04 μg/kg/min. The secretion remained stimulated for at least 180 min. So, it is possible to calculate the amount of histamine absorbed as "free" histamine during the 180 min. Since the dog weighed 20 kg and required 0.04 μg/kg/min for a threshold dose, he must have absorbed 0.8 μg/kg/min. The dog's secretion was stimulated for 180 min., so the total amount of histamine absorbed was 144 μg. But since the liver removes about half of the histamine given into the portal vein (LIVINGSTON and CODE, 1955), the actual total absorption was around 288 μg or 0.288 mg. Since 144 μg entered the systemic circulation, and 1.1 μg was excreted as "free" histamine in the urine, 0.8% of that absorbed appeared in the urine as "free" histamine. After 5 days of pretreatment with the sulfa drug, the output of acid, after the oral histamine, was 17.3 mEq compared with 0.3 mEq, and the output of urinary "free" histamine was 2.85 μg for 4 hours compared with 1.1 μg, or 2.6 times 1.1 μg. Since the 2.85 μg is equivalent to 0.8% of that which passed the liver, then roughly 360 μg passed the liver.

The experiment should be checked by the use of a C^{14}-histamine tracer, which may prove to be more sensitive. It should be done on a gastric pouch dog. The result would categorically establish that the agent, passing into the portal blood and general circulation to stimulate the gastric glands, was histamine and not a "gastrin" released from the mucosa as a result of the contact with it of histamine. *Otherwise, no stronger evidence than provided by this experiment of* IRVINE *et al. could be produced showing that the gastric secretory excitant absorbed* into the blood and stimulating the parietal cells was histamine. The C^{14}-histamine given orally could also be isolated as a small part in the gastric juice.

Knowing the uncontrollable variations which occur in this type of work, one would feel more certain regarding the interpretation of the results of such a well designed study, if more tests of each type were performed so that an average of at least 5 or 10 tests were available.

F. Absorption of histamine from the intestine

1. Portocaval shunt (Eck fistula)

Since 1932, considerable interest has been directed to a study of the hypersecretion which occurs in a HEIDENHAIN pouch before and after the production of an Eck Fistula or a portocaval shunt (LEBEDINSKAJA, 1932). The entire literature on this topic will not be reviewed. Only those reports which bear directly on the nature of the substance which gets into the systemic circulation to stimulate gastric secretion will be referred to. The hypersecretion is definite and is known to continue for at least two months. The agent supposed to be released by the pyloric mucosa by GREGORY could be histamine, KOMAROV's "gastrin", or some unknown agent. GREGORY suggested that normally it is removed by the liver. On the other hand it might be due to histamine, released or absorbed from the stomach and large intestine, in an amount which is not entirely removed by the liver, or to some metabolic change which follows a portocaval shunt. For example, the ammonia in the urine is increased after an Eck Fistula.

Recently GREGORY (1958) has published a physiological study in which he believed that the secretory excitant involved was an agent produced in the pyloric mucosa, and released by vagal excitation and its release was inhibited by acid applied to the pyloric or duodenal mucosa.

More recently the urine has been examined for the excretion of "free" histamine after the oral administration of histamine with and without the prior administration orally of succinylsulphathiazole. It was presumptively established that histamine was absorbed and in a sufficient quantity for some to pass the liver and to stimulate gastric secretion, and that the amount absorbed and passing through the liver was increased when the sulfa drug had been given (*vide infra*) (IRVINE et al., 1959 b). The same group, IRVINE et al. (1959 a), have performed another interestingly designed study on the absorption of histamine from the intestine.

As indicated elsewhere, IVY and JAVOIS (1924-25) and IVY et al. (1923) had found that oral histamine base, in doses of 33 to 66 mg, would stimulate secretion in a gastric pouch dog. LIM et al. (1925) had found that 50 mg of histamine di-HCl or 33 mg of the base applied to the pouch of the entire stomach would stimulate gastric secretion. IVY and MCILVAIN (1923) had found that the application of 50 ml of a 1:1000 aqueous solution of histamine di-HCl to a Thiry fistula of the jejunum would decidedly stimulate secretion in a gastric pouch. It was pointed out by IVY and collaborators that a small amount of histamine undoubtedly passes the intestinal and hepatic barrier when from 33 to 66 mg is brought into contact with the gastro-intestinal mucosa of the dog, 66 to 100 mg of the base being required in man. IRVINE et al. (1959 a) introduced various doses of histamine into the jejunum of three gastric pouch dogs. The doses were 333, 166, 83, 33, and 3.3 mg of histamine base in the form of the phosphate. They assayed the hourly output of urinary "free" histamine and of HCl from the pouch. In the fasting state from 0.1 to 0.9 μg of free histamine was excreted per hour. The acid secretory response to the 333 and 166 mg doses of the base were somewhat larger than to a meat meal given by mouth. However, the amount of urinary "free" histamine was definitely more with the histamine meal than with the meat meal. Significant amounts of acid were not secreted with oral doses of histamine base of less than 33 mg in the dogs. When 66 mg of histamine base was introduced into the rectum of the dogs, the output of free histamine increased, but the increase in acid output was not significant. The authors point out that the acid response of their dogs to the histamine or meal stimulus was unfortunately very variable[1]. Nevertheless their findings and those of IVY and JAVOIS check well. Both studies were not as quantitative as is desirable.

In two dogs with a gastric pouch (HEIDENHAIN), the introduction of 33 mg of histamine base into the jejunum caused a slight stimulation (0.3 to 0.5 mEq. HCl) of gastric secretion in 3 of 5 tests before portocaval shunt, and in all five tests after the shunt was made a decided stimulation occurred (0.6 mEq to 4.0

[1] In work of this sort where comparisons are to be made, we have found that gastric pouch dogs should be selected on the basis of small variation in response to a standard dose of histamine and a standard meal. Tests should not be started until 4 weeks after the pouch is made and then control tests (10 of each) with a standard meal and dose of histamine should be started. Since some pouch dogs develop a refractoriness, the control tests should be repeated to ascertain if the responsiveness of the pouch has changed.

mEq HCl). That this was not due to an increased sensitivity of the pouch to histamine was shown by repeating an intravenous infusion of histamine from time to time. When the two dogs were treated with aminoguanidine — a histaminase inhibitor — the gastric secretory response to the introduction of histamine in the jejunum was decidedly increased.

In three dogs with gastric pouches, the gastric secretory HCl output and the urinary output of "free" histamine was studied by infusing histamine into the portal and the femoral veins. In 12 tests on the 3 dogs it was found that to obtain a comparable HCl and free histamine output, the rate of infusion into the femoral vein had to be approximately one-half that into the portal vein. (See LIVINGSTON and CODE, 1955).

In view of the high dilution of the histamine absorbed into the portal blood, it would not be detectible by the older methods, though the most recent method of ADAM et al. (1957) might work. C^{14}-histamine as a tracer by the dilution technique should certainly prove that histamine and not some other highly conjectural substance, was absorbed.

G. Is release of histamine by alcohol the cause of the stimulation of gastric secretion?

1. Background

It has been known for a long time (1906) that alcohol, in concentrations of from 5 to 10%, stimulates gastric secretion when taken into the stomach as a test meal (ORBELI, 1906). It is known further that alcohol stimulates gastric secretion when given by any route. The literature up to 1940 has been rather completely reviewed by BEAZELL and IVY (1940-41). At that time a large literature had developed. It was pointed out that alcohol might stimulate gastric secretion (a) by an effect on the central vagus nucleus or local nervous mechanism in the stomach, (b) by acting directly on the parietal cells, since it passes from the blood into the gastric juice (like histamine), (c) by contacting the gastric and intestinal mucosa and causing the release of histamine or a "gastrin". At that time it had been demonstrated by DRAGSTEDT et al (1940) that alcohol in small dilutions released histamine from the perfused guinea pig lung. It increases the permeability of the intestinal mucosa to histamine. The effects of alcohol on gastric secretion are, in all known respects, the same as histamine and KOMAROV's "gastrin". This circumstantial evidence, along with the high histamine content of the gastric and intestinal mucosa, rendered the theory that alcohol stimulates by histamine release very attractive, and it has been widely accepted. But still there was circumstantial evidence indicating that a central action of alcohol was in part responsible.

2. Recent evidence

In 1956, HIRSCHOWITZ et al. gave from 10 to 40 ml of alcohol in saline solution intravenously to human subjects. After observing the effects of atropine, hexamethonium and vagotomy, it was concluded that alcohol acts in part centrally, like hypoglycemia, to stimulate gastric secretion. At that time no direct experimental evidence was available showing that alcohol in contact with the gastric or intestinal mucosa actually released histamine, or KOMAROV's "gastrin". Since then a few attempts have been made to obtain such evidence.

WOODWARD et al. (1957) observed that 5% alcohol in water applied to the mucosa of a HEIDENHAIN pouch dog or a pouch of the total corporic region, had little or no effect on acid output. The application of 5% alcohol to a pyloric pouch caused about 5.20 mEq of HCl secretion; a 10% concentration increased the acid output by 50% over that caused by a 5% solution. (The same 10% solution should have been applied to the total fundic pouch because of their refractoriness). *It was found that alcohol was not absorbed from the pyloric pouch.* If the alcohol was acidified (pH 1.2) and applied to the pyloric pouch no secretion occurred, due to "acid inhibition" of gastric secretion. Dilute alcohol given slowly intravenously (250 ml 5% alcohol in saline) during a 20-min period stimulated secretion. Bilateral vagotomy did not reduce the secretion to such an intravenous infusion. The same was true after surgical removal of the pyloric portion of the stomach. When alcohol (250 ml of 5%) was placed in a Thiry fistula, the stimulation was slight though the alcohol was well absorbed. This apparent discrepancy has no obvious explanation. The findings resulted in the conclusion, that alcohol stimulates gastric secretion almost entirely by the release of KOMAROV's "gastrin[1]" (or histamine) from the pyloric mucosa, and that stimulation does not occur if the pH of the gastric contents is as low as pH 1.2, because the acid releases an inhibitory agent or inhibits secretion reflexly. The secretion stimulated by intravenous alcohol must be due to the release of histamine from the general tissues. However, it may act on the vagus center. If this is true, there is no explanation for a failure of the alcohol absorbed from the intestine to stimulate. (More tests should have been done.) Furthermore, the failure of absorption of alcohol from the pyloric pouch requires confirmation, though it may be prevented by the "mucous barrier".

IRVINE et al. (1960), using dogs, obtained results much like those of WOODWARD et al. except for two important points. They found that intravenous alcohol stimulates the innervated and denervated gastric corporic mucosa equally well, and that the evidence indicates that alcohol intravenously does not cause a general tissue release of histamine. The absence of a general tissue release of histamine was based on the failure to find "free" histamine in the urine, whereas when histamine was infused "free" histamine increased in the urine.

3. Discussion

In the dog alcohol stimulates, when given intravenously, even though the vagi are cut and the pyloric gland area removed. When applied to the pyloric pouch it stimulates by releasing histamine or KOMAROV's "gastrin", since the alcohol apparently is not absorbed. When infused intravenously it stimulates secretion without "free" histamine output detectibly increasing in the urine. Here are two instances where C^{14}-L-histidine should help. If alcohol were applied to the pyloric mucosa of a C^{14}-L-histidine treated dog, then if histamine is released C^{14}-histamine will be released and appear in the blood and urine. If alcohol intravenously should release histamine from various tissues, then in a C^{14}-L-histidine treated animal, C^{14}-histamine should be released into the blood and urine. If alcohol applied to the pyloric pouch does not release C^{14}-histamine, then the observed stimulation may be due to the release of KOMAROV's "gastrin". The effect of alcohol on the release of ACh should also be considered. As indicated previously, hypoglycemia apparently stimulates HCl output without "free" histamine appearing in the urine. This may indicate that HCl output may be increased by a central action of alcohol on the vagal center. But, since alcohol stimulates after vagotomy and excision of the pyloric portion of the stomach, it is possible that alcohol acts either on cholinergic nerve endings in the acid secreting mucosa

[1] There is no reason why histamine should be omitted since the authors could not identify what agent was released.

or directly on the parietal cell. So it would be of interest to study the effect of alcohol on the local release of ACh in the corporic mucosa. The effect of alcohol on L-histidine decarboxylase should also be studied, since small amounts of alcohol may stimulate the activity of this enzyme, and thus release histamine locally in the corporic mucosa, or in the same manner that alcohol releases histamine from the lung. Since alcohol has an effect on adenosine triphosphate coenzyme, and perhaps other related enzymes, which may be concerned in the formation of HCl, it may stimulate HCl production by acting directly on the parietal cell. Then an increase in "free" histamine in the urine need not occur.

Irvine et al. (1961) performed an experiment, which was referred to and described, under attempts to find histamine in the gastric venous effluent when alcohol or insulin was introduced into the splenic artery. The experiment was directed to ascertain if circulating ethyl alcohol might release histamine at the parietal cell. They obtained no positive evidence that it did, but the hypothesis that histamine may be released is well worth exploring further, since it was not proven to be invalid as the authors pointed out, because the chemical method may not have been sensitive enough to have detected the small amounts of histamine which can be released and stimulate gastric secretion. Tests for ACh should be made on the venous effluent under such conditions. The mucosa should be pretreated with C^{14}-L-histidine which may be a more sensitive method than that of Adam et al. (1957).

It now appears to be generally agreed that circulating alcohol stimulates HCl output *in the dog* in the absence of the pyloric glandular area and pre-ganglionic vagal innervation. The evidence now indicates that alcohol may stimulate, by either acting at the level of the parietal cell or, by a general release of histamine too small to be detected in the plasma or the urine by the best direct chemical method that has been used to date. The use of C^{14}-L-histidine or the method of the "induced synthesis of histamine" should assist in the solution of this problem.

The variation in the effect of alcohol on gastric secretion in vagotomized patients, is probably due to complete or incomplete vagotomy and differences in the degree of refractoriness of the stomach as a consequence of the vagotomy. The variation in reports on atropine inhibition of alcohol stimulation are probably due to a difference in dosage effects. The variation in results when denervated pouches are used may be due to their variation in refractoriness. Perhaps more uniform results might be obtained if the refractoriness of the pouch is erased with a sub-threshold secretory dose of mecholyl.

H. Effect of local application of procaine on the release of histamine or Komarov's "gastrin"

Zeljony and Savich (1911-1912) found, that the application of a cocaine solution to the mucosa of a pyloric pouch, abolished the secretory response in the main stomach to the mechanical or chemical stimulation of the pyloric pouch. Lim et al. (1925) and Gregory and Ivy (1941), using a transplanted pouch, observed the same effect with procaine solution, it being shown that procaine intravenously did not stimulate the transplanted pouch. Procaine has the same effect when applied to a pouch of the entire stomach devoid of its pyloric portion.

Uvnäs (1942 b) has reported that when the vagi in cats are stimulated Komarov's "gastrin" (or histamine) is released, unless the pyloric mucosa is procainized.

There is agreement that local anesthetization prevents the release of "gastrin" (Komarov's "gastrin" or histamine) from the pyloric or corporic mucosa into the blood.

It should be emphasized that histamine and KOMAROV's "gastrin" are so much alike in their physiological effects on gastric secretion, that one cannot be differentiated from the other. Chemically, however, they are different.

It would appear that a nervous mechanism is involved in the release of histamine or KOMAROV's "gastrin", from the pyloric and corporic mucosa. If, as some report, there is no KOMAROV's "gastrin" in the corporic mucosa, *then only histamine could be the blood-borne agent released when the corporic mucosa is locally stimulated by meat juice and distension.* ACh could not be the blood borne agent in such experiments because eserine was not used and any ACh released would be destroyed by cholinesterase. It is very probable that ACh is released by vagal postganglionic nerve endings or by endings of the MEISSNER's plexus in the pyloric mucosa, and then it causes the release of histamine or KOMAROV's "gastrin". The cells which release this histamine may also be present in the corporic mucosa and release histamine on ACh stimulation.

I. Effect of atropine on histamine stimulated gastric secretion

1. Background

KEETON et al. (1920) found that "toxic" doses of atropine were required to abolish completely the gastric secretory effects of histamine and of their "gastrin" which was undoubtedly histamine. They suggested that "gastrin" or histamine is either liberated by secretory nerves in the mucosa, or that atropine works at one site in the secretory process and histamine at another. BABKIN (1950) postulated that the postganglionic endings of the vagus in the mucosa release ACh which in turn releases histamine to act on the parietal cell.

Everyone has found that histamine-stimulated gastric secretion is more difficult to inhibit with atropine than that due to a meal. It is also generally agreed that a dose of atropine which will cause drying of the mouth will decrease the volume output of secretion in man and in the dog. In those instances resistant to such doses of atropine, the best explanation is that histamine or KOMAROV's "gastrin" is being abnormally produced as the result of irritation or inflammation (IVY and BACHRACH, 1940).

It should be mentioned that a single dose of atropine begins to lose its effect after two hours. Some investigators do not take this fact into consideration in the interpretation of their results.

Since the literature is very large and has been reviewed in 1951 (CODE), we shall summarize the results of experiments made on dogs and cats which are most pertinent to the release and secretory action of histamine or KOMAROV's "gastrin". OBERHELMAN and DRAGSTEDT (1948) have made a study on patients.

2. Acetylcholine, or cholinergic mechanism

The fact that *acetylcholine and mecholyl* are very potent when injected into the arterial supply of the acid secreting mucosa, is too frequently forgotten in discussions of our subject.

BLOCK and NECHELES (1938) have found small amounts of acetylcholine in canine and human gastric juice. Their experiment has never been repeated. Further study may indicate that the presence of ACh in gastric juice is as important as the presence of histamine. Furthermore, there is good evidence showing that ACh stimulates directly the parietal cells (PEVSNER and GROSSMAN, 1955) and undoubtedly releases histamine or KOMAROV's "gastrin" from the pyloric mucosa (ROBERTSON et al., 1950 a; BENJAMIN et al., 1950). An arterial perfusion of 0.11 μg/kg/min of ACh will stimulate a good output of HCl (PEVSNER and

GROSSMAN, 1955). When the pyloric mucosa is bathed with a dilute solution of ACh or mecholyl, either histamine or KOMAROV's "gastrin" is released (ROBERTSON, 1950 a). This release occurs when an infusion of the arterial supply of a pyloric pouch is made with 0.06 μg/kg/min of ACh. So, ACh can stimulate the parietal cell directly, or by the release of histamine, or KOMAROV's "gastrin" from the pyloric or corporic mucosa.

3. Three physiologically active agents in gastric mucosa

So, there are *three physiologically active agents in the corporic and pyloric mucosa* which are very potent for the stimulation of gastric secretion. (a) *ACh,* which is liberated by postganglionic parasympathetic or vagal nerve endings. Whether there are cholinergic nerve endings in the nerve plexus of the mucosa is uncertain. ACh stimulates both HCl and pepsin output. (b) *Histamine* stimulates HCl output, and to a less extent pepsin output, some claiming none. (c) KOMAROV's *"gastrin"* acts like histamine, but some claim that it is only present in pyloric and duodenal mucosa (WOODWARD, 1960). It is not inactivated by histaminase (BAUER and UVNÄS, 1944). But, if KOMAROV's "gastrin" is not in the corporic or acid secreting mucosa, then histamine only remains as the blood borne agent that GREGORY and IVY (1941) have observed to be released from the corporic mucosa when that portion only of the stomach is distended (See GROSSMAN, 1961). [Local application of liver extract also stimulates a pouch of the total corporic mucosa in the dog (KIM and IVY, 1934).]

Because of the possible involvement of histamine, the effect of atropine on the various phases of gastric secretion will be briefly outlined.

4. Atropine and the phases of gastric secretion

Regarding the *cephalic phase*, atropine in doses which dry the mouth prevents secretion due to sham-feeding, hypoglycemia and vagal stimulation, all of which act on the stomach via the vagi. So, undoubtedly ACh is released by the postganglionic vagal nerve endings and, either directly or indirectly, stimulates the parietal and chief cells.

Regarding the *gastric phase, first,* the secretion which occurs on the distention of a total gastric pouch in the dog is prevented by atropine with or without the pyloric mucosa being present. *Second,* atropine prevents histamine-free extracts of liver from stimulating gastric secretion on slow intravenous infusion, but not if histamine is present. It is generally agreed that since the secretory response to a meal is less resistant to being decreased by atropine than to an analogous dose of histamine or KOMAROV's "gastrin", then atropine must act to retard or prevent their release in addition to blocking the ACh stimulation of secretion.

Quite recently GROSSMAN (1961) has found that the distention of a denervated corporic pouch sensitizes it to histamine and also to GREGORY's "gastrin", which indicates that distention acts like ACh or mecholyl.

Regarding the *intestinal phase,* the secretory response to food in the intestine is reduced or abolished by an adequate dose of atropine.

Therapeutic doses of atropine suppress but do not prevent the secretory response to alcohol; large doses do, especially in regard to volume of secretion. This shows that alcohol operates very peripherally, in part.

The increase in gastric secretion after thermal trauma is reduced but not abolished by ordinary amounts of atropine (CODE, 1951).

It is clear that if post-ganglionic fibers of the vagus are involved, then atropine in non-toxic doses, but doses which dry the mouth, should definitely depress secretion. The effect of atropine on the MEISSNER-AUERBACH's plexus in relation to the parietal cells is uncertain.

When the matter of *the release of histamine or* KOMAROV's *"gastrin"* only is involved, atropine usually abolished it completely. When atropine is used in such experiments, it has to be kept in mind that the reduction in secretory response may be due to the action of the drug on the release mechanism and on the secretory mechanism. This is true even after the preganglionic vagal fibers have been cut, because the postganglionic fibers are probably present but refractory.

The inhibitory effect of atropine on the release of histamine or KOMAROV's "gastrin" under local mechanical stimulation of the pyloric mucosa, or vagal stimulation is to be expected in view of their release when the pyloric mucosa is bathed with acetylcholine or mecholyl (ROBERTSON et al., 1950a). Also, secretion of acid by the corporic mucosa when the gastric artery is infused with ACh should be and is prevented or suppressed by atropine. The release of either histamine or KOMAROV's "gastrin", or both, when the arterial supply of the pyloric pouch is infused with ACh, should be depressed or prevented by atropine. This latter experiment has not been done, but the application of ACh to the pyloric mucosa releases gastrin, whatever its chemical nature may be.

As indicated above, some have expressed the view that atropine acts only to suppress the excitability of the parietal cell (GRAY, 1937). More recently JANOWITZ and HOLLANDER (1956) reported that if a dose of atropine is "tailored" to the dose of histamine, the secretion to large doses of histamine is completely suppressed in regard to volume output, but not acid concentration. Doses of atropine of 0.1 to 0.2 mg/kg were well tolerated, but a dose of 0.4 mg/kg was definitely toxic. The latter was the dose required to almost completely suppress the volume output. This phenomenon, of a greater suppression of volume output than of acid concentration, has been noted by most investigators.

The evidence would cause us to believe that when histamine is given, atropine first blocks the constant production of "tonic" amounts of ACh or produces a "chemical" vagotomy so far as the acid secreting mucosa is concerned. This renders the parietal cells less sensitive to histamine and the volume output decreases, since histamine very probably acts directly on the parietal cell. But, to obtain a further decrease in volume output, the dose of atropine must be such that the cell membrane or cytoplasm of the parietal cell is poisoned. Hypothetically the acid forming machinery inside the parietal cell is not so readily poisoned, as the cell membrane, since it still produces acid of high or normal concentration, but it can no longer get the water and chlorine to manufacture acid in good quantity or secretion in good volume. Here we have a situation similar to the salivary cells under atropine; the salivary cell can secrete very thick mucus at a stage of atropine action, but it cannot get water and electrolyte with which to dilute the mucin. This hypothesis can certainly be tested experimentally.

Summarizing, the evidence indicates that atropine acts to block the physiological release of histamine or GREGORY's "gastrin" in the pyloric and corporic mucosa and decreases the permeability of the membrane of the parietal cell without suppressing the acid secretory mechanism. Since an appropriate dose of atropine can block all the physiological stimuli of the parietal cell and cannot block the effect of an HCl-equivalent dose of exogenous histamine or GREGORY's "gastrin", either histamine and GREGORY's "gastrin" is not the physiological gastrin, or atropine prevents their release (GRAY, 1937; GRAY and IVY, 1937).

J. Effect of known metabolic derivatives of histamine on gastric secretion

In recent years the metabolic derivatives of histamine in different species, have been quite well identified by the use of C^{14}-histamine. It has been found that two major histamine metabolizing enzymes exist and operate to a variable extent in different species. One is diamine oxidase (DO) or histamine diamine oxidase (HDO) which is the same as histaminase. The other is a methylase which places a methyl group on the ring and renders histamine inactive. There may be others which are incompletely identified. There may be a methylase which replaces an H on the N of the side chain with a CH_3 group. Acetylation by an acetylase occurs in the intestine by bacteria, and, as indicated before, is called conjugated histamine and appears in the urine. Acetylhistamine has an acetyl group on the N of the side chain. In the rat the DO system predominates and in man and dog the methylating system (SCHAYER, 1959).

Table 8. *Effect of derivatives of histamine metabolism on basal gastric secretion* (IVY and LIEPINS, 1958)

Oxidative deamination HDO[1]	Methylation methylase + MO	Acetylation Acetylase
I. Histamine + HDO yields	I. Histamine + methylase yields	Histamine + Acetylase yields
II. Imidazole-4-acetaldehyde (Has not been synthesized)	IV. 1-Methyl-4-(aminoethyl) imidazole (Inactive)	VII. N-acetylhistamine: 4 (β-acetylaminoethyl) imidazole (Subcutaneously it is 1000 times less active than histamine)
+ Xanthine oxidase, or aldehyde oxidase + DPN yields	+ MO (or some DO's)[2] yields	
III. Imidazole-4-acetic acid (Inactive)	V. 1-Methylimidazole-4-acetaldehyde (Has not been synthesized) + Xanthine oxidase, or aldehyde oxidase + DPN yields	
IIIa. Imidazole-4-acetic acid riboside (Probably inactive) (Has not been synthesized)	VI. 1-Methylimidazole-4-acetic acid (Inactive)	

[1] HDO histamine diamine oxidase (histaminase).

[2] MO monoamine oxidase.

The information regarding the action of the various common metabolites of histamine on gastric secretion is summarized in Table 8 from IVY and LIEPINS (1958). It will be noted that all of the known metabolites which have been synthesized and are available for study, are inactive on gastric secretion.

There are two analogues of histamine in which the hydrogen on the side chain N is replaced by 1 or 2 methyl groups. They are discussed under analogues, but may be metabolites. They are not mentioned further here because at present we consider them to be only very interesting potential metabolites.

K. Analogues of histamine and gastric secretion

1. Stimulators

In 1915, CHIARI reported that pilocarpine, an imidazole, stimulated HCl and pepsin output. A further search for analogues of histamine was started by KOCH et al. in 1920. SCHNEDORF and IVY (1935) found that 4,(5) methylaminoethylglyoxaline[1] and histamine produced equal gastric secretory responses. This observation and that of VARTIAINEN (1935) showed that the amino group on the side chain need not be primary.

GROSSMAN et al. (1952) and ROBERTSON et al. (1950b) tested over 62 compounds closely related to histamine. The most interesting finding was that certain imidazoles, which had all the other biological actions of histamine, did not stimulate gastric secretion. The same was true of the methylated derivatives of ALLES et al. (1943). And, certain of the compounds, which had been studied by LEE and JONES (1949), did not stimulate acid secretion but had an effect on the guinea pig ileum and cat's blood pressure. Others which had no such effect stimulated acid secretion. In a group of compounds studied by CRAVER et al. (1951) and all of which stimulated salivary secretion, none stimulated gastric secretion. The foregoing results show that the action of histamine on the parietal cell is very specific and different from its other effects.

LEE and JONES (1949) stated that the compounds active on the blood pressure and ileal strip had one structural feature in common $-N=\overset{|}{C}-CH_2CH_2NH_2$ or $=N-\overset{\|}{C}-CH_2CH_2NH_2$ in which the group $-N=\overset{|}{C}-$ or $=N-\overset{\|}{C}-$ is part of an aromatic nucleus.

Among the 12 compounds found to stimulate gastric secretion, all but two had the foregoing structure, some with methyl substitutions on the side chain. The two exceptions were 4-beta-amino-ethyl pyrazole and 2-imidazole-2-benzyl (Priscoline).

2. Inhibitors

ROBERTSON and GROSSMAN (1952b) conducted a screening program on total gastric pouch dogs, to ascertain if a highly effective inhibitor of acid production stimulated by histamine might be found. The compounds were selected primarily on the basis of their chemical structure.

A submaximal continuous flow of gastric juice in the total gastric pouch dogs was maintained by the subcutaneous injection of 0.04 mg of histamine diphosphate every 10 min. The method in detail has been described by GROSSMAN (1951).

No inhibitor compounds as potent and specific as the acid secretory inhibitory fraction of enterogastrone and as urogastrone are known.

3. Comment

Some basic molecular characteristic of histamine, in relation to gastric secretion, would be expected and should be discoverable. It is possible that the secretory action is exerted primarily by one or more of the metabolites of histamine.

---

[1] Synthesized by PYMAN of Boots Drug Co., England; at that time the compound was called "methyl histamine."

4. N-Methyl and N-Dimethyl histamine

This latter possibility has been looked into by SCHNEDORF and IVY (1935) in 1935 when they found that N-methyl histamine [4, (5) methylaminoethyl glyoxaline[1]] was as active in stimulating gastric secretion and depressing blood pressure in the cat as histamine. Prof. PYMAN wrote one of us (A. C. I.) that it had the same oxytocic activity as histamine on the guinea pig uterus. This analogue, however, is not a well-known or established metabolite of histamine. KAPELLER-ADLER and IGGO (1957) found it in human urine, but it is not known whether it came from bacterial action in the intestine or whether it was produced in the body of her subjects. SCHAYER (1959) has suggested that the methylation of the amino group on the side chain of histamine might be a first step in the methylation process. He suggested further that some of the effects of aminoguanidine (antihistaminase) might be to prevent the histaminase from changing this N-methyl or N-dimethyl histamine into methyl imidazole acetic acid.

It is interesting that LIN et al. (1961; in press) have found that N-methyl and N-dimethyl histamine are about three times more potent on gastric secretion than histamine. Even more interesting, they are active when administered orally or by any route to denervated gastric pouch dogs. They are not oxidized by histaminase and their effect is not augmented by aminoguanidine. Since there appears to be a small amount of methylating enzyme in dog's gastric mucosa it would be of interest to study chemically, whether the gastric mucosa produces N-methyl-histamine from histamine. It may be that KOMAROV's "gastrin" is N-methyl-histamine attached to polypeptide or mucoprotein carriers (IVY et al., 1961; KATO, 1961; WOJCIECH and IVY, 1961). *This is especially pertinent since* BAUER and UVNÄS (1944) *have said that their "gastrin" is not destroyed by histaminase.* Antihistaminics ("Benadryl", "Histadyl" and "Pyronil") increased the effects of this N-methyl histamine on blood pressure and ileal strips, but did not block its effect on gastric secretion. These findings are of much theoretical and perhaps practical interest.

5. Aminoethyl-1,2,4-Triazole

Another histamine analogue has been discovered which is of interest from several viewpoints, namely, 3-beta-aminoethyl-1,2,4-Triazole. This compound was synthesized and reported on by AINSWORTH and JONES (1953). They stated that GROSSMAN had found it active on gastric secretion in a few tests. LIN informed one of the authors (A. C. I.) that the compound was active orally and was not a substrate for histaminase, which confirmed the finding of LINDELL and WESTLING (1957). A compound that acts directly on the parietal cell and is not a substrate for histaminase is of theoretical interest in relation to the gastrin problem (IVY, 1958c; IVY and LIEPINS, 1960). LIN et al. (1961) and IVY and LIEPINS (1960) have reported their findings on this analogue of histamine. The compound was active orally in dogs. Subcutaneously in dogs, histamine is about 1.5 times more potent gravimetrically than the triazole. On ileal strips the ratio of the activity of the triazole to histamine was 0.72 : 1, or histamine is 1.4 times more potent; on blood pressure histamine was 1.36 times more potent. The action of the triazole is more prolonged than that of histamine. The triazole acts additively with histamine (LIN and ALPHIN, 1959). Since aminoguanidine (AG) inhibits the destruction of histamine, AG augments the action of the triazole.

---

[1] Glyoxaline was the term used for imidazole in England in 1930.

6. Other analogues

LIN et al. (1961) have studied some 40 compounds consisting of imidazole, pyrazole, triazole analogues of histamine, a number of heterocylic nitrogen compounds with the beta-aminoethyl side chain. Their findings will be summarized. (A) Compounds with an imidazole ring are more potent on gastric secretion than those with a pyrazole or a triazole ring. (B) A side chain is required. The beta-aminoethyl group is the preferred side chain. Shortening the chain to a methylamine group abolishes the activity. Lengthening the chain reduces or abolishes the activity. (C) Substitution of the hydrogen atom of the primary amine with a methyl, benzyl, isopropyl or acetyl group decreases potency. Elimination of the amine with a hydroxyl group abolishes the activity. (D) The positions and number of nitrogens on the ring are important but not crucial, since imidazole, pyrazole and triazole (1,2,3 and 1,2,4) derivatives stimulate HCl secretion. (E) Substitution of the hydrogen attached to the nitrogen in the ring usually abolishes all activity. (F) There is no constant parallelism in the potency of the various compounds relative to the ileal strip, blood pressure reducing, and HCl stimulation activities of histamine.

7. Comment

We believe that a further study of analogues of histamine, both for their excitatory and inhibitory effects, is indicated. This will yield more information than we now possess regarding the chemical relation between histamine, its relation to cell membranes and structures and chemical blocking agents, such as "enterogastrone", after histamine has been released and causes physiological changes by entering or contacting cells.

L. Action of antihistamines

With few exceptions, all who have investigated the action of the numerous compounds classed as "antihistamines" or "histamine antagonists", are agreed that these compounds, while "blocking" all of the other physiological effects of histamine, do not significantly depress the gastric secretory response to histamine or to other stimuli for gastric secretion, or the basal secretion. This has been demonstrated in the human[1], the dog[2], the cat[3], the mouse[4] and the guinea pig[5]. Benadryl was reported to manifest a mild (REUSE, 1946; MCELIN and HORTON, 1945, 1946) or pronounced (MCGAVACK et al., 1946) depressing action on the histamine secretion in man, and various antihistamines were reported as having some inhibitory action on the histamine secretion (BOURQUE and LOEW, 1942—1943; LEHMANN and YOUNG, 1945; LOEW et al., 1946; LEHMANN and STEFKO, 1949) and on the cephalic and gastric phases (TAMARIT-TORRES et al., 1953) of gastric secretion in dogs. KHAYYAL et al. (1951) interpreted their finding of an inhibitory action in pigeons as indicating a species difference.

Not only do the antihistamines fail to inhibit gastric secretion, but it has been observed repeatedly that these compounds actually augment the basal secretion

[1] MOERSCH et al. (1946); BUNSE and JUNG (1948); HARTMAN and MOORE (1948); GILG (1948); DOSCHERHOLMEN (1949); ASHFORD et al. (1949); REITTER (1952); HIRVONEN (1952); KAY (1953); MASONI et al. (1957); FERRANDO and LOZZIO (1957); KOHOUT et al. (1960).

[2] LOEW and CHICKERING (1941); BURCHELL and VARCO (1942); LINDE (1950); PATON and SCHACHTER (1951); RAGINS et al. (1958).

[3] EMMELIN and FROST (1947); WOOD (1948); DUTTA (1949); WOOD (1950); DUTTA and TAMHANE (1953); HOWAT and SCHOFIELD (1954).

[4] DAVENPORT and CHAVRE (1950).

[5] GREGORY (1950b).

or intensify the histamine response in man[1], dog[2] and cat[3]. Among the explanations proposed for this effect are, that the antihistamines act synergistically with histamine on gastric secretion (GILG, 1948; EMMELIN and FROST, 1947), inhibit the breakdown of acetylcholine (REITTER, 1952), have less affinity for gastric gland cells than for other cells activated by histamine (142) (SANGSTER et al., 1946), release 'bound' histamine (LINDE, 1950), or prevent edema of the gastric mucosa which would in itself interfere with gastric secretion (PATON and SCHACHTER, 1951). STERN (1955) postulates that antihistaminics inhibit the action of diamine oxidase by competing with histamine for a receptor-coupling with the enzyme, and since diamine oxidase is present in all tissues except the gastric mucosa, the antihistamines cannot prevent secretion of gastric juice.

ROBERTSON and GROSSMAN (1952a) irrigated gastric pouches in histamine-stimulated dogs with solutions of antihistaminics to obtain a high local concentration of antihistamine. Inhibition occurred with all except one of the compounds used, but other evidence indicated that this was not a specific antihistaminic action. The fact that the pouch secretion after irrigation became mucoid and frequently bloody suggested that the inhibition was a result of direct irritation of the secretory glands. Evidence for true inhibition of histamine-stimulated canine pouches, by local application of antihistaminics, was subsequently claimed by KAY and FORREST (1956a) and JANOWITZ and HOLLANDER (1957), and of parasympathomimetically stimulated pouches by KAY and FORREST (1956b). The latter experiments were interpreted as indicating that cholinergic drugs evoke their gastric secretory effect through the mediation of histamine. However, the work of RAGINS et al. (1958) and BLAIR and FORREST (1960) supported the conclusion of ROBERTSON and GROSSMAN (1952a) that the inhibitory action of topical antihistaminics was attributable to mucosal injury. The problem is complicated to some extent by the fact that antihistaminics have local anesthetic and anticholinergic properties (JANOWITZ and HOLLANDER, 1957). The foregoing observations may explain why WOOD (1950) was able to reduce or abolish the gastric secretory response to intravenous infusions of histamine in anesthetized cats by injecting antihistamines retrograde into the ligated splenic artery to obtain a high concentration of the drugs in the gastric mucosa, whereas the same drugs had no inhibitory action when given intravenously. The high concentration may have caused injury.

M. Studies on histaminase inhibitors in relation to gastric secretion

Histaminase (HDO) inhibitors are considered to be potential new tools in the study of the physiology of gastric secretion. In fact, it is unfortunate that an inhibitor of the methylase, which probably exists in the gastric and intestinal mucosa, and is known to exist in the liver, is not available as a tool.

1. Aminoguanidine and other inhibitors

The information pertaining to the action of the inhibitors most commonly used, and their effect on gastric secretion (IVY and LIEPINS, 1960) is summarized in Table 9. A study of the table will show that aminoguanidine (AG) is the best one in the group because, *first*, of its potency and low toxicity and, *second*, it does not inhibit gastric histidine decarboxylase (SCHAYER and IVY, 1957, 1958; IVY,

---

[1] GILG (1948); DOSCHERHOLMEN (1949); REITTER (1952).
[2] LOEW and CHICKERING (1941); LINDE (1950); PATON and SCHACHTER (1951).
[3] EMMELIN and FROST (1947); WOOD (1948); DUTTA (1949); HOWAT and SCHOFIELD (1954).

1958c), *third*, it acts only on diamine oxidase (DO), and *fourth*, it is active by any route of administration.

SIRCUS in 1953, studied the effect of 2-methyl-5-amino-methyl-6-amino-pyrimidine (B_1-pyrimidine) in anesthetized or decerebrate cats and in unanesthetized dogs with gastric pouches on the gastric secretory response to insulin, carbachol, ethanol, histamine, vagal stimulation and feeding. An increase in volume output of secretion occurred after the intravenous injection of 50 mg per kilo of the chemical, B_1-pyrimidine. LIN et al. (1956) injected aminoguanidine (AG) slowly intravenously in a dose of 0.4 to 1.0 mg/kg/min into HEIDENHAIN and

Table 9. *Summarizing the action of inhibitors of histamine metabolism on gastric secretion*
From IVY and LIEPINS (1958)

Histamine metabolizing enzyme inhibitor	Effection			
	HDO	MO	Histidine decarboxylase	Gastric secretion
Aminoguanidine . .	marked	none	none (1)	augments
Iproniazid[1]	marked	marked	inhibits (1)	augments
B_1 pyrimidine . . .	moderate	?	none	augments[2]
Semicarbizide[1] . .	moderate	none	inhibits some (1, 2)	augments[2]
Isoniazid	moderate	none	?	augments

[1] High concentrations do not inhibit as much as smaller concentrations.
[2] Not very potent by weight (50—100 mg) required. (1) Inhibits rabbit's kidney histidine decarboxylase. (2) Inhibits rabbit's kidney and rat's stomach histidine decarboxylase. MO monoamine oxidase; HDO histamine diamine oxidase.

transplanted (IVY) pouch dogs and observed the appearance of free HCl in the basal secretion. The secretory response to a 0.05 mg dose of histamine diphosphate given subcutaneously every 10 min was augmented by intravenous AG. The effect was additive and a rough dose response curve occurred until the AG becomes toxic. To observe the augmentory effect, a minimal concentration of AG in the blood or body is required; also, the augmentation to histamine or a meal is not observable unless they are given in submaximal secretory amounts.

IVY, et al. (1956) observed that "Marsilid" (1-isonicotinyl-2-isopropylhydrazin) and "Rimifon" (isonicotinylhydrazine) would augment HCl output, but they were too toxic to use uniformly. More important they found that aminoguanidine augments the HCl output in response to a meal containing no histamine. Such a meal, of course, does not stimulate as much acid secretion in dogs as a meal of meat. A meat meal, especially if it is high in histamine content, very probably stimulates in part by the absorption of a very small amount of histamine (IRVINE et al., 1959a, b). FRAILE-OVEJERO and LLUCH-TRULL (1956) found that augmentation of secretion occurred after the administration of semicarbazide known to be an histaminase inhibitor by *in vitro* tests.

LIEPINS et al. (1958) found that AG and iproniazid (IPN) (Marsilid) and B_1-pyrimidine were active when given subcutaneously. AG and IPN were shown to be active orally also. IPN, which is a monoamine as well as a diamine oxidase inhibitor was about 75% as potent as AG in augmenting gastric secretion and on repeated administration manifested accumulative toxicity. Two of four dogs developed urticaria when a small dose of histamine (0.5 mg base) and a large dose of aminoguanidine was given with it. All four dogs manifested itching under high dosage. IPN had an accumulative toxic action; AG did not have this type of effect.

Aminoguanidine does not stimulate acid output by acting directly on the parietal cell, first, because the augmentation, as indicated above, is additive, not potentiating, and second, 3-β-aminoethyl 1,2,4-triazole, a very closely related histamine analogue (Ivy and Liepins, 1960; Lin et al., 1961), (see topic headed analogues), is not oxidized by histaminase and apparently acts directly on the parietal cell and, more importantly, in an additive and not potentiating manner. In other words, a dose of histamine and an histamine equivalent dose of 3-β-amino-ethyl-1,2,4-triazole act on the parietal cell as though one dose of histamine and a triazole equivalent dose of histamine had been given (Lin et al., 1961; Ivy and Liepins, 1960). There was no evidence of a true potentiation.

This evidence, we believe, shows that the action of AG on gastric secretion is only to reduce the destruction of histamine wherever it is being released and destroyed. The fact that AG causes free HCl to appear in the fasting secretion or causes an increased output of HCl in the basal secretion, shows that histamine is being released more or less continuously in the fasting state. This was sugge-ted by Ghosh and Schild (1958) and by Code (1956) on the basis of indirect evidence.

Where this *fasting release* of histamine is coming from is uncertain. Schayer and Ivy (1957) and Schayer (1957) injected rats and one dog with C^{14}-L-histidine and found C^{14}-histamine in the urine after the injection of aminoguanidine. Some of the urinary C^{14}-histamine comes from the renal decarboxylation of C^{14}-L-histidine (Schayer, 1957). But this is excreted in the urine, since it has been shown, as indicated in the section on urinary histamine, that the kidney has a high-grade capacity to take up arterial histamine. This means that a control urinary output has to be determined before a test procedure is applied. There is no evidence to show that any of the histamine produced by renal histidine decarb-oxylation enters the renal venous return (Lindell and Schayer, 1958). There is considerable histidine decarboxylase in the gastric and intestinal mucosa. As will be indicated later, there is no uncertainty regarding where the increased renal excretion of C^{14}-histamine comes from after feeding (See Topic V).

2. Oral administration of aminoguanidine

Liepins and Ivy (1959) and Liepins (1960) found that the oral administration of AG to dogs and human subjects secreting no free acid in their fasting secretion stimulated the output of HCl. Dogs were given orally 12 mg/kg of AG base as the hydrochloride in 50 ml of normal saline (pH 6.0). The same dose was given orally to dogs with a vagotomized total gastric pouch and an esophageal-jejunal anasto-mosis and it caused a decided secretion of HCl (440 mg HCl). When the same solution (12 mg/kg) was introduced into the vagotomized total gastric pouch for one hour, a decided stimulation of HCl secretion resulted (97 mg). The stomach pouch was washed with warm water to remove any histamine before the control basal secretion was collected. The introduction of the same AG solution into a large Heidenhain pouch (14 tests) for one hour had no effect. Increasing the concentra-tion of AG to 2.8 % also had no effect on the Heidenhain pouch (8 tests). (The pouch should have been sensitized with mecholyl or distension.) The subcutaneous injection of 12 mg/kg at one time produced 30 mg of HCl. The secretion stimulated by the application of the AG solution to the total stomach pouch for one hour, lasted for 6 to 18 hours, a most remarkable phenomenon. The introduction of 50 ml of saline solution as a control had no effect. Prior procainization of the pouch of the entire stomach prevented the secretion following the application of the aminoguanidine solution.

The results of this experiment show that an AG solution (0.4 % solution con-taining 12 mg AG base/kg; pH 6.0) applied to the pyloric mucosa releases a sub-stance from the mucosa which stimulates secretion. After the release mechanism has been in operation for one-half to one hour the initial stimulating agent may apparently be removed and the release mechanism continues to operate for 6 to 18 hours. The same release mechanism may operate when the AG solution is applied to the intestine. The agent released may be histamine or a "gastrin". If so, then much of the 440 mg of acid secreted when the AG was introduced into the intestine, was due to the release of the same agent, since the subcutaneous injection of 12 mg/kg of AG produced only 30 mg of HCl as compared to 440 mg of HCl.

The slow rise in the secretion (30 to 60 minutes) and the prolonged nature of the secretion suggests that the agent released is of the nature of "induced histamine" (newly synthesized histamine) or KOMAROV's "gastrin" and not of the nature of "bound histamine", as in the case of "mast cell histamine". The latter is released suddenly and for a short duration, and "bound histamine" is released more slowly and for a longer duration (SCHAYER, 1960c). Or, it suggests that time is required for the AG to penetrate the mucosa in sufficient quantity to overcome the inertia of the release mechanism.

IRVINE et al. (1959a) also found that the introduction of 10 mg/kg of AG into the jejunum of dogs, caused a decided increase in the basal output of acid and markedly augmented the secretory response to a threshold gastric secretory dose of histamine introduced into the jejunum. In our dogs no food had been ingested for 18 hours.

Since this is the only known instance in which AG has apparently released histamine or KOMAROV's "gastrin", from any tissue, the release is apparently quite specific. *By the use of C^{14}-L-histidine, it could readily be found whether C^{14}-histamine is released.*

3. Uptake of aminoguanidine (AG) by various tissues

With the idea of obtaining more precise knowledge about AG a chemical method was developed by LAWYER and LIEBER (1961). The method has been used in a preliminary manner to determine the relative extent to which the various tissues took up a dose of intravenously injected AG in rats and dogs (LAWYER and LIEBER, 1961). The glandular mucosa of the rat, which contains HDO, took up AG; whereas the mucosa of the corporic and pyloric mucosa of the dog, which contains none or only traces of HDO, did not take up AG. WELCH (1961) synthesized some C^{14}-aminoguanidine and administered it intravenously to four rats. The average mg of AG/gm of tissue was: Glandular stomach, 2.24; kidney, 1.22; liver, 1.06; small intestine, 0.88; skeletal muscle, 0.45; lung, 0.36; remainder of gut, 0.20; feces 0.16; blood, 0.04. To obtain normal values for the lung the animals were decapitated and bled head down, otherwise the lung is congested with blood. Decapitation was done 10 min. after the injection.

In the case of the observations of LAWYER and LIEBER and of WELCH, the uptake of AG correlated well with the values for histaminase found in tissues by BEST and MCHENRY (1930), EMMELIN (1951), ZELLER (1950-51), and WATON (1956). The glandular stomach of rodents differs from that of man and dog in regard to the presence and absence of urease, that of rodents containing none (SUMNER and SOMERS, 1953). This may be biochemically significant.

Aminoguanidine acts to augment gastric secretion by preventing the destruction of histamine wherever it is released. It does not act on or stimulate the parietal cell to secrete acid. When applied to the acid secreting mucosa in a low or relatively high concentration it does not stimulate the secretion of acid; if so, the secretion is in a very small amount. When applied to a denervated pouch of the entire stomach or introduced into the intestine, it stimulates markedly and for a long time (6 to 18 hours). Aminoguanidine applied to a pyloric pouch or to a pouch of the entire stomach, pretreated by the injection of C^{14}-L-histidine, should decide unequivocally whether histamine, KOMAROV's "gastrin", or both are being released.

IV. Relation of histamine to the gastric secretory mechanism

A. Summary

The role that histamine plays in the total gastric secretory picture as revealed by a large amount of experimental evidence is outlined in Table 10 and Figure 1. The subject has been reviewed by HEINZ and ÖBRINK (1954) and HAKKINEN (1960).

The summary in the Table makes no unsupportable assumptions of which we are aware; and, we believe there would be general agreement that the statements made are established by the presently available evidence.

There are three very important facts not mentioned in Table 10, and a fourth which is mentioned but requires emphasis. The *first* is that the gastric mucosa contains relatively a large amount of histamine, as much or more than any other normal tissue in some species, and it is located inside or in close relation to the acid forming or parietal cells. *Second*, the stomach of the dog and other species studied, except the rat, and perhaps the guinea pig, contains very little histamine destroying enzymes. *Third*, histamine is the most potent gastric secretory excitant now known in the body, acetylcholine ranking close. GREGORY's "gastrin" when purified further may be more potent. *Fourth*, because histamine is present in the gastric juice, and usually in proportion to the HCl output, it must be concluded either (a) that histamine is in some way involved in the secretion of hydrochloric acid, or (b) that the formation of HCl is in some way involved in histamine metabolism in the stomach. *As long as histamine remains in gastric juice, why it is there, will have to be explained.*

The precise cellular nature of the secretory mechanism for acid secretion is uncertain (BABKIN, 1950; EMMELIN and KAHLSON, 1944). It is hoped that histological historadiographs, using C^{14}-histamine and C^{14}-L-histidine may elucidate this problem.

The simplest view is that histamine is located in the parietal cell, that the formation of HCl can be brought about by the direct action on the cell of histamine, GREGORY's "gastrin", and acetylcholine released by postganglionic vagal and cholinergic nerve network endings. All three agencies may be involved. Anticholinergic drugs block ACh produced by nerve endings. There is only one need to assume the existence of special cells in the acid secreting mucosa which release histamine. That need arises when the corporic mucosa like the pyloric mucosa is releasing the hormone gastrin, whatever its chemical nature is. It is not very appropriate to suggest that the parietal cell releases the circulating agent into the gastric juice and blood; this is possible, however.

According to this view, the only ideal way to try to block the formation of HCl by the parietal cell is to obtain an agent that blocks the process in the parietal cell. Otherwise undesirable side reactions can be expected. The only such agents now known are (a) the gastric secretory fraction of properly made *enterogastrone* preparations and (b) of *urogastrone* from urine.

B. Gastric blood flow and histamine secretion

Some investigators have suggested that the secretory effect of histamine is accomplished by increasing the blood flow to the gastric mucosa (CONRAD and

Table 10. *Summary of theory of stimulation of gastric secretion*

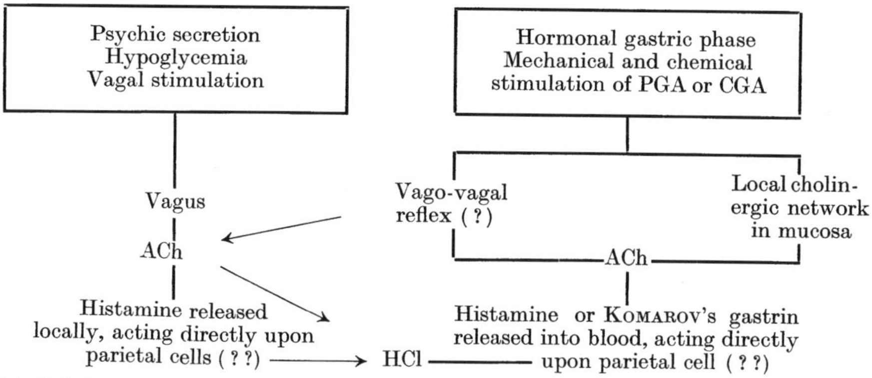

Gastric juice

Histamine: present

KOMAROV's gastrin: has not been looked for

ACh should be looked for

Urine

"Free histamine", not detected or studied well	"Free histamine" present after meat meal and after infusion of histamine

KOMAROV's gastrin has not been looked for

Action of atropine on mucosa

Blocks release of ACh	Blocks or definitely impaires response to ACh physiologically released

Procainization of mucosa

Has not been tried	Prevents release

Pre-treatment with non-stimulating dose of cholinergic drug makes vagotomized or denervated pouch more sensitive to histamine or GREGORY's gastrin	ACh injected in high dilution in saline into artery supplying the pyloric or corporic mucosa stimulates acid secretion in denervated pouch in the former instance and in the stomach with the vagi cut and the pyloric area removed. "ACh" juice contains histamine.

ACh acetylcholine. How alcohol stimulates is uncertain, since enough histamine release for free histamine detection in the urine does not occur; and, whether histamine is in alcohol stimulated juice has not been studied. (?) the effect of the vagus on the release of pyloric histamine or KOMAROV's "gastrin" is slight. (? ?) The release of histamine or KOMAROV's "gastrin" under sham feeding, hypoglycemia, or vagal stimulation has not been demonstrated in the absence of the pyloric mucosa. It is now probable that the vagus acts directly as shown in the first column (MILLICAN et al., 1949). Dogs secrete well but with a reduced volume when sham-fed after complete pylorectomy. ACh may act directly on the parietal cell to release histamine which stimulates secretion and enters the juice.
PGA = pyloric gland area; CGA = corporic gland area.

Kowalewski, 1949; Forrest and Code, 1954; Ziemlanski and Bierezowski, 1960). There can be no doubt that the increase in blood flow which occurs is favorable. But, that an increase in blood flow is the cause of the secretory effect of histamine is untenable, in view of the stimulation of HCl production by the isolated *in vitro* stomach of the frog and mouse. It is well-known that the presence of a small amount of "vasodilatin" in secretin increases its potency.

Nordgren and Öbrink (1956) found that "Priscol", an imidazol vasodilator chemically related to histamine, increased blood flow but did not stimulate acid production. Grossman, Robertson and Rosiere (203) found that Priscoline was 1/10th as potent as histamine when given subcutaneously to the total gastric pouch dog. Forrest and Code (1954) suggest that the inhibitory effect of norepinephrine on histamine-stimulated secretion in dogs, is exerted by its vasoconstrictor action; Harries (1956) on the other hand, while confirming the experimental findings, doubts this explanation. Not all vasoconstrictor drugs inhibit gastric secretion. Ivy and Javois (1924–1925) found that "Epinine", closely related chemically to epinephrine, stimulates gastric secretion very well.

Born and Vane (1953) attempting to explain the observation of Thompson and Vane (1953), found that as much histamine had to be infused directly into the gastric arteries in cats as was infused intravenously, to get the same secretion. They postulated that an interaction between histamine and blood may be necessary before secretion can occur and that this interaction requires time to become effective. The observations on the frog stomach *in vitro* renders this idea unacceptable.

Histamine certainly exerts its essential effect on the stimulation of the production of HCl. However, it can hardly be denied that vasodilation, active rather than passive in type, is essential in higher mammals, at least, for a copious secretion. Vasodilation may even enhance an already existing secretion (Nordgren and Öbrink, 1956). The question was studied in a rather crude manner in pouches of the entire stomach in unanesthetized dogs by Ivy et al. (1925). Dawson and Ivy (1926) emphasized that secretion stops abruptly after a rabbit is struck on the head and the blood pressure falls. The inhibitory effect of a passive hyperemia is easily seen in the cat when too much phenobarbital or chloralose-urethane is given and the blood pressure falls quickly or slowly to 70 or 80 mm Hg pressure.

V. The release of C^{14}-histamine from the glandular stomach and intestinal mucosa of the rat and dog

A. Introduction

Schayer (1952) has demonstrated that two mechanisms exist for rendering histamine available to the body. One is the release of "bound histamine" and the other is the new synthesis of histamine from L-histidine by histidine decarboxylase, the rate of which can be augmented by various stimuli. The latter type of histamine is referred to as "induced histamine", and, in order to study it, radioisotopic measurements are required.

Studies with radioisotopic techniques have shown that when C^{14}-histamine is injected subcutaneously as one dose, none can be found 12 to 24 hours later in any of the tissues. It has been metabolized, and the metabolic derivatives have been excreted in the urine. But, when C^{14}-2-L-histidine is injected subcutaneously, it as well as C^{14}-histamine is found in the organs for days, especially in the gastric and intestinal mucosa. The C^{14}-histamine is bound and released only in response to stimulation (Schayer, 1952, 1956 b, 1957; Schayer et al., 1954).

B. Experiments

Schayer and Ivy (1957) first undertook to determine if feeding caused the rat to release C^{14}-histamine from the gastric glandular mucosa. The rats were injected with C^{14}-L-histidine which is taken up and bound by the gastric and intestinal mucosa of the rat more than by any other tissue. The C^{14}-L-histidine is slowly changed, or may be stimulated to be changed more speedily by a decarboxylase into C^{14}-histamine which then may be released into the blood stream (Schayer 1956c, 1960 a,b,c; Schayer and Smiley, 1954; Schayer and Cooper, 1956; Schayer and Ganley, 1959; Schayer et al., 1958).

C. Experiment I

Six male rats with a chronic gastric fistula (Schayer and Ivy, 1957) were placed in individual restraining cages arranged so that urine and feces were not intermixed, the urine being collected in 6 N-HCl to prevent bacterial action. They were kept in the cage throughout the test. C^{14}-L-histidine was injected subcutaneously after a 12-hour fast when the rats weighed from 350 to 420 gm. Twenty-four hours later — 36 hours of fasting — 2 mg of aminoguanidine (AG) base was injected subcutaneously at a different site from the histidine site, hourly, day and night, for three additional days. Twenty-four hours after the start of AG, food was given for 12 hours, fasting followed for two 12-hour periods and then food was given again for 12 hours (Figure 8). The average urinary C^{14}-histamine counts for the first 12-hour control, 105; the second, 104; 12-hour feeding period 185 (78% increase); first 12-hour post-feeding period, 157; second post-feeding period, 68; final 12-hour feeding period, 106. It was calculated that the 78% increase in the six rats amounted to a decrease of 30% in the total C^{14}-histamine in the gastric and intestinal mucosa before feeding. Of course, this does not necessarily mean that 30% of the total histamine (non-labeled + labeled) in the mucosa was released as a result of feeding. Gastric secretion was followed because these were chronic fistula rats and, of course, it was stimulated by feeding (Lane et al., 1957).

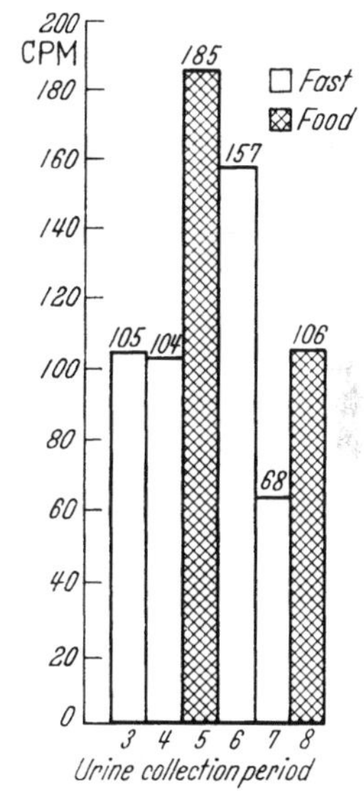

Fig. 8. Counts/min of C^{14}-histamine in the urine during urinary collection *periods 3, 4, 5, 6, 7* and *8*. *Period 1* started 12 hr after the withdrawal of food and when C^{14}-L-histidine was injected. *Period 3* started 24 hr after the injection of the histidine, fasting being continued, except as indicated. (From Schayer and Ivy, 1957)

1. Comment

Of course, in the interpretation of the results the presence of histamine in the food or histamine produced by bacteria in the intestine or the antihistaminase action of the AG are not involved. The only histamine involved is that derived from the decarboxylation of the C^{14}-L-histidine injected. The only possible other source of the increased C^{14}-histamine in the urine than the gastrointestinal mucosa, would be an increase in the decarboxylation of C^{14}-L-histidine in the liver, or kidney or skin. Such an interpretation, however, requires the assumption that eating a meal increases the release of C^{14}-histamine or histamine from the skin, liver and kidney.

D. Experiment II

Schayer and Ivy (1958) performed a second experiment to obtain more data on the source of the increase in the output of the C^{14}-histamine in the urine after feeding fasting rats. Twenty-four male rats were divided into two paired groups of equal body weight. The experiment was then continued as in the first experiment outlined above, except that one group was fed 48 hours after the withdrawal of food and the other group was fasted the entire 72 hour period.

Table 11. *C^{14}-Histamine in the glandular stomach and the small intestine of fasted and fed rats after administering C^{14}-2-L-Histidine.* From R. W. SCHAYER and A. C. IVY (1958)

Group	Rat No.		Weight, gm		Stomach, cpm[1]		Intestine, cpm[1]		Time of withdrawal of food to histidine + injection	Time from histidine[2] injection to feeding	Feeding interval	Total time	Total time after histidine
	Fed[3]	Not fed	Fed[3]	Fasted	Fed[3]	Fasted	Fed[3]	Fasted					
									hr	hr	hr	hr	hr
I	1	4	240	242	17	63	40	60					
	2	5	238	220	21	75	38	42					
	3	6	220	224	20	29	28	43	14	32	24	72	56
Av.			233	229	19	56	35	49					
II	1	4	315	270	44[4]	38	44[4]	48					
	2	5	247	260	16[4]	22	64[4]	52					
	3	6	200	230	36	31	44	70	16	32	18	66	50
Av.			254	253	31	30	50	57					
III	1	4	312	304	16	19	42	65					
	2	5	292	307	12	29	18	55					
	3	6	320	314	14	36	52	67	16	32	30	78	62
Av.			308	308	14	28	37	62					
IV	1	4	280	274	7	39	12	24					
	2	5	270	273	8	42	12	25					
	3	6	252	241	18	51	18	35	20	42	28	90	70
Av.			267	263	11	44	14	28					
Total av.					18.8	39.5	34.3	48.5[5]					

[1] cpm: Counts per minute/100 mg of benzenesulfonyl histamine.
[2] 0.35 mg of C^{14}-2-L-histidine, activity 10 μc/mg, given subcutaneously.
[3] Fasted and then fed.
[4] Rats 1 and 2 did not eat as well as 3.
[5] 18.8 vs. 39.5 = t_{22} = 3.70, sig. at a 1% level; 34.3 vs. 48.8 = t_{22} = 2.20, sig. at a 5% level.

Both groups were decapitated (Table 11). The C^{14}-histamine in the glandular stomach and small intestine was 52% and 30% less, respectively, in the 12 rats in the fed group. (39.5 − 18.8 = 20.7 ÷ 39.5 = 52%). (The differences in the averages were statistically significant.)

The total decrease of C^{14}-histamine in the stomach and intestine combined was 40% as compared to 30% in the first series of tests on chronic gastric fistula rats. (39.5 + 48.8 = 88.3; 34.3 + 18.8 = 53.1; 88.3 − 53.1 = 35.2 ÷ 88.3 = 40%) This difference of 10% is probably an experimental error since the loss of C^{14}-histamine from stomach and intestine is greater (40%) than the observed increase in the urine (30%). (The 10% loss may have been in the feces.)

However, when a balance sheet of the actual counts is composed, as in Table 12, the increase in the urinary excretion on feeding was 43% and the decrease in the C^{14}-histamine in the stomach and intestine is 40%. (Table 12; compare Experiment I, line D with Experiment II, line H).

Experiment I has been repeated on one dog. It was found that feeding caused a 190% increase in the output of C^{14}-methyl histamine in the urine after feeding, when AG and iproniazid were given subcutaneously to prevent the conversion of methyl histamine to methyl imidazoleacetic acid. (The opportunity to continue the study on dogs has not been available).

In view of these values, it is evident that the percentage loss of C^{14}-histamine from the combined gastric and intestinal mucosa checks well with the percentage increase in the urinary increase of C^{14}-histamine after feeding.

These values also show clearly that none of the increased urinary excretion comes from the effect of feeding on the liver, skin and kidney, or other tissues.

It is possible that some of the loss of C^{14}-histamine from the gastric and intestinal mucosa after feeding might be due to desquamation of the superficial cells.

Table 12. *Balance sheet of the increase in C^{14}-Histamine output in urine after feeding and the decrease in C^{14} in the stomach and intestine combined after feeding*

Experiment I. Increase in C^{14}-Histamine in urine	CPM[1]
A. Total excretion (CPM) of C^{14}-Histamine in the urine 12-hr feeding period	185
B. Prefeeding excretion of C^{14}-Histamine in the urine during control pre-feeding period	105
C. Increase in CPM as C^{14}-Histamine in urine as result of feeding	80
D. % Increase: 80:185 = 43	43%
Experiment II. Decrease in C^{14}-Histamine in stomach and intestine	
E. Total C^{14}-Histamine in stomach and intestine in 12-hr fed animals 48.8 + 39.5 =	88.3
F. Total C^{14}-Histamine in stomach and intestine in non-fed animals 34.3 + 18.8 =	53.1
G. Decrease in stomach and intestine as result of feeding	35.2
H. % Decrease: 35.2:88.3 = 40	40%

[1] CPM, counts/minute.

This possibility was considered in another study by IVY (1958a). It was found that a maximum of only 10% of the histamine loss in the gastric and 30% of that in the intestine could have been lost by desquamation. The rate of loss and renewal of the superficial cells in the intestine during 24 hours of realimentation after 48 hours of fasting was approximately three times faster than in the stomach (LEBLOND and WALKER, 1956). *That desquamation was not involved was more simply arrived at by the following observations: although the rate of desquamation of superficial cells is approximately twice as rapid in the intestine as in the stomach, the intestine showed only a 30% loss of C^{14}-histamine as compared to a 50% loss for the stomach.*

Further evidence supports the observations of SCHAYER and IVY to the effect that a meal increases the gastric mucosal metabolism of histamine and its excretion in the urine. BJURÖ (1963) found that a decrease in the intake of food by rats is associated with a decrease in the urinary excretion of histamine. BJURÖ (1963), on using C^{14}-histamine, concluded that the greater part of the urinary histamine in rats comes from the stomach. KAHLSON et al. (1963) reported that on feeding rats after 24 hours of fasting, an increase in the formation of C^{14}-histamine occured in the glandular stomach *in vitro*. The peak of the increased rate of formation was reached 3 or 4 hours after feeding. An increase in formation of C^{14}-histamine also occured after the injection of "non-histamine gastrin", indicating that this "gastrin" in some way releases histamine.

E. General comment

It is believed that it should first be made clear regarding what evidence is required to categorically prove that histamine is released into the blood by the gastric and intestinal mucosa during feeding in quantities sufficient to stimulate gastric secretion. When a transplanted gastric pouch in a dog secretes acid after feeding, that is categorical proof that something gets into the blood after eating which stimulates gastric secretion. When a denervated pyloric pouch is distended with a balloon, and a large transplanted pouch secretes, that is categorical proof that a chemical is released by the pyloric mucosa into the blood and that the chemical is not a secretagog absorbed from the food.

To prove categorically that histamine is released in the blood on feeding or mechanical stimulation of a pyloric pouch the following evidence would be required: (I) Histamine must be present in the gastric and/or pyloric mucosa in a labeled form. (II) It must be shown to be released into the blood in amounts adequate to stimulate the secretion of acid. (III) It must be seen to go to the surface or inside of the parietal cell. It is possible that these requirements shall never be met, and that we shall have to be satisfied with highly presumptive, circumstantial evidence.

Let us review the evidence briefly: I(A) There is plenty of histamine in both the corporic, pyloric, or intestinal mucosa to stimulate gastric secretion if it is released slowly into the blood. (B) Furthermore, new histamine can be produced in the mucosa as the old is released. (C) The histamine can be and has been labeled.

All the requirements for (I) have been met. But it is possible that the C^{14}-histamine produced by the decarboxylation of C^{14}-L-histidine is N-methyl or dimethyl histamine, and that the product is adsorbed to a polypeptide or mucoprotein carrier. The requirements for (II) have not been met by direct evidence. That is, the labeled histamine has not been actually detected in the blood but no such an attempt has yet been made, it being considered unnecessary until more important information was obtained. Neither has the concentration of unlabeled histamine in the blood been found by chemical and intestinal strip methods to be increased in the blood after feeding. But, since histamine is so potent, it could be released and stimulate HCl production without being detectible by any of the present chemical methods. However, since the kidney concentrates histamine, so far as the plasma is concerned, urine outputs of unlabeled and labeled histamine have been found to increase after feeding and certain other procedures which stimulate gastric secretion. In the case of rats and one dog, it has been found that *labeled histamine* in the urine increases after feeding. In rats it has been found that the increase of labeled histamine in the urine is approximately equal to the decrease in the gastric and intestinal mucosa. *So, the increase in the urine could have come only from the gastric and intestinal mucosa.* (C) Logically then, it is unnecessary to detect an increase of labeled histamine in the blood. *In the rat then the requirements for (II) have been logically met.* It might be pointed out that the use of AG was responsible in part for the increase in gastric secretion. It may have been for part of the increase. But a 52 % loss of the labeled histamine in the gastric and of 30 % in the intestinal mucosa is ample histamine along with the associated unlabeled histamine to stimulate gastric secretion over a 12-hour period without the assistance of AG (Lane et al., 1957). The direct measurement of an increase in labeled histamine in the urine after feeding which was equal to the loss in the gastric and intestinal mucosa shows circumstantially that the portion lost from the stomach had to go through the blood to reach the kidney. *All the requirements of (III) have been logically met.* It has been established that unlabeled and labeled histamine is in the gastric juice. It has not been established where it comes from, except when C^{14}-histamine was injected. It undoubtedly arises in or passes through the parietal cell. Histological C^{14}-histidine or C^{14}-histamine radioautographs should solve this problem of whether it makes the histamine it "secretes" when exogenous histamine is not injected.

In the rat and dog the evidence is strongly presumptive in support of the conclusion that either histamine or some unknown closely related substance is a gastric hormone. Aminoguanidine could act by augmenting, in an additive manner, the secretory response to histamine or a closely related substance, released after feeding, by the gastrointestinal mucosa. It could also augment the response to histamine absorbed from the intestine. But in the experiments outlined above any absorption from the intestine would not be detected because the histamine would be unlabeled except perhaps in traces.

VI. Non-histamine "gastrin"

A. Introduction

The subject calls for a brief consideration for two reasons. *First* whether the hormone, gastrin, is or is not histamine is a question which has received considerable attention in recent years. *Second*, it has been reported by SMITH (1954) that a "non-histamine gastrin" he made according to the method of UVNÄS, when injected into cats, released histamine from skin and skeletal muscle (SMITH, 1954). More recently, WADDELL et al. (1961) have reported that one of the non-histamine "gastrins" made from hogs by the method of GREGORY stimulates antibody production in rabbits. When anti-hog "gastrin" serum was reacted with hog, dog, and human "gastrin" *in vitro* and the reaction product was injected, a reduction in the gastric secretory potency of the "gastrin" occurred. KAHLSON et al. (1963) found that "non-histamine gastrin" increased the formation of C^{14}-histamine in the glandular stomach *in vitro* of fasting rats.

B. Observations

KOMAROV (1938, 1942) found a substance in the protein fraction of dog's pyloric mucosa free, or almost so, of histamine which on intravenous injection stimulated gastric secretion. Later UVNÄS (1942 a, 1944, 1945), HARPER (1946-1947), JALLING and JORPES (1946), and FRIEDMAN and KING (1947) reported on preparations of pyloric mucosa essentially free of histamine. HANSON and GROSSMANN (see GROSSMAN, 1950) made preparations by IVY's method for secretin which sometimes stimulated. More recently GREGORY and TRACY (1959, 1960, 1961) have prepared a non-histamine "gastrin" from hog's mucosa.

IVY (1958 b,c) has tried to produce preparations of "gastrin" from hog's mucosa, which were entirely free from histamine by the ileal strip method of testing, and still would stimulate gastric secretion when given intravenously to the anesthetized cat (UVNÄS 1942 a, 1944, 1945). He found that the methods of KOMAROV, UVNÄS, and JALLING and JORPES yielded "gastrin" preparations which would stimulate gastric secretion when given intravenously in the cat. But, they all contained enough histamine to stimulate a cat which is very susceptible to intravenous histamine (0.005 to 0.01 μg/kg/min; ave. 0.015 μg/kg/min). However, IVY (1958c) assayed a small sample of "gastrin" sent to him by Professor HARPER. It stimulated gastric secretion intravenously and failed to cause a contraction of ileal strips of the guinea pig.

In 1961, WOJCIECH and IVY, with KATO, prepared a "gastrin" from hog's pyloric mucosa by a method of their own which was especially designed to remove all free histamine (See Appendix A). When given to gastric pouch dogs (gastric fistula, vagotomized pouch of the entire stomach, and HEIDENHAIN pouch) which were standardized to a dose of histamine given intravenously and subcutaneously, the preparation stimulated secretion. The method has yielded an active product in 25 successive batches. The product produced 10 mg of HCl output when given subcutaneously or intravenously (10 min) to dogs in a dose of 8-10 mg. It was devoid of "free" histamine by blood pressure assay and by paper chromatography. It is interesting that with the IVY-WOJCIECH-KATO method one secretory unit (10 to 20 mg HCl) is obtained from 4 or 5 gm of mucosa, as observed by KEETON and KOCH (1915).

KATO (1961) working with IVY and WOJCIECH found that their "gastrin" preparation contained four different carriers of "gastrin". By isoelectric precipitation and paper chromatography two of the carriers were polypeptides and two were mucopolysaccharides. By paper chromatography and elution it was found that a "gastrin" could be separated from one of the mucopolysaccharides but not the polypeptides. ANDERSON et al. (1962) have also reported several isoelectrically precipitable "gastrins".

YUSEM (1961), working with an IVY-WOJCIECH-KATO preparation of "gastrin" and a chemical method which involved hydrolysis obtained a color reaction by the SHORE et al. (1959) chemical method for histamine, indicating the presence of a "bound histamine" or a substance closely related to histamine. Finding a chemical method for the reliable determination of very small quantities of histamine is a difficult problem.

It is of interest to indicate that WADDELL et al. (1961) studying a "gastrin" prepared by the GREGORY-TRACY method found one major antigenic component and at least three minor antigenic components. This recalls the four carriers of "gastrin" found by KATO (1961).

GROSSMAN (personal communication) has sent to the senior author (A.C.I.) a modification of GREGORY's method. This method is less complex than ours and that of GREGORY. It has yielded 28 active batches without a failure in our hands. With the GREGORY-GROSSMAN method WOJCIECH and IVY have obtained one dog unit (10 to 20 mg HCl) from 4 to 5 gm of mucosa. This is the same yield in the form of histamine we have obtained with the KEETON and KOCH method (1915) for hogs, pyloric mucosa.

C. Comment

An extract can be repeatedly made from hog's pyloric mucosa; also from the pyloric mucosa of dog, cat and man. On slow (15 sec.) intravenous injection or on subcutaneous injection, it stimulates gastric secretion. It is devoid undoubtedly of sufficient "free histamine" to stimulate gastric secretion especially when a gastric secretory dose is given subcutaneously. Enough is not known about its chemical nature to characterize it, except that it is in the non-heat coagulable protein fraction of the pyloric mucosa. The "gastrin" may be adsorbed or combined with a peptide or mucoprotein or both as a carrier. But, in one experiment it has been separated from its carrier. The IVY-WOJCIECH-KATO "gastrin" and the GREGORY-TRACY-GROSSMAN "gastrin" acts on the gastric glands like histamine but usually acts longer. It is not inactivated by histaminase (BAUER and UVNÄS, 1944).

If "non-histamine gastrin" releases histamine from the skin, as reported by SMITH (1954), then the stimulation of histamine metabolism in the gastric mucosa after a meal or after the injection of "non-histamine gastrin" (KAHLSON et al., 1963) is not a specific phenomenon. It is obviously important to determine whether "non-histamine gastrin" is quantitatively or qualitatively specific for the acid secreting mucosa.

"Non-histamine gastrin" may release histamine by acting on the "H-cells" or those cells in the acid secreting mucosa which hypothetically release histamine on stimulation by ACh. Or, it may release histamine by acting directly on the parietal cells. There is no evidence indicating that it acts on the parietal cells directly without the release of histamine into the gastric secretion.

Since the gastric hypersecretion in patients with a ZOLLINGER-ELLISON tumor disappears after the excision of the tumor, and since such tumors contain a "non-histamine gastrin", it would appear logically certain that "non-histamine gastrin" is at least quantitatively specific for the acid secreting mucosa, as regards the release of histamine. If not, then such a "gastrin" must act directly on the parietal cell without the release of histamine, which is contrary to the observations of EMMELIN and KAHLSON (1944) and KAHLSON et al. (1963) to the effect that histamine is in the gastric juice stimulated by the "non-histamine gastrin" of UVNÄS.

D. Concentration of histamine and "gastrin" in Zollinger-Ellison islet cell tumors of the pancreas without hypoglycemia

In the ZOLLINGER-ELLISON syndrome hypersecretion with peptic ulcer is found. It disappears after the removal of a tumor of the pancreas. The tumor is composed of cells which resemble the alpha-cells of the islets of LANGERHANS (ZOLLINGER and ELLISON, 1955; GREGORY et al., 1960; MARKS et al., 1961). Such tumors have been extracted by GREGORY and the extract prepared stimulated gastric secretion when given subcutaneously. The extracts contained less than 0.25 (GREGORY et al., 1960) and 0.01 (GROSSMAN et al., 1961) micrograms of histamine per gram of wet tissue and were 33 to 45 times (GREGOREY et al., 1960) more potent than the extract of 20 grams of hog's pyloric mucosa in stimulating gastric secretion. The method used to extract the tumors was that of GREGORY et al. (1960). This observation has been confirmed by GROSSMAN et al. (1961). CODE et al. (SUMMERSKILL et al., 1961) found a "gastrin" in an islet-cell tumor and also one human histologically "normal" pancreas. HALLENBECK et al., (1963) failed to obtain a detectible amount of a "gastrin" in normal pancreatic tissue of dogs, hogs and humans. They used a modified GREGORY method.

E. Comment

The gastric secretory activity of the GREGORY et al. extracts of these tumors is not due to free histamine, but to a substance analogous to KOMAROV's "gastrin". Similar non-tumorous cells may be the cells which produce KOMAROV's "gastrin" in the gastric mucosa.

VII. Histamine and HCl formation

Histamine in stimulating the parietal cell to secrete H^+, Cl^-, and water undoubtedly acts to increase the permeability of the cell to the Cl^- ion and water. It very probably increases the permeability of the cell to Na^+ ion also. Since the process of HCl formation may be exemplified as $NaCl + H_2CO_3 = NaHCO_3$ (plasma) + HCl (secreted), and since this reaction occurs spontaneously to the left, histamine must in some way excite the parietal cell to provide the energy for the reversal of the spontaneous process. The exciting action may be that histamine increases the permeability of the cell to NaCl. Then NaCl initiates an $Na^+-K^+-H^+$ exchange mechanism and a release of the energy required to reverse the spontaneous reaction referred to above. EYRING and DOUGHERTY (1955) have suggested that histamine serves as a mediator of sodium transport across the cell membrane.

VIII. Conclusions

Two apparently different substances which stimulate secretion of HCl by the gastric glands may be extracted from the pyloric mucosa. One is histamine. The second is unknown in regard to its chemical nature, except that it is found in what is usually called the polypeptide fraction of tissue extracts.

The second substance, usually called KOMAROV's "gastrin", may turn out (a) to be a substance closely allied chemically to histamine which is adsorbed or combined with peptides as carriers, or (b) to be a polypeptide as potent for gastric secretion as secretin is for pancreatic secretion or (c) to be a substance which releases histamine in the acid secreting mucosa near to or in the parietal cell.

A very large amount of strongly presumptive or circumstantial evidence indicates that histamine is physiologically involved as a circulating and a local tissue hormone in the process of gastric secretion. On the other hand, no evidence indicates that KOMAROV's "gastrin" is a circulating or a local tissue hormone, except its presence in pyloric mucosa, and perhaps in duodenal mucosa and in the ZOLLINGER-ELLISON Islet Cell Tumor. Since the gastric secretory effect of the tumor disappears after its removal, it is evident that the Islet Cell Tumor "gastrin" actually circulates.

In view of the very large amount of information available about histamine and the availability of radioisotopic techniques, it now appears that it will be very much easier to prove or disprove that histamine is a circulating or a local tissue hormone or both, than to prove that KOMAROV's "gastrin" is actually released by the pyloric mucosa and also perhaps by cells adjacent to the parietal cells.

All the established facts pertaining to the nature of the relation of histamine to the gastric secretory mechanism render such a reasonable physiological picture, that should it be found that histamine is in no way concerned, as a hormone, the problem of explaining the facts will be as difficult as it was to discover them. Since it appears from the literature that histamine or a histamine like substance is present in the gastric juice regardless of how the secretion is stimulated, since histamine in very small amounts stimulates acid secretion, since the urinary excretion of histamine is increased when gastric secretion is stimulated by various means, and since "non-histamine gastrin" apparently stimulates histamine metabolism in the gastric mucosa, it would appear that histamine is the final stimulus of the parietal cell. However, more evidence is required before such a conclusion can be considered as established.

Appendix

Production of "gastrins" devoid of free histamine from the pyloric mucosa of pigs

A. Method of IVY, WOJCIECH and KATO Applied to 25 successive batches of pyloric mucosa

1. The pyloric mucosa is washed gently, resected and frozen (dry ice) within 30 min post-mortem at the stockyards.

2. It is thawed by placing each specimen in 5 volumes boiling 0.12 N/HCl and then boiling for 5 to 10 min to destroy enzymes and bacteria.

3. The specimens are then passed through a meat grinder, and the ground material is placed in the acid fluid from step 2 and stirred for 30 min. The mixture is filtered through gauze.

4. Extract the ground material again with 3 vol. of 0.1 N/HCl and a third time with two volumes of 0.12 N/HCl.

5. Filter the combined extracts through gauze, if necessary, and centrifuge at 1800 r.p.m. for 20 min. (Supernatant is cloudy.) Discard the insoluble residue.

6. The supernatant is kept in the cold room (+ 5° C) for 16—20 hrs. (This is important to give a clear separation with NaCl precipitation.)

7. Add NaCl, 28 g/100 cc, to the supernatant. Allow the precipitate to harden at room temperature overnight.

8. The clear filtrate is siphoned out and the precipitate is collected on filter paper (Sargent & Co. No. 500). It is then dried using a fan.

9. The dried NaCl precipitate is decolorized partly and "defatted" with anhydrous acetone-ether (1:1). The extraction is repeated until a total of 15 to 20 volumes is used for 200—250 g of precipitate.

10. After defatting, the precipitate is weighed, and extracted with a solution made up of 85 parts of 95% ethanol and 15 parts of 0.12 N/HCl. Ten vol. is used for the first, and 5 vol. for the second and third extractions. Centrifugation instead of filtration is used to separate the fluid from the insoluble residue. Discard the residue.

11. The alcoholic extract is concentrated under vacuum in a N_2 atmospere at 20—25° C inside the flask. The concentration proceeds until the volume is approximately equal to that of the volume of the 0.12 N/HCl used.

12. The concentrate is made up to the initial volume of 0.12 N/HCl by adding distilled water and then placed *in sterile* (No-jax sausage) casings (Visking Co.) and dialyzed against running distilled water for 16 hrs. (During this procedure, a precipitate forms.)

13. The precipitate (A22) was separated from the supernatant (A23) by centrifuging. It is dried with half and half acetone and ether and weighed.

14. The supernatant (A23) has a pH of 3.9 to 4.0. This was tested by intravenous and subcutaneous injection in dogs. *It is active* in doses of 8—10 mg.

15. The dried precipitate (A22) was dissolved in 0.01 N/HCl, at a pH of approximately 2. This was tested by intravenous and subcutaneous injection in dogs. *It is active.*

Comment: The gastric secretory activity is approximately equally divided between A 22 and A 23. From 3 to 4 dog doses (threshold or minimal response doses) are obtained from each 40 gm piece of pyloric mucosa, depending on the dog. The gastric fistula dog with the vagi intact usually secretes more HCl in response to a unit dose than the dog with a pouch of the entire stomach with the vagi cut, or the HEIDENHAIN pouch dog.

The secretory response to this "gastrin" is usually more prolonged than that to free histamine, especially in the otherwise intact gastric fistula dog. *Psychic stimulation* must be carefully watched for and avoided in the gastric fistula dog with intact vagi.

No special attempt has yet been made by us to concentrate this "gastrin". We have been more interested to date in studying the solubility properties and in developing an easily repeatable or consistently reliable method. *The above method has not failed in* 10 *consecutive tests.*

The dog preparations used for assay consisted of two HEIDENHAIN pouches, two pouches of the entire stomach with vagi cut, and two gastric fistula dogs with vagi intact. Each dog was standardized to a threshold or minimal response dose of free histamine given intravenously (over 7—10 min.) and subcutaneously.

Like solutions of histamine, the solutions of A22 and A23 must be kept frozen, except when a sample is removed, to prevent deterioration.

When isoelectric precipitation is performed on the material soluble in the 80% acid ethanol after being made up to volume in Step 12 and before dialysis, three isoelectric proteins are found. One is insoluble at pH 2 to 1, one is insoluble at a pH of 5.4 to 5.5. One is insoluble at pH 8.4 to 8.5. These precipitates are all active, and some activity remains in the supernatant at pH 8.4 to 8.5. Drying the precipitate with half and half acetone and ether changes the isoelectric properties of the protein carriers of gastrin.

Chromatographic separation shows a fast moving (zone 4) and a slow moving (zone 3) carrier of "gastrin". A fast and slowly moving "gastrin" carrier is in the dried precipitate (A22) and the supernatant (A23). The fast moving carrier stains with toluidine blue like a mucopolysaccharide and the slow moving carrier stains with ninhydrin like a polypeptide. So, there are 4 different carriers of the "gastrin" we are studying, 2 are mucopolysaccharides and 2 are polypeptides.

We suspect that we are extracting the cells which contain a heparin-histamine complex and probably a polypeptide-histamine complex. The "gastrin" we are studying may be histamine or a compound which has color reactions like histamine.

It should be recalled that "heparin" is not a single compound but a group of several mucopolysaccharides.

More recently by paper chromatography the "gastrin" was separated from the mucopolysaccharide.

B. Method of R. W. Keeton and F. C. Koch for histamine "gastrin"

1. The stomach is obtained within 30 min after death at the abattoir, opened and washed with tepid water. The pyloric mucosa or lining is resected from the muscle wall and placed in about 5 times its weight of 0.4% aqueous HCl solution.

2. This material is taken to the laboratory where it is run through a meat grinder, returned to the acid solution and heated to 90°C on a steam bath, allowed to cool and stand for 12 hrs, after which it is heated again to 90°C and allowed to stand for 24 hrs.

3. The fluid is then filtered and its volume recorded.

4. The volume was then reduced under suction at not over 40—50°C to 1/15 its original volume.

5. Six volumes of 95% alcohol are added and the mixture allowed to stand 24 hrs, filtered and the filtrate evaporated under reduced pressure at not over 40—50°C.

6. The residue from "5" is dehydrated by adding some absolute alcohol and evaporated to dryness under reduced pressure. This is repeated 3 or 4 times.

7. The dehydrated residue from "6" is extracted 4 times with boiling absolute alcohol.

8. The hot absolute alcohol insoluble residue was dissolved in water and evaporated to dryness under reduced pressure. This was repeated until the odor of alcohol was gone.

9. The residue from "8" was dissolved in freshly distilled water so that 1 ml represented the extract of 4 to 5 g of the mucosa.

10. It can then be placed in tubes and sterilized. 1 cc is a gastric secretory dose if some error has not been made.

Comment: The recovery of added histamine has never been reported.

C. Method of Barsoum and Gaddum will also yield histamine "gastrin"

1. The pyloric linings are ground and placed in 2 volumes of 10% trichloracetic acid and thoroughly mixed. It is allowed to stand overnight.

2. The mixture is filtered and the precipitate washed 3 times with an equal volume of 5% trichloracetic acid.

3. The trichloracetic acid is removed by shaking with ether in a separatory funnel 4 or 5 times or until the aqueous phase is about neutral to Congo paper.

4. An equal volume of N/HCl is added to the aqueous extract which is then boiled for 1.5 hrs under a reflux condensor.

5. The extract is evaporated to dryness under reduced pressure at a temperature of 40—50°C.

6. Two volumes of 95% alcohol are added and the mixture evaporated at reduced pressure to remove the HCl. This is repeated two or three times and the pH checked with Congo paper.

7. The residue is extracted with 3 volumes of absolute alcohol 4 times. The alcohol extracts are combined and evaporated to dryness.

8. The residue from "7" is then dissolved in freshly distlled water or normal saline, placed in ampules, sterilized and kept in a refrigerator. Code, Hallenbeck, and Gregory (Am. J. Physiol. 151: 593, 1947) recovered 80% of added histamine by this method; Barsoum and Gaddum about 90% (J. Physiol. 85: 1, 1935).

D. Method of Gilman and Lindskog (1942) reported to recover 100% of added histamine

1. The fresh tissue is treated with an equal volume of 70% alcohol and thoroughly ground and macerated.

2. The mixture is placed in a bottle and enough 70% alcohol is added to make 15 volumes of alcohol to 1 of tissue. Enough HCl is added to the mixture to yield a 0.1 N solution. The bottle is then agitated in a mechanical shaker for 3 hrs.

3. The bottle is allowed to stand. The supernatant is decanted and filtered. The residuum is re-extracted 3 times with 2 volumes of 70% alcohol.

4. The supernatant was evaporated to dryness on a steam bath.
5. The residue can be kept in the refrigerator or desiccator as a powder to use as desired.

Comment: This is a very simple method. No one has repeated the method to confirm the 100% recovery of added histamine. But one of us knows from his personal experience with alcohol extraction of pyloric mucosa that the residue will contain "gastrin".

General Comment: A study of the foregoing methods will show that the last three methods were so constituted that histamine or some closely related substance would be the active principle of the extract. The first method, and those of KOMAROV and UVNÄS from the second step were designed to get rid of histamine as was the design in the secretin studies, and all other gastrointestinal hormones.

E. Method of GREGORY-TRACY-GROSSMAN for the production of a "gastrin" free of histamine from the pyloric mucosa of pigs

[I. E. GILLESPIE and M. I. GROSSMAN, Gastroenterology, **44**, 301 (1963)]. Forty different batches yielded an active preparation

1. The pyloric mucosa was removed from the muscularis externa within 30 min after death and was frozen with CO_2-ice. At the laboratory 1 kg of the frozen specimens was dropped one-by-one into distilled water (1000 ml) boiling briskly to coagulate protein and to destroy enzymes at 100° C for 1 min. The specimens were then ground, the water used for boiling being combined with the ground material.

2. The ground specimens were homogenized with a mechanical blendor for 2 min. The mixture was brought to a volume of 4 liters with distilled water. The mixture was boiled while stirring for 5 min and then cooled to 25° C. The solution was strained through a wire strainer and then through a linen cloth. The large particles were discarded and the fluid was centrifuged (2500 rpm, 5 min). The supernatant was decanted and brought to a pH 4.0 with glacial acetic acid, and then allowed to remain at 5° C for 24 hrs. The cloudy supernatant was removed by aspiration and discarded. The precipitate with some fluid was centrifuged (2000 rpm; 30 min). The cloudy supernatant was discarded.

3. The syrupy precipitate was placed in a 1 liter graduated cylinder and made up to the closest 100 ml mark (600 to 700 ml usually) with distilled water. A solution of 2.7% trichloracetic acid (TCA) in acetone was made up and 3 volumes (1800 to 2100 ml) of it was added while stirring to the syrupy fluid which has been transfered to a large beaker, so that the mixture could be stirred mechanically for 1 hr.

4. A BUCHNER funnel with a moistened coarse filter paper was prepared by suspending 2 g of Hyflo (JOHNS-MANSVILLE filter aid) in 200 ml of water with gentle suction to produce a pad. Five grams of Hyflo was added to the acetone-TCA mixture and allowed to settle. Then the Clearer portion was poured on the filter pad slowly and the sediment last. Gentle suction was applied until the filter pad cracked. The precipitate on the pad was discarded.

5. To the clear filtrate 1 ml of concentrated HCl was added for each 100 ml of filtrate. Then 2 volumes of ethyl ether were added to the filtrate, was shaken vigorously and allowed to stand for 15 min. (A large separatory funned may be used.) (The ether layer is discarded since it contains the TCA.) This extraction was repeated two more times.

6. The aqueous solution was transferred to an evaporating dish. The pH was adjusted to 3.0 by the addition of NaOH, first using a 50% and then a 2N solution. The mixture was heated to 75° C on a steam bath with stirring to remove the ether. The solution was then cooled to 20° C and transferred to a beaker, the volume being made up to 500 ml with water.

7. The solution was now treated with a 100% TCA (100 g TCA made up to 100 ml) by adding it dropwise while stirring. After standing for 15 min the mixture was added to a centrifuge tube (250 ml) and centrifuged (2500 rpm, 10 min), the centrifuging being repeated until all the precipitate was collected in the 250 ml tube.

8. The precipitate was now treated with 70 ml of a 0.15 N—HCl solution with stirring to obtain a complete dispersion. The TCA was then removed by filling the tube with ether and shaking and then aspirating or decanting the ether. The extraction of the TCA was repeated two more times. (This can be done in a separatory funnel.)

9. The acid aqueous phase was transferred to an evaporating dish, with the water washes used. The pH was adjusted to pH 8.0 with 2 N—NaOH, using 1 to 20 ml concentrated NH_4OH for the final adjustment. The mixture was heated at 75° C on a steam bath while stirring. The slightly cloudy fluid was made up to 100 ml with water and stored in a plastic bottle at —20° C.

10. This procedure yielded 1 ml of final solution for each 10 g of mucosa. Usually the dose of "gastrin" extract is expressed in grams of wet pyloric mucosa.

The protein content estimated by the absorption of ultraviolet light (280 mμ) using serum albumin as a standard was from 0.9 to 1.3 mg per gram weight of mucosa.

The histamine content when assayed on guinea pig ileum was less than 0.001 μg per gram of mucosa.

This preparation is referred to as "crude gastrin", or Stage II "gastrin".

11. A more purified product has been produced by GREGORY and TRACY [J. Physiol. **156**, 523 (1961)]. The "crude gastrin" is adsorbed on a column of calcium phosphate gel from which it is eluted with a solution disodium hydrogen phosphate. The protein concentration was 0.09 mg per gram weight of mucosa. (The foregoing method has been used successfully by the senior author.)

References

ABEL, J. J., and S. KUBOTA: On the presence of histamine (β-iminazolylethylamine) in the hypophysis, cerebri and other tissues of the body and its occurrence among the hydrolytic decomposition products of proteins. J. Pharmacol. exp. Ther. **13**, 243 (1919).

ACKERMAN, D., u. H. G. FUCHS: Zur Frage des Vorkommens von Histamin im normalen Harn. Z. Hoppe-Seylers physiol. Chem. **259**, 32 (1939).

ADAM, H. M.: Excretion of histamine in human urine. Quart. J. exp. Physiol. **35**, 281 (1950).

— W. I. CARD, M. J. RIDDELL, M. ROBERTS and J. A. STRONG: The effect of intravenous infusions of histamine on the urinary histamine and on gastric secretion in man. Brit. J. Pharmacol. **9**, 62 (1954a).

— — — — — and B. WOOLF: Dose-response curves for the effect of histamine on acid gastric secretion in man. Brit. J. Pharmacol **9**, 329 (1954b).

— D. C. HARDWICK and K. E. V. SPENCER: Method of estimating histamine in plasma. Brit. J. Pharmacol **12**, 397 (1957).

— R. B. HUNTER and T. W. KINNEAR: Observations on the urinary excretion of histamine in urticaria. Quart. J. exp. Physiol. **36**, 49 (1950—1951).

AINSWORTH, C., and R. G. JONES: 1,2,4-triazole analogs of histamine. J. Amer. chem. Soc. **75**, 4915 (1953).

ALLES, G. A., B. B. WISEGARVER and M. A. SHULL: Comparative physiological actions of some β-(imidazolyl-4-)alkylamines. J. Pharmacol. exp. Ther. **77**, 54 (1943).

ANDERSON, W. R., T. L. FLETCHER, C. L. PITTS and H. N. HARKINS. Isolation and assay of ovine gastrin. Nature **193**, 1286 (1962).

ANREP, G. V., M. S. AYADI, G. S. BARSOUM, J. R. SMITH and M. M. TALAAT: Excretion of histamine in urine. J. Physiol. (Lond.) **103**, 155 (1944).

ASHFORD, C. A., H. HELLER and G. A. SMART: Effect of antihistamine substances on gastric secretion in man. Brit. J. Pharmacol. **4**, 157 (1949).

ATKINSON, A. J., and A. C. IVY: The action of histaminase on the gastric secretory response to histamine and to a meal. Amer. J. Physiol. **107**, 168 (1934).

— — and V. BASS: Histaminase and gastric response to histamine. Amer. J. Physiol. **132**, 51 (1941).

BABKIN, B. P.: Secretory Mechanism of the Digestive Glands. New York: P. B. Hoeber 1944, 1950.

BAKER, T. W.: Histaminase in treatment of cold allergy. J. Amer. med. Ass. **114**, 1059 (1940).

BARGER, G., and H. H. DALE: β-iminazolylethylamine a depressor constituent of intestinal mucosa. J. Physiol. (Lond.) **41**, 499 (1911).

BARSOUM, G. S., and J. H. GADDUM: Pharmacological estimation of adenosine and histamine in blood. J. Physiol. (Lond.) **85**, 1 (1935).

BAUER, A., and B. UVNÄS: The activity of the gastric secretory excitant of the pyloric mucosa after treatment with histaminase. Acta Physiol. scand. **8**, 158 (1944).

BAYLISS, W. M., and E. H. STARLING: Mechanism of pancreatic secretion. J. Physiol. (Lond.) **28**, 325 (1902); **29**, 174 (1903).

BAZETT, H. C., J. C. SCOTT, M. E. MAXFIELD and M. D. BLITHE: Calculation of cardiac output from blood pressure measurements before and after meals. Amer. J. Physiol. **116**, 551 (1936).

BEAZELL, J. M., and A. C. IVY: The influence of alcohol on the digestive tract. Quart. J. Stud. Alcohol **1**, 45 (1940—1941).

BENJAMIN, F. B., C. E. ROSIERE and M. I. GROSSMAN: A comparison of the effectiveness of banthine and atropine in depressing gastric acid secretion in man and the dog. Gastroenterology **15**, 727 (1950).

BEST, C. H., and E. W. MCHENRY: Inactivation of histamine. J. Physiol. (Lond.) **70**, 349 (1930).

BIKICH, G., J. BORBOLA and G. HETENYI: Experimental approach to the role of histamine in peptic ulcer formation. Acta med. Acad. Sci. hung. **6**, 207 (1954).

BJURÖ, T.: Histamine metabolism in adrenalectomized rats. Acta Physiol. Scand **60**, Suppl. 220 (1963).
BLAIR, D. W., and A. P. M. FORREST: Effect of local antihistamines on gastric secretion in dogs. Brit. J. Surg. **47**, 428 (1960).
BLOCK, E., and H. NECHELES: Occurrence of acetylcholine in gastric juice. Amer. J. Physiol. **122**, 631 (1938).
BLOOMER, W. E.: Thesis Yale Univ. School of Medicine, 1942; cit. in Young (1948—1949).
BORBOLA, J., G. BIKICH and G. HETENYI: Determination of histamine in the gastric juice of man with special respect to duodenal ulcer in the active and inactive stage. Acta med. Acad. Sci. hung. **2**, 259 (1951).
BORN, G. V. R., and J. R. VANE: Gastric secretion induced by histamine. J. Physiol. (Lond.) **121**, 445 (1953).
BOURQUE, J. E., and E. R. LOEW: Histamine antagonists and gastric secretion. Amer. J. Physiol. **138**, 341 (1942—1943).
BROWN, C. L., and R. G. SMITH: An histamine-like substance in the gastric juice. Amer. J. Physiol. **113**, 455 (1935).
BUGAJSKI, J., and J. KAULBERSZ: Zawartosc Histaminy W Soku Zoladkowym Wydzielonym Po Pozornym Karmieniu. Histamine content in gastric juice secreted after sham feeding. Acta physiol. pol. **11**, 667 (1960).
BUNSE, W., u. F. JUNG: Hemmung der Histaminwirkung und Magensaftsekretion. Klin. Wschr. **26**, 345 (1948).
BURCHELL, H. B., and R. L. VARCO: The anti-histamine activity of thymoxyethyldiethylamine and N-ethyl-N'Dimethylaminoethylaniline as judged by the gastric response to histamine. J. Pharmacol. exp. Ther. **75**, 1 (1942).
CARNOT, P., W. KOSKOWSKI et E. LIBERT: Action de l'histamine sur les sucs digestifs chez l'Homme. C. R. Soc. Biol. (Paris) **86**, 670 (1922).
CHIARI, R.: Pharmakodynamische Erregung und Hemmung der Sekretion im Magen-Darmkanal. Ther. Mh. **29**, 202 (1915).
CODE, C. F.: Quantitative estimation of histamine in blood. J. Physiol. (Lond.) **89**, 257 (1937).
— Inhibition of gastric secretion. Pharm. Rev. **3**, 59 (1951).
— Histamine in blood. Physiol. Rev. **32**, 47 (1952).
— Histamine and gastric secretion. In: Ciba Foundation Symposium on Histamine. p. 189. Boston: Little, Brown and Co. 1956.
— G. A. HALLENBECK and R. A. GREGORY: Histamine content of gastric juice. Amer. J. Physiol. **151**, 593 (1947).
CONRAD, V., et K. KOWALEWSKI: Parallelisme entre les réactions thermiques cutanées et la sécrétion gastrique après injections d'extrait posthypophysaire et d'histamine. Acta gastro-ent. belg. **12**, 597 (1949).
CRAVER, B. N., W. BARRETT, A. CAMERON and E. HERROLD: Pharmacological actions of 35 derivatives of 4-methyl, 5-ethyl or 2-substituted imidazoles. Arch. int. Pharmacodyn. **87**, 33 (1951).
DALE, H. H., and P. P. LAIDLAW: The physiological action of β-iminazolyl-ethylamine. J. Physiol. (Lond.) **41**, 318 (1910); **43**, 182 (1911).
DAVENPORT, H. W., and V. J. CHAVRE: Conditions affecting acid secretion by mouse stomachs *in vitro*. Gastroenterology **15**, 467 (1950).
DAWSON, A. B., and A. C. IVY: Contributions to the physiology of the gastric secretion. X. Formation of hydrochloric acid by the gastric mucosa. Amer. J. Physiol. **76**, 158 (1926).
DOSCHERHOLMEN, A.: On the action of the antihistaminic agent Lergitin on the gastric secretion of hydrochloric acid. Acta med. scand. **135**, 195 (1949).
DOUGLAS, W. W., W. FELDBERG, W. D. M. PATON and M. SCHACHTER: Distribution of histamine and substance P in wall of dog's digestive tract. J. Physiol. (Lond.) **115**, 163 (1951).
DRAGSTEDT, C. A., J. S. GRAY, A. H. LAWTON and M. R. ARELLANO: Does alcohol stimulate gastric secretion by liberating histamine? Proc. Soc. exp. Biol. (N.Y.) **43**, 26 (1940).
DUTTA, N. K.: Some pharmacological properties common to antihistamine compounds. Brit. J. Pharmacol. **4**, 281 (1949).
—, and R. G. TAMHANE: Effect of atropine, pethidine, procaine, quinidine and prophenpyridamine maleate on the histamine-induced gastric acidity in cats. Indian J. med. Res. **41**, 45 (1953).
DWORETZKY, M., and C. F. CODE: Passage of histamine across wall of bowel. Amer. J. Physiol. **166**, 462 (1951).
EDKINS, J. S.: On the chemical mechanism of gastric secretion. Proc. roy. Soc. B **76**, 376 (1905).
— Chemical mechanism of gastric secretion. J. Physiol. (Lond.) **34**, 133 (1906).
—, and M. TWEEDY: The natural channels of absorption evoking the chemical mechanism of gastric secretion. J. Physiol. (Lond.) **38**, 263 (1909).

EHRMANN, R.: Physiologische und klinische Untersuchungen über die Magensaftsekretion. Int. Beitr. Path. Therap. Ernährungsstör. **3**, 382 (1911—1912).
EMMELIN, N.: On the presence of histamine in plasma in a physiologically active form. Acta physiol. scand. **11**, Suppl. 34 (1945).
— Disappearance of injected histamine from bloodstream. Acta physiol. scand. **22**, 379 (1951).
—, and J. FROST: Effect of β-dimethylaminoethyl benzhydryl ether hydrochloride on histamine-induced gastric secretion in cat. Acta physiol. scand. **13**, 75 (1947).
—, and G. S. KAHLSON: Histamine as a physiological excitant of acid gastric secretion. Acta physiol. scand. **8**, 289 (1944).
— — and F. WICKSELL: Histamine in plasma and method of its estimation. Acta physiol. scand. **2**, 123 (1941).
EMSMANN, O.: Über hämatogene Erregung von Magensekretion durch Salzsäureextrakte der großen drüsigen Organe des Körpers und des Darminhaltes. Int. Beitr. Path. Therap. Ernährungsstör. **3**, 117 (1911—1912).
EYRING, H., and T. F. DOUGHERTY. Molecular mechanisms in inflammation and stress. Am. Scientist **43**, 457 (1955).
FARRELL, J. I., and A. C. IVY: Contributions to the physiology of the pancreas: II. The proof of a humoral mechanism for external pancreatic secretion. Amer. J. Physiol. **78**, 325 (1926).
FAWCETT, G. G., J. ROGERS, J. M. RAHE and S. P. BEEBE: The active principles of different organs as shown in kymograph tracings. Amer. J. Physiol. **37**, 453 (1915).
FELDBERG, W.: On some physiological aspects of histamine. J. Pharm. Pharmacol. **6**, 281 (1954).
— Distribution of histamine. In: Ciba Symposium on Histamine, page 4. Boston: Little, Brown & Co. 1956.
—, and G. W. HARRIS: Distribution of histamine in mucosa of gastrointestinal tract of dog. J. Physiol. (Lond.) **120**, 352 (1953).
—, and B. HOLMES: The effect of muscular contractions and of curarine on acid gastric secretion in cats. J. Physiol. (Lond.) **99**, 3 (1941).
—, and J. TALESNIK: Reduction of tissue histamine by compound 48/80. J. Physiol. (Lond.) **120**, 550 (1953).
FERRANDO, R. J., e B. B. LOZZIO: Acción de los antihistaminicos sobre la secreción gastrica. Medicina (Parma) **17**, 235 (1957).
FORREST, A. P. M., and C. F. CODE: The inhibiting effect of epinephrine and norepinephrine on secretion induced by histamine in separated pouches of dogs. J. Pharm. exp. Ther. **110**, 447 (1954).
FRAILE-OVEJERO, A., and M. LLUCH-TRULL: Antihistaminases and gastric secretion stimulated by histamine in cats. Rev. esp. Fisiol. **12**, 347 (1956).
FRIEDMAN, M. H. F., and E. N. KING: Presence of a specific gastric hormone (gastrin) in the dog's pyloric mucosa. Fed. Proc. **6**, 107 (1947).
GADDUM, J. H.: Gefäßerweiternde Stoffe der Gewebe. Leipzig: Thieme 1936.
GAVIN, G., E. W. MCHENRY and M. J. WILSON: Histamine in canine gastric tissues. J. Physiol. (Lond.) **79**, 234 (1933).
GHOSH, M. N., and H. O. SCHILD: Continuous recording of acid gastric secretion in the rat. Brit. J. Pharmacol. **13**, 54 (1958).
GIBERTINI, G.: Il contenuto in istamina nella saliva, nel succo gastrico, nella bile. Soc. ital. Biol. Sper. (Boll.) **17**, 360 (1942).
GILG, E.: Effect of β-dimethylaminoethyl-benzhydryl-ether hydrochloride ("benadryl") on secretion of gastric juice. Acta pharmacol. (Kbh.) **4**, 81 (1948).
GILMAN, A., and G. E. LINDSKOG: The effect of pneumoccal lobar pneumonia on the histamine content of the lung. Yale J. Biol. Med. **14**, 387 (1942).
GRANT, R.: The effect of feeding on eosinophile counts in the gastric mucosa. Fed. Proc. **20**, 250 (1961).
GRAY, J. S.: The effect of atropine on gastric secretion and its relation to the gastrin theory. Amer. J. Physiol. **120**, 657 (1937).
—, and A. C. IVY: Effects of mecholyl on gastric secretion. Amer. J. Physiol. **120**, 705 (1937).
GREGORY, R. A.: Some factors influencing passage of fluid through intestinal loops in dogs. J. Physiol. (Lond.) **111**, 119 (1950a).
— The hormonal control of gastric secretion. Gastroenterologia **76**, 82 (1950b).
— Gastric secretory responses after portal venous ligation. J. Physiol. (Lond.) **144**, 123 (1958).
—, and A. C. IVY: The humoral stimulation of gastric secretion. Quart. J. exp. Physiol. **31**, 111 (1941).
—, and H. J. TRACY: The preparation and properties of gastrin. J. Physiol. (Lond.) **149**, 70 (1959).
— — The further purification of gastrin: secretory responses in a human subject. J. Physiol. (Lond.) **154**, 52 (1960).

GREGORY, R. A., and H. J. TRACY: The preparation and properties of gastrin. J. Physiol. (Lond.) **156**, 523 (1961).
— — J. M. FRENCH, and W. SIRCUS: Extraction of a gastrin-like substance from a pancreatic tumor in a case of Zollinger-Ellison syndrome. Lancet **1960 I**, 1045.
GROB, D., J. L. LILIENTHAL and A. M. HARVEY: On certain vascular effects of curare in man; "histamine" reaction. Bull. Johns Hopk. Hosp. **80**, 299 (1947).
GROSS, W.: Beitrag zur Kenntnis der Sekretionsbedingungen des Magens nach Versuchen am Hund. Arch. Verdau.-Kr. **12**, 507 (1906).
GROSSMAN, M. I.: Personal communications.
— Gastrointestinal hormones. Physiol. Rev. **30**, 33 (1950).
— Methods of assaying gastric secretory inhibitors. Meth. med. Res. **4**, 173 (1951).
— The pyloric gland area of the stomach; a brief survey. Gastroenterology **38**, 1 (1960).
— Stimulation of secretion of acid by distention of denervated fundic pouches in dogs. Gastroenterology **41**, 385 (1961).
—, and I. KOBAYASHI: Personal communication.
—, and C. R. ROBERTSON: Histamine and gastric secretion. Amer. J. Physiol. **153**, 447 (1948a).
— — Stimulation of gastric secretion by urticariogenic wetting agent (Tween 20) and its inhibition by benadryl. Proc. Soc. exp. Biol. (N. Y.) **68**, 550 (1948b).
— — and A. C. IVY: Hormone for gastric secretion. Amer. J. Physiol. **153**, 1 (1948).
— — and C. E. ROSIERE: The effect of some compounds related to histamine on gastric acid secretion. J. Pharm. exp. Ther. **104**, 277 (1952).
— H. J. TRACY and R. A. GREGORY: Zollinger-Ellison syndrome in a Bantu woman, with isolation of a gastrin-like substance from the primary and secondary tumors. II. Extraction of gastrin-like activity from tumors. Gastroenterology **41**, 87 (1961).
— J. R. WOOLEY, D. F. DUTTON and A. C. IVY: The effect of nausea on gastric secretion and a study of the mechanism concerned. Gastroenterology **4**, 347 (1945).
HAEGER, K., D. JACOBSEN and G. KAHLSON: Levels of histaminase and histamine in gastrointestinal mucosa and kidney of cat deprived of hypophysis or adrenal glands. Acta physiol. scand. **25**, 243 (1952).
—, and G. S. KAHLSON: Distribution of histamine and histaminase in gastrointestinal mucosa of fed and starved cats. Acta physiol. scand. **25**, 230 (1952a).
— — Disappearance of histaminase from whole body following adrenalectomy in cats. Acta physiol. scand. **25**, 255 (1952b).
HAKKINEN, I. P. T.: Histamine induced changes in the sulphate metabolism of the duodenum and prepyloric region of the stomach. Acta physiol. scand. **51**, Suppl. 177 (1960).
HALE, E. H., A. C. IVY and M. I. GROSSMAN: The comparative effects of water, carbonated water, sodium chloride solution, and sodium bicarbonate solution on gastric acid secretion in human subjects. J. Lab. clin. Med. **35**, 249 (1950).
HALLENBECK, G. A., C. F. CODE and D. C. MCILRATH: Absence of demonstrable gastric secretagogue in normal pancreatic tissue. Gastroenterology **44**, 627 (1963).
HANSON, M. E., and M. I. GROSSMAN: Unpublished Observations, 1946—1948. See: M. I. GROSSMAN 1950.
— — and A. C. IVY: Histamine and gastric secretion. Amer. J. Physiol. **153**, 242 (1948).
HARPER, A. A.: The effect of extracts of gastric and intestinal mucosa on the secretion of HCl by the cat's stomach. J. Physiol. (Lond.) **105**, 31 (1946—1947).
HARRIES, E. H. L.: Effect of noradrenaline on gastric secretory response to histamine in dog. J. Physiol. (Lond.) **133**, 498 (1956).
HARTMAN, W. J., W. G. CLARK and S. D. CYR: Histidine decarboxylase activity of basophils from chronic myelogenous leukemic patients. Origin of blood histamine. Proc. Soc. exp. Biol. (N. Y.) **107**, 123 (1961).
HARTMAN, S. A., and D. M. MOORE: Effect of tripelennamine hydrochloride (pyribenzamine) on gastric acidity of patients with peptic ulcer. Amer. J. dig. Dis. **15**, 271 (1948).
HEINZ, E., and K. J. ÖBRINK: Acid formation and acidity control in the stomach. Physiol. Rev. **34**, 643 (1954).
HILL, R. W., and C. F. CODE: Changes in concentration of histamine in canine gastric mucosa during secretion. Amer. J. Physiol. **197**, 5 (1959).
HIRSCHOWITZ, B. I., H. M. POLLARD, S. W. HARTWELL and J. LONDON: The action of ethyl alcohol on gastric acid secretion. Gastroenterology **30**, 244 (1956).
HIRVONEN, M.: Untersuchungen über die Wirkung einiger Antihistaminpräparate auf die Salzsäureproduktion. Ann. Med. intern. Fenn. **41**, 157 (1952).
HORTON, B. T., G. E. BROWN and G. M. ROTH: Hypersensitiveness to cold, with local and systemic manifestations of histamine-like character: its amenability to treatment. J. Amer. med. Ass. **107**, 1263 (1936).
HOWAT, H. T., and B. SCHOFIELD: The effect of urogastrone, enterogastrone and mepyramine maleate on gastric and pancreatic secretion. J. Physiol. (Lond.) **123**, 1 (1954).

IRVINE, W. T., and C. F. CODE: Gastric secretion and free histamine in urine. Amer. J. Physiol. **195**, 202 (1958).
— H. L. DUTHIE, H. D. RITCHIE and N. G. WATON: The liver's role in histamine absorption from the alimentary tract; its possible importance in cirrhosis. Lancet **1959 aI**, 1064.
— — and W. G. WATON: Urinary output of free histamine after a meat meal. Lancet **1959** b **I**, 1061.
— H. D. RITCHIE and H. M. ADAM: Histamine concentrations in the gastric venous effluent before and during acid secretion. Gastroenterology **41**, 258 (1961).
— D. B. WATKIN and E. J. WILLIAMS: The mechanism by which alcohol stimulates acid secretion. Gastroenterology **39**, 41 (1960).
IVY, A. C.: The role of hormone in digestion. Physiol. Rev. **10**, 282 (1930).
— Gastrointestinal changes in the rat on realimentation. Amer. J. Physiol. **195**, 216 (1958a).
— Proof that histamine is a gastric secretory hormone. Clin. Endocr. (Japan) **6**, 7 [July] (1958b).
— Proof that histamine is a gastric secretory hormone. Proc. World Congress of Gastroenterology, p. 102, Washington, D. C. (U.S.A.), May, 1958c.
—, and W. H. BACHRACH: An abnormal mechanism for the excitation of gastric secretion in the dog. Amer. J. dig. Dis. **7**, 76 (1940).
—, and J. I. FARRELL: Contributions to the physiology of gastric secretion. VIII. The proof of a humoral mechanism. A new procedure for the study of gastric physiology. Amer. J. Physiol. **74**, 639 (1925).
—, and A. J. JAVOIS: Contributions to the physiology of gastric secretion. VI. The stimulation of gastric secretion by amines and other substances. Amer. J. Physiol. **71**, 604 (1924—1925).
— H. KATO and R. WOJCIECH: Detailed report on purification of Komarov's "gastrin" distributed at the Federation meetings, Chicago (March) 1961.
—, and K. W. LIEPINS: Effect of derivatives and inhibitors of histamine metabolism on gastric secretion. Amer. J. Physiol. **195**, 521 (1958).
— — Effect of 1,2,4-triazole ethylamine on gastric secretion. Amer. J. Physiol. **198**, 614 (1960).
— R. K. S. LIM and J. E. MCCARTHY: Contributions to the physiology of gastric secretion. III. An attempt to prove that a humoral mechanism is concerned in gastric secretion by blood transfusion and cross-circulation. Amer. J. Physiol. **74**, 616 (1925).
—, and T. M. LIN: 1958. See IVY, 1958c.
— — E. K. IVY and E. KARVINEN: Effect of histaminase inhibitors on gastric secretion. Amer. J. Physiol. **186**, 239 (1956).
—, and J. L. MCILVAIN: The excitation of gastric secretion by application of substances to the duodenal and jejunal mucosa. Amer. J. Physiol. **67**, 124 (1923).
— — and A. J. JAVOIS: The stimulation of gastric secretion by histamine. Science **58**, 286 (1923).
—, and Y. OYAMA: Studies on the secretion of the pars pylorica gastrica. Amer. J. Physiol. **57**, 51 (1921).
— C. A. TANTURI, R. HERNANDEZ and E. BAROSO: Urticarial reaction induced in the dog by intravenous injection of sorbital monolaurate. Arch. Derm. Syph. (Chic). **58**, 659 (1948).
JALLING, O., and J. E. JORPES: On biological assay of gastrin. Acta physiol. scand. **13**, 231 (1946).
JANOWITZ, H. D., and F. HOLLANDER: Effect of atropine on histamine-stimulated gastric secretion in the dog. Amer. J. Physiol. **186**, 373 (1956).
— — Inhibition of histamine-stimulated secretion by topical application of antihistaminics to the canine mucosa. Proc. Soc. exp. Biol. (N. Y.) **95**, 320 (1957).
KAHLSON, G.: Nervous and humoral control of gastric secretion. Brit. Med. J. **1948 II,** 1091.
— ELSA ROSENGREN, D. SVAHN and R. THUNBERG. Increased formation of histamine in the gastric mucosa elicited by gastrin and food intake. J. Physiol. (Lond.) **167**, 45 (1963).
KALK, H.: Zur Frage der Existenz einer histaminähnlichen Substanz beim Zustandekommen des Dermographismus. Klin. Wschr. **8**, 64 (1929).
KAPELLER-ADLER, R., and B. IGGO: Histamine and its derivatives in human urine. Biochem. biophys. Acta (Amst.) **25**, 394 (1957).
KATO, H.: Chromatography of crude gastrin. Fed. Proc. **20**, 250 (1961).
KAY, A. W.: Effect of large doses of histamine on gastric secretion of HCl; augmented histamine test. Brit. med. J. **1953 II**, 77.
—, and A. P. M. FORREST: Inhibitory action of locally applied antihistaminics on canine acid gastric secretion induced by histamine. Brit. J. Surg. **43**, 522 (1956a).
— — Inhibitory action of locally applied antihistamine on canine gastric secretion induced by peripheral parasympathetic stimulation. Brit. J. Surg. **44**, 97 (1956b).
KEETON, R. W., and F. C. KOCH: The distribution of gastrin in the body. Amer. J. Physiol. **37**, 481 (1915).
— — and A. B. LUCKHARDT: Gastrin studies. III. The response of the stomach mucosa of various animals to gastrin bodies. Amer. J. Physiol. **51**, 454 (1920a).

KEETON, R. W., and A. B. LUCKHARDT and F. C. KOCH: Gastrin studies: IV. The response of the stomach mucosa to food and gastrinbodies as influenced by atropine. Amer. J. Physiol. **51**, 469 (1920b).

KHAYYAL, M., W. KOSKOWSKI et M. METAWI: Influence des substances antihistaminiques sur la sécrétion gastrique, provoquée par l'histamine chez le pigeon. C. R. Soc. Biol. (Paris) **145**, 1499 (1951).

KIM, M. S., and A. C. IVY: Mode of action of secretagogues in promoting gastric secretion. Mitt. med. Akad. Kioto **12**, 1015 (1934); also Thesis, Northwestern Univ. 1933.

KOBAYASHI, Y., and A. C. IVY: Histamine metabolizing activity of dog stomach and intestine. Amer. J. Physiol. **195**, 525 (1958).

— — Histamine metabolizing activity of the stomach and intestine of the rat. Amer. J. Physiol. **196**, 835 (1959).

— — Comparison of mono, di and triaminoguanidine and semicarbazide as *in vitro* diamino oxidase inhibitors. Amer. J. Physiol. [In Press].

KOCH, F. C., A. B. LUCKHARDT and R. W. KEETON: Gastrin studies. V. Chemical studies on gastrin bodies. Amer. J. Physiol. **52**, 508 (1920—1921).

KOHOUT, J., D. HOSCHLOVA, L. KORBOVA et S. NOVAK: Contribution à la thérapie de la maladie ulcéreuse par les substances antihistaminiques. Arch. Mal. Appar. dig. **49**, 787 (1960).

KOMAROV, S. A.: Action of nitrogenous bases of gastric juice on blood pressure, pancreatic secretion and flow of bile. Amer. J. Physiol. **115**, 604 (1936).

— Gastrin. Proc. Soc. exper. Biol. (N. Y.) **38**, 514 (1938).

— Studies on Gastrin: I. Methods of isolation of a specific gastric secretagogue from the pyloric mucous membrane and its chemical properties. Rev. Canad. Biol. **1**, 191 (1942); **2**, 377 (1942).

KOSKOWSKI, W.: Les propriétés dynamiques du sang au cours de la digestion et leurs changements dans différentes conditions experimentales. J. Physiol. (Paris) **31**, 697 (1933).

—, et P. KUBIKOWSKI: Sécrétion du suc gastrique après injection d'histamine et présence de cette substance dans le sang. C. R. Soc. Biol. (Paris) **100**, 292, 1240, 1243 (1929).

LANE, A., A. C. IVY and E. K. IVY: Response of the chronic gastric fistula rat to histamine. Amer. J. Physiol. **190**, 221 (1957).

LAWYER, C. B., and E. LIEBER: Chemically determined uptake of intravenously injected aminoguanidine by various organs. Fed. Proc. **20**, 250 (1961).

LEBEDINSKAJA, S. I.: Über die Magensekretion bei Eckschen Fistelhunden. Z. ges. exp. Med. **88**, 264 (1932).

LEBLOND, C. P., and B. E. WALKER: Renewal of cell populations. Physiol. Rev. **36**, 255 (1956).

LEE, H. M., and R. G. JONES: Histamine activity of some β-aminoethyl heterocylic nitrogen compounds. J. Pharmacol. exp. Ther. **95**, 71 (1949).

LEHMANN, G., and P. L. STEFKO: Action of thephorin upon histamine-induced gastric secretion in dogs and on gastric ulcer formation in rats. J. Lab. clin. Med. **34**, 372 (1949).

—, and J. W. YOUNG: Anti-histamine activity of di-ethyl aminoethyl-dihydroanthracene-carboxylate and other substances. J. Pharmacol. exp. Ther. **83**, 90 (1945).

LIEPINS, K. W.: Site of gastric secretory stimulating action of aminoguanidine in the alimentary tract. Fed. Proc. **19**, 191 (1960).

—, and A. C. IVY: Effect of oral aminoguanidine on gastric secretion. Physiologist **2**, August (1959).

— — and R. SUZUKI: Effect of certain histaminase inhibitors on gastric secretion. Amer. J. Physiol. **195**, 209 (1958).

LIM, R. K. S., A. C. IVY and J. E. MCCARTHY: Contributions to physiology of gastric secretion. II. The intestinal phase of gastric secretion. Quart. J. exp. Physiol. **15**, 13 (1925).

LIN, T. M., and R. S. ALPHIN: Comparative study of histamine and 3 β-aminoethyl-1,2,4-triazole on gastric secretion. Fed. Proc. **18**, 416 (1959).

— — F. G. HENDERSON and K. K. CHEN: 3-β-aminoethyl-1,2,4-triazole, a potent stimulant of gastric secretion. J. Pharmacol. exp. Ther. **134**, 88 (1961).

— D. N. BENSLAY and F. G. HENDERSON: Comparative study of histamine and histamine metabolites on gastric secretion. Fed. Proc. **20**, 251 (1961).

— F. G. HENDERSON, K. K. CHEN and D. N. BENSLAY: Structure-Activity and Enzyme-Substrate relationships of histamine, histamine metabolites and analogues in stimulation of gastric secretion. Proc. 1st. Intern. Pharmacol. Meet., Stockholm 1961. (1963 publ.)

— A. C. IVY, E. KARVINEN and E. K. IVY: Effect of an histaminase inhibitor (aminoguanidine) on the gastric secretory response to exogenous histamine. Amer. J. Physiol. **186**, 231 (1956).

LINDE, S.: Studies on stimulation mechanism of gastric secretion. Acta physiol. scand. **21**, Suppl. 74 (1950).

LINDELL, S. E., and R. W. SCHAYER: The renal removal of injected C^{14} histamine from the blood of dogs. Brit. J. Pharmacol. **13**, 44 (1958).
—, and H. WESTLING: Enzymic oxidation of some substances related to histamine. Acta physiol. scand. **39**, 370 (1957).
LIVINGSTON, R. H., and C. F. CODE: Role of the liver in the conjugation of histamine in intact animals. Amer. J. Physiol. **181**, 428 (1955).
LOEW, E. R., and O. CHICKERING: Gastric secretion in dogs treated with histamine antagonist, thymoxyethyldiethylamine. Proc. Soc. exp. Biol. (N. Y.) **48**, 65 (1941).
— R. MACMILLAN and M. E. KAISER: The anti-histamine properties of benadryl,β-dimethylaminoethyl benzhydryl ether hydrochloride. J. Pharmacol. exp. Ther. **86**, 229 (1946).
LUCKHARDT, A. B., R. W. KEETON, F. C. KOCH and V. LA MER: Gastric studies. II. Further studies on the distribution and extraction of gastric bodies. Amer. J. Physiol. **50**, 527 (1919—1920).
MCELIN, T. W., and B. T. HORTON: Clinical observations on use of benadryl; new antihistamine substance. Proc. Mayo Clin. **20**, 417 (1945).
— — Clinical observations on the use of benadryl: Its effect on histamine-induced gastric acidity in man. Gastroenterology **7**, 100 (1946).
MCGAVACK, T. H., H. ELIAS and L. J. BOYD: The influence of Benadryl. (Dimethylaminoethylbenzhydryl ether hydrochloride) on gastric acidity. Gastroenterology **6**, 439 (1946).
MCHENRY, E. W., and G. GAVIN: Histaminase. Biochem. J. **26**, 1365 (1932).
MACINTOSH, F. C.: Histamine as normal stimulant of gastric secretion. Quart. J. exp. Physiol. **28**, 87 (1938).
MALLIK, K. C. B., and B. K. BHATTACHARYA: Blood histamine in peptic ulcer. J. Indian med. Ass. **30**, 275 (1958).
MARKS, I. N., G. SELZER, J. H. LOUW and S. BANK: Zollinger-Ellison syndrome in a Bantu woman, with isolation of a gastrin-like substance from the primary and secondary tumors. I. Case report. Gastroenterology **41**, 77 (1961).
MASONI, A., L. LOSITO e V. LATTANZIO: Azione del dimenidrinati sulla secrezione gastrica basale e da istamina. Arcisped. S. Anna Ferrara **10**, 13 (1957).
MATHESON, A. R., and S. E. AMMON: Observations on the effect of histamine on the human gastric secretion. Lancet **1923I**, 482.
MAYDELL, B. E.: Zur Frage der Magensekretion. Pflügers Arch. ges. Physiol. **150**, 390 (1913).
— On gastric secretion. Physiol. Abstr. **2**, 415 (1917—1918).
MELLANBY, J.: Secretion of pancreatic juice. J. Physiol. **61**, 419 (1926).
MILLICAN, R. C., S. M. ROSENTHAL and H. TABOR: On metabolism of histamine; urinary excretion following oral administration: conjugation *in vitro*. J. Pharmacol. exp. Ther. **97**, 4 (1949).
MITCHELL, R. G., and C. F. CODE: Effect of diet on urinary excretions of histamine. J. Appl. Physiol. **6**, 387 (1954).
MODRAKOWSKI, G.: Über die Grunderscheinungen des anaphylaktischen Schocks. Naunyn-Schmiedebergs Arch. exp. Path. Pharmak. **69**, 67 (1912).
MOERSCH, R. U., A. B. RIVERS and C. G. MORLOCK: Some results of the gastric secretory response of patients having duodenal ulcer noted during the administration of benadryl. Gastroenterology **7**, 91 (1946).
MONGAR, J. L., and H. O. SCHILD: A comparison of the effects of anaphylactic shock and of chemical histamine releasers. J. Physiol. (Lond.) **118**, 461 (1952).
MOTA, I., W. T. BERALDO, A. G. FERRI and L. C. U. JUNQUEIRA: Action of 48/80 on the mast cell population and histamine content of the wall of the gastrointestinal tract of the rat. In: Ciba Symposium on Histamine, pg. 47. Boston: Little, Brown and Co., 1956.
NECHELES, H., and R. K. S. LIM: Isolation of gastric and pancreatic secretory excitants from circulation by vivi-dialysis. Chin. J. Physiol. **2**, 415 (1928).
NEUGEBAUER, K., u. J. SCHMID: Über die Histaminbindungsfähigkeit des Magenschleims. Wien. Z. inn. Med. **30**, 383 (1949).
NORDGREN, B., and K. J. ÖBRINK: Effect of vasodilator (priscol) on gastric secretion. Acta physiol. scand. **37**, 177 (1956).
OBERHELMAN, H. A., JR., and L. R. DRAGSTEDT: Effect of vagotomy on gastric response to histamine. Proc. Soc. exp. Biol. (N. Y.) **67**, 336 (1948).
ÖBRINK, K. J.: Some relations in gastric stimulation by intravenous injection of histamine. Acta physiol. scand. **12**, 213 (1946).
— Kinetical studies on the parietal secretion of the stomach. Acta physiol. scand. **15**, Suppl. 51 (1948).
ORBELI, L. A.: De l'activité des glandes à pepsine avant et après la section des nerfs pneumogastriques. Arch. Sci. Biol. (St. Petersburg) **12**, 71 (1906).
PARROT, J.-L., et J. REUSE: Rôle physiologique et physiopathologique de l'histamine. J. Physiol. (Paris) **46**, 99 (1954).

Parrot, J.-L., et B. Vasseur: Étudec ritique du rôle physiologique de l'histamine dans la stimulation de la sécrétion gastrique. J. Physiol. (Paris) **52**, 185 (1960).
Parsons, E.: Histamine as a constituent of secretion preparations. Amer. J. Physiol. **71**, 479 (1925).
Paton, W. D. M., and M. Schachter: Influence of antihistamine drug on release of histamine in unanesthetized dog. Brit. J. Pharmacol. **6**, 509 (1951).
Pevsner, L., and M. I. Grossman: The mechanism of vagal stimulation of gastric acid secretion. Gastroenterology **28**, 493 (1955).
Popielski, L.: Über das peripherische reflektorische Zentrum der Magendrüsen. Zbl. Physiol. **16**, 121 (1902).
— Über die physiologischen und chemischen Eigenschaften des Peptons Witte. Pflügers Arch. ges. Physiol. **126**, 483 (1909); **152**, 168 (1913).
— β-imidazolyläthylamin und die Organextrakte. Erster Teil. β-imidazolyläthylamin als mächtiger Erreger der Magendrüsen. Pflügers Arch. ges. Physiol. **178**, 214 (1920).
Ragins, H., E. T. Benditt, H. B. Greenlee and L. R. Dragstedt: Studies of the parenteral and topical effects of antihistamines on gastric secretion. Gastroenterology **35**, 1 (1958).
Reitter, H.: Die Mechanismen der Magensekretion dargestellt am Beispiel der Beeinflussung durch sog. Antihistaminica. Z. klin. Med. **149**, 553 (1952).
Reuse, J.: Substances antagonistes de l'histamine et fonction gastrique. C. R. Soc. Biol. (Paris) **140**, 1237 (1946).
Riley, J. F.: "The Mast Cells". London: E & S. Livingston, Ltd. 1959.
—, and G. B. West: Presence of histamine in tissue mast cells. J. Physiol. (Lond.) **120**, 528 (1953).
Roberts, M., and H. M. Adam: New methods for the quantitative estimation of free and conjugated histamine in body fluids. Brit. J. Pharmacol. **5**, 526 (1950).
Robertson, C., and M. I. Grossman: Inhibition of histamine induced gastric acid secretion by irrigation of antihistaminics into gastric pouches in dogs. Arch. int. Pharmacodyn. **90**, 223 (1952a).
— — Results of a screening program for inhibitors of gastric acid secretion. Arch. int. Pharmacodyn. **91**, 1 (1952b).
— K. Langlois, C. G. Martin, G. Slezak and M. I. Grossman: Release of gastrin by Ach. Amer. J. Physiol. **163**, 37 (1950a).
— C. E. Rosiere, D. Blickenstaff and M. I. Grossman: The potentiating action of certain xanthine derivatives on gatric acid secretory responses in the dog. J. Pharmacol. exp. Ther. **99**, 362 (1950b).
Rogers, J., J. M. Rahe, G. G. Fawcett and G. S. Hackett: The effects upon the gastric secretion of organ extracts. Amer. J. Physiol. **39**, 345 (1915).
Rose, B.: Production of symptoms by subcutaneous injection of histamine without increase of blood histamine. Science **92**, 454 (1940).
— Studies on blood histamine in cases of allergy; blood histamine during wheal formation. J. Allergy **12**, 327 (1941).
—, and J. S. L. Browne: Fate of intravenously injected histamine. Amer. J. Physiol. **124**, 412 (1938).
— — Histamine content of tissues after adrenalectomy. Amer. J. Physiol. **131**, 589 (1940 to 1941).
—, and S. Karady: Histamine metabolism in the adrenalectomized rat. Amer. J. Physiol. **126**, 614 (1939).
— — and J. S. L. Browne: Histaminase content of tissues. Amer. J. Physiol. **129**, 219 (1940).
Rosenthal, S. M., and H. Tabor: Improved colorimetric method for estimation of histamine. J. Pharm. exp. Ther. **92**, 425 (1948).
Roth, G. M., and B. T. Horton: Physiologic effects of histaminase and histamine. J. Amer. med. Ass. **114**, 522 (1940).
Rothlin, E., et R. Gundlach: Étude expérimentale de l'influence de l'histamine sur la sécrétion gastrique. Internat. Cong. Physiol., Paris, 1920; also Arch. int. Physiol. **17**, 59 (1921).
Sacks, J., A. C. Ivy, J. P. Burgess and J. E. Vandolah: (1932a). Cit. in Sacks, J., A. C. Ivy, J. P. Burgess and J. E. Vandolah (1932b).
— — — — Histamine as the hormone for gastric secretion. Amer. J. Physiol. **101**, 331 (1932b).
Sangster, W., M. I. Grossman and A. C. Ivy: The effect of two new histamine antagonists (benadryl and compound 63) on histamine stimulated gastric secretion in the dog. Gastroenterology **6**, 436 (1946).
Schayer, R. W.: Biogenesis of histamine. J. biol. Chem. **199**, 245 (1952).
— Formation and binding of histamine by free mast cells of rat peritoneal fluid. Amer. J. Physiol. **186**, 199 (1956a).

SCHAYER, R. W.: Formation and binding of histamine by rat tissues *in vitro*. Amer. J. Physiol. **187**, 63 (1956b).
— The metabolism of histamine in various species. Brit. J. Pharmacol. **11**, 472 (1956c).
— Histidine decarboxylase of rat stomach and other mammalian tissues. Amer. J. Physiol. **189**, 533 (1957).
— Catabolism of physiological quantities of histamine *in vivo*. Physiol. Rev. **39**, 116 (1959).
— Relationship of induced histidine decarboxylase activity and histamine synthesis to shock from stress and from endotoxin. Amer. J. Physiol. **198**, 1187 (1960a).
— Relationship of stress-induced histidine decarboxylase to circulatory homeostasis and shock. Science **131**, 226 (1960b).
— Significance of induced synthesis of histamine in physiology and pathology. Chemotherapia **3**, 128 (1960c).
—, and J. A. D. COOPER: Metabolism of C^{14} histamine in man. J. appl. Physiol. **9**, 481 (1956).
— K. J. DAVIS and R. L. SMILEY: Binding of histamine *in vitro* and its inhibition by cortisone. Amer. J. Physiol. **182**, 54 (1955).
—, and O. H. GANLEY: Adaptive increase in mammalian histidine decarboxylase activity in response to nonspecific stress. Amer. J. Physiol. **197**, 721 (1959).
—, and A. C. IVY: Evidence that histamine is a gastric secretory hormone in the rat. Amer. J. Physiol. **189**, 369 (1957).
— — Release of C^{14}-histamine from stomach and intestine on feeding. Amer. J. Physiol. **193**, 400 (1958).
— Z. ROTHSCHILD and P. BIZONY: Increase in histidine decarboxylase activity of rat skin following treatment with compound 48/80. Amer. J. Physiol. **196**, 295 (1958).
—, and R. L. SMILEY: Binding and release of radioactive histamine in intact rats. Amer. J. Physiol. **177**, 401 (1954).
— K. Y. T. WU and R. L. SMILEY: Sources of urinary histamine in the rat. Amer. J. Physiol. **179**, 481 (1954).
SCHNEDORF, J. G., and A. C. IVY: Effect of methylhistamine and hydroxyethylglyoxaline on gastric secretion and blood pressure in the dog. Proc. Soc. exp. Biol. (N. Y.) **32**, 777 (1935).
SHEARD, C., E. E. MCCRAKEN and H. E. ESSEX: The circulation time of the blood in dogs before and during the digestion of food. Amer. J. Physiol. **109**, 96 (1934).
SHORE, P. A., A. BURKHALTER and V. H. COHN: A method for the fluorometric assay of histamine in tissues. J. Pharmacol. exp. Ther. **127**, 182 (1959).
SIRCUS, W.: Effect of B_1 pyrimidine on gastric secretion. Quart. J. exp. Physiol. **38**, 25 (1953).
SMITH, A. N.: Effect of compound 48/80 on acid gastric secretion in cat. J. Physiol. (Lond.) **119**, 233 (1953a).
— Release of histamine by histamine liberator compound 48/80 in cats. J. Physiol. (Lond.) **121**, 517 (1953b).
— Gastrin and histamine release. J. Physiol. (Lond.) **123**, 71 (1954).
— The distribution and release of histamine in human gastric tissues. Clin. Sci. **18**, 533 (1959).
STEGGERDA, F. R., H. E. ESSEX and F. C. MANN: The inactivation of histamine in perfused organs. Amer. J. Physiol. **112**, 70 (1935).
STERN, P.: Interpretation of inefficacy of antihistaminics upon secretion of gastric juice. J. Allergy **26**, 268 (1955).
SUMMERSKILL, W. H., C. F. CODE, G. A. HALLENBECK and J. T. PRIESTLEY: Intractable peptic ulcer in hereditary endocrine-ulcer disease: "gastrin" content of endocrine tissues. Proc. Mayo Clin. **36**, 611 (1961).
SUMNER, J. B., and G. F. SOMERS: Chemistry and Methods of Enzymes. 3rd ed. New York: Academic Press, Inc. 1953.
TABOR, H., and E. MOSETTIG: Isolation of acetylhistamine from urine following oral administration of histamine. J. biol. Chem. **180**, 703 (1949).
TAMARIT-TORRES, J., F. DELLA CRUZ CARO y F. JR. ENRIQUEZ DE SALAMANCA: Acción sobre la función gastrica de un nuevo antihistaminico de síntesis. Arch. Med. exp. (Madr.) **16**, 83 (1953).
THOMPSON, J. E., and J. R. VANE: Gastric secretion induced by histamine and its relationship to the rate of blood flow. J. Physiol. (Lond.) **121**, 433 (1953).
TOMASZEWSKI, Z.: I. Über die sekretorische Tätigkeit der Magendrüsen unter dem Einflusse des Liebigextraktes. Zbl. Physiol. **27**, 627 (1913).
— Über die chemischen Erreger der Magendrüsen. Pflügers Arch. ges. Physiol. **171**, 1 (1918).
TRACH, B., C. F. CODE and O. H. WANGENSTEEN: Histamine in human gastric mucosa. Amer. J. Physiol. **141**, 78 (1944).
TSUKAMOTO, M.: Effects of histamine, compound 48/80, atropine, and diamox, administered to gastric submucosa, on acid secretion in the rat. Gastroenterology **41**, 572 (1961).
UNGAR, G.: Effet de l'excitation du bout périphérique des nerfs sensitifs sur la sécrétion gastrique; transmission neuro-humorale histaminique. C. R. Soc. Biol. (Paris) **118**, 620 (1935).

UPDIKE, E. H., C. F. CODE and G. A. HALLENBECK: Excretion of free histamine in urine during gastric secretion stimulated by humoral mechanisms. Amer. J. Physiol. **195**, 197 (1958).

URBACH, K. F.: Nature and probable origin of conjugated histamine excreted after ingestion of histamine. Proc. Soc. exp. Biol. (N. Y.) **70**, 146 (1949).

UVNÄS, B.: The part played by the pyloric region in the cephalic phase of gastric secretion. Acta physiol. scand. 4 (Suppl. 13) (1942b).

— Further studies on the gastric secretory excitant from the pyloric mucosa. Acta physiol. scand. **4**, Suppl. 13 (1942a); **7**, 289 (1944).

— The presence of a gastric secretory excitant in the human gastric and duodenal mucosa. Acta physiol. scand. **10**, 97 (1945).

VALETTE, G., H. HUIDOBRO et Y. COHEN: Le pouvoir d'inactivation du rein vis-à-vis de l'histamine *in vivo*. J. Physiol. (Paris) **47**, 292 (1955).

VANDOLAH, J., and A. C. IVY: Unpublished, 1928.

— — Effect of adenylic acid on gastric secretion, 1928—1929. Cit. in SACKS et al., 1932b; see also Proc. Soc. exper. Biol. (N. Y.) **31**, 28 (1933).

VARTIAINEN, A.: Action of certain new histamine derivatives. J. Pharmacol. exp. Ther. **54**, 265 (1935).

VOLBORTH, G. W.: The presence of secretion in the intestinal juice. Amer. J. Physiol. **72**, 331 (1925).

WADDELL, W. R., J. P. LYTHGOE and A. P. MONACO: Immunological studies of gastrin. Science **134**, 2099 (1961).

WATON, N. G.: Studies on mammalian histidine decarboxylase. Brit. J. Pharmacol. **11**, 119 (1956).

WEAVER, M., A. B. LUCKHARDT and F. C. KOCH: Preparation of potent vasodilatin-free pancreatic secretion J. Amer. med. Ass. **87**, 640 (1926).

WEISS, S., G. P. ROBB and L. B. ELLIS: Systemic effects of histamine in man, with special reference to responses of cardiovascular system. Arch. intern. Med. **49**, 360 (1932).

WELCH, H. H.: Uptake of intravenously injected C^{14} aminoguanidine by rat tissues. Fed. Proc. **20**, 174 (1961).

WOJCIECH, R., and A. C. IVY: Method for preparation of a "gastrin" containing no "free histamine". Fed. Proc. **20**, 250 (1961).

WOOD, D. R.: Effect on gastric secretion of different rates of histamine infusiou and of "neo-antergan". Brit. J. Pharmacol. **3**, 231 (1948).

— Inhibition of experimental gastric secretion by histamine antagonists. J. Physiol. (Lond.) **111**, 38 (1950).

WOODWARD, E. R.: The role of the gastric antrum in the regulation of gastric secretion. Gastroenterology **38**, 7 (1960).

WOODWARD, E. D., C. R. ROBERTSON, H. D. RUTTENBERG and H. SCHAPIRO: Alcohol as a gastric secretory stimulant. Gastroenterology **32**, 727 (1957).

WRIGHT, R. D., and E. R. TRETHEWIE: Histamine of the reptilian stomach and lung. Nature (Lond.) **178**, 546 (1956).

YOUNG, L. E.: The extractable histamine content of gastric mucosa and lung before and after parenteral histamine administration. Yale J. Biol. Med. **21**, 499 (1948—1949).

YUSEM, M.: Chemical estimation of histamine in "gastrin". Fed. Proc. **20**, 250 (1961).

ZELJONY, G. P., and V. V. SAVICH: Concerning the mechanism of gastric secretion. Proc. Soc. Russ. Phyns, St. Petersburg (Russian), Jan.-May, 1911—1912.

ZELLER, E. A.: Diamin-Oxydase. Advanc. Enzymol. **2**, 93 (1942). — In: The Enzymes, Chemistry and Mechanism of Action. Edited by J. B. SUMNER and K. MYRBÄCK. New York: Academic Press 1950—1951.

ZIEMLANSKI, S., and W. BIEREZOWSKI: Smiany Temperatury Beony Sluzowez Zoeadka W Pohistaminowyn Wydzielaniu Soku Zoladkowego. Temperature changes in the gastric mucosa during gastric juice secretory reactions to the administration of histamine. Acta physiol. pol. **11**, 930 (1960).

ZOLLINGER, R. M., and E. H. ELLISON: Primary peptic ulcerations of jejunum associated with islet cell tumors of pancreas. Arch. Surg. **142**, 709 (1955).

Section C

The Relation of Histamine to Inflammation

By

P. STERN

With 2 Figures

Inflammation is a complex process involving many biochemical changes with the participation of several mediators (MENKIN, 1956; RAJKA, 1959; UNGAR, 1952). MEIER (1959) and MEIER et al. (1956) have recently discussed the biochemistry of the inflammatory process and its causal connections in an excellent review. Since a number of factors should be considered, it is difficult to speak of the role of a single mediator in the development of inflammation. It has been demonstrated that histamine plays an important role, but its action could not account for the whole set of events (HAAS, 1951; FELDBERG, 1954; ROCHA E SILVA, 1955). Yet, thanks to the availability of histamine liberators we may at present discern the part played by histamine better than in the past. The function of any naturally occurring agent can be better recognized by eliminating it from the organism in order to gain insight into its real physiological tasks. This method has rendered excellent service in the fields of vitamins and hormones where it has long been in use. FELDBERG (1956) reviewing the mediators participating in the development of the inflammatory processes stated: "Nowadays we have the possibility of depleting a tissue of its histamine. Unfortunately this has so far been achieved only in some species and in some tissues, but by comparing, as ZWEIFACH has done, the inflammatory vascular reaction in a normal and in a histamine-depleted tissue, we might perhaps obtain more precise information about the role of released histamine in the histamine-like vascular reactions of inflammation."

Since then, we have performed such an experiment which led to a better appraisal of the role played by histamine in the course of inflammation (STERN et al., 1956). Later on, further experiments on inflammation from our laboratory confirmed the results of our basic experiments.

In order to solve the question about the actions of histamine, we (STERN et al., 1956) made use of the granuloma pouch method described by SELYE (1953) in the rat previously depleted of histamine with the histamine liberator Compound 48/80 (a condensation product of p-methoxyphenylethylamine and formaldehyde). The histamine-depleted tissue was, after a definite time interval, subjected to microscopical examination and the histological picture compared to that of a granuloma pouch wall containing normal amounts of histamine.

Methods: 25 cc. of air was injected under the skin of the back of a rat and the pouch so obtained received an injection of 0.5–1 cc. of a 1% aqueous suspension of *Ol. crotonis*. The inflammation reaches a maximum after 6 days. Afterwards, a slow healing process sets in spontaneously. The animals were killed on the sixth day, the wall of the pouch examined histologically and its thickness measured. By transillumination of the intact pouch one can easily see the free exudate. The quantity of exudate may be accurately determined by punction before sacrificing the animal. The histamine liberator was applied intraperitoneally in the following dosage: each animal received an initial dose of 150 μg, and then, on every subsequent day, the dose was increased by 50 μg until a dose of 350 μg. The dissected pouch was fixed in 4% formalin and embedded in paraffin. Tissue slices were stained with eosin hemalum, or according to HAITINGER (1938), after a previous fixation in Carnoy's fluid. This treatment allows a better view of proteins outflowing to extracellular spaces.

Results: Rats treated with compound 48/80 show the following changes: after 24 hours the subcutaneous connective tissue on the edge of the pouch is somewhat loosened. Fibres and fat cells are slightly pulled apart and among them there are numerous granules of protein stained pink with eosin. In HAITINGER preparations the granules show a red-brown fluorescence which also indicates their origin from plasma proteins. The tissue of the pouch wall is lined with a layer of polymorphonuclear and eosinophilic leucocytes, among which some lymphocytic elements can be found. In deeper layers, adjacent to the dorsal muscles the inflammatory exudation is much stronger and inflammatory cells also occur between muscle fibres.

Forty eight hours following the application of the croton oil there appear in the exudate some younger connective tissue elements in addition to those formerly described.

During the next days, up to the sixth, the productive changes in the inflamed region develop progressively. There is still a great number of leucocytes, but the most striking feature is the presence of fibrillar connective tissue elements which, in addition to that of young cells, is indicative of organization of the exudate.

Untreated controls show a very similar picture to that of the experimental animals when observed the first day. During the subsequent days however, the course of the inflammatory reactions become significantly different for each group. One finds extensive damaging processes to leucocytes and collagen fibres in the subcutaneous tissue which sometimes goes as far as to necrosis. Quantitatively the number of polymorphonuclear and eosinophilic leucocytes is much greater in controls than in the treated rats.

The appearance of productive elements (blood vessels and fibres) does not occur so early in controls, and when they appear, after 3–4 days, they are by far less abundant than in the histamine-depleted animals. Such a development, poor in productive events, holds on up to the sixth day. By comparative examination of the experimental and control series one gains the impression that the qualitative alteration leading to the described differences of the exudates in both series sets in from the second to the third day after the beginning of the inflammation. IRINO (1958) obtained equivalent results using also the granuloma pouch method in his experiments.

The differences in the histological pictures with normal and histamine-depleted animals are illustrated by Figs. 1 and 2.

From this experiment one might conclude that the role played by histamine in the development of the inflammatory process is quite considerable. Its real function in the process will be dealt with later. JAQUES (1953) has shown, some years ago, that there is less histamine in the edematous fluid of a histamine-depleted tissue than in a tissue containing the normal amount of histamine. In order to obtain additional evidence of histamine function in inflammation, animals were treated with methylthiouracyl (IGNJAČEV et al., 1956). Hypothyroidosis is known to produce a decrease of histamine in the skin in man and rat (FELDBERG and LOESER, 1954). In our experiments the same histological changes were obtained as in those treated with the histamine releaser. since the effect was. in fact. the same,

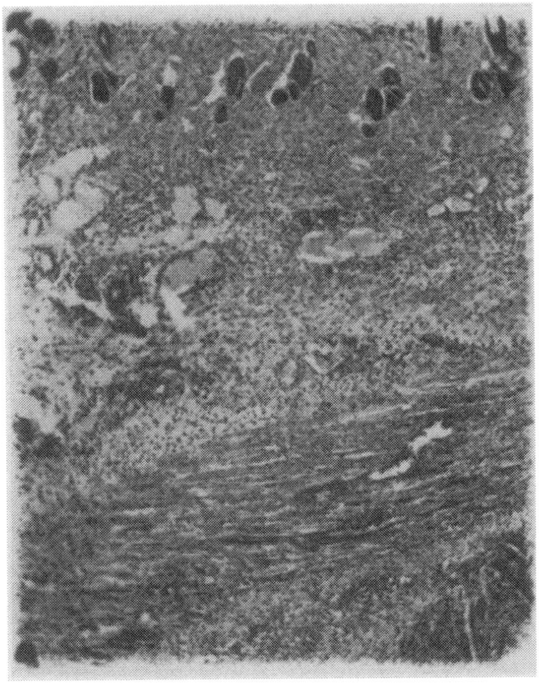

Fig. 1. Granuloma-pouch of rat sacrificied after 2 days

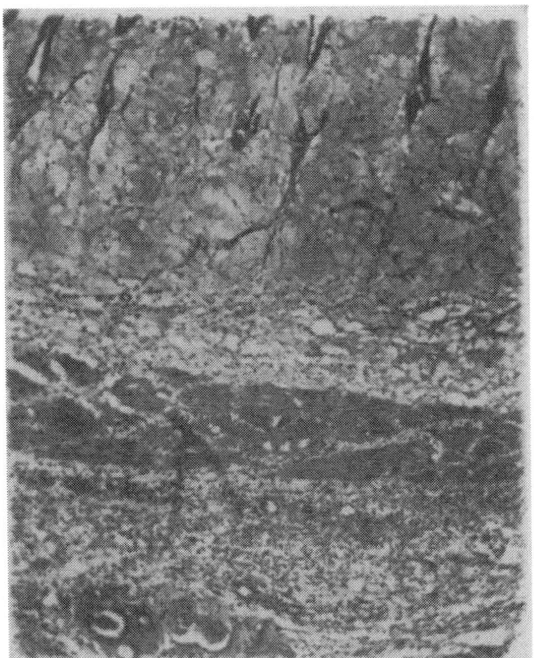

Fig. 2. Granuloma-pouch of a histamine-liberator-treated rat sacrificied after 2 days

viz. a reduction of the histamine content of the skin. A histological examination of the thyroid glands in the animals treated with methylthiouracyl showed that they had really developed a hypothyroid condition.

Since we had shown earlier that azulenes inhibit the release of histamine, *i.e.* that they act as antagonists of the histamine releaser 48/80 (Stern, 1951) we attempted to use them for this reason in our experiments (Stern and Milin, 1956; Stern and Nikulin, 1957). The antiphlogistic action of drugs containing azulenes has been known for ages. Rats were treated with an aqueous solution of Azulen SN (10, 20, and 40 mg/kg) for a six-day period during the development of inflammation. Again we could demonstrate histologically the same changes as those occurring in consequence of a pre-treatment with the histamine liberator. There was but little necrosis and exudation, the pouch wall was thinner and the healing tendency much more marked than in the controls. Thus it is irrelevant whether the organism is depleted of histamine previously, or its release into an active form inhibited. Supporting evidence was obtained by Ferluga et al. (1963) who administered ε-aminocaproic acid, a well-known inhibitor of proteolytic enzymes (Sherry et al., 1959). Ungar (1952) suggested long ago that inhibiting the conversion of profibrinolysin into fibrinogen should have an antiphlogistic effect, since it blocks the release of histamine.

Finally we have also found that subtivaccine (an autolysate from *B. subtilis* and *B. megatherium*) is a very slowly acting histamine liberator and accordingly it does not elicit adverse side effects like other, more rapidly acting, releasers, when applied in man. We therefore studied the development of inflammation after a 10-day treatment with daily intracutaneous doses of 0.05 cc. of subtivaccine. The results were the same as after treatment with compound 48/80 (CIGLAR, 1958; STERN, 1959).

The question to be asked now is about how does raised tissue histamine influence the course of the inflammatory process. Already CIGLAR et al. (1958) have shown that depleting rat tissues of Ca^{++}, and thereby increasing the capillary permeability, aggravates the inflammation by causing more edema and necrosis, and less granulation tissue. The same situation should be expected with increased histamine. HUKOVIĆ and STERN (1962) succeeded in increasing rat skin histamine levels by means of As_2O_3. With such animals NIKULIN et al. (1962) observed in the granuloma pouch similar histological pictures as in Ca^{++}-depleted animals. The inflammation was considerably more serious than in controls. In allergic skin inflammation STERN (1956) and RAAB (1962) both found an identical relationship between histamine levels and intensity of inflammation.

Discussion: The treatment with the histamine liberator 48/80, methylthiouracyl, azulene, and subtivaccine always led to the same tissue response. Inflammation in animals treated with these agents was never as severe as in animals with a normal amount of tissue histamine. Conversely, the increase in capillary permeability due to high tissue histamine or to depletion of Ca^{++} aggravates inflammatory processes. Thus a quantitative relationship exists between the histamine concentration at the site of inflammation and the seriousness of the inflammatory reaction. The more histamine present, the worse the inflammatory response: there is more edema and more necrosis, and less granulation tissue, and *vice versa*. An explanation of such an influence of histamine upon the amount of granulation tissue might be seen in its action on histidine decarboxylase: a decrease of tissue histamine induces a rise of the enzyme activity which, in turn, enhances the formation of collagen (SANDBERG, 1962).

Because of these findings there necessarily arises not only the question about the role of histamine in the inflammatory process, but also the question whether histamine is the actual damaging factor and therefore whether it should be desirable to eliminate it in order to alleviate the course of the inflammation. It is well known that histamine is easily released even after the slightest damages or bruises (PATON, 1958; see also other Sections of this Handbook). This is absolutely plausible if we recall the participation of histamine in the transmission of pain sensations (ROSENTHAL and MINARD, 1939; STERN and HUKOVIĆ, 1956), and its nociceptive function (SPECKMANN, 1953). Every injury to tissues causing an inflammatory reaction, be it the invasion of bacteria, the action of bacterial toxins or mechanical trauma, will release histamine which, in turn, will produce strong vasodilatation in the region where it has been released. Inflammation does not mean definite tissue damage, but represents its response to a lesion. According to ZWEIFACH (1953) and FELDBERG (1956) the function of histamine in the inflammatory process consists in causing strong vasodilatation and increased capillary permeability, this being probably its only task in the development of inflammation. All that follows in the further course of the inflammatory process is merely a consequence of this basic action. Histologically every inflammatory process is accompanied by a transient vasoconstriction of capillaries, but this quickly changes into the opposite phenomenon, a powerful vasodilatation with stasis and exudation into intercellular spaces. One of the common causes of all these events is histamine, regardless of the origin of inflammation. Histamine is the most powerful capillary dilatating agent known so far, with the exception, perhaps, of bradykinin (ROCHA E SILVA,

1960; FRIMMER, 1961; WILHELM, 1962), and it acts directly on the capillaries independently of their innervation. We need not stress the uniformity of the inflammatory process in its biochemical and, partly, its morphological manifestations no matter the cause of it. There are several varieties of the process, of course, depending mainly on its localization and the type of the tissue concerned, but the basic process is always biochemically and morphologically the same.

The first, and most uniform phase which is independent of the location or type of tissue affected or the causative factors, is due to the action of histamine. This substance is the plug to spark the motor of inflammation. In addition, histamine by way of axonal reflexes, produces a dilatation of arterioles in the surroundings of the inflamed region. ZWEIFACH (cit. in FELDBERG, 1956) demonstrated a dilatation of capillaries as the consequence of applying small doses of histamine to the mesentery of the rat, while a microlesion, in addition, produced sticking of leucocytes and thrombocytes to capillary walls, an effect which the small doses of histamine needed to produce vasodilatation were unable to call forth. Nevertheless, during an inflammatory process histamine is released in great excess which may be responsible for changes requiring more than small amounts of the amine. In our experiments with histamine depleted rats, we could observe all the basic elements of inflammation, though not as strongly marked as in tissues with a normal histamine content. It should be kept in mind that it is impossible to deplete the tissues completely of histamine, but that there remain about 10% of the initial amount after treatment with the histamine releaser. This amount is sufficient for triggering the primary inflammatory reactions. Menkin's substances are released as a result of a cell lesion, and the latter might be caused by an excess of histamine. The fact that there is much less necrosis in inflamed tissue in histamine-depleted rats speaks in favor of this view. The results of KRAMER's experiments using ricin as phlogogen also point in the same direction (KRAMER, 1958). Hence we can say that without histamine the inflammation would probably not take the morphological course which is observed regularly, but the presence of an excess of histamine induces many additional morphological changes like necrosis, very strong exudation, *etc.*

Such reactions take place only in living tissue, still capable of responding to injury. That this is really so we could verify in experiments on the tuberculin reaction in the skin of guinea pigs (MISIRLIJA et al., 1956). We produced the tuberculin reaction in tuberculous guinea pigs choosing the retroauricular and the flank regions, the latter containing 10 times less histamine than the former (FELDBERG and MILES, 1953). It is well known that necrosis in the tuberculin reaction is the result of an antigen-antibody interaction, so histamine should no longer have the opportunity of producing further morphological changes. The tuberculin reaction, therefore, shows identical symptoms in both the retroauricular and the flank regions. We think that the antiphlogistic activity of cortisone may be interpreted in the same way, since this substance interferes with the release of histamine. Apparently the role of histamine is the same not only in the common, but also in the allergic inflammation.

What would be the course of the inflammatory process in a tissue completely devoid of histamine is difficult to tell, since at present we are unable to obtain such a state. The effect of cortisone, perhaps, mimics this picture most closely. We know that too feeble a production of proliferative tissue (SELYE, 1953) occurs in this case, which is detrimental to the carrier organism. Along with histamine, however, bradykinin plays a similar role and very probably takes part in the earliest phase of inflammation. Our own results show that bradykinin produces in the granuloma pouch a similar picture as croton oil; but in histamine-depleted tissue bradykinin causes a less intense inflammatory response than in controls with normal histamine. The release of bradykinin, however, begins later than that of histamine so the polypeptide cannot have, for the initial stage of the inflammatory process, such a meaning as the amine (STERN et al., 1962).

It must be underlined that 5-hydroxytryptamine does not possess the significance for the inflammatory process attributed to this substance before. In the first place 5-hydroxytryptamine hardly occurs in the skin of man (LEWIS, 1958). In other organs its concentration is inferior to that of histamine. In the rat, 5-hydroxytryptamine is plentifully found in the skin, but our results have shown that the tissue depleted of 5-hydroxytryptamine by means of reserpine exhibits still stronger morphological inflammatory symptoms than control tissue (STERN and GMAZ-NIKULIN, 1960). Thus it may be justified to say that 5-hydroxytryptamine plays probably no important role in the inflammatory process. 5-Hydroxytryptamine may be found in edematous fluid, *e.g.* in the fluid taken from joints during anaphylactoid reaction. It must be pointed out, however, that anaphylactoid reactions produced by dextran, egg albumin, *etc.* are no good models of inflammation (BÜCH and WAGNER-JAUREGG, 1960). In such cases there is no cellular reaction and many other factors characterizing inflammation are lacking. The granuloma pouch method is certainly better suited than edema of the snout or paws produced by the above mentioned agents.

Conclusions: Tissues depleted of histamine react differently to inflammatory injury as those with normal histamine contents. Histamine-depleted tissue shows less necrosis, less edema, milder lesions, and a greater healing tendency than control tissue. In tissues with high histamine levels the process develops in exactly the opposite direction.

Histamine probably plays a basic role in the beginning of the inflammatory process by dilatating the capillaries and increasing their permeability. Very small amounts of histamine suffice to produce these phenomena. The excess of histamine released during the development of an inflammatory reaction causes further lesions of the tissue. The inflammatory process would possibly develop faster and more favorably to the subject if no further release of histamine would occur.

References

BÜCH, O., u. TH. WAGNER-JAUREGG: Zur Problematik antiphlogistischer Teste. Arzneimittel-Forsch. **10**, 834—836 (1960).

CIGLAR, M.: Über die Freisetzung histaminartiger Stoffe durch kutane Verabreichung eines Autolysates aus aeroben Erdbazillen (B. subtilis und B. megatherium). Z. Rheumaforsch. **17**, 2—7 (1958).

— Ž. IGNJAČEV, A. MISIRLIJA, A. NIKULIN u. P. STERN: Beitrag zur Wirkungsweise des Kalziums im Entzündungsprozeß. Arch. int. Pharmacodyn. **113**, 360—366 (1958).

FELDBERG, W.: On some physiological aspects of histamine. J. Pharm. Pharmacol. **6**, 281—301 (1954).

— The role of mediators in the inflammatory tissue response. Int. Arch. Allergy **8**, 15—31 (1956).

—, and A. A. LOESER: Histamine content of human skin in different clinical disorders. J. Physiol. (Lond.) **126**, 286—292 (1954).

—, and A. A. MILES: Regional variations of increased permeability of skin capillaries induced by a histamine liberator and their relation to the histamine content of the skin. J. Physiol. (Lond.) **120**, 205—213 (1953).

FERLUGA, J., A. NIKULIN u. P. STERN: Die antiphlogistische Wirkung der Epsilon-Amino-Kapronsäure. Allergie u. Asthma **9**, 18—22 (1963).

FRIMMER, M.: Beeinflussung der Durchlässigkeit von Blut-Capillaren der Kaninchenhaut für Makromoleküle durch biogene gefäßaktive Substanzen. Naunyn-Schmiedebergs Arch. exp. Path. Pharmak. **242**, 390—402 (1961).

HAAS, H.: Histamin und Antihistaminica, I—II. Aulendorf: Verl. Cantor 1951.

HAITINGER, M.: Fluorescenz-Mikroskopie. Leipzig 1938.

HUKOVIĆ, S., i P. STERN: Količina histamina u tkivima pod utjecajem arsen-trioksida. Acta med. iugosl. **16**, 43—50 (1962).
IGNJAČEV, Ž., A. NIKULIN, P. STERN, A. MISIRLIJA u. M. CIGLAR: Hypothyreoidismus und entzündliche Reaktion. Acta endocr. (Kbh.) **23**, 426—432 (1956).
IRINO, S.: Granuloma pouch and skin histamine. Acta med. Okayama **12**, 112—125 (1958).
JAQUES, R.: Das Thalassinödem der Ratte und seine Beeinflussung durch verschiedene Pharmaka. Helv. physiol. pharmacol. Acta **11**, C55—C57 (1953).
KRAMER, M.: Zur antiphlogistischen Wirkung des Histaminliberators 48/80, einiger Antihistaminica und einiger Antirheumatica. Naunyn-Schmiedebergs Arch. exp. Path. Pharmak. **233**, 125—133 (1958).
LEWIS, G.: 5-Hydroxytryptamine. New York — London — Paris — Los Angeles: Pergamon Press 1958.
MEIER, R.: Biochemische Kausalzusammenhänge des Entzündungsvorgangs. In: Medizinische Grundlagenforschung, Band II (BAUER, K. FR., Ed.). Stuttgart: G. Thieme Verlag 1959.
— P. DESAULLES u. B. SCHÄR: Analyse der biochemischen Ursachen der entzündlichen Zellreaktion. Verh. Naturf. Ges. (Basel) **67**, 447—478 (1956).
MENKIN, V.: Biochemical Mechanisms in Inflammation. Springfield, Ill.: Charles C. Thomas Publ. 1956.
MISIRLIJA, A., P. STERN i S. HUKOVIĆ: Značenje histamina i nervnog sistema za tuberkulinsku reakciju. Tuberkuloza **8**, 102—105 (1956).
NIKULIN, A., J. FERLUGA i P. STERN: Uticaj količine tkivnog histamina na tok upalnog procesa. Acta med. iugosl. **16**, 182—188 (1962).
PATON, W. D. M.: The Release of Histamine. Progress in Allergy **5**, 79—148. New York-Basel: S. Karger 1958.
RAAB, W.: Die Beeinflussung des experimentellen Dinitrochlorbenzolekzems des Meerschweinchens durch den Histaminliberator 48/80. Arch. klin. exp. Derm. **214**, 307—318 (1962).
RAJKA, E.: Allergie und allergische Erkrankungen. Bd. I, Allgemeiner Teil. Budapest: Akadémia Kadó 1959.
ROCHA E SILVA, M.: Histamine: Its Role in Anaphylaxis and Allergy. Springfield, Ill.: Charles C. Thomas, Publ. 1955.
— Biochemistry and Pharmacology of Bradykinin. In: Polypeptides. Oxford-London-New York-Paris: Pergamon Press 1960.
ROSENTHAL, S. R., and D. MINARD: Experiments on histamine as the chemical mediator for cutaneous pain. J. exp. Med. **70**, 415—425 (1939).
SANDBERG, N.: Accelerated collagen formation and histamine. Nature (Lond.) **194**, 183 (1962).
SELYE, H.: Use of "granuloma pouch" technique in the study of antiphlogistic corticoids. Proc. Soc. exp. Biol. (N. Y.) **82**, 328—333 (1953)
SHERRY, S., A. P. FLETCHER, NORMA ALKJAERSIG, and W. D. SAWYER: ε-aminocaproic acid "a potent anti-fibrinolytic agent". Trans. Ass. Amer. Phycns. **72**, 62—70 (1959).
SPECKMANN, K.: Histamin als Regulator nervös gesteuerter Abwehrgänge in der Peripherie. Verh. Deutsch. Ges. innere Med., 59. Kongr. München: Verl. J. F. Bergmann 1953.
STERN, P.: Antiallergische Wirkung der Azulene. 1st Internat. Congr. for Allergy, Zürich. Basel-New York: S. Karger 1951.
— Die Bedeutung des Histamins in der Entstehung des Ekzems. Arch. int. Pharmacodyn. **105**, 279—284 (1956).
— Studies in animals on the effect of subtivaccin, an autolysate from B. Subtilis and B. Megatherium, on the permeability of inflammatory tissues and on that of the central nervous system. Acta physiol. pharmacol. neerl. **8**, 457—465 (1959).
—, u. S. HUKOVIĆ: Die Rolle des Histamins in der Übertragung des Schmerzempfindens Arch. int. Pharmacodyn. **108**, 273—278 (1956).
—, u. R. MILIN: Die antiallergische und antiphlogistische Wirkung der Azulene. Arzneimittel-Forsch. **6**, 445—450 (1956).
—, u. A. NIKULIN: Über die entzündungshemmende Wirkung der Azulene. Ärztl. Forsch. **11**, I/495—I/498 (1957).
— —, and J. FERLUGA: The role of histamine and bradykinin in the inflammatory process. Arch. int. Pharmacodyn. **140**, 528—538 (1962).
— — A. MISIRLIJA u. M. CIGLAR: Histamin im Entzündungsprozeß. Naunyn-Schmiedebergs Arch. exp. Path. Pharmakol. **227**, 522—527 (1956).
—, u. EDITA GMAZ-NIKULIN: 5-Hydroxytryptamin und Histamin im Entzündungsprozeß. Int. Arch. Allergy **16**, 157—162 (1960).
UNGAR, G.: Inflammation and its control. A biochemical approach. Lancet **1952 II**, 742.
WILHELM, D. L.: The mediation of increased vascular permeability in inflammation. Pharmacol. Rev. **14**, 251—280 (1962).
ZWEIFACH, B. W.: Symposium on the Mechanism of Inflammation. Montreal: Ed. G. JASMIN and A. ROBERT. ACTA Inc. 1953.
— cited from FELDBERG (1956).

Section D

L'histamine dans l'allergie humaine

Par

Umberto Serafini

Avec 3 Figures

I. Introduction

Les recherches expérimentales de Dale et Laidlaw (1910) qui, les premiers, ont mis en évidence les analogies qui existent entre le choc anaphylactique et le choc histaminique, ont eu le grand mérite d'ouvrir un nouveau et vaste domaine d'études dont l'intérêt a été démontré par le grand nombre de travaux d'ordre biologique sur l'importance de l'histamine dans la pathogénèse des phénomènes anaphylactiques.

Du point de vue expérimental, grâce à ces recherches on est parvenu à démontrer la libération de l'histamine préformée dans les organes de choc des animaux de laboratoire, à la suite de la réaction antigène-anticorps. Ces travaux, qui sont à la base de la théorie histaminique de l'anaphylaxie, ont été par la suite étendus aux manifestations allergiques humaines, en vue des analogies de plus en plus évidentes entre les syndromes allergiques et les manifestations anaphylactiques chez l'animal d'expérience ainsi que celles entre les réactions allergiques générales et locales et les réactions à l'histamine.

Il faut remarquer à cet égard qu'au cours des vingt dernières années, l'intérêt des recherches concernant le rôle physiologique et physiopathologique de l'histamine a été soutenu grâce surtout à des découvertes fondamentales telles que celle des antihistaminiques de synthèse (Bovet et Staub, 1937), celle des rapports étroits établis entre l'histamine et les mastocytes (Riley et West, 1953; West, 1956) et celle des substances histamino-libératrices (Paton, 1951), comme le 48/80, au même temps qu'on a démontré que des substances actives différentes de l'histamine sont libérées ou activées au cours de l'anaphylaxie, comme la 5-hydroxytryptamine, la bradykinine, les *slow reacting substances* (Erspamer, 1954; Rocha e Silva et al., 1949; Rocha e Silva, 1955, et d'autres).

Ces acquisitions, qui sont le fruit d'un grand nombre de recherches dans le domaine expérimental, donnent désormais la possibilité d'approfondir et d'étendre nos connaissances sur le rôle joué par l'histamine dans la physiopathologie chez l'homme et, en particulier, de préciser l'importance de l'histamine dans la pathogénie de cet ensemble de manifestations cliniques, si important du point de vue théorique et pratique, qui constitue l'allergie humaine.

Il faut cependant, tout de suite, affirmer que les recherches concernant le rôle de l'histamine dans l'allergie humaine ont donné des résultats sans aucun doute moins significatifs que ceux obtenus dans le domaine des phénomenes anaphylactiques expérimentaux. Toutefois ces résultats sont fort nombreux et revêtent un intérêt certain, si bien qu'on est en mesure d'affirmer qu'ils constituent un chapitre bien défini pouvant être traité séparément.

Eu égard à l'ampleur et à la complexité du problème de «l'histamine dans l'allergie humaine», il nous semble préférable de nous borner à examiner séparément les aspects, à notre avis, les plus importants, et précisément: les aspects *pathogéniques*, les aspects *diagnostiques* et les aspects *thérapeutiques*.

II. Aspects pathogéniques

A. Libération de l'histamine au cours des réactions allergiques

Dans le domaine de l'allergie clinique, les recherches sur le rôle joué par l'histamine se sont orientées au début surtout sur les variations de l'histaminémie et, plus exactement, sur le taux d'histamine dans le sang chez les sujets allergiques, soit au cours des manifestations cliniques, soit dans les intervalles. Le développement de ces recherches a été favorisé par la possibilité de doser l'histamine dans le sang et dans les humeurs soit par la méthode de CODE (1937) et celles qui en dérivent, soit par les métodes chimiques (LOWRY et coll., 1954 et d'autres).

L'appréciation de ces résultats est rendue d'ailleurs assez problématique par la variabilité de l'histaminémie normale qui oscille entre 2 et 7,5 γ par 100 cc de sang (HAWORTH et MACDONALD, 1937; ROSE et BROWNE, 1940). D'après certains Auteurs il semblerait que chez le même individu il se manifesterait dans le temps une certaine stabilité du taux d'histamine, ce qui constituerait une constante individuelle (HAWORTH et MACDONALD, 1937).

Il est cependant nécessaire de rappeler que beaucoup de ces recherches (et pratiquement toutes celles qui ne sont pas récentes) ont été effectuées sur le sang *in toto*, alors que l'on ne peut considérer «active» que l'histamine libre dissoute dans le plasma, étant donné que la fraction histaminique contenue dans les cellules sanguines, et spécialement dans les leucocytes et dans les plaquettes, n'engendre pas le moindre trouble ou symptôme.

D'après les données les plus fidèles, au cours des *périodes de rémission des symptômes*, l'histaminémie est à peu près normale (CERQUA, 1936; ROSE, 1941a et b; HJORT et coll., 1950; COLLI et QUACCI, 1949). D'après ROSE (1941b) et SERAFINI (1948) par contre, chez un même sujet allergique, il se produit des variations du contenu histaminique du sang plus marquées que chez les sujets normaux. D'après MAAS et coll. (1956) celà serait moins en rapport avec une variabilité individuelle qu'avec le fait que certains malades présentent un niveau élevé et d'autres un niveau bas de l'histaminémie.

L'analyse des variations du taux de l'histamine *pendant les manifestations allergiques* n'a pas donné de résultats définitifs; alors que certains Auteurs, en effet, ont vu dans ces conditions une augmentation de l'histamine du sang dans l'asthme (CERQUA, 1936; HAWORTH et MACDONALD, 1937; PARROT et REUSE, 1954; CAPUANI, 1939; RANDOLPH et RACKEMANN, 1941; COLLI et QUACCI, 1949), dans l'urticaire (CERQUA, 1936; FIESSINGER et GAJDOS, 1937; ROSE, 1941a et b, dans un seul cas sur 8 examinés; GATÉ et PELLERAT, 1947), dans l'oedème de Quincke (BUSINCO, 1939), dans les maladies du sérum (LECOMTE, 1956), dans le choc anaphylactique dû aux médicaments; d'autres Auteurs, au contraire, ont constaté une diminution de l'histamine dans l'oedème de Quincke (ROSE, 1941a et b, dans 7 cas sur 8), dans l'urticaire (NILZEN, 1947), dans le choc provoqué par le sérum (CERQUA, 1936); d'autres encore n'ont pas constaté la moindre modification (HJORT et coll., 1950) et d'autres enfin n'ont pas eu de résultats uniformes (CECCARINI et RICCIARDI, 1946; STRENGERS et coll., 1947).

Il faut rappeler à ce propos que l'histaminémie ne peut donner qu'un tableau très approximatif de ce qui se passe dans les tissus. L'effet de l'histamine est essentiellement local; une partie seulement de la substance libérée se déverse dans la circulation et est en mesure de provoquer des phénomènes d'ordre général. D'autre part, l'augmentation de l'histaminémie peut n'être qu'extrêmement fugace et le taux peut redevenir rapidement normal (1–2 minutes) (Serafini et Giunchi, 1946). Différents Auteurs (Beall et van Arsdel, 1960; Helander et coll., 1961) ont montré, grâce à une histamine marquée en C^{14} que l'histamine en excès est rapidement éliminée de la circulation (dans un délai de 1 à 2 minutes). Cela peut expliquer les résultats négatifs ou discordants obtenus au cours de certaines manifestations allergiques (Rose et coll., 1950).

Dans l'ensemble, l'avis des Auteurs (Jimenez Diaz, 1944; Gaté et Pellerat, 1947; Rose, 1941a et b) est presque unanimement négatif quant à la signification d'une augmentation de l'histaminémie rapportée à l'état allergique.

Sur les données de la littérature nous avons donc le droit de conclure, en accord avec ce qu'ont affirmé Giunchi et Serafini (1942, 1944), qu'il n'est pas possible d'établir des rapports bien définis et concordants entre les variations de l'histaminémie et l'état allergique. Les données fondamentales qui nous amènent à cette conclusion et qu'il est nécessaire de garder présentes à l'esprit, peuvent se résumer ainsi: un taux normal d'histamine peut être observé chez des sujets par ailleurs certainement allergiques aussi bien dans des périodes normales qu'au cours des crises de la maladie (Giunchi et Serafini, 1942, 1944; Rose, 1941a et b, et d'autres); un taux élevé d'histamine peut être retrouvé même dans des conditions pathologiques n'ayant aucun rapport avec l'allergie comme, par exemple, la leucémie à cause de l'augmentation des leucocytes, dans les états d'anoxémie suivant une décompensation cardiaque.

Cette affirmation n'exclut pas naturellement la possibilité d'un mécanisme histaminique localisé et n'implique pas que l'on nie *a priori* la valeur d'une augmentation de l'histaminémie au cours d'une crise allergique suivant des valeurs normales, au cours de périodes de répit de la symptomatologie (que l'on se rappelle, toutefois, la possibilité d'une diminution de l'histaminémie aux cours des manifestations allergiques (Rose, 1941a et b), mais sert surtout à limiter la signification que l'on peut attribuer à une augmentation de l'histaminémie – dans un seul dosage –, que certains Auteurs ont considérée non seulement comme un argument en faveur de l'intervention d'un mécanisme histaminique dans différentes formes morbides mais qu'ils ont estimée comme le signe d'un état allergique, en identifiant histamine et allergie.

Mieux que l'étude de l'histaminémie, les recherches sur «l'épreuve de surcharge d'histamine» (Serafini et Biozzi, 1946a et b; Serafini, 1948) pourraient donner des résultats plus intéressants. Cette épreuve consiste à mesurer l'histaminémie à des intervalles de temps déterminés (1, 2, 3, 5, 7, 10 minutes) à la suite d'une injection sous-cutanée d'l mg d'histamine. Les variations de l'histaminémie qu'on observe par cette méthode sont très différentes selon qu'il s'agisse de patients allergiques ou normaux. Alors que chez ces derniers l'injection d'histamine ne provoque aucune variation ou alors une très légère diminution du taux d'histamine, chez les asthmatiques, au contraire, l'histaminémie augmente généralement dans les minutes qui suivent immédiatement la piqûre. Chez les malades atteints d'urticaire, de rhinopathie vasomotrice et de migraine, on observe des oscillations comparables à celles que l'on retrouve chez les asthmatiques mais moins constantes. Dans les cas où l'épreuve est négative, il est possible de penser que les phénomènes allergiques sont plus étroitement limités à l'organe de choc et que la méthode n'est pas en mesure de mettre en évidence l'altération du métabolisme.

Une démonstration ultérieure de l'altération du métabolisme de l'histamine chez les sujets allergiques a pu être donnée par les recherches de Serafini et Biozzi (1946c) sur les modifications de l'histaminémie suivant une fatigue physique.

Un excercice physique capable d'engendrer une fatigue réelle, a déterminé, dans un groupe de malades atteints de pollinosis, une augmentation de l'histaminémie, alors que chez des sujets normaux il n'a pas été observé la moindre variation. Chez un malade souffrant de rhinite et d'asthme on a observé, en plus d'une augmentation marquée de l'histaminémie, une attaque d'asthme.

Ces observations pourraient être mises en rapport avec celles très récentes qui ont démontré chez des asthmatiques et en général chez des allergiques le manque du pouvoir histaminopexique du sérum, alors que cette propriété existerait chez les individus normaux grâce à la présence d'une fraction particulière de γ globulines (PARROT et LABORDE, 1953, 1961; BONET-MAURY et coll., 1960; BENDA et coll., 1959). D'après ces Auteurs ce phénomène serait une propriété caractéristique et importante de ce que l'on appelle «terrain allergique». Ces recherches ne semblent cependant pas susceptibles de mener à une conclusion définitive car il ne manque pas de résultats négatifs ou opposés (KAPLAN et DAVIS, 1953; GEDDA et TEODORI, 1961).

Il ne faut pas oublier enfin les recherches effectuées sur le contenu en histamine des cellules sanguines. En ce qui concerne les *cellules éosinophiles*, on a observé une augmentation du taux d'histamine chez des sujets qui présentaient une éosinophilie marquée (CODE et MACDONALD, 1937; RANDOLPH et RACKEMANN, 1941; VALENTINE et LAWRENCE, 1948; et d'autres) et, bien que l'on n'ait pas pu mettre en évidence un parallélisme entre l'histamine du sang et le nombre des éosinophiles (ECKERT et TOTTERMAN, 1950; et d'autres) on a affirmé que les cellules éosinophiles possèdent, entre autres fonctions, celle de transporteurs de l'histamine du sang (PARROT et GABE, 1945; PARROT et REUSE, 1954). Malgré les difficultés techniques, certains Auteurs (CODE, 1952; PARROT et GABE, 1945; HUMPHREY et JAQUES, 1954) ont pu démontrer que les plaquettes contiennent des quantités importantes d'histamine.

Par ailleurs dans des recherches toutes récentes sur les rapports étroits entre le contenu en histamine du sang et la présence de basophiles, RILEY et WEST (1953) ont remarqué qu'il y avait un taux élevé d'histamine dans les mastocytes tissulaires et GRAHAM et coll. (1955) ont précisé que la moitié de l'histamine du sang est contenue dans les basophiles. Dans la basopénie expérimentale (CODE et MITCHELL, 1957) et pathologique (RORSMAN, 1958), on a observé un contenu en histamine effectivement très bas. Il faut noter également que les *mastzellen* de différentes espèces, y compris l'homme, forment l'histamine qu'ils contiennent (SCHAYER, 1956).

En dehors du sang, le comportement de l'histamine a été étudié dans d'*autres milieux biologiques*: ainsi JIMENEZ DIAZ et ARJONA (1953) ont constaté une augmentation du contenu en histamine dans les *fèces* des asthmatiques. Ces derniers Auteurs ont également souligné que les fèces des asthmatiques ont une plus grande capacité de former de l'histamine si on les incube avec de l'histidine. D'autre part, on a observé chez des asthmatiques (ROSE, 1941a et b), chez des malades atteints d'urticaire (ADAM et coll., 1950) et dans certains états pathologiques avec éosinophilie marquée (DUNÉR et PERNOW, 1956, 1958), que l'*élimination urinaire* d'histamine est nettement supérieure à celle que l'on rencontre chez des individus normaux. Certains Auteurs (DUNÉR et PERNOW, 1956, 1958; MITCHELL et coll., 1954) ont d'autre part obtenu chez des sujets asthmatiques en période normale, des résultats négatifs. MITCHELL (1959) également, après avoir observé les taux d'histamine libre dans l'excrétion urinaire chez des enfants allergiques et normaux, suivant l'injection sous-cutanée d'histamine, a déduit que pour l'asthme, on n'enregistre pas de variations significatives en ce qui concerne l'élimination ou la rapidité de destruction de l'histamine.

Toujours dans le cadre des recherches sur les rapports entre histamine et allergie, des données d'un intérêt particulier nous sont fournies par les résultats de l'analyse de certains *phénomènes allergiques provoqués* «in vivo» et «in vitro».

Il faut rappeler à ce sujet les observations classiques de LEWIS (1927) qui, se basant sur de nombreuses recherches fort bien documentées, a conclu que les manifestations d'urticaire produites par différents stimuli peuvent déterminer la libération d'histamine ou plus généralement de substances H.

Au cours des manifestations provoquées par l'«*urticaria factitia*» SERAFINI et GIUNCHI (1946) ont mis en évidence, au bout de quelques minutes du frottis, une augmentation de l'histaminémie qui a été considérée comme une conséquence de la libération d'histamine à l'endroit de la stimulation cutanée. De même au cours des réactions cutanées allergiques, il se libère de l'histamine (KATZ, 1942). L'expérience rapportée par SERAFINI et GIUNCHI (1946) est assez significative à cet égard, dans un cas d'asthme provoqué par des pellicules de cheval où, après avoir provoqué des manifestations importantes par 54 intradermo-réactions avec une dilution à 1/10.000 de l'allergène, les Auteurs ont pu mettre en évidence une augmentation marquée de l'histaminémie, après l'application du stimulus (Fig. 1).

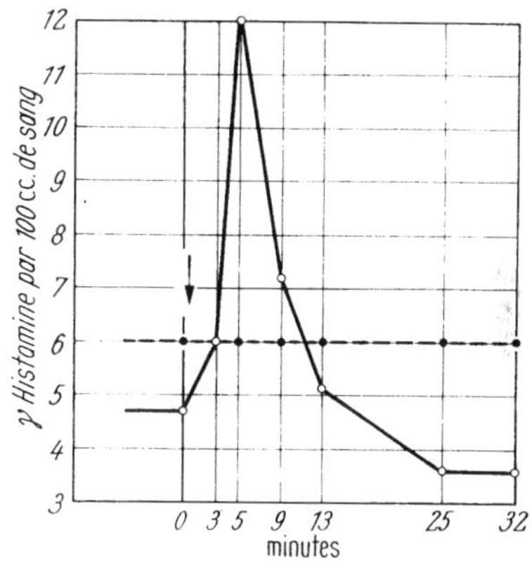

Fig. 1. Variations du taux de l'histamine sanguine consécutives à l'injection d'antigène à un sujet sensible aux pellicules de cheval. 54 intradermo-réactions au moyen de l'allergène spécifique ont provoqué des réactions cutanées très intenses et un accroissement de l'histaminémie (exprimée en μg d'histamine-base p. 100 cc.). (SERAFINI, 1948)

Dans l'«*urticaria a frigore*», on est parvenu à démontrer, d'abord par voie indirecte, en vue de l'augmentation de la sécrétion gastrique, de l'hypotension et des symptômes généraux (HORTON et BROWN, 1929; MARTINETTI, 1943) puis par voie directe (MCELIN et HORTON, 1945; PELLERAT, 1945), la libération d'histamine au cours des manifestations engendrées par le froid. Il ne faut pas oublier non plus les résultats en grande partie négatifs en ce qui concerne une augmentation d'histamine chez des sujets sensibles au froid, obtenus récemment par DUNÉR et coll. (1960) et par SPUZIC et IVKOVIC (1961).

Dans l'*urticaire provoquée par la fatigue*, en outre, SERAFINI (1951) a pu démontrer une augmentation marquée de l'histaminémie pendant les manifestations provoquées par l'effort physique. Chez un de ces sujets l'histaminémie a atteint les valeurs maxima parallèlement au maximum des manifestations cutanées (Fig. 2). Chez le même malade, l'injection d'un antihistaminique peu avant l'effort, a inhibé complètement l'apparition de l'urticaire.

D'autre part PELLERAT et MURAT (1946) ont pu démontrer une baisse marquée du taux d'histamine dans la peau à la suite d'un traitement par le chlorure d'éthyle; ces mêmes Auteurs ont également observé que le taux d'histamine diminue dans la peau si l'urticaire et l'eczéma se manifestent. De même NILZEN (1947) a observé une diminution de l'histamine de la peau après frottis et sur le lieu des papules chez des malades atteints d'urticaire.

Les intéressantes recherches de KATZ et COHEN (1941) ont démontré comment en additionnant au sang d'un malade atteint de pollinosis l'antigène spécifique on provoque (en accord avec ce que KATZ (1940) avait constaté dans des expériences similaires avec du sang de lapin sensibilisé) la libération d'une quantité très importante d'histamine dans le plasma (avec une augmentation de 169 a 900 %). Ces recherches ont été confirmées par NOAH et BRAND (1954). VAN ARSDEL et coll.

(1958) ont récemment entrepris des recherches analogues avec des résultats comparables à ceux que nous venons de rapporter et ont en outre signalé un fait singulier, à savoir, que l'excès d'antigène provoque sur la libération d'histamine un effet inhibiteur.

Il faut aussi rappeler les travaux de certains Auteurs (ROSA et BARBIERI, 1951; SCHILD et coll., 1951) qui ont mis au point une méthode pour étudier les bronches humaines isolées. ROSA et BARBIERI (1951) ont poursuivi des recherches sur les bronches d'un asthmatique sensibilisé à la farine, soumis à une intervention de pneumectomie en raison d'un cancer du poumon droit. En ajoutant 1 cc de solution de l'antigène spécifique (farine) aux 10 cc du bain de perfusion contenant un fragment du tissu bronchique, on a obtenu une contraction accentuée et durable de la préparation. Un dosage qualitatif a montré que le liquide de perfusion contractait l'utérus isolé du cobaye, baissait la pressions anguine chez le chat et que ces effets étaient inhibés par des antihistaminiques. Des recherches quantitatives ont en outre révélé la libération d'une très grande quantité d'histamine, jusqu'à 3–4 γ par gramme de tissu en 10 minutes.

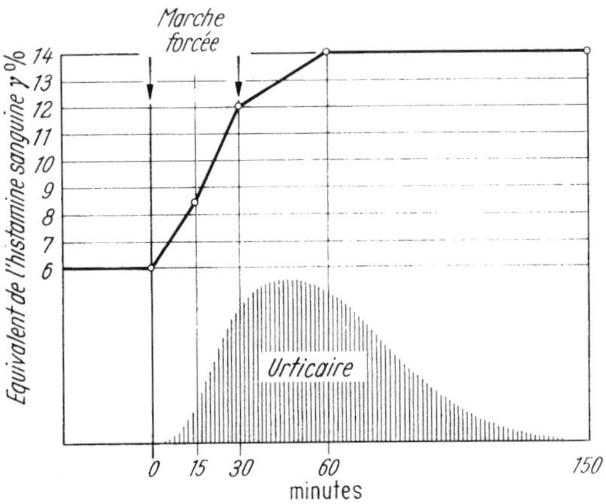

Fig. 2. Variations du taux de l'histamine sanguine au cours des manifestations urticariennes provoquées par l'effort (marche rapide durant 30 min). Le tracé supérieur correspond à l'histaminémie (exprimée en μg d'histamine-base p. 100 cc.); le tracé inférieur, à l'évolution des manifestations cliniques, prurit et sensation de chaleur, jusqu 'à l'acmé de l'éruption urticarienne qui se produit entre la 30e et la 60e minute. (SERAFINI, 1951)

SCHILD et coll. (1951) après avoir démontré qu'une préparation de bronche isolée d'un asthmatique allergique se contracte quand elle est mise en contact avec son antigène spécifique, ont en outre observé la libération d'une grande quantité d'histamine, supérieure (en microgrammes par gramme de tissu) à celle libérée par le poumon du cobaye soumis au choc anaphylactique. Ils ont également souligné la nécessité d'employer des doses élevées d'antihistaminiques pour inhiber la contraction d'une bronche allergique engendrée par l'antigène spécifique.

Dans ce même domaine il faut souligner l'affirmation de ROSE, ENTIN et BAXTER (1950) d'après laquelle le contenu en histamine du tissu pulmonaire est, chez les asthmatiques, beaucoup plus élevé que chez des témoins (en moyenne 115 γ au lieu de 15–35 γ par gramme de tissu).

Il faut rappeler enfin que FORTUNATO (1948) a observé que les altérations de la muqueuse nasale produites chez le lapin par l'histamine, sont analogues à celles que l'on retrouve dans l'allergie clinique.

De l'ensemble de ces observations, dont nous n'avons rappelé ici que celles qui nous paraissent avoir un intérêt réel, il découle qu'il y aurait de nombreux arguments en faveur de la conception d'après laquelle l'histamine est libérée au niveau des tissus au cours de certaines manifestations allergiques chez l'homme sous l'effet de la réaction antigène-anticorps ou d'autres stimuli.

B. D'autres médiateurs chimiques

Pour une meilleure compréhension du rôle pathogénique de l'histamine il ne faut pas non plus oublier les récentes acquisitions sur la *multiplicité des médiateurs chimiques* en mesure d'être libérés ou activés au cours des réactions allergiques.

L'intérêt présenté par la connaissance de ces substances réside principalement dans le fait qu'elles sont libérées très probablement dans une mesure plus ou moins grande suivant les différentes éspèces animales et qu'elles peuvent présenter chez l'homme une importance pathogénétique différente suivant la localisation de l'organe de choc. Ces acquisitions se basent sur de nombreuses observations dont nous ne citerons ici que les plus significatives dans le cadre de l'allergie clinique.

En ce qui concerne l'*acétylcholine*, il a été démontré que chez l'homme l'injection de 20–40 mg de cette substance provoque fréquemment des accès d'asthme, seulement toutefois chez des sujets spontanément asthmatiques. On doit signaler encore que dans le sang des asthmatiques, on trouve un taux extrèmement élevé d'acétylcholine (WENNER et BUHRMESTER, 1937; SCUDAMORE et coll., 1951) alors que des extraits provenant de morceaux de peau eczémateuse et frappée d'herpès, donneraient des réactions de type acétylcholinique (ROTHMAN et COON, 1940).

Au cours de ces dernières années d'autres substances actives sur les vaisseaux ont été découvertes.

La *5-hydroxytryptamine*, qui est une substance très bien étudiée du point de vue expérimental à la suite des recherches de HUMPHREY et JAQUES (1954), intervient vraisemblablement de façon très limitée au cours des manifestations cliniques chez l'homme. On connaît bien toutefois les manifestations asthmatiques qui peuvent se produire dans des cas de carcinoïdes du grêle (THORSON et coll., 1954). Il faut remarquer que même l'administration intradermique provoque une vasodilatation intense; la zone erythémateuse est douloureuse plus que prurigineuse. CHRISTENSSON et EKWALL (1960), ont noté une augmentation de l'acide hydroxyindolacétique dans l'urine de deux patients sur les 15 chez lesquels on avait provoqué des phénomènes de rhinite. Il faut enfin ajouter que la butanolamide de l'acide methyl-1-lysergique antisérotoninique, semble, d'après SICUTERI (1959 c), fort efficace dans la migraine.

Nous avons précédemment rappelé la libération de «slow reacting substances» (BROCKLEHURST, 1956), au cours de la réaction antigène-anticorps d'une bronche humaine isolée.

Il faut enfin signaler la possibilité d'une intervention, même chez l'homme, d'*héparine* qui est libérée des mastocytes en même temps que l'histamine et la sérotonine, et de la *bradykinine* (ROCHA E SILVA et coll., 1949) laquelle, avec d'autres polypeptides présentant des propriétés analogues, peuvent être groupés sous l'appelation de «plasmakinines».

C. Evidences indirectes sur la participation de l'histamine dans les phénomènes allergiques

En dehors des recherches que nous venons de rapporter tendant principalement à démontrer, spécialement par la méthode directe, le rôle de l'histamine dans la pathogénie des manifestations allergiques, il est nécessaire de rappeler ici trois groupes de recherches qui pourraient apporter d'autres éléments, même s'ils sont moins significatifs et nets que les précédents, à l'hypothèse qui attribue à l'histamine un rôle prépondérant dans beaucoup de syndromes allergiques.

Les groupes de recherches se rapportent: 1) à la possibilité de reproduire des symptômes de type allergique à la suite d'une administration d'histamine; 2) à l'action thérapeutique positive dont font preuve les antihistaminiques dans certaines formes allergiques; 3) à la possibilité de provoquer chez l'homme des syndrômes typiquement allergiques au moyen de substances histamino-libératrices.

En ce qui concerne le premier groupe, il faut remarquer, comme il est bien connu, que l'administration d'histamine, quelle que soit la voie d'introduction, (sous-cutanée, intraveineuse, par aérosol) détermine chez les asthmatiques une crise de broncho-sténose d'une intensité particulière. Il faut remarquer que cette crise est d'autant plus intense et prolongée que la forme d'asthme est plus grave et plus invétéré, indépendamment de l'existence précédente d'une sensibilisation allergique. Les récentes recherches pharmacodynamiques de TIFFENEAU (1958) ont permis en effet de prouver l'existence d'une réactivité bronchique particulière, bien distincte de la réactivité allergique. Ces recherches ont mis en évidence une «hypersensibilité cholinergique histaminique» particulière (aux doses «seuil») chez tous les asthmatiques (et tendant à s'accentuer au fur et à mesure que l'asthme devient plus intense) et qui représente, d'après cet Auteur, l'expression d'un substrat fondamental de l'asthmatique. L'allergie pulmonaire, au contraire, n'est intense que dans un tiers des cas et tend à diminuer avec l'âge et la gravité de l'asthme. Une «allergie pulmonaire» n'est pas asthmogène si l'hypersensibilité cholinergique-histaminique est faible (asthme latent, asthme récent).

Sur la base de ces recherches il est donc possible d'affirmer que, même dans l'éventualité de crises asthmatiques où il ne serait pas possible de démontrer un mécanisme de réaction antigène-anticorps, les substances vaso-actives surmentionnées peuvent revêtir une importance pathogénique; et cette affirmation ne perd pas son importance à cause du fait que le mécanisme à travers lequel on parvient à une réactivité bronchique particulière n'est pas facile à prouver sans que l'on assiste apparemment à une sensibilisation précédente. A cet égard on peut toujours suggérer que différents facteurs constitutionnels et acquis (en particulier des inflammations, etc.) sont en mesure de provoquer, même sans le concours d'anticorps, une altération de la réactivité des tissus bronchiques qui se traduirait par l'acquisition de la part de ces tissus, d'une forte capacité de réponse des récepteurs à l'histamine, qu'elle soit d'origine exogène ou endogène.

Les recherches de TIFFENEAU (1958) amènent à admettre une hyperexcitabilité des effecteurs moteurs pulmonaires (muscles lisses des bronches et des vaisseaux, glandes) vis-à-vis de leurs médiateurs cholinergo-histaminiques, peuvent en outre rendre vraisemblable que l'apparition des manifestations cliniques se vérifie même quand la libération d'histamine et d'autres médiateurs chimiques suivant la réaction antigène-anticorps est minime. Dans l'absence d'une telle hyperexcitabilité des effecteurs il n'apparaît pas de symptômes cliniques et la réaction antigène-anticorps peut être considérée comme latente (SPOUJITCH, 1960).

LECOMTE (1956) a récemment observé que l'application de poudre d'histamine dans la muqueuse nasale de malades souffrant de rhume des foins saisonnier, au cours d'une période de guérison clinique apparente, provoque du prurit, des éternuements et de l'oedème, démontrant ainsi que la muqueuse nasale du malade est plus sensible que celle d'un sujet normal.

Les recherches sur la dermatose allergique ne sont pas tellement démonstratives. L'urticaire en effet, d'après certains Auteurs, sérait déchaînée par l'injection d'histamine ou bien, suivant d'autres, d'histamine et d'acétylcholine. Nos recherches sur cette dernière possibilité, néanmoins, n'ont pas pu confirmer les observations précédentes.

Des remarques intéressantes ont été faites dans le domaine des céphalées médicales. Dans les céphalées d'origine inflammatoire le seuil histaminique est assez bas, comme d'ailleurs dans les cas de céphalée histaminique de HORTON.

En conclusion l'affirmation de JONEZ (1952) que l'injection d'une quantité suffisante d'histamine chez un individu allergique est capable de produire les symptômes dont celui-ci souffre habituellement, ne saurait être admise que sous certaines réserves: elle ne peut être vérifiée en effet que pour certaines manifestations cliniques d'origine allergique.

Quant au deuxième argument plaidant en faveur de l'importance du rôle pathogénique de l'histamine, il faut rappeler que l'introduction en thérapeutique des *antihistaminiques de synthèse* (et en particulier de certains d'entre eux comme le Néo-Antergan) avait tout au début fait songer qu'on aurait pu en tirer des conclusions certaines et définitives quant à la nature des différentes manifestations cliniques.

D'une façon générale, on peut dire que les antihistaminiques exercent une action bienfaisante dans les formes cutanées, et surtout, pour les formes prurigineuses, dans l'urticaire et dans certains eczémas; leur action est au contraire minime, presque négligeable, dans l'asthme bronchique et dans la plus grande partie des autres manifestations attribuées à l'allergie. Il n'est guère facile de relier les résultats thérapeutiques à l'hypothèse du rôle joué par l'histamine, comme on le voit.

Il faut toutefois avoir présent à l'esprit plusieurs possibilités: il est essentiel, comme nous l'avons dit plus haut, de savoir à quelle forme de réaction allergique on a à faire, étant donné que les formes à développement immédiat réagissent souvent favorablement aux antihistaminiques, contrairement à celles à développement tardif. Il ne faut pas oublier non plus que suivant l'organe de choc et la réactivité différente des patients, il est possible qu'il se libère une quantité considérable d'histamine dépassant, si l'on veut, l'effet antagoniste de l'antihistaminique ou éventuellement l'insuffisance de la dose de l'antihistaminique. Ceci a son importance, à notre avis, et doit être pris en considération pour interpréter les résultats si différents, des plus positifs jusqu'aux négatifs, obtenus dans des cas cliniques identiques. Il faut enfin rappeler l'hypothèse très intéressante de DALE (1948). Cet Auteur a, en effet, émis l'hypothèse que dans le cas des réactions cutanées, l'histamine est libérée à une certaine distance des effecteurs représentés par les muscles lisses des vaisseaux; par conséquent l'histamine pourrait être bloquée par le médicament avant d'avoir atteint son lieu d'action. Inversement, au cours de l'asthme bronchique, l'histamine, libérée dans le voisinage immédiat des effecteurs pourrait exercer directement son action en se trouvant dans un certain sens à l'abri de l'action protectrice du médicament.

En ce qui concerne le troisième groupe, il faut rappeler que l'administration de *substances histamino-libératrices* (1935 L et 48/80) chez des sujets normaux engendre, selon la voie d'introduction et les doses employées, une symptomatologie différente inhérente aux propriétés pharmacologiques de ces dérivés.

Les données qui présentent le plus d'intérêt pour nous sont celles provenant des recherches effectuées sur l'effet des substances histamino-libératrices dans certaines affections pathologiques considérées comme d'origine allergique.

Chez les asthmatiques, par exemple, l'administration de quelques microgrammes d'un histamino-libérateur détermine une crise de bronchosténose d'une intensité particulière. Conformément à ce qui a été observé chez ces mêmes malades à la suite d'une injection d'histamine, le «seuil asthmogène» est d'autant plus bas et l'accès d'asthme d'autant plus intense et prolongé que la forme asthmatique dont les malades souffrent est plus grave et invétérée (état de mal asthmatique).

Le mécanisme à travers lequel l'histamino-libérateur détermine la crise doit sans aucun doute être relié à une action histaminique représentée essentiellement par la congestion et l'oedème de la muqueuse ainsi que par le spasme des muscles lisses des bronches: tous ces phénomènes peuvent faire nous rendre compte de la rapidité extraordinaire avec laquelle s'installe la manifestation clinique.

Les observations auxquelles nous venons de faire allusion sur la plus grande gravité des symptômes provoqués par l'histamino-libérateur dans les formes asthmatiques graves et invétérées (SICUTERI, 1959a et b), en accord avec ce que TIFFENEAU (1958) avait déjà signalé pour l'histamine, peut faire apparaître comme vraisemblable qu'avec l'aggravation de la symptomatologie asthmatique il se produise dans l'organe de choc (appareil bronchique) un état d'hyperexcitabilité des récepteurs en vertu de quoi des doses même minimes d'histamine libérées par l'histamino-libérateur, sont en mesure de déclencher une symptomatologie imposante.

Il faut remarquer que l'hypothèse d'une réactivité en excès des effecteurs du tissu bronchique pourrait de même expliquer la raison pour laquelle de nombreux stimuli exogènes ou endogènes sont en mesure de déterminer la symptomatologie.

La constatation, ensuite, que la réactivité cutanée des asthmatiques à l'égard des histamino-libérateurs ne s'éloigne pas des données que l'on retrouve chez des sujets normaux, rend probable le fait que l'hypersensibilité des effecteurs est localisée au tissu bronchique, démontrant ainsi avec une précision assez grande l'un des caractères les plus particuliers de ce que l'on appelle organe de choc ou de réaction.

SICUTERI et coll. (1960) ont effectué en outre une recherche assez poussée sur le seuil des céphalées dues à l'histamino-libérateur 48/80 chez des malades présentant des céphalées inflammatoires, constatant que l'injection intraveineuse de doses très petites du 48/80, incapable par elles-mêmes de provoquer des réactions vasculaires, donnait lieu à des crises de céphalées avec tout le caractère des souffrances habituelles, et prouvant ainsi qui ce test s'avérait plus sensible que celui de l'histamine.

En conclusion, bien que la preuve de l'intervention de l'histamine dans la genèse des phénomènes définis comme allergiques, en accord avec ce qui a été constaté pour l'anaphylaxie n'ait pas encore été donnée, il paraît hors de doute que, tout au moins dans beaucoup de manifestations allergiques, et en particulier dans les plus typiques à caractère immédiat, l'histamine joue un rôle important.

Sans entrer dans le détail des mécanismes qui interviennent dans la libération d'histamine et pour lesquels nous renvoyons le lecteur aux autres Chapitres, il nous semble possible, sur la base de la revue que nous venons de faire et qui, faute de place, est forcément incomplète, que l'importance et la signification de l'histamine dans l'allergie puissent se résumer comme suit:

1) l'histamine constitue une substance active des plus importantes parmi celles libérées par les organes de choc sous l'effet des réactions antigène-anticorps ou d'autres stimuli.

2) L'histamine est libérée dans une mesure plus ou moins grande suivant le *genre* et le *lieu* des manifestations allergiques.

Dans l'allergie clinique, en effet, comme nous l'avons déjà dit, nous assistons à deux types de réactions: les «réactions à développement immédiat» du genre des réactions urticariennes où il se produit un mécanisme de réaction antigène-anticorps analogue à celui de l'anaphylaxie et où la libération d'histamine paraît avoir un rôle important (pollinosis, urticaire, asthme allergique) et les «réactions à développement tardif» au cours desquelles, à travers un mécanisme immunologique différent, l'intervention de l'histamine apparaît plus négligeable (dermatites, eczémas, réactions vasculaires allergiques particulières, réactions tuberculiniques). Il faut remarquer en outre que même dans les réactions du premier type, la part de l'histamine peut varier en rapport avec la diversité du siège de la manifestation: ainsi, par exemple, on peut admettre qu'elle est plus grande dans les formes urticariennes et dans les formes nasales, moindre dans les formes asthmatiques. Dans les formes engendrées par les auto-anticorps, l'intervention de l'histamine apparaît, dans l'état actuel de nos connaissances, des plus douteux.

3) La libération d'histamine représente l'étape finale d'une série de réactions dont on ne connaît pas complètement les différentes phases. Cette libération trouve son origine dans une lésion cellulaire produite par différents stimuli mais en premier lieu par la réaction antigène-anticorps qui constitue un facteur de l'étiologie et de la pathologie toutàfait fondamental au cours des réactions allergiques. L'histamine libérée, parfois en quantité considérable, à cause même de la lésion cellulaire, peut revêtir une signification pathologique et déterminer des effets importants.

D'un autre côté, et ceci est une mise au point importante à laquelle on est parvenu au cours de ces toutes dernières années, même la libération de quantités d'histamine minimes peut déterminer des manifestations cliniques quand il existe une hyperexcitabilité particulière des effecteurs.

4) Afin d'évaluer de la façon la plus exacte possible le rôle de l'histamine dans la genèse des états pathologiques il faut enfin souligner:

a) que l'existence d'un mécanisme pathogénétique dû à l'histamine a été démontré au cours de très nombreuses manifestations de nature non allergique, ce qui nous amène à admettre que l'intervention de l'histamine ne se borne pas exclusivement aux manifestations allergiques mais s'étend à une série de phénomènes qui n'ont aucun rapport avec l'allergie.

b) Qu'il paraît désormais démontré qu'en dehors de l'histamine, les substances intervenant dans les phénomènes allergiques et anaphylactiques et ayant un effet microvasculaire et sur la musculature lisse (sérotonine, bradykinine, substances à réaction lente) sont nombreuses et revêtent une signification différente dans les différentes espèces animales et chez le même individu suivant l'organe qui est le siège des manifestations pathologiques et aussi, vraisemblablement, suivant les différents facteurs les ayant provoquées.

III. Aspects diagnostiques

Dans le domaine général l'histamine a trouvé, comme on le sait, différentes applications diagnostiques telles que, par exemple, celles se rapportant à la localisation du siège d'une obstruction artérielle des membres (par voie intradermique), à l'étude de la sécrétion gastrique (par voie sous-cutanée), à la révélation de l'existence de phéochromocytome (par voie intraveineuse) et enfin celles se référant au temps de circulation.

Les applications diagnostiques qui nous intéressent ici concernent la pathologie de certains états allergiques.

En ne parlant que de la valeur diagnostique de l'*histaminémie* pour déterminer un état allergique, nous avons plus haut appelé l'attention sur les données qui nous amènent à conclure qu'il n'est pas possible d'établir des rapports bien définis et univoques entre les variations de l'histaminémie et les états allergiques. Nous avons même fait allusion à la nécessité de recherches ultérieures pour préciser la valeur réelle diagnostique de la détermination du *pouvoir histaminopexique du sérum*.

La *réactivité cutanée histaminique* a été également particulièrement étudiée. Cette réactivité qui se manifeste au bout de 10 minutes, est représentée par les éléments de la triple réponse dite de Lewis (dilatation des capillaires à l'endroit de l'injection d'histamine, érythème diffus, papule oedémateuse). Des données très utiles pour l'étude soignée de la réactivité histaminique peuvent être obtenues au moyen d'injections intradermiques de solutions croissantes d'histamine (Serafini et Mené, 1947; Biozzi, 1947 et d'autres). Grâce à ce procédé il devient possible de préciser le point exact à partir duquel commence à se manifester la sensibilité cutanée histaminique des malades examinés *(seuil cutané histaminique)*. A ce propos il est possible d'affirmer que les sujets normaux manifestent de façon évidente la réaction cutanée caractéristique déjà pour une dilution de 1/500.000. La réaction persiste jusqu'à la dilution de 1/1.000.000. Les sujets normaux réagissant à des dilutions de 1/5.000.000 apparaissent comme extrèmement rares (SOLLMANN et PILCHER, 1917; BIOZZI, 1947 et d'autres).

Les nombreuses recherches se basant sur ces techniques pour poser un diagnostique général d'allergie ont permis d'établir que chez les sujets allergiques la réactivité histaminique revêt fréquemment une intensité plus grande que celle rencontrée chez des sujets normaux; les données, toutefois, ne sont pas constantes (MURPHY et COBE, 1932; MCCONNELL, 1933; GUICHARDOT, 1946 et d'autres).

Même si l'on se rapporte aux recherches effectuées avec l'emploi de dilutions croissantes d'histamine par BIOZZI (1947), il semble que le seuil de la sensibilité histaminique et l'importance de la réponse aux différentes dilutions (de 1/10.000 à 1/1.000.000) n'atteignent pas de façon constante un niveau plus élevé chez des sujets allergiques que chez des sujets normaux. Si l'on compare les réponses cutanées à une même dose d'histamine dans quatre groupes de malades (normaux, asthmatiques, patients atteints d'urticaire ou de pollinosis) on remarque que les asthmatiques et les malades atteints d'urticaire présentent généralement des réactions semblables ou à peine supérieures à celles des sujets normaux tandis que chez les malades atteints de pollinosis les réactions cutanées sont nettement plus intenses que chez les témoins.

Les recherches d'ATKINSON (1945) tendant à prouver dans les cas des syndrômes de Menière, l'hypothèse d'une différence entre les deux groupes par rapport à la réactivité cutanée plus ou moins grande envers l'histamine, n'ont pas été confirmées par la suite (HAGGIE, 1951).

Tout ce que nous venons d'exposer nous amène à conclure négativement en ce qui concerne le problème qui nous intéresse plus spécialement, à savoir, si l'intradermoréaction à l'histamine peut constituer un élément digne de foi pour diagnostiquer l'existence d'un état allergique. Une telle conclusion est en accord avec celle à laquelle sont parvenus différents Auteurs (FARMER, 1948; BIOZZI, 1947 et d'autres).

En ce qui concerne l'asthme bronchique et la migraine, de nombreuses recherches ont été effectuées.

La constatation que nous venons de rappeler sur l'hyperexcitabilité particulière de patients atteints d'*asthme bronchique* à l'histamine, présente un intérêt diagnostique certain, surtout quand cette hyperexcitabilité, comme l'a montré TIFFENEAU (1957), peut préceder les premiers symptômes de la maladie.

L'épreuve peut s'effectuer par aérosol (TIFFENEAU, 1957). La sensibilité pulmonaire à l'histamine est exprimée comme la plus petite dose d'histamine (0,5—40 γ) capable de produire une variation dans la ventilation appréciable au moyen d'un spiromètre *(effet-seuil)*. Si elle est positive cela témoigne de l'existence d'une hyperexcitabilité des effecteurs moteurs du poumon (muscles lisses des bronches et des vaisseaux, glandes) à l'égard de l'histamine (et même de l'acétylcholine) qui semble particulièrement évidente dans l'asthme grave et invétéré et sérait l'expression, d'après TIFFENEAU (1957), d'un substratum local et fondamental de la maladie asthmatique.

Le seuil asthmogène histaminique peut être étudié également grâce à une injection rapide par voie intraveineuse (SICUTERI, 1959b) d'une solution d'une concentration variable mais toujours dans un volume déterminé, contenant de 0,1 à 1,5 γ/kg d'histamine. Il nous parait intéressant de rappeler ici que le seuil asthmogène a été précisé par SICUTERI (1959b) même, au moyen d'une injection intraveineuse d'une solution de 48/80 (de 2 à 30 γ/kg). La crise de bronchosténose dérivant de l'administration de l'histamino-libérateur, s'installe avec un plus grand retard que celle obtenue par l'administration d'histamine.

Dans le domaine des *céphalées* il faut rappeler que certains malades, et en particulier ceux qui présentent des céphalées d'origine inflammatoire dans les structures meningo-vasculaires de la base du crâne, présentent une sensibilité pouvant être mesurée par la méthode des doses progressive. Dans la migraine l'histamine à petites doses peut provoquer une sensation caractéristique de picotement aux tempes, tout le long du vaisseau généralement atteint. À des doses plus

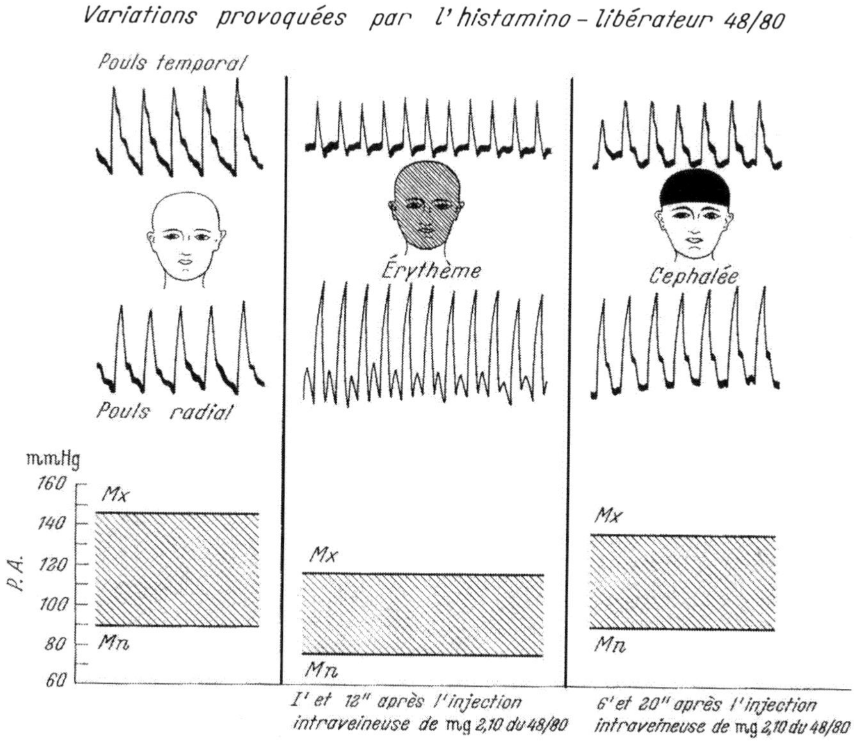

Fig. 3. Variations provoquées par l'histamino-libérateur 48/80 (d'aprés SICUTERI et coll. 1961)

élevées (1 mg par voie intramusculaire) elle peut déclencher la crise de migraine avec le phénomène caractéristique de la phase de latence, comme on l'observe dans la céphalée histaminique de Horton (SICUTERI et coll., 1957); une crise retardée peut également être observée si l'histamine est injectée localement au voisinage de l'artère temporale.

Les modifications sphygmo-piézographiques des artères temporales, radiales et du pouls oculaire, étudiées au moyen de l'appareil de Bovet et Gatti, vont de pair avec la chute des niveaux de la pression, comme l'ont démontré BOVET et GATTI (1957), et aussi SICUTERI et coll. (1961).

L'emploi de 48/80 dans les céphalées (SICUTERI et coll., 1961) a permis de préciser que dans les céphalées inflammatoires le seuil douloureux avec le 48/80 apparaît comme très bas; parfois 2–3 γ/kg sont suffisants pour réveiller la douleur typique sans que l'on assiste à des réactions vasculaires appréciables (Fig. 3). SICUTERI (1959a) a en outre signalé que les doses de 48/80 engendrant la symptomatologie douloureuse sont nettement inférieures à celles nécessaires pour provoquer des phénomènes vasomoteurs, ce qui n'est jamais le cas avec l'histamine, même quand les conditions de l'expérience sont identiques.

Il semble donc que tandis que le seuil histaminique dans la migraine peut essentiellement être expliqué comme un moyen vasculo-mécanique pour stimuler et par conséquent pour mesurer le degré de sensibilité des effecteurs, l'emploi du 48/80 permet, au delà du contrecoup vasomoteur localisé, d'étudier plus directement, au moyen de la libération locale d'histamine et d'autres substances, les phénomènes physiopathologiques tissulaires qui apparaissent comme le substrat fondamental de ces états pathologiques.

D'un point de vue diagnostique il faut enfin rappeler le phénomène de la «réactivation histaminique» observée par TZANCK et SIDI (1950) dans les états pathologiques dûs aux dermatoses de contact. Les expériences des Auteurs ont prouvé que l'injection d'histamine est en mesure de rendre positives les cuti-réactions pratiquées avec des allergènes auxquels les malades étaient certainement sensibles alors que ces mêmes essais ont un caractère négatif en l'absence de l'histamine.

IV. Aspects thérapeutiques

La connaissance des rapports existants entre l'histamine et l'allergie revêt pour le praticien une grande importance puisqu'il s'y rattache certaines applications d'ordre thérapeutique. Vu son importance nous examinerons en premier lieu le problème de l'*histaminothérapie*.

En injectant dans l'organisme des doses minimes d'histamine, le but que l'on se propose est d'obtenir une diminution de la sensibilité à l'égard de cette substance qui est libérée dans les tissus des sujets allergiques à la suite de la réaction antigène-anticorps ou d'autres stimuli.

Ce traitement est basé sur des recherches expérimentales qui ont mis en évidence comment l'administration répétée d'histamine engendre chez l'animal une diminution de la sensibilité à l'histamine elle-même et des phénomènes anaphylactiques, (FARMER, 1948; FABINYI et SZEBEHELYI, 1949; et d'autres) et chez l'homme une réduction des phénomènes provoqués par l'injection intradermique d'histamine (LEWIS, 1927).

Le traitement par l'histamine a été employé par plusieurs Auteurs pour un groupe assez vaste de syndrômes allergiques et non allergiques. Des résultats positifs ont été obtenus dans 20–80 % des cas, suivant les différentes formes pathologiques et la voie d'introduction, dans beaucoup de formes de nature allergique (BUSINCO, 1939; FORTUNATO, 1948; STAFFIERI, 1946; VANNUCCHI et MANCI, 1946) et tout spécialement dans les rhinites vasomotrices, dans l'asthme bronchique, dans la migraine et dans les céphalées. Dans les céphalées histaminiques du type Horton on obtient constamment des résultats positifs, ainsi, que nous avons nous-mêmes pu le constater.

Tout récemment WALKER (1955) a rapporté, avec l'introduction de l'histamine par électrophorèse, les pourcentages suivants de résultats positifs: 55 % dans l'asthme bronchique sans emphysème; 45 % dans l'asthme accompagné d'emphysème; 60 % dans les pollinosis; 44 % dans l'urticaire; 70 % dans les eczémas des enfants; 45 % dans les eczémas des adultes; 70 % dans les migraines.

Les doses d'histamine administrées varient suivant la tolérance du sujet, la voie d'introduction et la méthode de traitement employée. La méthode rapide s'effectue avec une injection intraveineuse, en administrant 1 mg d'histamine (base) dans 250 cc de solution physiologique dans un délai de 2 à 6 heures et en répétant l'injection un jour sur deux pendant au moins 10 jours, ou alors tous les jours pendant six jours. La méthode généralement adoptée est l'injection sous-cutanée au moyen de doses progressivement croissantes; l'on commence par la dose de 0,01 mg d'histamine (base) par voie intradermique; les doses successives sont injectées par voie sous-cutanée et augmentées jusqu'à une dose de 100 à 500 γ. 25 injections sont généralement suffisantes.

En relation aux voies d'introduction, en dehors des voies sous-cutanées et intradermiques qui sont les plus couramment employées, on a suggéré également un traitement par scarification, par voie orale, par voie intraveineuse, par ionisation par injection dans la muqueuse nasale ou par aérosol.

Les recherches de GREPPI (1951) sur l'*«histaminothérapie protégée»* mènent à ce propos un intérêt particulier. La thérapie consiste en l'introduction quotidienne par aérosol, ou par voie intramusculaire ou intraveineuse, de doses élevées et progressives d'histamine, dont les effects toxiques sont préalablement inhibés par l'administration d'un antihistaminique par voie intraveineuse. Après ce traitement les malades présentent, avec une amélioration clinique indiscutable, une diminution de la sensibilité céphalalgique et asthmogène à l'histamine. Pour expliquer le mécanisme à travers lequel s'effectue cette amélioration, ces Auteurs émettent l'hypothèse que l'histamine introduite à des doses élevées, même si elle est bloquée dans ses effets par l'administration simultanée d'un antihistaminique de synthèse, est en mesure de provoquer, grâce à la posologie suffisante d'un point de vue thérapeutique, le phénomène d'accoutumance.

Bien que l'efficacité du traitement soit substantiellement imputable à l'action pharmacologique de l'histamine, il n'a pas été encore établi s'il s'agit d'une action indirecte qui stimule le pouvoir antihistaminique de l'organisme, ou plutôt d'un effet capable de provoquer une augmentation de la tolérance des tissus.

Il faut rappeler cependant que l'histaminothérapie peut présenter certains *inconvenients* en déterminant, bien que rarement, des réactions d'ordre général désagréables et en provoquant parfois l'apparition ou l'augmentation des symptômes d'asthme et de l'ulcère gastro-duodénal. Cette dernière éventualité, qui doit être reliée sans aucun doute au pouvoir excito-sécréteur marqué de l'histamine, doit être présente à l'esprit, surtout quand on injecte aux malades des doses élevées, comme par exemple c'est le cas au cours de l'histaminothérapie *«protégée»*.

Dans l'ensemble, cette thérapie témoigne d'une activité appréciable et dans certains cas véritablement frappante, bien que limitée à certaines formes telles que la migraine, la rhinopathie vasomotrice, certains syndrômes de Menière, l'eczéma. L'adoption de la protection antihistaminique est – par notre propre expérience – un artifice technique des plus utiles. Dans presque toutes les autres allergopathies, et en particulier dans l'asthme, on n'obtient généralement pas de résultats favorables.

Nous ne jugeons pas opportun de traiter ici les *antihistaminiques de synthèse* dont les résultats thérapeutiques, que l'on peut obtenir au cours des manifestations allergiques, et en particulier de celles du type immédiat, ont été évoqués, bien que brièvement, dans les pages qui précèdent.

Nous désirons par contre mentionner quelques récentes applications thérapeutiques, telles que l'association *histamine-gammaglobulines humaines*, experimentés avec des résultats satisfaisants par quelques Auteurs (BARRÉ et coll., 1960; CASTAÑO, 1961; GRONEMEYER et coll., 1961; GELFAND et coll., 1961) et *l'administration des histamino-libérateurs* (SICUTERI et coll., 1961) à des doses élevées, sous la protection des antihistaminiques, au cours de différentes formes pathologiques (asthme bronchique, céphalées de plusieurs espèces, dermatoses).

Il n'est pas encore possible de porter un jugement définitif sur ces nouveaux procédés thérapeutiques qui doivent encore être soumis à une plus vaste experimentation clinique.

Bibliographie

ADAM, H. M., R. B. HUNTER, and T. W. G. KINNEAR: Observations on the urinary excretion of histamine in urticaria. Quart. J. exp. Physiol. **36**, 49 (1950).
ATKINSON, M.: Ménière's syndrome; validity of intradermal histamine test. Ann. Otol. (St. Louis) **54**, 201 (1945).
BARRÉ, E., A. DANRIGAL, J. L. RICHIER et F. LE BRANCHU: Un complexe histamine globuline. Premiers résultats cliniques obtenus dans le traitement de l'asthme. Presse méd. **68**, 29 (1960).
BEALL, G. N., and P. P. VAN ARSDEL JR: Histamine metabolism in human disease. J. clin. Invest. **39**, 676 (1960).
BENDA, R., E. ORINSTEIN et L. F. MIRAVET: Pouvoir histamino-protecteur (ou histamino-phylactique) de certains sérums humains. Acta allerg. (Kbh.) **13**, 315 (1959).
BIOZZI, G.: La reattività cutanea all'istamina in varie malattie allergiche. Riv. Clin. Med. (Marginalia Dermatol.) **47**, 270 (1947).
BONET-MAURY, P., N. FLAVIAN, J.-L. PARROT et M. PROVOST: Démonstration de l'histaminopexie sérique à l'aide de l'histamine marqué en C_{14}. J. Physiol. (Paris) **52**, 29 (1960).
BOVET, D., e G. L. GATTI: Azione dei farmaci sullo sfigmogramma temporale nell'uomo e suo significato nelle cefalee sperimentali e nell'emicrania. Settim. med. **44**, 6 (1957).
—, et A. M. STAUB: Action protective des éthers phénoliques au cours de l'intoxication histaminique. C. R. Soc. Biol. (Paris) **124**, 547 (1937).
BUSINCO, L.: Prime osservazioni sopra l'istaminemia e la istaminolisi nella malattia di Quincke. Boll. Soc. ital. Biol. sper. **14**, 646 (1939).
BROCKLEHURST, W. E.: A slow reacting substance in anaphylaxis "SRS-A". *In:* Histamine. Ciba Foundation Symposium. Londre: J. et A. Churchill Ltd. 1956.
CAPUANI, G. F.: Istaminemia nell'asma bronchiale. Rif. med. **55**, 1539 (1939).
CASTAÑO, I. R.: Thérapie d'allergie respiratoire par le complexe d'histamine-gamma globuline. Fourth International Congress of Allergology. Excerpta med. (Amst.) n° **42**, October 15—20 (1961), p. 13.
CECCARINI, F., e L. RICCIARDI: Effetti terapeutici dei cosiddetti antistaminici sintetici in dermatologia. Attualità di terapia antiallergica. Milano: Libreria Vinciana 1946.
CERQUA, S.: L'equivalente istaminico nel sangue in diverse condizioni patologiche. Minerva med. **27**, 542 (1936).
CHRISTENSSON, B., and B. EKWALL: Urinary excretion of 5-Hydroxyindolacetic acid (5 H I AA) in provoked allergic rhinitis. Acta allerg. (Kbh.) **15**, 425 (1960).
CODE, C. F.: The quantitative estimation of histamine in the blood. J. Physiol. (Lond.) **89**, 257 (1937).
— Histamine in blood. Physiol. Rev. **32**, 47 (1952).
—, and A. D. MAC DONALD: The histamine-like activity of blood. Lancet **1937 II**, 730.
—, and R. G. MITCHELL: Histamine, eosinophils and basophils in the blood. J. Physiol. (Lond.) **136**, 449 (1957).
COLLI, A., e G. QUACCI: Istaminemia ed asma bronchiale. Arch. Sci. Med. **87**, 157 (1949).
DALE, H. H.: Antihistamine substances. Brit. med. J. **1948 II**, 281.
—, and P. P. LAIDLAW: The physiological action of β-iminazolylethylamine. J. Physiol. (Lond.) **41**, 318 (1910).
DUNÉR, H., and B. PERNOW: The urinary excretion of histamine in case of Loeffler'syndrome. Acta med. scand. **156**, 313 (1956).
— — Urinary excretion of histamine in bronchial asthma. Acta med. scand. **161**, 361 (1958).
— —, and G. STERKY: The histamine concentration of the blood on exposure to cold and heat. Acta allerg. (Kbh.) **15**, 417 (1960).
ECKERT, D., and G. TOTTERMAN: On histamine content of white blood corpuscles, with special reference to eosinophils. Scand. J. clin. Lab. Invest. **2**, 58 (1950).
ERSPAMER, V.: Il sistema cellulare enterocromaffine e l'enteramina. R. clin. Sci. Milano: Farmitalia 1954.
FABINYI, M., and J. SZEBEHELYI: The mechanism of desensitization with histamine. Acta allerg. (Kbh.) **2**, 233 (1949).
FARMER, L.: Experiments on histamine refractoriness. III° The effect of histamine pretreatment on the establishment of active sensitization. J. Allergy **19**, 358 (1948).
FIESSINGER, N., et A. GAJDOS: Urticaire et histamine. Paris: Vigot ed. 1937.
FORTUNATO, V.: Allergia del naso e dei seni paranasali. Relaz. 37° Congr. Soc. It. ORL. Perugia: Donnini Ed. 1948.
FRUGONI, C., et U. SERAFINI: État actuel de la question de l'asthme en Italie. *In:* « L'Asthme ». Rapports du 2e Congrés International de l'Asthme, Le Mont-Dore, 3—5 juin 1950. L'Expansion Scient. Franç. Ed. (1950).

GATÉ, J., et J. PELLERAT: L'histamine cutanée. Son rôle en dermatologie. Les composés antihistaminiques de synthèse. Indications et résultats thérapeutiques en dermatologie. Congrès Français de Medécine. XXVIe Session. Paris: Masson et Cie Editeurs 1947.
GEDDA, L., e U. TEODORI: Genetica delle allergopatie. Rel. Congresso Soc. Ital. Allergol. Pisa, 2—3 ottobre 1961. Folia allerg. (Roma) **8**, 373 (1961).
GELFAND, H. H., J. CINDER, S. F. GRANT, and M. SOIFFER: Preliminary report on histaglobin — a new approach to immunization against histamine. Fourth International Congress of Allergology. Excerpta med. (Amst.) n° **42**. October 15—20 (1961), p. 13.
GIUNCHI, G., e U. SERAFINI: L'equivalente istaminico del sangue in varie condizioni fisiopatologiche. Studio comparativo di alcuni metodi di determinazione dell'equivalente istaminico nel sangue (e.i.s.). L'e.i.s. nei soggetti normali. Diagn. e Tecn. Lab. **13**, 121 (1942).
— — L'equivalente istaminico del sangue in varie condizioni fisiopatologiche: l'equivalente istaminico del sangue (e.i.s.) nella pollinosi. Policlinico, Sez. med. **51**, 81 (1944).
GRAHAM, H. T., O. H. LOWRY, F. WHEELWRIGHT, M. A. LENZ, and H. H. PARISH: Distribution of histamine among leukocytes and platelets. Blood **10**, 467 (1955).
GREPPI, E.: Cefalee ed allergia. Premier Congrès International d'Allergie Basel: S. Karger 1951.
GRONEMEYER, W., E. FUCHS, and M. BRÜCKNER: The possibility of affecting allergic reactions by a new type of histamine-γ globulin compound. Fourth International Congress of Allergology. Excerpta med. (Amst.) n° **42**, October 15—20 (1961), p. 13.
GUICHARDOT, P.: Exploration de la réaction cutanée à l'histamine en dermatologie. Lyon: Molin Ed. 1946.
HAGGIE, M.: Value of histamine skin tests in Ménière's disease. Brit. med. J. **1951 II**, 1057.
HAWORTH, E., and A. D. MACDONALD: On histamine in cotton, dust and in blood of cotton workers. J. Hyg. **37**, 234 (1937).
HELANDER, E., C. G. HELANDER, S.-E. LINDELL, B. SODERHOLM, and H. WESTLING: The elimination of C_{14} labelled histamine from the blood in man. Fourth International Congress of Allergology. Excerpta med. (Amst.) n° **42**, October 15—20 (1961).
HJORT, A. M., A. S. WORDEN, and J. HOGLE: Evaluation of histamine and cholinesterase in allergic phenomena. Ann. intern. Med. **32**, 217 (1950).
HORTON, B. T., and G. E. BROWN: Systemic histamine-like reactions in allergy due to cold: 6 cases. Amer. J. med. Sci. **178**, 191 (1929).
HUMPHREY, J. H., and R. JAQUES: The histamine and serotonin content of the platelets and polymorphonuclear leucocytes of various species. J. Physiol. (Lond.) **124**, 305 (1954).
JIMENEZ DIAZ, C.: Algunos problemas de la patologia interna. Madrid: Editorial Cientifico Medica 1944.
—, et E. ARJONA: Le rôle de l'infection dans la génèse des maladies allergiques. Acta allerg. (Kbh.) Suppl. III°, 105 (1953).
JONEZ, H. D.: Use of histamine in treatment of allergic diseases. Ann. Allergy **10**, 455 (1952).
KAPLAN, E. H., and Z. DAVIS: Binding of histamine by animal proteins. Proc. Soc. exp. Biol. (N. Y.) **84**, 218 (1953).
KATZ, G.: Histamine release from blood cells in anaphylaxis in vitro. Science **91**, 221 (1940).
— Histamine release in the allergic skin reaction. Proc. Soc. exp. Biol. (N. Y.) **49**, 272 (1942).
—, and S. COHEN: Experimental evidence for histamine release in allergy. J. Amer. med. Ass. **117**, 1782 (1941).
LECOMTE, J.: Contribution clinique et expérimentale à l'étude du rôle de l'histamine dans certains phénomènes anaphylactiques. Rev. belge Path. **25**, Suppl. XI, (1956).
LEWIS, T.: The blood vessels of the human skin and their responses. Londre: Shaw and Sons Ed. 1927.
LOWRY, O. H., H. T. GRAHAM, F. B. HARRIS, M. K. PRIEBAT, A. R. MARKS, and R. U. BREGMAN: The chemical measurement of histamine in blood plasma and cells. J. Pharmacol. exp. Ther. **112**, 116 (1954).
MAAS, J. W., G. A. FEHMERS, and T. STRENGERS: Some aspects of blood histamine in normal, allergic and tuberculous children. Acta allerg. (Kbh.) **10**, 170 (1956).
MARTINETTI, R.: Edema cutaneo quale manifestazione allergica « a frigore ». Settim. med. **31**, 281 (1943).
MCCONNELL, F. S.: Observations on formation of wheals; response of normal and allergic individuals. J. Allergy **4**, 177 (1933).
MCELIN, T. W., and B. T. HORTON: Clinical observations on the use of Benadryl. A new antihistamine substance. Proc. Mayo Clin. **20**, 417 (1945).
MITCHELL, R. G.: Excretion of injected histamine by asthmatic children. J. Allergy **30**, 506 (1959).
— G. B. LOGAN, G. A. PETERS, and L. L. HENDERSON: Urinary excretion of histamine in patients having asthma and hay fever. Observations on changes produced by administration of cortisone. J. Allergy **25**, 504 (1954).

Murphy, J. A., and H. M. Cobe: Histamine: reactive substance in human dander. J. Allergy **3**, 161 (1932).
Nilzen, A.: Studies in histamine (H-substance) with special reference to conditions obtaining in urticaria and related skin changes. Acta dermat. vener. (suppl. 17) **27**, 1 (1947).
Noah, J. W., and A. Brand: Release of histamine in the blood of ragweed-sensitive individuals. J. Allergy **25**, 210 (1954).
— — Correlation of blood histamine release and skin test response to multiple antigens. J. Allergy **26**, 385 (1955).
Parrot, J.-L., et M. Gabe: Sur la répartition de l'histamine dans les éléments constitutifs du sang humain. C. R. Soc. Biol. (Paris) **139**, 965 (1945).
—, et C. Laborde: Le pouvoir histaminopexique du sérum sanguin. Son absence chez les sujets allergiques. Presse méd. **61**, 1267 (1953).
— — L'histaminopexie plasmatique en allergie. Méd. et Hyg. (Genève) **19**, 27 (1961).
—, et J. Reuse: Rôle physiologique et physiopathologique de l'histamine. J. Physiol. (Paris) **46**, 99 (1954).
Paton, W. D. M.: Compound 48/80: potent histamine liberator. Brit. J. Pharmacol. **6**, 499 (1951).
Pellerat, J.: Recherches sur l'histamine et les antihistaminiques de synthèse. Thèse doct. Sciences nat., Lyon (1945).
—, et M. Murat: Action des antihistaminiques de synthèse sur l'histaminémie. C. R. Soc. Biol. (Paris) **140**, 297 (1946).
Randolph, T. G., and F. M. Rackemann: The blood histamine level in asthma and in eosinophilia. J. Allergy **12**, 450 (1941).
Riley, J. F., and G. B. West: Presence of histamine in tissue mast cells. J. Physiol. (Lond.) **120**, 528 (1953).
Rocha e Silva, M.: Histamine. Its Role in Anaphylaxis and Allergy. Springfield (Ill.) USA: Thomas Publ. 1955.
— W. T. Beraldo, and G. Rosenfeld: Bradykinin, hypotensive and smooth muscle stimulating factor released from plasma globulin by snake venoms and by trypsin. Amer. J. Physiol. **156**, 261 (1949).
Rorsman, H.: Basophil leucocytes in urticaria, asthma and atopic dermatitis. Acta allerg. (Kbh.) **12**, 205 (1958).
Rosa, L., e L. Barbieri: Liberazione di istamina dal bronco umano isolato di allergopatico. Quad. dell'allergia **9**, 164 (1951).
Rose, B.: Studies on blood histamine in cases of allergy. I. Blood histamine during wheal formation. J. Allergy **12**, 327 (1941a).
— Studies on blood histamine in patients with allergy. II. Alterations in the blood histamine in patients with allergic disease. J. clin. Invest. **20**, 419 (1941b).
—, and J. S. L. Browne: Alterations in the blood histamine in shock. Proc. Soc. exp. Biol. (N. Y.) **44**, 182 (1940).
— M. Entin, and H. Baxter: Cit. *in* Feinberg, S. M., Malkiel, S. and Feinberg, A. R. The antihistamines. The Year Book Ed. Chicago: 1950.
— I. Rusted, and I. A. Fownes: Intravascular catheterization. Studies of bronchial asthma. Histamine levels in arterial mixed venous blood of asthmatic patients before and during induced attacks. J. clin. Invest. **29**, 1113 (1950).
Rothman, S., and J. M. Coon: Studies on liberation of acetylcholine in skin. J. invest. Derm. **3**, 99 (1940).
Schayer, R. W.: Formation and binding of histamine by free mast cells of rat peritoneal fluid. Amer. J. Physiol. **186**, 199 (1956).
Schild, H. O., D. F. Hawkins, J. L. Mongar, and H. Herxheimer: Reactions of isolated human asthmatic lung and bronchial tissue to a specific antigen. Histamine release and muscular contraction. Lancet **1951 II**, 376.
Scudamore, H. H., L. I. Vorhaus, and R. M. Kark: Acetylcholine and cholinesterase in blood of patients suffering with bronchial asthma. J. Lab. clin. Med. **37**, 860 (1951).
Serafini, U.: Studies on histamine and histamine antagonists. J. Allergy **19**, 256 (1948).
— Sull'importanza dell'istamina nella patogenesi dell'orticaria da fatica fisica. Gazz. int. Med. Chir. **55**, 341 (1951).
— e G. Biozzi: La prova di carico con istamina. Nota 1, — Curve istaminemiche da carico nei normali e negli asmatici. Policlinico, Sez. prat. **53**, 985 (1946a).
— — La prova di carico di istamina in alcune malattie allergiche (Primi Risultati). Clin. nuova **2**, 142 (1946b).
— — L'equivalente istaminico del sangue dopo fatica fisica nei normali e nei pollinosici. Clin. nuova **2**, 357 (1946c).
— e G. Giunchi: L'equivalente istaminico del sangue in varie condizioni fisiopatologiche. Nota III. La liberazione di istamina durante le reazioni cutanee allergiche. G. Clin. med. **27**, 702 (1946).

SERAFINI, U., e G. MENÉ: Studi sugli antistaminici sintetici. Nota IVa. Azione di vari antistaminici sintetici per via orale e per via endovenosa sulla reattività cutanea alla istamina ed agli allergeni. Boll. Soc. ital. Biol. sper. **23**, 778 (1947).

SICUTERI, F.: Introduzione alla conoscenza biologica e clinica degli istaminoliberatori. Rass. Fisiopat. clin. ter. **31**, 995 (1959a).

— La intolleranza degli asmatici all'istamina ed all'istaminoliberatore 48/80 valutata con il criterio della «Soglia asmogena». Progr. med. (Napoli) **15**, 165 (1959b).

— Prophylactic and therapeutic properties of 1-Methyl-lysergic acid butanolamide in migraine. Int. Arch. Allergy **15**, 300 (1959c).

— M. RICCI e G. FRANCHI: Biologia e clinica della liberazione di istamina. La Settimana Medica Ed. Firenze: 1961.

— — R. MONFARDINI and M. FICINI: Experimental headache with endogenous histamine. Acta allerg. (Kbh.) **11**, 188 (1957).

— —, and E. ROMAGNOLI: Behaviour of pressure and pulse of cerebrospinal fluid in man during release of histamine by compound 48/80. Acta allerg. (Kbh.) **13**, 222 (1960).

SOLLMANN, T., and J. D. PILCHER: Endermic reactions. J. Pharmacol. exp. Ther. **9**, 309 (1917).

SPOUJITCH, V.: The complexity of allergic reactions. Acta allerg. (Kbh.) suppl. VII°, 112 (1960).

SPUZIC, I., and L. IVKOVIC: Histamine in plasma in induced urticaria due to cold. Acta allerg. (Kbh.) **16**, 228 (1961).

STAFFIERI, M.: Istaminoterapia locale delle allergie nasali. Arch. ital. Otol. **57**, 277 (1946).

STRENGERS, T., I. C. M. VERSCHURE, and A. C. M. LIPS: Treatment of bronchial asthma with antihystamine-preparation "antergan" under control of histamine-level of blood. Acta med. scand. **129**, 193 (1947).

THORSON, A., G. BIÖRCK, G. BJÖRKMAN, and J. WALDENSTRÖM: Malignant carcinoid of small intestine with metastases to liver, valvular disease of right side of heart (pulmonary stenosis and tricuspid regurgitation without septal defects), peripheral vasomotor symptoms, bronchoconstriction, and unusual type of cyanosis. Clinical and pathologic syndrome. Amer. Heart J. **47**, 795 (1954).

TIFFENEAU, R.: Examen pulmonaire de l'ashmatique. Déductions diagnostiques, prognostiques et thérapeutiques. Paris: Masson Ed. 1957.

— Hypersensibilité cholinergo-histaminique pulmonaire de l'asthmatique. Acta allerg. (Kbh.) suppl. V°, 187 (1958).

TZANCK, A., et E. SIDI: Les dermatoses allergiques. Paris: Masson Ed. 1950.

VALENTINE, W. N., and J. S. LAWRENCE: Studies on blood histamine before and after clotting in health and disease states. Amer. J. med. Sci. **216**, 619 (1948).

VAN ARSDEL, P. P. JR., E. MIDDLETON JR., W. B. SHERMAN, and H. BUCHWALD: A quantitative study on the in vitro release of histamine from leucocytes of atopic persons. J. Allergy **29**, 429 (1958).

VANNUCCHI, V., e F. MANCI: Terapia istaminica a microdosi nella corizza vasomotoria. Riv. clin. Med. (suppl. 2 Marg. Otolaring.) **5**, 426 (1946).

WALKER, V.: Communications au 2e Congrès International d'Allergie, Rio de Janeiro (1955).

WENNER, W. M. F., and C. C. BUHRMESTER: Potassium and acetylcholine of the blood of rabbit in anaphylactic shock. J. Allergy **9**, 85 (1937).

WEST, G. B.: Histamine and mast cells. *In:* Ciba Foundation Symposium on Histamine. London: J. & A. Churchill Ltd. 1956.

Section E

Histamine and Experimental Asthma of the Guinea Pig

By

ERNESTO MENDES

The respiratory symptoms produced in sensitized guinea pigs submitted to inhalations of the specific antigen were called by RATNER (1953) "respiratory anaphylaxis". Since those symptoms have sufficient analogy with the human asthmatic syndrome, we prefer to call them "experimental asthma". KALLÓS and PAGEL (1937) also concluded that inhalation of the homologous antigen elicits in the allergic guinea pig attacks which clinically, roentgenologically, pharmacologically and immunologically simulate human bronchial asthma. Furthermore, according to MALKIEL (1951), ACTH and cortisone do not protect guinea pigs against fatal anaphylaxis, in spite of the great improvement obtained with these hormones in human asthma. FEINBERG et al. (1953) have demonstrated that ACTH and cortisone markedly inhibited experimental asthma in guinea pigs passively sensitized with aerosol of crystallized ovalbumin. A similar inhibitory effect could not be obtained in the bronchospasm of the guinea pig produced by an aerosol of histamine.

Our study was conducted in order to investigate and evaluate the action of Prednisone on the experimental asthma of the guinea pig and on bronchospasm provoked by inhalation of histamine or serotonin in the same species. From these experiments (MENDES, 1957) we have drawn the following conclusions:

1. Prednisone, given orally, in daily amounts of 5–10 mg during the last 6 days of sensitization, prevents experimental asthma produced by egg white in the guinea pig.

2. A similar inhibitory effect was not obtained, with the same doses of Prednisone, upon bronchospasm of the guinea pig, elicited by aerosols of histamine or serotonin.

3. The mode of action of the hormone upon these types of reaction is not sufficiently clear, but several possibilities may be discussed.

The effect of Prednisone upon guinea pigs sensitized to egg albumin appeared quite obvious, since the drug inhibited experimental asthma. Only 2 guinea pigs presented tachypnoea, after 10–11 minutes of nebulization, in sharp contrast with the control group, not treated with Prednisone. All the untreated guinea pigs manifested fatal asthma after 1–2 minutes. With the suppression of Prednisone, its inhibitory effect had nearly disappeared, after 7 days, for most guinea pigs had typical asthma or tachypnoea after 2–3 minutes of inhalation and only one animal was free of symptoms. This inhibitory effect of Prednisone upon experimental asthma due to aerosol of egg albumin has the same significance as that obtained by several authors, using ACTH or cortisone (FEINBERG and

MALKIEL, 1952). Cortisone and ACTH do not protect guinea pigs against common direct anaphylaxis, but do inhibit a definite proportion of inverse anaphylactic shock with Forssman antigen (ARBESMAN et al., 1951). FEINBERG et al. (1953) confirmed the inhibitory effect of ACTH, cortisone, Pyribenzamine, localized chemical inflammation, sodium nucleate and human serum against guinea pig asthma elicited by aerosols of antigens. This effect could be partially explained by the stimulus of the pituitary-adrenal axis, according to the concepts of SELYE (1950). Bilateral adrenalectomy, however, does not prevent the inhibitory effect of sodium nucleate upon experimental asthma; BENAIN et al. (1955) admit that such "stress" is not mediated by pituitary-adrenocortical stimulation. HERXHEIMER and ROSA (1952) demonstrated that ACTH or cortisone, when administered during the period of antibody formation, resulted in a prolonged reaction time, when the animals were exposed to aerosol; they explained this fact by the interference of the hormones with antibody formation. Considerable work has been done about the relationship between cortisone and ACTH, and liberation of histamine, but the reports do not always agree (ROSE, 1958).

In our experiments, Prednisone did not protect guinea pigs against bronchospasm induced by aerosol of histamine, since the animals died with asphyxic convulsions, within 60–70 seconds after starting the nebulization; this period was the same as in the control group. Identical observations were made by FEINBERG et al. (1953) using ACTH and cortisone.

Similar results were obtained with serotonin (MENDES, 1960). Prednisone did not protect guinea pigs against bronchospasm provoked by aerosols of 5-hydroxytryptamine creatinine sulphate.

According to CARRYER and CODE (1952), FRIEDLAENDER and FRIEDLAENDER (1950), SCHILD et al. (1951) there is no evidence that ACTH and cortisone inhibit the liberation of histamine under experimental conditions or that they affect its action once it has been released. These hormones apparently do not interfere with the actions of histamine, injected or after liberation, but they seem to inhibit the biogenesis of histamine. The basis for such an assumption can be found in some experiments by SELYE (1950) and HALPERN (1956). SELYE (1950) mentioned that cortisone and ACTH inhibit anaphylactoid reactions of the rat, due to parenteral administration of egg white, which can be related, at least in part to a liberation of histamine (ROCHA E SILVA, 1955). HALPERN (1956) thinks that cortisone interferes with the biogenesis of histamine, since after depletion by dextran the return of the histamine stocks in tissues is greatly delayed by the hormones. It is logical to assume that cortisone also interferes with the biogenesis of serotonin. ROCHA E SILVA (1954) suggested that certain polysaccharides were able to activate the histamine releasing agent (anaphylatoxin) present in blood, in such a way that the favorable effect of the adrenocorticoids might be due to interference with the mechanism of anaphylatoxin formation.

In addition to these possible ways of action, ACTH and cortisone can modify unspecifically the capillary permeability. BENDITT et al. (1950) noted that the previous administration of these hormones for 5 days inhibits the signs of increased capillary permeability, produced by hyaluronidase. Similar observations were made by HAYES and BRIDGMAN (1951). The "spreading activity" of hyaluronidase is partially prevented by anti-histaminics (MAYER, 1950).

Notwithstanding the great amount of work done (HALPERN, 1956; SCHAYER – see Chapter 4, Section D) there are only indirect evidences that adrenocortical hormones would act by inhibiting the biogenesis of histamine. It is also probable that they do not influence the effects of histamine which has already been released, excepting perhaps, those effects due to disturbances of capillary permeability.

Anaphylatoxin and experimental asthma

Anaphylatoxin is known since 1910, after the work of FRIEDBERGER (1910) who prepared it, by adding the immune precipitate to the guinea pig serum. BORDET (1913) obtained it by adding polysaccharides instead of the immune precipitate, and NOVY and DE KRUIF (1917) by diluting the serum with destilled water.

Interest in anaphylatoxin had disappeared with the acceptance of the histamine theory of anaphylaxis. However, in recent years, this interest was again aroused, after the demonstration that anaphylatoxin is a releaser of histamine.

HAHN and OBERDORF (1950) demonstrated that antihistaminics prevent fatal shock caused by anaphylatoxin. ROCHA E SILVA et al. (1951) verified that the isolated lung of the guinea pig liberates considerable amounts of histamine when perfused with anaphylatoxin, this suggesting that the fatal shock provoked by it follows bronchospasm due to histamine liberation. DALE (1956) suggested that under the effect of anaphylatoxin, the release of histamine would occur in the endothelium, whereas in anaphylactic shock it would take place more deeply in the smooth muscle itself. Recent experiments by GIERTZ et al. (1961) indicate some qualitative differences in the way histamine is released by anaphylatoxin or in anaphylaxis.

ROCHA E SILVA (1954) discusses the participation of a blood born factor in anaphylactic shock, this explaining recent interest in anaphylatoxin, inasmuch as it would conciliate the humoral and cellular theories of anaphylaxis. Nevertheless, there are many obscure points to be clarified before participation of anaphylatoxin in allergic phenomena might be accepted. This is the opinion of several authors. A thorough discussion of this problem is presented by GIERTZ and HAHN in another part of this book (see Chapter 3, Section E).

Anaphylatoxin prepared with rat's serum is a strong liberator of histamine in the guinea pig when given by the intracardiac route or flooded through the isolated lung. It also stimulates fragments of the isolated guinea pig ileum by a release of histamine. In view of these facts we decided to verify whether anaphylatoxin inhalation in the guinea pig was able to induce bronchial spasm the same way as histamine did. Besides, we tried to find out whether anaphylatoxin could provoke experimental asthma in guinea pigs previously sensitized to it as antigen, and whether this method would be suitable to differentiate the immunological reactions to anaphylatoxin and to normal rat serum (MENDES, 1959).

From these experiments we have concluded: 1) guinea pigs submitted to inhalations with rat's anaphylatoxin did not present bronchospasm or other symptoms, although this substance provoked fatal shock of the histaminic type when applied by the intracardiac route. 2) It is possible to sensitize guinea pigs to anaphylatoxin by means of intraperitoneal and intramuscular injections and provoke, afterwards, experimental asthma by inhalations of the same material. 3) When anaphylatoxin and normal rat's serum were used to induce experimental asthma, a different immunological behaviour could be observed with either agent.

Although ROCHA E SILVA (1954) had obtained strong contractions of isolated smooth muscle in the guinea pig, when in contact with anaphylatoxin, we did not observe any sign of contraction of the bronchiolar muscle, as indicated by dispnea in animals sprayed for the first time. This fact appeared to suggest that anaphylatoxin probably does not affect directly the bronchiolar muscles demanding previous contact with some humoral factor, in order to liberate histamine. Furthermore, the mucous membranes seem to act as a barrier, inasmuch as intraperitoneal injections of 4 to 5 ml of anaphylatoxin did not cause any effect in the guinea pig. As a matter of fact, during the process of sensitizing the animals, we have used the intraperitoneal and intramuscular routes, and no symptoms were observed.

UNGAR (1956) reported that the isolated sensitized guinea pig lung, when treated with the antigen plus normal serum, releases more histamine than when flooded by the antigen alone. For this reason, in our experiments, some guinea pigs were submitted previously to an inhalation of normal guinea pig serum, with the purpose of boosting the action of anaphylatoxin. Notwithstanding this artifice no response has been obtained. It is true that the amount of anaphylatoxin that may be sprayed within 30–40 minutes is approximately 4–6 ml for each group of animals, the amount inhaled by each animal being smaller than the one used by intracardiac route, which usually provokes bronchospasm. Besides, it is interesting to recall the diversity of results in the same kind of animal, when anaphylatoxin is flooded or inhaled. In the first case, ROCHA E SILVA (1954) had obtained remarkable quantities of histamine, much larger than those which occur in anaphylactic shock, and therefore able of producing bronchospasm whereas no sign of histamine release is obtained through inhalation. This apparent discrepancy according to the route used, may explain our results. When animals are not sensitized, the inhalation of anaphylatoxin will not provoke symptoms in the guinea pigs, although it liberates great amounts of histamine when injected directly into the blood stream.

Nevertheless, anaphylatoxin was capable of sensitizing guinea pigs and provoke bronchospasm afterwards when sprayed in the same animal. There were indications that, immunologically, anaphylatoxin and normal rat serum may behave like different antigens when experimental asthma of the guinea pig is used as a method. This experimental procedure could be conveniently utilized, in order to verify whether the transformation of rat's normal serum into anaphylatoxin would cause immunological changes capable of making them antigenically different. Indeed, it appeared that some animals sensitized by anaphylatoxin would not present asthma when sprayed with normal rat serum, suggesting a different immunological behaviour.

A refractory period was also verified which usually occurs after the induction of dyspnea by a certain antigen. Some guinea pigs showed this refractory period when sprayed with normal rat serum and not with anaphylatoxin, this probably signifying that one antigen will not exhaust the antibodies for the other.

However, these observations would demand future investigations by employing different and more accurate methods.

References

ARBESMAN, C. E., E. NETER, and L. F. BERTRAM: The effect of ACTH and cortisone on certain immunologic mechanisms including reversed anaphylaxis. J. Allergy **22**, 340—349 (1951).

BENAIN, C., S. M. FEINBERG, and L. A. STERNBERG: Stresses and hypersensitivity. J. Allergy **26**, 481—489 (1955).

BENDITT, E. P., S. SCHILLER, H. WONG, and A. DORFMAN: Influence of ACTH and cortisone upon alteration in capillary permeability induced by hyaluronidase. Proc. Soc. exp. Biol. (N. Y.) **75**, 782—784 (1950).

BORDET, J.: Gélose et anaphylatoxine. C. R. Soc. Biol. (Paris) **74**, 877 (1913).

CARRYER, H. M., and C. F. CODE: Release of histamine during hemolytic reactions in the blood rabbits. Proc. Soc. exp. Biol. (N. Y.) **73**, 452—455 (1952).

DALE, H. H.: (1953). In: Histamine. Ciba Foundation, Symposium. London: J. & A. Churchill 1956.

FEINBERG, S. M., and S. MALKIEL: Protective effect of cortisone on induced asthma in guinea-pig. Proc. Soc. exp. Biol. (N. Y.) **81**, 104—105 (1952).

— —, and F. C. MCINTIRE: The effect of stress factors on asthma induced in guinea pigs by aerosolized antigens. J. Allergy **24**, 302—308 (1953).

Friedberger, E.: Weitere Untersuchungen über Eiweißanaphylaxie, IV. Mitt. Z. Immun.-Forsch. **4**, 636 (1910).
Friedlaender, S., and A. S. Friedlaender: Effect of pituitary adrenocorticotrophic hormone (ACTH) on histamine intoxication and anaphylaxis in guinea pig. J. Allergy **21**, 303—309 (1950).
Giertz, H., F. Hahn, I. Jurna u. W. Schmutzler: Vergleichende Untersuchungen über den anaphylaktischen und den Anaphylatoxinschock am intakten Meerschweinchen. Naunyn-Schmiedebergs Arch. exp. Path. Pharmak. **242**, 65 (1961).
Hahn, F., u. A. Oberdorf: Antihistaminica und anaphylaktoide Reaktionen. Z. Immun.-Forsch. **107**, 528—538 (1950).
Halpern, B. N.: Histamine release by long chain molecules. In Histamine: Ciba Foundation Symposium, p. 92. London: J. & A. Churchill 1956.
Hayes, M. A., and R. M. Bridgman: Dermal spreading of hyaluronidase as influenced by prolonged local treatment with certain steroid hormones. Proc. Soc. exp. Biol. (N. Y.) **77**, 597—599 (1951).
Herxheimer, H., and L. Rosa: The action of cortisone in the anaphylactic shock of the guinea pig. J. Physiol. (Lond.) **118**, 7 (1952).
Kallós, P., u. W. Pagel: Experimentelle Untersuchungen über Asthma bronchiale.Acta med. scand. **91**, 292—305 (1937).
Malkiel, S.: Influence of ACTH and cortisone on histamine and anaphylactic shock in guinea pig. J. Immunol. **66**, 379—384 (1951).
Mayer, R. L.: Antihistamine agents in allergy; activity of pyribenzamine and related compounds with special reference to their mode of action. Ann. N. Y. Acad. Sci. **50**, 1127—1141 (1950).
Mendes, E.: Action of prednisone on experimental asthma of guinea pig. Acta allerg. (Kbh.) **11**, 181—187 (1957).
— Experimental asthma in the guinea-pig provoked by anaphylatoxin. Acta allerg. (Kbh.) **13**, 8—18 (1959).
— Ácidos aminados essenciais (Histidina e Triptofano) e vitaminas (ácido ascórbico) na alergia. Rev. paul. Med. **56**, 305—318 (1960).
Novy, F. G., and P. H. De Kruif: Anaphylatoxin and anaphylaxis. J. infect. Dis. **20**, 618 (1917).
Ratner, B.: Temporal and quantitative factor influencing the development of experimental asthma in the guinea-pig. J. Allergy **24**, 316—325 (1953).
Rocha e Silva, M.: Anaphylatoxin and histamine liberation. Quart. Rev. Allergy **8**, 220 (1954).
— Histamine. Its role in anaphylaxis and allergy. Springfield: Charles C. Thomas 1955.
— O. Bier, and M. Aronson: Histamine release by anaphylatoxin. Nature (Lond.) **168**, 465—466 (1951).
Rose, B.: Hormone and allergic responses. In: Schaeffer, J. W., G. A. Lo Grippo and M. W. Chase: Mechanisms of hypersensitivity. London: J. & A. Churchill 1958.
Schild, H. O., D. F. Hawkins, J. L. Mongar, and H. Herxheimer: Reactions of isolated human asthmatic lungs and bronchial tissue to specific antigen; histamine release and muscular contraction. Lancet **1951 II**, 376—382.
Selye, H.: Stress. Montreal, Acta Inc. (1950).
Ungar, G.: In Histamine: Ciba Foundation Symposium, p. 431. London: J. & A. Churchill 1956.

Author Index

Page numbers in *italics* refer to the bibliography

Subject Index

D

F

H

M

N

Q

R

FSC
www.fsc.org
MIX
Papier | Fördert
gute Waldnutzung
FSC® C083411

Kolibri 360 GmbH
Ferdinand-Jühlke-Straße 7
99095 Erfurt, Deutschland
produktsicherheit@kolibri360.de